LOVELL AND WINTER'S

PEDIATRIC ORTHOPAEDICS

FIFTH EDITION

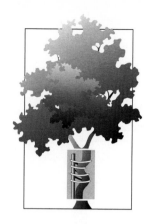

LOVELL AND WINTER'S

PEDIATRIC ORTHOPAEDICS

FIFTH EDITION

VOLUME 1

Edited by

RAYMOND T. MORRISSY, M.D.

*Chief
Department of Orthopaedics
Children's Healthcare of Atlanta
at Scottish Rite
Clinical Professor of Orthopaedics
Emory University
Atlanta, Georgia*

STUART L. WEINSTEIN, M.D.

*Ignacio V. Ponseti Chair of Orthopaedic Surgery
Department of Orthopaedic Surgery
University of Iowa Hospital
Iowa City, Iowa*

With 43 Contributors

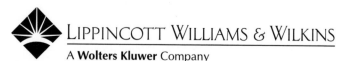

LIPPINCOTT WILLIAMS & WILKINS
A **Wolters Kluwer** Company

Philadelphia • Baltimore • New York • London
Buenos Aires • Hong Kong • Sydney • Tokyo

Acquisitions Editor: Robert Hurley
Developmental Editor: Brian Brown and Sonya L. Seigafuse
Production Editor: Deirdre Marino
Manufacturing Manager: Tim Reynolds
Cover Designer: Co. Laborative Design
Compositor: Maryland Composition Company, Inc.
Printer: Maple Press

© **2001 by LIPPINCOTT WILLIAMS & WILKINS**
530 Walnut Street
Philadelphia, PA 19106 USA
LWW.com

Printed in the USA

Library of Congress Cataloging-in-Publication Data

Lovell and Winter's pediatric orthopaedics.—5th ed. / editors, Raymond T. Morrissy,
Stuart L. Weinstein.
    p. ; cm.
   Includes bibliographical references and index.
   ISBN 0-7817-2582-8
     1. Pediatric orthopedics. I. Title: Pediatric orthopaedics. II. Lovell, Wood W., 1915–
III. Winter, Robert B., 1932– IV. Morrissy, Raymond T. V. Weinstein, Stuart L.
   [DNLML: 1. Orthopedics—Adolescence. 2. Orthopedics—Child. 3. Orthopedics—Infant.
WS 270 L911 2000]
RD732.3.C48 P43 2000
618.92′7—dc21
                                     00-042433

10 9 8 7 6 5 4 3 2 1

*To Orthopaedic Residents and Fellows
that through continued inquiry and learning
they may find medicine to be fun for a lifetime*

➡ **Cross-references to the *Atlas of Pediatric Orthopaedic Surgery, Third Edition***

In this edition of **Lovell and Winter's Pediatric Orthopaedics,** we have taken some time and inserted cross-references to surgical procedures in the **Atlas of Pediatric Orthopaedic Surgery.** In order to make these references visible but not intrusive, we have used a simple back-arrow symbol followed by the procedure number in the third edition of the atlas. Thus, "➡ 2.9" refers the reader to the ninth procedure in Chapter 2 of the atlas, which illustrates placement of segmental hook and pedicle screw instrumentation for scoliosis.

We feel that this intermeshing of the content of the atlas and the textbook greatly enhances the value of both to the reader by making the pair more user-friendly and more comprehensive. These references are also used as hot-links on the CD-ROM, which contains both the textbook and the atlas. We hope that you find this new feature useful.

RTM
SLW

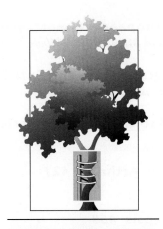

CONTENTS

VOLUME 2

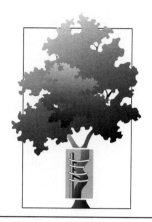

CONTRIBUTING AUTHORS

Behrooz A. Akbarnia, M.D.
Clinical Professor
Department of Orthopaedics
University of California–San Diego
9500 Gilman Drive
La Jolla, California 92093
Medical Director
San Diego Center for Spinal Disorders
8010 Frost Street
San Diego, California 92123

Benjamin A. Alman, M.D., F.R.C.S.C.
Assistant Professor
Department of Surgery
University of Toronto
Orthopaedic Surgeon and Scientist
Department of Orthopaedic Surgery/Developmental
    Biology
The Hospital for Sick Children
555 University Avenue
Toronto, Ontario M5G 1X8
Canada

David D. Aronsson, M.D.
Professor
Department of Orthopaedics and Rehabilitation and
    Pediatrics
University of Vermont College of Medicine
Robert T. Stafford Hall
Burlington, Vermont 05405
Chief, Pediatric Orthopaedics
Department of Orthopaedics and Rehabilitation and
    Pediatrics
Fletcher Allen Health Care
111 Colchester Avenue
Burlington, Vermont 05401

Frank R. Berenson, M.D.
Clinical Assistant Professor
Department of Pediatrics
Mercer University
1550 College Street
Macon, Georgia 31207
Child Neurologist
Department of Pediatrics
Children's Healthcare of Atlanta at Scottish Rite
1001 Johnson Ferry Road Northeast
Atlanta, Georgia 30342

Michael T. Busch, M.D.
Vice-Chief of Orthopaedics
Director of Sports Medicine
Department of Orthopaedics
Children's Healthcare of Atlanta at Scottish Rite
5455 Meridian Mark Road
Atlanta, Georgia 30342

Robert M. Campbell, Jr., M.D.
Associate Professor
Department of Orthopaedics
University of Texas Health Science Center at San
    Antonio
7703 Floyd Curl Drive
San Antonio, Texas 78229
Staff Physician
Principal Investigator for Titanium Rib Project
Department of Pediatric Orthopaedics
Christus Santa Rosa Children's Hospital
519 West Houston Street
San Antonio, Texas 78207

William G. Cole, M.D.
Professor of Surgery and Genetics
University of Toronto
Head, Division of Orthopaedics
The Hospital for Sick Children
555 University Avenue
Toronto, Ontario M5G 1X8
Canada

Leonard P. Connolly, M.D.
Assistant Professor
Department of Radiology
Harvard Medical School
25 Shattuck Street
Staff Radiologist
Department of Radiology
Children's Hospital
300 Longwood Avenue
Boston, Massachusetts 02115

Colleen Coulter-O'Berry, M.S., P.T., P.C.S.
Team Leader, Limb Deficiency
Physical Therapist IV
Department of Orthotics and Prosthetics
Children's Healthcare of Atlanta at Scottish Rite
5445 Meridian Mark Road
Atlanta, Georgia 30342

Jon R. Davids, M.D.
Assistant Consulting Professor
Department of Orthopaedic Surgery
Duke University Medical Center
Durham, North Carolina 27710
Director, Motion Analysis Laboratory
Shriners Hospital
950 West Faris Road
Greenville, South Carolina 29605

Dennis P. Devito, M.D.
Department of Orthopaedics
Children's Healthcare of Atlanta at Scottish Rite
5445 Meridian Mark Road
Atlanta, Georgia 30342

Frederick R. Dietz, M.D.
Professor
Department of Orthopaedic Surgery
University of Iowa
Division of Pediatric Orthopaedics
University of Iowa Hospitals and Clinics
200 Hawkins Drive
Iowa City, Iowa 52242

Alain Diméglio
Service d'Orthopedie Pediatrique
Hôpital Lapeyronie
371 Avenue du Doyen Gaston Giraud
34295 Montpellier
Cedex 5, France

Peter G. Gabos, M.D.
Assistant Clinical Professor
Department of Orthopaedic Surgery
Jefferson Medical College
Thomas Jefferson University Hospital
Philadelphia, Pennsylvania 19107
Pediatric Orthopaedic Surgeon
Department of Orthopaedic Surgery
Alfred I. duPont Hospital for Children
1600 Rockland Road
Wilmington, Delaware 19899

Mark C. Gebhardt, M.D.
Frederick W. and Jane M. Ilfield Professor of
    Orthopaedic Surgery
Department of Orthopaedic Surgery
Harvard Medical School
Boston, Massachusetts 02115
Associate Orthopaedic Surgeon
Orthopaedic Service
Massachusetts General Hospital
55 Fruit Street
Boston, Massachusetts 02114

Brian J. Giavedoni, B.Sc., C.P.(C)
Clinical Supervisor for Prosthetics
Department of Orthotics and Prosthetics
Children's Healthcare of Atlanta at Scottish Rite
5445 Meridian Mark Road
Atlanta, Georgia 30342

Michael J. Goldberg, M.D.
Henry H. Banks Professor and Chairman
Department of Orthopaedics
Tufts University School of Medicine
Orthopaedist-in-Chief
Department of Orthopaedics
New England Medical Center
750 Washington Street
Boston, Massachusetts 02111

Walter B. Greene, M.D.
Chairman
Department of Orthopaedic Surgery
University of Missouri Health Science Center
One Hospital Drive
Columbia, Missouri 65212

Diego Jaramillo, M.D.
Associate Professor
Department of Radiology
Harvard Medical School
25 Shattuck Street
Boston, Massachusetts 02115
Chief, Division of Pediatric Radiology
Department of Radiology
Massachusetts General Hospital
55 Fruit Street
Boston, Massachusetts 02114

Douglas K. Kehl, M.D.
Associate Clinical Professor
Department of Orthopaedic Surgery
Emory University School of Medicine
69 Butler Street Southeast
Atlanta, Georgia 30303
Department of Orthopaedic Surgery
Children's Healthcare of Atlanta at Scottish Rite
1001 Johnson Ferry Road Northeast
Atlanta, Georgia 30342

Richard E. Lindseth, M.D.
Professor and Chairman
Department of Orthopaedic Surgery
Indiana University School of Medicine
541 Clinical Drive
Indianapolis, Indiana 46202

Randall T. Loder, M.D.
Clinical Professor
Department of Orthopaedics
University of Minnesota
420 Delaware Street Southeast
Minneapolis, Minnesota 55455
Chief of Staff
Shriners Hospital
2025 East River Parkway
Minneapolis, Minnesota 55414

John E. Lonstein, M.D.
Clinical Professor
Department of Orthopaedic Surgery
University of Minnesota
Minneapolis, Minnesota 55455
Staff Physician
Twin Cities Spine Center
913 East 26th Street
Minneapolis, Minnesota 55404

William G. Mackenzie, M.D.
Clinical Assistant Professor
Orthopaedic Department
Thomas Jefferson Medical College
1015 Walnut Street
Philadelphia, Pennsylvania 19107
Pediatric Orthopaedic Surgeon
Department of Orthopaedics
Alfred I. duPont Hospital for Children
1600 Rockland Road
Wilmington, Delaware 19803

José A. Morcuende, M.D., Ph.D.
Department of Orthopaedic Surgery
University of Iowa
Iowa City, Iowa 52242

Raymond T. Morrissy, M.D.
Chief
Department of Orthopaedics
Children's Healthcare of Atlanta at Scottish Rite
5445 Meridian Mark Road
Clinical Professor of Orthopaedics
Emory University
Atlanta, Georgia 30342

Vincent S. Mosca, M.D.
Associate Professor and Chief
Pediatric Orthopaedics
Department of Orthopaedics
University of Washington School of Medicine
Seattle, Washington 98195
Director, Department of Orthopaedics
Children's Hospital and Regional Medical Center
4800 Sand Point Way Northeast
Seattle, Washington 98105

Colin F. Moseley, M.D., C.M.
Clinical Professor
Department of Orthopaedics
University of California–Los Angeles
1010 Westwood Boulevard
Chief of Staff
Shriners Hospital for Children
3160 Geneva Street
Los Angeles, California 90020

Peter O. Newton, M.D.
Assistant Clinical Professor
Department of Orthopaedic Surgery
University of California–San Diego
Director, Scoliosis Service
Department of Orthopaedic Surgery
Children's Hospital and Health Center
3030 Children's Way
San Diego, California 92123

Jonathan H. Phillips, M.D.
Department of Orthopaedics
Nemours Children's Clinic
83 West Columbia Street
Orlando, Florida 32806

Charles T. Price, M.D.
Surgeon in Chief and Chief of Orthopaedics
Nemours Children's Clinic
83 West Columbia Street
Orlando, Florida 32806

Thomas S. Renshaw, M.D.
Professor
Department of Orthopaedic Surgery
Yale University
800 Howard Avenue
New Haven, Connecticut 06520
Attending Physician
Department of Orthopaedic Surgery
Yale–New Haven Hospital
20 York Street
New Haven, Connecticut 06510

Margaret M. Rich, M.D., Ph.D.
Assistant Chief of Staff
Shriners Hospital for Children
2001 South Lindbergh Boulevard
St. Louis, Missouri 63131

Perry L. Schoenecker, M.D.
Professor
Department of Orthopaedic Surgery
Washington University School of Medicine
#1 Barnes-Jewish Plaza
St. Louis, Missouri 63110
Chief of Staff
Shriners Hospital for Children
2001 South Lindbergh Boulevard
St. Louis, Missouri 63131

Paul D. Sponseller, M.D.
Associate Professor
Orthopaedic Surgery
Johns Hopkins Medical Institutions
Head, Division of Pediatric Orthopaedics
Department of Orthopaedic Surgery
Johns Hopkins Hospital
601 North Caroline Street
Baltimore, Maryland 21287

Dempsey S. Springfield, M.D.
Professor and Chairman
Leni and Peter W. May Department of Orthopaedics
Mount Sinai School of Medicine
Chief of Service
Department of Orthopaedics
Mount Sinai Hospital
1 Gustave L. Levy Place
New York, New York 10029

George H. Thompson, M.D.
Professor
Department of Orthopaedic Surgery and Pediatrics
Case Western Reserve University
Director, Pediatric Orthopaedics
Rainbow Babies and Children's Hospital
11100 Euclid Avenue
Cleveland, Ohio 44106

William C. Warner, Jr., M.D.
Associate Professor
Department of Orthopaedics
University of Tennessee
956 Court Avenue
Memphis, Tennessee 38163
Staff Physician
Campbell Clinic
1400 South Germantown Road
Germantown, Tennessee 38138

Peter M. Waters, M.D.
Associate Professor
Orthopaedic Surgery Department
Harvard Medical School
Clinical Director
Hand and Upper Extremity Surgery
Children's Hospital
300 Longwood Avenue
Boston, Massachusetts 02115

Stuart L. Weinstein, M.D.
Ignacio V. Ponseti Chair of Orthopaedic Surgery
Department of Orthopaedic Surgery
University of Iowa Hospital
Iowa City, Iowa 52245

Dennis R. Wenger, M.D.
Clinical Professor
Department of Orthopaedic Surgery
University of California–San Diego
Director, Pediatric Orthopaedics
Children's Hospital and Health Center
3030 Children's Way
San Diego, California 92123

Dowain A. Wright, M.D., Ph.D.
Clinical Assistant Professor
Department of Pediatrics
University of California–San Francisco School of
    Medicine at Fresno
Department of Rheumatology and Immunology
Valley Children's Hospital
9300 Valley Children's Place
Madera, California 93638

David J. Zaleske, M.D.
Associate Professor
Department of Orthopaedics
Harvard Medical School
Boston, Massachusetts 02115
Chief, Pediatric Orthopaedics Unit
Massachusetts General Hospital
15 Parkman Street
Boston, Massachusetts 02114

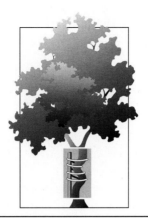

PREFACE TO THE FIRST EDITION

The field of pediatric orthopaedics has changed significantly in recent years. In the main, textbooks have kept abreast of change, to the extent that there is now a broad and useful literature addressed to the techniques of treatment of the orthopaedic disorders of children. The editors believe, however, that their fellow surgeons will have increasingly shared the desire for a work focused especially upon the decision-making process that precedes and governs the selection of surgical technique. Basic research and clinical specialization have had a dual effect upon clinical decision making. They have broadened the field of choice, and at the same time have made judicious choice more difficult.

Chapters that will aid the reader at the critical junctures at which decisions must be made have been contributed by authorities of eminence, persons who have long and successful experience dealing with the conditions about which they have written. The reader will notice that each topic is covered in depth, and that the emphasis on decision making will facilitate his assessment of the indications and contraindications for a particular treatment approach.

Although we have attempted to match depth with breadth, children's fractures have not been included because the subject is well covered in other textbooks that have recently appeared.

We would like to state that our task has been made not only worthwhile but pleasurable by the continued thoughtful and kind cooperation of the contributors whose names appear in the pages of this book. They have our deepest thanks.

Wood W. Lovell, M.D.
Robert B. Winter, M.D.

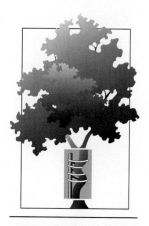

PREFACE

The fifth edition of *Lovell and Winter's Pediatric Orthopaedics* is appearing at the beginning of a new millenium and in the same year that the World Health Organization is launching the Bone and Joint Decade, aimed at improving the quality of life for people with musculoskeletal conditions, and at advancing understanding and treatment of these conditions through research, prevention, and education.

In looking through the first edition of the book—published 25 years ago—the tremendous changes in the orthopaedic care of infants, children, and adolescents is striking. However, as we read through the chapters of the fifth edition we are also struck by how much remains unknown. There are significant gaps in our knowledge of the natural history of many of the common orthopaedic conditions of childhood, the biologic basis of many of these conditions, and the long-term effectiveness of our current treatments. This fifth edition, with all of its new knowledge, is still testimony to the purpose of the Bone and Joint Decade—to improve the quality of life for those affected with musculoskeletal conditions through research, prevention, and education.

As the fifth edition is published we are in the midst of a scientific revolution that will have a profound effect on pediatric orthopaedics. While surgical techniques continue to advance, they are far outpaced by the advances in molecular genetics, where key discoveries are made weekly. As we edited the final proofs, authors were making changes to incorporate new genetic discoveries relevant to the diagnosis and mechanism of diseases for which there was no such information when they submitted their manuscripts a few short months before, let alone when the fourth edition was published five years ago. As these discoveries are applied to the clinical setting, our practice will change at an ever-increasing pace.

In this fifth edition of *Pediatric Orthopaedics,* we have tried to keep pace with the rapid advances in basic research as applied to clinical medicine by presenting discussions of the knowledge about each condition as it currently exists. Twelve chapters are written by new authors, and five previous contributors have added coauthors for this edition. Each author was carefully chosen for his expertise in a designated area. An important new chapter on the growth of the child, long overdue, has been added. All chapters summarize the current information on the natural history of a condition when known and the outcomes of standard treatments.

The contributors have indicated their evidence-based preferences for treatment when such evidence exists, and have clearly pointed out the lack thereof with other treatment alternatives. The editors have entered into a give-and-take dialogue with each contributor to identify controversial areas and to present a balanced view of them. New with this edition are cross-references to the third edition of the *Atlas of Pediatric Orthopaedic Surgery,* which link the detailed surgical techniques with the indications in the textbook.

The editors realize that some readers of this edition will be among the leaders of the new generation of orthopaedic surgeons who will fill in the gaps in our knowledge and improve the orthopaedic care of children. Patients and parents both expect and deserve their physicians to provide them with the latest evidence regarding their condition and its treatment so they can make informed choices. This is a significant burden for a parent who is deciding on the course of treatment for their child; the treatment may have significant consequences for their child in the decades ahead. We hope that this edition will provide the latest and best information for the pediatric orthopaedic surgeon practicing in the new millenium.

Raymond T. Morrissy
Stuart L. Weinstein

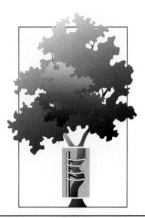

ACKNOWLEDGMENTS

The editors would like to acknowledge the great fortune that we have had to practice our profession in the finest medical system in the world during a period of unprecedented advances in research and innovation combined with extraordinary cross-fertilization provided by our scientific societies and publishers. This text stands as testimony to these advances and provides an information base for our colleagues that physicians of past generations would certainly envy.

We would like to give special thanks to those who have contributed to this book. These individuals were selected because they have worked hard to attain their knowledge and expertise and have the special talent of being able to relate the knowledge and expertise to others. In addition, we readily acknowledge the work of all of our colleagues in orthopaedics and other fields of medicine who have contributed to our knowledge.

Finally, we acknowledge the opportunity to be involved in teaching residents and fellows. Their stimulating inquiries have been a large part of what has made orthopaedic surgery fun and exciting for us over the past two decades.

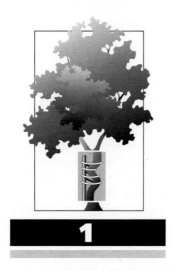

1

EMBRYOLOGY AND DEVELOPMENT
OF THE MUSCULOSKELETAL
SYSTEM

FREDERICK R. DIETZ
JOSÉ A. MORCUENDE

The development of an adult organism from a single cell is an unparalleled example of integrated cell behavior. The single cell divides many times to produce the trillions of cells of the organism, which form structures as complex and varied as the eyes, limbs, heart, or the brain. This amazing achievement raises a multitude of questions: How are the body's tissues and organs are formed? How do the different patterns form in the embryo that tell different parts what to become? How do individual cells become committed to particular development fates? Increased knowledge in developmental biology comes from the understanding of how genes direct those developmental processes. In fact, developmental biology is one of the most exciting and fast-growing fields of biology, and has become essential for understanding many other areas of biology and medicine.

Embryology at the level of gross anatomy and microscopic anatomy is fairly well described. Manipulation of experimental animals, mainly the chick and mouse, have provided insights into the relationship of tissues involved in

F. R. Dietz: Department of Orthopaedic Surgery, University of Iowa; Division of Pediatric Orthopaedics, University of Iowa Hospitals and Clinics, Iowa City, Iowa 52242.

J. A. Morcuende: Department of Orthopaedic Surgery, University of Iowa, Iowa City, Iowa 52242.

normal growth and differentiation. Molecular mechanisms underlying developmental events are being discovered. An integration of the approaches of genetics, molecular biology, developmental biology, and evolutionary biology is taking place, resulting in an explosion in understanding of the importance of individual genes and interactions of cells and tissues in specifying development of complex organisms from single cells. One of the major reasons for the synthesis and complementariness of these varying disciplines is the existence of homology, both within organisms and between species. Genes and their gene products are often very similar in structure and function in fruit flies, chickens, mice, and men. For example, *HOX* genes, which convey body/plan positional information, are conserved among species, and are similar in structure and function, i.e., homologous. In complex organisms, the same gene is often used at different times in development, and in different areas of the body, to perform similar functions.

The picture is as yet fragmented. Genes and gene products are being identified as important for development through the timing and location of their activation, the effects of their ectopic expression, and the consequences of their inactivation. However, "upstream" and "downstream" causes and effects of gene activity are often complex and may be key to manipulating biology in the service of disease and disorder prevention and correction. The mechanisms of gene actions and tissue interactions, which truly regulate and direct development, will be clearer in the coming several decades.

This chapter describes the early stages of embryonic development, followed by the descriptive anatomy of limb development and the formation of the vertebral column. It also examines bone formation and growth, and emphasizes progress in the understanding of the cellular and molecular mechanisms involved in these aspects of development. Concluding each section are observations that relate developmental anatomy to the clinical problems faced by orthopaedic surgeons.

DEVELOPMENTAL ANATOMY OF EARLY EMBRYOGENESIS AND ORGANOGENESIS

Embryogenesis has been traditionally divided into the embryonic period and the fetal period. The embryonic period is considered the time from fertilization to the end of the eighth week. During this period, the body plan is completed and all major organs are established. The stages of the embryonic period include fecundation, cleavage, gastrulation, neurulation, and organogenesis. By the eighth week of gestation, the organism's shape is fully formed, and the remaining of the gestation will involve the growth and the maturation of the organ functions.

Cleavage: Creating Multicellularity

The first stage of development after fertilization is a series of cleavage divisions in which the zygote divides in an ordered

pattern to produce a ball of much smaller cells, called a blastula. This starts the production of a multicellular organism. Cleavage is a very well-coordinated process under genetic regulation. The specific type of cleavage depends upon the evolutionary history of the species and on the mechanism used to support the nutritional requirements to the embryo. The pattern and symmetry of cell cleavage particular to a species is determined by the amount and distribution of the cytoplasm (yolk), and by those factors in the cytoplasm influencing the angle of the mitotic spindle and the timing of its formation. In most species (mammals being the exception), the rate of cell division and the placement of the blastomeres with respect to one another is completely under the control of proteins and mRNA stored in the mother oocyte. The zygote DNA is not used in early cleavage embryos. In addition, the differential cellular cleavage provides the embryo with axis information, dividing the cell into an animal pole (where the nucleus is frequently found) and a vegetal pole.

In mammals, the protected uterine environment permits an unusual style of early development. It does not have the same need as the embryos of most other species to complete the early stages rapidly. Moreover, the development of the placenta provides for nutrition from the mother, so that the zygote does not have to contain large stores of material such as yolk. Thus, cleavage has several specific characteristics. First, it is a relatively slow process. Each division is approximately 12 to 24 hours apart. A frog egg, for example, can divide into 37,000 cells in just 43 hours. Second, there is a unique orientation of the cells with relation to one another. The first cleavage is a meridional division, but in the second division, one pair of cells divides meridionally and the other equatorially (Fig. 1-1). This type of cleavage is called rotational cleavage (1). Third, there is an asynchrony in the early divisions. Cells do not divide at the same time. Therefore, embryos do not increase evenly from 2- to 4- to 8-cell stages, but frequently contain an odd number of cells. Fourth, the zygotic genome is activated early during cleav-

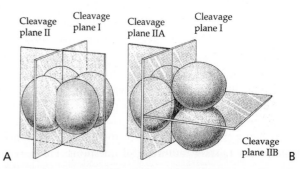

FIGURE 1-1. Comparison of early cleavage divisions in the sea urchin and in mammals. **A:** The plane of cell division in the sea urchin is perpendicular to cells. In mammals (**B,** rabbit) in the second division, one of the two blastomeres divides meridionally and the other divides equatorially. Early cell division in mammals is asynchronous—not all cells divide at the same time. (From ref. 2, with permission.)

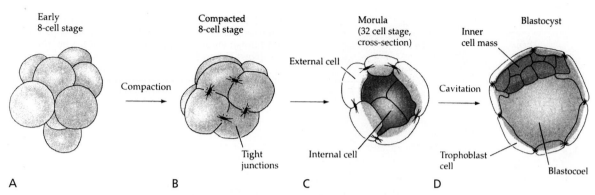

FIGURE 1-2. The cleavage of a mouse embryo, up to blastocyst. **A:** Early 8-cell stage with loose cell arrangement. **B:** Compacted 8-cell stage. During the process of compaction, cells suddenly huddle together, maximizing their contacts. Tight junctions, sealing off the inside of the sphere, stabilize outside cells. The inner cells develop gap junctions, which enables the passing of small molecules and ions. **C:** Morula with differentiation between the external cells and the inner cell mass. **D:** Blastocyst before implantation. (From ref. 2, with permission.)

age divisions to produce the proteins needed for the process to occur (3). Finally, the most crucial difference from other species is the phenomenon of compaction. At the 8-cell stage, blastomeres form a loose arrangement of cells, but after the third division, the cells cluster together and form a compact ball, with the outside cells stabilized by tight junctions and the inner cells developing gap junctions that enable the passing of small molecules and ions (Fig. 1-2).

Up to the 8-cell stage, the embryo is remarkably adaptable, and each of its cells can form any part of the later embryo or adult. One example is seen in the development of a pair of identical twins from a single fertilized egg. Similarly, this embryonic cell potential can be demonstrated experimentally by using chimeras. These are animals made by combining individual cells from early embryos of genetically different strains of animals, then the reaggregated cells are implanted in foster mothers. Analysis of the genetic composition of the tissues of the developed animal shows that the single cells from the 4-cell stage can participate in forming many different parts of the animal; they are said to be totipotent (4,5).

In mammals, the next stage in development is the generation of the cells that will form the placenta and the membranes that surround the developing embryo. The cells of the compacted embryo divide to produce a 16-cell morula. This morula consists of a small group (1 or 2) of internal cells surrounded by a larger group of external cells (Fig. 1-2C) (6). The position of a cell at this stage determines whether it will form extraembryonic structures or contribute to the embryo proper. Inner cells will form the embryo and most of the external cells will form the trophoblast. This structure will enable the embryo to get oxygen and nourishment from the mother, and will secrete hormones and regulators of the immune response so that the mother will not reject the embryo. Experimentally, this separation of cell activities also has been shown with chimeras. Cells from different strains of mouse can be arranged so that the cells of one strain surround the cells of the other strain. The

development of such cell-aggregates shows that only the cells on the inside contribute to mouse development (7). By the 64-cell stage, the inner cell mass and the trophoblast have become separate cell layers, neither of which contributes cells to the other group. Thus, the distinction between these two cell types represents the first differentiation event in mammalian development.

Implantation and Gastrulation: Organizing the Embryonic Cells to Form Tissues and Organs

In human beings, implantation begins 1 or 2 days after the blastocyst enters the uterus, approximately on day 7 (Fig. 1-3A). At the time of implantation, the exposed surface of the uterine lining, the endometrium, is a single-layered epithelial sheet, which forms numerous tubular glands. Having adhered to the epithelium, the trophoblastic cells penetrate it and erode it (Fig. 1-3B). The endometrium responds by a dramatic increase in vascularity and capillary permeability, the so-called "decidual reaction" (Fig. 1-4). These processes are apparently mediated by estrogens produced by the blastocyst and estrogen receptors in the wall of the uterus. In addition, the trophoblast initiates the secretion of human chorionic gonadotropin, which will maintain the production of progesterone by the ovaries, essential for the maintenance of the pregnancy. Human chorionic gonadotropin is detectable in the blood and urine, and serves as the basis of pregnancy tests.

The next phase of development—gastrulation—involves a remarkable process in which the ball of cells of the blastula turns itself into a multilayered structure and rearranges to form the three embryonic tissue layers known as endoderm, ectoderm, and mesoderm. In addition, during gastrulation, the body plan of the organism is also established. Gastrulation thus involves dramatic changes in the overall structure of the embryo, converting it into a complex three-dimensional structure.

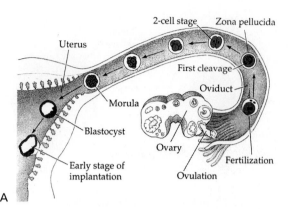

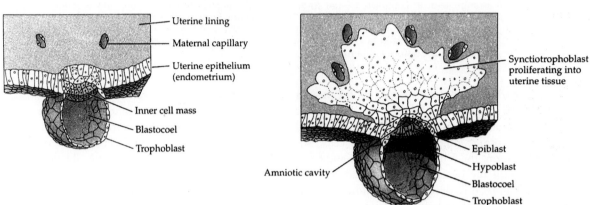

FIGURE 1-3. **A:** Development of human embryo from fecundation to implantation (blastocyst at 7 days). **B:** Tissue formation of human embryo between days 7 and 8. The inner cell mass will give rise to the embryo proper, and the trophoblast to the placenta. The distinction between those two groups of cells represents the first differentiation event in embryonic development. (From ref. 2, with permission.)

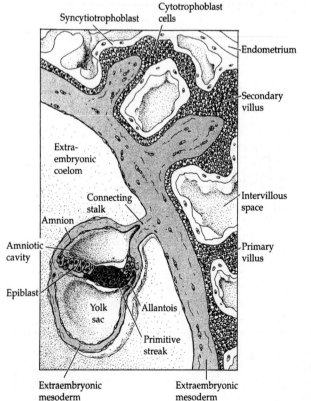

FIGURE 1-4. Placenta development in the human embryo at the end of the third week of gestation. The trophoblast cells forming the placenta are coming into contact with the blood vessels of the uterus. The endometrium responds by a dramatic increase in vascularity and capillary permeability, the so-called decidual reaction. The trophoblast divides into the cytotrophoblast, which will form the villi, and the syncytiotrophoblast, which will ingress into the uterine cavity. The actual embryo forms from the cells of the epiblast. (From ref. 11, with permission.)

The mechanics of gastrulation in mammals are not well understood. In sea urchins and insects, the phenomenon of gastrulation can be compared to what happens if a ball is punctured, then kicked: the ball collapses and the inner surface on one side makes contact with the other side, making a large dimple. In the embryo, a large area of cells on the outside of the embryo is brought to lie inside it by a complicated invagination. Subsequent development depends on the interactions of the outer ectoderm, middle mesoderm, and inner endoderm layers of cells. The ectoderm will give rise to the epidermis of the skin and to the nervous system; the mesoderm will give rise to connective tissues, including the bones, muscle, and blood; and the endoderm will give rise to the lung and the lining of the gut and associated organs.

In addition, during gastrulation, the cells are positioned according to the body plan appropriate to the species, and there is a process of differentiation of the functional characteristics required of each part of the body plan. Specification of the axes in mammals does not involve any maternal component. The dorsoventral axis is established by the interaction between the inner cell mass and the trophectoderm, whereas the anteroposterior axis may be set only at implantation. The generation of the left–right asymmetry is under genetic control. This vertebrate body plan will be maintained thereafter as the embryo grows.

The movements of gastrulation involve the entire embryo. Cell migration in one part of the embryo must be intimately coordinated with other cell movements occurring simultaneously elsewhere. However, gastrulation depends on a relatively simple repetition of basic cell activities. Cells can change their shape by extending or contracting. They can group or separate by forming or breaking their adhesions to neighboring cells or to the extracellular matrix.

They can secrete extracellular matrix that constrains or guides their location or movement. These activities, together with cell proliferation, underlie almost all morphogenetic activities during gastrulation. The special problem posed in early embryonic development is to understand how these and other elementary cell activities are coordinated in space and time.

Recent experiments have suggested that the maternal and paternal genomes (imprinting) have different roles during mammalian gastrulation. Mouse zygotes can be created that have only sperm-derived or oocyte-derived chromosomes. The male-derived embryos die without embryo proper structures, but with well-formed chorionic structures. Conversely, the female-derived embryos develop normally, but without chorionic structures (8,9). This observation also has been confirmed using mouse chimeras (10). Therefore, the maternal and paternal genomic information may have distinct functions during early development.

Early Organogenesis in Vertebrate Development: Neurulation and Mesoderm Segmentation

During gastrulation, the germ layers (ectoderm, mesoderm, and endoderm) move to the positions in which they develop into the structures of the adult organism. The anteroposterior body axis of the vertebrate embryo emerges, with the head at one end and the future tail at the other. During the next stage of development, the main organs of the body begin to emerge gradually (11). A major set of interactions takes place between the mesodermal cells and the ectoderm in the dorsal midline (Hensen's node) so that the ectoderm cell layer will form the nervous system (Fig. 1-5). At the

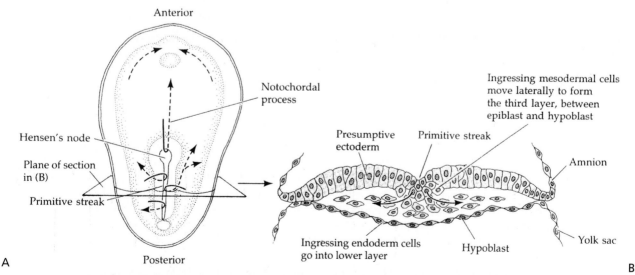

FIGURE 1-5. Cell movements during the gastrulation stage. **A:** Surface view of cells migrating through Hensen's node which travel anteriorly to form the notochord. Cells traveling through the primitive streak will become the precursors of mesoderm and endoderm. **B:** Transverse section of the embryo. (From ref. 11, with permission.)

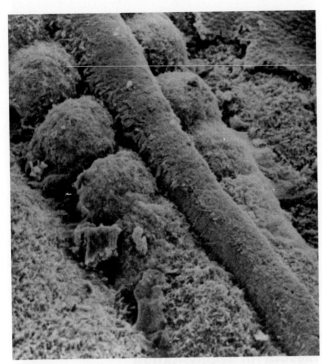

FIGURE 1-6. Scanning electron microscopy showing the neural tube and the well-formed somites with paraxial mesoderm that has not yet separated into distinct somites. (Courtesy of K. W. Tosney.)

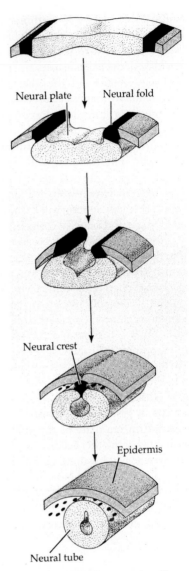

FIGURE 1-7. Diagrammatic representation of neural tube formation. The ectoderm folds in at the most dorsal point, forming a neural tube that is connected by neural crest cells, and an outer epidermis. (From ref. 11, with permission.)

same time, the mesoderm on either side of the middle breaks up into blocks of cells to form the somites, a series of repeated segments along the axis of the embryo (Fig. 1-6) (12). The interactions between the dorsal mesoderm and its overlying ectoderm are one of the most important of all development. The action by which the flat layer of ectodermal cells is transformed into a hollow tube is called neurulation (Fig. 1-7). The first indication of neurulation is a change in cell shape in the ectoderm. Midline ectodermal cells become elongated, whereas cells destined to form the epidermis become flattened. The elongation of the cells causes this region to rise above the surrounding ectoderm, thus creating the neural plate. Shortly thereafter, the edges of the neural plate thicken and move upward to form the neural folds, which subsequently will fuse to form the neural tube beneath the overlying ectoderm. The formation of the neural tube does not occur all at once. It starts near the anterior end of the embryo and proceeds anteriorly and posteriorly. The two open ends are called anterior and posterior neuropores (Fig. 1-8). In mammals, failure to close the anterior neuropore results in anencephalia, and the posterior neuropore in spina bifida. Neural tube defects can be detected during pregnancy by ultrasonography and chemical analysis of the amniotic fluid.

The process of neurulation is intimately linked to changes in cell shape generated by the cytoskeleton (microtubules and microfilaments). Differential cell division seen in different regions of the neural plate would also contribute

to the size and shape of this region. In addition, those cells directly adjacent to the notochord and those cells at the hinges of the neural groove will also help to mold the neural tube. Separation of the neural tube from the ectoderm that will form the skin requires changes in cell adhesiveness. Although molecules that can induce neural tissue, such as noggin protein, have been identified, induction of neurulation is due to inhibition of bone morphogenetic protein (BMP) activity. Positional identity of cells along the anteroposterior axis is encoded by the combinatorial expression of genes of the four *HOX* complexes.

The cells at the dorsalmost portion of the neural tube become the neural crest. These cells will migrate through the embryo, and will give rise to several cell populations.

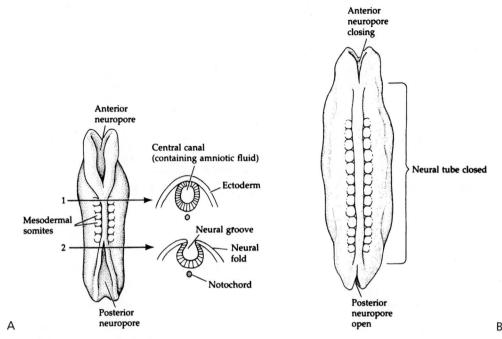

FIGURE 1-8. Neural tube formation in human embryos does not occur simultaneously throughout the ectoderm. **A:** At the initial stages, both anterior and posterior neuropores are open. **B:** Closing of the neural tube proceeds both cranially and caudally. Failure to close the posterior neuropore at day 27 results in spina bifida, the severity of which depends upon how much of the spinal cord remains open. Failure to close the anterior neuropore results in lethal anencephaly. (From ref. 11, with permission.)

Although derived from the ectoderm, the neural crest has sometimes been called the fourth germ layer because of its importance. It gives rise to the neurons and supporting glial cells of the sensory, sympathetic, and parasympathetic nervous systems; the melanocytes of the epidermis; and the cartilage and connective tissue components of the head. Although not well understood, the mechanisms of neural crest migration are not random but rather follow precise pathways specified by the extracellular matrix. Differences in adhesiveness between the anterior and posterior halves of the somites result in the neural crest being prevented from migrating over the posterior halves. Thus, presumptive dorsal ganglia cells collect adjacent to anterior halves, giving them a segmental arrangement.

The formation of mesodermal structures does not occur subsequent to that of the neural tube, but simultaneously. The brain and spinal cord must develop in the correct relationship with other body structures, particularly the mesoderm. Five regions of mesoderm can be identified at the neurula-stage embryo (Fig. 1-9): the chordamesoderm, which will generate the notochord, a transient organ whose functions include inducing neural tube formation and establishing the body axis; the dorsal (somitic) mesoderm, which will produce many of the connective tissues of the body; the intermediate mesoderm, which will form the urinary system and genital ducts; the lateral plate mesoderm, which will give rise to the heart, blood vessels and blood cells, and the body lining cavities; and lastly, the head mesoderm, which will contribute to the connective tissues and muscles of the face.

At the neural stage, the body plan has been established and the regions of the embryo that will form limbs, eyes, heart, and the other organs have been determined. But although the positions of various organs are fixed, there is no overt sign yet of differentiation. The potential to form a given organ is now confined to specific regions. Each region has, however, considerable capacity for regulation, so that, if a part of the region is removed, a normal structure can still form. In later sections, limb and axial skeleton formation will be discussed in more detail.

Conceptual Insights of Embryogenesis and Early Organogenesis

Development is essentially the emergence of organized and specialized structures from an initially very simple group of cells. Thus, the cells of the body, as a rule, are genetically alike (they all have the same DNA content) but phenotypically different—some are specialized as muscle, others as neurons, and so on. During development, differences are generated between cells in the embryo that lead to spatial organization, changes in form, and the generation of different cell types. All these features are ultimately determined

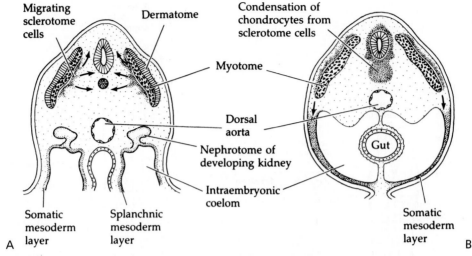

FIGURE 1-9. Mesoderm formation in human embryo. Diagram of a transverse section through the trunk of an early 4-week (**A**) and late 4-week embryo (**B**). Sclerotome cells migrate from the somite, and these cells ultimately become chondrocytes. The remaining dermatome cells will form the dermis. The myotome will give rise to the striated muscle of both the back and limbs. (From ref. 11, with permission.)

by the DNA sequence of the genome. Each cell must act according to the same genetic instructions, but it must interpret them with regard to time and space.

Multicellular organisms are very complex, but they are generated by a limited repertoire of cell activities. In the same way that an artist moves from one part of a sculpture to another to achieve first the overall figure's shape, then the specific anatomic features, using a selected number of instruments over and over again, nature also displays a comparable economy in choosing processes and molecular tools. The key to understanding development lies in cell biology, in the processes of signal transduction, and in the control of gene expression that results in changes of cell state, movement, and growth. The single most important fact in development is based on the surprising finding that the developmental control genes are maintained through evolution. Thus, for many genes discovered in the invertebrate systems, homologue genes have been identified in vertebrates. These have similar developmental roles in species ranging from the fruit fly to fish to mouse to human.

It is convenient to distinguish three main developmental processes, even though they considerably overlap with, and influence, one another. These are the emergence of pattern, cell differentiation, and change in form or morphogenesis.

Pattern Formation

Pattern formation is the process by which spatial and temporal arrangements of cell activities are organized within the embryo, so that a well-defined structure develops. Pattern

formation is critical for the proper development of every part of the organism. In the developing limb, for example, pattern formation enables the cells to know whether to make the upper arm or the fingers, and where the muscles should form.

Pattern formation in many animals is based on a mechanism in which the cells first acquire a positional identity, which determines their future behavior. The ability of cells to sense their relative positions within a limited population of cells, and to differentiate according to this position, has been the subject of intense research. Pattern formation in many systems has similar principles, and, more striking, similar genes. Many of the so-called homeotic genes that determine segment identity in *Drosophila* have turned up in vertebrates, and appear to play similar roles in segmentation of structures such as the brain or the vertebral column.

Homeotic genes are like embryonic switches, analogous to switches of railroad yards that direct trains into one path rather than another. Homeotic genes are involved in specifying regional identity along the anteroposterior axis. The name comes from the fact that mutations in some of these genes result in what is called a homeotic transformation, in which one body structure replaces another. For example, in mice in whom *HOXD11* is mutated, anterior sacral vertebrae are transformed into lumbar vertebrae. Homeotic genes in all systems work similarly: They code for proteins called transcription factors, which control gene expression. In vertebrates and *Drosophila*, the order of homeotic genes on the chromosome corresponds to their temporal and spatial expression on the anteroposterior axis of the embryo.

Cell Differentiation

Cell differentiation is the process in which cells become structurally and functionally different from each other, ending up as distinct types, such as muscle, bone, or cartilage. Because each cell of the organism has the same genetic material, the achievement and persistence of the differentiation state depends on a series of signals that ultimately control the transcription of specific genes. In humans, the zygote gives rise to about 250 clearly distinguishable types of cells. One of the major goals of developmental biology is to discover how these differences emerge from the fertilized oocyte.

In any organism, differentiation leads to the production of a finite number of discrete kinds of cells, each with its peculiar repertory of biochemical activities and possible morphological configurations. When cells achieve a distinctive state of differentiation, they do not transform into cells of another type. Differentiation leads to a stable, irreversible set of cellular activities. At the organ level, once an embryonic part is capable of realizing its prospective fate in the absence of the conditions that established that capability, it is said to be determined. Determination is thus a step that limits the subsequent development of the part to a specific tissue and cellular differentiation.

Pattern formation and cell differentiation are very closely interrelated, as can be seen by considering the difference between the upper and lower extremities. Both contain the same tissues—muscle, cartilage, bone, and so on—yet the patterns in which they are arranged are different. It is essentially pattern formation that makes human beings different from rabbits or chimpanzees.

Morphogenesis

Although vertebrate morphogenesis—change in form—is far from completely understood, developmental biology supports the findings that the same family of molecules and pathways that guide the earliest stages of embryogenesis, setting up such basic elements of body pattern as the head-to-tail and dorsoventral axis, also help out in morphogenesis. What is more, these molecules and pathways have been conserved over the course of evolution. Morphogenesis relies on a rather restricted number of cellular activities and encompasses the formation of all tissues and organs from the first embryonic tissue layers to the finished limb, spine, or brain. However, before any tissue or organ can form, earlier steps must occur, steps that tell cells who they are and what tissues they should form. Those early steps take place in the "control room" for development, and morphogenesis is then what happens on the "factory floor"—the actual assembly of the tissues and organs that make up the organism. In addition, spatial patterns of cell proliferation, folding of cell groups, rearrangement of cells, and cell migration make important contributions to morphogenesis, the process that shapes the embryo. Finally, as the embryo develops, cells become different, and this process culminates in the specialization of cells for particular functions. Therefore, during development, morphogenesis gives rise to structures appropriate to their position within the embryo, and, within these structures, the differentiation of individual cells and their interactions are spatially ordered.

Clinical Significance

Broadly defined, birth defects or congenital abnormalities occur in 6% of all live births. Twenty percent of infant deaths are due to congenital anomalies. Approximately 3% of newborns have significant structural abnormalities. At present, the cause of approximately 50 to 60% of birth defects is unknown: chromosomal abnormalities cause 6 to 7%, specific gene mutations cause 7 to 8%, environmental teratogens are responsible for 7 to 10% of defects, and combined genetic predisposition with environmental factors cause the remaining 20 to 25% of congenital abnormalities.

Starting from a single cell, the embryo can spawn all the new cells and tissues needed to provide an organism with its correct complement of organs. Many of the molecules and pathways known to control cell differentiation and growth during organ formation in the embryo do not become obsolete in the adult. They do help maintain and repair tissues and regulate their response to external environment signals. Some of these proteins are or will soon be in clinical use, such as erythropoietin, which triggers red blood cell production; platelet-derived growth factor (PDGF) for diabetic skin ulcers; and BMP for bone and cartilage regeneration. Finally, in malignant disease, the control of cell activities, such as proliferation, differentiation, and migration, appears to break down. An understanding of the way in which cell behavior is coordinated in embryos could therefore give insights into bone and cartilage regeneration and cancer biology.

DEVELOPMENTAL ANATOMY OF THE LIMB

At 26 days after fertilization, the upper limb is evident as a slight elevation on the ventrolateral body wall at the level of the pericardial swelling. The lower limb elevation appears 2 days later, just caudal to the level of the umbilical cord, and develops similarly, but slightly later than the upper limb (Fig. 1-10). At this time, the neural tube is closed, all somites are present, and the anlage of the vertebrae and intervertebral discs is present. The limb bud initially consists of loose mesenchymal tissue enclosed in an epithelial ectodermal sheath. The limb bud is formed from mesenchymal cells of the lateral plate, then augmented by cells from the adjacent somites. The skeletal elements and tendons develop from the lateral plate mesenchyme, whereas limb muscle arises from somitic mesenchymal cells that migrate into the limb bud.

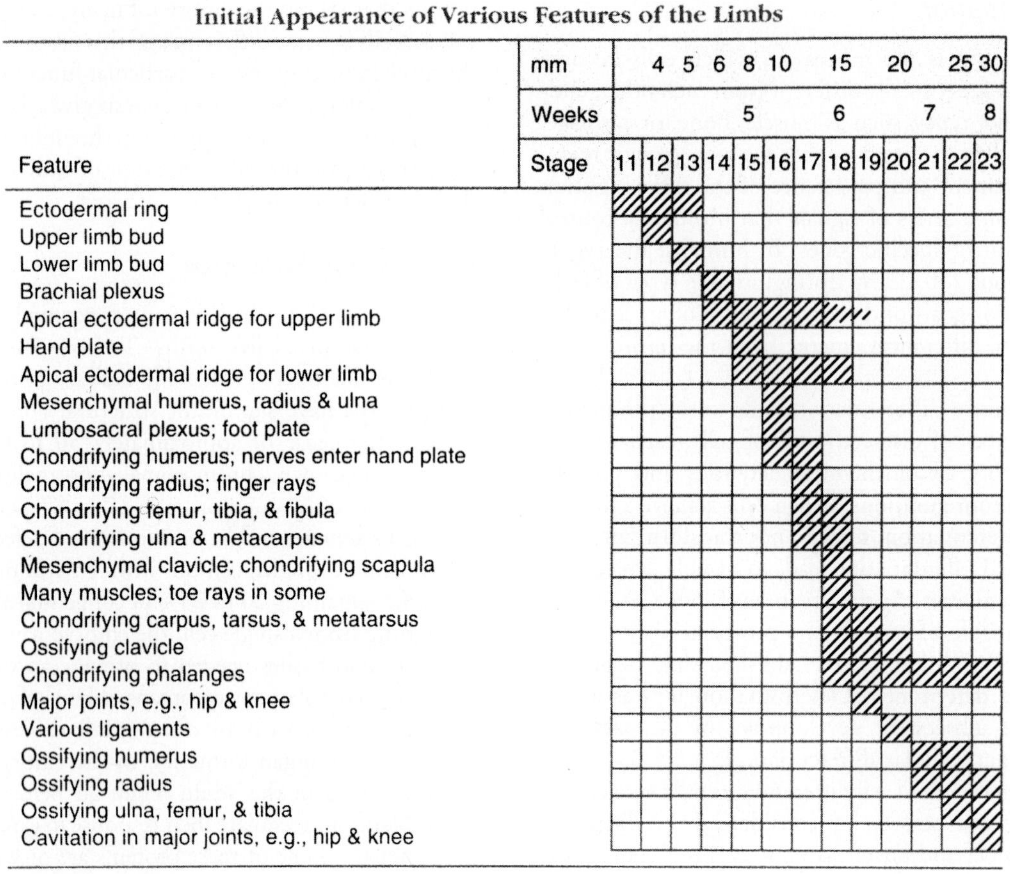
Initial Appearance of Various Features of the Limbs
Feature
mm
4 5 6 8 10 15 20 25 30
Weeks
5 6 7 8
Stage
11 12 13 14 15 16 17 18 19 20 21 22 23
Ectodermal ring
Upper limb bud
Lower limb bud
Brachial plexus
Apical ectodermal ridge for upper limb
Hand plate
Apical ectodermal ridge for lower limb
Mesenchymal humerus, radius & ulna
Lumbosacral plexus; foot plate
Chondrifying humerus; nerves enter hand plate
Chondrifying radius; finger rays
Chondrifying femur, tibia, & fibula
Chondrifying ulna & metacarpus
Mesenchymal clavicle; chondrifying scapula
Many muscles; toe rays in some
Chondrifying carpus, tarsus, & metatarsus
Ossifying clavicle
Chondrifying phalanges
Major joints, e.g., hip & knee
Various ligaments
Ossifying humerus
Ossifying radius
Ossifying ulna, femur, & tibia
Cavitation in major joints, e.g., hip & knee

FIGURE 1-10. Timing of the appearance of limb features. (From ref. 83, with permission.)

This mesenchymal swelling is covered by ectoderm, the tip of which thickens and becomes the apical ectodermal ridge (AER) (Fig. 1-11). Underlying the AER are rapidly proliferating, undifferentiated mesenchymal cells that are called the progress zone (PZ). Proliferation of these cells causes limb outgrowth. Cells begin to differentiate only after leaving the PZ. The interaction between the AER and the undifferentiated mesenchymal cells underlying it is crucial for limb development. Experimental procedures on chick embryos reveal the following about the limb bud mesenchyme: (i) if removed, no limb develops; (ii) when grafted under the ectoderm at a location other than the normal limb area, an AER is induced and a limb will develop; (iii) lower limb mesoderm will induce leg formation when placed under an upper limb AER. Grafting experiments with the AER reveal that: (i) AER removal aborts further limb development. The later in limb development the AER is removed, the less severe is the resulting limb truncation (limb elements develop from proximal to distal); (ii) an extra AER will induce a limb bud to form supernumerary limb structures; (iii) nonlimb mesenchymal cells placed beneath the AER will not result in limb development, and the AER withers (13).

The implications of these experiments are that the AER is necessary for the growth and development of the limb, whereas the limb bud mesenchyme induces, sustains, and instructs the AER. In addition to biochemical influence on the PZ, the tightly packed columnar cells of the AER perform a mechanical function, directing limb shape by containing these undifferentiated cells in a dorsoventrally flattened shape. The length of the AER controls the width of the limb, as well. When all limb elements have differentiated, the AER disappears.

The three axes of limbs—anteroposterior (AP: thumb to small finger), dorsoventral (DV: back of hand to palm), and proximal-distal (PD)—are specified very early in limb development. The AP and DV axes are fixed before morphological differentiation of limb components occurs. The PD axis is determined as the limb grows out. The AP axis is set first, followed by the DV axis, then the PD axis. This has been shown by rotation of transplanted limb buds from their normal position and finding, at different stages, whether the limb bud retained the axis orientation of its original limb position or developed the orientation of the host bud (10,14,15).

AP axis determination is under the control of an area of

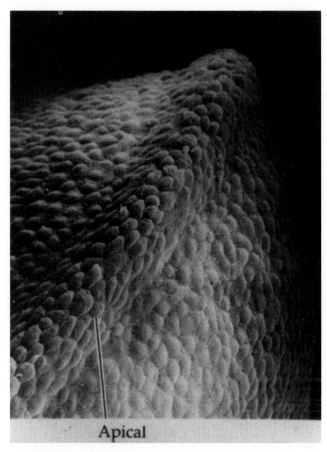

Apical

FIGURE 1-11. Scanning electron photomicrograph of an early chick forelimb bud, with the apical ectodermal ridge at the tip of the limb bud. (Courtesy of K. W. Tosney.)

tissue in the posterior aspect of the limb bud called the zone of polarizing activity (ZPA), or polarizing region. If this tissue is grafted onto the anterior aspect of a limb bud, a duplication of digits in a mirror image to the normally present digits occurs (16). Cells for the new digits are recruited from the underlying mesoderm, and the distal part of the limb widens, as does the AER. If less tissue from the polarizing region is grafted, fewer new digits develop (17). This and other experiments suggest that a morphogenic gradient of a diffusible signal originating from the ZPA determines AP axis. This is discussed in the section on the molecular biology of limb development.

The DV axis is under the control of both the mesoderm and ectoderm of the limb bud at different stages of development. The mesoderm specifies the axis initially, but, very early after limb bud formation, the ectodermal orientation becomes preeminent. If the ectoderm of a right limb bud is transplanted onto the mesenchyme of a left limb bud, the distal limb that develops will be that of a right limb, with respect to muscle pattern and joint orientation (14,15).

The PD axis seems to be determined by the length of time a mesodermal cell remains at the tip of the limb bud

in the progress zone under the influence of the AER. Once a cell leaves the tip, its position in the limb is fixed. Young tips grafted onto older limb buds will duplicate existing limb elements, whereas older tips grafted on young buds will only form distal elements. The best hypothesis as to how this information is passed is that the number of rounds of cell division that occur while under the influence of the AER determines the PD fate of a cell. Support for this hypothesis comes from experiments in which the limb bud is irradiated. The surviving cells of the irradiated tip have to undergo several extra rounds of mitosis before they can escape the influence of the AER and thereby gain positional determination. In these experiments, intermediate limb elements are not formed, only the preexisting proximal elements and newly formed distal elements (18).

Cellular differentiation of the homogenous, undifferentiated-appearing mesenchymal cells in the limb bud results from signals different than those conveying the axis/positional information as described above. The center of the limb bud develops a condensation of cells that prefigures the skeletal elements—the chondrogenic core, which begins at the body wall and progresses distally with limb elongation. A rich vascular bed surrounds the chondrogenic core. Immediately adjacent to the vascular bed is a thick avascular zone that extends to the ectodermal sheath of the limb bud. Although the signaling mechanism has not been discovered, the ectoderm appears to control initial mesodermal differentiation by maintaining the adjacent mesenchymal cells in a flattened configuration, which prevents differentiation into chondrogenic cells. The central mesenchymal cells assume a rounded shape and form the chondrogenic core (17,19). This process of differentiation occurs from proximal to distal. Early in the 7th week, cartilage anlage of the entire upper limb skeletal elements, with the exception of the distal phalanges, is present. Paddle-shaped hand plates have formed by the end of the 6th week, and condensations of cells have formed identifiable digital rays in the hand. The same is true of the foot 1 week later. The cells between the digital rays are a loose mesenchyme that undergoes programmed cell death (apoptosis) to create the separated fingers and toes.

After the chondrogenic anlagen of the future skeletal structures and the vascular bed develop, the ingrowth of nerves develops, followed immediately by the development of muscle tissue. All bones are prefigured in mesenchyme, followed by cartilage, then bone. Actual bone appears toward the end the embryonic period, first in the clavicle, mandible, and maxilla, between the 6th and 7th weeks. Ossific centers appear soon after in the humerus, radius, femur, tibia, and ulna, in that order. Just prior to birth, ossific centers appear in the calcaneus, talus, cuboid, distal femoral epiphysis, and proximal tibial epiphysis.

The mechanisms controlling the development and patterning of the vasculature are not well worked out. Vascular cells are believed to have an intrinsic capacity to form vessels and to branch, which is controlled by inhibitory signals extrinsic to the angiotrophic tissues. Well-developed veins develop on the postaxial border of the limb buds and persist as the fibular and saphenous veins, permitting identification of the embryonic postaxial border, even in mature organisms. The early preaxial veins, the cephalic and great saphenous veins, develop secondarily. The initial arterial supply to the limb bud organizes into a single axial artery. In the arm, this artery becomes the subclavian, axillary, brachial, and anterior interosseous arteries. In the leg, the axial artery comes from the umbilical artery and becomes the inferior gluteal, sciatic, proximal popliteal, and distal peroneal arteries. The femoral and tibial arteries develop secondarily.

The brachial and lumbosacral plexuses and the major peripheral nerves are present by the 5th week. They progressively invade their target tissues, and by the 7th week have innervated the muscles and cutaneous tissues in the adult pattern. Each dermatome represents a single dorsal root's sensory fibers. From cranial to caudal, the dermatomes of the limbs descend along the preaxial border and ascend along the postaxial border of the limb. Overlapping and variability among individuals make assessment of dermatomal sensation nonspecific for single nerves (Fig. 1-12).

Mesenchymal cells that are to become limb muscles migrate from the somatic layer of the lateral mesoderm during the 5th week, and surround the chondrogenic core of the limb bud. They develop into dorsal and ventral groups from an undifferentiated mass and individual muscles gradually become distinct, again in a proximal/distal sequence. Most anatomically distinct adult muscles are identifiable in the eighth week. Mesenchymal cells develop into myoblasts (activation of a single gene, *MyoD1,* is sufficient to turn a fibroblast into a myoblast phenotype in tissue culture), which then elongate, form parallel bundles, and fuse into myotubes. Muscle-specific contractile proteins, actin and myosin, are synthesized, and the myotubes form sarcomeres. By the 8th week, both myotube development and innervation are sufficiently advanced for movement to begin. By 12 weeks the cross-striations of the myofibrils are apparent in myotube cytoplasm. Most muscle cells are formed prior to birth, with the remaining cells developing in the first year of life. Enlargement of muscles results from an increase in diameter with the creation of more myofilaments and elongation with the growth of the skeleton. Ultimate muscle size results from genetic programming, exercise, and the hormonal milieu.

Development of the synovial joints commences in the 6th week of development. A condensation of cells in which the joint develops is called the interzone. The interzone cells differentiate into chondrogenic cells, synovial cells, and central cells. The chondrogenic cells are adjacent to the mesenchymal cells, and form the articular cartilage. The central cells form the intraarticular structures. The synovial cells differentiate into both the tough fibrous capsule and the loose, vascular synovium. Programmed cell death (apoptosis) results in cavitation that produces the joint per se. Motion is necessary for normal joint development, as the host of conditions causing arthrogryposis demonstrate, as well as animal experiments that create joint anomalies by paralyzing the developing fetus.

During the embryonic period, all four limbs are similar,

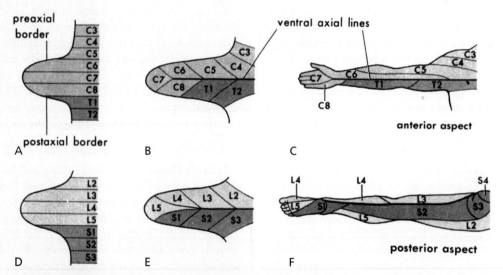

FIGURE 1-12. Development of the dermatome pattern in the limb. **A** and **D:** Diagram of the segmental arrangement of dermatomes in the 5th embryonic week. **B** and **E:** The pattern is shown one week later as the limb bud grows. **C** and **F:** The mature dermatome pattern is shown. The original ventral surface becomes posterior in the mature leg and anterior in the mature arm, due to the normal rotation of the limbs. (From ref. 20, with permission.)

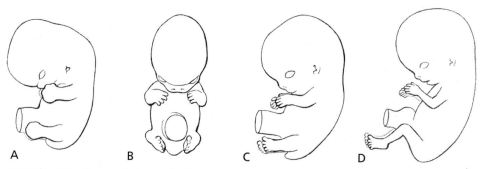

FIGURE 1-13. Normal limb rotation is depicted. **A:** 48 days, the hand and foot plates face each other. **B:** 51 days, elbows are bent laterally. **C:** 54 days, the soles of the feet face each other. **D:** lateral rotation of the arms and medial rotation of the legs result in caudally facing elbows and cranially facing knees. (From ref. 20, with permission.)

with parallel axes. The preaxial borders are cephalad and the postaxial borders are caudad. The thumb and hallux are preaxial; the radius/tibia and ulna/fibula are homologous bones occupying the same positions in the limb bud. The longitudinal axis at this stage passes through the long finger and the second toe. During the fetal period, the upper limb rotates 90 degrees externally (laterally), and the lower limb rotates 90 degrees internally (medially). The forearm flexors come to lie medially and the forearm extensors, laterally. The leg extensors lie ventrally, and the leg flexors lie dorsally (Fig. 1-13).

Thus, by the 8th week, the task of tissue differentiation is largely completed and growth is the major task ahead.

Molecular Insights of Limb Development

The explosion in molecular biology and molecular genetic techniques has revealed much about how an individual gene's activation at specific moments in development can cause the events that create complex organisms from single cells. The story is incomplete, and this section highlights presently known or suspected molecular mechanisms that underlie development. The development of organs employs mechanisms of cell growth, differentiation, and patterning similar to those that occur in earlier development of the basic body plan. The mechanisms for differentiation and patterning are remarkably conserved from fruit flies to chicks to mice and to humans.

The limb is one of the best-studied body structures and much information is available from the study of nonhuman animals, especially chicks, mice, and fruit flies. Much knowledge is inferred from the observations that certain genes and gene products are present at crucial moments in development. Often, many different genes and molecules are expressed simultaneously or in a closely overlapping sequence, and the complex interactions that control development are not fully worked out. The information presented in this section is based on study of limb development in the chick, except where noted. Most other information

comes from gene "knock out" experiments in mice, wherein a specific gene is rendered nonfunctional and the effects on development are noted.

Limb Bud Outgrowth and Proximal-distal Patterning (Fig. 1-14)

As discussed previously, the AER is required for limb bud outgrowth. The AER is a band of cells at the limb bud tip, lying between the dorsal and ventral limb ectoderm. Although the stimulus for AER formation, which resides in the mesoderm, is unknown, some of the molecular signals that are important in specifying the location of the AER have been identified. Engrailed-1 (En-1) is a homeobox-containing transcription factor whose expression is limited to the ventral limb ectoderm (21). Radical fringe (r-Fng) is a secreted factor that modulates signaling that is expressed only in the dorsal ectoderm (22). Radical fringe is a homolog of the *Drosophila* gene *fringe*, which helps specify dorsal–ventral boundaries in the fruit fly (23,24).

Excision of the AER results in truncation of the limb. The earlier the excision, the more proximal is the truncation. Limb bud outgrowth can be sustained after excision of the AER, by insertion of beads carrying fibroblast growth factors (FGF). Fibroblast growth factors are a group of similar proteins that affect cell proliferation, differentiation, and motility. During development, they have in common a role in mediating mesenchymal–epithelial tissue interaction. To obtain the most normal limb development, two FGF-soaked beads must be placed so that the polarizing region is mimicked, as well as the AER (25). The absence of the mechanical flattening of the limb bud by the AER results in a bulbous limb bud and bunching of the digits. Nevertheless, fully differentiated limb skeletal structures can be produced.

FGF2, -4, and -8 are expressed in the AER, and each is able by itself to sustain limb bud outgrowth (probably because of the ability of different FGFs to activate the same

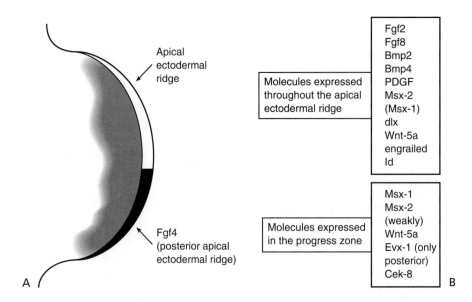

FIGURE 1-14. A diagram of the tip of the limb bud showing the apical ectodermal ridge and progress zone (**A**) and some of the molecules that are expressed in these tissues (**B**). (Adapted from ref. 83, with permission.)

receptors) (26–28). *In vivo* FGF-8 is found in the entire AER, whereas FGF-4 expression is limited to the posterior portion of the AER. FGF-10 and 8 are the critical FGFs expressed during the initiation of limb bud outgrowth. FGF-10 is expressed first in the lateral plate mesoderm at the site of the future limb bud. FGF-10 induces FGF-8 expression in ectodermal cells that will become the AER. Some experiments suggest that FGF-8 and FGF-10 act in a positive feedback loop; that is, the expression of each supports and promotes the expression of the other. Mice in whom FGF-10 function is eliminated develop normally, except for the complete absence of limbs and failure of normal pulmonary development (29).

Proximal-distal positional information is engraved upon individual cells in the progress zone based on the length of time (number of mitoses?) the cell spends in the progress zone as discussed in the section Developmental Anatomy of the Limb in this chapter (30,31). Some experimental work suggests that transforming growth factor β (TGF-β) acts in a gradient from the AER to increase cell adhesion by activating integrins, which are mediators of cell adhesion. Perhaps the longer a cell is in the progress zone, the more TGF-β it sees, and the more integrins are activated, the greater the cell adhesion, and ultimately, the more distal is the limb positional information programmed into the cell.

Anterior-Posterior Axis Determination/Zone of Polarizing Activity (Fig. 1-15)

The ability of a small piece of tissue excised from the posterior and proximal limb bud to induce duplication of digits, when grafted to an anterior position on another limb bud,

suggested that this region of polarizing activity synthesized a morphogen, acting by a gradient to specify anterior-posterior limb elements (16). If acting through a morphogenic gradient, the zone of polarizing activity should give different digit patterns when transplanted to different areas of the limb bud, which it does (32). Furthermore, if a physical barrier is placed between the anterior and posterior parts of the limb bud, a normal number and order of digits is formed in the posterior portion of the limb bud, and no digits are formed anteriorly (33).

By serendipity, retinoic acid was found to cause reduplication of limbs in amputated salamanders (34). Subsequently, retinoic acid was identified in the limb bud, with a high concentration posteriorly and a low concentration anteriorly. Retinoic acid on filter paper, placed anteriorly, induces mirror-image digits to those formed from the natural posterior gradient (35). Nevertheless, retinoic acid is not a simple morphogen acting through a gradient. Bathing an entire limb bud in retinoic acid should eliminate the gradient, but instead mirror-image reduplication occurs. Also, when retinoic acid concentration is at a minimum, the zone of polarizing activity is at a maximum. The action of retinoic acid is complex and includes several classes of nuclear retinoic acid receptors and retinoic-binding proteins in the cytoplasm. These different receptors and binding proteins are present in different amounts in various parts of the developing limb, suggesting a very complex role for retinoic acid. If retinoic acid synthesis is blocked, limb bud outgrowth does not occur or is severely stunted. At present, it appears that retinoic acid acts by regulating the cells that can express a protein called sonic hedgehog (shh) (36). It is likely that

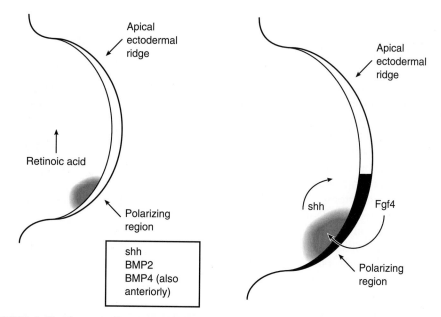

FIGURE 1-15. The two diagrams of the tip of the limb bud illustrate some of the molecules involved in the interaction between the polarizing region and mesenchyme of the progress zone that specify the anteroposterior axis of the limb. On the left, the arrow shows the direction of the decreasing concentration of retinoic acid. Retinoic acid acts by regulating cell production of sonic hedgehog (*shh*). shh, in turn, stimulates bone morphogenetic protein2 (*BMP2*) which is a homologue of a *Drosophila* segment polarity-specifying gene. *BMP4* expression overlaps that of BMP2, and is, therefore, probably involved in anteroposterior axis determination, as well. The diagram on the right shows the feedback loop between shh and fibroblast growth factor-4 (*FGF4*), an ectodermally expressed protein, that appears to maintain the apical ectodermal ridge. (Adapted from ref. 83, with permission.)

an *HOX* gene is an intermediate that is stimulated by retinoic acid and the *HOX* gene expression specifies the shh-expressing cells. If retinoic acid receptors are blocked after shh expression has been established, limb malformations still occur, suggesting some additional role in limb patterning, perhaps through its effect on *HOX* genes (36). Retinoic acid is interesting and important, not only for its role in normal development, but because it is a powerful teratogen. Various retinoids, which are derivatives of vitamin A, have been used in pharmacological doses, mainly to treat dermatologic conditions, such as types of acne, psoriasis, exfoliative dermatitis, and disorders of keratinization. The retinoids have been associated in animals and humans with multiple different birth defects. Because of the prolonged elimination half-life of systemic retinoids, pregnancy is not recommended for 2 years after discontinuing their usage (37).

Liver and central nervous system toxicity, as well as anemia and hyperlipidemia, may occur with systemic retinoid use. These problems usually resolve with discontinuation of retinoid therapy. Rheumatologic complications of retinoid use include hyperostosis, arthritis, myopathy, vasculitis, and a condition mimicking seronegative spondyloarthropathy (38).

The shh gene is expressed in the zone of polarizing activity. Activation of this gene through cell transfection in anomalous locations in the limb bud, will cause digit duplication in the same manner as transplantation of the zone of polarizing activity tissue (39). It appears that shh stimulates the gene for bone morphogenic protein 2 (BMP2) (40). The gene activation of both occurs in the same cells, with shh preceding that of BMP2. The bone morphogenic proteins are members of the TGF-β superfamily, and BMP2 is, specifically, a homolog of a fruit fly gene that specifies segment polarity, making it a good candidate for an axis-determining gene. BMP2 is secreted from cells, and, therefore, its action extends over a larger area than just the cells in which it is produced. BMP4 expression overlaps that of BMP2, and it is probably involved in anteroposterior axis specification as well. shh in the mesenchyme also appears to participate in a positive feedback loop with FGF-4 in the ectoderm, which may be important in maintaining the AER and supporting continued limb outgrowth and patterning (41). BMP2 and BMP4 also function in regulating the size and shape of long bones. Overexpression of these genes appears to cause an increase in the quantity of mesenchymal cells that differentiate into the chondrogenic precursors of the skeleton.

It appears that BMP2 and BMP4 are involved as well in the molecular mechanisms of joint formation. If noggin, a

BMP inhibitor, is not present, joints do not form. Present evidence suggests that members of the HOXA and HOXD families are regulators of BMP and growth and differentiation factor 5 (GDF-5). GDF-5 (a BMP-related protein) is expressed specifically in the prospective joint region. If noggin is not present, GDF-5 is not expressed and BMP2 and BMP4 are not inhibited, resulting in a continuous, jointless skeleton. A balance of activating and inhibiting signals seems to be necessary for normal joint cavitation (42,43).

Some experimental work suggests that cell–extracellular matrix interactions are involved in the mechanism of joint cavitation. Specifically, CD44s, an isoform of a cell surface receptor that interacts with hyaluronan, is found in a single layer of cells outlying the presumptive joint cavity in rats (44). One hypothesis is that the creation of a hyaluronan-rich, but proteoglycan- and collagen II–poor extracellular matrix results in a loss of cell adhesion and allows joint cavity formation (44).

Dorsal-ventral Axis Patterning/Ectodermally Controlled Patterning

Experiments in which limb bud ectoderm is transplanted onto mesoderm, with reversal of its dorsal-ventral axis, reveal that digits, muscles, and tendons conform to the axis of the overlying ectoderm (14). Several genes involved in dorsal-ventral specification have been identified. Evidence suggests that Wnt-7A, a secreted signaling protein, confers the dorsal character to the ectoderm and stimulates Lmx-1 (45). Lmx-1 is a homeobox-gene that encodes a transcription factor that dorsalizes mesoderm. The ventral limb expresses the homeobox-containing transcription factor engrailed (En-1). En-1 appears to suppress Wnt-7A expression, thereby limiting the activity of Lmx-1 to the dorsal mesenchyme (46).

The actions of several genes are important in determining more than a single axis. For example, Wnt-7A expression is necessary for normal anteroposterior digit formation and shh is necessary for limb outgrowth, proximal-distal, in addition to anteroposterior patterning. The coordinated development of all three axes is believed to be regulated by interactions of several signaling genes. Wnt-7A, shh, and FGF-4 are promising candidates for this role (47,48).

Both the AER and the ZPA activate *HOXA* and *HOXD* genes. *HOX* genes are the vertebrate homologs of the fruit fly homeogenes, which specify body segment identity. *HOXD* genes are expressed in an overlapping, nested fashion in the anteroposterior axis of the developing limb (49) (Fig. 1-16). *HOXD* genes can also be activated by shh alone. *HOXA* genes have an overlapping expression along the dorsal axis, suggesting a role in specifying limb components. *HOX* genes have specifically been shown to affect the growth of cartilage and precartilaginous condensations (50,51). They may be important in determining the length, segmentation, and branching of limb elements. *HOX* genes are not

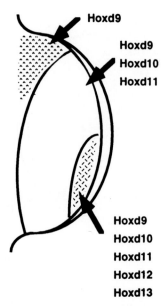

FIGURE 1-16. The pattern of expression of the HOXD genes is shown. The overall HOXD expression is sequential from the anterior to posterior aspect of the limb buds; however several individual HOXD genes have clustered expression patterns. The pattern of HOXD gene expression can be altered by polarizing signals, implicating the Hoxd genes in limb pattern determination. (From ref. 83, with permission.)

expressed strictly along AP or DV axes, and their position of expression differs in various areas of the limb. Human limb malformations caused by mutations in *HOX* genes have been identified, and will be discussed in the section on clinical significance. The activity of *HOX* genes overlaps, and is sufficiently redundant that a mutation of a single *HOX* gene generally results in a minor limb anomaly.

The specific signals and mechanisms that control muscle, ligament, and tendon development have not been identified. Exploration of these mechanisms may ultimately be of great clinical utility.

Clinical Significance

Limbs are extremely susceptible to anomalies, probably because of their complex developmental biology and their exposed position outside of the body wall. Nearly all teratogens and chromosomal anomalies have ill effects on limb development. A large number of single gene mutations disturb the normal development of limbs, as well. Rapid advances in molecular genetics are resulting in the identification of the gene(s) responsible for many Mendelian disorders. Developmental molecular biologists are identifying genes that create limb deformities in animals, whose homologous human genes may be responsible for other specific limb defects.

Limb deficiencies occur in 3 to 8 of 1,000 live births (52). One-half of limb deficiencies occur as isolated defects and the other half occur with associated malformations (52). Associated malformations may be life-threatening. The most common associated malformations are musculoskeletal, head and neck, cardiovascular, gastrointestinal, and genitourinary.

As discussed previously, destruction of the AER or the progress zone, or failure of expression of critical signaling molecules, can result in truncation or absence of limb development. Although specific defects have not been identified in humans, there are several inherited disorders with limb deficiencies that may well have a mutation in a specific signaling molecule. These include Roberts syndrome with phocomelia, acheiropodia (Brazil type) with absent hands and feet, Buttiens distal limb deficiencies syndrome, and CHILD syndrome with variable transverse and longitudinal deficiencies. A mouse mutant with a single digit has been found to have a mutation in the *HOXA-13* gene (53). Human split-hand/split-foot deformity (lobster claw deformity) is characterized by a failure of central ray formation, and at least one causative gene has been localized, but not yet identified (54).

Vascular anomalies or accidents probably cause some limb deficiencies by prohibiting limb outgrowth or by causing necrosis of already differentiated limbs (55,56). Amniotic bands result in amputation by interfering with vascular supply (52).

Intercalary limb deficiencies, with absence of proximal structures, may result from a temporary injury to the progress zone as discussed in the section Developmental Anatomy of the Limb.

Synostoses are failures of joint formation or separation of adjacent bone, such as the radius and ulna, with a single exception. That exception is distal syndactyly, which is caused by amniotic bands (57). The vast majority of synostoses are inherited, but only a few of the mutated genes have been identified. Identification of the causative genes is likely in the near future, and will shed much light on the mechanisms of normal joint formation and of normal bone modeling from the mass of undifferentiated mesenchymal cells that prefigure the skeletal elements. Nearly 100 disorders have synostosis as a feature (see ref. 52, pp. 721–724). The mouse mutant-limb deformity gives a flavor for the kind of causation of these deformities. Limb-deformity mice are characterized by fusion of adjacent bones, such as the radius and ulna. The limb bud is narrow and the AER is patchy (58). A decrease in shh expression and an absence of Fgf-4 expression have been found (59).

Teratogens, such as thalidomide and alcohol, can cause synostoses in humans. Retinoic acid creates synostoses in animals when applied during chondrogenesis of developing limbs (60).

Failure of programmed cell death may be an important factor in causing some disorders with synostosis as a feature. A failure of aphotic cell death in the interdigital mesenchyme is presumed to be the cause of some syndactyly.

Excessive partitioning of skeletal elements are usually inherited conditions. Triphalangeal thumb is the most common of these disorders. The abnormality has been linked to a region on chromosome 7 in several affected families, but the gene has not been identified (61,62). Other families do not link to this locus, implying that more than one gene mutation causes triphalangeal thumb.

Polydactyly, whether isolated or associated with other anomalies, is usually an inherited condition. Given the complex interactions that occur in limb pattern specification, it is not surprising that a number of causes of this condition are being found.

Grieg cephalopolysyndactyly is an autosomal dominant disorder characterized by postaxial polysyndactyly of the hands and preaxial polysyndactyly of the feet and dysmorphic facies. A DNA-binding transcription factor, named GLI 3, is the cause of this disorder (63). The expression of GLI 3 is restricted to the interdigital mesenchyme and joint-forming regions of the digits. A mouse mutant with a defect in the homologous gene has ectopic expression of both shh and FGF-4 in the anterior limb bud (64). Another mutation causing human polydactyly is in the *HOXD* cluster of homeobox genes that has been implicated in digit specification. Synpolydactyly is caused by a mutation of *HOXD-13* (65). Smith-Lemli-Opitz syndrome is characterized by a variety of birth defects, including postaxial polydactyly and brachydactyly. Cholesterol synthesis is defective in children with this syndrome and shh utilizes cholesterol as a transport molecule. It is possible that the limb anomalies in this syndrome result from a distortion of the normal shh gradient due to cholesterol insufficiency.

Skeletal dysplasias are a heterogeneous group of disorders whose genetic causes are rapidly being discovered, giving insight into the mechanisms of normal and disordered skeletal development (see Chapter 8).

Many single and group congenital anomalies that occur sporadically are believed to result from vascular disturbances in the embryo or fetus. The best-developed of the vascular causation hypotheses is the subclavian artery disruption sequence, which seeks to explain Klippel-Feil syndrome, Poland anomaly, Mobius syndrome, absence of the pectoralis major, terminal transverse limb deficiencies, and Sprengel deformity. A disruption occurs when a normal embryo suffers a destructive process with cascading consequences. Because all the tissues affected in these various disorders receive their major blood supply from the subclavian artery, it is hypothesized that a defect of arterial formation or an injury to existing arteries causes these defects. The location and extent of tissue abnormality is determined by the extent, location, and timing of the interruption of normal blood supply. The observation underlying this hypothesis is that the disorders listed above often occur together in various combinations.

Possible mechanisms resulting in arterial ischemia include vessel occlusion from edema, thrombus, or embolus; extrinsic vessel compression caused by surrounding tissue edema, hemorrhage, cervical ribs, aberrant muscles, amniotic bands, or uterine compression; abnormal embryologic events, including delayed or abnormal vessel formation and disruption of newly formed vessels; and environmental factors such as infection, hyperthermia, hypoxia, vasculitis, or drug effects. It is possible that some fetuses suffer ischemia due to normal embryologic events that are idiosyncratically not well tolerated, such as the rapid descent of the heart and great vessels.

The vascular accident hypothesis is attractive in explaining combinations of congenital anomalies and their usually sporadic occurrence. However, there are often combinations of anomalies that are difficult to relate to a single vascular event, and the question of whether the anomalies resulted in, rather than being caused by, vascular abnormalities is not easily resolved.

Amniotic bands or constriction rings cause a large portion of nonhereditary congenital limb anomalies. Constriction rings are diagnosed by the occurrence of a soft tissue depression encircling a limb or by injury from amputations or disruptions. Constriction rings are commonly multiple and may be broad or narrow. The depth of the ring determines whether the limb distal to the ring is normal, hypoplastic, engorged (from venous or lymphatic obstruction), or amputated (from vascular insufficiency). Syndactyly, clubfoot, and clubhand have also been associated with constriction rings.

The origin of constriction rings is uncertain. The mechanisms by which amniotic strands might form are disputed (66–69). One hypothesis holds that amnion adheres to areas of preoccurring hemorrhage and by themselves are not pathogenic (70). Nonetheless, the syndrome is common, affecting one in 5,000 to 15,000 births. Recurrence risks of this syndrome are low (52).

DEVELOPMENTAL ANATOMY OF THE VERTEBRAL COLUMN

The vertebral column, be it cartilage or bone, defines the species of the subphylum of vertebrates. Evolution of a vertebral column to replace the notochord allows a strength, flexibility, and protection to the neural tube that conferred many advantages to vertebrate species. Minor and even major anomalies of the vertebral column are compatible with life and good function. Vertebral column development depends on the appropriate prior development of the notochord and somites.

While the mesoderm is forming during gastrulation, a mass of ectodermal cells proliferates and forms the archenteron, a tube that migrates cranially in the midline between the ectoderm and the endoderm. The floor of the archenteron forms the notochordal plate. For a short time, there is a direct connection between the primitive gut and the amniotic cavity, since the endodermal floor is not continuous and the blastopore (the opening of the archenteron) communicates with the amniotic cavity. This connection is obliterated by the end of the 3rd week and remnants of this connection are presumed to be responsible for diastematomyelia.

The notochord arises from cells in the primitive streak, which come from the ingress of cells from the epiblast during gastrulation and, later, from the caudal eminence. This ingress of cells forms the endoderm as well as the notochord and the paraxial mesoderm (segmental plate). The notochord develops from cranial to caudal by adding cells as it develops. It is initially a solid rod in which a small central canal develops. The notochord induces the formation of the neural groove, which gradually closes to form a tube with a central canal. By the 23rd day, the neural groove is closed, except at its most cranial and caudal ends. These openings are termed the neuropores, which close by the end of the 4th week. Closure of the neural tube progresses cranially to caudally. Failure to close properly is hypothesized to be the cause of neural tube defects such as myelomeningocele.

The somites also develop from cells that are internalized through the primitive streak. These cells form the paraxial mesoderm that will become the somites, and ultimately become the vertebrae. Presomitic cells cluster by increased adhesion into distinct balls of epithelial cells surrounding mesenchymal cells, giving the embryo its first segmental organization. Positional information is programmed into the somites by the time they are morphologically distinct. For example, a thoracic somite will still form a rib when transplanted into the cervical region. The positional information is imparted during gastrulation (69,70). Somites do not depend on interaction with the neural tube or notochord for development and fated cells will develop into somites *in vitro*.

Four occipital, 8 cervical, 12 thoracic, 5 lumbar, 5 sacral, and 4 or 5 coccygeal pairs of somites will develop. The first somites are evident at $3\frac{1}{2}$ weeks and 30 pairs are present at $4\frac{1}{2}$ weeks. Not all of the somites are visible simultaneously. Somites develop a complex internal organization. The somite begins as a ball of pseudostratified epithelium surrounding a central cavity, the somitocoel. The central cavity becomes filled with mesenchymal cells. Some of these cells, along with cells in the medioventral portion of the somite, become the sclerotome. Cells from the sclerotome will form the vertebral bodies and vertebral arche and emerge without the epithelial portion of the sclerotome to surround the neural tube. In addition to contributing to the sclerotome, cells from the central cavity migrate to become the intervertebral discs and contribute to rib formation. The dorsolateral wall of the somite is called the dermomyotome. It separates into the dermatome laterally and the myotome lying between the dermatome and the sclerotome. The dermatome gives rise to the dermis of the skin, and the myotome supplies cells for muscle, tendons, and fascia (Fig. 1-17).

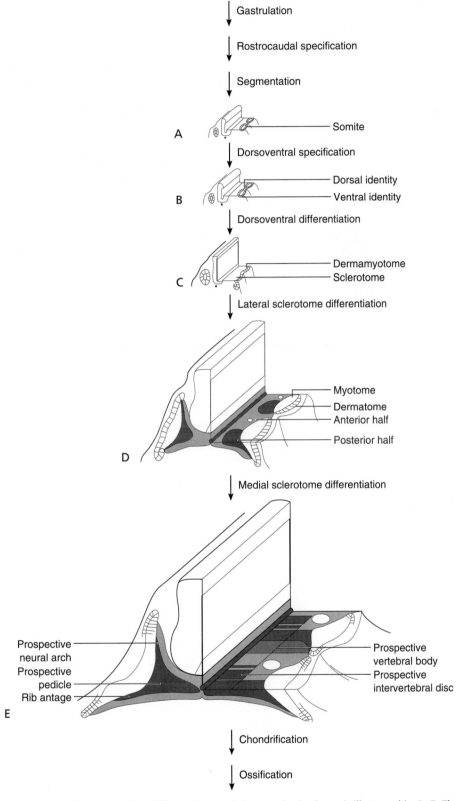

FIGURE 1-17. The progressive differentiation of the vertebral column is illustrated in **A–E**. The dark areas in **D** and **E** demonstrate the portion of the sclerotome that develops into the neural arch, the vertebral body, rib anlage, and the intervertebral disc. (Adapted from ref. 83, with permission.)

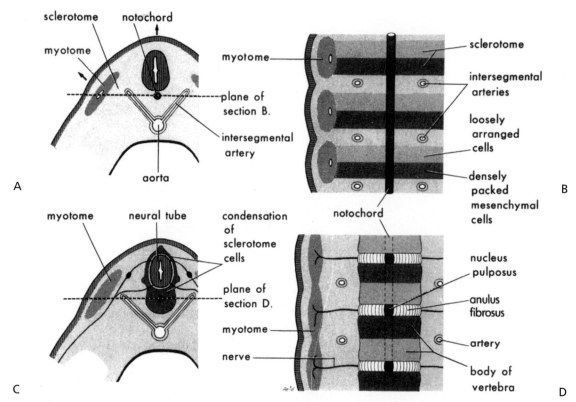

FIGURE 1-18. A: Transverse section through a 4-week embryo. The top arrow shows the direction of the growth of the neural tube, and the side arrow shows the dorsolateral growth of the somite remnant. **B:** Coronal section of the same-stage embryo, showing the condensation of sclerotomal cells around the notochord, with loosely packed cells cranially and densely packed cells caudally. **C:** A transverse section through a 5-week embryo, depicting the condensation of sclerotome cells around the notochord and neural tube. **D:** Coronal section illustrating the formation of the vertebral body from cranial and caudal halves of adjacent sclerotomes, resulting in the segmental arteries crossing the bodies of the vertebrae and the spinal nerves lying between the vertebrae. (From ref. 20, with permission.)

The sclerotomal cells from the paired somites migrate medially, meeting around the notochord and separating it from the dorsal neural tube and the ventral gut. The continuous perichordal sheath is distinct from the more lateral, segmented sclerotomes. Between the adjacent somites lies the transverse intersegmental arteries. The segmental spinal nerves originally exit at the midportion of the somitic sclerotomal mass. Resegmentation of the sclerotomic tissues occurs at $4\frac{1}{2}$ weeks (Fig. 1-18). This process of resegmentation occurs by variable-rate mitosis, which results in each somitic sclerotome's thinning cranially and condensing caudally. The transverse intersegmental arteries and spinal nerves traverse the cellularly loose cranial portion of the sclerotome. The dense caudal portion of each sclerotome unites with the cranial, less-condensed part of the next sclerotome, to form the primordium of the vertebrae. Thus, the skeletal portions of the somites no longer correspond to the original segmentation. The segmental spinal nerves that originally were in midsomite now lie at the level of the disc. The intersegmental arteries located between somites come to lie at the midportion of the vertebral bodies, and the myotomes bridge the vertebrae. The densely cellular, caudal portion of the sclerotome gives rise to the vertebral arch. The initially continuous notochordal sheath segments into loosely cellular cranial, and densely cellular caudal, portions. The cranial portion becomes the vertebral centrum, and the dense, caudal portion becomes the intervertebral disc. The vertebral centrum surrounds the notochord and forms the vertebral body. Notochordal cells in the vertebral centrum degenerate, although some remnants of the notochord may remain. Rests of notochordal cells persisting in the sacral or cervical areas may give rise to chordomas in later life. The neural arches develop from ventral to dorsal, enclosing the neural tube, and unite in the fetal period. The spinal nerves and the dorsal root ganglia arise at the level of the somite and enter the myotome at the beginning of the 6th week. The presence of ganglia are necessary for normal neural arch segmentation. Although somites form from cranial to caudal, resegmentation progresses from midspine cranially and caudally.

Neural crest cells (a specialized region of neuroectoderm) accumulate just before closure of the neural tube cranially, and are situated between the neural tube and somites. These cells become the peripheral nervous system sensory cells and nerve fibers, as well as the Schwann cells and melanocytes. Peripheral nerve afferents and preganglionic fibers of the autonomic nervous system develop from the neural tube, as do the brain and spinal cord. At each cervical, thoracic, and lumbar somite, a corresponding ganglion develops.

Molecular Insights of Vertebral Column Development

HOX genes are expressed in an overlapping fashion in the developing spinal column, and evidence suggests that they specify individual vertebrae's morphology (73). Transgenic mice, with out-of-sequence activation of certain *HOX* genes, can be created that transform the atlas into a cervical vertebra with a body, and lumbar vertebrae can become like thoracic vertebrae with rib formation (74,75). Conversely, *HOX* gene inactivation can transform the axis into an atlas-appearing vertebra (76). Overlapping, redundant expression of *HOX* genes occurs and inactivation of more than one adjacent *HOX* gene has been found necessary to alter vertebral morphology in some regions of the vertebral column (77). Retinoic acid application can alter the normal expression patterns of *HOX* genes, and it can create varying morphologic abnormalities, depending on the timing and location of its application. A particular retinoic acid receptor (the gamma receptor) is expressed only in prebone tissue, and its inactivation causes transformation of the axis to an atlas and C7 to C6 (78).

PAX genes are a family of genes containing a DNA-binding domain, and are expressed in the sclerotome at high levels during sclerotome condensation. Some evidence suggests that a defect in specific *PAX* genes, or genes they modify, may result in failure of formation of vertebral elements (79). The homeobox gene *MSX2* is necessary for spinous process development in mice (80). Clearly, the interactions of genes and tissues involved in vertebral column formation are complex.

Clinical Significance

The vertebral column represents the central characteristic skeletal structure of vertebrates, and it is remarkable how even severe vertebral abnormalities are so well tolerated by the organisms. Because vertebral column development has been highly conserved during evolution, most if not all the vertebral abnormalities seen in vertebrates can also be found in humans. In fact, mouse genetics had led to the identification of probably all types of vertebral abnormalities (81,82).

Defects at different stages of embryo development will result in different vertebral malformations. In general, the earlier the disruption in the developmental process, the more severe will be the phenotype. The developmental processes that can be affected include mesoderm formation during gastrulation, axial patterning, notochordal mesoderm induction, somite formation, sclerotome condensation, neural tube closure, and axial identity specification. Although disorders in pattern formation result in specific prevertebral phenotypes, general disorders of mesenchyme condensation, cartilage, or bone formation affect composition, and therefore morphology, of the skeleton. Misspecifications of vertebral identity, called homeotic transformations, are characterized by the presence of all vertebral components, but with shapes characteristic of usually the adjacent vertebra.

Disruption of the allocation of the mesodermal cells during gastrulation leads to a block in the whole vertebral column formation. Because gastrulation also generates the other two germ layers, the embryo will have multiple congenital abnormalities and will not survive (83). Defects during sclerotome formation are compatible with life and typically result in segmental vertebral agenesis. Because sclerotome formation depends on the inductive activity of the notochord, it is mainly notochord mutants that are found within this category. In the affected region, somite ventralization is hindered, and the corresponding vertebrae appear to be deleted.

Although disruptions of gastrulation and sclerotome formation lead to absence, truncation, or interruption of vertebral column formation, disorders of somatogenesis are compatible with vertebral development. However, multiple vertebral components can be lacking or fused. Variations on number, shape, and position of vertebrae are common developmental anomalies. Most columns have 24 segments, including 7 cervical, 12 thoracic, and 5 lumbar vertebrae. However, columns with 23 or 25 elements are commonly seen, and they are most likely related to differences in the number of elements of the lumbar spine. This number difference may be due to the last lumbar vertebra being incorporated into the sacrum (sacralization) or the first sacral vertebra being freed (lumbarization).

Developmental anomalies that affect vertebral shape are varied. The most common conditions are spina bifida, hemivertebra and wedge vertebrae, and vertebral bars. Spina bifida occulta is a failure in the completion of the neural arch, but without neurological compromise. Failure of the neural arch to fuse in the cervical spine, and sometimes in the upper thoracic spine, is seen shortly after birth, but spina bifida is most commonly seen at the level of the lumbosacral spine. This is a normal finding in children at 2 years of age, in 50% at 10 years, and in approximately 20% of adults. Neural tube defects (NTDs) can be subdivided into four subgroups. The first, a meningocele, is a cyst that involves only the meninges but not the neural elements. The second, a myelomeningocele, includes the neural elements as part of the sac. The third, a lipomeningocele, is a deformity in which there is a sac containing a lipoma that is intimately involved with the sacral nerves. The fourth, rachischisis, is a complete absence of skin and sac, with exposure of the muscle and dysplastic spinal cord.

Closure of the neural tube progresses cranially to caudally. Failure to close properly is widely believed to be the cause of most cases of myelomeningocele (84). This hypothesis is supported by observations of early fetuses with myelomeningocele and is consistent with animal models of neural tube defects (85). The competing hypothesis, championed by Gardner, suggests that overdistension and rupture of a closed neural tube causes NTDs (86,87). Myelomeningocele has multiple causes, resulting in a common phenotype. An inherited predisposition to NTDs appears to be present in some cases, based on an increased incidence of NTDs in some families and a variation in prevalence in different ethnic groups (86). Furthermore, a mouse model of NTD has been shown to result from a mutation in the gene *Pax-3*. *Pax-3* is a homeobox gene that has been shown to be involved in the fusion of the dorsal neural tube, as well as in neutral crest cell migration and dermomyotome development (85). Environmental factors are responsible for some proportion of NTDs, and multiple teratogens have been identified that interfere with neurulation. Examples include vinblastine, which disrupts actin microfilaments, and calcium channel blockers, which interfere with microfilament contraction (88,90). Retinoic acid, hydroxyurea, and mitomycin C interfere with the timing of neuroepithelial development and cause NTDs in animal models (91). Folate supplements taken during pregnancy decrease the risk of NTD in subsequent children when a prior child has been affected, as well as decreasing the incidence of NTDs in pregnancies without a prior history of NTD (84). The mechanism of the effect of folate on NTDs is unknown. The interaction of genes and environment that act to cause myelomeningoceles, as well as the molecular pathology, is under active investigation (85).

Defects of vertebrae formation or segmentation include hemivertebra and vertebral bars. Hemivertebra appears as a wedge, usually situated laterally between two other vertebrae. As a consequence, a lateral curvature of the spine develops. Vertebral bars are due to localized defects in segmentation and are observed most frequently in the posterolateral side of the column, resulting in absence of growth in that side. The outcome is a progressive lordosis and scoliosis. When located anteriorly, vertebral bars lead to progressive kyphosis. Klippel-Feil sequence is regarded as a defect in cervical segmentation. Clinically, there is a short, broad neck, low hairline, limited range of motion of the head and neck, and multiple vertebral abnormalities.

Finally, other congenital abnormalities may be observed. Diastematomyelia is a longitudinal splitting of the spinal cord associated with a bony or fibrocartilaginous spicule or septum arising from the vertebral body, which is believed to result from remnants of the early connection between the primitive gut or the amniotic cavity. It is commonly associated with skin changes and abnormalities of the lower extremities. A chordoma is a neoplasm that arises from noto-chordal rests, and is found especially in the sacrococcygeal region. Sacrococcygeal teratoma is a neoplasm composed of multiple embryonic tissues that can undergo malignant transformation.

DEVELOPMENTAL ANATOMY OF THE NERVOUS SYSTEM

The neural tube is pivotal in development, and has been discussed in the section Developmental Anatomy of the Vertebral Column. The neural tube becomes the central nervous system (the brain and spinal cord), and the neural crest develops into most of the peripheral nervous system. The spinal cord develops from the portion of the neural tube that is caudal to the four occipital somites. The neural tube forms from the folding of the neural groove and begins at the brain/spinal cord junction. As the neural groove fuses, so does the neural fold. Neural crest cells begin their migration from neural-fold tissue, just after neural tube closure occurs in the spinal regions. Neural crest cells migrate either beneath the surface ectoderm or between the neural tube and the somite. Migration occurs through extracellular matrix along relatively cell-free paths. Neural crest cells form the pia mater, the spinal ganglia, and the sympathetic trunks and ganglia.

As the neural tube closes, the dorsal region, called the alar laminae, is separated from the ventral basal laminae by a shallow groove—the sulcus limitans. A thin bridge of tissue persists to connect the two halves of the alar and basal laminae, named the roof and floor plates. The alar plate develops into the sensory pathways (dorsal columns), and the basal plate develops into the motor pathways (ventral horns). The notochord is necessary for floor plate induction, and the floor plate appears to specify the dorsoventral organization of cell types in the developing spinal cord.

The ventral horn neurons develop axons that form the ventral roots. The dorsal root ganglia develop from neural crest cells. The axons of the ganglion cells form central processes, which become the dorsal roots and peripheral processes that end in sensory organelles.

Spinal cord development proceeds in a rostral-caudal direction, and motor neurons develop neural capabilities before sensory nerves. Autonomic nerve function is established last (44). Movement is visible by ultrasound 5½ weeks postfertilization. The spinal cord extends the entire length of the vertebral column during the embryonic period. During fetal development, the vertebral column grows more rapidly than the spinal cord. Coupled with some loss of caudal spinal cord tissue, the caudal tip of the spinal cord ends at the 2nd or 3rd lumbar vertebra in newborns. In the adult, the spinal cord terminates at the inferior portion of the first lumbar vertebra. Thus, the lumbar and sacral nerve roots have an oblique course below the conus medullaris, before their exit from their intervertebral foraminae, resulting in the formation of the cauda equina (Fig. 1-19).

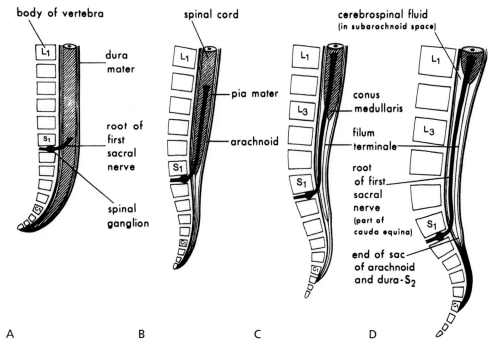

FIGURE 1-19. Illustration of the position of the spinal cord and meninges in relation to the vertebral column at 8 weeks (**A**), 24 weeks (**B**), birth (**C**), and adult (**D**). (From ref. 20, with permission.)

Myelination of peripheral nerve axons begins in the fetal period and continues during the first year after birth. Schwann cells myelinate peripheral nerves, whereas ligodendrocytes myelinate the axons within the spinal cord.

Molecular Insights of Nervous System Development

The molecular basis of nervous system formation is not well understood, but probably will be in the next decade. There is an intimate relationship between the notochord and the neural plate and tube, which is necessary for differentiation of the floor plate or the spinal cord, and for specification of ventral structures in the developing spinal cord. Hepatocyte nuclear factor-3 appears to regulate shh (an important axis-specifying gene in the limb as well), which can induce ventral structures (92). *PAX* genes have dorsoventrally restricted expression in the developing spinal cord. Dorsal structures can develop without the notochord, but specific molecules may be necessary for complete dorsal specification. For example, dorsalin-1, a TGF-β family member, can induce neural crest cell differentiation (93). The transcription factor genes, *Pax-3* and *Gli-3,* are necessary for neural tube closure (94). The large number of NTDs suggests that neural tube closure does not have a large redundancy in it developmental regulation.

Clinical Significance

Multiple anomalies of the brain occur and have orthopaedic implications because of disordered control of limbs, but will not be discussed here. Failure of closure of the caudal neuropore may result in myelomeningocele. Other evidence suggests that increased cerebral spinal fluid pressure causes rupture of an already closed neural tube at its weakest point—where it closed last. At least ten genes have been identified in mutant animals that result in NTD. Multiple teratogens, such as valproic acid and vitamin A, or exposure to hypothermia, can cause NTD. Although the mechanism is unknown, perifertilization folic acid decreases the incidence of NTD in humans.

Myeloschisis is a rare condition in which the neural groove fails to form a neural tube. Myelomeningocele has uncovered neural tissue that has herniated into the dysraphic area of the spine. Meningocele, in which the neural elements remain in their normal location, is probably a primary defect of the vertebral column development, rather than a primary neural defect. Ten percent of people have spina bifida occulta in which the vertebral neural arch fails to fully develop and fuse, usually at L5 or S1.

BONE FORMATION AND GROWTH

An examination of the human skeleton reveals the numerous sizes and shapes of bones, which have precise functions of locomotion and protection of vital organs, are major sites for hematopoiesis, and participate in calcium hemostasis and storage of phosphate, magnesium, potassium, and bicarbonate. The molecular composition of the bone is remarkably constant. Regardless of the animal species or the bone considered, bone is always a two-phase composite substance made up of two very different materials. The two major components of bone are the organic matrix, or osteoid, and the inorganic matrix. Various calcium salts, primarily hydroxyapatite, are deposited in crystals within and between the matrix. These inorganic crystals give bone its rigidity, hardness, and strength to compression.

Connective tissue, cartilage, and bone all differentiate from that type of diffuse mesoderm known as mesenchyme. Mesenchyme arises primarily from the primitive streak and secondarily from mesodermal segments and the lateral somatic and splanchnic mesodermal layers (see Fig. 1-9). In early embryos, the mesenchyme acts as an unspecialized "packing" material, but soon differentiates into various tissues and organs.

There are two mechanisms of bone formation (osteogenesis), and both involve the transformation of a preexisting connective tissue into bone tissue. The transformation of fibrous primitive connective tissue into bone is called intramembranous ossification. The replacement of cartilage by bone is called "endochondral ossification." Except for the clavicle and the flat bones of the skull, all bones of the appendicular and axial skeleton form by endochondral ossification.

Intramembranous Ossification

Intramembranous ossification occurs by mesenchymal cells derived from the neural crest that interact with the extracellular matrix secreted by the epithelia cells arising from the head. If the mesenchymal cells do not contact this matrix, no bone will be developed (95,96). The mechanism responsible for the conversion of mesenchymal cells to bone is still unknown. However, bone morphogenetic proteins may play a significant role in this process.

During intramembranous ossification, the mesenchymal cells proliferate and condense into packed nodules. Some of these cells differentiate into capillaries and others change their shape to become osteoblasts. These cells are capable of secreting osteoid, the organic extracellular matrix that subsequently will become mineralized. High levels of alkaline phosphatase and the appearance of matrix vesicles mark the commencement of ossification. The cells will eventually be surrounded by calcified matrix and become osteocytes.

Endochondral Ossification

By far the most common mechanism of ossification is cartilaginous (or endochondral). The process begins with the formation of a cartilage precursor or template. Mesenchyme cells condense and proliferate, but, instead of turning into osteoblasts, as in intramembranous ossification, they become chondroblasts. These cells will then secrete the cartilage extracellular matrix. Soon after the cartilaginous model is formed, the cells in the center become hypertrophic and secrete a matrix that will subsequently be invaded by capillaries. As this matrix is degraded and the chondrocytes die, osteoblasts carried by the blood vessels begin to secrete bone matrix. Eventually, all cartilage is replaced by bone (Fig. 1-20). This process appears to be dependent on the mineralization of the extracellular matrix. A special, condensed mesenchymal tissue, the perichondrium, surrounds the cartilage model. This tissue is essentially the same as that surrounding the intramembranous centers of ossification, but in the perichondrium, the osteoprogenitor cells remain dormant for a time, while the cartilage model is enlarged by the chondrocytes.

Ossification begins at the primary center, within the shaft, and proceeds outward from the medullary cavity and inward from the periosteum, in a repetitive sequence. As the cartilage model is replaced by bone, extensive remodeling occurs. First, the medullary cavity is created and enlarged by resorption of the bony struts and spicules. Second, the developing bone continues to enlarge by both interstitial and appositional growth. The same repetitive sequence of events occurs in the epiphyseal centers of ossification. Once the shaft and epiphyses are ossified, leaving the cartilage physeal plates between them, each skeletal segment increases in size until maturity. The initiation of the endochondral ossification process, as well as the highly ordered progression of the chondrocytes through the growth plate, must be under strict spatial and temporal control. In view of the complexity of the process, it is remarkable that the human bones in the limbs can grow for some 15 years independently of each other, and yet eventually match to an accuracy of 0.2 percent.

Growth Plate Structure and Development

Growth of the different parts of the body is not uniform, and different bones grow at different rates. Patterning of the embryo occurs while the organs are still very small. For example, the limb has its basic structure established when its size is approximately 1 cm long. Yet, it will grow to be hundreds of times longer. How is this growth controlled? Most of the evidence suggests that the cartilaginous elements in the limb have their own individual growth programs. These growth programs are specified when the elements are initially patterned and involve both cell proliferation and extracellular matrix secretion. An understanding of the processes of bone formation, growth, and remodeling is fundamental in pediatric orthopaedics.

The process of endochondral ossification, which occurs in all growth plates, is unique to the immature skeleton. Once the growth plates have been formed, longitudinal growth of the bones occurs by appositional growth of cells

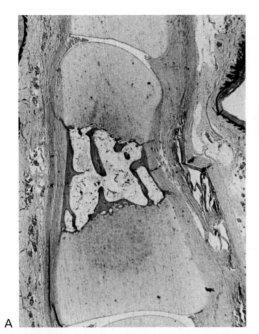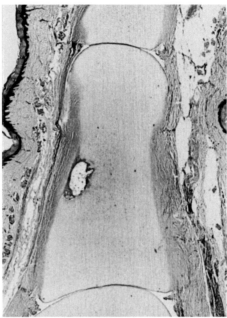

FIGURE 1-20. **A:** Formation of the primary ossification center of a phalanx. Note the central location with bone and bone marrow formation. **B:** Delayed ossification center formation in a case of digital duplication. (From ref. 97, with permission.)

and extracellular matrix from within the growth plate, and new bone formation on the metaphyseal side. The rate of increase in the length of a long bone is equal to the rate of new cell production per column multiplied by the mean height of the enlarged cell. The rate of proliferation depends on the time the cells take to complete a cell cycle in the proliferative zone, and the size of this zone. Generally, the greater the number of chondrocytes and the higher the plate, the faster the growth rate of the bone (Fig. 1-21). In addition, total longitudinal growth for the life span of the growth plate depends on the total number of progenitor cell divisions and the number of divisions of each daughter cell. The number of cell divisions is genetically determined, but the rate is influenced by hormonal and metabolic factors.

The function of the growth plate is related to its structure as an organ, which depends on the integrated function of three distinct components. The first component is the physeal cartilage, which is divided into three histologically recognizable zones: resting, proliferative, and hypertrophic. The second component is the metaphysis, which is the region in which calcified cartilage is replaced by bone. The third component is the circumferential structures known as the perichondrial ring of LaCroix and the groove of Ranvier. Each of these components has its unique cellular architecture and extracellular matrix biochemistry; their integrated functioning results in longitudinal and latitudinal bone growth. Interestingly, although cartilage lacks blood vessels, to a large extent the metabolic activity of each zone depends on the blood supply system around the physis.

Physeal Cartilage

Resting Zone. The resting zone, located just below the secondary center of ossification, contains chondrocytes that are widely dispersed in an abundant matrix. The cells contain abundant endoplasmic reticulum characteristic of protein synthesis, but low intracellular and ionized calcium content. The function of these cells is not well understood, but data indicate that the resting zone is relatively inactive in cell or matrix turnover, although it may be a source for the continuous supply of chondrocytes to the proliferative zone.

Proliferative Zone. The proliferative zone is characterized histologically by longitudinal columns of flattened cells parallel to the long axis of the bone. The cells contain glycogen stores and significant amounts of endoplasmic reticulum. The total calcium is similar to the resting zone, but the ionized calcium is significantly greater. The oxygen tension is high in this zone (57 mm Hg), and, together with the presence of glycogen, suggests an aerobic metabolism. Of the three zones, it has the highest rate of extracellular matrix synthesis and turnover.

Hypertrophic Zone. The hypertrophic zone is characterized by enlargement of the cells to five to seven times their original size in the proliferative zone. Electron microscopy studies suggest that these cells maintain cellular morphology compatible with active metabolic activity. Biochemical studies have demonstrated that mitochondria of the hypertrophic chondrocyte are used primarily to accumulate and

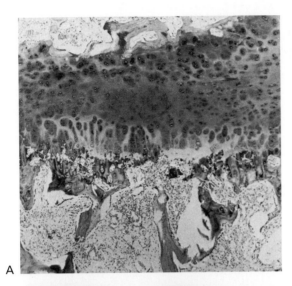

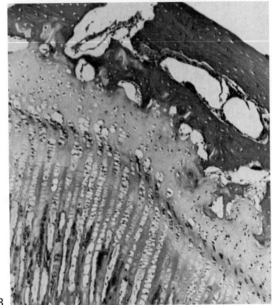

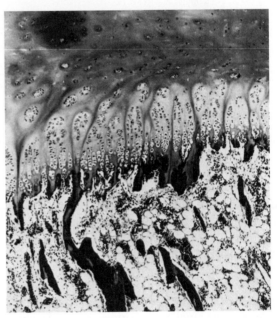

FIGURE 1-21. Variations on growth plate morphology. **A:** Limited column formation in a slow-growing physis. **B:** Elongated cell columns in a fast-growing physis (distal femur). **C:** Some physis form clusterlike groups divided by longitudinal cartilaginous columns. (From ref. 97, with permission.)

release calcium, rather than for ATP production. In addition, the cells have the highest concentration of glycolytic enzymes and synthesize alkaline phosphatase, neutral proteases, and type X collagen, thereby participating in mineralization. Because the growth plate is radially constrained by the ring of LaCroix, its volume changes are expressed primarily in the longitudinal direction. In the last part of this zone there is a provisional calcification of the cartilage.

Metaphysis

The metaphysis functions in the removal of the mineralized cartilage of the hypertrophic zone, and in the formation of the primary spongiosa. Bone formation begins with the invasion of the hypertrophic lacunae by vascular loops, bringing with them osteoblasts that begin the synthesis of bone. The osteoblasts progressively lay down bone on the cartilage template. Subsequently, the initial woven bone and cartilage of the primary trabeculae are resorbed by osteoblasts and replaced by lamellar bone to produce the secondary spongiosa.

Perichondral Ring of Lacroix and Groove of Ranvier

Surrounding the periphery of the physis there is a wedge-shape structure, the groove of Ranvier, and a ring of fibrous tissue, the ring of LaCroix. The groove of Ranvier has active proliferative cells that contribute to the increase in diameter, or latitudinal increase, of the growth plate. The ring of

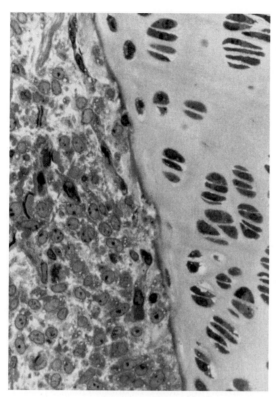

FIGURE 1-22. Photomicrograph of the zone of Ranvier, demonstrating the demarcation between the cells of the growth plate and the mesenchymal cells of the zone of Ranvier. (From ref. 97, with permission.)

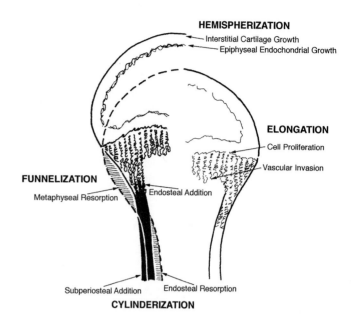

FIGURE 1-23. Diagrammatic representation of the remodeling process of bone during growth. Bone resorption and deposition result in longitudinal growth and shape changes of the epiphysis, metaphysis, and diaphysis. (From ref. 98, with permission.)

LaCroix contains a thin extension of the metaphyseal cortex and fibrous portion of the groove of Ranvier, and periosteum that provides it with a peripheral supporting girdle around the growth plate (Fig. 1-22).

Vascular Anatomy of the Growth Plate

There are three major vascular systems that supply the growth plate. The epiphyseal arteries enter the secondary ossification center, and the terminal branches pass through the resting zone and terminate at the uppermost cell of the proliferative cells. The nutrient artery of the diaphysis supplies the extensive capillary loop network at the junction of the metaphysis and growth plate. Finally, the perichondral arteries supply the ring of LaCroix and the groove of Ranvier. Capillaries from this system communicate with the epiphyseal and metaphyseal systems, in addition to the vessels of the joint capsule.

Bone grows in thickness in addition to length. Because the metaphysis is larger than the diaphysis, some of it must be trimmed during the process of remodeling. This process is called funnelization. In the area termed the cut-back zone, osteoclasts resorb the peripheral bone of the metaphysis. In this way, the metaphysis gradually narrows to the width of the diaphysis. The epiphysis also grows in circumference by a process called hemispheration, which is a process similar to that occurring in the growth plate. Thus, the bone acquires its final shape by a combination of intramembranous ossification, at the diaphyseal level, and endochondral ossification, at the epiphysis and growth plate, with process of elongation, funnelization, hemispherization, and cylinderization (Fig. 1-23).

Glossary

Allele   A particular form of a gene. One allele is inherited from each parent in diploid organisms (thus, two alleles of each gene are present), which may or may not be the same.

Apical ectodermal ridge   A ridgelike thickening of the ectoderm at the tip of the developing limb bud in chicks and mammals. This structure interacts with the underlying mesoderm of the progress zone in the development of the limb bud.

Apoptosis   Programmed cell death. This type of cell death is unlike necrotic cell death in that no damage to surrounding tissue occurs. It is characterized by fragmentation of the DNA and shrinkage of the cell, and occurs widely during development.

Blastocyst   Stage of mammalian development that corresponds to the blastula stage of other animal embryos. It is the stage at which the embryo implants in the uterine wall.

Blastula   Hollow ball of cells, composed of an epithelial layer of small cells enclosing a fluid-filled cavity—the blastocoel.

Body plan   Describes the overall organization of an organism, and, in most animals, is organized around two main axes, the anteroposterior axis and the dorsoventral axis, with a plane of bilateral symmetry, where it exists.

Cell differentiation   Process by which cells become structurally and functionally different from one another and become distinct cell types, e.g., muscle, bone, cartilage cells.

Cell motility   The ability of cells to change shape and move.

Chimera   An organism made up of cells from two or more different species.

Cleavage   Stage in development that occurs after fertilization, and consists of a series of rapid cell divisions without growth, which divides the embryo into a ball of much smaller cells called a blastula. This stage is the beginning of a multicellular organism.

Compaction   Process in which the blastomeres undergo a change in behavior and maximize their contact to form a compact ball of cells. Perhaps the most crucial difference between mammalian cleavage and all other types of animal cleavage.

Dermatome   The region of the somite that gives rise to the dermis.

Dermomyotome   The region of the somite that gives rise to both muscle and dermis.

Determination   A stable change in the internal state of a cell, such that its eventual cell type (or group of cell types) is fixed. A determined cell will not alter its eventual cell type, even when grafted into other regions of the embryo.

Embryonic stem cells (ES cells)   Cells derived from the inner cell mass of a mammalian embryo that can be indefinitely maintained in culture.

Epiblast   Group of cells within the blastocyst (mouse) or blastoderm (chicken), which gives rise to the embryo proper. In the mouse, it develops from cells of the inner cell mass.

Gastrulation   Process in which the blastula turns itself into a multilayered structure and rearranges to form the three embryonic germ layers. In addition, during gastrulation, the body plan of the organism is also established.

Gene knock-out   The inactivation of a specific gene in a transgenic organism.

Genotype   The exact genetic make-up of a cell or organism in terms of the alleles it possesses for any given gene(s).

Germ layers   Regions of the early animal embryo that will give rise to distinct types of tissue. Most animals have three germ layers—ectoderm, mesoderm, and endoderm.

Haploid   Cells containing only one set of chromosomes (half the diploid number of chromosomes), and thus containing only one copy of each gene. In most animals, the only haploid cells are the gametes—the sperm or egg.

Hensen node   Condensation of cells at the anterior end of the primitive streak that will give rise to the notochord. It corresponds to the Spemann organizer in amphibians.

Homeobox   A region of DNA in a homeotic gene, encoding a DNA-binding domain called the homeodomain. The homeodomain is present in a large number of transcription factors that are important in development, and are conserved—present with relatively minor variations—in a large number of species of animals from fruit flies to mice to humans.

Homeotic gene   A type of gene that was originally identified in *Drosophila* (fruit fly), which is important in specifying body-segment identity during development, for example, specifying thorax vs. abdomen.

Homologous genes   Genes in different animals that share a significant similarity in their nucleotide sequence and are derived from a common ancestral gene, often, but not always, with similarity in function.

HOX genes   A group or "family" of homeobox-containing genes that are present in all animals, and are involved in patterning the anteroposterior axis.

Induction   A process whereby one group of cells signals (or induces) another group of cells to develop in a particular way.

Inner cell mass   Group of cells in the early mammalian embryo, derived from the inner cells of the morula, which form a discrete mass of cells in the blastocyst. Some of the cells of the inner cell mass give rise to the embryo proper.

Invagination   Local inward movement of a sheet of embryonic epithelial cells to form a bulgelike structure, as in early gastrulation.

Lateral plate mesoderm   In vertebrate development, a group of cells that lies lateral and ventral to the somites, and gives rise to the tissues of the heart, kidney, gonads, and blood.

Mesenchyme   Term describing loose connective tissue, usually of mesodermal origin, whose cells are capable of migration. Some epithelia of ectodermal origin, such as the neural crest, undergo an epithelial to mesenchymal transition.

Mesoderm Germ layer that gives rise to the skeletomuscular system, connective tissues, the blood, and internal organs, such as the kidney and heart.

Morphogen A substance that effects pattern formation based on its local concentration—often a gradient or threshold effect.

Morula Solid ball of cells in the very early stage in mammalian development, resulting from the process of cleavage.

Myotome The part of the somite that gives rise to muscle.

Neural crest cells Cells derived from the edge of the neural plate that migrate to different regions of the body and give rise to the autonomic nervous system, the sensory nervous system, melanocytes, and some cartilage of the head.

Neurulation The process in which the neural plate develops folds and forms the neural tube, which becomes the brain and spinal cord.

Notochord A rodlike structure of mesodermal origin that runs from head to tail, and lies beneath the future central nervous system.

Ontogeny Development of an individual organism.

Organizer or **organizing region** Signaling center that directs the development of part of the embryo or the whole embryo. In amphibians, the organizer usually refers to the Spemann organizer.

Organogenesis Stage of development when the main organs of the body begin to emerge gradually.

Pattern formation The process by which cells in a developing embryo acquire identities that lead to a well-ordered spatial pattern of cell activities.

PAX **genes** Genes encoding proteins that regulate DNA transcription and contain both a homeodomain and another protein motif, the "paired" motif. *PAX* genes are related to the pair-rule genes in *Drosophila,* which are expressed in transverse stripes in the blastoderm, each pair-rule gene being expressed in alternate parasegments.

Phenotype The observable characteristics of a cell or an organism, as distinguished from the genotype, which includes alleles that are not expressed in the phenotype of the cell or organism.

Phylogeny Evolutionary history of a species or group.

Progress zone Undifferentiated mesenchymal cells at the tip of the bud, which result in limb outgrowth and are under regulatory control of the apical ectodermal ridge.

Segmentation Division of the body of an organism into a series of morphologically similar units or **segments.**

Somites Segmented balls of mesoderm that lie on both sides of the notochord. They give rise to muscles, the vertebral column, and the dermis.

Stem cell Cell type found in certain adult tissues that is both self-renewing and also gives rise to differentiated cell types.

Transcription factor A protein that initiates or otherwise regulates transcription of a gene into RNA by binding to specific regions of the DNA.

Transgenic An organism that has been genetically altered by the artificial introduction or removal of a gene or genes.

Zone of polarizing activity An area at the posterior margin of the limb bud that has been identified in mice and chicks, and is critical in specifying the anteroposterior axis in the developing limb.

References

Developmental Anatomy of Early Embryogenesis and Organogenesis

1. Gulyas BJ. A reexamination of the cleavage pattern in eutherian mammalian eggs: rotation of the blastomere pairs during second cleavage in the rabbit. *J Exp Zool* 1975;193:235.
2. Gilbert SF. *Developmental biology*, 4th ed. Sunderland, MA: Sinauer Associates, 1994:178.
3. Piko L, Clegg KB. Quantitative changes in total RNA, total poly(A), and ribosomes in early mouse embryos. *Dev Biol* 1982;89:362.
4. McLaren A. *Mammalian chimeras*. Cambridge: Cambridge University Press, 1976.
5. Kelly SJ. Studies of the developmental potential of 4- and 8-cell stage mouse blastomeres. *J Exp Zool* 1977;200:365.
6. Barlow P, Owen DA, Graham C. DNA synthesis in the preimplantation mouse embryo. *J Embr Exp Morphol* 1972;27:432.
7. Hillman N, Sherman MI, Graham CF. The effect of spatial arrangement of cell determination during mouse development. *J Embryol Exp Morphol* 1972;28:263.
8. McGrath J, Solter D. Completion of mouse embryogenesis requires both maternal and paternal genomes. *Cell* 1984;37:179.
9. Surani MAH, Barton SC, Norris ML. Development of reconstituted mouse eggs suggests imprinting of the genome during gametogenesis. *Nature* 1984;308:548.
10. Saunders JF, Errick J. Inductive activity and enduring cellular constitution of a supernumerary apical ectodermal ridge grafted to the limb bud of the chick embryo. *Dev Biol* 1976;50:16.
11. Gilbert SF. *Developmental biology*, 3rd ed. Sunderland, MA: Sinauer Associates, 1991.
12. Keynes RJ, Stern CD. Mechanisms of vertebrate segmentation. *Development* 1988;103:413.

Developmental Anatomy of the Limb

13. Saunders JF. The experimental analysis of chick limb bud development. In: Ede DA, Hinchliffe JR, Balls M, eds. *Vertebrate limb and somite morphogenesis*. Cambridge: Cambridge University Press, 1977:1.
14. MacCabe JA, Errick J, Saunders JW. Ectodermal control of the dorsoventral axis in the leg bud of the chick embryo. *Dev Biol* 1974;39:69.
15. Akita, K. The effect of the ectoderm on the dorsoventral pattern of epidermis, muscles and joints in the developing chick leg: a new model. *Anat Embryol* 1996;193:377.

16. Saunders JW, Gasseling MT. Ectoderm-mesenchymal interactions in the origin of the wing symmetry. In: Fleischmajer R, Billingham RE, eds. *Epithelial-mesenchymal interactions.* Baltimore, MD: Williams and Wilkins, 1968:78.

17. Solursh M, Singley CT, Reiter RS. The influence of epithelia on cartilage and loose connective tissue formation by limb mesenchyme cultures. *Dev Biol* 1981;86:471.

18. Wolpert L, Tickle C, Sampford M. The effect of cell killing by X-irradiation on pattern formation in the chick limb. *J Embryol Exp Morphol* 1979;50:175.

19. Zanetti N, Solursh M. Control of chondrogenic differentiation by the cytoskeleton. *J. Cell Biol* 1984;99:115.

20. Moore KI, Persaus TVN. *Before we are born. Essentials of embryology and birth defects,* 4th ed. Philadelphia: WB Saunders, 1993:266.

21. Davis CA, Holmyard DP, Millen KJ, et al. Examining pattern formation in mouse, chicken and frog embryos with an En-specific antiserum. *Development* 1991;111:287.

22. Johnston SH, Rauskolb C, Wilson R, et al. A family of mammalian Fringe genes implicated in boundary determination and the Notch pathway. *Development* 1997;124:2245.

23. Wu JY, Wen L, Zhang WJ, et al. The secreted product of *Xenopus* gene lunatic Fringe, a vertebrate signaling molecule. *Science* 1976;273:355.

24. Cohen B, Bashirullah A, Dagnino L, et al. Fringe boundaries coincide with Notch-dependent patterning centers in mammals and alter Notch-dependent development in *Drosophila. Nature Genet* 1997;16:283.

25. Niswander L, Tickle C, Vogel A, et al. FGF-4 replaces the apical ectodermal ridge and directs outgrowth and patterning of the limb. *Cell* 1993;75:579.

26. Ohuchi H, Nakagawa T, Yamamoto A, et al. The mesenchymal factor, FGF10, initiates and maintains the outgrowth of the chick limb bud through interaction with FGF8, an apical ectodermal factor. *Development* 1997;124:2235.

27. Ohuchi HTN, Yamauchi T, Ohata T, et al. An additional limb can be induced from the flank of the chick embryo by FGF-4. *Biochem Biophys Res Commun* 1995;209:809

28. Cohn MJ, Izpisua-Belmonte JC, Abud H, et al. Fibroblast growth factors induce additional limb development from the flank of chick embryos. *Cell* 1995;80:739.

29. Min H, Danilenko DM, Scully SA, et al. *Fgf-10* is required for both limb and lung development and exhibits striking functional similarity to *Drosophila branchless. Genes Dev* 1998;12:3156.

30. Summerbell D, Lewis, JH, Wolpert L. Positional information in chick limb morphogenesis. *Nature Lond* 1973;244:492.

31. Summerbell D, Lewis JH. Time, place, and positional value in the chick limb-bud. *J Embryol Exp Morphol* 1975;33:621.

32. Tickle C, Summerbell D, Wolpert L. Positional signalling and specification of digits in chick limb morphogenesis. *Nature Lond* 1975;254:199.

33. Summerbell D. The zone of polarizing activity: Evidence for a role in normal chick limb morphogenesis. *J Embryol Exp Morphol* 1979;50:217.

34. Maden M. Vitamin A and pattern formation in the regenerating limb. *Nature Lond* 1982;295:672.

35. Summerbell D. The effect of local application of retinoic acid to the anterior margin of the developing chick limb. *J Embryol Exp Morphol* 1983;78:269.

36. Thaller C, Eichele G. Retinoid signaling in vertebrate limb development. In: Crombrugghe B, Horton WA, Olsen BR, et al., eds. *Molecular and developmental biology.* New York: Ann NY Acad Sci 1996;785:1.

37. Monga M. Vitamin A and its congeners. *Semin Perinatol* 1997;21:135.

38. Nester G, Zuckner J. Rheumatologic complications of vitamin A and retinoids. *Semin Arthritis Rheum* 1995;24:291.

39. Riddle R, Johnson R, Laufer E, et al. Sonic hedgehog mediates the polarizing activity of the ZPA *Cell* 1993;75:1401.

40. Francis P, Richardson M, Brickell P, et al. Bone morphogenetic proteins and a signalling pathway that controls patterning in the chick limb. *Development* 1994;120:209.

41. Niswander L, Jeffrey S, Martin GR, et al. A positive feedback loop coordinates growth and patterning in the vertebrate limb. *Nature* 1994;371:609.

42. Brunet LJ, McMahon JA, McMahon AP, et al. Noggin, cartilage morphogenesis, and joint formation in the mammalian skeleton. *Science* 1998;280:1455.

43. Dickman S. Growing joints use their noggins. *Science* 1998;280:1350.

44. Noonan KJ, Reiter RS, Kurriger GL, et al. Spatial and temporal expression of CD44 isoforms in the developing and growing joints of the rat limb. *J Orthop Res* 1998;16:100.

45. Dealy CN, Roth A, Ferrari D, et al. *Wnt-5a* and *Wnt-7a* are expressed in the developing chick limb bud in a manner suggesting roles in pattern formation along the proximodistal and dorsoventral axes. *Mech Dev* 1993;43:175.

46. Riddle RD, Ensini M, Nelson C, et al. Induction of the LIM homeobox gene Lmxl by Wnt7a establishes dorsoventral pattern in the vertebrate limb. *Cell* 1995;83:631.

47. Parr, BA, McMahon AP. Dorsalizing signal Wnt-7a required for normal polarity of D-V and A-P axes of mouse limb. *Nature* 1995;374:350.

48. Yang Y, Niswander L. Interaction between the signaling molecules Wnt7a and SHH during vertebrate limb development: dorsal signals regulate anteroposterior patterning. *Cell* 1995;80:939.

49. Izpisua-Belmonte JC, Ede DA, Tickle C, et al. Mis-expression of posterior Hox-4 genes in Talpid (ta³) mutant wings correlates with the absence of anteroposterior polarity. *Development* 1992b;114:959.

50. Duboule D. Vertebrate Hox genes and proliferation: an alternative pathway to homeosis? *Curr Opin Genet Dev* 1995;5:525.

51. Goff DJ, Tabin CJ. Analysis of HoxD-13 and HoxD-11 misexpression in chick limb buds reveals that Hox genes affect both bone condensation and growth. *Development* 1997;124(3):627.

52. Stevenson RE, Hall JG, Godoman RM. Human malformations and related anomalies: vol II. In: *Oxford monographs on medical genetics,* no. 27. New York: Oxford University Press, 1993.

53. Mortlock DP, Post LC, Innis JW. The molecular basis of hypodactyly (Hd): a deletion in Hoxal 3 leads to arrest of digital arch formation. *Nature Genet* 1996;13:284.

54. Raas-Rothschild A, Manouvrier S, Gonzales M, et al. Refined mapping of a gene for split hand-split foot malformation (SHFM3) on chromosome 10q25. *J Med Genet* 1996;33:996.

55. Hoyme HE, van Allen MI, Benirschke K. Vascular pathogenesis of transverse limb reduction defects. *Pediatrics* 1982;101:839.

56. Van Allen MI, Hoyme HE, Jones KL. Vascular pathogenesis of limb defects. I. Radial artery anatomy in radial aplasia. *J Pediatr* 1982;101:832.

57. Torpin R. Fetal malformation caused by amnion rupture during gestation. Springfield, IL: Charles C Thomas, 1968.

58. Zeller R, Jackson-Grusby L, Leder P. The limb deformity gene is required for apical ectodermal ridge differentiation and anteroposterior limb pattern formation. *Genes Dev* 1989;3:1481.

59. Chan DC, Wynshaw-Boris A, Leder P. Formin isoforms are differentially expressed in the mouse embryo and are required for normal expression of *fgf-4* and *shh* in the limb bud. *Development* 1995;121:3151.

60. Kochhar DM. Cellular basis of congenital limb deformity induced in mice by vitamin A. In: Bergsma D and Lenz W, eds.

Morphogenesis and malformation of the limb, vol. 13. Birth Defects Original Article Series. New York: Liss, 1977:111.

61. Heutink P, Zguricas J, van Oosterhout L, et al. The gene for triphalangeal thumb maps to the subtelomeric region of chromosome 7q. *Nature Genet* 1994;6:287.

62. Radhakrishna U, Blouin J-L, Solanki JV, et al. An autosomal dominant triphalangeal thumb: polysyndactyly syndrome with variable expression in a large Indian family maps to 7q36. *Am J Med Genet* 1996;66:209.

63. Hui CC, Joyner AL. A mouse model of Greig cephalopolysyndactyly syndrome: the *extra-toes* mutation contains an intragenic deletion of the *Gli3* gene. *Nature Genet* 1993;3:241.

64. Masuya H, Sagai T, Wakana S, et al. A duplicated zone of polarizing activity in polydactylous mouse mutants. *Genes Dev* 1995;9:1645.

65. Muragaki Y, Mondlos S, Upton J, et al. Altered growth and branching patterns in synpolydactyly caused by mutations in HOXD 13. *Science* 1996;272:548.

66. Lockwood C, Ghidini A, Romero R, et al. Amniotic band syndrome: reevaluation of its pathogenesis. *Am J Obstet Gynecol* 1989;160:1030.

67. Patterson TS. Congenital ring construction. *Br J Plast Surg* 1961;14:1.

68. Streeter GL. Focal deficiencies in fetal tissues and the relation to intra-uterine amputation. *Contrib Embryol* 1930;22:41.

69. Van Allen MI, Curry C, Gallagher L. Limb body wall complex: I. Pathogenesis. *Am J Med Genet* 1987;28:529.

70. Houben JJ. Immediate and delayed effects of oligohydramnios on limb development in the rat: chronology and specificity. *Teratology* 1984;30:403.

Developmental Anatomy of the Vertebral Column

71. Chevallier A. Role due mesoderme somitique dans le developpement de la cage thoracique de l'embryon d'oiseau. *J Embryol Exp Morphol* 1975;33:291.

72. Chevallier A, Kieny M, Mauger A, et al. Developmental fate of the somitic mesoderm in the chick embryo. In: Ede DA, Hinchliffe JR, Balls M, eds. *Vertebrate limb and somite morphogenesis.* Cambridge: Cambridge University Press, 1977:421.

73. Kessel M, Gruss P. Homeotic transformations of murine vertebrae and concomitant alteration of Hox codes induced by retinoic acid. *Cell* 1991;67:89.

74. Kessel M, Balling R, Gruss P. Variations of cervical vertebrae after expression of a *Hox-1.1* transgene in mice. *Cell* 1990;61:301.

75. Pollock RA. Altering the boundaries of *Hox-3.1* expression: evidence for anipodal gene regulation. *Cell* 1992;71:911.

76. Ramirez SR. Hoxb-4 (Hox-2.6) Mutant mice show homeotic transformation of a cervical vertebra and defects in the closure of the sternal rudiments. *Cell* 1993;73:279.

77. Chisaka O, Capecchi MR. Regionally restricted developmental defects resulting from targeted disruption of the mouse homeobox gene *hox-1.5. Nature* 1991;350:473.

78. Kessel M. Reversal of axonal pathways from rhombomere 3 correlates with extra Hox expression domains. *Neuron* 1993;10:379.

79. Dietrich S, Gruss P. Undulated phenotypes suggest a role of *Pax-1* for the development of vertebral and extravertebral structures. *Dev Biol* 1995;167:529.

80. Takahashi Y, Monsoro-Burq A-H, Bontoux M, et al. A role for Qhox-8 in the establishment of the dorsoventral pattern during vertebrate development. *Proc Natl Acad Sci USA* 1992;89:10,237.

81. Gruneberg H. *The pathology of development.* Oxford: Blackwell Scientific, 1963.

82. Lyon MF, Seale AG. *Genetic variations and strains of the laboratory mouse.* Oxford: Oxford University Press, 1989.

83. Dietrich S, Kessel M. The vertebral column. In: Thorogood P, ed. *Embryos, genes and birth defects.* New York: John Wiley and Sons, 1997.

84. Dias MS. Myelomeningocele. In: Choux M, DiRocco C, Hockley AD, et al., eds. *Pediatric neurosurgery.* London: Churchill Livingstone, 1997:32.

85. George TM, McLone DG. Mechanisms of mutant genes in spina bifida: a review of implications from animal models. *Pediatr Neurosurg* 1995;23:236.

86. Gardner WJ. Diastematomyelia and the Klipper-Feil syndrome. Relationship to hydrocephalus, syringomyelia, meningocele, meningomyelocele, and iniencephalus. *Clev Clin Q* 1964;31:19.

87. Gardner WJ. The dysraphic states from syringomyelia to anencephaly. Amsterdam: *Excerpta Medica,* 1973.

88. Partington MD, McLone DG. Hereditary factors in the etiology of neural tube defects. *Pediatr Neurosurg* 1995;23:311.

89. Papalopula N, Kintner CR. Molecular genetics of neurulation. In: Bock G, Marsh J, eds. *Neural tube defects.* Ciba Foundation Symposium No. 181. Chichester, UK: John Wiley, 1994:299.

90. Schoenwolf GC, Smith JL. Mechanisms of neurulation: traditional viewpoint and recent advances. *Development* 1990;109:243.

91. Copp AJ, Brook FA, Estibeiro P, et al. The embryonic development of mammalian neural tube defects. *Prog Neurobiol* 1990;35:363.

Developmental Anatomy of the Nervous System

92. Echelard Y, Epstein DJ, St-Jacques B, et al. Sonic hedgehog, a member of a family of putative signaling molecules, is implicated in the regulation of CNS polarity. *Cell* 1993;75:1417.

93. Basler K, Edlund T, Jessell TM, et al. Control of cell pattern in the neural tube: regulation of cell differential by *dorsalin-1,* a novel TGFβ family member. *Cell* 1993;73:687.

94. Copp AJ, Bernfield M. Etiology and pathogenesis of human neural tube defects insights from mouse models. *Curr Opin Pediatr* 1994;6:624.

Bone Formation and Growth

95. Tyler MS, Hall BK. Epithelial influence on skeletogenesis in the mandible of the embryonic chick. *Anat Rec* 1977;206:61.

96. Hall BK. The embryonic development of bone. *Am Sci* 1988;76:174.

97. Ogden JA. *Pediatric orthopaedics,* 3rd ed. Philadelphia: JB Lippincott, 1990.

98. Ham AW. Some histophysiologic problems peculiar to calcified tissue. *J Bone Joint Surg Am* 1952;34:701.

Lovell & Winter's Pediatric Orthopaedics, fifth edition, edited by Raymond T. Morrissy and Stuart L. Weinstein.
Lippincott Williams & Wilkins, Philadelphia © 2000

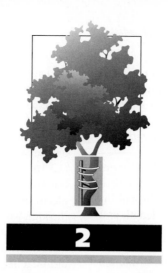

2

GROWTH IN PEDIATRIC ORTHOPAEDICS

ALAIN DIMÉGLIO

BASIC CONCEPTS

It is growth that distinguishes adult from pediatric orthopaedics. It is this ongoing 17-year adventure, punctuated by upheavals and accidents along the way, and jolted by seismic shocks, that gives this discipline its originality and makes it so interesting. Growth analysis is the evaluation of the effects of time in the growing child. Growth is a complex and well-synchronized phenomenon with a hierarchical pattern that organizes the different types and rates of growth in various tissues, in various organs, and in various individuals through time (1).

Growth can be considered as "microgrowth," which is mainly growth at the cellular level, e.g., in the growth plate. Even though the histological structure is the same, each growth plate has its own characteristics and dynamics (1). The study of height, weight, and body proportions may

A. Diméglio: Service d'Orthopedie Pediatrique, Hôpital Lapeyronie, 34295 Montpellier Cedex 5, France.

be considered as the study of "macrogrowth." This is the culmination of all of the effects of microgrowth on the individual: the meeting point of growth of the lower limbs, growth of the trunk, growth of the upper limbs, increase in weight, etc. (2–5). It is this latter form of growth that this chapter deals with.

The scope of this process called growth, and the changes it brings, are made more palpable by some facts. From birth onward, height will increase by 350% and weight will increase 20-fold; the femur and tibia will triple in length and the spine will double in length (2,6,7). This requires an enormous amount of energy.

The energy requirements in the first 3 years of life are much greater than those of the adult: calories, 110 versus 40 calories per kilogram per day; protein, 2 versus 1 grams per kilogram per day; water, 150 versus 5 milliliters per kilogram per day. Skeletal mineralization alone requires storage of 1 kg of calcium between birth and adulthood (8).

In pediatric orthopaedics, the effects of various diseases, disorders, and injuries are best analyzed on the basis of past growth, whereas treatments often are planned mostly based on assumptions about future or remaining growth of various parts of the body. Growth is an essential element in the natural history of any orthopaedic disorder in the growing child (9). It would be a mistake to assume that only growth in height is important. It is equally important to consider the manner in which the skeletal system develops, i.e., the timing of growth in various parts of the body and the changing proportions of various body segments (5,8,10). In addition, the orthopaedist must not lose sight of other aspects of growth, such as growth of the nervous system.

The orthopaedist will need to know the normal values for many parameters and how to measure them (11–15). He or she will need to know the significance of these values, e.g., the significance of bone age on the growth of the lower limb in a girl with a bone age of 13 years, or the effect of a ten-level spinal fusion in a boy with a bone age of 10 years. Bone age, Tanner classification of the stages of puberty, and measurement of the upper and lower portions of the body are all parameters that may need to be considered in the analysis of any particular case (2,16).

Knowledge of the synchronization of the various events in growth will also allow the orthopaedist to anticipate certain events, e.g., the onset of the increase in growth velocity in a girl with early breast development. However, these values vary with the individual, and average values may not apply to a particular individual. What is most important is the pattern and rate of growth for the particular individual. It is the rate of growth that will influence orthopaedic decisions, more than the final height. Likewise, a change in direction, of one of the parameters, which alters its synchronization with other parameters, may signal an abnormality, a return to normal, or the onset of a normal phase of growth. For this reason, a sequence of measurements of the important parameters is far superior to a single measurement.

The problem often raised about growth data is that such data are ethnically specific, and that it is difficult to transfer parameters from one population to another. For example, bone age atlases are not transferable between populations, nor are growth curves transferable from one country to another. Comparing data from children in England (13–15), Switzerland (17), France (18), and the United States (12,16,19) reveals no significant differences in final heights, bone ages, or other parameters of growth. Looking beyond racial diversity, there are growth constants, i.e., stages through which every child must pass, regardless of age, that are the same in all ethnic groups.

A few simple tools are required at the time of the consultation: a height gauge, scales, a metric tape, and a bone age atlas. With these tools, the specialist will be able to perform rapid mental arithmetic and reach a reasonable decision. A few simple questions will guide the orthopaedist to the information that is required (2).

How tall is the child?
What is the child's sitting height?
How long is the subischial leg length?
What is the child's chronological age? What is the bone age?
How much has the child grown in a single year?
How much growth does the child have left in the trunk and in the lower limbs?
Exactly what point has the child reached on his or her developmental path?
Where is the child in relation to puberty?
Are the child's proportions within normal limits?
How much does the child weigh?

BIOMETRIC MEASUREMENTS

There is not much useful data that can be obtained from a single measurement. A single measurement can be an error, two measurements constitute an indication, and three measurements define a tendency.

In any child with a disturbance of growth, whether generalized or localized to a particular part of the body, measurements of growth should be taken at regular intervals (3,11–15,20,21). Examples would be children with skeletal dysplasia (22), spinal deformity (23), limb-length discrepancy (24), or paralytic conditions (25–27). Birthdays are a convenient reminder for annual evaluations such as measurements of growth. At every clinic, the first response must be to measure the different anthropometric parameters. Checking the child every 6 months, preferably once around his or her birthday, allows an easy assessment of the growth velocity of the child and the different body segments (2). These measurements provide a real-time image of growth, and, carefully recorded in a continually updated "growth notebook," they provide charts that make decisions easier (2,7). Growth velocity is an excellent example, because it provides the best indicator of the beginning of puberty, on which so many decisions rest. The first sign of puberty is the increase in growth to more than 0.5 cm per month or 6 cm per year.

The orthopaedic surgeon must be familiar with the measurement of these parameters. He or she should be able to perform these measurements and teach the correct method to others. It is often useful and possible to instruct the family or the primary physician how to obtain necessary data.

Standing Height

The height gauge is to the orthopaedic specialist what the stethoscope is to the cardiologist (2). In children younger than 5 years of age, standing height is measured with the child lying down, because in this age group it is both easier and more reliable (15).

Between birth and maturity, the body will grow approximately 1.20, or even 1.30, meters. Growth is brisk before the age of 5 years. After that, it slows considerably until the onset of puberty, which is around 11 years in girls and 13 years in boys. At 5 years of age, standing height is 60% of the adult height; it reaches 80% of the final height by the age of 9 years. At puberty, standing height increases more rapidly.

Standing height is a global marker, and it is composed of two more specific measurements known as subischial height (the growth of the lower limbs) and sitting height (the growth of the trunk) (7,15). These two different regions often grow at different rates at different times, which is valuable information for decisions in orthopaedics. Values for the standing heights of girls and boys at various ages are given in Tables 2-1 and 2-2. The percentages of standing

TABLE 2-1. STANDING HEIGHTS OF GIRLS AT VARIOUS AGES

| Age (yr) | Height (cm) | | | | | | | SD | 50th Centile as Percentage of Adult Height |
	3rd	10th	25th	50th	75th	90th	97th		
0.08	49.2	50.4	51.6	53.0	54.4	55.6	56.8	2.00	32.7
0.25	54.9	56.2	57.5	59.0	60.5	61.8	63.1	2.16	36.4
0.50	61.1	62.5	63.9	65.5	67.1	68.5	69.9	2.34	40.4
0.75	65.5	67.0	68.6	70.2	72.0	73.5	74.9	2.52	43.3
1.00	69.1	70.8	72.4	74.2	76.0	77.7	79.3	2.69	45.7
1.25	72.2	73.9	75.7	77.6	79.5	81.2	82.9	2.85	47.8
1.50	74.9	76.7	78.5	80.5	82.6	84.4	86.2	3.01	49.7
1.75	77.2	79.1	81.1	83.2	85.3	87.2	89.1	3.15	51.3
2.00	79.4	81.3	83.4	85.6	87.8	89.8	91.8	3.30	52.8
2.0	78.4	80.3	82.4	84.6	86.8	88.8	90.8	3.30	52.1
2.5	82.2	84.3	86.5	88.9	91.3	93.5	95.6	3.57	54.8
3.0	85.7	88.1	90.4	93.0	95.6	97.9	100.2	3.83	57.3
3.5	89.2	91.6	94.1	96.8	99.6	102.0	104.5	4.07	59.7
4.0	92.3	94.9	97.5	100.4	103.3	105.9	108.5	4.30	61.9
4.5	95.4	98.1	100.8	103.8	106.9	109.7	112.4	4.52	64.0
5.0	98.2	101.1	104.0	107.2	110.3	113.2	116.1	4.74	66.1
5.5	101.0	104.0	107.0	110.3	113.7	116.7	119.6	4.94	68.0
6.0	103.8	106.8	110.0	113.4	116.9	120.0	123.1	5.14	69.9
6.5	106.4	109.6	112.8	116.4	120.0	123.2	126.4	5.31	71.8
7.0	109.1	112.4	115.7	119.3	123.0	126.3	129.6	5.46	73.6
7.5	111.7	115.0	118.4	122.2	126.0	129.4	132.8	5.60	75.3
8.0	114.2	117.6	121.1	125.0	128.9	132.4	135.8	5.75	77.1
8.5	116.7	120.3	123.8	127.8	131.8	135.3	138.8	5.87	78.8
9.0	119.3	122.9	126.6	130.6	134.6	138.3	141.9	6.00	80.5
9.5	121.9	125.6	129.3	133.5	137.6	141.3	145.0	6.14	82.3
10.0	124.5	128.3	132.1	136.4	140.6	144.5	148.3	6.31	84.2
10.5	127.1	131.1	135.0	139.5	143.9	147.9	151.8	6.56	86.1
11.0	129.5	133.7	138.0	142.7	147.4	151.6	155.8	6.97	88.1
11.5	132.0	136.5	141.0	146.1	151.1	155.6	160.1	7.47	90.1
12.0	135.0	139.6	144.2	149.3	154.4	159.1	163.6	7.61	92.0
12.5	139.0	143.3	147.7	152.5	157.4	161.8	166.1	7.21	94.0
13.0	142.6	146.7	150.9	155.5	160.2	164.4	168.5	6.90	95.9
13.5	145.4	149.4	153.4	157.9	162.3	166.3	170.3	6.61	97.3
14.0	147.6	151.4	155.3	159.6	163.9	167.8	171.6	6.38	98.4
14.5	149.4	153.1	156.9	161.1	165.3	169.0	172.7	6.20	99.3
15.0	150.3	153.9	157.6	161.7	165.8	169.5	173.2	6.09	99.8
15.5	150.6	154.2	157.9	162.0	166.1	169.7	173.4	6.04	99.9
16.0	150.9	154.5	158.2	162.2	166.2	169.9	173.5	6.00	100.0

(From ref. 15, with permission.)

TABLE 2-2. STANDING HEIGHTS OF BOYS AT VARIOUS AGES

| Age (yr) | Height (cm) | | | | | | | SD | 50th Centile as Percentage of Adult Height |
	3rd	10th	25th	50th	75th	90th	97th		
0.08	50.2	51.4	52.7	54.0	55.4	56.6	57.8	2.00	30.9
0.25	56.6	57.9	59.2	60.7	62.1	63.4	64.7	2.16	34.7
0.50	63.8	65.2	66.6	68.2	69.7	71.2	72.6	2.34	39.0
0.75	67.9	69.4	71.0	72.7	74.4	75.9	77.4	2.52	41.6
1.00	71.2	72.8	74.5	76.3	78.1	79.7	81.4	2.69	43.7
1.25	74.0	75.7	77.4	79.4	81.3	83.0	84.7	2.85	45.4
1.50	76.5	78.3	80.1	82.1	84.2	86.0	87.8	3.01	47.0
1.75	78.7	80.6	82.5	84.6	86.7	88.7	90.5	3.15	48.4
2.00	80.7	82.7	84.7	86.9	89.1	91.1	93.1	3.30	49.8
2.0	79.7	81.7	83.7	85.9	88.1	90.1	92.1	3.30	49.2
2.5	83.5	85.6	87.8	90.2	92.6	94.8	96.9	3.57	51.6
3.0	87.0	89.3	91.6	94.2	96.8	99.1	101.4	3.83	53.9
3.5	90.4	92.8	95.3	98.0	100.8	103.2	105.7	4.07	56.1
4.0	93.5	96.1	98.7	101.6	104.5	107.1	109.7	4.30	58.2
4.5	96.5	99.2	102.0	105.0	108.1	110.8	113.5	4.52	60.1
5.0	99.4	102.2	105.1	108.3	111.5	114.4	117.2	4.74	62.0
5.5	102.2	105.2	108.2	111.5	114.8	117.8	120.8	4.94	63.8
6.0	104.9	108.0	111.1	114.6	118.1	121.2	124.3	5.14	65.6
6.5	107.6	110.8	114.0	117.6	121.2	124.4	127.6	5.31	67.3
7.0	110.3	113.5	116.8	120.5	124.2	127.5	130.8	5.46	69.0
7.5	112.9	116.2	119.6	123.4	127.2	130.6	133.9	5.60	70.6
8.0	115.4	118.8	122.3	126.2	130.0	133.5	137.0	5.73	72.2
8.5	117.9	121.4	125.0	128.9	132.9	136.4	139.9	5.85	73.8
9.0	120.4	124.0	127.6	131.6	135.7	139.3	142.9	5.98	75.4
9.5	122.8	126.5	130.2	134.3	138.4	142.1	145.8	6.10	76.9
10.0	125.1	128.8	132.6	136.8	141.0	144.8	148.5	6.24	78.3
10.5	127.2	131.0	135.0	139.3	143.6	147.6	151.4	6.44	79.8
11.0	129.4	133.3	137.4	141.9	146.4	150.4	154.4	6.67	81.3
11.5	131.7	135.8	140.0	144.7	149.4	153.6	157.8	6.95	82.7
12.0	133.7	138.0	142.4	147.3	152.2	156.6	160.9	7.24	84.1
12.5	136.3	140.7	145.3	150.3	155.4	159.9	164.4	7.48	85.5
13.0	138.7	143.4	148.2	153.4	158.7	163.5	168.2	7.82	87.1
13.5	141.5	146.4	151.3	156.8	162.3	167.2	172.0	8.11	89.1
14.0	145.0	150.0	155.0	160.7	166.3	171.3	176.2	8.31	92.0
14.5	148.4	153.4	158.4	164.0	169.6	174.6	179.6	8.30	94.6
15.0	152.3	157.1	161.9	167.3	172.7	177.6	182.4	8.00	96.6
15.5	155.9	160.4	165.0	170.1	175.2	179.8	184.3	7.55	97.9
16.0	158.9	163.1	167.4	172.2	177.0	181.3	185.5	7.08	98.8
16.5	160.7	164.8	168.9	173.5	178.0	182.1	186.2	6.77	99.4
17.0	161.7	165.7	169.8	174.3	178.8	182.8	186.8	6.67	99.8
17.5	162.0	166.0	170.0	174.5	179.0	183.0	187.0	6.66	99.9
18.0	162.2	166.2	170.2	174.7	179.2	183.2	187.2	6.65	100.0

(From ref. 15, with permission.)

and sitting heights attained for various ages are given in Table 2-3. Values for sitting heights and subischial lengths for girls and boys are given in Figures 2-1 and 2-2.

Sitting Height

In children younger than 2 years of age, sitting height is measured with the child lying down, for the same reasons that standing height is measured supine in this age group (7,15) (Fig. 2-3). After age 2 years, the child should be placed on a stool or table at a convenient height. The most important consideration of all is that the child should always be measured under the same conditions using the same measuring instruments. The sitting height averages 34 cm at birth and averages 88 cm for girls and 92 cm for boys at the end of growth.

In patients with scoliosis, it can be instructive to follow the sitting height rather than the standing height (7,28). If one is treating a girl at age 6 years with juvenile scoliosis, her sitting height will be approximately 64 cm, and will grow to about 88 cm. Thus, one will have to control the curve while her trunk grows 24 cm. The measurement of

TABLE 2-3. PERCENT OF STANDING AND SITTING HEIGHT ATTAINED EACH YEAR

Age (yr)	Girls' Standing Height (%)	Girls' Sitting Height (%)	Girls' Subischial Leg Length (%)	Boys' Standing Height (%)	Boys' Sitting Height (%)	Boys' Subischial Leg Length (%)
0	31	37	25	29	35	23
1	46	53	37	43	50	35
2	52	58	44	50	55	41
3	57	63	50	54	59	47
4	62	67	56	58	63	52
5	66	70	61	64	66	57
6	70	73	66	65	69	61
7	73	76	70	69	67	65
8	77	78	75	72	74	69
9	80	81	79	75	76	73
10	84	84	83	78	78	77
11	88	87	89	81	81	81
12	92	90	94	84	83	84
13	96	95	98	87	86	89
14	98	98	100	92	90	93
15	100	99	100	96	95	98
16	100	100	100	98	98	100
17	100	100	100	99	99	100
18	100	100	100	100	100	100

(From ref. 15, with permission.)

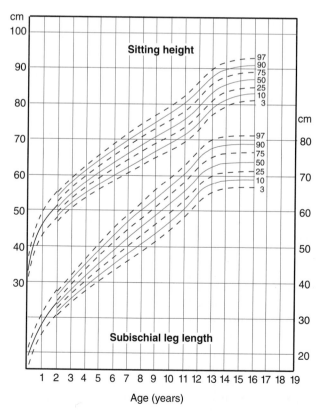

FIGURE 2-1. Normal values for sitting height and subischial leg length (stature minus sitting height) in girls. (Adapted from ref. 15, with permission.)

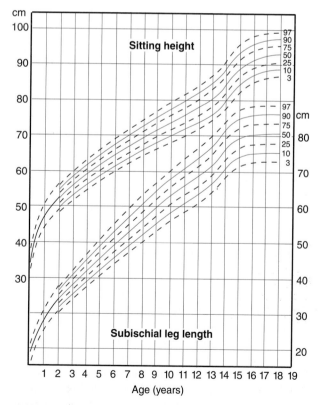

FIGURE 2-2. Normal values for sitting height and subischial leg length (stature minus sitting height) in boys. (Adapted from ref. 15, with permission.)

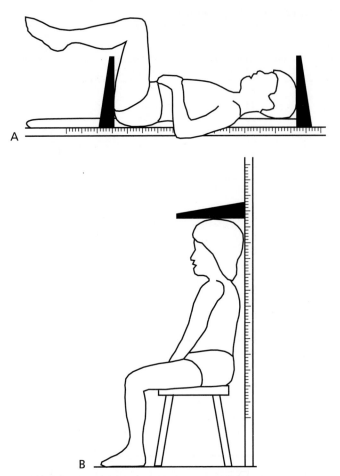

FIGURE 2-3. **A:** Measurement of sitting height. **B:** Once the child is able to sit reliably, measurement with a sitting height gauge can be accurately accomplished by sitting the patient on a firm table or stool at a convenient height.

sitting height can also be useful in anticipating the onset of puberty (7). In an average population, puberty starts at about 75 cm sitting height in girls and 78 cm in boys. At 84 cm sitting height, 80% of girls have menarche (2,7,29).

Subischial Limb Length

The segment of the body made up of the legs is measured to determine the subischial leg length. As implied by the name, it is measured by subtracting the sitting height from the standing height (15).

At birth, the subischial leg length averages 18 cm. At the completion of growth, it will average 81 cm in boys and 74.5 cm in girls. This 63 cm of growth in boys and 56.5 cm of growth in girls contributes a far greater percentage of growth in height than does the trunk (15). This accounts for the changing proportions of the body during growth (Fig. 2-4).

Arm Span

The arm span provides an indirect way to control the standing height. Combining these two measurements avoids virtually all errors. To measure the arm span, the patient simply raises the arms to a horizontal position, and the distance between the tips of the middle fingers is measured with a tape measure (30,31). There is an excellent correlation between the arm span and the standing height. The standing height is about 97% of the arm span (30). In 77% of normal children, the arm span will be 0 to 5 cm greater than the standing height; in 22%, it will be 5 to 10 cm greater; and in 1%, it will be 10 cm or more greater. This relationship remains throughout puberty, with the arm span tending to be slightly greater in proportion to standing height in boys than in girls. If the trunk is normal, i.e., without deformity, its length will equal about 52% of the arm span, and the lower limbs will be equal to about 48%, or the same as their proportions in the standing height (2).

The relationship of arm span to standing height is useful in determining what would be the normal height of a child who is in a wheelchair; this allows calculation of the normal height and weight (25–27,30). It is routinely used for any child who has a spine deformity, e.g., scoliosis, to calculate the normal values for pulmonary function. This relationship also is useful in diagnosing certain disorders characterized by a disproportion between the limbs and the trunk, e.g., Marfan syndrome, in which the arm span is usually 5 cm greater than the standing height. In children with spinal deformity, the arm span is a good estimate of what the standing height would be if there were no scoliosis.

Weight

Weight must always be brought into the equation when making a surgical decision, whether one is dealing with a case of idiopathic scoliosis, paralytic scoliosis, or lower limb osteotomy. Children should always be weighed at consultations (2,12,13). There may be striking morphological changes from one year to the next. If weight evaluation becomes an integral part of each consultation, changes will become obvious, and can be incorporated into the orthopaedic specialist's deliberations. A simple rule for a boy's weight is: 18 to 20 kg at age 5 years; 30 kg at age 10 years; and 60 kg at age 17 years (2). Note that weight doubles between 10 and 17 years of age. At age 5 years, the weight has reached 32% of the final normal weight (2,15).

Weight that is greater than 10% of normal for the patient may be part of the reason that a scoliosis brace is no longer correcting the curve as it did before or may account for the fact that a hip deformed by Perthes disease is now symptomatic, or that the child cannot walk or run as far. Weight can explain delayed menarche, because girls generally need to reach 40 kg for menarche to occur. If the patient's weight (obesity) becomes a problem that aggravates the orthopaedic

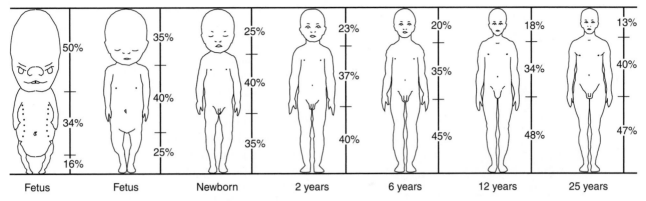

FIGURE 2-4. The proportions of the body as they change during growth. The head and trunk together constitute the sitting height. The segment below is the subischial leg length. (Adapted from ref. 8, with permission.)

condition, it is useful to have objective measurements to document the problem for the patient and his or her parents. A generally accepted estimate of body fat is expressed in Quetelet's body mass index: weight (kg)/height (m²) (31). In this index, 20 to 25 kg/m² is normal; 25 to 30 kg/m² is moderate obesity; 30 to 40 kg/m² is major obesity; and more than 40 kg/m² is morbid obesity.

CHRONOLOGY

Intrauterine Development

Growth does not start at birth. During the first trimester of gestation, the systems are busy organizing themselves, and are developing at a brisk pace (32–35). During this period, the fetus makes daily progress, reaching a weight six million times greater than that of the egg by the time the infant is born. By the second month of life, sitting height is increasing at a rate of 1 mm daily, which subsequently increases to 1.5 mm per day. Were this rate of growth to continue until the age of 10 years, the child would stand 6 m tall (2).

From the third month onward, the embryo becomes a fetus, and turns into a miniature adult. At the end of the second trimester of gestation, the fetus has reached 70% of its size, measuring 30 cm, but has achieved no more than 20% of birth weight (approximately 800 g). It is during the third trimester that the fetus gains weight at the highest rate (700 g per month). This means that various stages of growth do not occur simultaneously during intrauterine life. Length increases steadily and rapidly during the first 6 months *in utero*, whereas weight gain is most rapid during the final 3 months of gestation.

Today, with high-resolution ultrasonography, it is possible to follow the growth of the fetus and to detect the slight-est abnormality. Several good references are available regarding these measurements (36,37). It can be anticipated that many orthopaedic conditions characterized by disproportionate or abnormal growth will be diagnosed prenatally.

After birth, not only does the overall rate of growth vary at different ages, but the rates at which various segments of the body grow differ, as well. For example, during the first 5 years of life, sitting height and subischial leg length increase at about the same rate; from age 5 years to puberty, the sitting height accounts for one-third of the gain and the subischial leg length accounts for two-thirds; from puberty to maturity, the ratio is reversed, with the sitting height accounting for two-thirds of the gain in height and the subischial leg length accounting for one-third (2; Fig. 2-4). The amounts of increase in sitting height and subischial leg length for various ages are shown for girls and boys in Figures 2-5 and 2-6.

From Birth to 5 Years

Birth marks a very obvious transition in the growth of the child. At birth, standing height for the neonate is 30% of the final height (50 to 54 cm). By the age of 5 years, the standing height has increased to 108 cm, which is double the birth height and 62% of the final height. The first year of life sees particularly vigorous growth rates, with the infant's height increasing by 25 cm (2). This means that the height gain during a single year is as great as it is during the entire surge of puberty. At the age of 1 year, the growth rate starts to slow down, but remains strong, with the infant growing another 10 cm between 1 and 2 years of age and 7 cm between 3 and 4 years of age (2).

At birth, the sitting height of the neonate is approximately 34 cm, which is roughly two-thirds of the standing height and 37% of the final sitting height. By the age of 5 years, the sitting height will have increased to 62 cm,

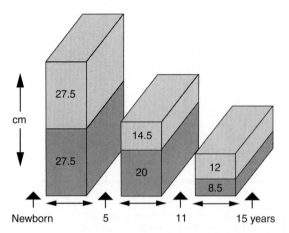

FIGURE 2-5. The growth in sitting height (*top bars*) and subischial leg length (*bottom bars*) at various ages in girls. These data are from our studies, and are in agreement with the figures of Tanner (15).

approximately 66% of the final sitting height, with only about 30 additional centimeters to grow (7,38). This information is useful in anticipating the effects of the deformity and the consequences of arthrodesis in spinal deformity in young patients.

Increase in the subischial leg length follows a pattern almost identical to that for sitting height. At birth, the lower limbs are relatively small, compared with the trunk (only 18 cm). By the age of 5 years, the subischial leg length will have increased by an average of 28 cm, to about 46 cm, representing more than 50% of the final length. At age 5 years, the subischial leg length will increase by about another 35 cm in boys and 28.5 cm in girls, before growth ceases; this is a considerable amount of growth, but less than occurred in the first 5 years (2).

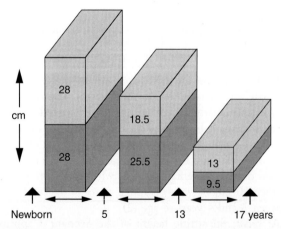

FIGURE 2-6. The growth in sitting height (*top bars*) and subischial leg length (*bottom bars*) at various ages in boys. These data are from our studies, and are in agreement with the figures of Tanner (15).

At birth, the weight is between 3,000 and 3,500 g, 5% of the final figure. At 5 years, the weight averages 18 to 20 kg, 32% of the final adult weight. In 5 years, the weight gain is 15 to 17 kg.

During the first 5 years of growth after birth, the proportions change. The cephalic end of the body becomes relatively smaller, whereas the subischial leg length increases (Fig. 2-4). It is now readily appreciated why any congenital limb deformity or chondrodystrophy has such a dramatic onset during this period of rapid growth. Similarly, any limb paralysis occurring during the first years of life will usually result in severe shortening, not only because so much growth remains, but also because its effects are felt when growth is extremely rapid.

During this period, growth is not only a vertical, but also a volumetric phenomenon. Birth weight triples in a single year, and quadruples by the age of 3 years. The circumference of the chest is 32 cm at birth, but increases 25 cm, to reach 57 cm by the age of 5 years (2,7,38). Chest morphology has undergone dramatic changes. There has been neurological growth: the head circumference is 35 cm at birth and increases by 12 cm in the first year, reflecting the growth of the nervous system. Any neurological assault on the infant during this period can have serious effects on neurological development. By the time the child has reached 5 years of age, sitting height has approximately 26 to 30 cm of growth left (38). This figure demonstrates how difficult the decisions about the management of scoliosis can be during childhood (7). The lower limbs have approximately 35 cm of growth left. This indicates a need for great caution whenever predictions are being made concerning inequality of length.

From 5 to 10 Years of Age

Between 5 and 10 years of age, there is a marked deceleration in growth, with standing height increasing at approximately 5.5 cm per year. Two-thirds of this growth (3.5 cm) occurs in the lower limb, and one-third (2 cm) occurs in the sitting height (7). The trunk is now growing at a slower rate, whereas the lower limbs are growing faster than the trunk, thus changing the proportions of the body (Fig. 2-4). During this 5-year period, standing height will increase by 26% (almost 28 cm), sitting height by 13% (10 cm), and subischial leg length by 20% (18 cm) (Figs. 2-5 and 2-6).

At the age of 10 years, approximately 38 cm of growth remains in standing height for boys and 24 cm for girls, made up of 20 cm in sitting height and 18 cm in the lower limb for boys and 16 cm in sitting height and 10 cm in the lower limb for girls. At the age of 10 years, the average weight is 30 kg, which represents an increase of 12 kg from 5 to 10 years of age, or approximately 2.5 kg per year. The weight at age 10 years represents only 48% of the final average weight at maturity. At this age, in contrast, the standing height is 78% of the final standing height for boys and 83% for girls. Thus, at age 10 years, the child has attained more than 75% of his or her height, but less than 50% of his or her weight (2,12–14).

Puberty

Although age is a poor indicator of puberty, we may start anticipating puberty at age 10 years in girls and age 12 years in boys. It is the acceleration in the velocity of growth that best characterizes the beginning of puberty. From a clinical viewpoint, puberty will be recognized by a combination of factors other than growth: sexual development, chronological age, and bone age. After the age of 10 years, the growth of boys and girls proceeds differently. On average, girls will experience the onset of puberty at 11 years, boys at 13 years. Puberty and its accompanying rapid growth is a period of great importance to the orthopaedic surgeon. Thus, it is important to recognize the period just before puberty (2,9,10,12–15,17,28,39–43).

There are four main characteristics that dominate the phase of growth called puberty:

- a dramatic increase in stature (2);
- changing of the proportions of the upper and lower body segments (8,10,31);
- change in overall morphology: biachromial diameter, pelvic diameter, fat distribution, etc. (30); and
- development of sexual characteristics (15,39,40).

The picture during puberty (from 11 to 13 years in girls and from 13 to 15 years in boys) is dominated by a return to a dramatic increase in the growth rate. However, this time the growth is far more noticeable in the trunk than in the lower limbs. During puberty, annual growth rates for the different parts of the body reverse: two-thirds for sitting height, one-third for subischial leg length.

It is during this period that boys surpass girls in height. On average, boys are 13 cm taller than girls. This is accounted for by two factors. First, boys have approximately 2 more years of growth than girls. Second, boys have a slightly greater increase in the rate of growth during puberty than girls, accounting for approximately 2 cm of additional height.

During puberty, the standing height increases by approximately 1 cm per month. At the onset of puberty, boys have 14% ($\pm$1%) of their remaining standing height to grow. This is approximately 22.5 cm ($\pm$1 cm), made up of 13 cm in sitting height and 9.5 cm in subischial leg length. Girls have 12% ($\pm$1%) of their standing height to grow. This is approximately 20.5 cm ($\pm$1 cm), made up of 12 cm in sitting height and 8.5 cm in subischial leg length.

The peak in the growth rate during puberty occurs between 13 and 15 years of bone age in boys and between 11 and 13 years of bone age in girls (2,5,15,31,39,40,42). By the time girls and boys have passed bone ages of 13 and 15

years, respectively, lower limb growth virtually ceases, with all remaining growth (4.5 cm) taking place in sitting height. This is an extremely important factor to consider in the treatment of many disorders, especially scoliosis and limb-length discrepancy.

These figures, ratios, and rates provide only a partial reflection of the growth phenomenon. Precise evaluation of the characteristics of puberty, using the Tanner classification, the onset of menstruation, and the Risser sign, is something that needs to be undertaken with a great deal of care. One of the major problems with using only the onset of menarche and the Risser sign is that they occur after the growth of puberty has begun to slow.

Secondary Sexual Characteristics

Secondary sexual characteristics develop throughout the course of puberty; the first appearance of pubic hair, the budding of the nipples, and the swelling of the testes are the first physical signs to signal the onset of puberty (2,15,39,40). The first physical sign of puberty in boys, testicular growth in 77% (31), occurs on average 1.7 years before the peak height velocity and 3.5 years before attaining adult height. The bone age will be approximately 13 years at the onset of puberty; the Risser sign is 0, and the triradiate cartilage is open. At this age, girls have well-developed secondary sexual characteristics, and their rate of growth is decelerating.

In 93% of girls, the first physical sign of puberty is breast budding, which occurs about 1 year before peak height velocity (31). This averages 11 years in bone age. The Risser sign is still 0, and the triradiate cartilage is still open at the onset of puberty. Menarche occurs about 2 years after breast budding, and final height is usually achieved 2.5 to 3 years after menarche. After menarche, girls will gain the final 5% of their standing height, about 3 to 5 cm (7,29,43). The appearance of axillary hair, although variable, often signals the peak of the pubertal growth curve.

The secondary sexual characteristics generally develop in harmony with bone age, but there are discrepancies in 10% of cases (2,5,7,15,31). In these circumstances, it is best to believe the bone age. Puberty may be accelerated and growth can end more quickly than usual, catching the unaware physician off guard. In fact, it has been demonstrated that it is not uncommon to see an acceleration of the bone age during puberty (31).

Pubertal Diagram

Using all of these landmarks, it is possible to draw a diagram relating the events occurring during puberty (Figs. 2-7 and 2-8). Even if one indicator is missing or does not match the other, it is still possible to have a good idea of where the child is on his or her own way through puberty (2,7). By plotting the gains in standing height and sitting height

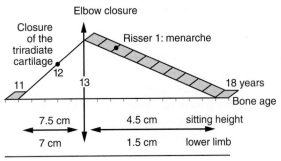

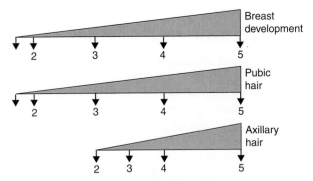

FIGURE 2-7. Top: The pubertal growth curve in girls, illustrating the relationship between the various landmarks. **Bottom:** The corresponding clinical Tanner stages. (Adapted from ref. 7, with permission.)

every 6 months, a picture of the period of puberty is developed. It is also easy to divide this into two parts. The first phase, i.e., the ascending limb of the growth curve, is characterized by an increase in the velocity of growth, and is the major portion of the pubertal growth spurt. The second phase, i.e., the descending limb of the growth curve, is characterized by a slowing of the rate of growth (2,7).

Although the peak of this curve is fleeting, it can be roughly identified by accurate assessment of certain skeletal markers at 6-month intervals. Triradiate cartilage closure occurs about halfway up the ascending limb of the pubertal curve. This closure corresponds to an approximate bone age of 12 years for girls and 14 years for boys. After closure of the triradiate cartilage, there is still a significant amount of growth remaining: greater than 12 cm of standing height for girls and more than 14 cm for boys.

The closure of the olecranon apophysis in the elbow is a very good skeletal marker for the peak of the growth spurt (7). The closing of the growth centers of the elbow (discussed below) divides the ascending and descending phases of puberty, and, as such, is useful in assessing further growth. It is especially useful, because this is a period when there are few changes occurring in the bones of the hand and wrist, as used in the Greulich and Pyle atlas (G&P) (16).

Menarche usually occurs after closure of the olecranon

apophysis, on the descending limb of the growth curve, when the rate of growth is slowing. This is usually between bone ages of 13 and 13.5 years, and corresponds to Risser I on the iliac apophysis (28,29,44–46). At this stage, the average girl will gain an additional 4 cm of sitting height and 0.6 cm of subischial leg length. The menarche is not as precise as many other indicators during puberty. Forty-two percent of girls experience menarche before Risser I, 31% at Risser I, 13% at Risser II, 8% at Risser III, and 5% at Risser IV (7).

The first phase of the pubertal growth spurt is the ascending phase, which corresponds to the acceleration in the velocity of growth. This phase lasts 2 years, from approximately 11 to 13 years of bone age in girls and from 13 to 15 years of bone age in boys. The gain in standing height for girls during this phase is about 14.5 cm, made up of 7.5 cm in sitting height and 7 cm in subischial leg length. The gain in standing height for boys during this phase is about 16.5 cm, made up of 8.5 cm in sitting height and 8 cm in subischial leg length. During this first phase of the pubertal growth spurt, the sitting height contributes 53% and the subischial leg length contributes 47%. Thus, more

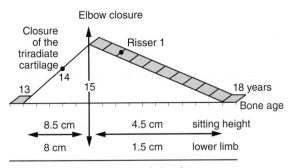

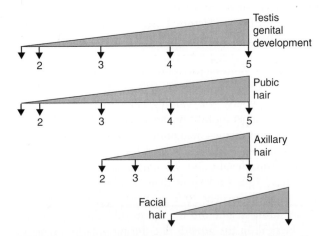

FIGURE 2-8. Top: The pubertal growth curve in boys, illustrating the relationship between the various landmarks. **Bottom:** The corresponding clinical Tanner stages. (Adapted from ref. 7, with permission.)

growth comes from the trunk than from the legs during this phase of growth (7).

The second phase of the pubertal growth spurt is a period of deceleration in the rate of growth. This phase lasts 2.5 years, from 13 to 15.5 years of bone age in girls and from 15 to 17.5 years of bone age in boys. During this phase, boys and girls will gain about 6 cm in standing height, with 4.5 cm coming from an increase in sitting height and 1.5 cm coming from an increase in subischial leg length. During this phase, the increase in sitting height contributes 80% of the gain in the standing height (7).

At skeletal maturity, the average weight for boys is 63 kg, with a standing height of 174 cm (±1 cm), and the average weight for girls is 56 kg, with a standing height of 166 cm (±1 cm). From 10 to 20 years of age, the gain in weight averages 33 kg in boys and 26 kg in girls. During the growth spurt of puberty, the average gain in weight each year is 5 kg (2).

RADIOLOGICAL STUDY

In pediatric orthopaedics, chronological age is of no significance. Everything turns on bone age. Personal data indicate that about 50% of children have a bone age that is significantly different from their chronological age. In some disorders, this is characteristic: delayed bone age in Perthes disease (47,48), slipped capital femoral epiphysis (49–51), severe cerebral palsy, and rickets with nephropathy. Whether it is a case of Legg-Calvé-Perthes disease, limb-length discrepancy, or chondrodystrophy, all reasoning, analysis, forecasting, and decision-making must be based on bone age.

Accurate assessment of bone age is not easy (7,52–56). The younger the child, especially before puberty, the more difficult it is to determine future growth, making errors more likely. In addition, children are often bone age mosaics. Bone age determinations for the hands, elbows, pelvis, and knees will not always agree with one another (2,7).

Often, the bone age determination is made too quickly and with too little information. The standard deviations for determining bone age must be understood, as well as the nuances of what to look for in the interpretation of the radiograph. When using a particular method, e.g., the Greulich and Pyle atlas (16), it is important to read the entire book to understand what to look for and to know the standard error, and not simply to compare radiographs. If there is a major decision to be made, it is better to have two interpretations of the child's bone age, and to enlist the support of pediatric radiologists with experience in bone age determination (55,56).

Cundy and colleagues (56) demonstrated that four radiologists' interpretations of skeletal age differed by more than 2 years in 10% of patients. Carpenter and Lester (54) evaluated bone age in children younger than 10 years of

age. It was shown that separate readings of the distal radius and ulna, the carpal bones, the metacarpals, and the phalanxes could magnify these errors, and that the age of the carpal bones and the distal radius and ulna often lagged behind the age of the metacarpals and phalanxes. In Legg-Calvé-Perthes disease, discrepancy in maturation between carpal bone and metacarpal bone is frequent (48). This means that excessive haste in reading the bone age can result in fatal strategic errors.

There are several different methods to evaluate bone age. Knowledge of these methods and their limitations is important to the orthopaedist, especially in difficult cases (16,57–59). Like the goniometer, the Greulich and Pyle atlas (16) forms an essential part of the tool kit for the orthopaedic specialist. Our use of this atlas enabled us to compare it with its French counterpart, the Sempé and Pavia atlas (18). We learned that there is no major significant difference between these two atlases. The Tanner and Whitehouse method, although accurate, is very time-consuming and difficult, making it impractical for daily use (58). Therefore, the Greulich and Pyle atlas is sufficient for clinical decision-making in orthopaedic practice, when used by physicians knowledgeable in the method.

One of the weaknesses of the Greulich and Pyle atlas is that there are few changes in the hand during the critical time of puberty. For this reason, the author has found the Sauvegrain method (59) to be of enormous value during puberty (Fig. 2-9). This method evaluates the anteroposterior and lateral views of the elbow, assigning a value to the epiphyses, which is then plotted on a chart to give the bone age. It is reliable and based on the skeletal maturation of the elbow, which occurs during a 2-year period corresponding with the ascending limb of the growth velocity curve. Thus, it is extremely helpful in boys aged 13 to 15 years and in girls aged 11 to 13 years, a period in which many of the clinical decisions involving future growth are made. In addition, it shows good correlation with the Greulich and Pyle atlas but is much easier to use.

At the beginning of puberty, the growth centers of the elbow are wide open, but 2 years later, when the peak velocity of the pubertal growth spurt is reached and growth begins to slow, they are all completely closed. This complete closure occurs 6 months before Risser I. There is great value in analysis of olecranon ossification (7). At the start of puberty, at bone age 11 years for girls and 13 years for boys, two ossification centers appear (Fig. 2-10). Six months later (bone age 11.5 years for girls and 13.5 years for boys), they merge to form a half-moon shape. By bone age 12 years for girls and 14 years for boys, the olecranon apophysis has a rectangular appearance. Six months later (bone age 12.5 years for girls and 14.5 years for boys), the olecranon apophysis begins to fuse with the ulna, a process that takes another 6 months, being completed by the bone age of 13 years in girls and 15 years in boys. The radiographic appearance of

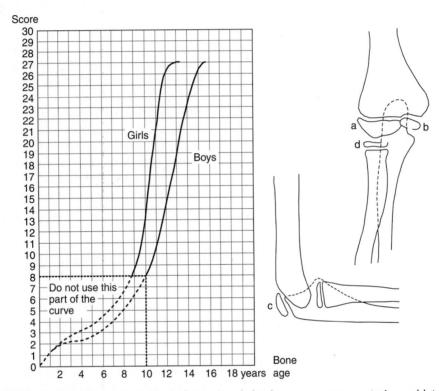

FIGURE 2-9. The Sauvegrain method of assessing skeletal age uses anteroposterior and lateral radiographs of the elbow. It is useful only in boys at ages 11 to 15 years and in girls at ages 9 to 13 years. The condyle and epicondyle, the trochlea, the olecranon, and the head of the radius are compared with the drawings, and each part is assigned the corresponding coefficient marked on the drawing, which represents the radiograph. Next, the overall summed value is plotted on the y axis of the chart. A horizontal line through this point intersects the line of the curve for either boys or girls, thus giving the corresponding bone age. (Adapted from ref. 59, with permission.)

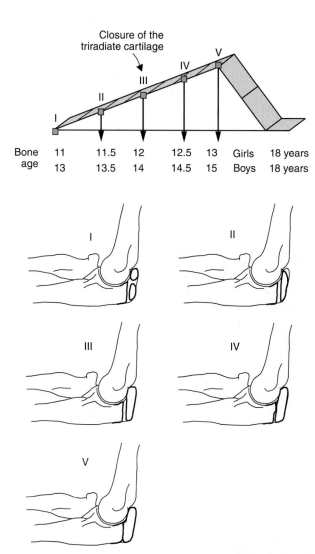

Closure of the triradiate cartilage

Bone age	11	11.5	12	12.5	13	Girls	18 years
	13	13.5	14	14.5	15	Boys	18 years

FIGURE 2-10. A simplification of the Sauvegrain method using only the stages of closure of the olecranon apophysis and its relationship to the pubertal growth curve and the Risser sign. *I:* 11 years in girls; 13 years in boys; double ossific nucleus. *II:* 11 years, 6 months in girls; 13 years, 6 months in boys; semi-moon shape. *III:* 12 years in girls; 14 years in boys; quadrangular shape. *IV:* 12 years, 6 months in girls; 14 years, 6 months in boys; beginning of fusion. *V:* 13 years in girls; 15 years in boys; complete fusion.

the hand and elbow at the peak of the pubertal growth curve is shown in Figure 2-11.

The Risser sign is one of the most commonly used markers of skeletal maturation, especially in the treatment of scoliosis (7,28,60–62). It appears on the radiograph of the pelvis, which is often seen in the assessment of this disorder, thus obviating the need for an additional radiograph. The duration of excursion of the Risser sign is also variable, and may range from 1 to 3 years (44,45). However, the value of this sign for accurate decision making has been questioned. Little and Sussman (63) concluded that, all things considered, it is better to rely on chronological age. Al-

though this author does not agree with their conclusions, when important decisions are made the Risser sign should be augmented with the bone age, as determined by the method of Greulich and Pyle (16). Figures 2-12 and 2-13 show theses correlations.

There are several useful relationships between the events of puberty and the Risser sign. What is important to understand, first, is that the Risser sign is 0 for the first two-thirds of the pubertal growth spurt. This period of Risser 0 is important in the decision-making for many conditions; thus, it is necessary to have more precise markers of the stage of puberty (growth) during this period. Ideally, Risser 0 would be a sign of the period corresponding to the ascending limb of the growth-acceleration curve, but the child is Risser 0 for years before the onset of puberty. Therefore, Risser 0 gives little information other than to indicate that the peak of the growth velocity curve has not been reached. The author has recommended dividing this period of the ascending limb of the pubertal growth curve, characterized by Risser 0, into three periods, based on the triradiate cartilage and the closure of the olecranon apophysis: triradiate cartilage open, triradiate cartilage closed but olecranon open, and olecranon closed (7) (Fig. 2-12).

Risser I heralds the beginning of the descending slope of the pubertal growth peak. It generally appears after the olecranon apophysis is united to the ulna (Fig. 2-12), and when the epiphyses of the distal phalanges (II, III, IV, V) of the hand fuse (Fig. 2-13). The rate of growth in sitting height and standing height decreases abruptly. Axillary hair generally appears during this period (Figs. 2-7 and 2-8).

At Risser II, the greater trochanteric apophysis unites to the femur. This corresponds to a bone age of 14 years in girls and 16 years in boys (Fig. 2-12). There is approximately 3 cm left to grow in sitting height. The proximal phalangeal epiphyses fuse in the hand (Fig. 2-13). At Risser II, there is still a 30% risk of progression (5 degrees or more) for a 30-degree curve and a 2% risk for a 20-degree curve (64).

At Risser III, there is 1 year of growth remaining. This corresponds to bone ages of 14.5 years for girls and 16.5 years for boys. Sitting height will increase about 2 cm. The phalangeal epiphyses of P1-2 fuse during this period (Figs. 2-12 and 2-13). At this point, there is a 12% risk of a curve of 20 degrees or greater progressing 5 degrees or more (7).

Risser IV corresponds to a bone age of 15 years for girls and 17 years for boys. The distal epiphysis of the ulna is united to the shaft. The trunk still has to grow 1 cm, and the risk of the progression of scoliosis is markedly decreased, although, for boys, a slight risk remains (65).

Risser V is very much like Risser 0: it is a long period that does not provide much information to the clinician. The distal radial epiphysis generally unites around the time of Risser V. The iliac apophysis may fuse at age 22 or 23 years, but in some cases it never fuses. Thus, it would be futile, if not naive, to wait until the iliac crest is completely ossified, before discontinuing the treatment of scoliosis (53).

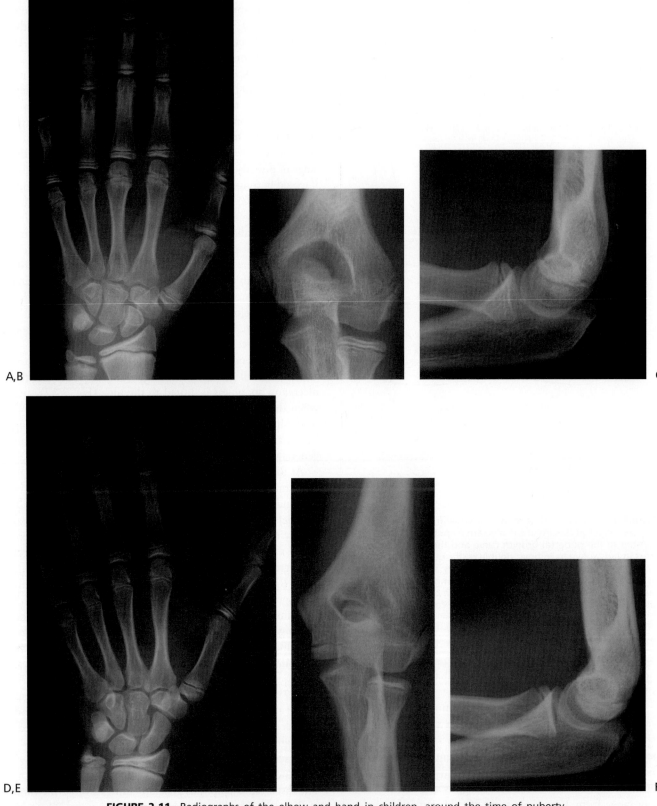

FIGURE 2-11. Radiographs of the elbow and hand in children, around the time of puberty, illustrate the appearance at various bone ages. These figures can be used to compare the method of Sauvegrain (Fig. 2-9), the simpler method of Diméglio, using only the olecranon apophysis (Fig. 2-10), and the Greulich and Pyle atlas (16). **A–C:** Girls 10 years, 9 months; boys 12 years, 9 months (3 months before puberty). **D–F:** Girls 11 years; boys 13 years (beginning of puberty).

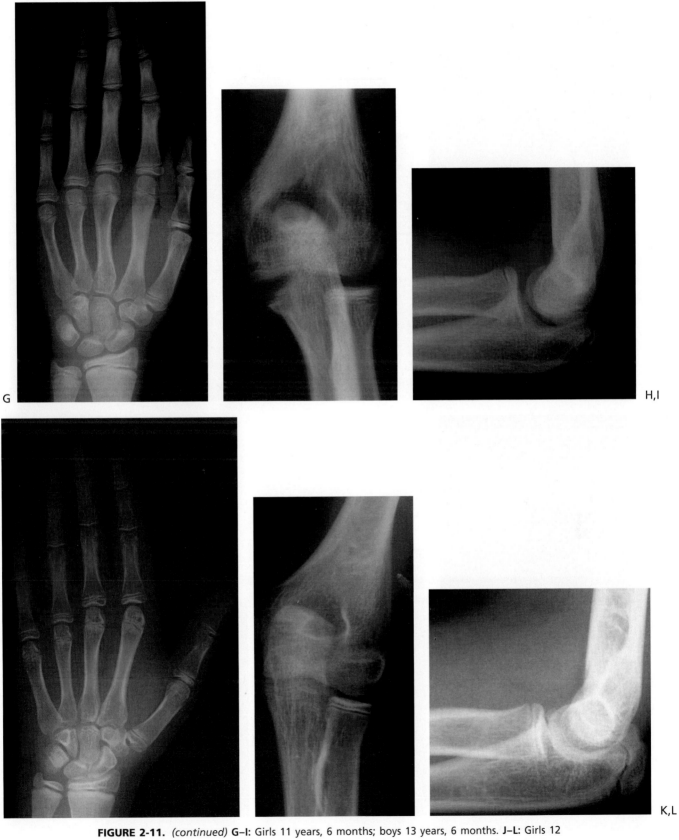

G

H,I

J

K,L

FIGURE 2-11. *(continued)* **G–I:** Girls 11 years, 6 months; boys 13 years, 6 months. **J–L:** Girls 12 years; boys 14 years.

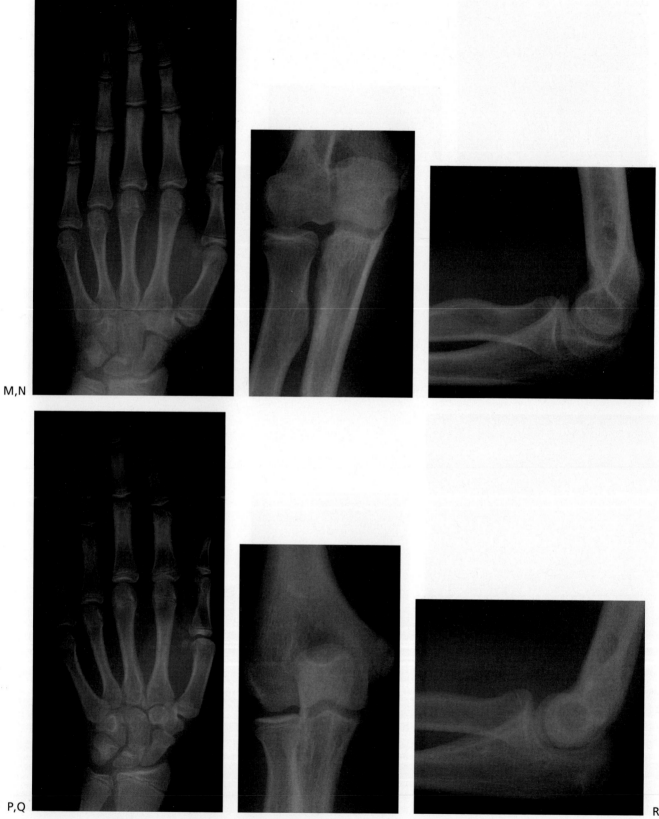

M,N

O

P,Q

R

FIGURE 2-11. *(continued)* **M–O:** Girls 12 years, 6 months; boys 14 years, 6 months. **P–R:** Girls 12 years, 9 months; boys 14 years, 9 months.

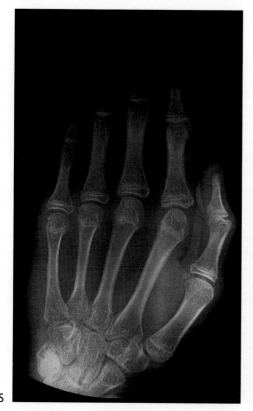
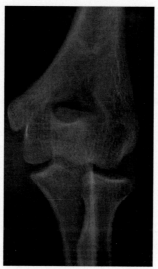
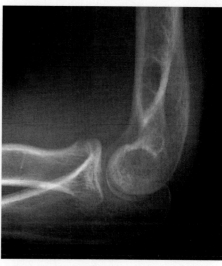

S T,U

FIGURE 2-11. *(continued)* **S–U:** Girls 13 years, 6 months; boys 15 years, 6 months (elbow closure and fusion of the distal phalanx of the thumb).

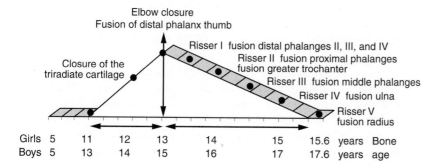

Elbow closure
Fusion of distal phalanx thumb

Risser I fusion distal phalanges II, III, and IV

Closure of the
triradiate cartilage

Risser II fusion proximal phalanges
fusion greater trochanter

Risser III fusion middle phalanges

Risser IV fusion ulna

Risser V
fusion radius

Girls	5	11	12	13	14	15	15.6	years	Bone
Boys	5	13	14	15	16	17	17.6	years	age

FIGURE 2-12. The relationship between the closure of the olecranon apophysis, the Risser sign, and the bone age, from the Greulich and Pyle atlas (16). The closure of the olecranon apophysis occurs before Risser I at the peak of the pubertal growth curve, and, at the same time, there is fusion of the distal phalanx of the thumb.

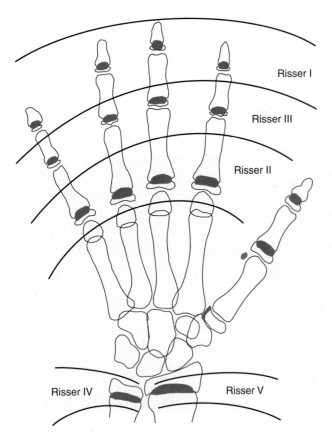

FIGURE 2-13. The correlation between the closure of the physes in the hand and the Risser sign that occurs in 80% of adolescents. The thumb is a special zone. The distal phalanx of the thumb fuses just as the olecranon apophysis closes, or at a Sauvegrain score of 27. This is bone age 13 years in girls and 15 years in boys. The Risser sign will still be 0. The sesamoid ossifies at the beginning of puberty.

GROWTH OF TRUNK AND THORAX

Growth in the Spinal Column

Measurement of sitting height provides an indirect reflection of spinal growth. The spine makes up 60% of the sitting height, whereas the head represents 20%, and the pelvis represents 20% (6,7,66). If we accept the fact that there are at least three growth zones per vertebra (sometimes four), the resulting morphology of the spinal column is the product of 100 growth plates. The pattern of growth in the posterior arch, where closure is linked in particular to the presence of the neural stem, differs from that seen in the body of the vertebrae, which behaves like a long bone (6,7,23).

If you held any of the vertebrae of a newborn in your hand, you would find very little morphological variation between them. The process by which cervical, thoracic, and lumbar vertebrae acquire their individual identities is gradual. In the vertebral body, ossification first appears in the

dorsal region, which forms a hub from which it radiates to the cranial and caudal parts of the spine. The process of ossification is extremely slow, and does not finish until the 25th year of life.

The lumbosacral vertebrae are relatively smaller at birth than the thoracic and cervical vertebrae. However, during the first years of growth, they grow more rapidly. Between 3 and 15 years of age, the lumbar vertebrae and their disks increase about 2 mm per year, whereas the thoracic vertebrae and their disks increase 1 mm. The disks account for approximately 30% of the height of the spinal segment at birth. At maturity, this figure will decrease to 25%, with the disks constituting 22% of the cervical spine, 18% of the thoracic spine, and 35% of the lumbar spine (6,7).

The anterior and posterior portions of the vertebrae do not grow at the same rate. In the thoracic region, the posterior components grow at a faster pace than their anterior counterparts. The reverse occurs in the lumbar region. Growth potential thus varies from one level to the next, differing from anterior to posterior. Also, as the vertebrae develop, there is a constant remodeling of the anatomic organization of the spine, e.g., the articular apophyses change in both morphology and direction (7,23,24).

The height of the spine will nearly triple from birth to adulthood. The average adult spine is approximately 70 cm long in men, with the cervical spine measuring 12 cm, the thoracic spine 28 cm, the lumbar spine 18 cm, and the sacrum 12 cm. The average female spine is approximately 65 cm long at maturity. At birth, the vertebral column is approximately 24 cm long. In the newborn, only 30% of the spine is ossified, and, as mentioned above, there is little significant difference in morphology from one vertebra to another. The height of a thoracic vertebra is about 7.6 mm, and a lumbar vertebra is about 8 mm in height (6,7).

Cervical Spine

At birth, the cervical spine measures 3.7 cm; it will grow about 9 cm, to reach the adult length of 12 to 13 cm. The length of the cervical spine will nearly double by 6 years of age, and will gain an additional 3.5 cm during the pubertal growth spurt. The cervical spine represents 22% of the C1-S1 segment and 15 to 16% of the sitting height (6,7).

The diameter of the cervical spinal canal varies with location, typically decreasing in width from C1 to C7 or from C1 to C3, then widening slightly. These differences are important in the clinical setting, because the room available for the spinal cord can be very consequential. It should be remembered that, regardless of the size of the child, e.g., in dwarfing conditions, the spinal cord will attain the usual adult diameter. The average width of the cervical cord is 13.2 mm, and the average anteroposterior depth is 7.7 mm (6,7). Therefore, the transverse and sagittal diameters of the cervical canal are important. In the adult, at C-3, the normal

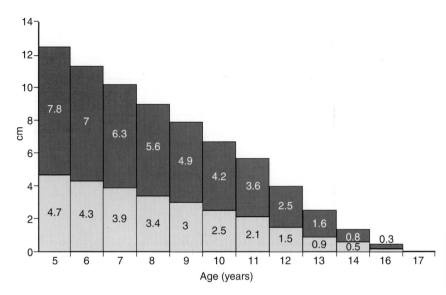

FIGURE 2-14. Growth remaining in the spine for both thoracic spine (*top bars*) and lumbar spine (*bottom bars*) segments in girls at various ages. (Adapted from ref. 7, with permission.)

transverse diameter is 27 mm and the average sagittal diameter is approximately 19 mm (6,7).

T1-S1 Segment

The T1-S1 segment is very important, because the most frequent disorders of the spine during growth will originate in this segment. The T1-S1 segment measures about 19 cm at birth and 45 cm at the end of growth in the average man and 42 to 43 cm in the average woman (6,7,66). This segment makes up 49% of the sitting height at maturity. Knowledge of the effects of arthrodesis on this segment of the spine require precise knowledge of the growth remaining at various ages (7) (Figs. 2-14 and 2-15).

Thoracic Spine (T1-12)

The thoracic spine is about 11 cm long at birth, and will reach a length of about 28 cm in boys and 26 cm in girls at the end of growth. Its length more than doubles from birth to the end of the growth period. The growth of the thoracic segment has a rapid phase from birth to 5 years of age (7 cm), a slower phase from 5 to 10 years of age (4 cm), and rapid growth through puberty (7 cm) (6,7).

The T1-12 segment represents 30% of the sitting height, so a single thoracic vertebra and its disc represents 2.5% of the sitting height. By knowing the amount of growth that each vertebra contributes to the final height, the effect of a circumferential arthrodesis, which stops all growth in the vertebrae and discs, can be calculated (Figs. 2-14 to 2-17).

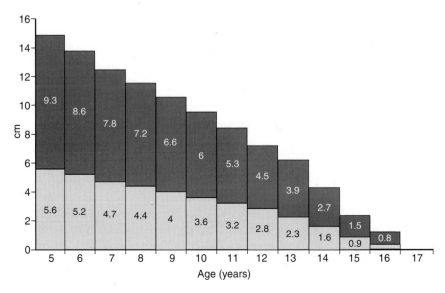

FIGURE 2-15. Growth remaining in the spine for both thoracic spine (*top bars*) and lumbar spine (*bottom bars*) segments in boys at various ages. (Adapted from ref. 7, with permission.)

If you perform a circumferential arthrodesis of six thoracic vertebrae in a 10-year-old boy, you will lose about 3 cm of sitting height:

the remaining growth in sitting height is about 20 cm
the remaining growth from T1 to S1 is about 10 cm
the remaining growth of T1-12 is 30% of the sitting height: (20 cm × 30)/100 = 6 cm
for six thoracic vertebrae, 6 × 2.5% = 15%: (20 cm × 15)/100 = 3 cm

On the other hand, posterior arthrodesis results in only one-third of this deficit (2.5% of sitting height for each thoracic vertebra), about 0.8% of final sitting height.

The thoracic spinal canal is narrower than either the lumbar or the cervical canal. The fifth finger may be intro-

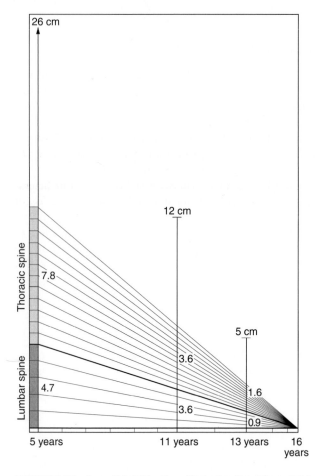

FIGURE 2-16. From this table, the effect of a circumferential fusion of the spine in girls can be calculated. The numbers at the top of the vertical lines represent the remaining sitting heights at various ages. The numbers on the horizontal lines represent the amount of growth remaining in each spinal segment during various periods of growth. To determine the effect of circumferential arthrodesis on five thoracic vertebrae at age 7 years, divide 7.8 cm by 12 thoracic vertebrae, and multiply the answer by 5. For a posterior arthrodesis, divide values by 3. (Adapted from ref. 7, with permission.)

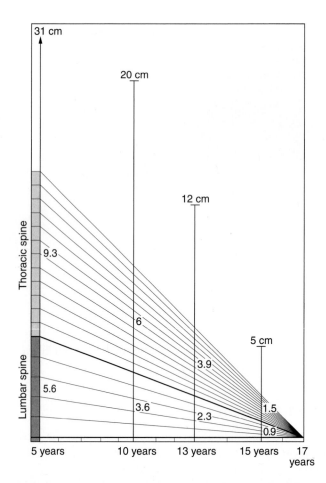

FIGURE 2-17. From this table, the effect of a circumferential fusion of the spine in boys can be calculated. The numbers at the top of the vertical lines represent the remaining sitting heights at various ages. The numbers on the horizontal lines represent the amount of growth remaining in each spinal segment during various periods of growth. To determine the effect of circumferential arthrodesis on five thoracic vertebrae at age 7 years, divide 9.3 cm by 12 thoracic vertebrae, and multiply the answer by 5. For a posterior arthrodesis, divide values by 3. (Adapted from ref. 7, with permission.)

duced into this canal at age 5 years, when it has attained its maximum volume. The average transverse and antero-posterior diameter at T7 is about 15 mm.

Lumbar Spine (L1-5)

The L1-5 lumbar spine is approximately 7 cm in length at birth, and it grows to approximately 16 cm in males and 15.5 cm in females. As in the thoracic spine, growth is not linear: there is rapid growth from 0 to 5 years of age (gain of about 3 cm); slow growth from 5 to 10 years of age (gain of about 2 cm); and rapid growth again from 10 to 18 years of age (gain of about 3 cm). The height of the lumbar spine doubles from birth to maturity (6,7).

The lumbar spine represents 18% of the sitting height,

and a single lumbar vertebra and its disc account for 3.5% of the sitting height. Values for the remaining growth of the lumbar segment at various ages are given in Figures 2-14 and 2-15. A circumferential arthrodesis, stopping all the growth of one lumbar vertebra at 10 years of age, results in a 3.5% deficit in the final sitting height. On the other hand, a posterior vertebral arthrodesis results in a deficit only one-third this great, a bit more than 1% of the final sitting height (6,7).

At the skeletal age of 10 years, the lumbar spine has reached 90% of its final height, but only 60% of its final volume. The medullar canal in the lumbar spine is wider than that in the thoracic spine. The forefinger can be introduced. At birth, the spinal cord ends at L3, and at maturity, it ends between L1 and L2.

Thoracic Perimeter

The growth of the thorax represents the fourth dimension of the spine (7). The thoracic circumference is a rough but valuable indicator of this fourth dimension of spinal growth. The thorax has a circumference of 32 cm at birth, and it will grow 56 cm in boys and 53 cm in girls, to almost three times its size at birth. The thoracic circumference is approximately 96% of the sitting height (7).

In boys, the thoracic circumference is 36% of its final size at birth, 63% at age 5 years, 73% at 10 years, 91% at 15 years, and 100% at 18 years. From birth to 5 years, the thoracic circumference grows exponentially and increases by 24 cm. From age 5 to 10 years, the increase is slower, and the thoracic perimeter is 66 cm at 10 years, which means that it grew only 10 cm in 5 years. It then is at 73% of its final value. Another acceleration occurs from age 10 to 18 years, particularly during puberty. The thoracic circumference then increases by 23 cm, i.e., as much as from birth to 5 years.

The thoracic circumference equals 96% of sitting height. These do not grow simultaneously, especially during puberty. At age 10 years, the thoracic circumference is at 74% of its final size, whereas sitting height is almost at 80% of its value at the end of growth. The transverse and anteroposterior diameters, which can be measured with obstetrical calipers, are two more parameters to assess the growth of the thorax. At the end of growth, the thorax has an anteroposterior diameter of about 21 cm and a transverse diameter of 28 cm in boys. In girls, the respective values are 17 cm and 24 cm. Thus, the transverse diameter has increased by 14 cm and the anteroposterior diameter has increased by 9 cm since birth. The addition of the values for the transverse and anteroposterior diameters of the thorax should equal 50% or more of the sitting height (7).

It is easy to note in all of these growth data the nonparallel but well-synchronized growth of the various parts of the body.

Scoliosis and Puberty

The sitting height plays an essential part in the treatment of scoliosis (7); unfortunately, it is not recorded often enough. Gain in sitting height always needs to be compared with angular development (7,9). This relationship is all that is needed for the proper assessment of treatment efficacy. If the increase in sitting height is accompanied by stable angulation, the treatment is definitely working well (7,9,67). If, on the other hand, it is accompanied by deterioration of angulation, the treatment needs to be reconsidered.

When we treat scoliosis, we must also think of growth. In congenital scoliosis, the intrauterine growth, and that occurring in the first few years of life, can reveal a great deal about the future behavior of the curve. In idiopathic infantile and juvenile scoliosis, the growth during the first 10 years of life can be very important, and may give clues to the behavior of the curve during the pubertal growth spurt (7,67). However, in adolescent idiopathic scoliosis, the most common form of scoliosis, there is no information before the curve begins in puberty. The ultimate outcome of the curve will be determined during the pubertal growth spurt. Thus, monitoring the behavior of a curve during this short and decisive period gives the only clues to the natural history of the curve. To detect these clues, it is necessary to know the onset of puberty (7).

The natural history of the curve can be judged during the first 7-cm increase of sitting height in girls and during the first 8-cm increase in boys, just after the start of the increased velocity of growth that marks the onset of puberty. Any curve increasing by 1 degree each month (12 degrees per year) during the ascending phase of the pubertal peak is likely to be a progressive curve that will require treatment. Any curve increasing by 0.5 degree each month during this phase must be monitored closely. Any curve gaining less than 0.5 degree each month during this phase can be considered mild (7). This observation of the natural history of the curve during the early part of puberty gives information about the behavior of the curve during the last phase of puberty, as growth is slowing, and thus can give guidance regarding the frequency of follow-up visits and the duration of bracing.

However imprecise and approximate the Risser sign may be, it is widely used as a deciding factor in many reports of brace treatment or surgery, and can be very useful if its limitations are understood. The data of Lonstein and Carlson (64), relating Risser sign and curve magnitude, have been discussed. As was pointed out above, because two-thirds of the pubertal growth spurt occurs before the appearance of Risser I, and because of its often ambiguous relationship to bone age, its value in both clinical decision-making and research should be questioned. Bone age, the growth rate, and secondary sexual characteristics are the most reliable parameters. Risser stages must not be regarded as a first-choice indicator; they must always be compared with bone age, especially when making decisions that will have major consequences, such as ordering or removing a brace or scheduling vertebral fusion (7).

Evaluation of the vertebral ring apophyses has been recommended by Blount (68) and G. Duval-Beaupère (personal communication), as another way to judge the remaining growth of the spine and thus the risk of progression of the curve. Although there may be some value in this radiological sign, it is important to know that in some patients these apophyses may not close until after 20 years of age (53).

A frequent question asked by parents, and considered by physicians, is how much will a spinal fusion for scoliosis decrease the final height of the child. To determine the answer to this question, the surgeon needs to know the remaining growth in sitting height and the contribution to that height made by the vertebrae that will be fused (7,69). After a bone age of 13 years in girls, when there is only 4 cm of future growth in sitting height, and a bone age of 15 years in boys, when there is only 5 cm of remaining growth in sitting height, there is little need for concern about final height. Figures 2-14 and 2-15 show the growth remaining in the spine at various ages, and Figures 2-16 and 2-17 show the effects of arthrodesis at various ages.

However, arthrodesis for deformity is often required before these ages. Faced with deformity in a developing spine, the specialist may be best advised to carry out a vertebral arthrodesis to prevent progression of a severe deformity (70). It may be better to have a short spine that is straight than to have a longer but crooked spine with the same sitting height (69). In addition, the vertebrae in many cases of congenital scoliosis will not grow normally, and thus arthrodesis of these vertebrae does not alter the height as much as it would in a normal spine. Arthrodesis of five vertebral bodies, at the age of 3 years, will result in an approximately 12-cm deficit in sitting height. Other examples are discussed above.

The crankshaft effect on the spine, after arthrodesis for scoliosis, was described by Dubousset and colleagues in 1989 (71). The crankshaft phenomenon occurs when there is a solid posterior arthrodesis with sufficient anterior growth remaining to produce a rotation of the spine and trunk with progression of the curve. Thus, it is very important for the surgeon to consider the state of skeletal maturity and the amount of growth remaining in the portion of the spine that is to be fused (72,73).

Roberto et al. (74) reviewed 86 immature patients who underwent posterior arthrodesis at Risser 0 or I. They found that 72% of the patients progressed less than 10 degrees, 21% progressed 11 to 15 degrees, and seven patients progressed more than 16 degrees. Patients in Tanner stage I, with open triradiate cartilage, had the greatest increase in the curve, and the crankshaft phenomenon decreased with greater maturity. There was no correlation between the amount of curve progression and subjective patient satisfaction.

Sanders and colleagues (75) performed a retrospective study of posterior spinal instrumentation with fusion in 43 patients with idiopathic scoliosis, who were at Risser 0 at the time of surgery. The triradiate cartilage was open in 23 patients and closed in 20 patients. The crankshaft effect was observed in 10 of the 23 patients with open triradiate cartilage, and in 1 patient with a closed triradiate cartilage.

These studies emphasize the problem with using only one factor in determining the remaining growth of the spine, which is difficult at best. They also emphasize the fact that, for much of the decision-making required in the treatment of scoliosis, the Risser sign is not useful, because so much of the spinal growth occurs before Risser I. The last spurt of puberty predominantly involves the growth of the thorax, which may completely change the evolution of idiopathic scoliosis (7,72). The growth of the thorax, a largely ignored factor, can explain some surgical results. In addition, the greater the residual curve, the greater the chance of significant crankshaft development (7,72).

In paralytic scoliosis, in which the curve is severe or rapidly progressive, circumferential fusion with segmental instrumentation is the best strategy to avoid the crankshaft phenomenon. The greater the magnitude of the curve, the more complex and hazardous is the surgery, and the more unlikely it is to correct the curve to 0 degrees. In such cases, there is no reason to wait for the pubertal spurt (7). Puberty can only worsen the situation. The deficit in sitting height caused by such early fusion is largely compensated by the correction of the curve. A loss of sitting height by early arthrodesis at 10 years of age is not significant for the patient who will live, at least most of the time, in a wheelchair. At age 5 years, the spinal canal has grown to 95% of its definitive size; therefore, circumferential arthrodesis will have no influence on the size of the spinal canal (7).

In congenital scoliosis, the first 5 years of life are the golden period to perform hemiepiphysiodesis (38,76,77). A gain in angulation of 10 to 15 degrees for each vertebral segment can be obtained.

LOWER LIMB GROWTH

The lower limb grows more than the trunk. The femur and tibia combined grow about 55 cm in girls and 63 cm in boys from birth to the end of growth. The cycle of growth in the lower limb is very regular: a strong increase in growth during the first 5 years of life, a steady and slower growth from 5 years of age to the beginning of puberty, a slight growth spurt during the accelerated velocity of growth at the beginning of puberty, and early cessation after the velocity peak (78–81). The femur grows more than the tibia.

The relation between the femur and the tibia is constant throughout growth. The proportions are set as early as age 5 years. The difference in length between the two bones is 2 cm at birth and 10 cm at the end of growth. The length

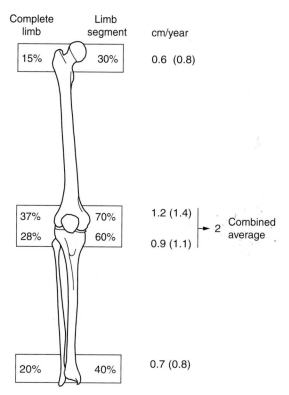

Complete limb · Limb segment · cm/year

15% · 30% · 0.6 (0.8)

37% · 70% · 1.2 (1.4)
28% · 60% · 0.9 (1.1) — 2 Combined average

20% · 40% · 0.7 (0.8)

FIGURE 2-18. A diagrammatic illustration of the contributions of the various growth plates to the length of the lower limb and its individual bones as a percentage, and in centimeters, of growth per year. The numbers in parentheses represent the increased growth seen during the first year of puberty in the growth plates. All other numbers are averages for the remaining period of growth.

of the tibia is 80% that of the femur. This is a useful ratio to remember when balancing lower limb lengthening. The relation between the tibia and the fibula is also constant. The length of the fibula is 98% that of the tibia, i.e., there is no significant difference. The contributions of the various growth plates to the length of the lower limb and its individual bones are shown in Figure 2-18.

Femoral Growth

The femur is approximately 9 cm long at birth and will undergo a fivefold increase in length, to 45 cm by the time growth has finished. Growth is particularly vigorous during the first 5 years of life, with the femur doubling in length by 4 years of age, and reaching 60% of the final length by 5 years of age (79).

Between birth and 5 years of age, the femur grows 15 cm (±1 cm). From 5 years of age until puberty, femoral growth slows to a steady rate of less than 2 cm per year, increasing to more than 2.5 cm during puberty. The proximal femoral physis of the femur accounts for 30% of femoral growth, or approximately 10 cm. The distal and

proximal femoral growth plates grow roughly 1 cm and 0.7 cm, respectively, each year. At puberty, this rate of growth increases to approximately 1.2 cm for the distal femur and 0.8 cm for the proximal femur.

Tibial Growth

The tibia is 7 cm long at birth, and grows at a slower rate than the femur. By the time it has stopped growing, it will be 35 cm long, having also increased practically fivefold in length. By the age of 4 years, the tibia will have nearly doubled its length, and it will have attained 50% of its final length by age 5 years. The tibial and femoral growth profiles are almost identical, with vigorous growth during the first 5 years of life, which then slows to about 1.3 cm each year until puberty, when growth increases to 1.6 cm per year.

The proximal tibial physis accounts for about 60% of the length of the tibia, or about 15 cm. This occurs at a rate of roughly 0.9 cm per year. The distal tibial physis grows slower, and accounts for about 40% of growth potential, equivalent to 10 cm. The proximal physis grows about 0.7 cm each year from age 5 years until puberty, when it increases to 0.9 cm per year. The distal physis grows about 0.5 cm from age 5 years until puberty, when it increases to 0.7 cm per year (78–81).

The growth of the tibia and the fibula is interdependent, and perfect harmony is necessary. Excessive growth in the fibula, which happens in cases of achondroplasia, may lead to genu varum. Similarly, resection of the fibula during growth may result in ankle valgus. These clinical examples demonstrate how important it is to restore continuity, length, and growth to either bone if deformity is to be avoided.

Knee Growth

Consideration of the growth of the distal femur and the proximal tibia together illustrates the importance of injury to both of these growth centers. Any serious injury to the growth centers around the knee during the early years of life is likely to result in severe shortening of the lower limb. The knee undergoes the greatest growth of all. From birth to maturity, the knee grows about 40 cm in boys (25 cm for the femur and 15 cm for the tibia) and 35 cm in girls (22 cm for the femur and 13 cm for the tibia). The knee accounts for two-thirds of growth (65%) in the lower limb (37% for the femur and 28% for the tibia) (78–81).

Stated another way, the knee grows about 2 cm per year from age 5 years onward, with slightly more than 1 cm (1.2 cm) of growth in the femur and slightly less than 1 cm (0.8 cm) in the tibia. The ratio between the length of the femur and the length of tibia is 1.04, and this remains constant after 5 years of age. When the growth of the femur and the tibia are combined, total growth in the lower limb averages around 3.5 cm per year, with the femur accounting for 54% of growth and the tibia accounting for 46%.

Foot Growth

When the sizes of the fetal foot and the lower limb are compared, the ratio is 1.41 at 8 weeks, 0.9 at birth, and 0.6 in adults. This means that the length of the foot is relatively great during intrauterine life and decreases throughout growth. At birth, the foot is about 7.5 cm long, i.e., 40% of its final size. At age 10 years, a girl's foot will grow about 3.5 cm and a boy's foot will grow about 5.5 cm. At that age, a girl's foot has attained about 91% of its final length and a boy's foot has attained about 85% of its final length (5,82).

The foot is the first organ of the musculoskeletal system that begins to grow at puberty (5). The growth spurt of the foot occurs a few months before the start of puberty, i.e., at the time of the increase in size of the testes and the appearance of the sesamoid bone in the thumb. Although it is the first to start growing during puberty, the foot is also the first musculoskeletal structure that stops growing. Growth of the foot stops at bone age 12 years in girls, i.e., 3 years before the end of growth, and at bone age 14 years in boys (82).

This makes the foot unique among the musculoskeletal structures in that its rate of growth mostly declines during puberty. When puberty begins, at approximately bone age 11 years in girls, the foot is already 22 cm long, and has only 1.6 cm or 2% of its growth left. When puberty starts in boys, around age 13 years, the foot is about 24 cm long, and has 2 cm or 2.5% of its growth remaining. Thus, arthrodesis at the beginning of puberty will have no significant impact on the length of the foot.

The foot represents 15% of the standing height in both girls and boys at skeletal maturity. This illustrates the importance of using clinical measures of limb-length discrepancy, along with the scanogram data, in decision-making. Conditions that affect the size of the foot can affect the total limb length, and this additional amount will not be reflected on the scanogram.

Growth and Limb-length Discrepancy

Although there are many methods for prediction, an understanding of the growth of the limbs gives the physician important information, both in predicting limb-length discrepancy and in more accurately applying the information from the various methods, e.g., the Moseley straight-line graft (80).

Contrary to widespread belief, there is more growth in the trunk or in sitting height during puberty than there is in the subischial length or growth of the limbs (2). The growth spurt in the lower limbs occurs during the first year of puberty, and, after bone age of 12.6 years in girls and

14.6 years in boys, the growth of the limbs decreases rapidly (43,83). The following examples give some idea of the timing of epiphysiodesis for different amounts of correction.

5 to 6 cm. Both tibia and femur at the beginning of puberty. Bone age 11 years in girls and 13 years in boys.

4 cm. Both tibia and femur 6 months after the onset of puberty. The elbow is useful for this determination.

3 cm. Only femur at the beginning of puberty or both tibia and femur at bone age 12 years in girls and 14 years in boys.

2 cm. Only femur at bone age 12 years in girls and 14 years in boys.

When performing an epiphysiodesis at the beginning of puberty or later, the risk of overcorrection is relatively small. The risk of undercorrection is greater, but, because the discrepancy is decreased if not totally corrected, the patient is often happy with the result. The growth of the limbs is complete at Risser I, or at bone age 13.6 years in girls and 15.6 years in boys (43,83). In the Greulich and Pyle atlas (16), this corresponds to fusion of the distal phalangeal physis of the index and middle fingers. The amounts of growth remaining at the various growth plates in the lower extremity are given in Figures 2-19 and 2-20.

With knowledge of the growth of the lower limbs (expressed as a percentage), it is easy to make a quick prediction of limb inequality at skeletal maturity (79). It can be assumed that the leg discrepancy at age 3 years will double for girls and at age 4 years for boys, if the inhibition of growth remains constant. Thus, a boy with a 4-cm discrepancy at age 4 years will have an 8-cm difference at the end of growth. At 9 years, the lower limb still has an average of 20% of its growth to attain in girls, and 27% of its growth to attain in boys. So a 4-cm discrepancy at that age will increase to 4.8 cm in girls and 5.08 cm in boys. At the onset of puberty, 10% average of the growth of the lower limb remains, so the final length discrepancy will be around 4.4 cm (2,79). A general rule for a quick prediction of limb-length discrepancy, for a problem such as congenital short femur, is to multiply the discrepancy at certain ages by a factor, e.g., multiply the discrepancy by 3 at age 1 year, by 2 at 4 years, by 1.8 at 5 years, by 1.4 at 9 years for boys and by 1.2 at 9 years for girls, and by 1.1 at the beginning of puberty for both boys and girls.

Such predictions are general, and should be used with caution. For the final decision in complex cases, it is best to use all of the information possible—standing height, sitting height, Hechard-Carlioz chart (84), Moseley chart (80), and Lefort residual coefficient (85)—while considering the bone age to lessen the margin of error. The younger the patient, the higher the risk of inaccurate prediction (86).

Thanks to the Green and Anderson tables (78) and to the Moseley, Hechard-Carlioz, and Lefort charts, limb-length discrepancy can be predicted. These forecasts do not need to be interpreted with mathematical strictness, because there

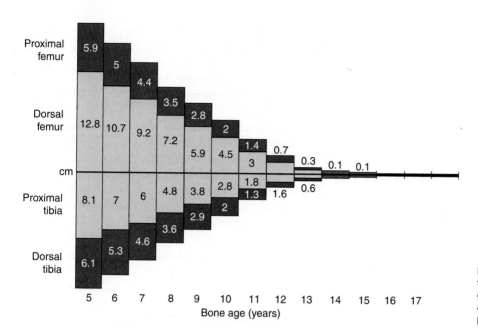

FIGURE 2-19. The remaining growth in the lower limbs of girls at the four growth plates, between the ages of 5 and 17 years. (Adapted from ref. 79, with permission.)

is a reasonable margin for error (2,86). Furthermore, these forecasts are best suited to cases of malformation and injury in which the difference in the rate of growth between the two limbs remains constant. Other causes of limb-length discrepancy, such as poliomyelitis, vascular malformation, and chronic arthritis, may not follow a constant curve and are more difficult to evaluate (87).

A decision for lengthening versus epiphysiodesis often depends on the final height of the child. Predicting the final height before puberty is inexact (20). Approximately 80% of children will remain in the same percentile for height after age 5 years. Tables to make these predictions from bone age are found in the Greulich and Pyle atlas (16). The timing of epiphysiodesis remains a controversial subject.

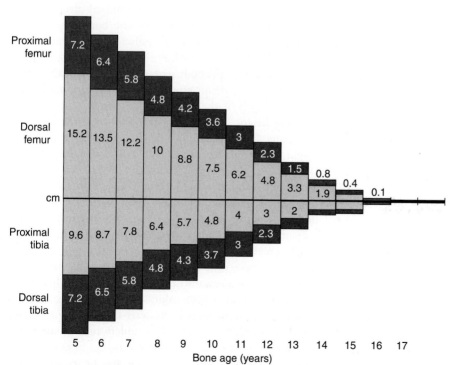

FIGURE 2-20. The remaining growth in the lower limbs of boys at the four growth plates, between the ages of 5 and 17 years. (Adapted from ref. 79, with permission.)

The main problem with this procedure is to reduce the margin of error (79,88,89).

UPPER LIMB GROWTH

Upper limb growth follows the same pattern as lower limb growth (2). The first 5 years of life are characterized by an acceleration of growth velocity, between 5 years and the beginning of puberty there is a plateau, and at the very beginning of puberty there is a slight spurt in growth (2,90–92). At birth, the length of the upper limb is 20 cm: the humerus makes up 7.5 cm, the ulna 6.5 cm, and the hand 6 cm. The upper limb grows 10 cm during the first year, 6 cm during the second year, approximately 5 cm during the third year, and 3.5 cm in the fourth year. After the age of 5 years, the rate of growth decreases. The contributions of the various growth plates to the length of the upper limb and its individual bones are shown in Figure 2-21 (2,3,93).

The upper limb grows about 3 cm annually from age 5 years to puberty, when it grows about 3.5 cm each year until the end of growth. This growth is made up of approximately 1.3 cm in the humerus, 1.1 cm in the ulna, 1 cm in the radius, and 0.7 cm in the hand. The length of the upper limb bones nearly doubles by 3 years of age. By 5 years of age, the bones of the upper extremity have reached half their final length (2,92).

The maturity gradient in the upper limbs is similar to that in the lower limbs. The hand shows its relatively slight acceleration of growth about 6 months before the forearm, and the forearm reaches its peak growth velocity about 6 months before the upper arm (94). The proximal humerus reaches its maximal growth rate at approximately the same time as the trunk.

Proportions among the various bones of the upper and lower limbs are established by 5 years of age (2). Thus, the ulna is eight-tenths the size of the humerus, and the humerus represents 70% of the length of the femur. Study of these indices is extremely valuable in assessing retarded growth during the course of chondrodystrophy (rhizomelic and mesomelic dwarfism) (2,95).

There are growth charts and curves that help to predict inequality (2,3,92). Surgical lengthening of the upper limbs may be rare, but it is feasible.

Growth in the Paralytic Child

The growth pattern is abnormal in many children with paralytic disorders, e.g., cerebral palsy, spina bifida, and poliomyelitis. In these children, therefore, it is essential to record and follow the parameters of growth closely to establish a surgical indication with as much accuracy and safety as possible (25–27,96,97). There are two problems that make it difficult to measure and evaluate the parameters of growth in such children. First, contractures and deformities make morphometric measurements difficult to impossible. Second, reference values that pertain to normal children are not applicable to these children.

Nevertheless, it is still possible to gain valuable information about growth if the child is scrutinized carefully from head to foot. The length of only one bone more or less spared by the deficit could be sufficient to determine the standing height of the child. For example, after age 8 years, the proportions of the body segments remain the same; thus, the length of the femur represents 28% of standing height, and the length of the tibia and fibula represents 24% of standing height. For the upper extremities, the humerus represents 19% of standing height and 36.5% of sitting height, the radius represents 14.5 and 27.8%, respectively, and the ulna represents 15.5 and 29.5%, respectively (2).

Weight is an important parameter to take into consideration. Many children, especially those with cerebral palsy, have a deficit of 20 to 30 kg. Surgical procedures are not the same for children who weigh 20, 40, and 60 kg. Underweight creates a risk of infection after surgery, when it reflects malnutrition (98–100). There are many parameters that are used to assess nutritional status, e.g., measuring the triceps and the subscapular skinfold, or measuring the total lymphocyte count. Whichever tests the surgeon relies on should be used before surgery on underweight children, especially those with chronic conditions.

On the other hand, obesity can also be a problem in

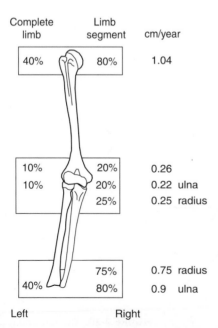

FIGURE 2-21. A diagrammatic illustration of the contributions of the various growth plates to the length of the upper limb and its individual bones as a percentage and in centimeters of growth per year.

surgery. The obesity of children with muscular dystrophy or spina bifida may restrict the choice of surgical approaches and instrumentation. The gain in weight during puberty is the major enemy of the diplegic or ambulatory quadriplegic child (2,101).

The assessment of bone age is more difficult with paralyzed children. Bone age retardation can be very severe in cerebral palsy. These patients sometimes display a wide range of bone ages, with the bone age of the hand not matching that of the elbow or the pelvis (personal experience). The real bone age, therefore, must be approximated. This information must be correlated with the results of anthropometric measurements (25–27). These measurements are based on radiographs that measure the bone length, but they can also be obtained during a clinical examination. For the tibia, a simple measurement is possible from the medial joint line of the knee to the inferior rim of the medial malleolus (102).

LESSONS LEARNED FROM GROWTH

Charts and diagrams are only models or templates (2). They do not by themselves define a true age. They define trends and outline the evolution of growth. They should be taken as just what they are: a convenient means to map the route through puberty. They record ephemeral points in the processes of growth and anticipate the events that lie in the future. Their use helps the surgeon to avoid uncertain or unnecessary treatments, and aids in successful strategies. Nothing can produce worse results than decisions leading into uncharted territory (2,9).

Percentages provide an extremely valuable and objective tool for evaluating residual growth, particularly with respect to the proportions between the lengths of various segments of the limbs and the limbs and the trunk (2,7). However diverse their ethnic origins, and even though stature has been increasing in succeeding generations over the centuries, boys of all generations and ethnic backgrounds will always have approximately 14% of outstanding growth in sitting height and 10% of length of the femur or tibia remaining at the beginning of puberty. Neither the percentage nor the proportions change, and even the ratios are stable. The humerus makes up, and will always make up, about 20% of sitting height and 38% of standing height (2,4,95,103,104).

A figure in isolation is meaningless; a ratio is more reliable. For instance, the length of the femur in relation to standing height, or the length of the thoracic segment in relation to sitting height, provides more objective values. To gain this information, the examiner should try to obtain a general overview of the child's growth, and to plot the child's anthropometric chart.

The ratios of the various body segments are important in many conditions, especially the various types of dwarfism. The ratio of sitting height to subischial leg length is essential when analyzing chondrodystrophy. Special curves can be used to follow these patients (105,106). Dwarfism can be divided into two families: short-trunk dwarfism, the prime example of which is represented by Morquio syndrome, and normal-trunk dwarfism, in which mainly the limbs are shorter than normal. The prime example here is achondroplasia (2). In this disease, the weight is an important parameter to consider, and obesity is a frequent cause of complications (107).

The various processes that make up growth are well synchronized, organized, and interdependent, but they vary widely in the time during growth when they occur. For instance, the growth of the trunk accounts for the majority of increase in standing height during the last part of puberty. Also, weight gain lags behind growth in length until puberty, when the percentage gain in weight far exceeds the percentage gain in height. All changes are gradual. Growth itself is a succession of phases, periods of deceleration or acceleration, spurts, and alternating processes. However intellectually comfortable it may be to believe that the limbs grow linearly, checking growth curves every 6 months reveals that there are breaks and phases during which growth alternates between the proximal and distal parts of a limb.

Treatment of children often requires a consideration of remaining growth. Puberty is the time when most of these decisions will be made. Treatment is easiest when it is done in anticipation of future growth. Puberty is a short period of about 2 years with rapid changes in growth. The milestones that mark the path during this short period must be noted and understood by the orthopaedic surgeon. Measurements at one period of time, e.g., the Risser sign or the length of the femur, are of limited value. Thus, in children in whom growth disturbance is anticipated, it is best to record several parameters over time to have an accurate picture of growth.

References

Basic Concepts

1. Buckwalter JA, Ehrlich MG, Sandell LJ, et al. *Skeletal growth and development: clinical issues and basic science advances.* Rosemont, IL: American Academy of Orthopaedic Surgeons, 1997.
2. Diméglio A. *La croissance en orthopédie.* Montpellier, France: Sauramps Médical, 1987.
3. Exner GU. *Normalwerte in der kinderorthopädie: wachstum und entwicklung.* Stuttgart, Germany: Georg Thieme Verlag, 1990.
4. Godin P. *Recherches anthropologiques sur la croissance des diverses parties du corps de 13 à 18 ans.* Maloine A, ed. Paris: 1903.
5. Marschall WA. *Human growth and its disorders.* London: Academic, 1977.
6. Diméglio A, Bonnel F. Growth of the spine. In: Raimondi AJ, Choux M, Di Rocco C, eds. *Principles of pediatric neuro-surgery: the pediatric spine, development and the dysraphic state.* New York: Springer-Verlag, 1989;9:39.
7. Diméglio A, Bonnel F. *Le rachis en croissance.* Paris: Springer-Verlag, 1990.

8. Lowrey GH. *Growth and development of children*, 6th ed. Chicago: Mosby–Year Book, 1973.

9. Duthie R. The significance of growth in orthopaedic surgery. *Clin Orthop* 1959;14:7.

10. Sinclair D. *Human growth after birth*, 2nd ed. London: Oxford University Press, 1969.

11. Hensinger RN. *Standards in pediatric orthopedics: charts, tables and graphs illustrating growth*. New York: Raven, 1986.

12. Tanner JM, Davies PSW. Clinical longitudinal standards for height and height velocity for North American children. *J Pediatr* 1985;107:317.

13. Tanner JM, Whitehouse RH, Takaishi M. Standards from birth to maturity for height, weight, height velocity and weight velocity: British children 1965, parts I and II. *Arch Dis Child* 1966; 41:454.

14. Tanner JM, Whitehouse RH. Clinical longitudinal standards for height, weight, height velocity and weight velocity and the stages of puberty. *Arch Dis Child* 1976;51:170.

15. Tanner JM. Physical growth and development. In: Forfar JO, Arneil GC, eds. *Textbook of paediatrics*, 2nd ed. New York: Churchill Livingstone, 1978;7:249.

16. Greulich WW, Pyle SI. *Radiographic atlas of skeletal development of the hand and wrist*, 2nd ed. Stanford, CA: Stanford University Press, 1959:50.

17. Prader A, Largo RH, Molinari L, et al. Physical growth of Swiss children from birth to 20 years of age: first longitudinal study of growth and development. *Helv Paediatr Acta* 1989;52 [Suppl].

18. Sempé M, Pavia C. *Atlas de la maturation squelettique*. Paris: SIMEP, 1979.

19. Hamill PVV, Drizd TA, Johnson CL, et al. National Center for Health Statistics percentiles. *Am J Clin Nutr* 1979;32: 607.

Biometric Measurements

20. Bailey DK, Pinneau S. Tables for predicting adult height from skeletal age. *J Pediatr* 1952;40:421.

21. Cheng JCY, Leung SSF, Chiu BSK, et al. Can we predict body height from segmental bone length measurements? A study of 3,647 children. *J Pediatr Orthop* 1998;18:387.

22. Goldberg MJ. *The dysmorphic child: an orthopedic perspective*. New York: Raven, 1983.

23. Lonstein JE. Embryology and spine growth. In: Lonstein JL, Bradford DS, Winter RB, et al., eds. *Moes' textbook of scoliosis and other spinal deformities*, 3rd ed. Philadelphia: WB Saunders, 1995:23.

24. Moseley CF. Growth. In: Lovell WW, Winter RB, eds. *Pediatric orthopaedics*, 2nd ed. Philadelphia: Lippincott–Raven, 1986:25.

25. Miller F, Koreska J. Height measurement of patients with neuromuscular disease and contractures. *Dev Med Child Neurol* 1992;34:55.

26. Stevenson RD. Measurement of growth in children with developmental disabilities. *Dev Med Child Neurol* 1996;38: 855.

27. Stevenson RD. Use of segmental measures to estimate stature in children with cerebral palsy. *Arch Pediatr Adolesc Med* 1995; 149:658.

28. Duval-Beaupère G. Les repères de maturation dans la surveillance des scolioses. *Rev Chir Orthop* 1970;56:59.

29. Duval-Beaupère G. Croissance résiduelle de la taille et des segments après la première menstruation chez la fille. *Rev Chir Orthop* 1976;62:501.

30. Jarzem PF, Gledhill RB. Predicting height from arm measurement. *J Pediatr Orthop* 1993;13:761.

31. Buckler J. *A longitudinal study of adolescent growth*. New York: Springer-Verlag, 1990.

Chronology

32. O'Rahilly R, Meyer DB. The timing and sequence of events in the development of the human vertebral column during the embryonic period proper. *Anat Embryol* 1979;157:167.

33. Ounsted M, Ounsted C. On fetal growth rate: its variations and their consequences. *Clin Dev Med* 1973;46:1.

34. Uhthoff HK. *The embryology of the human locomotor system*. New York: Springer-Verlag, 1990.

35. Gruenwald P. Growth of the human foetus. *Am J Obstet Gynecol* 1966;94:1112.

36. Jeanty P, Kirkpatrick C, Dramaix-Wilmet M, et al. Ultrasonic evaluation of fetal limb growth. *Radiology* 1981;140:165.

37. Mahony BS. Ultrasound evaluation of the fetal musculoskeletal system. In: Callen PW, ed. *The ultrasonography in obstetrics and gynecology*. Philadelphia: WB Saunders, 1994:254.

38. Diméglio A. Growth of the spine before age 5 years. *J Pediatr Orthop Br* 1993;1:102.

39. Marshall WA, Tanner JM. Variation in the pattern of pubertal changes in girls. *Arch Dis Child* 1969;44:291.

40. Marshall WA, Tanner JM. Variations in the pattern of pubertal changes in boys. *Arch Dis Child* 1970;45:13.

41. Staheli LT. *Fundamentals of pediatric orthopedics*. New York: Raven, 1992:1.1.

42. Terver S, Kleinman R, Bleck EE. Growth landmarks and the evolution of scoliosis: a review of pertinent studies on their usefulness. *Dev Med Child Neurol* 1980;22:675.

43. Duval-Beaupère G, Combes J. Segments supérieur et inférieur au cours de la croissance physiologique des filles: etude longitudinale de la croissance de 54 filles. *Arch Fr Pediatr* 1971;28: 1057.

44. Caffey J. *Pediatric x-ray diagnosis*, 7th ed. Chicago: Mosby–Year Book, 1978.

45. Ozonoff MB. *Pediatric orthopedic radiology*, 2nd ed. Philadelphia: WB Saunders, 1992.

46. Buric M, Moncilovic MD. Growth pattern and skeletal age in school girls with idiopathic scoliosis. *Clin Orthop* 1982;10: 238.

Radiological Study

47. Harrison MHM, Turner MH, Jacobs P. Skeletal immaturity in Perthes disease. *J Pediatr Orthop Br* 1976;58:37.

48. Kristmundsdottir F, Burwell RG, Hall DJ. A longitudinal study of carpal bone development in Perthes' disease: its significance for both radiologic standstill and bilateral disease. *Clin Orthop* 1986;209:115.

49. Loder RT, Farley FA, Herzenberg JE, et al. Narrow window of bone age in children with slipped capital femoral epiphyses. *J Pediatr Orthop* 1993;13:290.

50. Exner GU. Growth and pubertal development in slipped capital femoral epiphysis: a longitudinal study. *J Pediatr Orthop* 1986; 6:403.

51. Exner GU. Slipped capital femoral epiphysis and puberty. *Mapfre Medicina* 1999;10[Suppl 1]:22.

52. Anderson M. Use of the Greulich-Pyle "Atlas of Skeletal Development of the Hand and Wrist" in clinical context. *Am J Phys Anthropol* 1971;35:347.

53. Bunch W, Dvonch V. Pitfalls in the assessment of skeletal immaturity: an anthropologic case study. *J Pediatr Orthop* 1983; 3:220.

54. Carpenter CT, Lester EL. Skeletal age determination in young

children: analysis of three regions of the hand/wrist film. *J Pediatr Orthop* 1993;13:76.

55. Graham CB. Assessment of bone evaluation: methods and pitfalls. *Radiol Clin North Am* 1972;10:185.

56. Cundy P, Paterson D, Morris L, et al. Skeletal age estimation in leg length discrepancy. *J Pediatr Orthop* 1988;8:513.

57. Acheson RM. The Oxford method of assessing skeletal maturity. *Clin Orthop* 1957;10:19.

58. Frisch H, Riedl S, Waldhört T. Computer-aided estimation of skeletal age and comparison with bone age evaluations by the method of Greulich-Pyle and Tanner-Whitehouse. *Pediatr Radiol* 1996;26:226.

59. Sauvegrain J, Nahm H, Bronstein N. Etude de la maturation osseuse du coude. *Ann Radiol* 1962;5:542.

60. Biondi J, Weiner DS, Bethem D, et al. Correlation of Risser's sign and bone age determination in adolescent idiopathic scoliosis. *J Pediatr Orthop* 1985;5:697.

61. Dhar S, Dangerfield PH, Dorgan JC, et al. Correlation between age and Risser's sign in adolescent idiopathic scoliosis. *Spine* 1993;18:14.

62. Risser JC. The iliac apophysis: an invaluable sign in the management of scoliosis. *Clin Orthop* 1958;11:111.

63. Little DG, Sussman MD. The Risser sign: a critical analysis. *J Pediatr Orthop* 1994;14:569.

64. Lonstein JE, Carlson JM. The prediction of curve progression in untreated idiopathic scoliosis during growth. *J Bone Joint Surg Am* 1984;1061.

65. Karol LA, Johnston CE, Browne RH, et al. Progression of the curve in boys who have idiopathic scoliosis. *J Bone Joint Surg Am* 1993;75;1804.

Growth of Trunk and Thorax

66. Nehme AEE, Riseborough EJ, Reed RB. Normal spine growth. In: Zorab PA, Siegler S, eds. *Scoliosis.* London: Academic, 1980:103.

67. Duval-Beaupère G, Dubousset J, Queneau P. Pour une théorie unique de l'évolution des scolioses. *Presse Med* 1970;78:1141.

68. Blount WP. Use of the Milwaukee brace. *Orthop Clin North Am* 1972;3:1.

69. Winter RW. Scoliosis and spinal growth. *Orthop Rev* 1977,6:17.

70. Risser J, Agostini S, Sampaio J, et al. The sitting-standing height ratio as a method of evaluating early spine fusion in the growing child. *Clin Orthop* 1973;24:7.

71. Dubousset J, Herring JA., Shufflebarger HL. The crankshaft phenomenon. *J Pediatr Orthop* 1989;9:541.

72. Shufflebarger HL, Clark CE. Prevention of crankshaft phenomenon. *Spine* 1991;16[Suppl 8]:S409.

73. Richards BS. The effects of growth on the scoliotic spine following posterior spinal fusion. In: Buckwalter JA, Ehrlich MG, Sandell LJ, et al., eds. *Skeletal growth and development: clinical issues and basic science advances.* Rosemont, IL: American Academy of Orthopaedic Surgeons, 1997;3:577.

74. Roberto RF, Lonstein JE, Winter RB, et al. Curve progression in Risser stage 0 on patients after posterior spinal fusion for idiopathic scoliosis. *J Pediatr Orthop* 1997;17:718.

75. Sanders JO, Herring JA, Browne RH. Posterior arthrodesis and instrumentation in the immature (Risser-grade-0) spine in idiopathic scoliosis. *J Bone Joint Surg Am* 1995;77:39.

76. Roaf R. The treatment of progressive scoliosis by unilateral arrest. *J Bone Joint Surg Br* 1963;45:637.

77. Winter RB. Convex anterior and posterior hemiarthrodesis and hemiepiphysiodesis in young children with progressive congenital scoliosis. *J Pediatr Orthop* 1989;1:361.

Lower Limb Growth

78. Anderson M, Green WT, Messner MB. Growth and predictions of growth in the lower extremities. *J Bone Joint Surg Am* 1963;45:1.

79. Diméglio A, Bonnel F. Growth and development of the knee. In: De Pablos J, ed. *The immature knee.* Barcelona: Biblio Stm, 1998:3.

80. Moseley CF. A straight-line graph for leg length discrepancies. *J Bone Joint Surg Am* 1977;59:174.

81. Tupman GS. A study of bone growth in normal children and its relationship to skeletal maturation. *J Bone Joint Surg Br* 1962;44:42.

82. Blais MM, Green WT, Anderson M. Lengths of the growing foot. *J Bone Joint Surg Am* 1956;38:998.

83. Duval-Beaupère G, Sayet A. Contribution respective des segments supérieur et inférieur à la croissance des garçons. *Arch Fr Pediatr* 1979;36:369.

84. Hechard P, Carlioz H. Méthode pratique de prévision des inégalités de longueur des membres inférieurs. *Rev Chir Orthop* 1978;64:81.

85. Lefort J. Utilisation du coefficient de croissance résiduelle dans le calcul prévisionnel des inégalités de longueur des membres inférieurs. *Rev Chir Pediatr Orthop* 1981;67:753.

86. Kasser JR, Jenkins R. Accuracy of leg length prediction in children younger than 10 years of age. *Clin Orthop* 1997;338:9.

87. Shapiro F. Developmental patterns in lower extremity length discrepancies. *J Bone Joint Surg Am* 1982;64:95.

88. Little DG, Nigo L, Aiona MD. Deficiencies of current methods for the timing of epiphysiodesis. *J Pediatr Orthop* 1996;16:173.

89. Menelaus MB. Correction of leg length discrepancy by epiphysial arrest. *J Bone Joint Surg Br* 1966;48:336.

Upper Limb Growth

90. Maresh MM. Growth of major long bones on healthy children: a preliminary report on successive roentgenograms of the extremities from early infancy to twelve years of age. *Arch Dis Child* 1943;66:227.

91. Maresh MM. Linear growth of long bones of extremities from infancy through adolescence: continuing studies. *Am J Dis Child* 1955;89:725.

92. Pritchett JW. Growth and prediction of growth in the upper extremity. *J Bone Joint Surg Am* 1988;70:520.

93. Pritchett JW. Growth-plate activity in the upper extremity. *Clin Orthop* 1991;268:235.

94. Flatt A. Growth, size, function of the hand. In: *The care of congenital hand anomalies.* St. Louis: Mosby, 1977:16.

95. Aldegheri R, Agostini S. A chart of anthropometric values. *J Bone Joint Surg Br* 1983;75:86.

96. Spender QW, Cronk CE, Charney EB, et al. Assessment of linear growth of children with cerebral palsy: use of alternative measures to height or length. *Dev Med Child Neurol* 1989;31:206.

97. Belt-Niedballa BJ, Ekvall SW, Cook CM, et al. Linear growth measurement: a comparison of single-arm lengths and armspan. *Dev Med Child Neurol* 1986;28:319.

98. Jensen JE, Jensen TG, Smith TK, et al. Nutrition in orthopaedic surgery. *J Bone Joint Surg Am* 1982;64:1263.

99. Klein JD, Garfin SR. Nutritional status in the patient with spinal infection. *Orthop Clin North Am* 1996;27:33.

100. Szoke GM, Lipton G, Miller F, et al. Wound infection after

spinal fusion in children with cerebral palsy. *J Pediatr Orthop* 1998;18:727.

101. Samilson RL, Green WT, Jones M, et al. Orthopaedic aspects of cerebral palsy. *Clin Dev Med* 1975;52/53:71.

102. Zorab PA, Prime FJ, Harrison A. Estimation of height from tibial length. *Lancet* 1963;1:195.

Lessons Learned from Growth

103. Godin P. Lois de la croissance basées sur 2 000 observations d'enfants. *Comptes Rendus Acad Sci* 1914;(July):99.

104. Mahmoud Y, El-Najjar. Reconstruction of the individual from the skeleton. In: *Forensic anthropology.* Springfield, IL: Charles C Thomas, 1978:55.

105. Horton WA, Hall JG, Scott CI Jr, et al. Growth curves for height for diastrophic dysplasia, spondyloepiphyseal dysplasia congenita, and pseudoachondroplasia. *Am J Dis Child* 1982; 136:316.

106. Horton WA, Rotter JI, Rimoin DL, et al. Standard growth curves for achondroplasia. *J Pediatr* 1978;93:435.

107. Hecht JT, Hood OJ, Schwartz RJ, et al. Obesity in achondroplasia. *Am J Med Genet* 1988;31:597.

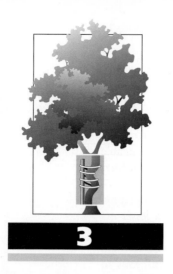

IMAGING TECHNIQUES AND APPLICATIONS

DIEGO JARAMILLO
LEONARD P. CONNOLLY

Imaging of the pediatric skeleton has changed dramatically over the last decade. Although plain films remain the main-

D. Jaramillo: Department of Radiology, Harvard Medical School, Boston, Massachusetts 02115; Division of Pediatric Radiology, Massachusetts General Hospital, Boston, Massachusetts 02114
L. P. Connolly: Department of Radiology, Harvard Medical School; Department of Radiology, Children's Hospital, Boston, Massachusetts 02115.

stay of orthopaedic practice, magnetic resonance (MR) imaging and ultrasonography now allow visualization of cartilaginous structures and, more recently, their blood supply. Various techniques to investigate the biochemical and metabolic composition of the cartilage are being developed, and may soon be clinically useful. The revolution in image processing allows reconstruction of an imaging data set in multiple projections. It is now possible to generate curved reformations, maximal intensity projections, computer-simulated disarticulations, and even computer-simulated surgery. Most images, with the exception of conventional radiographs, are now in digital format, and it is possible to transmit, store, and manipulate data with increasing ease. The information is not only more readily available and less often lost, but results can become standardized and quantified. Some techniques are being replaced by less-invasive or easier approaches. Conventional tomography, diagnostic angiography, myelography, and, to a lesser extent, arthrography, are used much less. Unfortunately, the newer imaging modalities remain costly, and access to them is still limited. The expertise of orthopaedic surgeons in the use and interpretation of these modalities has increased remarkably. This chapter provides an overview of the imaging modalities, their mechanisms of contrast, some information about normal appearances and variations, a discussion of risks and limitations, and an overview of costs and trends in utilization. Radiation exposure and sedation for the more complex examinations is discussed at the end of the chapter.

RADIOGRAPHIC TECHNIQUES: PLAIN RADIOGRAPHS, ARTHROGRAPHY, CONVENTIONAL TOMOGRAPHY, COMPUTED TOMOGRAPHY

Basis of Radiographic Contrast

Radiographic density depends on the relative absorption of an x-ray beam by the structures being imaged. There are five main radiographic densities: heavy metal, calcium, water and water-density tissues, fat, and air. In the bones, radiographic density primarily reflects calcium content. The relative content of water and fat in the marrow has much less influence on the radiographic density. In the soft tissues, the relative concentrations of fat and water are the main determinants of density. The fat around the joints, in between the muscles, and underneath the skin is detectable on routine radiographs. Analysis of soft tissue abnormalities, such as displacement or effacement of fat planes or fat pads, is crucial in the radiographic detection of subtle injury or infection.

In the newborn, the skeleton is made up of woven bone, which is very radiopaque (Fig. 3-1). The newly formed bone of the metaphysis is particularly sclerotic. There is little differentiation between cortex and medulla. With age, the marrow cavity becomes larger, and the woven bone becomes lamellar bone (1); this transformation and the fatty conversion of the marrow (2) result in a skeleton with clear differentiation between cortical bone and the much less dense medullary cavity.

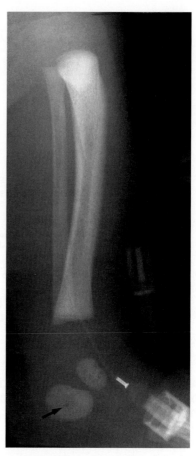

FIGURE 3-1. Normal radiographic appearance of bones in the newborn. The bones are sclerotic and the perichondral regions are prominent. The calcaneal nutrient foramen is normally prominent (*arrow*).

Intravenous and Arthrographic Contrast Materials

Iodinated contrast material is used intravenously for computed tomography (CT) examinations and for arthrography and myelography. Radiographic contrast materials are iodine-based compounds, and can be ionic or nonionic. Nonionic agents are several times as expensive, but deliver a smaller osmolar load, and are associated with less morbidity and mortality (3). When administered intravenously, ionic agents have a 5 to 12% incidence of side effects (vomiting, pain, and allergic reactions), compared with 1 to 3% for nonionic agents. The rate of fatal outcomes for all contrast media studies is approximately 0.9 per 100,000 (4), but less than 5% of these occur in children (5).

When administered arthrographically, reactions to contrast agents are infrequent, but nonionic contrast materials are associated with less pain and a greater persistence in the joint (6). Epinephrine, particularly in the knee, slows loss of contrast from the joint and prevents dilution due to influx of fluid. Air, which allows double contrast, is a safe adjunct, but is infrequently used in pediatric hip arthrography.

Normal Age-related Changes and Variants

Although ossification normally occurs in a very predictable pattern, the variation in some areas can resemble disease. Normal variants are often bilateral, but reassuring symmetry is not always present. It is, therefore, important to become familiar with the most common normal variants of the growing skeleton.

Epiphyseal and Apophyseal Variants

Distal Femoral Epiphyseal Irregularity. The secondary center of ossification of the distal femur can be very irregular throughout childhood. Irregularity is found in approximately two-thirds of boys and 40% of girls (Fig. 3-2). The irregularity, when present, involves both condyles in 44% of cases, only the lateral condyle in 44%, and only the medial condyle in 12% (7). Accessory centers of ossification are

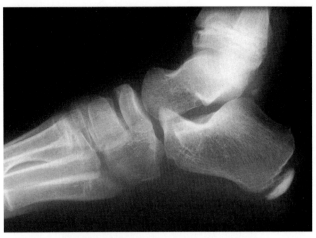

FIGURE 3-3. Normal calcaneal sclerosis in a 9-year-old girl. The density of the calcaneal apophysis is much greater than that of the rest of the calcaneus.

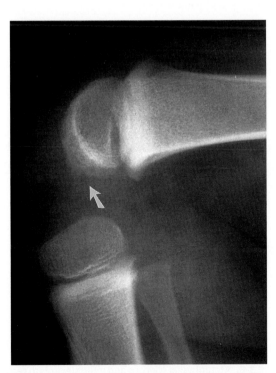

FIGURE 3-2. Femoral epiphyseal irregularity. Lateral radiograph of a 17-month-old boy shows abnormality of the contour of the posterior aspect of the epiphysis (*arrow*), a normal variant. Incidentally noted is the normal sclerosis of the metaphysis of the distal femur and proximal tibia.

more conspicuous in the posterior femoral condyles, and are almost always later incorporated into the parent bone.

Irregularity of the Tibial Tubercle. The tibial tubercle ossifies between 8 and 12 years of age in girls and 9 and 14 years of age in boys (8). During this time, normal irregularity of ossification must be differentiated from Osgood-Schlatter disease. In the latter, the child has local pain and inflammation. Edema anterior to the tubercle and patellar tendon thickening are readily detectable by soft tissue radiography, sonography, and magnetic resonance (MR) imaging. Osgood-Schlatter disease, however, is diagnosed clinically, rather than by imaging.

Calcaneal Sclerosis. The calcaneal apophyseal center ossifies in girls at 4 to 6 years of age, and in boys at 4 to 9 years of age. Ossification is uneven and asymmetric, and neither fragmentation nor sclerosis indicates disease (Fig. 3-3). Normal calcaneal sclerosis decreases with disuse of the foot or after a month of not bearing weight (9). The diagnosis of Sever's disease (calcaneal apophysitis) is primarily clinical. Soft tissue swelling on radiographs or cross-sectional images, and increased scintigraphic activity, may provide supportive evidence; imaging evaluation, however, is not necessary (10).

Physeal Variants

Pseudofracture Due to Physeal Obliquity. When the radiographic beam penetrates the physis obliquely, one end of the physeal disc is projected above the other, which suggests a fracture. This pseudofracture is easily recognized in

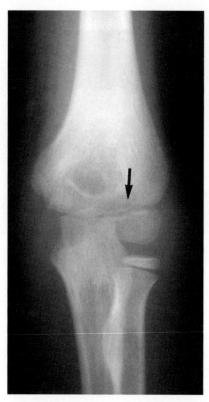

FIGURE 3-4. Physeal obliquity resembling a fracture in an 8-year-old boy. The physis of the capitellum is projected over the metaphysis of the distal humerus (*arrow*), creating the false impression of a lateral condylar fracture.

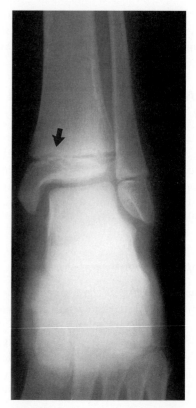

FIGURE 3-5. Normal physeal closure of the distal tibial physis in an 11-year-old girl who sprained her ankle. Cephalad to the medial talar hump is a physeal "hump" (*arrow*), which corresponds to the area of normal physeal closure.

the proximal humerus. In the distal humerus, however, it can be confused with a lateral condylar fracture (Fig. 3-4).

Poland's Hump of Distal Tibia. The distal tibial physis closes asymmetrically. An undulation, known as Poland's hump (or Kump's bump), is located just above the medial talar hump. The physis becomes thinner and closes first here (Fig. 3-5). The obliquity of this area may give the false impression of early physeal closure.

Metaphyseal Variants

Transverse Metaphyseal Bands. The juxtaphyseal metaphysis of weight-bearing bones can be sclerotic during childhood (11) (Fig. 3-6). Metaphyseal sclerosis is normal between 2 and 6 years of age. Unlike this normal density, the metaphyseal band of lead intoxication affects both weight-bearing and nonweight-bearing bones (such as the fibula). Increased density in chronic lead poisoning is not due to metal deposition, but to osteoclastic dysfunction, which results in failure of resorption of the trabecula of the metaphyseal spongiosa.

Following a fracture or a period of slower growth due

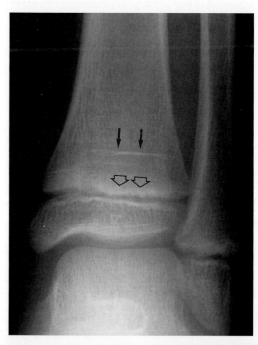

FIGURE 3-6. Metaphyseal sclerosis and multiple growth recovery (Harris) lines in a 7-year-old girl. The most prominent Harris line is outlined by the two *closed arrows*. This parallels the growth plate, which has migrated away from the line since the time of the growth slowdown. The *open arrows* denote a normal metaphyseal sclerosis of the distal tibia.

to disease, a disc of sclerotic bone forms in the metaphysis next to the physis. A growth recovery line, or Harris line, is formed when the physis migrates away from this disc (Fig. 3-6). Before it becomes separated from the metaphysis, however, the growth recovery line and the metaphyseal spongiosa overlap and create a spurious metaphyseal density.

Apparent metaphyseal sclerosis can result from resorption of the metaphyseal trabecula, with preservation of the zone of provisional calcification. This can be seen in neonates under stress, and in children with leukemia or methotrexate osteopathy (12).

Avulsive Cortical Irregularity. Sites of tendinous insertions at metadiaphyseal junctions have thin cortices. Because these areas are prone to repeated minor avulsive injury, the cortex can become irregular, and new bone formation can be mistaken for a neoplasm (13). This is most prominent in the posterior aspect of the distal femur, at the insertion of the medial head of the gastrocnemius muscle (Fig. 3-7). The cortex is thin or absent in this region, such that, on a frontal radiograph, a cortical defect appears as a rounded lucency. Tangential radiographs show irregularity or discontinuity of the cortex.

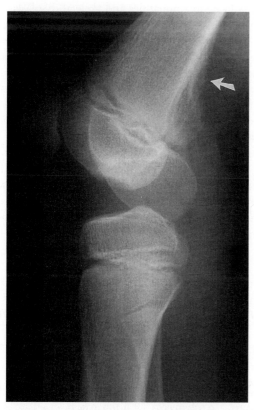

FIGURE 3-7. Normal distal femoral metaphyseal cortical irregularity (*arrow*) at the insertion of the medial head of the gastrocnemius muscle. In this radiograph, a slight obliquity accentuates the normal variant.

If a cortical irregularity has a characteristic radiographic appearance, no further imaging is needed. When there is uncertainty about the nature of the lesion, a limited CT can be used to confirm the diagnosis, by showing a typical defect in the posterior cortex and no soft tissue mass. MR imaging is not indicated unless there is a strong suspicion for a tumor. A large cortical defect encountered incidentally during an MR study of the knee may be confused with a marrow lesion on coronal images, but analysis of the entire data set clarifies the potential pitfall (14).

Round Bone Variant

Tarsal Navicular Fragmentation. The navicular is the last tarsal bone to ossify (see scintigraphic normal variants in the section Skeletal Scintigraphy below). There are normally two ossification centers, but multiple irregular, dense centers can develop, fusing close to age 20. Normal navicular fragmentation and sclerosis differs from aseptic necrosis of the navicular, or Kohler's disease, which affects older children, and is associated with pain (15).

Main Applications and Specific Technical Considerations

Plain Radiographs

General Principles. Coning (decreasing the area exposed to x-rays) reduces scatter radiation, improves image quality, and reduces radiation exposure. Coning is easy and always beneficial. When multiple anatomic areas need to be imaged, it is better to obtain multiple coned-down radiographs, rather than a single large radiograph. Whenever possible, gonads and breasts should be shielded. When examining the hips, however, one of the radiographs must be obtained without gonadal shielding, because the shield can hide abnormalities of the sacrum in girls and the pubis in boys. Radiation dose considerations are discussed at length at the end of this chapter and in Tables 3-1 and 3-2. Good positioning is crucial, particularly when obtaining lateral projections of the elbow, wrist, and ankle.

The soft tissues should be well-depicted on properly exposed radiographs. The subcutaneous fat is more lucent than the deeper muscles and ligaments. The deep soft tissues have fat planes between the muscles that are also discernible radiographically. The analysis of soft tissue abnormalities is crucial in the evaluation of early osteomyelitis, because deep soft tissue swelling is present as early as 3 days after the beginning of the infection. In effusions in the elbow and ankle, displacement of periarticular fat pads is often the first indicator of occult fractures. Effacement or displacement of the fat planes around the bones is important in the evaluation of fractures of the navicular (navicular fat pad sign),

TABLE 3-1. RADIATION DOSES FOR COMMON RADIOGRAPHIC PROCEDURES

Patient Age	Estimated Midline Doses (mrad)
Posteroanterior Chest (400-speed)	
10–15 yr	2.3
6–10 yr	2.2
3–6 yr	2.1
1–3 yr	1.8
3-Foot Spine Posteroanterior (1,100-speed)	
25–30 cm	17
20–25 cm	15
17–20 cm	15
13–17 cm	12
3-Foot Spine Lateral (1,100-speed)	
35–40 cm	35
30–35 cm	29
27–30 cm	26
23–27 cm	22
Anteroposterior Pelvis and Hips (400-speed)	
10–15 yr	11
6–10 yr	6.4
3–6 yr	4.7
1–3 yr	4.5
Anteroposterior Hand (100-speed)	
10–15 yr	3.0
6–10 yr	2.6
3–6 yr	2.6
1–3 yr	2.6

(Adapted from ref. 16, with permission.)

and fractures of the distal radius (pronator quadratus sign). Evaluation of superficial soft tissues is useful in evaluation of cellulitis and in the detection of foreign bodies. Specific radiographic exposures for the evaluation of soft tissues can be obtained, if necessary; with digital imaging it is possible to modify the window and level of the image to depict primarily the soft tissues.

Evaluation of Skeletal Maturity. Determination of skeletal maturity, or bone age, is of great importance, and consti-

tutes nearly 1% of pediatric imaging examinations (17). Skeletal age is usually determined during the evaluation of metabolic disorders, skeletal dysplasias, and short stature. Bone age is also estimated during assessment of residual growth, which is crucial to time spine fusion for scoliosis and epiphysiodesis for limb-length discrepancy.

The most widely used technique is to compare the radiographic appearance of the physes and secondary centers of ossification of the left hand to radiographic standards, usually those of Greulich and Pyle (18). The book of Greulich and Pyle provides standard deviations for each chronological age obtained by the Brush foundation study. A bone age that differs more than two standard deviations from the chronological age is considered abnormal.

In young children, the bone age determination is based on whether the ossification centers have appeared. In older children, as the ossification centers become elongated, the width of the epiphyseal ossification center approaches that of the metaphysis. In late childhood and puberty, the physes become progressively undulated, and the epiphyses begin to cap the metaphyses. In adolescence, physeal closure becomes the most important feature. Carpal bones should not be analyzed during routine evaluation of patients who are relatively normal, because including the carpal bones makes the evaluation less consistent. Carpal bones, however, are more sensitive indicators of dysfunctional maturation such as occurs in endocrinopathies and skeletal dysplasias.

In the first year of life, when the hand epiphyses and carpal bones are solely cartilaginous, other techniques can be applied. The best is to radiograph the knee and ankle, and use the standards of Pyle and Hoerr (19,20), in a fashion similar to those described for the hand. Alternatively, skeletal maturity can be determined by the Sontag method (21), based on counting the number of ossification centers in the hemiskeleton.

There has been growing concern about the generalizability of the standards of Greulich and Pyle (G&P). These standards were derived from white children of upper socioeconomic status in the 1930s, and may not be exactly applicable to children of other ethnic groups or socioeconomic conditions. Recently, preadolescent and adolescent black

TABLE 3-2. ESTIMATED RADIATION DOSES FROM BONE SCINTIGRAPHY BY AGE [rad/mCi (mGy/MBq)]

Target Organ	Newborn	1 Year	5 Years	10 Years
Kidneys	0.340 (0.092)	0.137 (0.037)	0.077 (0.021)	0.052 (0.014)
Ovaries	0.115 (0.031)	0.055 (0.015)	0.033 (0.009)	0.022 (0.006)
Bone surfaces	5.92 (1.6)	1.813 (0.49)	0.777 (0.21)	0.444 (0.12)
Red marrow	0.592 (0.16)	0.208 (0.056)	0.104 (0.028)	0.059 (0.016)
Testes	0.010 (0.027)	0.048 (0.013)	0.027 (0.007)	0.169 (0.047)
Urinary bladder wall	1.48 (0.40)	0.629 (0.17)	0.34 (0.091)	0.225 (0.061)
Effective dose equivalent*	0.407 (0.11)	0.154 (0.042)	0.077 (0.021)	0.052 (0.014)

* rem/mCi (mSv/MBq).

and Hispanic girls and Asian and Hispanic boys have been found to have a skeletal age (determined by G&P standards) that exceeds the chronological age by approximately 9 months (22,23). The skeletal age of Pakistani children (as determined by G&P standards), on the other hand, is estimated to be 6 months to a year lower than the chronological age (24), whereas that of central European children can be evaluated accurately by those standards (25). Interobserver variability studies show an average spread of 1 year for the G&P method (26). A recent study depicts the G&P method as very inaccurate, with 95% confidence intervals of −2.5 to 2.2 years (27). All these reservations notwithstanding, the method continues to be the standard against which all other techniques are measured, and the most disseminated way of determining skeletal maturity. The Tanner-Whitehouse method (28), based on assigning a maturity score to each bone of the hand and wrist, is more comprehensive and reproducible, but its determination takes four times longer (26). There are computer programs that can be used to aid in the evaluation, but these are not widely available (29).

Also included in the book by Greulich and Pyle are the standards of Bayley and Pinneau. These allow the estimation of the final height of the patient, based on the current height and the chronological age. A recent evaluation of the technique showed that it remained reliable, although height is underestimated early in life and overestimated when predicted closer to maturity (30).

Investigation of Child Abuse. Plain film radiography is the most important tool for evaluating child abuse. Most fractures of child abuse, particularly the characteristic metaphyseal fractures, are subtle, and are often undetected unless great attention is paid to the technical details of imaging (31). In a small infant, including most of the skeleton in a single large film is tempting, but is likely to lead to missed diagnoses. Most subtle injuries are found only when there is appropriate collimation (which reduces unwanted scatter radiation), and when the x-ray beam is centered on the area evaluated. Only high-detail film screen combinations should be used (32). A complete skeletal survey needs to be obtained in every case. This includes anteroposterior (AP) and lateral views of the skull and thorax, a lateral view of the spine, AP views of the abdomen and pelvis, oblique views of the hands, and AP views of each of the other segments of the extremities (32).

Digital Radiography. Digital radiography is becoming the most widely used technique to obtain x-ray images of the skeleton (33). Digital radiographs can be manipulated electronically, archived digitally, and transmitted with great ease. In children, the use of an air gap between the extremity and the detector further improves musculoskeletal computed imaging by reducing scatter (34).

Most large radiology departments in the United States are implementing picture archiving and communication systems (PACS), of which digital radiography is an integral part. Many departments record images only digitally. Such "filmless" departments are likely to become the norm over the next decade (35,36). Integration of multiple modalities has become possible because there is now a standard for network interfaces, the Digital Imaging and Communications in Medicine (DICOM) (1). Most modern imaging equipment is DICOM-compatible.

Computed radiography results in dose reduction, because exposure is decreased (less milliampere seconds), and because there are less repeat radiographs related to exposure errors. Other advantages of computed musculoskeletal radiography include improved contrast resolution, ability to enhance images after acquisition, and elimination of film screen contact problems (33). Disadvantages of digital radiography include higher initial costs and lower resolution than conventional radiography, which is particularly noticed in the detection of subtle fractures.

Arthrography

Despite advances in cross-sectional imaging of the hip, arthrography remains a valuable diagnostic technique for children with developmental dysplasia of the hip (DDH) and Legg-Calvé-Perthes (LCP) disease (37). In both, arthrography depicts the femoroacetabular relationship in different anatomic positions. This information is not currently provided by conventional MR imaging, in which the hips are studied in a neutral position, or with CT or sonography (38). In children, arthrography is usually performed intraoperatively, prior to immobilization or corrective surgery.

Technique. Arthrography is performed by introducing a needle under fluoroscopic or sonographic guidance. If done fluoroscopically, the needle can be introduced 1 cm distal to the proximal femoral physis, and 1 cm medial to the lateral aspect of the femoral head (39,40), avoiding the femoral artery. Alternatively, the needle can be placed inferior to the adductor muscle, and directed superiorly into the joint space, under fluoroscopic control. This medial adductor approach minimizes degradation of the image by extraarticular contrast, when the initial injection fails, because contrast material in the soft tissues does not overlap with the femoral head.

Once the needle hits the bone, it is withdrawn 1 mm so that it rests in the joint space. A small trial injection is important to confirm the intraarticular location of the needle, and to minimize extraarticular contrast material. Nonionic contrast material is infused into the joint until mild capsular distention is attained. In general, it is best to dilute the contrast material (e.g., 5 mL of contrast material in 5 mL of normal saline solution). The contrast material should be just enough to coat the anatomic structures adequately. Too much contrast leads to overdistention, which distorts the normal articular relationships and obscures the anatomic landmarks. In the infant hip, 1 to 2 mL of this mixture is adequate for joint depiction (41), but the volume varies significantly with age and with the laxity of the joint. Once the joint space is opacified, images are obtained with the hip held in various positions, such as neutral, abduction, mild adduction, abduction with flexion and external rotation (frog lateral or Lauenstein projection), and abduction with internal rotation (Von Rosen projection) (38, 42,43).

Normal Anatomy. In infants and children, there is usually a large discrepancy between the contour of the bones and the cartilaginous structures outlined arthrographically. The structures depicted on arthrography include the cartilaginous and ossified femoral head, the acetabulum, and the labrum. The acetabulum should be concave inferiorly; its lateral extent is defined by the fibrocartilaginous acetabular labrum, which is also radiolucent. The capsule extends just cephalad to the labral tip, creating a recess between the superior surface of the labrum and the capsule. This recess resembles a rose thorn, when filled with contrast material, surrounding the tip of the labrum (40) (Fig. 3-8). The acetabular cartilage has a smooth surface, and has a radius of curvature appropriate to the size of the child. The width of

the acetabular cartilage is increased in DDH. The normal femoral cartilaginous head is smooth, and fits tightly within the acetabulum. Any pooling of contrast between the femoral head and the acetabulum is abnormal. The contrast agent collects around the femoral head and metaphysis, but is contained by the orbicular ligament, forming a waist known as the "zona orbicularis."

Developmental Dysplasia of the Hip. Arthrography is indicated during reduction of dislocation of the hip, to indicate the position of the femoral head during the reduction maneuvers, and to identify any obstacles to reduction (2). Arthrography ensures that the reduction has been adequate, and that it is maintained after the placement of a spica cast. It shows the medial joint space after reduction, showing whether the femoral head is properly seated.

Obstacles to reduction (43) include structures that may get interposed between the articular surfaces, such as a pulvinar (Latin for "cushion"), a hypertrophied ligamentum teres, a redundant capsule with areas of infolding, a hypertrophied transverse acetabular ligament, and a psoas tendon indenting the capsule between the acetabulum and the femoral head. The pulvinar is seen as a radiolucent structure with irregular borders, located in the depth of the acetabulum. This fibrofatty tissue usually recedes after the hip is located. A redundant, large ligamentum teres is outlined by contrast, and is usually easy to identify. Psoas interposition is not reliably detected by arthrography, and capsular and transverse ligament interpositions may be difficult to detect. There is some controversy about the relative importance of these obstacles to reduction.

Another important factor interfering with reduction is an abnormal configuration of the acetabulum (44) and the acetabular labrum ("inverted labrum" or "limbus") (45). Histologic studies suggest that, rather than being a mere labral inversion, this abnormality consists of a true cartilaginous ridge within the acetabular concavity, creating two separate acetabular chambers (4). Imaging in the abduction and internal rotation (Von Rosen) position differentiates between a subluxated hip with intervening soft tissues and a dysplastic hip with increased femoral anteversion. With increased anteversion, medial pooling of contrast resolves in the Von Rosen position (2).

Legg-Calvé-Perthes Disease. Arthrography is often performed in severe LCP disease to decide whether the hips require bracing or surgery (osteotomies), and to assess the best position for immobilization (5–8). It helps assess *containment* of the femoral head by the acetabulum, *congruency* of the femoral head and the acetabulum, and *deformity* of the cartilaginous femoral head. It helps to determine the optimal position of the femoral head for immobilization

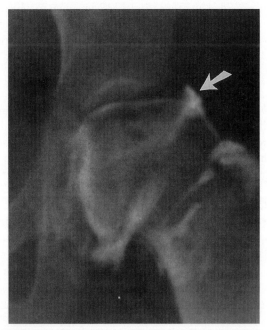

FIGURE 3-8. Arthrography of the hip in a 7-year-old boy with Legg-Calvé-Perthes disease. Anteroposterior arthrogram in the neutral position shows that the deformed femoral head is flattened and incompletely contained by the acetabulum. The *arrow* points to the "rose thorn," the capsular recess surrounding the lateral aspect of the acetabular labrum.

during the process of epiphyseal healing (46). In order to maximize containment (9), it is important to document which positions lead to the greatest percentage of the femoral head being covered by the acetabulum (Fig. 3-8). On the other hand, it is desirable to place the head in a position in which the acetabulum and femoral head are congruent. When the contours of the acetabulum and the femoral head are parallel, only minimal contrast should come between the articular surfaces. Lack of congruity is seen as pooling of contrast between the flattened portions of the femoral head and the acetabulum. Unfortunately, the maneuvers that increase containment, such as abduction, also increase the pool of contrast material between the femoral head and the acetabulum. In summary, arthrography is performed to detect causes of decreased containment, and to show positional changes in the joint (47,48).

In LCP disease, lateral displacement of the femoral head is usually multifactorial. The epiphyseal cartilage is abnormally thick, and there is hypertrophy of the synovium and of the ligamentum teres. Occasionally, increased joint fluid may contribute to the subluxation. With severe flattening of the femoral head, the abducted femur can hinge on the lateral acetabular margin. This "hinge abduction" (49) separates the femoral head from the acetabulum, simultaneously reducing containment and congruity (5). Arthrography can also be used to detect irregularity of the articular cartilage, which is important prognostically (50).

Conventional Tomography

Conventional tomography is a radiographic technique to show fine detail of structures within a specific anatomic plane. This is accomplished by blurring the structures below and above a certain plane by moving the radiographic tube (10). The more complex the motion (hypocycloidal, trispiral), the better the detail: the wider the arc of motion, the thinner the slice. The widespread use of CT and MR imaging has almost eliminated the need for tomography, and most major hospitals no longer have complex motion units. Linear tomography is the only technique still widely available, but its resolution is less than that of complex motion tomography, because the blurring is less optimal. The most important use of conventional tomography in pediatric orthopaedic imaging is in the evaluation of pseudoarthrosis after spinal fusion, when orthopaedic hardware may produce severe artifacts on CT or MR imaging.

Computed Tomography

CT is an extension of plain radiography, but its contrast resolution is 100 times greater. CT can detect changes in radiologic attenuation as small as 0.1% (51). CT displays various musculoskeletal structures; pixel brightness represents x-ray attenuation. The attenuation of muscle and cartilage is very similar, so that the main contribution of orthopaedic CT is to outline the contour of the bony structures. CT also provides tomographic display and allows digital manipulation and storage of the data. Multiplanar and three-dimensional (3D) reconstructions can be performed with great ease, if the images are acquired appropriately. There are many image reconstruction packages that can be used on a conventional workstation; alternatively, the vendors of CT units also market workstations with proprietary software. Most can generate a 3D image with surface or volume rendering in one or two minutes. In complex cases, it is advisable for the orthopaedic surgeon and the radiologist to review the images jointly on the workstation, because significant information can be gained from options, such as simulated disarticulation, color display, and cine-loop, to display the objects in motion.

The image is acquired by rotating an x-ray beam around the patient and detecting the attenuated beam after it traverses the patient. The data from the detectors is sent to a computer, which reconstructs it into an axial (transaxial) image. With conventional CT, the motion of the x-ray beam is circular, and single slices are obtained at predetermined increments. With helical (spiral) CT, the source-detector system rotates continuously as the patient is advanced through the gantry, so that the scanning motion is spiral. This helical method of scanning is faster and acquires a continuous set of data. The interval between slices, and the location of the center of the slice, can be modified after imaging, if the raw data is still available (52). Although helical CT can deliver a lower radiation dose in examinations of the chest and abdomen, for the high spatial resolution required for most musculoskeletal studies, the radiation doses for helical and conventional CT are essentially equal (52). Most orthopaedic studies are performed with a slice thickness of 1 to 3 mm. Coronal and sagittal reconstructions can be obtained routinely, and are very helpful.

The main disadvantage of spiral CT is that it produces blurring and stair-step artifacts. Helical CT is also slightly less sensitive than conventional CT for detecting subtle fractures (53). In children, however, the loss of sensitivity is more than offset by the reduction of artifacts caused by motion. Spiral CT is faster, and provides better images and reconstructions than conventional CT in almost every pediatric application.

Indications. Trauma is one of the main indications for CT. CT scanning is used extensively to evaluate fragment separation in triplane and Tillaux fractures, clearly demonstrated by multiplanar reconstructions. In patients with scaphoid fractures, CT can demonstrate subtle fractures and subsequent nonunion. In slipped capital femoral epiphysis, CT demonstrates the physeal irregularity, the degree of infe-

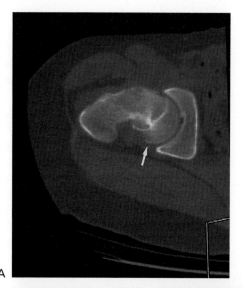

A

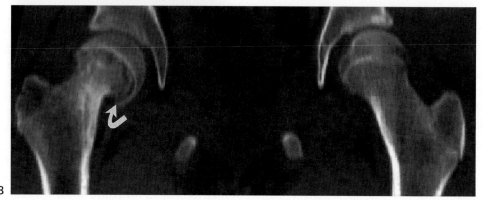

B

FIGURE 3-9. CT evaluation of a slipped capital femoral epiphysis. A 13-year-old girl with several months of right hip pain, which has exacerbated recently. The data set was obtained with 3-mm collimated slices, and reconstructed at 1-mm intervals. **A:** Axial oblique reconstruction, to display the entire length of the femoral neck, shows that there is a gentle posterior curve of the femoral neck indicating chronic slippage. In addition, the physis is wide and irregular, indicating a superimposed, more acute component. The femoral head (*arrow*) is very displaced posteriorly. **B:** Coronal reconstruction shows the physeal widening of the right hip (*curved arrow*). By comparison to the degree of posterior slippage, the degree of inferior displacement is relatively minor.

rior and posterior displacement of the femoral head (Fig. 3-9), and the retroversion of the contralateral femur. In acetabular fractures, 3D reconstructions better demonstrate the relationships between fragments.

In infants with hip dislocation who have undergone reduction and placement of the hips in an abduction spica cast, CT can be used to assess the position of the femoral heads (54). A cross-sectional technique is very useful in this setting, because frontal radiographs fail to show posterior redislocation. The assessment of the position of the femoral head can be done with less than five CT sections (Fig. 3-10). If a low mAs technique is used, the total ovarian dose can be as low as 112 mrad (1.12 mGy) (53). In adolescents and young adults with undetected hip dysplasia, CT with 3D reconstructions demonstrates the configuration and containment of the femoral head, the acetabular architecture, and the narrowing of the joint space (Fig. 3-11). In the spine, vertebral abnormalities and intervertebral fusions are easily demonstrated with CT.

CT can be used for measurements of the orientation of various skeletal structures. *Glenoid version* is the angle be-

tween the main axis of the scapula and the glenoid (55). *Femoral anteversion* is determined by obtaining slices from the femoral head to the lesser trochanter, and slices through the distal femoral condyles. A line through the main axis of the femoral neck and another along the posterior surfaces of the distal femoral condyles form the angle of femoral anteversion. The angle of anteversion is 32 degrees at birth and 16 degrees by age 16 years (56). A more recent study found a mean angle for children of 34 degrees and 22.2 degrees for adults, using CT, and angles of 23.2 degrees and 15.7 degrees, respectively, using MR imaging (57). *Tibial torsion* is determined by obtaining a single slice through the widest portion of the proximal tibial epiphysis and another one through the malleoli. The angle of tibial torsion is formed by a line through the center of the epiphysis (representing the main axis of the proximal tibia), and a line connecting the distal tibial malleolus. External tibial torsion determined by physical examination is normally 4 degrees at birth, and 14 degrees at 10 years of age (58,59). Using CT, a study of 50 adults revealed an external tibial torsion of 37.5 degrees in females and 40.5 degrees in males (60).

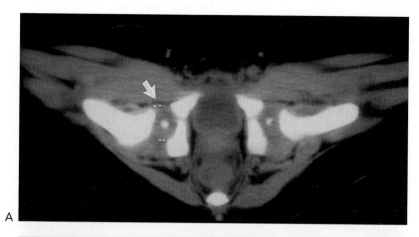

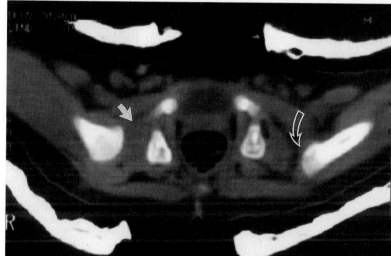

FIGURE 3-10. CT scanning to verify the position of a hip after dislocation of reduction and spica cast placement in two different infant girls. **A:** Normal anatomy. Both hips are located concentrically. The ossification centers are present. *Dotted lines* partially outline the contour of the right cartilaginous epiphysis. **B:** Redislocation of the left hip. The right hip is located concentrically (*closed arrow*). The left hip has redislocated posteriorly. The *open curved arrow* points to the left metaphysis, because the unossified epiphysis is not visible on this slice.

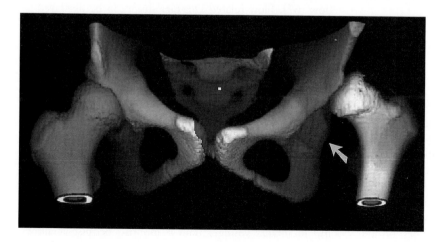

FIGURE 3-11. 3D-CT evaluation of developmental dysplasia of the hip. Surface transparent rendering of a 3D reconstruction of a helical CT in a 10-year-old girl with developmental dysplasia of the left hip shows a poorly developed acetabulum, which is empty (*arrow*). There is also superior subluxation of the femoral head and irregularity of the contour of the capital femoral epiphysis. The data set was obtained with 3-mm collimated slices, and reconstructed at 1-mm intervals.

We were unable to find a systematic large study of tibial torsion in children using CT, which may reflect the decreasing use of these measurements.

Tarsal coalition is evaluated by obtaining thin sections through the hindfoot. The subtalar joint, usually difficult to depict on radiographs, is imaged in the coronal plane. The patient lies horizontally, with the hips and knees in flexion and the ankles in plantar flexion, so that the feet are flat on the CT table. Coronal imaging optimizes the evaluation of talocalcaneal coalitions. Both feet should be studied, because bilateral abnormalities can be seen in up to 81% of patients (61). CT images demonstrate a complete osseous fusion if the coalition is bony, or irregularity of the articular surfaces of the anterior and middle facets if it is fibrous. The subtalar joint is reoriented in an inferomedial direction (62). Calcaneonavicular coalitions, which are usually evident on oblique radiographs, are best seen on sagittal reconstructions (63).

If a calcaneonavicular coalition is found on radiographs, we routinely do not obtain a CT. A recent large series, however, showed that multiple tarsal coalitions may be more frequent than previously thought, with an incidence of 20% (64) and not 5 to 10%, as previously believed. This would argue for obtaining CT studies more often. The accuracy for detecting tarsal coalitions is comparable for CT and MR imaging (65). CT allows easier evaluation of both feet, and it is less expensive and more readily available; we prefer to use CT for the initial evaluation of talocalcaneal coalitions.

Risks and Limitations. The main limitation of CT is that it delivers a high radiation dose (see section on Radiation). Most body parts can only be imaged axially, but with high detail reconstructions, this is a less important limitation.

Utilization Trends. CT has replaced conventional tomography for most applications. In musculoskeletal imaging, CT is the modality of choice whenever evaluation of bony contours is the most important goal.

ULTRASONOGRAPHY

Mechanisms of Contrast

Sonography is based on the application of high-frequency sound pulses and the detection of the reflected echoes. The intensity of the echoes depends on the differences in speed of sound transmission at tissue interfaces. A structure that reflects most of the ultrasound beam is termed highly echogenic, and is bright on ultrasonographic display. Sound-transmitting structures, such as water, allow the passage of the ultrasound beam, and are darker (free of echoes) on the display screen. Higher-frequency sound beams have greater resolution, but less penetration. In musculoskeletal imaging, it is very useful to image the contralateral side, because sub-

tle increases in echogenicity or thickening of soft tissues may be detectable only by comparison. Superficial lesions are sometimes difficult to detect because the ultrasound transducers themselves deform the contour of the structures, but they can be imaged successfully through a soft standoff pad.

Ultrasonography is safe (11), easy to perform, and relatively inexpensive. Images are displayed in real time, and joint motion can be analyzed. Most units are unable to display large fields of view, which limits the depiction of large lesions. The sound beam is wholly reflected by bone, and the cortex is seen as a bright interface with complete shadowing beyond it. Fat, ligaments, and tendons have high echogenicity, but less than that of bone. Cartilage and muscle are of low echogenicity. Articular cartilage is uniformly hypoechoic, whereas epiphyseal cartilage has many internal echoes, which represent the epiphyseal vascular canals. These canals form a parallel array of echogenic lines at birth, but later they tend to converge toward the ossification center. The muscle fibers have a striated appearance, separated by the echogenic epimysium and perimysium (66). Fluid-filled collections, whether filled with watery contents (cysts) or blood (aneurysms), are hypoechoic. Gas is highly echogenic, and is suggested by the "comet tail artifact," a series of echoes that trail a bright echo. The distinctive parallel lines of tendons represent individual echogenic fibers (66). Tissue calcification can produce significant increases in echogenicity. Edema also increases echogenicity because of an increased number of interfaces in the swollen tissues.

Doppler Sonography

When a sound beam hits moving objects, such as blood cells, the frequency of the reflected beam increases when the object is moving toward the transducer, and decreases when the object moves away from the transducer. This is the Doppler effect. Its frequency shifts can be used to assess flow (67). Flow-related Doppler shifts can be displayed as a spectral time-frequency graph, or by superimposing the Doppler information on the gray scale imaging, as occurs with color Doppler and power Doppler sonography. With color Doppler sonography, flow toward the transducer is typically encoded red, whereas flow away from it is encoded blue (12). With power Doppler sonography, only the amplitude of the Doppler signal is shown. Power Doppler sonography has a greater sensitivity to slow flow, but it lacks directional information (13).

Normal Sonographic Anatomy of the Hip

Sonography is a fundamental modality for evaluation of the hip in infants younger than 6 months, because it allows dynamic assessment of articular relationships and depicts the nonosseous structures without radiation exposure (68). Five major structures are displayed: the hypoechoic carti-

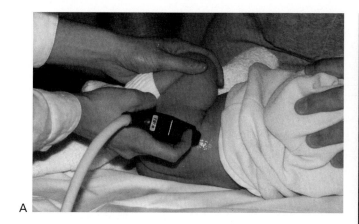

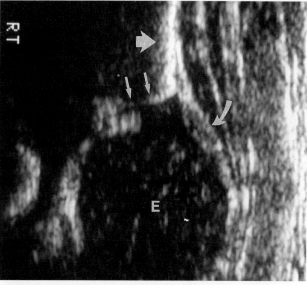

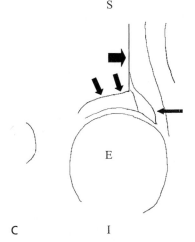

FIGURE 3-12. Normal coronal hip ultrasound on a 6-week-old girl with family history of developmental dysplasia of the hip. **A:** Photograph showing the performance of sonography in the coronal plane. The transducer is oriented vertically, parallel to the iliac wing. (From ref. 70, with permission.) **B:** Coronal sonogram. The ultrasound image is oriented like an anteroposterior radiograph, with the head on top. *Large arrow,* straight iliac wing; *double arrows,* bony acetabulum; *curved arrow,* fibrocartilaginous labrum and capsule; *E,* unossified proximal femoral epiphysis. **C:** Diagram outlining the salient features of the sonogram in Figure 3-12**B.** The labeling is the same as that of the sonogram. The epiphysis is labeled *E.* The single, *thin arrow* points to the cartilaginous labrum. The *double arrows* point to the bony acetabulum, and the single, *thick arrow* points to the iliac wing. *S,* superior; *I,* inferior.

lages of the proximal femoral epiphysis and acetabulum; the very echogenic bones of the proximal femoral metaphysis and acetabulum; and the echogenic fibrocartilaginous labrum (Fig. 3-12).

Sonography of hip dysplasia is based primarily on coronal and transverse views (69). Both are obtained with the transducer placed lateral to the joint (Figs. 3-12 to 3-14). Graf and Schuler described the coronal view, comparable to a frontal radiograph, to show the morphology of acetabular structures (71). With proper positioning of the transducer, the lateral edge of the iliac bone is depicted as a straight line. The bony acetabular roof is an oblique, slightly concave, much shorter line. Sonograms in which the iliac bone is curved are either too anterior or too posterior, are technically inadequate, and may spuriously enlarge or reduce the size of the acetabular roof. The angle between the iliac wing and the bony acetabulum (the alpha angle) is approximately 60 degrees in normal newborns (72).

The sonolucent cartilaginous acetabulum is more concave than the bony roof, and it is in direct contact with the cartilaginous epiphysis. It blends laterally with the fibrocartilaginous labrum. Cephalad and lateral to the labrum is the thin echogenic capsule. Superomedially, the capsule is continuous with the fibrous perichondrium, which is attached to the ilium (73). The femoral epiphysis is sonographically homogeneous at birth. The ossification center is seen with sonography several weeks earlier than with radiographs (74). The junction between the cartilage and bone of the proximal femoral metaphysis is an interrupted line. When imaged in internal rotation, the cartilages of the greater trochanter and femoral head are continuous.

Harcke and Grissom have developed the transverse view to examine hip motion and detect subluxation dynamically (75). It is usually obtained with the hip in mild flexion, when the femoral metaphysis obscures the anterior acetabulum. The ischial portion of the acetabulum is a short echogenic line just posterior to the femoral epiphysis. The femoroacetabular relationships can be assessed during abduction and adduction, and during the Barlow maneuver. Alternatively, the transverse view can be obtained with the hip extended, allowing visualization of the pubic component of the acetabulum. The anterior axial view is used to detect adequacy of reduction. The two hips are easily compared. Other views have been useful in specific situations.

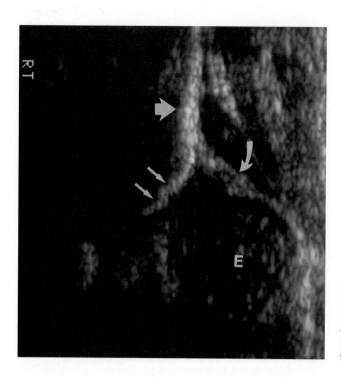

FIGURE 3-13. Coronal sonogram in a 1-month-old girl with bilateral hip dysplasia; only one side is displayed. The femoral head is incompletely covered by the acetabulum. The acetabulum is shallow and has a vertical orientation. There is an echogenic pulvinar deep to the femoral head. *Large arrow,* straight iliac wing; *double arrows,* bony acetabulum; *curved arrow,* fibrocartilaginous labrum and capsule; *E,* unossified proximal femoral epiphysis.

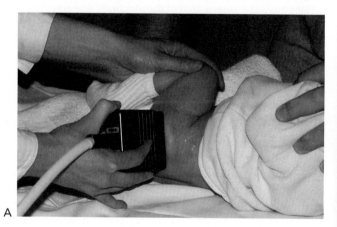

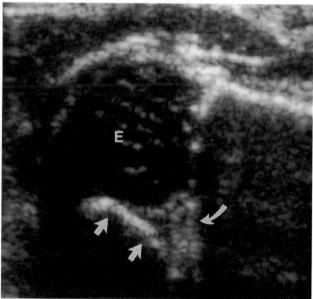

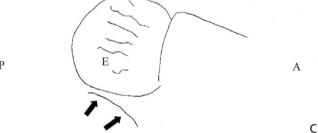

FIGURE 3-14. Transverse sonogram in a 1-month-old girl with hip dysplasia. **A:** Photograph showing the performance of sonography in the transverse plane. The transducer is oriented horizontally, perpendicular to the iliac wing. In this case, the examination is being done with the hip in flexion, but it can also be done in the neutral position. (From ref. 70, with permission.) **B:** Axial sonogram shows the unossified proximal femoral epiphysis (*E*) being displaced posteriorly with respect to the ischium (*double arrows*). An echogenic pulvinar (*curved arrow*) displaces the femoral head laterally. **C:** Line diagram outlining the salient features of Fig. 3-14B. The labeling is the same as that of the sonogram. The unossified epiphysis is marked *E.* It is continuous with the metaphysis. The two *arrows* point to the ischium. *A,* anterior; *P,* posterior.

Main Applications

Developmental Dysplasia of the Hip

In infants less than 6 months of age, we use ultrasonography as the first imaging study performed to detect hip dysplasia. The value of hip sonography is dependent on the experience and skill of the individual performing the study; when an expert operator is not available, a radiograph of the hip is preferred as the initial study. In some parts of Europe, sonography is used to screen the entire newborn population. In Coventry, England, screening of more than 14,000 newborns detected a 6% incidence of sonographic abnormalities. Of these, nearly 80% were normal by 4 weeks and 90% by 8 weeks (76); uncritical acceptance of sonographic abnormalities in the first weeks of life can lead to overtreatment. In the United States, however, hip sonography is usually performed when the physical examination is abnormal or when there are risk factors (77). These include a positive family history, breech delivery, oligohydramnios, and conditions sometimes caused by uterine crowding, such as torticollis, clubfoot, or metatarsus adductus.

Graf has divided hips into various types according to (a) the angle between the acetabulum and the iliac wing (alpha), (b) the angle between the fibrocartilaginous labrum and the iliac wing (beta), (c) the characteristics of the bony roof (good, deficient, or poor), and (d) the appearance of the acetabular rim (angular, round, or flat) (72). Under 3 months of age the hip can appear slightly dysplastic due to immaturity, but any infant hip with an alpha angle under 50 degrees, a beta angle over 70 degrees, or subluxability on the dynamic examination is clearly abnormal. Before 2 weeks of age, hormonally induced ligamentous laxity can confound the evaluation of hip stability; up to 6 mm of posterior displacement of the femoral head with the Barlow maneuver is normal (75). Hip sonography for evaluation of dysplasia should only be performed after this period, when any displacement during the dynamic study is considered abnormal. Graf and Harcke have recommended a unified study in which evaluation of acetabular morphology, primarily done coronally, is done in tandem with the dynamic assessment of joint stability (77). Sonography is of little value when hip dislocation is clinically obvious. When the femoral head is dislocated, the acetabular concavity cannot be adequately depicted, and it is very difficult to align the femoral head with the midplane of the acetabulum. Infants with successfully treated dysplasia should be evaluated with a radiograph at 6 months of age to ensure that the acetabular abnormality has indeed been resolved.

Other Applications

Sonography can also detect femoral head ischemia and hip effusion. Doppler sonography in any plane has been used to show the vascularity of the femoral head of infants and

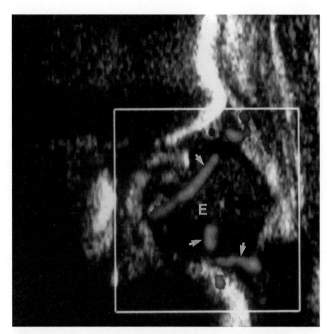

FIGURE 3-15. Power Doppler sonography of the normal hip. In this coronal view, there is clear depiction of flow in the vascular canals (*arrows*) of the proximal femoral epiphysis (*E*).

newborns (78) (Fig. 3-15). There are, unfortunately, many pitfalls. Blood flow may be difficult to detect when the infant is moving significantly. Usually, only a few vessels are detected; it is difficult to differentiate normal perfusion from ischemia limited to a portion of the head. The main limitation, however, is that ultrasound cannot be performed through a cast; infants in spica casts, who would be the ideal candidates, cannot be readily examined sonographically.

The evaluation of joint fluid is performed using an anterior approach with the transducer placed in the groin along the femoral neck (Fig. 3-16). The metaphysis, physis, and epiphysis are well seen. An effusion makes the capsule and the joint fluid between the capsule and the femoral neck clearly visible (79). This technique detects as little as 1 cc of joint fluid. There is no relationship between the amount of echogenicity of the joint fluid and its likelihood of being infected. Absence of fluid on sonography speaks strongly against septic arthritis. On Doppler sonography, increased flow in the capsule is sensitive, but not specific for infection (80). Ultimately, if septic arthritis is suspected and fluid is detected, the hip should be tapped and the fluid analyzed. This should be done expeditiously; some prefer to use sonography for confirmation and guidance, whereas others elect to go directly to aspiration and obtain imaging guidance when osteomyelitis is suspected.

Utilization Trends

The use of sonography is increasing rapidly. Sonography is one of the main modalities for evaluation of hip dysplasia.

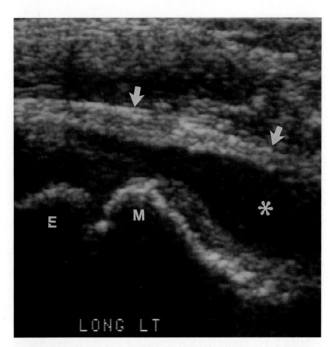

FIGURE 3-16. Large hip effusion in a 3-year-old boy with juvenile rheumatoid arthritis. Ultrasound evaluation reveals a large effusion (*asterisk*) contained by a thick capsule (*arrows*). *E*, epiphyseal ossification center; *M*, metaphysis.

It is also the most important imaging study in the evaluation of a septic hip. Sonography has become increasingly important in the evaluation of other joints, particularly to show relationships in various positions. The role of sonography in the evaluation of superficial masses in the extremities is expanding; it is commonly used to determine whether masses are cystic, and to evaluate the vascularity of malignant bone tumors. There is also increasing interest in its use for evaluation of complications of osteomyelitis, such as subperiosteal or soft tissue abscess (81). Sonography is particularly useful in patients with metallic hardware suspected of osteomyelitis, in whom MR imaging, CT, and even scintigraphy would have limitations (82). It should be used with caution in osteomyelitis, however, because pus can be isoechoic with normal soft tissues and difficult to detect, and because sonography cannot depict the intramedullary extension of the infection. There has been significant progress in imaging tendinous and ligamentous abnormalities in adults, but little has been done in children.

MAGNETIC RESONANCE IMAGING

Mechanisms of Contrast

MR imaging relies on the application of a radiofrequency pulse to induce resonance in certain nuclei, usually hydro-

gen (83). In order to resonate, the protons need to be aligned in a magnetic field. Following the application of the radiofrequency pulse, the protons relax and emit a radio signal, which is processed to generate an image.

The radiofrequency pulse causes protons, which are aligned longitudinally in the direction of the magnet, to flip 90 degrees into the transverse plane. Once the pulse is discontinued, the protons return to their original state of longitudinal alignment with the main magnetic field. There are two mechanisms of relaxation: T1 relaxation, related to recovery of magnetization in the longitudinal plane; and T2 relaxation, related to decay of magnetization in the transverse plane.

During T1 relaxation, the magnitude of the longitudinal magnetization increases exponentially. The rate of relaxation differs among tissues. The hydrogen protons in fat relax faster than those in water, for example. Contrast on T1-weighted images reflects these differences in relaxation. Because protons in fat relax rapidly, their longitudinal magnetization, and thus their signal intensity, will increase at a faster rate than those in water. On a T1-weighted image, therefore, fat has a high signal intensity, and appears bright. Protons in water, on the other hand, will not have relaxed to the same degree. Thus, on T1-weighted images, water is of low signal intensity, and appears dark (Fig. 3-17).

When the radiofrequency pulse is applied, all the protons are aligned in the transverse plane, and emit signal together. Transverse magnetization is greatest at this time. Subsequently, the protons lose their alignment (dephase) along the transverse plane, losing transverse magnetization and therefore signal intensity. T2 relaxation is the decay in transverse magnetization due to dephasing of the protons. Protons in water relax more slowly than those in fat, so their signal decays at a slower rate. Thus, on an image that reflects differences in T2 relaxation time, the signal intensity of water is greater than that of fat.

Intermediate images (often called proton-density images) are obtained at a time when the signal increase due to T1 relaxation is greatest and the signal decay due to T2 relaxation is smallest. These images have maximal signal, but less contrast.

Other factors affecting contrast include magnetic susceptibility and flow. *Magnetic susceptibility* reflects distortion of the magnetic field due to tissue inhomogeneity. In the skeleton, for example, multiple interfaces between marrow fat and bony trabeculae decrease the signal from bones. Magnetic susceptibility accounts for much of the image degradation due to metallic artifacts.

Flow results in decrease in signal, intensity in slower sequences. On most MR images of the skeleton, therefore, vessels appear dark. Paradoxically, in faster sequences, the flow of unsaturated protons into the imaged slice of tissue produces flow-related enhancement.

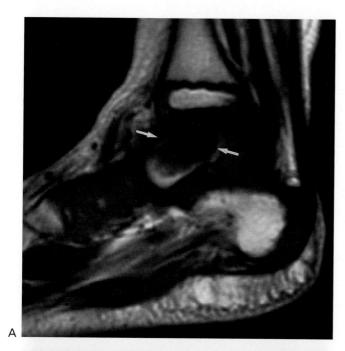

A

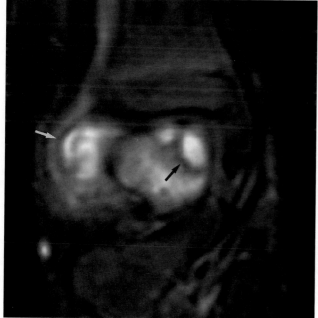

B

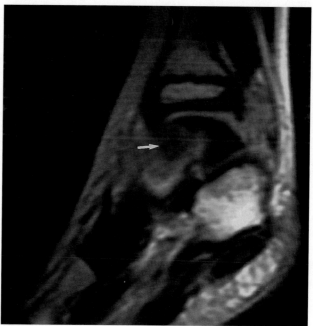

C

FIGURE 3-17. Osteomyelitis of the talus in a 2-year-old boy presenting with foot pain and fever. **A:** Sagittal T1-weighted image of the foot shows decreased signal intensity in the talus (*arrows*). This reflects marrow edema, and suggests osteomyelitis. **B:** Coronal fat-suppressed, T2-weighted image of the same ankle shows that there are two discrete areas of higher signal intensity within the talar dome (*black arrow*). The signal of the marrow of the entire talus is abnormal. There is a joint effusion (*white arrow*). **C:** Sagittal T1-weighted image following the administration of gadolinium shows that most of the talus enhances. The center of the talus, however, does not enhance, indicating a small abscess (*arrow*).

Clinical Use of Pulse Sequences

Many pulse sequences have been devised over the past several years. Because they are so numerous, and because many have peculiarities that are vendor-specific, it is impossible to review pulse sequences adequately in this setting (84). T1-weighted images are the best to determine the intramedullary extent of a tumor. They are anatomically informative, and can depict marrow edema. T2-weighted images are more sensitive than T1-weighted images for detection of increased water content, as is seen in infection, trauma, or tumor (Fig. 3-17). Obtaining T2-weighted images takes longer, and therefore they are almost exclusively acquired using fast spin-echo techniques. Intermediate (proton density)-weighted images are the best for depiction of anatomy, but provide little contrast resolution. Gradient-recalled echo images are good for evaluating ligaments and cartilage. Spoiled gradient-recalled echo images allow excellent differentiation between cartilage and bone, and show cartilaginous abnormalities well (Fig. 3-18). Short tau inversion recovery (STIR) images are very sensitive to marrow lesions (Fig. 3-19). Fat suppression can be used with any of the sequences mentioned above to maximize optical visual contrast between the lesion and the adjacent tissues.

Contrast Materials

Gadolinium (Gd) is the most widely used contrast agent for musculoskeletal MR imaging. The element with the most unpaired electrons in its outer shell, Gd distorts the local magnetic field. This distortion hastens T1 and T2 relaxation. As mentioned previously, a faster T1 relaxation increases signal intensity on T1-weighted images. After Gd administration, signal intensity on T1-weighted images will be increased in hyperemic areas and decreased in ischemic regions.

Gd is used in ionic and nonionic forms. There is little difference in safety between them, and the images obtained are almost indistinguishable. There is, however, one important difference: nonionic Gd diffuses freely into cartilage, whereas ionic Gd does not. Negatively charged ionic Gd is bound to diethylenetriamine pentaacetic acid (DTPA) to form $Gd(DTPA)^{2-}$. $Gd(DTPA)^{2-}$ penetrates cartilage only when the similarly charged glycosaminoglycan molecules break down. This suggests that ionic Gd can map glycosaminoglycan content in cartilage (85).

Gd compounds are not nephrotoxic. Serious adverse events have been reported at a rate of 1/20,000 (86) in adults, but are probably much less frequent in children. The only absolute contraindication for use of $Gd(DTPA)^{2-}$ is pregnancy. There is some *in vitro* evidence suggesting that Gd may predispose to erythrocyte sickling. Contrast, however, has been used to evaluate patients with sickle cell disease, without complications (87).

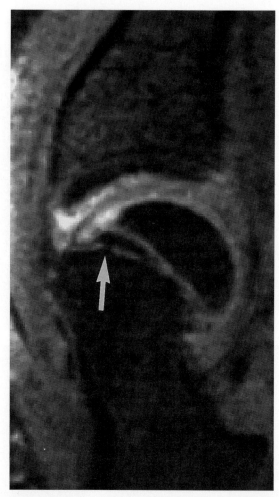

FIGURE 3-18. MR evaluation of a Salter-Harris type 1 fracture of the proximal femur. This 14-year-old boy had a severe trauma to the hip. Sagittal reconstruction of a 3D, fat-suppressed, spoiled gradient-recalled echo acquisition reveals a posterior displacement of the femoral head. The separation of the femoral physis from the metaphysis is seen as a dark cleft (*arrow*).

Intravascular Gd diffuses rapidly into the intracellular space. It shows increased vascularity in inflamed synovium, infected marrow, traumatized bone, and active tumor. It is perhaps most useful in showing areas devoid of blood flow, such as an abscess in bone or soft tissues, necrotic tumor, or an ischemic femoral head. When injected intravenously, Gd can also be used to obtain MR angiographic images of the arterial and venous systems (Fig. 3-19).

Injected intraarticularly, Gd leads to MR arthrographic images (Fig. 3-20). MR arthrography has revolutionized imaging of the shoulder and hip, and is the most reliable way to diagnose labral tears in these joints.

Normal Age-related Changes and Variants

Age-related transformations of cartilage to bone, and of hematopoietic to fatty marrow, strongly influence the MR

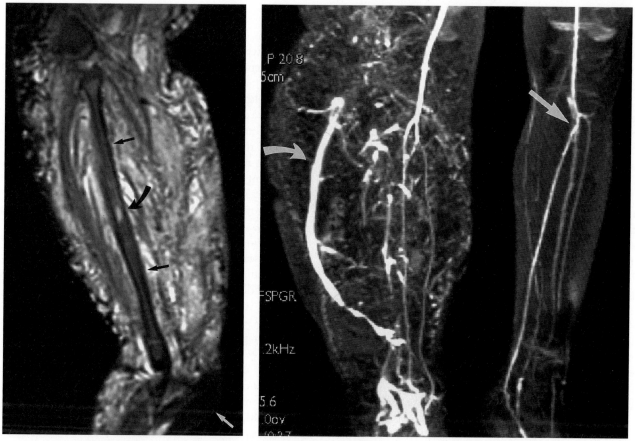

FIGURE 3-19. Marked deformity of the right limb of a 3-year-old boy with Klippel-Trenaunay syndrome. **A:** Sagittal fast short tau inversion recovery (STIR) image at the level of the fibula (*straight black arrows*) shows that there is extensive involvement of the subcutaneous tissues, sparing the heel (*white arrow*). The marrow of the midfibula is abnormal (*curved black arrow*). **B:** 3D contrast-enhanced magnetic resonance angiography shows that the major arteries are intact, but that there is a large superficial draining vein (*curved arrow*). The normal trifurcation of the contralateral side is clearly shown (*straight arrow*).

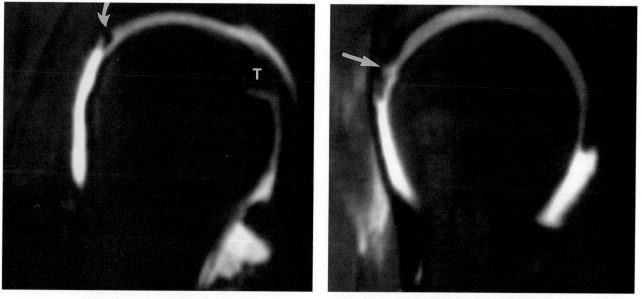

FIGURE 3-20. MR arthrography in a 25-year-old woman with hip dysplasia and hip pain. **A:** Coronal fat-suppressed, T1-weighted image after the intraarticular administration of gadolinium shows the ligamentum teres (*T*) and the transverse ligament. There is irregularity of the superior labrum (*arrow*). **B:** Oblique sagittal image of the same patient shows that the irregularity extends to the anterior labrum (*arrow*).

appearance of the growing skeleton. Epiphyseal cartilage is of homogeneous signal intensity at birth; it has intermediate signal intensity on T1-weighted images and low signal intensity on T2-weighted images and STIR images. During the first years of life, epiphyseal cartilage becomes hypointense in weight-bearing regions. Later, signal intensity increases in areas of active ossification (88). The secondary ossification center is initially spherical, but becomes hemispherical as the ossification center abuts the physis.

Epiphyseal vascular canals are visible after the intravenous administration of gadolinium (89). Enhancement of these vascular canals excludes epiphyseal ischemia. The physis is of high signal intensity on most pulse sequences. It is a few millimeters thick, and becomes progressively undulated as the child matures. With physeal closure, the cartilage loses signal intensity and ultimately disappears (90).

Because of its high water content, normal hematopoietic marrow is of low signal intensity on T1-weighted images, intermediate signal intensity on conventional T2-weighted and STIR images, and high signal intensity on fast spin-echo T2-weighted images and STIR images (91). These imaging characteristics closely resemble those of diseased fatty marrow. It is therefore important to know the normal distribution of hematopoietic marrow, which changes greatly with age. Conversion of hematopoietic to fatty marrow begins in the epiphyses and diaphysis, then advances from the diaphysis into the metaphyses. In the extremities, conversion begins in the fingers and toes, and ends in the proximal humeral and femoral metaphyses. In the axial skeleton, hematopoietic marrow persists throughout life (2).

Main Applications

Spinal Disorders

MR imaging depicts the vertebral bodies, disc spaces, spinal cord, epidural space, and nerve roots, in excellent detail. In infants, it evaluates abnormalities of segmentation very well. The normal conus medullaris is at the L2 level. If the conus is caudal to it, the cord may be tethered. Infections and tumors involving the epidural and subarachnoid spaces are best demonstrated with Gd-enhanced imaging. MR imaging is the best modality for evaluating protrusion or herniation of the discs, spinal stenosis, and nerve root compression, all of which are uncommon in the first decade.

Joint Disorders

MR imaging demonstrates the contour of the cartilaginous structures and the marrow, and can detect synovial abnormalities. In complicated cases of DDH, MR imaging depicts the position of the femoral head before and after reduction,

and detects obstacles to reduction (pulvinar, interposed psoas tendon, deformed labrum, or capsular infolding) (92–95). This can be done less invasively than with arthrography, although arthrography remains the best technique for guidance during the operative procedure. After placement of the hip in a cast, the reduction of the hip can be verified without the radiation required for a CT. Gd-enhanced MR imaging may detect ischemia related to abduction during treatment for DDH (96,97). If it becomes cheaper and more available, MR imaging may become the procedure of choice for evaluating many of the complex problems in hip dysplasia.

MR imaging can also be useful in the early diagnosis of LCP disease. Although radiographs are often diagnostic at presentation, MR imaging can be helpful when the clinical presentation is unclear. Marrow edema is seen early on MR images; suspected avascular necrosis can be confirmed by lack of Gd enhancement of the femoral epiphysis (98). At a later stage of the disease, MR imaging can be useful prognostically by showing physeal and metaphyseal abnormalities (99) and the extent of marrow involvement (100–102). In advanced disease, MR imaging shows the containment of the femoral head and the congruity of the articular surfaces (38). These factors can be best assessed when imaging in multiple positions, similar to those studied during arthrography (103).

Osteomyelitis

MR imaging has been shown to have sensitivity and specificity greater than 90% for detecting bone infection in children (104). It is useful for detection of marrow abnormality by showing edema and increased blood flow in the infected bone (Fig. 3-17). Any MR imaging of osteomyelitis should include Gd enhancement to ascertain whether the infected volume contains drainable pus. An abscess is seen as a non-enhancing (dark) center (the collection of pus) surrounded by a ring of enhancing tissue in the abscess wall (105). In spinal osteomyelitis, MR imaging is crucial for detecting epidural abscess and extension of the infection into the paraspinal soft tissues. MR imaging is preferable to scintigraphy (106,107) in pelvic osteomyelitis, where bony geometry is complex and soft tissue involvement is often the most important component of the infection. MR imaging is also recommended in patients who do not begin to respond after 48 hours of antibiotic therapy to exclude a subperiosteal or soft tissue abscess. It is useful in osteomyelitis involving the physis, in which adequate mapping of the infection is important to minimize physeal damage during surgical drainage.

The question of when to use MR imaging for osteomyelitis is not resolved (108). MR imaging is superior to scintigraphy in that it shows whether there are drainable collections in the bone, subperiosteal space, and soft tissues. The main advantage of scintigraphy over MR imaging is that it can show the entire skeleton. We recommend MR imaging whenever the disease is localized, and scintigraphy when the affected area cannot be defined (as in a difficult-to-examine infant or young child), or when the disease has a high likelihood of being multifocal (as in a newborn).

Disorders of the Epiphysis, Physis, Articular Cartilage, and Meniscus

MR imaging helps in the evaluation of epiphyseal separation related to birth trauma or child abuse (109,110). MR imaging also detects extension of a lateral or medial condylar fracture into the unossified epiphysis of the elbow (111–115). A patellar sleeve fracture is shown by MR imaging as a separation between the cartilage and bone of the lower pole of the patella (116). MR imaging can show occult fractures in children and adolescents; just like with infections, it is better to use MR imaging, a more specific test, whenever the symptoms are localized. On the other hand, scintigraphy is preferable when the clinical picture is less well-defined, as in the limping young child.

Repeated trauma to the physis of young gymnasts may produce focal areas of physeal widening, and sometimes transphyseal bridging. These are demonstrated well on MR images (117). Distal radial physeal dysfunction results in positive ulnar variance. In these patients, MR imaging can show associated tears of the triangular fibrocartilage complex. Other sports-related injuries can affect other physes in the same manner. Similar chronic physeal injury can be seen in ambulatory meningomyelocele patients in whom impaired sensation and continued motion result in repeated physeal damage.

In patients with a suspected posttraumatic bony bridge, MR imaging can define the size and location of the bridge, as well as the percentage of the physis affected by the abnormality (111,118,119). A 3D, fat-suppressed, spoiled gradient-recalled echo sequence provides most, if not all, of the information required to assess growth arrest (120,121). The ratio between the area of the bridge and the area of the physis can be calculated on an axial map (122), to ascertain the resectability of the bridge.

In osteochondritis dissecans, MR imaging can show whether the articular cartilage overlying the osteochondral injury is ruptured, the size of the osteochondral fragment, the stability of the fragment, and the presence of loose bodies. High-signal-intensity fluid, on T2-weighted images between the parent bone and the fragment, indicates that the fragment is unstable, even if the overlying cartilage appears to be intact (123).

Meniscal and ligamentous injuries have a similar MR imaging appearance in children and adults (124). Meniscal tears, which are usually vertical in children (125), should not be confused with the intrameniscal nutrient vessel. Meniscal vessels are horizontal, central, originate from the capsular attachment, and do not extend to the articular surface (126).

Tumors

The length of an intramedullary tumor is best depicted on T1-weighted images with a large field of view (Fig. 3-21). T1-weighted images also depict skip lesions and metastases or multifocal disease in the contralateral extremity (127). Higher-resolution postcontrast images show involvement of the epiphysis and joint space. Extension into the joint, although uncommon, is generally extrasynovial. In the knee, it is shown by MR images along the cruciate ligaments (128). Axial images show whether the lesion arises in the medullary cavity, in the surface of the bone (cortex or periosteum), or in the soft tissues. They also help detect involvement of the vessels (particularly the popliteal vessels) and of adjacent muscles (Fig. 3-21).

The dimensions of the tumor should be measured in orthogonal planes. For planning of surgery or radiation therapy, it is important to measure the distances between the tumor and the nearest articular surface, and between the tumor and the adjacent physis (129).

Risks and Limitations

There are no known harmful physiologic effects on human beings of magnetic fields as high as 10 T (most clinical magnets have field strengths ranging from 0.5 to 1.5 T (130). Switched gradient fields can produce peripheral nerve stimulation, but this is not seen in routine clinical practice, and is not considered harmful (131). The real dangers in MR imaging come from metallic devices and pieces of metal in the body (132). Pacemakers are an absolute contraindication to MR imaging. MR imaging is also contraindicated in patients with shrapnel, bullets, or other metallic objects. Most orthopaedic hardware can be imaged safely, because these devices are not ferromagnetic, and they are well-secured in the body. External fixators, however, are usually contra-indicated. Detailed information about the safety of devices and objects in the MR environment is available in the excellent publications (periodically updated) by Schellock and Kanal (133) and at their web site (http://Kanal.arad.upmc.edu/mrsafety.html). Orthopaedic hardware can cause significant artifact that limits the evaluation of adjacent tissues. The artifact is less with titanium hardware, with hollow objects, or if the orthopaedic devices are aligned with the magnetic field. Some pulse sequences minimize metallic artifacts (134).

Perhaps the greatest limitation of MR imaging is its cost (Table 3-3). The greater the field, the stronger the signal resonating from the protons, but the more expensive the equipment.

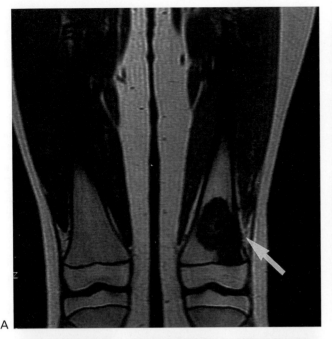

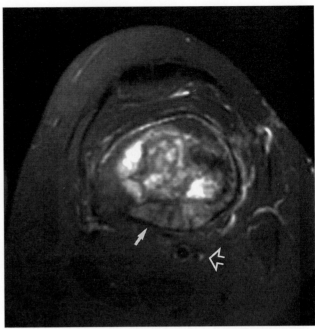

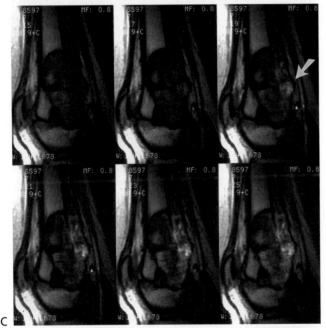

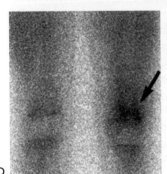

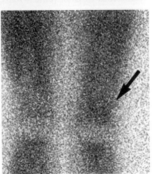

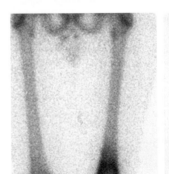

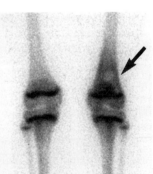

FIGURE 3-21. Osteogenic sarcoma in a 14-year-old boy evaluated by MR imaging and scintigraphy. **A:** Coronal T1-weighted image of the entire femur confirms a tumor with well-defined margins (*arrow*) and no skip metastases. The very low signal intensity area within the tumor corresponds to a cement plug after biopsy. **B:** Axial fat-suppressed, T2-weighted images show that the tumor extends posteriorly underneath the periosteum (*closed arrow*). The popliteal vessels (*open arrow*) are spared. **C:** Dynamic fast spoiled gradient echo images, obtained at 3-second intervals, show that the subperiosteal component of the lesion enhances rapidly (*arrow*), indicating persistence of active tumor in this region. This scan was performed after therapy. **D:** Thallium-201 scan before (**left**) and after (**right**) therapy shows that the intense radiotracer uptake in the tumor (*arrow*) in the initial study decreases markedly after therapy. **E:** Tc-99m methylene diphosphonate (MDP) scan after therapy shows that there is increased radiotracer uptake in the tumor (*arrow*). There is no evidence of skip metastasis, and the remainder of the study did not show metastatic disease.

TABLE 3-3. RELATIVE COSTS OF RADIOGRAPHIC PROCEDURES (NORMALIZED TO CONVENTIONAL RADIOGRAPHS)

MR	
Enhanced	8
Unenhanced	6
CT	
Enhanced	5
Unenhanced	4
Bone scintigraphy	
3-Phase with magnification	6.5
SPECT	3.5
Hip ultrasound	1.3
Radiography: 2 views of hip	1

SPECT, single-photon emission computed tomography.

Utilization Trends

MR imaging is the main cross-sectional imaging modality for evaluating the pediatric skeleton. Joint pathology, particularly in the knee, shoulder, elbow, and ankle, is almost exclusively evaluated with MR imaging. Its use in the hip is increasing. MR imaging is the most important modality for detecting tumor extent, and is increasingly used in musculoskeletal infection and trauma. In a child with complex trauma or suspected osteomyelitis needing imaging beyond radiographs, we recommend the following. If the symptoms and signs are poorly defined, or if the disease has a high likelihood of being multifocal (e.g., child abuse or multifocal osteomyelitis), scintigraphy is preferred. If the disease can be localized MR imaging is usually the best modality because of its superior resolution and its capability to show cartilage and soft tissues in addition to bone.

NUCLEAR MEDICINE

Mechanism of Contrast

Radiation emitted by a radiopharmaceutical within a patient is imaged in nuclear medicine studies. Most radiopharmaceuticals consist of a radionuclide bound to a ligand whose distribution reflects a physiologic function. The vast majority of clinical applications rely on detection of gamma rays emitted during decay of technetium-99m (Tc-99m), iodine-123 (I-123), iodine-131 (I-131), gallium-67 (Ga-67), and indium-111 (In-111) or x-rays emitted during decay of thallium-201 (Tl-201). Radionuclides that emit positrons, which then interact with free electrons in matter to produce gamma rays, are also used. Positron emission tomography (PET) uses radionuclides, such as fluorine-18 (most often bound to glucose), and isotopes of oxygen, nitrogen, and carbon to assess regional tissue physiology. The use of positron-emitting radionuclides has mostly been limited to centers with immediate access to a cyclotron. Recent improvements in regional distribution methods for these unstable short-lived radionuclides, along with advances in imaging technology, promise to greatly change the practice of nuclear medicine over the next decade.

The primary imaging instrument used in nuclear medicine is the gamma camera. In a gamma camera, scintigraphic images are produced by gamma rays or x-rays as they strike a detector. The field of view of a typical gamma camera is 40 cm × 50 cm. Dynamic images may be obtained by continuous image acquisition, before a radiopharmaceutical becomes fixed to its target tissue, or while a radiopharmaceutical is being excreted. Static images show the distribution of a radiopharmaceutical at a particular point in time. These are usually obtained after tissue fixation. Scintigraphic imaging is most often displayed two-dimensionally (planar imaging), but can also be performed in a way that enables 3D tomographic display.

Skeletal Scintigraphy

Skeletal scintigraphy is performed with Tc-99m-labeled diphosphonates. Diphosphonates are analogs of pyrophosphate, a normal constituent of bone. Within 4 hours of intravenous administration, 40% to 60% of administered radiopharmaceutical localizes in the skeleton, concentrating in amorphous calcium phosphate and crystalline hydroxyapatite. The remainder is excreted by the kidneys.

In determining the radiopharmaceutical dose to be administered for pediatric skeletal scintigraphy, the goal is to keep the child's absorbed radiation dose at a minimum, while retaining the ability to obtain a study of diagnostic quality. Pediatric doses of radiopharmaceuticals are generally calculated by adjusting recommended adult doses according to body weight or body surface area. For neonates and infants, the minimal total dose, below which a study will be inadequate, is given. The minimal total dose is determined by the type of examination, the time over which the examination is to be performed, and the characteristics of the imaging system being used (135). The units of administered doses are the curie (radioactivity of a sample decaying at a rate of 3.7×10^{10} disintegrations per second), or its newer Système Internationale (SI) equivalent, the becquerel (radioactivity of a sample decaying at a rate of 1 disintegration per second). For scintigraphy with Tc-99m methylene diphosphonate (MDP), we administer a dose of 0.2 millicuries (mCi) per kg, or 7.4 megabecquerels (MBq), per kg. The minimum dose administered is 1.0 mCi (37 MBq) when only skeletal-phase images are obtained, and 2.0 mCi (74 MBq), when multiphase imaging is indicated. The maximum administered dose is 20 mCi (740 MBq).

At our institution, simple immobilization techniques have proven sufficient, and sedation is rarely required for skeletal scintigraphy in children. This is true even in young children, provided that the imaging team takes time to gain the trust and allay the anxieties of the child and the parents.

Skeletal scintigraphy may include angiographic-phase, tissue-phase, and skeletal-phase imaging. When all three phases are obtained, the study is referred to as a three-phase bone scan. Skeletal-phase imaging is performed for all indications. The need to include radionuclide angiography- and tissue-phase imaging depends on the clinical question. A three-phase bone scan is routinely performed when musculoskeletal infection is suspected, and may help evaluate benign and malignant bone tumors and some traumatic injuries.

For radionuclide angiography, the patient is positioned so that the region of highest clinical concern is within the field of view. Recording begins immediately after the administration of a radiopharmaceutical as a rapid bolus and continues for 60 seconds. During the angiographic phase, radiopharmaceutical distribution reflects regional perfusion. Immediately following the radionuclide angiogram, static tissue-phase imaging may be performed of the regions of interest. Tissue-phase images, sometimes referred to as "blood pool images," depict tracer in the blood vessels and soft tissue. Early tracer localization in bone, particularly at sites of active bone formation, is also shown. Static skeletal-

phase imaging is performed between 2 and 4 hours after radiopharmaceutical administration, depending on the specific Tc-99m-labeled diphosphonate used. By this time the tracer has almost completely cleared from the blood and soft tissues, and is seen principally in the skeleton and, in variable amounts, in the kidneys and bladder. More delayed skeletal-phase images may be useful when clearance from the blood and soft tissues is slow. This is rare in children. The highest skeletal-phase localization of Tc-99m-labeled diphosphonates occurs in areas of high blood flow, active bone growth, and high osteoblastic activity.

Optimal performance of skeletal scintigraphy in children requires the ability to depict normal and abnormal Tc-99m-labeled diphosphonate distribution in anatomically small structures, in anatomically small regions within larger structures, and in metaphyseal bone adjacent to the highly diphosphonate-avid physis. The choice of collimator, which is the component of the gamma camera that projects the emitted gamma rays or x-rays onto the detector, is therefore extremely important. Skeletal scintigraphy of children should be performed with high-resolution or ultrahigh-resolution collimators. "All-purpose" collimators, which are appropriately used for imaging adult patients, do not provide the resolution needed for pediatric studies.

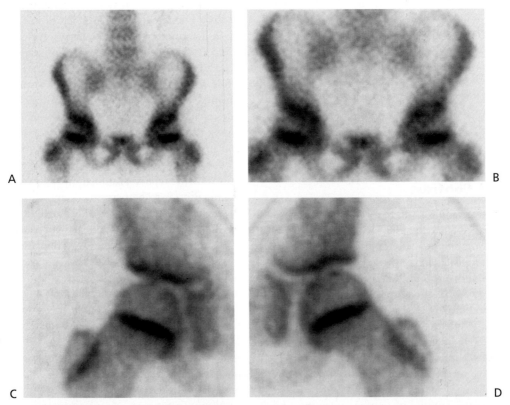

FIGURE 3-22. Comparison of high-resolution planar imaging of the pelvis without (**A**) and with (**B**) postprocess zoom, and pinhole imaging of the hips (**C,D**). Anatomic detail is best demonstrated with pinhole images, but the field of view is restricted.

Magnification is useful when resolution superior to that provided by high-resolution or ultrahigh-resolution collimators is required for skeletal-phase imaging. Two general magnification methods are available to nuclear medicine practitioners. *Electronic magnification* includes acquisition and postprocess zoom. Acquisition zoom limits an acquired image to a portion of a gamma camera's field of view, thereby concentrating more pixels on an object of interest. Postprocess zoom is performed on display systems by increasing the size, but not the number, of pixels in the central portion of a gamma camera's field of view. *Collimator magnification* involves the use of a pinhole or converging collimator. Collimator magnification, unlike electronic magnification, improves system resolution. A pinhole collimator is capable of providing substantial improvements in system resolution, whereas relatively modest gains are provided by a converging collimator (Fig. 3-22). Pinhole collimation provides the highest spatial resolution (1.5–2.0 mm) attainable in clinical nuclear medicine (136). This level of resolution is often crucial in assessing small structures, such as the femoral capital epiphyses (Figs. 3-23 and 3-24), and in evaluating metaphyseal bone abutting the physes. A pinhole

collimator is an essential component of nuclear medicine imaging systems that are used in children.

The pinhole collimator must be close to the object of interest, at or just above the skin surface, for most clinical studies. This limits the field of view and increases imaging time. Imaging a single hip using a pinhole collimator will typically require 10 to 20 minutes. In contrast, the acquisition time for an image of both hips and the entire pelvis obtained using a high-resolution parallel hole collimator is typically approximately 5 minutes. Despite this limitation, pinhole images should be obtained when high-resolution or ultrahigh-resolution planar imaging is equivocal for indicating or excluding abnormalities in small structures or metaphyseal bone. Pinhole imaging should also be strongly considered when the clinical suspicion of pathology at one of these sites is high, and high-resolution or ultrahigh-resolution planar imaging appears normal.

Using similar principles to those employed in MR imaging and CT, the gamma camera system can be rotated around the patient to obtain tomographic images. This technique, single-photon emission computed tomography (SPECT), provides better 3D lesion localization and greater

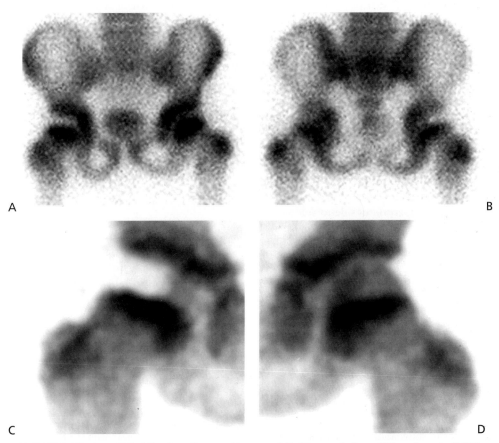

FIGURE 3-23. Legg-Calvé-Perthes disease. Absence of Tc-99m methylene diphosphonate (MDP) uptake in the right femoral capital epiphysis is identifiable on high-resolution images (**A,** anterior; **B,** posterior projection). This is shown unequivocally by anterior projection pinhole imaging (**C,** right hip; **D,** normal left hip). (From ref. 136, with permission.)

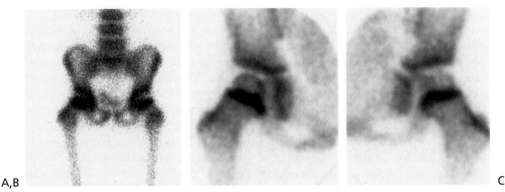

A,B   C

FIGURE 3-24. Transient synovitis with vascular tamponade. Preserved, but decreased Tc-99m methylene diphosphonate (MDP) uptake in the left femoral capital epiphysis is shown less convincingly on the high-resolution image (**A**) than with pinhole magnification imaging: normal right hip (**B**), left hip (**C**). (From ref. 136, with permission.)

contrast than does planar imaging. For evaluating complex structures, such as the spine and pelvis, the 3D properties of SPECT more than compensate for a spatial resolution slightly lower than that of planar imaging.

Familiarity with the normal distribution of Tc-99m-labeled diphosphonates, within the skeleton at different ages, is essential to differentiate normal variations from pathologic conditions (137,138). Uptake of Tc-99m diphosphonate is high in long-bone physes and in physeal equivalents of the flat bones. This high, but physiologic, uptake decreases gradually with age, but may persist even after the growth centers appear closed radiographically. A structure that has not begun ossification has no Tc-99m diphosphonate uptake. For example, absent uptake is normal (if symmetrical) in the femoral capital epiphyses during the first 6 months of life. Similarly, the tarsal navicular, which ossifies between the ages of 1 and 3.5 years in girls and between 3 and 5.5 years in boys, is also not visualized when cartilaginous; absence of uptake should not be misinterpreted for Köhler disease (130,139). Comparison of side-to-side symmetry of Tc-99m-labeled diphosphonate localization is valuable, but will not always prevent mistaking the normal for the abnormal. In the ischiopubic synchondroses, which typically ossify between the ages of 4 and 12 years, asymmetric ossification and Tc-99m-labeled diphosphonate localization common (140,141).

Main Applications

There are numerous indications for skeletal scintigraphy in children. Skeletal scintigraphy derives its value from a high sensitivity for detecting osseous pathology and an ability to evaluate the entire skeleton with relative ease.

Skeletal scintigraphy can show abnormalities within diseased or injured bone, well before radiographic changes become apparent. This is particularly important with osteomyelitis, which typically produces abnormal Tc-99m-

labeled diphosphonate uptake within 24 to 48 hours (Fig. 3-25), whereas radiographic osseous manifestations are seen after 7 to 10 days. The high sensitivity of skeletal scintigraphy enables diagnosis of avascular necrosis, detection of skeletal metastases, and identification of traumatic injuries, before radiographic manifestations develop. Among traumatic injuries, skeletal scintigraphy is most important for identifying lower-extremity injuries of toddlers and stress injuries of young athletes. A higher sensitivity of skeletal scintigraphy, compared to radiography, for rib fractures and diaphyseal injuries in abused infants and children, makes skeletal scintigraphy useful when child abuse is suspected. For this indication, it must be emphasized, however, that the radiographic skeletal survey is the imaging study of choice, because scintigraphy often fails to detect linear skull fractures and certain metaphyseal injuries. In child abuse, skeletal scintigraphy complements the radiographic skeletal

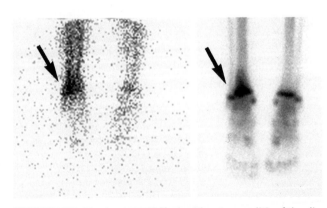

A,B

FIGURE 3-25. Twelve-year-old boy with osteomyelitis of the distal right tibia seen on a Tc-99m methylene diphosphonate (MDP) scan. **A:** Radionuclide angiogram shows increased perfusion of the entire tibia, most noticeable in the distal tibial metaphysis (*arrow*). **B:** Static image demonstrates the increased radiotracer uptake in the distal tibia compatible with osteomyelitis (*arrow*).

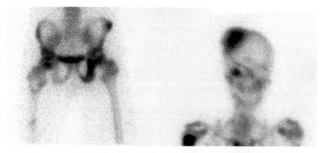

FIGURE 3-26. Metastatic osteosarcoma in a 17-year-old adolescent male. Tc-99m methylene diphosphonate (MDP) scan shows areas of increased uptake in the left ileum, left ischium, skull, face, and proximal humerus, compatible with bony metastases.

survey (142,143), being most valuable when radiographs are negative, or when the demonstration of additional injuries to those shown radiographically would significantly increase diagnostic certainty.

Skeletal scintigraphy allows evaluation of the entire body without increasing radiation exposure relative to that delivered by a limited examination. This is not the case when a radiographic examination is extended from a limited to a wide area. The ability to provide a whole-body evaluation is also an advantage of scintigraphy over MR imaging because sensitive, practical methods of evaluating the entire skeleton with a single MR imaging examination have not been established. Coupled with the high sensitivity described above, the ability to provide a whole-body evaluation has resulted in skeletal scintigraphy playing an essential role in staging and surveillance of a number of pediatric malignancies, most notably osteosarcoma, Ewing's sarcoma, and neuroblastoma (Fig 3-26). Imaging of the entire skeleton is useful when acute osteomyelitis may be multifocal, as in newborns (144,145), and in assessing some other benign conditions, such as chronic recurrent multifocal osteomyelitis. The ability to extend the examination beyond a limited area is invaluable in evaluating children with poorly localized skeletal pain or limping, and in identifying sites of pathology that present with referred pain.

The main limitation of skeletal scintigraphy is a lack of specificity. Many different bone diseases lead to increased Tc-99m-labeled diphosphonate uptake. This limitation requires that scintigraphy be interpreted with close consideration of clinical and other imaging findings. The anatomic resolution of skeletal scintigraphy is poorer than that provided by other imaging modalities. Information regarding the soft tissues is very limited with skeletal scintigraphy.

Risks

Radiopharmaceuticals administered for clinical use, including the Tc-99m-labeled diphosphonates, deliver radiation doses that are considered safe and acceptable (146). Ab-

sorbed doses vary with a patient's age and weight, physiologic status, and pathologic condition. They also vary slightly with the specific diphosphonate used.

Pediatric radiation dosimetry per unit of administered radioactivity of Tc-99m diphosphonate, as estimated by Stabin (147), is summarized in Table 3-2. The highest dose is delivered to the bone surfaces, with the actual dose varying with the abovementioned factors. For example, the bone surfaces of an infant administered our minimal dose of 1.0 mCi (37 MBq), would absorb 5.92 rads (59.2 mGy), whereas the bone surfaces of a 15-year-old weighing 50 kg would absorb 2.81 rads (28.1 mGy), following an administered dose of 10 mCi. The effective dose equivalent for the body would be 0.407 rem (4.07 mSv) for the infant and 0.33 rem (3.33 mSv) for the 15-year-old.

Utilization Trends

Skeletal scintigraphy is likely to remain a mainstay of orthopaedic diagnosis, despite advances in other imaging modalities. The complementary roles of skeletal scintigraphy and other modalities are increasingly apparent. Scintigraphy is preferable when more than a limited area must be imaged, when metallic artifacts interfere with CT or MR imaging, or when specific physiologic information is desired.

Other scintigraphic techniques may assume increasing importance. Nuclear medicine researchers have placed particular emphasis on developing radiopharmaceuticals and techniques that assess tumoral viability and chemotherapeutic response. Available methods relevant to pediatric orthopaedics include the use of Tl-201, Tc-99m-hexakis-2-methoxyisobutylisonitrile (MIBI), and [fluorine-18] fluorodeoxyglucose (FDG) in assessing skeletal malignancies, as well as I-131 or I-123 metaiodobenzylguanidine (MIBG) and In-111 octreotide for evaluating neuroblastoma. In regards to FDG, it is worth noting that increased access to FDG, and the commercial availability of gamma cameras capable of imaging both positron-emitting and conventional radiopharmaceuticals, will make PET widely available to clinical practitioners. An additional area in which considerable efforts have been applied in nuclear medicine is infection. Diagnosis of infection in bone already affected by another condition that causes abnormal uptake of Tc-99m-labeled diphosphonates can be assisted by studies performed with radiolabeled (In-111 or Tc-99m) leukocytes or Ga-67 citrate.

BONE DENSITOMETRY

Modern techniques for measuring bone density are based on measuring the attenuation of a beam of energy as it passes through bone. They include dual energy x-ray absorptiometry (DEXA), and quantitative CT (QCT). Techniques measuring radiographic attenuation mostly reflect the inorganic component (hydroxyapatite crystals) of the bone (148). Other modalities that do not use radiation are being developed. Quantitative ultrasound measures the change in velocity and energy of sound waves as they are attenuated by bone. Measurement of bone density by MR imaging, based on the magnetic susceptibility induced, is still an experimental technique (149). Bone density is frequently evaluated in adults. In children, bone densitometry is difficult because of lack of dedicated pediatric equipment and a paucity of normal data. Whether the evaluation should be of trabecular or cortical bone is not clear. Turnover is faster in trabecular than in cortical bone, but cortical bone density does not change with age.

Techniques

Dual-energy X-ray Absorptiometry

DEXA is the most common technique for measuring bone density. An x-ray tube produces a photon beam, and a computer determines the attenuation of the beam and converts the result into a value for bone mineral content or bone mineral density (150,151). The result is expressed as gm/cm^3 of ashed bone or equivalent hydroxyapatite. The study takes 2 to 15 minutes, depending on whether the whole body, the lumbar spine, or the proximal femur are examined. Sedation is often necessary in the youngest patients, because motion can increase the projected bone area by nearly 10% (41,152).

DEXA is limited because density measurements are based on a two-dimensional projection of the body, and thus depend on both the mass and the size of the bone being examined (152). Size varies considerably in children, and DEXA does not allow for bone size, which leads to significant error. Other problems include the marked variation in normal values reported in children and the variation in results due to the changing composition of bone marrow and overlying soft tissues.

Despite its limitations, the use of DEXA in children continues to grow because of its availability, low radiation dose (see below), and low cost. DEXA can measure total body fat, as well as density of bone. This is important for certain metabolic studies.

Quantitative Computerized Tomography

QCT is the most accurate technique for evaluating bone density, because it can assess both the size of a bone and its density (153). Radiographic attenuation values of the bone determined by CT scanning are compared to those of a reference phantom. QCT allows cortical and trabecular density to be measured separately, and can provide a measurement of the cross-sectional area of a vertebral body (152). QCT is generally performed in a conventional CT unit, and, therefore, unlike DEXA, does not require addi-

tional equipment purchases or siting costs. The capability of QCT to measure cortical and cancellous bone separately is important, because cortical bone density in the appendicular skeleton varies little with age, size, gender, race, or the passage of puberty. There is also abundant data about normals (154–156). QCT, however, is used less than DEXA, because of its higher cost and greater radiation dose.

Main Applications of Bone Densitometry

There is increasing interest in the clinical evaluation of bone density (150). Assessment of bone density is justified to evaluate loss or lack of bone mineral content (osteopenia). In children, this can be due to osteoporosis (lack of both collagen matrix and mineral content); rickets (osteomalacia, lack of mineral content only); or abnormal bone formation in conditions such as osteogenesis imperfecta and several chondrodysplasias (152).

It is sometimes useful to know the bone density of a patient being evaluated for scoliosis, or who has had surgery for this disease. Children often receive therapy that decreases bone mineral content, such as steroids for rheumatoid arthritis or inflammatory bowel disease. Children with eating disorders are sometimes evaluated with bone densitometry. There is great interest in identifying children who are likely to develop osteoporosis as adults; intervention may be more fruitful at a young age.

Risks, Limitations, and Utilization Trends

Radiation exposure is less with DEXA than with CT. One DEXA study results in an effective dose of 0.1 mrem (1 microSv) for lumbar spine measurements and 0.4 mrem for measurements of the entire body. QCT exposes the body to a total equivalent dose of 4–9 mrems. Although this is 10 to 20 times the DEXA dose, it is still much lower than the exposure for conventional CT or for ordinary radiographs. For reference, it is useful to consider that a child on a round-trip transcontinental flight in North America is exposed to 6 to 8 mrems of ionizing radiation (152). DEXA has become the dominant modality, because of convenience and lower radiation exposure.

RADIATION EXPOSURE: PRACTICAL ISSUES

Patients and parents frequently ask about the risks of examinations that utilize ionizing radiation (radiography, CT, nuclear medicine). It is important for orthopaedic surgeons to understand these risks, and to communicate them clearly. In order to do this, the physician must be familiar with the radiation effects, the way in which radiation dose is measured, and the way in which radiation risks are estimated and prevented.

Radiation Effects

The effects of radiation are classified as stochastic or nonstochastic (or deterministic). Stochastic effects include carcinogenesis and mutagenesis; their *probability of occurrence* is a function of dose, and any radiation exposure increases risk. For nonstochastic effects, *severity* of the effect varies with dose; examples include cataract formation, bone marrow cellular depletion, and nonmalignant skin damage. The threshold for nonstochastic effects is higher than would be expected to be delivered with diagnostic examinations.

When a patient or parent asks whether an examination is safe, they are primarily asking about risk of cancer, which is the main late somatic effect of radiation, and the risk of genetic mutations. The most common radiation-induced malignancies are leukemia, thyroid, and lung in both sexes, and the breast in women. The minimum latent period following radiation exposure is 2 to 10 years. The data from radiation carcinogenesis comes from exposure to large doses such as nuclear accidents; how this data can be extrapolated to clinical data is unclear.

Dosimetry

Radiation dosimetry is described in either traditional units or SI units. The traditional unit, by which radiation absorbed by tissue is quantified, is the rad. The SI unit for absorbed dose is the gray (Gy), which is equivalent to 100 rads. Because the biological effectiveness of the various types of ionizing radiation differs, the concept of dose equivalent has been introduced to quantify radiation dose. The traditional unit for dose equivalent is the rem, and SI unit is the sievert (Sv). For diagnostic imaging, the dose equivalent in rems or sieverts is numerically equal to the absorbed dose in rads or grays (157).

Radiation effect varies according to the tissues exposed. Some tissues, such as the breasts and gonads, are much more susceptible to radiation damage than the tissues of the extremities (157). Children are more susceptible to the deleterious effects of radiation than are adults. Additionally, the potential for damage from a radiation dose distributed uniformly over the entire body, as resulted from atomic bomb detonations, is greater than that of the same dose received by only a part of the body, as occurs with diagnostic radiographs. Finally, a given dose has less potential for damage when absorbed over months or years, than when absorbed over seconds, minutes, or hours.

Relationship between Radiation Dose and Effect

Based on epidemiological studies of groups such as survivors of the atomic bombs dropped during World War II, the risk of developing a fatal malignancy secondary to low doses of radiation has been estimated as 5% per Sv (0.05% per rem) and the risk for developing a nonfatal malignancy has been estimated as 1% per Sv (0.01% per rem) (158,159). For children, the risk of developing a fatal malignancy may be 10% per Sv (160). The mutagenic potential of radiation is difficult to assess because of a fairly high rate of spontaneously occurring mutations in man; the estimated risk of a severe genetic effect in all succeeding generations has been estimated as 1% per Sv (0.01% per rem) (158,159). Because the general population includes individuals who are past their reproductive years, this risk is higher in children. It is important to emphasize that although the above numbers sound precise, they are rough approximations of risk that have been derived from methods in which the level of uncertainty is high.

Radiation Exposure and Diagnostic Examinations

Table 3-1 provides entrance doses at our institution for some commonly performed studies. It can be readily seen that the risk of these studies is small. This is made more apparent when it is noted that the risk estimations discussed above are based on uniform radiation of the entire body. The exposure to structures outside the x-ray beam (e.g., the lungs of a child whose foot is being imaged), and of internal structures within the x-ray beam, are less than the reported skin entry dose. Exposure from nuclear medicine studies is expressed in terms of the radiation to specific structures, and in terms of the equivalent dose.

When communicating risks of radiation to patients or their parents, it is essential that they understand the rationale for performing an examination, and how the results of the examination are to be used in guiding management. They need to be aware of the risk implied by not obtaining the examination, so that this risk can be weighed against that of radiation. The patient and/or parent should also be made aware that, although many epidemiological and animal studies have assessed the risk of low-level radiation, none is conclusive, and that whatever risk assessment is provided is an opinion. Sometimes, it is useful to put the risk assessment in the context of easily comprehended numbers or daily risks. Using the risk estimations described previously, each 0.00001 Sv (10 uSv or 1 mrem) dose equivalent delivered to a child could be considered to impart a one in one million risk of death from fatal malignancy. This is roughly equivalent to the risk of death from driving 47 miles by car (160). It also is useful to compare radiation related to diagnostic imaging with that of natural background radiation resulting from cosmic radiation, radioactive deposits within the earth surface, radon gas, and other sources. Yearly average background radiation exposure in the United States is approximately 0.003 Sv (3 mSv or 300 mrem). This is about equivalent to what an adult might receive from 15 to 20 chest radiographs for which the dose equivalent range is 0.15 to 0.20 mSv (15 to 20 mrem) (161). The risk of developing cancer, and dying as a result of irradiation received from a chest radiograph, is equivalent to the risk of death by cancer from flying 1000 miles by jet or living two months in Denver (because of the increased exposure to solar irradiation at higher altitudes) (162,163). The risk from diagnostic studies involving the appendicular skeleton is likewise low.

The effects of examinations that result in irradiation of the pelvis or breasts may be more significant; these studies should be requested with more caution. According to the National Radiological Protection Board of the United Kingdom, one x-ray of the hip, for example, is equivalent to 7 weeks of natural background radiation. An x-ray of the pelvis is equivalent to 4 months, and an x-ray of the lumbar spine is equivalent to 7 months. A CT of the abdomen and pelvis approximates 4.5 years of natural background radiation [http://www.nrpb.org.uk/Qmedical.htm].

One study of scoliosis patients indicated that each patient received a mean of 14.1 single x-ray exposures over a mean of 44 months. The ovaries received a mean total cumulative dose of 183 uSv over the time period study, indicating that an improvement in ovarian protection needs to be made (164). In a study of dose distribution to the spine in children, lumbar spine examinations caused the highest mean entrance surface doses (2.6 mGy, anteroposterior projection; 6.7 mGy, lateral projection), with the female gonads receiving the highest dose. The mean entrance surface doses were lower for thoracic spine examinations (2.1 mGy, frontal view; 6.1 mGy, lateral view), with the breasts, thyroid, lungs, and esophagus receiving the highest dose (165). In a study of adolescents with idiopathic scoliosis, it was found that a three- to sevenfold reduction in cumulative doses to the thyroid gland and female breast could be achieved by replacing anteroposterior views with posteroanterior views. This leads to a three- to fourfold reduction in the lifetime risk of breast cancer, and halves the lifetime risk of thyroid cancer (166).

Practical Steps to Reduce Radiation Exposure

The presence of some risk, and an inability to precisely quantify that risk, requires that every effort be made to limit the potential for radiation effects. There are many concrete steps that physicians can take in order to reduce radiation risks and damage to their patients. The best way to reduce radiation exposure from diagnostic studies is to avoid unnecessary examinations. If the study is indicated, however, the main goal should be to maximize the diagnostic information. Obtaining a suboptimal study to reduce exposure may require a repeat examination and defeat the effort to minimize radiation dose. Imaging teams that deal with children need to be adept at immobilization techniques to prevent unnecessary exam repetition. X-ray beams should be restricted to the area of interest. Gonadal shielding should

be carefully positioned for radiographic studies in which the gonads are within the radiated field (unless this would obscure the area of clinical concern), or outside, but within 5 cm of the radiated field.

Proper use of fluoroscopy reduces dosage to patients and operators. Use of the smallest field possible reduces overexposure to adjacent areas of the patient's body, and reduces scattered radiation, producing higher-quality images. The greater the distance between the patient and the fluoroscopic x-ray source, the greater the decrease in radiation dosage to the patient. Radiation dosage can also be reduced by decreasing the distance between the patient's body and the image receptor/intensifier. Unfortunately, this creates a greater amount of scattered radiation, which results in poorer image quality. Reduction of beam-on time also reduces dosage to the patient. Short and intermittent, rather than continuous and extended, exposures should be used. This is facilitated by systems that can display the last image of the patient, even after the beam has been disengaged. Finally, magnification can be both useful and necessary, but does contribute to a higher dosage. Electronic magnification causes less radiation dosage than geometric magnification (167).

Occupational radiation exposure is of great concern to orthopaedic surgeons who may have to use lengthy fluoroscopic guidance during complex surgical cases. The dose to an individual standing 1 meter from the patient is approximately 0.02% of the entrance dose to the patient, or 0.3 to 0.9 mrad (0.003 to 0.009 mGy) per minute (168). Aprons reduce radiation levels by a factor of 20 to 100. Because radiation intensity falls off with the square of the distance, any surgeon not involved in directly holding the patient can reduce the exposure by a factor of 4, simply by stepping back 2 m from the fluoroscopic unit. Direct exposure to the hands can result in exposures of 40 to 100 rads (0.4 to 1 Gy). In order to reduce exposure, the surgeon's hands should not be in the field when the beam is on, and, when possible, should be kept on the exit side of the patient. Fluoroscopy is not contraindicated during pregnancy, but every possible precaution to minimize radiation to the conceptus should be taken, including the use of double aprons, and strict monitoring of exposure.

CT examinations deliver high doses of radiation. Because a higher beam energy increases the dose, the peak kilovoltage should be kept at appropriate and limited levels. The type of filter used in the x-ray beam, collimation of the x-ray beam, reducing the number and spacing of adjacent sections, and allowing more statistical noise can also reduce the patient dose, but often at the expense of image quality (167).

SEDATION FOR IMAGING

Most imaging procedures require patients to remain still. MR imaging, for example, requires the child to remain still for 45 minutes to an hour. In most institutions, sedation is performed routinely for all MR imaging, for most CT studies, and for some nuclear medicine examinations and bone density studies of children under the age of 5 years. General radiography and ultrasonography seldom require sedation.

Close monitoring of the sedated child during the procedure is essential. This requires pulse oximetry, electrocardiographic monitoring, and, sometimes, capnometry. When performing MR imaging, it is important to verify that all monitoring devices are MR-compatible, in order to avoid burns (from heating of the wires) or accidents. Fiberoptic systems are being increasingly used, in order to avoid the risk of these complications.

Sedation is performed under strict compliance with the guidelines of the American Academy of Pediatrics (169–172). A limited sedation formulary facilitates reproducibility, familiarity with the medications and their complications, and quality control. Chloral hydrate is commonly used for children less than 1 year of age; intravenous sodium pentobarbital is used for older children. The sedation protocol of the Department of Radiology at Children's Hospital in Boston includes the following recommendations: For children under 1 year of age, oral chloral hydrate is given in a dose of 50 mg/kg, repeated after 30 minutes, if needed. In other institutions, doses in the 80 to 100 mg/kg range (maximum, 2.5 g) have given a 96% success rate for pediatric MR imaging (173–175). For children 1 to 5 years old, intravenous sedation is recommended, because it is reliable, fast, and easily controlled. Our protocol includes diluted sodium pentobarbital at a dose of 3 to 6 mg/kg (maximum, 200 mg). In general, intravenous sedatives are administered in small increments, in order to avoid oversedation. If the patient is not adequately sedated after receiving the total of 6 mg/kg of sodium pentobarbital, an additional 2 mcg/kg of fentanyl may be administered intravenously.

References

Radiographic Techniques: Plain Radiographs, Arthrography, Conventional Tomography, Computed Tomography

1. Ogden J. Anatomy and physiology of skeletal development. In: Ogden J, ed. *Skeletal injury in the child*. Philadelphia: WB Saunders, 1990:23.
2. Kricun M. Red-yellow marrow conversion: its effect on the location of some solitary bone lesions. *Skeletal Radiol* 1985;14:10.
3. Cohen MD. A review of the toxicity of nonionic contrast agents in children. *Investigative Radiology* 1993;28[Suppl 5]:S87.
4. American College of Radiology. *Manual on iodinated contrast material*. Reston, VA: American College of Radiology, 1991.
5. Shehadi WH. Death following intravascular administration of contrast media. *Acta Radiol [Diagn] (Stockh)* 1985;26:457.
6. Obermann WR , Bloem JL, Hermans J. Knee arthrography: comparison of iotrolan and ioxaglate sodium meglumine. *Radiology* 1989;173:197.
7. Caffey J, Madell SH, Royer C, et al. Ossification of the distal femoral epiphysis. *J Bone Joint Surg Am* 1958;40:647.
8. Ogden J. Radiology of postnatal skeletal development: X. Patella and tibial tuberosity. *Skeletal Radiol* 1984;11:246.
9. Shopfner C, Coin C. Effect of weight-bearing on the appearance and development of the secondary calcaneal epiphysis. *Radiology* 1966;86:201.
10. Lawson JP. Symptomatic radiographic variants in extremities. *Radiology* 1985;157:625.
11. Laor T, Jaramillo D. Metaphyseal abnormalities in children: pathophysiology and radiologic appearance. *AJR Am J Roentgenol* 1993;151:1029.
12. Ecklund K, Laor T, Goorin AM , et al. Methotrexate osteopathy in patients with osteosarcoma. *Radiology* 1997;202:543.
13. Keats T, Joyce J. Metaphyseal cortical irregularities in children. *Skeletal Radiol* 1984;12:112.
14. Yamazaki T, Maruoka S, Takahashi S, et al. MR findings of avulsive cortical irregularities of the distal femur. *Skel Radiol* 1995;24:43.
15. Schmidt H Freyschmidt J. *Köhler/Zimmer Borderlands of normal and early pathologic findings in skeletal radiography*, 4th ed. Stuttgart: Thieme, 1993.
16. Godderidge C. *Pediatric imaging*. Philadelphia: WB Saunders, 1995.
17. Laor T, Jaramillo D, Oestreich AE. Musculoskeletal system. In: Kirks DR, Griscom NT, eds. *Practical pediatric imaging: diagnostic radiology of infants and children*. 3rd ed. Philadelphia: Lippincott-Raven, 1998:327.
18. Greulich W, Pyle S. *Radiographic atlas of skeletal development of the hand and wrist*, 2nd ed. Stanford: Stanford University Press, 1959.
19. Hoerr N, Pyle S, Francis C. *Radiographic atlas of skeletal development of the foot and ankle*. Springfield, IL: Charles C Thomas, 1962.
20. Pyle S, Hoerr N. *A radiographic standard of reference for the growing knee*. Springfield, IL: Charles C Thomas, 1969.
21. Sontag L, Snell D, Anderson M. Rate of appearance of ossification centers from birth to the age of five years. *Am J Dis Child* 1939;58:949.
22. Ontell FK, Ivanovic M, Ablin DS, et al. Bone age in children of diverse ethnicity [see comments]. *Am J Roentgenol* 1996;167:1395.
23. Loder R, Estle D, Morrison K, et al. Applicability of the Greulich and Pyle skeletal age standards to black and white children of today. *AJDC* 1993;147:1329.
24. Shaikh AH, Rikhasor RM, Qureshi AM. Determination of skeletal age in children aged 8–18 years. *J Pak Med Assoc* 1998;48:104.
25. Groell R, Lindbichler F, Riepl T, et al. The reliability of bone age determination in central European children using the Greulich and Pyle method. *Br J Radiol* 1999;72:461.
26. King DG, Steventon DM, O'Sullivan MP, et al. Reproducibility of bone ages when performed by radiology registrars: an audit of Tanner and Whitehouse II versus Greulich and Pyle methods. *Br J Radiol* 1994;67:848.
27. Bull RK, Edwards PD, Kemp PM, et al. Bone age assessment: a large scale comparison of the Greulich and Pyle, and Tanner and Whitehouse (TW2) methods. *Arch Dis Child* 1999;81:172.
28. Tanner JM, Whitehouse RH, Cameron N, et al. *Assessment of skeletal maturity and prediction of adult height (TW2 method)*, 2nd ed. London: Academic Press, 1983.
29. Tanner JM, Gibbons RD. A computerized image analysis system for estimating Tanner-Whitehouse 2 bone age. *Hormone Res* 1994;42:282.

30. Kahleyss S, Hoepffner W, Keller E, Willgerodt H. [The determination of bone age by the Greulich-Pyle and Tanner-Whitehouse methods as a basis for the growth prognosis of tall-stature girls]. *Padiatr Grenzgeb* 1990;29:137.

31. Kleinman PK. Skeletal imaging strategies. In: Kleinman PK, ed. *Diagnostic imaging of child abuse*. St. Louis: Mosby, 1998:237.

32. Belanger PL. Quality assurance and skeletal survey standards. In: Kleinman PK, ed. *Diagnostic imaging of child abuse*. St. Louis: Mosby, 1998:418.

33. Kottamasu SR, Kuhns LR, Stringer DA. Pediatric musculoskeletal computed radiography. *Pediatr Radiol* 1997;27:563.

34. Kottamasu SR, Kuhns LR. Musculoskeletal computed radiography in children: scatter reduction and improvement in bony trabecular sharpness using air gap placement of the imaging plate. *Pediatr Radiol* 1997;27:119.

35. Huang HK. Display, picture archiving and communicating systems, and teleradiology. *Acad Radiol* 1995;2[Suppl 2]:S103.

36. Huang HK, Wong ST, Pietka E. Medical image informatics infrastructure design and applications. *Med Inform Lond* 1997;22:279.

37. Aliabadi P, Baker ND, Jaramillo D. Hip arthrography, aspiration, block, and bursography. *Radiol Clin North Am* 1998;36:673.

38. Kaniklides C. *Diagnostic radiology in Legg-Calvé-Perthes disease*. Uppsala: Uppsala University, 1996.

39. Wilkinson R. Hip arthrography in children. In: Dalinka M, ed. *Arthrography*. New York: Springer-Verlag, 1980:119.

40. Ozonoff M. *The hip. Pediatric orthopedic radiology*, 2nd ed. Philadelphia: W.B. Saunders, 1992:164.

41. Harcke HT. Imaging techniques and applications. In: Morrissy RT, Weinstein SL, eds. *Lovell & Winter's Pediatric Orthopaedics*, 4th ed, vol. 1. Philadelphia: Lippincott-Raven, 1996:25.

42. Lonnerholm T. Arthrography of the hip in children; technique, normal anatomy and findings in unstable hip joints. *Acta Radiol* 1980;21:279.

43. Drummond D, O'Donnell J, Breed A, et al. Arthrography in the evaluation of congenital dislocation of the hip. *Clin Orthop* 1989;243:148.

44. MacEwen GD, Mason B. Evaluation and treatment of congenital dislocation of the hip in infants. *Orthop Clin North Am* 1988;19:815.

45. Ponseti IV. Morphology of the acetabulum in congenital dislocation of the hip. *J Bone Joint Surg Am* 1978;60:586.

46. Herring JA. The treatment of Legg-Calvé-Perthes disease. *J Bone Joint Surg Am* 1994;76:448.

47. Gershuni DH, Axer A, Hendel D. Arthrographic findings in Legg-Calvé-Perthes disease and transient synovitis of the hip. *J Bone Joint Surg Am* 1978;60:457.

48. Kamegaya M, Moriya H, Tsuchiya K, et al. Arthrography of early Perthes' disease; swelling of the ligamentum teres as a cause of subluxation. *J Bone Joint Surg Br* 1989;71:413.

49. Reinker KA. Early diagnosis and treatment of hinge abduction in Legg-Perthes disease. *J Ped Orthop* 1996;163:3.

50. Gallagher J, Weiner D, Cook A. When is arthrography indicated in Legg-Calve-Perthes disease? *J Bone Joint Surg Am* 1983;65:900.

51. Chung T, Kirks DR. Techniques. In: Kirks DR, Griscom NT, eds. *Practical pediatric imaging: diagnostic radiology of infants and children*, 3rd ed. Philadelphia: Lippincott-Raven, 1998:1.

52. White K. Helical/spiral CT scanning: a pediatric radiology perspective. *Pediatr Radiol* 1996;26:5.

53. Link TM, Meier N, Rummeny EJ, et al. Artificial spine fractures: detection with helical and conventional CT. *Radiology* 1996;198:515.

54. Eggli KD, King SH, Boal DKB, et al. Low-dose CT of developmental dysplasia of the hip after reduction: diagnostic accuracy and dosimetry. *Am J Roentgenol* 1994;163:1441.

55. Waters PM, Smith GR, Jaramillo D. Glenohumeral deformity secondary to brachial plexus birth palsy. *J Bone Joint Surg Am* 1998;80:668.

56. Ruby L, Mital MA, O'Connor J, et al. Anteversion of the femoral neck: comparison of methods of measurements in patients. *J Bone Joint Surg Am* 1979;61:46.

57. Tomczak RJ, Guenther KP, Rieber A, et al. MR imaging measurement of the femoral antetorsional angle as a new technique: comparison with CT in children and adults. *Am J Roentgenol* 1997;168:791.

58. Ritter MA, DeRosa GP, Babcock JL. Tibial torsion? *Clin Orthop* 1976;120:159.

59. Staheli LT, Engel GM. Tibial torsion: a method of assessment and a survey of normal children. *Clin Orthop* 1972;86:183.

60. Reikeras O, Hoiseth A. Torsion of the leg determined by computed tomography. *Acta Orthop Scand* 1989;60:330.

61. Leonard MA. The inheritance of tarsal coalition and its relationship to spastic flat foot. *J Bone Joint Surg Br* 1974;56:520.

62. Laor T. Helical CT applications in musculoskeletal disorders. In: Marilyn J, Siegel MD, eds. *Special course in pediatric radiology: current concepts in body imaging at the millennium*. Chicago, 1999:247.

63. Wechsler RJ, Schweitzer ME, Deely DM, et al. Tarsal coalition: depiction and characterization with CT and MR imaging. *Radiology* 1994;193:447.

64. Clarke DM. Multiple tarsal coalitions in the same foot. *J Pediatr Orthop* 1997;17:777.

65. Emery KH, Bisset GS, Johnson ND, et al. Tarsal coalition: a blinded comparison of MRI and CT. *Pediatr Radiol* 1998;28:612.

Ultrasonography

66. Erickson SJ. High-resolution imaging of the musculoskeletal system. *Radiology* 1997;205:593.

67. Merritt C. Physics of ultrasound. In: Rumack C, Wilson S, Charboneau J, eds. *Diagnostic ultrasound*, vol. 1. St. Louis: Mosby–Year Book, 1998:3.

68. Grissom L, Harcke HT. The pediatric hip. In: Rumack C, Wilson S, Charboneau J, eds. *Diagnostic ultrasound*, vol. 2. St. Louis: Mosby–Year Book, 1998:1799.

69. Graf R. Advantages and disadvantages of various access routes in sonographic diagnosis of dysplasia and luxation in the infant hip. *J Pediatr Orthop B* 1997;6:248.

70. Share JC, Teele RL. Ultrasonography of the infant hip: a practical approach. *Appl Radiol* 1992:27.

71. Graf R, Schuler P. *Sonography of the infant hip: an atlas*. Weinheim: VCH Verlagsgesellschaft, 1986.

72. Graf R. *Guide to sonography of the infant hip*. New York: Thieme, 1987.

73. Graf R, Fronhofer G. [Redefinition of the proximal perichondrium and perichondrial gap in hip ultrasound imaging.] *Orthopade* 1997;26:1057.

74. Harcke HT, Lee MS, Sinning L, et al. Ossification center of the infant hip: sonographic and radiographic correlation. *Am J Roentgenol* 1986;147:317.

75. Harcke HT, Grissom LE. Performing dynamic sonography of the infant hip. *Am J Roentgenol* 1990;155:837.

76. Marks DS, Clegg J, al-Chalabi AN. Routine ultrasound screening for neonatal hip instability. Can it abolish late-presenting congenital dislocation of the hip? *J Bone Joint Surg Br* 1994;76:534.

77. Harcke HT. Screening newborns for developmental dysplasia of the hip: role of sonography. *Am J Roentgenol* 1994;162:395.

78. Bearcroft P, Berman L, Robinson A, Butler G. Vascularity of the neonatal femoral head: in vivo demonstration with Power Doppler US. *Radiology* 1996;200:209.

79. Miralles M, Gonzalez G, Pulpeiro JR, et al. Sonography of the painful hip in children: 500 consecutive cases. *Am J Roentgenol* 1989;152:579.

80. Strouse PJ, DiPietro MA, Adler RS. Pediatric hip effusions: evaluation with power Doppler sonography. *Radiology* 1998; 206:731.

81. Mah ET, LeQuesne GW, Gent RJ, Paterson DC. Ultrasonic features of acute osteomyelitis in children [see comments]. *J Bone Joint Surg Br* 1994;76:969.

82. Bureau NJ, Chhem RK, Cardinal E. Musculoskeletal infections: US manifestations [In Process Citation]. *Radiographics* 1999; 19:1585.

Magnetic Resonance Imaging

83. Balter S. An introduction to the physics of magnetic resonance imaging. *Radiographics* 1987;7:371.

84. Nitz WR. MR imaging: acronyms and clinical applications. *Eur Radiol* 1999;9:979.

85. Bashir A, Gray ML, Boutin RD, et al. Glycosaminoglycan in articular cartilage: in vivo assessment with delayed Gd(DTPA)2-enhanced MR imaging. *Radiology* 1997;205:551.

86. Prince MR. Contrast-enhanced MR angiography: theory and optimization. *Magn Reson Imaging Clin North Am* 1998;6:257.

87. Bonnerot V, Sebag G, Montalembert MD, et al. Gadolinium-DOTA enhanced MRI of painful osseous crises in children with sickle cell anemia. *Pediatr Radiol* 1994;24:92.

88. Jaramillo D, Shapiro F. Growth cartilage: normal appearance, variants and abnormalities. *Magn Reson Imaging Clin North Am* 1998;6:455.

89. Barnewolt CE, Shapiro F, Jaramillo D. Normal gadolinium-enhanced MR images of the developing appendicular skeleton: Part I. Cartilaginous epiphysis and physis. *Am J Roentgenol* 1997;169:183.

90. Chung T, Jaramillo D. Normal maturing distal tibia and fibula: changes with age at MR Imaging. *Radiology* 1995;194:227

91. Babyn PS, Ranson M, McCarville ME. Normal bone marrow: signal characteristics and fatty conversion. *Magn Reson Imaging Clin North Am* 1998;6:473.

92. Suzuki S, Kashiwagi N, Seto Y, et al. Location of the femoral head in developmental dysplasia of the hip: three-dimensional evaluation by means of magnetic resonance image. *J Pediatr Orthop* 1999;19:88.

93. McNally EG, Tasker A, Benson MK. MRI after operative reduction for developmental dysplasia of the hip [see comments]. *J Bone Joint Surg Br* 1997;79:724.

94. Kashiwagi N, Suzuki S, Kasahara Y, et al. Prediction of reduction in developmental dysplasia of the hip by magnetic resonance imaging. *J Pediatr Orthop* 1996;16:254.

95. Suzuki S. Deformity of the pelvis in developmental dysplasia of the hip: three-dimensional evaluation by means of magnetic resonance image. *J Pediatr Orthop* 1995;15:812.

96. Jaramillo D, Villegas-Medina OL, Doty DK, et al. Gadolinium-enhanced MR imaging demonstrates abduction-caused hip ischemia and its reversal in piglets. *Am J Roentgenol* 1996;166: 879.

97. Jaramillo D, Villegas-Medina O, Laor T, et al. Gadolinium-enhanced MR imaging of pediatric patients after reduction of dysplastic hips: assessment of femoral head position, factors impeding reduction, and femoral head ischemia. *Am J Roentgenol* 1998;170:1633.

98. Bos CFA, Bloem JL, Bloem RM. Sequential magnetic resonance imaging in Perthes disease. *J Bone Joint Surg Br* 1991;73: 219.

99. Jaramillo D, Kasser JR, Villegas-Medina OL, et al. Cartilaginous abnormalities and growth disturbances in Legg-Calvé-Perthes disease: evaluation with MR imaging. *Radiology* 1995;197:767.

100. Ducou le Pointe H, Haddad S, Silberman B, et al. Legg-Perthes-Calvé disease: staging by MRI using gadolinium. *Pediatr Radiol* 1994;24:88.

101. Sebag G, Pointe HDL, Klein I, et al. Dynamic gadolinium-enhanced subtraction MR imaging—a simple technique for the early diagnosis of Legg-Calve-Perthes disease: preliminary results. *Pediatr Radiol* 1997;27:216.

102. Sebag GH. Disorders of the hip. *Magn Reson Imaging Clin North Am* 1998;6:627.

103. Jaramillo D, Galen TA, Winalski CS, et al. Legg-Calve-Perthes disease: MR imaging evaluation during manual positioning of the hip—comparison with conventional arthrography. *Radiology* 1999;212:519.

104. Mazur J, Ross G, Cummings R, et al. Usefulness of magnetic resonance imaging for the diagnosis of acute musculoskeletal infections in children. *J Pediatr Orthop* 1995;15:144.

105. Dangman B, Hoffer F, Rand F, et al. Osteomyelitis in children: gadolinium enhanced MR imaging. *Radiology* 1992;182:743.

106. Gylys-Morin VM. MR imaging of pediatric musculoskeletal inflammatory and infectious disorders. *Magn Reson Imaging Clin North Am* 1998;6:537.

107. Jaramillo D, Treves ST, Kasser JR, et al. Osteomyelitis and septic arthritis in children: appropriate use of imaging to guide therapy. *Am J Roentgenol* 1995;165:399.

108. Harcke HT. Role of imaging in musculoskeletal infections in children [Editorial]. *J Pediatr Orthop* 1995;15:141.

109. Lazar RD, Waters PM, Jaramillo D. The use of ultrasonography in the diagnosis of occult fracture of the radial neck. A case report. *J Bone Joint Surg Am* 1998;80:1361.

110. Nimkin K, Kleinman PK, Teeger S, et al. Distal humeral physeal injuries in child abuse: MR imaging and ultrasound findings. *Pediatr Radiol* 1995;25:562.

111. Jaramillo D, Hoffer F, Shapiro F, et al. MR imaging of fractures of the growth plate. *Am J Roentgenol* 1990;155:1261.

112. Jaramillo D, Hoffer FA. Cartilaginous epiphysis and growth plate: normal and abnormal MR imaging findings. *Am J Roentgenol* 1992;158:1105.

113. Beltran J, Rosenberg ZS, Kawelblum M, et al. Pediatric elbow fractures: MR evaluation. *Skeletal Radiol* 1994;23:277.

114. Beltran J, Rosenberg ZS. MR imaging of pediatric elbow fractures. *MRI Clin North Am* 1997;5:567.

115. Gordon I, Peters A, Gutman A, et al. Tc-99m bone scans are more sensitive than I-123 MIBG scans for bone imaging in neuroblastoma. *J Nucl Med* 1990;31:129.

116. Bates GD, Hresko MT, Jaramillo D. Patellar sleeve fracture: demonstration with MR imaging. *Radiology* 1994;193:825.

117. Shih C, Chang C, Penn I, et al. Chronically stressed wrists in adolescent gymnasts: MR imaging appearance. *Radiology* 1995; 195:855.

118. Rogers L, Poznanski A. Imaging of epiphyseal injuries. *Radiology* 1994;191:297.

119. Havranek P, Lizler J. Magnetic resonance imaging in the evaluation of partial growth arrest after physeal injuries in children. *J Bone Joint Surg Am* 1991;73:1234.

120. Disler DG. Fat-suppressed three-dimensional spoiled gradient-recalled MR imaging: assessment of articular and physeal hyaline cartilage. *Am J Roentgenol* 1997;169:1117.

121. Borsa JJ, Peterson HA, Ehman RL. MR imaging of physeal bars. *Radiology* 1996;199:683.

122. Craig JG, Cramer KE, Cody DD, et al. Premature partial closure and other deformities of the growth plate: MR imaging and three-dimensional modeling. *Radiology* 1999;210:835.

123. De Smet A, Fisher DA, Graf BK, et al. Osteochondritis dissecans of the knee: value of MR imaging in determining lesion stability and the presence of articular cartilage defects. *Am J Roentgenol* 1990;155:549.

124. Zobel MS, Borrello JA, Siegel MJ, et al. Pediatric knee MR imaging: patterns of injuries in the immature skeleton. *Radiology* 1994;190:397.

125. Busch MT. Meniscal injuries in children and adolescents. *Clin Sports Med* 1990;9:661.

126. Al-Otaibi L, Siegel MJ. The pediatric knee. *Magn Reson Imaging Clin North Am* 1998;6:643.

127. Laor T, Chung T, Hoffer F, et al. Musculoskeletal magnetic resonance imaging: how we do it. *Ped Radiol* 1996;26:695.

128. Schima W, Amann G, Stiglbauer R, et al. Preoperative staging of osteosarcoma: efficacy of MR imaging in detecting joint involvement. *Am J Roentgenol* 1994;163:1171.

129. Jaramillo D, Laor T, Gebhardt MC. Pediatric musculoskeletal neoplasms. Evaluation with MR imaging. *Magn Reson Imaging Clin North Am* 1996;4:749.

130. Budinger TF. MR safety: past, present, and future from a historical perspective. *Magn Reson Imaging Clin North Am* 1998;6:701.

131. Schaefer DJ. Safety aspects of switched gradient fields. *Magn Reson Imaging Clin North Am* 1998;6:731.

132. Price RR. The AAPM/RSNA physics tutorial for residents. MR imaging safety considerations. Radiological Society of North America. *Radiographics* 1999;19:1641.

133. Shellock FG, Kanal E. *Magnetic resonance, bioeffects, safety, and patient management.* Philadelphia: Lippincott-Raven, 1994.

134. Eustace S, Shah B, Mason M. Imaging orthopedic hardware with an emphasis on hip prostheses. *Orthop Clin North Am*, 1998;29:67.

Nuclear Medicine

135. Treves ST. *Pediatric nuclear medicine*, 2nd ed. New York: Springer-Verlag, 1995.

136. Connolly LP, Treves ST, Connolly SA, et al. Pediatric skeletal scintigraphy: applications of pinhole magnification. *Radiographics* 1998;18:341.

137. Connolly L, Treves ST. *Pediatric skeletal scintigraphy with multimodality imaging correlations.* New York: Springer-Verlag, 1997.

138. Hahn K, Fischer S, Gordon I. *Atlas of bone scintigraphy in the developing paediatric skeleton.* Berlin: Springer-Verlag, 1993.

139. Connolly L, Treves ST. *Pediatric skeletal scintigraphy.* New York: Springer-Verlag, 1998.

140. Cawley KA, Dvorak AD, Wilmot MD. Normal anatomic variant scintigraphy for the ischiopubic synchondrosis. *J Nucl Med* 1983;24:14.

141. Kloiber R, Pavlosky W, Portner O, et al. Bone scintigraphy of hip joint effusions in children. *Am J Roentgenol* 1983;140:995.

142. Nimkin K, Kleinman PK. Imaging of child abuse. *Pediatr Clin North Am* 1997;44:615.

143. Conway JJ, Collins M, Tanz RR, et al. The role of bone scintigraphy in detecting child abuse. *Semin Nucl Med* 1993;23:321.

144. Aigner RM, Fueger GF, Ritter G. Results of three-phase bone scintigraphy and radiography in 20 cases of neonatal osteomyelitis. *Nucl Med Commun* 1996;17:20.

145. Bressler E, Conway J, Weiss S. Neonatal osteomyelitis examined by bone scintigraphy. *Radiology* 1984;152:685.

146. Adelstein S. Radiation risk. In: Treves ST, ed. *Pediatric nuclear medicine*, 2nd ed. New York: Springer-Verlag, 1995:17.

147. Stabin MG. *Internal dosimetry in pediatric nuclear medicine.* In:

Treves ST, ed. *Pediatric nuclear medicine*, 2nd ed. New York: Springer-Verlag, 1995:556.

Bone Densitometry

148. Weiner S, Traub W. Bone structure: from angstroms to microns. *FASEB J* 1992;6:879.

149. Majumdar S, Kothari M, Augat P, et al. High-resolution magnetic resonance imaging: three-dimensional trabecular bone architecture and biomechanical properties. *Bone* 1998;22:445.

150. Genant HK. Current state of bone densitometry for osteoporosis. *Radiographics* 1998;18:913.

151. Jergas M, Genant HK. Spinal and femoral DXA for the assessment of spinal osteoporosis. *Calcif Tissue Int* 1997;61:351.

152. Gilsanz V. Bone density in children: a review of the available techniques and indications. *Eur J Radiol* 1998;26:177.

153. Kovanlikaya A, Loro ML, Hangartner TN, et al. Osteopenia in children: CT assessment. *Radiology* 1996;198:781.

154. Gilsanz V, Skaggs DL, Kovanlikaya A, et al. Differential effect of race on the axial and appendicular skeletons of children [see comments]. *J Clin Endocrinol Metab* 1998;83:1420.

155. Gilsanz V, Boechat MI, Gilsanz R, et al. Gender differences in vertebral sizes in adults: biomechanical implications [see comments]. *Radiology* 1994;190:678.

156. Gilsanz V, Roe TF, Mora S, et al. Changes in vertebral bone density in black girls and white girls during childhood and puberty [see comments]. *N Engl J Med* 1991;325:1597.

Radiation Exposure: Practical Issues

157. Sorenson J, Phelps M. Radiation safety and health physics. In: Sorenson J, Phelps M, eds. *Physics in nuclear medicine.* Philadelphia: WB Saunders, 1987:519.

158. International Commission on Radiation Protection. 1990 recommendations of the International Commission on Radiation Protection. ICRP Publication 60. *Ann ICRP* 1991;21:1.

159. Gibbs S. Basic mechanism of radiation injury–somatic and genetic. In: American College of Radiology Commission on Physics and Radiation Safety Committee on Radiologic Units S, and Protection. *Radiation risk: a primer.* Reston: American College of Radiology, 1996.

160. Poznanski A. Approaches to minimizing risk in pediatric radiology. In: American College of Radiology Commission on Physics and Radiation Safety Committee on Radiologic Units S, and Protection. *Radiation risk: a primer.* Reston: American College of Radiology, 1996:19.

161. Tolbert D. Sources of radiation exposure. In: American College of Radiology Commission on Physics and Radiation Safety Committee on Radiologic Units S, and Protection. *Radiation risk: a primer.* Reston: American College of Radiology, 1996: 3.

162. Kelsey CA, Mettler FA Jr, Sorenson JA, et al. Health care workers' perceptions of risks. *Health Phys* 1987;53:541.

163. Sorenson JA. Perception of radiation hazards. *Semin Nucl Med* 1986;16:158.

164. Palmer SH, Starritt HC, Paterson M. Radiation protection of the ovaries in young scoliosis patients. *Eur Spine J* 1998;7: 278.

165. Almen AJ, Mattsson S. Dose distribution at radiographic examination of the spine in pediatric radiology. *Spine* 1996;21:750.

166. Levy AR, Goldberg MS, Mayo NE, et al. Reducing the lifetime

risk of cancer from spinal radiographs among people with adolescent idiopathic scoliosis. *Spine* 1996;21:1540, 1548.

167. Parry RA, Glaze SA, Archer BR. The AAPM/RSNA physics tutorial for residents. Typical patient radiation doses in diagnostic radiology. *Radiographics* 1999;19:1289.

Sedation for Imaging

168. Wagner LK. *Radiation bioeffects and management test and syllabus*, vol. 32. Reston: The American College of Radiology, 1991.
169. American Academy of Pediatrics. Guidelines for monitoring and management of pediatric patients during and after sedation for diagnostic and therapeutic procedures. *Pediatrics* 1992;89:1110.
170. Thompson JR, Schneider S, Ashwal S, et al. The choice of sedation for computed tomography in children: a prospective evaluation. *Radiology* 1982;143:475.
171. Strain JD, Harvey LA, Foley LC, et al. Intravenously administered pentobarbital sodium for sedation in pediatric CT. *Radiology* 1986;161:105.
172. Strain JD, Campbell JB, Harvey LA, et al. IV Nembutal: safe sedation for children undergoing CT. *Am J Roentgenol* 1988;151:975.
173. Greenberg SB, Faerber EN, Aspinall CL. High dose chloral hydrate sedation for children undergoing CT. *J Comput Assist Tomogr* 1991;15:467.
174. Greenberg SB, Faerber EN, Aspinall CL, et al. High-dose chloral hydrate sedation for children undergoing MR imaging: safety and efficacy in relation to age. *Am J Roentgenol* 1993;161:639.
175. Greenberg SB, Faerber EN, Radke JL, et al. Sedation of difficult-to-sedate children undergoing MR imaging: value of thioridazine as an adjunct to chloral hydrate. *Am J Roentgenol* 1994;163:165.
176. Stabin MG. Internal dosimetry in pediatric nuclear medicine. In: Treves ST, ed. *Pediatric nuclear medicine*, 2nd ed. New York: Springer-Verlag, 1995:556.

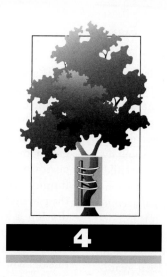

4

THE PEDIATRIC ORTHOPAEDIC EXAMINATION

DAVID D. ARONSSON

D. D. Aronsson: Department of Orthopaedics and Rehabilitation and Pediatrics, University of Vermont College of Medicine, Burlington, Vermont 05405; Department of Orthopaedics and Rehabilitation and Pediatrics, Fletcher Allen Health Care, Burlington, Vermont 05401.

The pediatric orthopaedic examination may vary depending on the age of the child, the chief complaint, and the magnitude of the problem. In all cases, it is important for the clinician to respect the dignity of the child, the parents or legal guardian, and any other health care professionals that accompany the patient. The clinician begins by washing his or her hands and introducing himself or herself to the child, parents or legal guardian, and other health care professionals, and shaking their hands. If a resident physician accompanies the clinician into the examination room, it is important to introduce the resident and explain why he or she is present. The clinician then sits down and slowly takes an accurate history from the child and parents or legal guardian, while simultaneously making eye contact with them. These basic principles of respect for the child, parents or legal guardian, and other health care professionals are followed in all situations.

Although a short, focused history and limited physical examination may be appropriate for a 5-year-old boy sustaining a torus fracture, a thorough history and physical examination are required to evaluate a 2-year-old boy with developmental delay and inability to walk. The history begins with the chief complaint in the words of the child, or, if the child is not yet talking, in the words of the parents or legal guardian. The history of present illness includes details concerning when and how the problem developed, how it has evolved, whether it has been treated, and any situations that aggravate or relieve the symptoms. The developmental history includes the birth history, with details concerning the pregnancy, delivery, and perinatal course. The developmental history also includes developmental milestones, such as when the child first sat independently, pulled to standing, cruised, walked independently, and developed handedness. The past medical history includes any allergies, hospitalizations, operations, major illnesses, and if the patient is taking any medication. The family history includes the siblings, parents, grandparents, and any other relatives who had a similar problem or any major illness. The review of systems includes general questions about each system, such as the gastrointestinal system or the musculoskeletal system, to detect any problems that may or may not be associated with the history of present illness. The personal and social history reviews the living situation of the patient and any habits that he or she may have, such as smoking.

The physical examination includes the height and weight of the patient, and a thorough examination of the skin, spine, and upper and lower extremities, as well as a neurologic examination. The pediatric orthopaedic examination does not typically include the vital signs or a detailed examination of the head, eyes, ears, nose, throat, chest, heart, or abdomen. These aspects of the physical examination are usually performed by the child's pediatrician, but if concerns about these areas arise during the examination, they are examined in detail.

The history and physical examination also vary with the age of the patient, because infants and young children are unable to give a history, whereas older children will often give a more accurate history than their parents or legal guardian. The teenage boy with a postural round back deformity may have a benign history with no concerns, but the parents or legal guardian may be concerned that he will develop a kyphotic deformity with osteoporosis, like his grandmother. Many pediatric orthopaedic disorders develop only in certain age groups, such as Legg-Calvé-Perthes disease, which typically develops in 4- to 10-year-old boys. As a result, discussion of the pediatric orthopaedic examination in this chapter is divided into three sections, according to the age of the patient.

The first section includes newborns, infants, and young children from birth to 4 years of age. These patients are usually unable to give an accurate history, so the majority of the history is obtained from the parents or legal guardian. Such young patients are often apprehensive about going to the doctor, and are not interested in being examined; so some type of user-friendly materials, such as toys or stickers, may be necessary to earn their trust, so that they will allow the examiner to perform an accurate and thorough physical examination. The majority of the physical examination of an infant often can be done in the mother's lap. For pertinent parts of the examination, the infant can be placed on the examining table; if he or she is upset or uncooperative, bottle-feeding during this part of the examination can calm the infant. The 2-year-old child, in the "terrible twos," is often very apprehensive about going to the doctor and being placed in an examination room. The clinician should not burst into the room, conduct a brief history, and then perform a physical examination on an upset and combative child. At first, the parents will often try to help the clinician if the child is uncooperative, but if the clinician perseveres with the examination in the face of an uncooperative child, the parents will usually side with their child. In this situation, the parents may themselves become uncooperative and not volunteer any new information, just to get out of the examination room as quickly as possible. As a result, rather than leaving the office with the knowledge and confidence that the clinician has solved the problem, they leave with the impression that the problem is not resolved, and that the clinician was hurried, uncaring, and not interested in helping their child. Some clinicians believe that the problem is "the white coat," whereas others believe that it involves the entire situation of taking an apprehensive 2-year-old child to the doctor, being placed in an examination room, then having a stranger come in who expects to conduct a physical examination. These issues can be avoided if the clinician can gain the respect and trust of the child before embarking on the physical examination. This can be achieved by sitting down with the child while conducting the history with the parents or legal guardian, and by simultaneously engaging the child in the conversation and taking short interruptions to entertain or play with the child. Once the history is completed, the physical examination can then be initiated in a nonthreatening manner.

The second section includes children from 4 to 10 years of age. These patients are usually interested in participating in the examination, and will often correct their parents if the information given is incorrect. They like receiving stickers, playing with toys in the examination room, and playing with the water at the sink. As a result, they are usually calm and not threatened by the clinician, and will typically cooperate during the physical examination. Many children between 4 and 10 years of age do not like removing their clothes and putting on a johnny or hospital gown. This situation can be avoided if they wear a pair of shorts and a T-shirt for the examination. In this age group, some children with special health needs will be particularly resistant to anyone attempting to conduct a physical examination on them. In this situation, it is often helpful to tell the parents or legal guardian what you would like to accomplish. For example, if you would like to examine the child for possible scoliosis, and to perform an Adams

forward-bending test, this can easily be explained to the parents or legal guardian. Once explained, they will often be able to get the child into the correct position, so that you can perform the test.

The third section includes children and adolescents from 10 to 18 years of age. These patients are usually very motivated to get better, and will give an accurate history, believing that the doctor can indeed help them to get better. Teenagers are often very concerned about removing their clothes, so it is reassuring to them to know that they do not need to remove their shorts or underwear. If conducted appropriately and in a manner that respects their privacy, teenagers will typically allow the clinician to perform a complete physical examination.

In all age groups, it is often beneficial to begin with a patient profile, which is filled out by the parents or legal guardian (ages birth to 4 years old), the parents or legal guardian with help from the patient (ages 4 to 10 years old), or the patient with help from the parents or legal guardian (ages 10 to 18 years old) before the actual examination (Fig. 4-1). The patient profile includes the chief complaint and history of present illness, with details concerning the birth and developmental history. It also lists any allergies, medications that the patient is taking, previous hospitalizations, or

Name of patient _____

Age: Years _____ Months _____

Brothers _____

_____

_____

Height of mother _____

Referring physician _____

Birthdate _____

Grade in school _____

Sisters _____

_____

_____

Height of father _____

Family physician _____

What is the reason for today's visit? _____

When did the problem first start? _____

Is it better or worse than when you first noticed it? _____

Is there a family history of this problem? _____
Have you had any treatment? _____

If yes, please list treating physician(s) and treatment _____

Past history:
Major illnesses?   Yes _____   No _____   If yes, please list _____

Operations?   Yes _____   No _____   If yes, please list _____

FIGURE 4-1. Patient profile.

Past history:
Medications?   Yes _____ No _____   If yes, please list _____

Allergies?   Yes _____ No _____   If yes, please list _____

Drug allergies?   Yes _____ No _____   If yes, please list _____

Birth history of patient:
Premature?   Yes _____ No _____   Reason? _____

Problems?   Yes _____ No _____   Reason? _____

Breech?   Yes _____ No _____   Reason? _____

Cesarean?   Yes _____ No _____   Reason? _____

Birth place: Hospital? _____   Birth weight: _____ lb _____ oz

Developmental milestones of the patient:
   At what age did the child: Roll over? _____ months

                                  Sit up? _____ months

                                  Walk? _____ months

Would you like a copy of our medical report to be sent to anyone?
If yes, please list name and address:

_____

_____

_____

Signature of parent or guardian: _____

FIGURE 4-1. *(continued)*

operations. The patient profile includes the family history as well as a release signature to mail a copy of the office note to the parents, legal guardian, or referring pediatrician or family physician.

THE ORTHOPAEDIC EXAMINATION FROM BIRTH TO 4 YEARS OF AGE

A 1-month-old Girl Is Referred for Evaluation of a Hip Click

A hip click may be a benign click that reflects a popping sensation as the iliopsoas tendon slides over the anterior hip capsule with internal and external rotation of the hip, or it may indicate a subluxation or dislocation reflecting developmental dysplasia of the hip (DDH). To distinguish between these two very different entities, the clinician focuses on certain aspects of the history and physical examination that are associated with DDH. The history begins with a review of the pertinent findings from the patient profile with the parents or legal guardian. The most important information, the hip click, is documented in the chief complaint and history of present illness. For an infant with a hip click, it is important to document when and how it was first de-

tected. If the infant has DDH, the type of treatment and the prognosis will vary, depending on the age of the patient and the magnitude of the DDH. The birth history is important in this case, because DDH is associated with primigravida mothers, oligohydramnios, breech presentations, congenital muscular torticollis, and certain types of foot deformities, such as metatarsus adductus. The breech presentation is the most important of these findings because even if born by cesarean section, if the infant was in the frank (single) breech presentation, the frequency of DDH is 20 to 30%. The developmental history is also important; if the child has a neuromuscular disorder, such as arthrogryposis multiplex congenita, the infant may have a teratologic, rather than a typical, DDH. A patient with a teratologic DDH usually requires a completely different treatment approach than a patient with a typical DDH. The family history may reveal DDH in the parents, siblings, cousins, or aunts and uncles. This information may be crucial in evaluating the patient, because the incidence of DDH is higher when other family members have the disorder. It is also important to ask about any previous treatment that has been rendered by clinicians or paramedical personnel, because this may influence patient management.

The examination of a 1-month-old infant with a hip click can be started with the infant in the mother's lap. In this position, the infant is comfortable and not threatened, and the clinician can examine the range of motion of the hands, wrists, elbows, and shoulders. The neck can be examined to look for a congenital muscular torticollis with a contracture of the sternocleidomastoid muscle, a condition that is seen in association with DDH. With the infant in the same position, the knees, ankles, and feet can be examined to look for a metatarsus adductus deformity, another condition that is seen in association with DDH. The infant can then be placed prone over the mother's shoulder, similar to the position for burping the infant, while the clinician examines the spine and looks for a sacral dimple, hairy patch, or anal problems. A sacral dimple or hairy patch may be a sign of an underlying tethered spinal cord or lipomeningocele. These disorders can cause varying degrees of paralysis of the lower extremities that may result in a paralytic dislocation of the hip with a positive hip click. Finally, after the majority of the physical examination has been completed and the infant and parents or legal guardian are comfortable with the clinician, the infant can be placed on a firm surface to thoroughly examine the hips.

The key to the early diagnosis of DDH is the physical examination. The examination should be performed on a firm surface with the infant relaxed. If the infant is crying or upset, the DDH may not be detected. In this situation, allow the parent or legal guardian to feed or calm the infant and begin the examination as soon as the infant is happy and comfortable. The examination begins with the hips and knees flexed to 90 degrees. The examiner places the thumb along the medial thigh and the long finger laterally along the axis of the femur. Gentle pressure is applied to the knee in a posterior direction, while the examiner palpates a "clunk" as the hip dislocates out of the acetabulum. If the hip subluxates rather than dislocates, the examiner may note only a sensation of sliding as the femoral head slides over the posterior lip of the acetabulum. This telescoping maneuver is often termed the "Barlow provocative test," which represents a "sign of exit" as the hip dislocates from the acetabulum (Fig. 4-2A). With the hip in the dislocated or subluxated position, the examiner then gently abducts the hip, while pushing anteriorly with the long finger over the greater trochanter, and palpates another clunk as the hip slides over the posterior lip and into the acetabulum. This is a positive Ortolani maneuver, which represents a "sign of entry" as the hip reduces into the acetabulum (Fig. 4-2B). The original Barlow test was actually a two-part test: the first part included an Ortolani maneuver to determine if the hip was dislocated. The second part, or the Barlow provocative test, was performed to determine if the hip could be dislocated or subluxated. The Barlow and Ortolani tests detect ligamentous laxity and instability, and although they are valuable during the neonatal period, they usually become negative by 3 months of age (1).

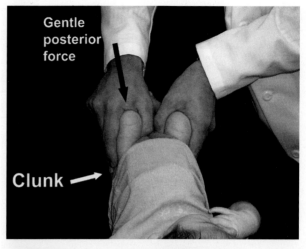

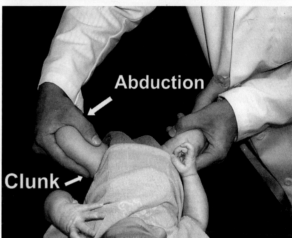

FIGURE 4-2. A: The Barlow test is performed in two parts to determine if the hip is located and stable, located and able to be subluxated or dislocated, dislocated and able to be located, or dislocated and not able to be located. The first part of the test is an Ortolani maneuver to determine if the hip is dislocated. The second part, or the Barlow provocative test, is performed with the hips flexed to 90 degrees; the clinician places the thumb along the medial thigh and the long finger along the lateral axis of the femur. Gentle pressure in a posterior direction is applied to the knee, while the clinician palpates a "clunk" as the hip dislocates or subluxates out of the acetabulum. **B:** The Ortolani maneuver is performed by gently abducting the hip, while pushing anteriorly with the long finger over the greater trochanter; the clinician palpates another clunk as the hip slides over the posterior lip and into the acetabulum.

Once the infant is 3 months old, the ligamentous laxity has usually resolved, and if the hip is subluxated or dislocated superolaterally, the adductor and flexor muscles become tight, causing an adduction contracture. At this age, the most common physical finding is limited abduction of the hip (Fig. 4-3). The superolateral subluxation of the hip causes a limb-length discrepancy that may be detected by examining the overall limb lengths. The shortening of the thigh causes an increased number of thigh folds compared with the other thigh, and if the hips are flexed to 90 degrees,

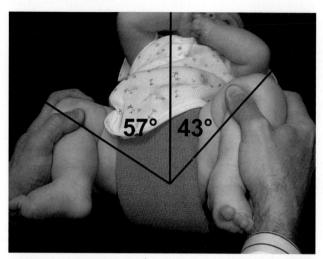

FIGURE 4-3. Once the infant is 3 months old, the ligamentous laxity usually disappears and the hip develops an adduction contracture. The most common physical finding in a patient with developmental dysplasia of the hip at this age is limited abduction of the hip, compared with the uninvolved side.

the knee of the involved hip will be lower than the opposite side (Galeazzi sign) (Fig. 4-4).

A 2-year-old Boy Is Referred for Evaluation of Intoeing and Tripping over His Feet

In this case, the clinician focuses on certain aspects of the history and physical examination to determine if the child

is developing satisfactorily and tripping like most 2-year-old children, or if there is evidence of developmental delay. If there is a delay in development, there may be associated problems with coordination or retention of primitive reflexes. The clinician begins by reviewing the chief complaint and history of present illness. If the intoeing is physiologic and represents a normal developmental variation, it will often first be noted by the grandparents, parents, or legal guardian when the child begins walking, and it will usually be symmetric. The clinician asks if the parents believe that the intoeing is originating from the hips, thighs, legs, or feet. A unilateral problem, involving a foot with intoeing and tripping over the foot, may indicate a mild clubfoot or a neurologic problem such as a tethered spinal cord. The clinician also reviews the pertinent findings in the birth history and developmental history in the patient profile with the parents or legal guardian. Most children who are developing satisfactorily will sit independently (without hand support) by 6 to 9 months of age, cruise (walk with assistance) by 10 to 14 months of age, and walk independently by 8 to 18 months of age (Table 4-1).

If there is concern about possible developmental delay, it is important to verify the details concerning the birth history to determine if the infant was premature, or if there were any perinatal complications. Premature infants born after 25 to 30 weeks of gestation, with a birth weight of 750 to 1500 g, have an increased incidence of cerebral palsy, particularly spastic diplegia. The first sign of this disorder may be noted by the parents when they discover that their child is delayed in walking or having trouble with intoeing and tripping over his or her feet. While verifying the developmental history with the parents or legal guardian, it is valuable to ask if the infant is ambidextrous, right-handed,

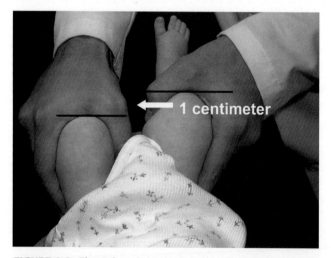

FIGURE 4-4. The Galeazzi sign is elicited by flexing the hips and knees to 90 degrees, with the patient supine. If there is superolateral subluxation of the femoral head with shortening of the thigh segment, the knee of the involved hip will be lower than the opposite side.

TABLE 4-1. AVERAGE DEVELOPMENTAL ACHIEVEMENT BY AGE

Age	Achievement
1 month	Partial head control in prone position
2 months	Good head control in prone position; partial head control in supine position
4 months	Good head control in supine position; rolls over prone to supine
5 months	Rolls over supine to prone
6 months	When prone, lifts head and chest with weight on hands; sits with support
8 months	Sits independently; reaches for toys
10 months	Crawls; stands holding onto furniture
12 months	Walks independently or with hand support
18 months	Developing handedness
2 years	Jumps; knows full name
3 years	Goes upstairs alternating feet; stands momentarily on one foot; knows age and gender
4 years	Hops on one foot; throws ball overhand
5 years	Skips; dresses independently

or left-handed. Children who are developing satisfactorily will usually remain ambidextrous until 18 months to 2 years of age (Table 4-1). If the child is 2 years old and strongly right-handed or left-handed, the birth and developmental history may reveal a previous intrauterine cerebral vascular accident, and the handedness may be one of the early signs of cerebral palsy with spastic hemiplegia.

For a 2-year-old boy with intoeing and frequent falling, the examination will usually proceed in a different fashion than it would for a 1-month-old girl with a hip click. Before beginning the physical examination, the clinician needs to remember that infants and young children enjoy being with their parents, and are often not particularly interested in being examined. They do not understand why they are trapped in an examination room with the door closed and why a stranger in a white coat wants to "wiggle" their legs. This awkward situation can be overcome if the clinician can gain the respect and trust of the child and the child's parents or legal guardian before embarking on anything that the child may perceive as threatening, such as a physical examination. The clinician can sit down with the child and parents or legal guardian and review the chief complaint, history of present illness, and the exact details about the birth and developmental history, while taking frequent breaks to talk and play with the child. Once the history is completed and everyone is more at ease, particularly the child, the physical examination can be initiated in a non-threatening manner.

It is often beneficial with a 2-year-old child to begin the physical examination by opening the door and asking the child and parents or legal guardian if they would like to take a walk down the hall. This is a very nonthreatening way to begin the examination, and there is nothing that the child wants to do more than get out of the room. The clinician will find that most toddlers are more comfortable walking away from than walking toward the clinician. The clinician can stay in the room for a moment, then look out the door as the family is walking down the hall to observe the child's gait pattern and the foot-progression angle (2). The foot-progression angle compares the axis of the foot, a line connecting a bisector of the heel with the center of the second metatarsal head, with an imaginary straight line drawn on the floor (Fig. 4-5). The normal foot-progression angle in children 1 to 4 years of age can vary from 40 degrees of inward rotation to 40 degrees of outward rotation. The gait pattern can also vary considerably in this age group, but usually it will be relatively symmetric, with a similar amount of time being spent in the stance phase (60% of the gait cycle) and the swing phase (40% of the gait cycle) between the two extremities. The degree and location of any rotational variations or torsional deformities can be documented by creating a rotational profile (Fig. 4-6). The rotational profile includes the foot-progression angle, internal rotation of the hips, external rotation of the hips, the thigh–foot angle, and any foot deformities. The

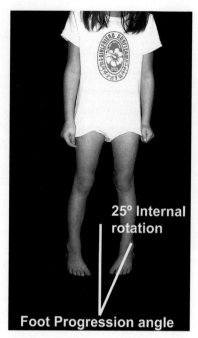

FIGURE 4-5. While the patient is walking, the foot-progression angle compares the axis of the feet with an imaginary straight line drawn on the floor.

foot-progression angle measures the degree of intoeing or outtoeing compared with an imaginary straight line drawn on the floor. The internal and external rotation of the hip measures the femoral version or torsional deformity of the femur (Fig. 4-7). The thigh–foot angle is the angle between the axis of the thigh and the axis of the foot, with the knee bent to 90 degrees (Fig. 4-8). This angle measures the tibial version or torsional deformity of the tibia (3). The foot examination records the amount of metatarsus adductus or any other foot deformity that may be contributing to the intoeing or outtoeing. Once the profile is filled out, it gives an objective view of the location and magnitude of any rotational variations or torsional deformities of the lower

	Right	Left
FPA		
MR		
LR		
TFA		
Foot		

FIGURE 4-6. Rotational profile.
FPA, foot-progression angle; MR, hip medial rotation; LR, hip lateral rotation; TFA, thigh–foot angle. Record angles in degrees, and describe foot deformity.

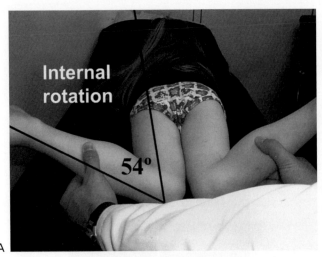
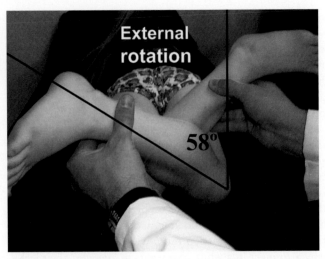

FIGURE 4-7. The internal and external rotation of the hips can be measured in the supine or the prone position. **A:** Standing at the foot of the bed, with the patient prone, the clinician uses gravity to allow the hips to fall into internal rotation. The angle between the leg and a line perpendicular to the tabletop measures the internal rotation. **B:** With the patient in the same position, the clinician uses gravity to allow the hips to fall into external rotation. The angle between the leg and a line perpendicular to the tabletop measures the external rotation.

extremities. The rotational profile can then be used as a baseline while following the child to document that the deformity does indeed improve with growth. Two-year-old boys often have persistent internal femoral or internal tibial torsional deformities that cause them to walk with the feet turned in, or pigeon-toed.

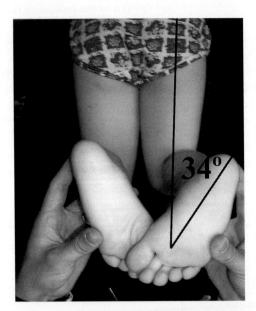

FIGURE 4-8. Standing at the foot of the bed, with the patient prone, the clinician measures the angle between the axis of the thigh and the axis of the foot, with the foot held in a neutral position. This angle, termed the "thigh–foot angle," measures the amount of tibial torsion.

An 18-month-old Boy Is Referred for Developmental Delay and Inability to Walk

The chief complaint and history of present illness reveals that the parents are concerned that their son is unable to walk. On further questioning, it is revealed that the parents first suspected that their son might be delayed when he was 4 months old and was still having difficulty with head control. They became more concerned when he was still unable to sit independently at 10 months of age. He just recently began pulling to standing, and he is unable to walk. The birth history reveals that he was born after a 28-week gestation, with a birth weight of 1100 g. He had perinatal respiratory difficulties, and was hospitalized in the neonatal intensive care unit for 2 months. He developed a seizure disorder at 1 year of age, and his seizures are now under good control with medication.

In this case, the boy is developmentally delayed, so the physical examination will focus on the neurologic examination and developmental progress. It is often convenient to begin the physical examination with the boy in the supine position; the clinician grasps his hands and gradually pulls him into the sitting position, while looking for head and trunk control. An infant will usually have head control by 3 to 4 months of age and trunk control by 6 to 8 months of age (Table 4-1). Delayed head and trunk control may indicate overall developmental delay, which, if associated with prematurity and a low birth weight, may indicate cerebral palsy. In infants there are a series of primitive reflexes, including the Moro, grasp, neck-righting, symmetric tonic neck, and asymmetric tonic neck reflexes, which are often

TABLE 4-2. PRIMITIVE AND POSTURAL REFLEXES

Primitive Reflex	Age When It Disappears
Grasp	3 months
Moro	6 months
Asymmetric tonic neck	6 months
Symmetric tonic neck	6 months
Neck-righting	10 months

Postural Reflex	Age When It Appears
Foot-placement	Early infancy
Parachute	12 months

present at birth, then gradually disappear with normal growth and development by 4 to 10 months of age (Table 4-2). If these reflexes persist beyond 6 to 10 months of age, it may be an early sign of a neuromuscular disorder.

The Moro reflex is present at birth, and is elicited by introducing a sudden extension of the neck. The shoulders abduct and the upper limbs extend, with spreading of the fingers, followed by an embrace (Fig. 4-9). The Moro reflex usually disappears by 6 months of age (4). The grasp reflex is elicited by placing a finger in the infant's palm from the ulnar side. The infant's fingers will firmly grasp the examiner's finger. If traction is applied to the hand, the grasp reflex is so strong that the examiner can lift the infant's shoulder from the table (Fig. 4-10). The grasp reflex usually disappears by 3 months of age. The neck-righting reflex is elicited by turning the head to one side, and is positive if the trunk and limbs turn toward the same side. This reflex usually disappears by 10 months of age (4). The symmetric

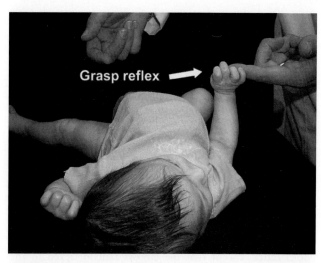

FIGURE 4-10. The grasp reflex is elicited by introducing the clinician's finger into the infant's palm from the ulnar side. The infant's fingers will flex and firmly grasp the clinician's finger. If traction is applied, the muscles of the arm and shoulder girdle contract, allowing the clinician to temporarily suspend the infant by grasp reflex.

tonic neck reflex is elicited by flexion of the neck, which causes flexion of the upper limbs and extension of the lower limbs. Similarly, extension of the neck causes extension of the upper limbs and flexion of the lower limbs. The asymmetric tonic neck reflex is elicited by turning the head to the side, which results in extension of the upper and lower extremities on the side toward which the head is turned, and flexion of the upper and lower extremities on the opposite side (the "fencing" position) (Fig. 4-11). The symmetric and asymmetric tonic neck reflexes usually disappear by 6 months of age. The extensor thrust, an abnormal reflex, is

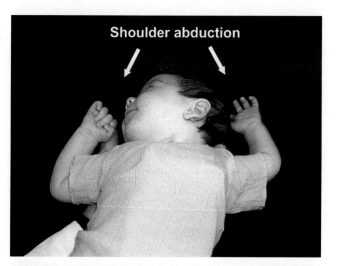

FIGURE 4-9. The Moro reflex is elicited by gently lifting the infant with the clinician's right hand under the upper thoracic spine and the left hand under the head. The clinician then drops the left hand to allow sudden neck extension; the infant abducts the upper limbs, with spreading of the fingers, followed by an embrace.

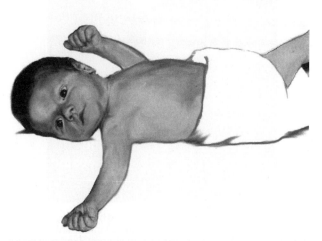

FIGURE 4-11. In the supine position, the asymmetric tonic neck reflex is elicited by turning the head to one side, then the other. A positive response is extension of the upper and lower limbs on the facial side and extension on the occipital side (the "fencing" position). (From ref. 5, with permission.)

elicited by holding the infant under the arms and touching the feet to the floor, which causes a rapid extension of the joints of the lower limb, progressing from the feet to the trunk (Fig. 4-12). A normal infant will flex rather than extend the lower extremities when placed in this position. All of these primitive reflexes need to resolve with development before it is possible for the child to walk independently.

There is another group of reflexes that disappear at different stages of development, including the rooting, startle, gallant, and Landau reflexes. The rooting reflex is elicited by touching the corner of the mouth, which results in the mouth and tongue turning toward the side that was stimulated. The startle reflex is elicited by making a loud noise, which results in a mass myoclonic response resembling a Moro reflex, except that the elbows remain flexed in the startle. The startle reflex may persist until late childhood. The gallant reflex is elicited by stroking the side of the trunk, which results in the infant bending the spine toward the side that was stimulated. The Landau reflex is elicited by supporting the infant by the trunk in the horizontal prone position; the typical response is extension of the neck and spine. If the infant collapses into an upside-down U, it may indicate hypotonia.

There is another group of postural reflexes that gradually

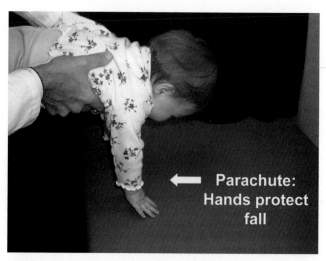

FIGURE 4-13. The parachute reflex is elicited by holding the infant in the air in the prone position, then suddenly lowering or tipping the infant headfirst toward the table. The reflex is positive if the infant extends the upper extremities and places the hands on the tabletop.

appear as a result of development of the nervous system, including the parachute reflex and the foot-placement reaction (Table 4-2). The parachute reflex is elicited by holding the infant in the air in the prone position, then suddenly lowering the infant headfirst toward the table, simulating a fall. The reflex is positive if the infant extends the upper extremities as if to break the fall (Fig. 4-13). This reflex usually appears by 12 months of age, and remains until late adulthood. The foot-placement reaction is elicited by holding the infant under the arms, then gently lifting the infant, so that the dorsum of the foot comes up against the underside of the table. It is positive if the infant picks up the extremity as if to step up onto the table (Fig. 4-14). The foot-placement reaction usually develops early in infancy, and may persist until the age of 3 or 4 years.

Bleck (4) studied 73 infants and children who were 12 months of age or older and were still not yet walking independently. He used seven tests to develop a prognosis for walking to predict if an infant would subsequently walk. One point was assigned if the primitive reflexes were still present, and one point was assigned if the normal postural reflexes were still absent (Table 4-3). A score of two points or more indicated a poor prognosis for walking, a one-point score indicated a guarded prognosis (might walk), and a zero-point score indicated a good prognosis.

Analysis of these different reflexes gives the clinician a general idea of the magnitude of the developmental delay. The examination can then proceed by evaluating the spine for any scoliosis or kyphosis. An examination of the upper and lower extremities is performed to assess range of motion of the joints and to document any contractures. If any con-

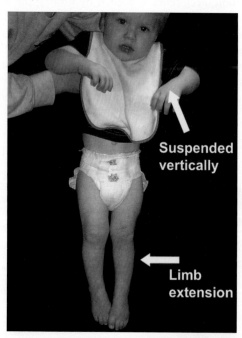

FIGURE 4-12. The extensor thrust is elicited by holding the infant under the arms and gradually lowering the infant until the feet touch the floor. An extensor thrust is an abnormal reflex in which there is progressive extension of the lower limbs, progressing superiorly from the feet to the trunk. The typical response in a normal infant is flexion of the lower extremities.

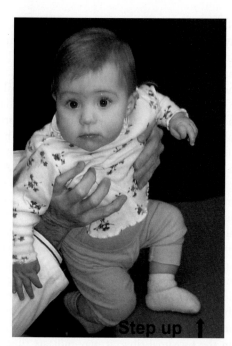

FIGURE 4-14. The foot-placement reaction is elicited by holding the infant under the arms, then gently lifting the infant so that the dorsum of the foot or the anterior surface of the tibia comes up against the underside of the table. It is positive if the infant picks up the extremity as if to step up onto the table.

tractures or deformities are identified the clinician attempts to passively correct the contracture or deformity to determine if it is flexible or rigid. The reflexes are tested, including the Babinski reflex, because children with spastic cerebral palsy and developmental delay may have hyperreflexia with a positive Babinski reflex. If the child is spastic with adduction and flexion contractures of the hips, an anteroposterior pelvis radiograph is beneficial, because many of these children with increased tone may have subluxated hips.

TABLE 4-3. PROGNOSIS FOR WALKING

Reflex	Points
Primitive reflex	
Asymmetric tonic neck	1
Neck-righting	1
Moro	1
Symmetric tonic neck	1
Extensor thrust	1
Postural reflex	
Parachute	1 if absent
Foot-placement	1 if absent

Prognosis for walking: 2 points, poor; 1 point, guarded (might walk); 0 points, good.
(From ref. 2, with permission.)

A 2-month-old Girl Is Referred for Evaluation Because She Is Not Moving Her Left Arm Like She Moves the Right Arm

In this case, the examination will focus on the upper extremities, comparing the paralyzed left side with the right side, and looking for any asymmetry. It is important to distinguish traumatic brachial plexus neuropathy, a true paralysis of the upper extremity, from osteomyelitis, septic arthritis, or birth fractures, which can cause a pseudoparalysis of the extremity. The treatment for each of these conditions is different, and delay in diagnosis in infants with osteomyelitis and septic arthritis can be devastating. An infant with osteomyelitis, septic arthritis, or a birth fracture will usually have swelling at the site, whereas an infant with traumatic brachial plexus palsy will usually have no swelling or swelling may be detected in the neck. In an infant with traumatic brachial plexus palsy or birth fracture of the humerus, the paralysis is usually noted at birth, whereas an infant with osteomyelitis or septic arthritis will often use the arm normally, then suddenly develop the pseudoparalysis. It is important to ask the parents or legal guardian the exact time that the paralysis was noted, whether it has changed with time, and if there was any associated swelling. Traumatic brachial plexus palsy is one of the most common birth injuries, often seen in cases of primigravida mothers with large babies after difficult deliveries. It occurs because of traction and lateral tilting of the head to deliver the shoulder, or, if in the breech presentation, by traction and lateral tilting of the trunk and shoulders to deliver the head. There are three types of brachial plexus palsies, depending on which part of the brachial plexus is affected.

The Erb type affects the upper roots, typically C5 and C6; the Klumpke type affects the lower roots, typically C8 and T1; and the total plexus involvement type affects all of the roots in the brachial plexus. The prognosis for recovery depends on the magnitude of the injury and the time of recovery of certain key muscles (e.g., biceps). In an infant with upper brachial plexus palsy (Erb type), the clinical picture is easily recognized by the absence of active motion of the involved extremity in the Moro reflex. Paralysis of C5 and C6 causes the shoulder to be held in adduction and internal rotation, with the elbow and wrist in extension and the fingers flexed, a position not seen in an infant with a birth fracture involving the humerus. In an infant with lower brachial plexus palsy (Klumpke type), the clinical picture is recognized by an absence of the grasp reflex in the involved extremity. The hand is flaccid, with little or no voluntary control. When there is total plexus involvement, the entire extremity is flaccid, and the Moro and grasp reflexes are both absent. In all types of brachial plexus palsies, after the birth there may be swelling in the supraclavicular area and an associated fracture of the clavicle or humerus, particularly if it was a difficult delivery. The supraclavicular swelling usually disappears by the time the infant is referred to the orthopaedist.

A 3-year-old Girl Is Referred for Evaluation of Bowed Legs (Genu Varum)

In developing the history of present illness, the clinician asks who first noted the deformity and exactly when it was first noted. It is also valuable to ask if the problem has changed since it was first detected, because a developmental variation will usually improve with growth, but a deformity may get worse over time. In a girl with bowed legs, the birth history and developmental history are typically unremarkable, so the history and physical examination will focus on the lower extremities, in a search for asymmetry between the limbs. The terms "varus" and "valgus" refer to the orientation of the distal fragment compared with the midline of the body. For example, in a child with a bowleg deformity, the distal fragment (the tibia) is angulated toward the midline, so it is termed "genu varum" (Fig. 4-15). In a child with a knock-knee deformity, the distal fragment (the tibia) is angulated away from the midline, so it is termed "genu valgum." Genu varum (bowed legs) and genu valgum (knock-knees) can be developmental variations that correct spontaneously with growth, or they can be actual deformities that are associated with other medical problems (6).

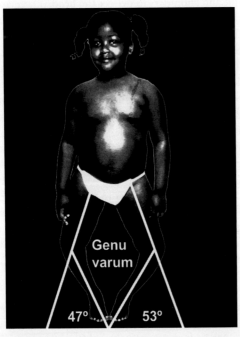

FIGURE 4-15. Varus and valgus deformities are named by how the distal segment is positioned, compared with the proximal segment. In a child with a bowleg deformity, the distal segment (the tibia) is positioned toward the midline, compared with the proximal segment (the femur), so it is termed "genu varum."

The family history may be relevant in this situation, because there may be several family members with short stature and genu varum. The review of systems may also be relevant in this situation, if the clinician discovers that there have been kidney problems in the past, and the girl has renal rickets with genu varum. It is important to remember that most infants have genu varum, and that it gradually corrects to neutral alignment by 18 to 24 months of age. The lower extremities then gradually develop a genu valgum, which reaches a maximum between 3 and 5 years of age. After the age of 5 years, the genu valgum gradually improves to reach the normal adult tibiofemoral alignment of 7 degrees of genu valgum by the end of growth.

On physical examination, it is important to record the height and weight of the child, and whether either one is more than two standard deviations from the mean. Short stature may be associated with nutritional rickets or another metabolic disorder that is associated with the genu varum. The limbs are closely inspected to determine exactly where the deformity is located. If the genu varum deformity is located in the proximal tibia, it may indicate tibia vara or Blount's disease. If the genu varum deformity appears to involve the entire limb in a symmetric fashion, it may indicate physiologic bowing, a developmental variation (6). The spine and upper extremities are examined for any findings that may be associated with a metabolic disorder or a particular syndrome, such as spondyloepiphyseal dysplasia. If the boy was referred for genu varum, the deformity or developmental variation is documented by measuring the intercondylar distance. To measure the intercondylar distance, the child is placed in the supine position, with the lower extremities in extension. The feet are brought together until the medial malleoli are just touching, and the magnitude of the genu varum deformity is recorded in centimeters as the distance between the femoral condyles (Fig. 4-16). Similarly, if the girl was referred for genu valgum, the deformity or developmental variation is documented by measuring the intermalleolar distance. The child is again placed in the supine position, with the lower extremities in extension. The feet are brought together until the femoral condyles are just touching, and the magnitude of the genu valgum deformity is recorded, in centimeters, as the distance between the medial malleoli (Fig. 4-17).

A 2-year-old Boy Is Referred for a Limp of the Right Lower Extremity That Developed after He Fell Down the Basement Stairs Earlier That Day

In this case, the history and physical examination will proceed in a different manner. This problem may be the result of a contusion or fracture, so a careful history is obtained from the parents or legal guardian. Details concerning the mechanism of injury and the child's method of coping with the injury are solicited from the parents or legal guardian.

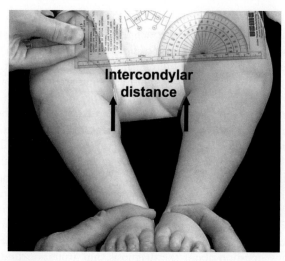

FIGURE 4-16. To measure the intercondylar distance, the child is placed supine, with the lower extremities in extension. The feet are brought together until the medial malleoli are just touching, and the intercondylar distance is the distance between the femoral condyles.

The clinician asks if there are any other injuries, such as a head contusion or laceration. The past medical history may reveal that the boy has had multiple previous fractures, causing the clinician to consider the diagnosis of osteogenesis imperfecta. If the history is not consistent with the magnitude of the physical findings, it is important to remember the possibility of a battered child syndrome. Each year, more than 2.5 million children in the United States sustain injuries that are inflicted by their parents, legal guardians, or caregivers. Although possible, it is unusual for a child

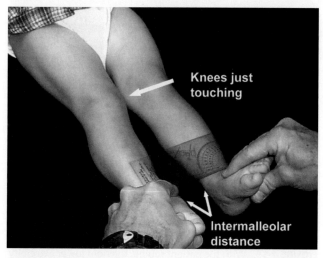

FIGURE 4-17. To measure the intermalleolar distance, the child is placed supine, with the lower extremities in extension. The feet are brought together until the femoral condyles are just touching, and the intermalleolar distance is the distance between the medial malleoli.

younger than 2 years of age to sustain a fracture of the femur or humerus in a normal fall. The examining clinician must keep this in mind when examining infants and children with these injuries. If the child has a fracture or contusion, there will be focal pain and swelling at the site. This can often be demonstrated by squeezing the noninjured side and observing the reaction of the child, then squeezing the injured side at the site of the fracture or contusion and observing the reaction of the child. If there is a fracture or contusion, the child will usually grimace or react to the painful stimulus. If there is focal tenderness and swelling indicating a possible fracture, anteroposterior and lateral radiographs of the involved bone will usually document the fracture.

A 3-year-old Boy Is Referred Because He Was Limping on the Right Side for 2 Days, Then Awoke That Morning and Refused to Walk

This is a typical history for a patient with toxic synovitis involving the hip, but it is also typical for a patient with septic arthritis of the hip, or osteomyelitis involving the proximal femur. Although less common, the history is also consistent with an acute attack of juvenile rheumatoid arthritis, or an early sign of acute lymphoblastic leukemia. A 3-year-old boy will often be interested in showing the clinician exactly where it hurts. If steered in the appropriate direction, the child may point to the groin area, the distal femur, or the knee when describing the pain. It is important to remember that pain can be referred, and hip disorders presenting as knee pain are a classic example of referred pain. The parents or legal guardian can expand on the history to include the exact time of onset and whether the pain is constant or intermittent. A patient with acute septic arthritis involving the hip would typically have a history of 1 to 2 days of severe and constant pain, whereas a patient with juvenile rheumatoid arthritis may have had intermittent low-grade pain for months, then recently developed severe pain. The pain associated with juvenile rheumatoid arthritis is often worse in the morning, which is not usually seen with the other disorders. If the patient has toxic synovitis involving the hip joint, a detailed history from the parents or legal guardian will often reveal that the child had an upper respiratory infection or sore throat 1 to 2 weeks before developing the limp and inability to walk. The history may reveal that the patient had chicken pox 2 weeks before developing the limp and inability to walk. In this case, the clinician may question the possibility of a *Streptococcus* infection. If the patient has been ill with decreased appetite and weight loss, the clinician may want to order blood tests to evaluate for leukemia.

In beginning the physical examination, the clinician remembers that, although the history revealed that the patient refused to walk, that does not necessarily mean that he will

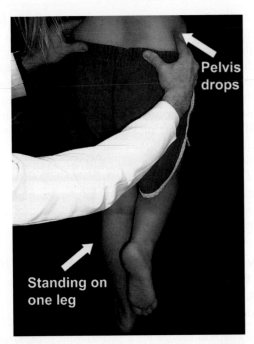

FIGURE 4-18. The clinician palpates the iliac crests while the patient stands on the left lower extremity. When a child stands on the left lower extremity the right iliac crest normally rises because the left hip abductor muscles contract to support the pelvis. The Trendelenburg test is positive if the right iliac crest drops, indicating weakness of the left hip abductor muscles. A trunk shift toward the weightbearing limb also indicates abductor weakness.

not want to walk now. The door can be opened and the parents asked if they would like to go for a walk with the child. The child is observed to see if he will stand and walk, and if successful, the gait is observed to determine if it is symmetric. If the child has an antalgic (painful) gait on one side, with a shortened stance phase, the clinician observes to determine the location of the pain. If the child will not walk, but will stand, he can be asked to stand on one leg, then on the opposite leg. When standing on one leg, the hip abductor muscles (gluteus medius) flex to hold the pelvis up on the opposite side, increasing the hip joint reactive forces. If the hip is irritable, the increased joint reactive forces are so painful that the patient will not contract the hip abductor muscles, causing the pelvis to drop on the opposite side—a positive Trendelenburg test (Fig. 4-18).

It is important to palpate the spine, pelvis, and lower extremities, beginning with the uninvolved side. If the patient has osteomyelitis involving the spine, sacroiliac joint, or distal femur, the clinician will appreciate focal increased pain and swelling to palpation. The hips are examined with the child relaxed in the supine position, and the clinician looks for any asymmetry as the hips are taken through a range of motion. A 3-year-old boy will typically remain relaxed as the hips are taken through a full range of motion. In a 3-year-old boy, the hips should easily flex to 130 degrees, extend to 0 degrees, abduct to 80 degrees, adduct to

30 degrees, internally rotate to 75 degrees, and externally rotate to 75 degrees. If the patient has an irritable hip, he will guard and contract his muscles, not allowing the clinician to take the hip through a full range of motion. This is noted particularly in attempting to internally and externally rotate the hip, with the hip in 90 degrees of flexion. If the hip is irritable, it is important to distinguish toxic synovitis, a benign self-limiting disorder of the hip, from septic arthritis, which can have devastating long-term consequences. The patient with septic arthritis involving the hip will typically be ill, with decreased appetite and a fever. The clinical findings are usually more pronounced, with severe pain occurring with any range of motion, whereas the patient with toxic synovitis will usually allow the clinician to flex and extend the hip through a limited range of motion. If there is any question about the diagnosis, hip aspiration under fluoroscopic control is recommended.

After examining the hip, the limb can then be placed in the figure-4 position, with the hip in flexion, abduction, and external rotation (FABER test) (Fig. 4-19). In this position, if the knee is pushed toward the examination table, it transmits a tensile force to the sacroiliac joint. If there is septic arthritis or inflammation involving the sacroiliac joint, it will be painful during the FABER test.

The knees are also examined in the supine position by palpating for any focal areas of tenderness. The clinician evaluates for an effusion or fluid in the knee by gently milking the suprapatellar pouch and lateral aspect of the knee, and observing a fluid wave on the medial aspect (Fig. 4-20). If there is a large effusion, the patella can be balloted against the femoral condyles when the knee is in extension.

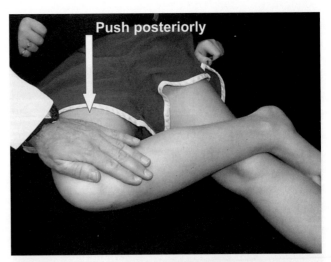

FIGURE 4-19. With the patient supine, the right lower extremity is placed in the figure-4 position with the hip in flexion, abduction, and external rotation (FABER test). In this position, if the knee is pushed toward the examination table, it transmits a tensile force to the sacroiliac joint that can cause pain if the sacroiliac joint is inflamed.

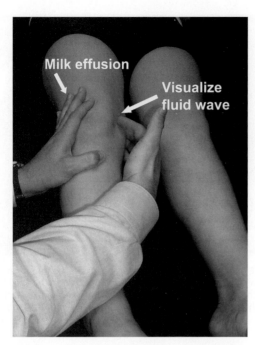

FIGURE 4-20. To palpate for an effusion of the right knee, the clinician's left hand milks the suprapatellar pouch and the lateral aspect of the knee. An effusion is easily visualized as a fluid wave on the medial aspect of the knee.

If the patient has septic arthritis or juvenile rheumatoid arthritis involving the knee, there will typically be an effusion that is easily detectable on clinical examination.

A 4-month-old Girl Is Referred for Evaluation Because She Has an Extra Finger on the Right Hand

Polydactyly occurs when there are more than five digits on the hand or foot; it is one of the more common congenital deformities in newborns. It is common to have polydactyly involving both the hands and feet in the same infant, and polydactyly is often seen in association with syndactyly, in which case it is termed polysyndactyly. The history begins by verifying the pertinent data from the patient profile. The clinician asks when the extra digit was first noted and whether the parents or legal guardian believe that it is functioning properly. This helps the clinician understand whether the parents or legal guardian are mainly concerned about functional limitations, cosmesis, or both. The birth and developmental history are typically unremarkable in a patient with polydactyly. The family history is important, because polydactyly is typically inherited as an autosomal dominant trait. If other members of the family had polydactyly, the clinician asks if any of them had treatment for the disorder. In polydactyly, if the extra digit is located on the radial side of the hand or the tibial side of the foot, it is termed preaxial polydactyly. If the extra digit involves the

index, long, and ring fingers, or the second, third, and fourth toes, it is termed central polydactyly. If the extra digit is located on the ulnar side of the hand or the fibular side of the foot, it is termed postaxial polydactyly. In the review of systems, it is important to ask about other medical problems, because postaxial polydactyly is associated with a number of syndromes, such as trisomy 13 (7).

On physical examination, the polydactyly is not always obvious, but if the clinician looks specifically at the hands or feet, the extra digit is noted. The extra digit should be closely observed while the child plays with a toy, and it should be taken through a full range of motion to determine if there are any functional limitations of the digit. Watching the child play is probably the best way to detect functional limitations. When the infant is 4 to 6 months of age, an occupational therapy evaluation is often valuable for the parents or legal guardian to obtain more information about the function of the hand.

THE ORTHOPAEDIC EXAMINATION FROM 4 TO 10 YEARS OF AGE

A 4-year-old Boy Is Referred Because He Is Walking on His Toes

The history reveals that the parents first noted that the child walked on his toes when he began walking independently at 2 years of age. If asked, he is able to walk with his feet flat on the floor, but, if he is not thinking about it, he returns to walking on his toes. He has continued to walk on his toes about 95% of the time since he was 2 years old. The birth history reveals that he was born after a 28-week gestation, when his mother spontaneously went into labor. The birth was by emergency cesarean section, and the birth weight was 1400 g. The perinatal course was complicated, and the patient was hospitalized in the neonatal intensive care unit for 6 weeks because of pulmonary problems. The developmental history reveals that he first sat at 11 months of age and first walked independently at 2 years of age. The family first noted that he was right-handed at 12 months of age when he preferred to play with toys using the right hand. The past history and family history are unremarkable, and the child is being evaluated to determine if he should begin kindergarten this fall or wait until next year.

The child wore his own shorts and T-shirt for the physical examination to avoid having to wear a johnny or hospital gown. The clinician begins by asking the patient to walk in the hallway, and notes that he is walking on his toes. There is no heel strike, foot flat, or toe-off, but he remains on his toes. This type of gait pattern is termed a toe-toe gait pattern, in contrast to the typical heel-toe gait pattern. In the typical gait pattern, the stance phase begins with heel strike, followed by foot flat (the first rocker), then, in mid-stance, there is forward rotation of the tibia over the foot (the second rocker), and, at terminal stance, there is plantar flexion of the foot and ankle at push-off (the third rocker), beginning the swing phase of the gait cycle. In this patient, because he ambulates with a toe-toe gait pattern, there is a loss of the first rocker and a decrease of the second and third rockers. The clinician also notes that the gait pattern is asymmetric, because he spends more time in the stance phase on his right side, compared with the left (8). This is an important observation, because patients with myopathy or idiopathic toe-walking will typically have a symmetric gait pattern. During gait, it is also noted that, at the end of the swing phase, the knees do not extend completely, and, at the end of the stance phase, the hips do not extend completely. When he is asked to walk at a faster pace, the child tends to posture both upper extremities, left more than right, with the elbows in flexion, the forearms in pronation, and the wrists in flexion. This is also an important observation, because posturing of the upper extremities during gait is commonly seen in patients with cerebral palsy. While he is walking, he is noted to have a foot-progression angle of 10 degrees of inward rotation on the left and 5 degrees of inward rotation on the right.

After observation of the patient's gait pattern the physical examination begins with the spine and continues with the upper and lower extremities. The spine is examined from the back with the patient standing while the clinician looks for any asymmetry. The clinician's hands are placed on the patient's iliac crests, and the right iliac crest is 5 mm higher than the left, indicating a slight limb-length discrepancy, with the right longer than the left. The patient is then asked to bend forward at the waist, as if he is touching his toes, and the examiner observes for a rib or lumbar prominence, indicating a rotational deformity of the spine, as is often seen in patients with scoliosis (the Adams forward-bending test). In this case, there is a left lumbar prominence that measures 6 degrees by scoliometer at L3 (3). This prominence may reflect a structural scoliosis or a postural scoliosis secondary to the limb-length inequality. The spinous processes are palpated to determine if there is any tenderness in the spine.

The patient is then asked to sit on the examination table for examination of the upper extremities. The patient is asked to pick up an object, to determine if there is hand preference, and to determine if he can do it with both hands. Grasp strength of both hands is tested simultaneously by having the patient squeeze the clinician's index and long fingers of both hands at the same time. Pinch strength is tested by having the patient pick up a pen or small object between the index finger and the thumb. Stereognosis is tested by placing a known object, such as a coin, into the hand, and asking the patient to identify the object without looking at it. The shoulders, elbows, forearms, and wrists are taken through a full range of motion, to determine if there are any contractures. In this patient, no weakness or contractures were noted. Patients with spastic cerebral palsy will often have adduction contractures of the shoulders, flex-

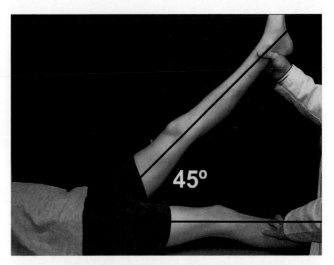

FIGURE 4-21. With the patient supine on the examination table, the clinician gradually raises one lower extremity by flexing the hip with the knee in extension. The straight-leg-raising test measures the angle between the lower limb and the tabletop.

ion contractures of the elbows, pronation contractures of the forearms, flexion contractures of the wrists, and a thumb-in-palm contracture of the hand.

The patient is then placed supine on the examination table, and a straight-leg-raising test is performed, demonstrating 45 degrees of straight-leg raising on the left and 50 degrees on the right (Fig. 4-21). If limited straight-leg raising is noted, it often indicates contracture of the hamstring muscles, but it may indicate radiculopathy with nerve root compression. This can be differentiated by observing the popliteal angle, which may cause some discomfort if there is contracture of the hamstring muscles, but may cause shooting pains down the leg if there is radiculopathy (Fig. 4-22). In this case, the popliteal angles are 64 degrees on the left and 45 degrees on the right. In the supine position, the hips are taken through a full range of motion. Patients with spastic cerebral palsy will often have flexion and adduction contractures of the hips. A flexion contracture is demonstrated by flexing one hip completely so that the knee is against the chest, and observing the amount of flexion of the other hip. Placing the knee against the chest flattens the lumbar spine and levels the pelvis, so that gravity will allow the other hip to extend. Any residual flexion of the other hip is recorded in degrees; this patient has a flexion contracture of 64 degrees on the left and 20 degrees on the right (Thomas test) (Fig. 4-23). A hip flexion contracture can also be demonstrated by placing the patient in the prone position with the lower extremities flexed over the end of the table. This position flattens the lumbar spine and levels the pelvis. One hip remains flexed while the clinician gradually extends the other hip; as soon as the pelvis moves, the amount of residual hip flexion is the flexion contracture (prone Staheli test) (9) (Fig. 4-24). With the patient in the

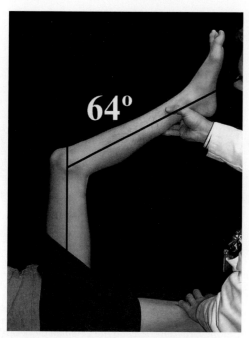

FIGURE 4-22. With the patient supine on the examination table, the clinician gradually raises one lower extremity by flexing the hip and knee to 90 degrees. The hip is kept at 90 degrees of flexion, and the knee is gradually extended as far as is comfortable. The popliteal angle is the angle between a line drawn along the leg and a line drawn along the axis of the thigh.

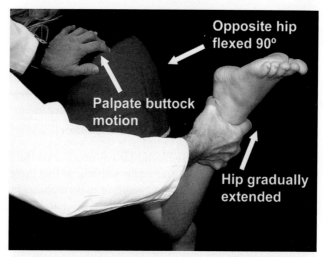

FIGURE 4-24. The prone Staheli test is another technique to measure a hip flexion contracture. The patient is placed prone, with the lower extremities flexed at the hips over the end of the table. This position flattens the lumbar spine and corrects the anterior pelvic tilt. One hip remains flexed, while the clinician gradually extends the other hip until motion is detected in the pelvis. The amount of hip flexion that is present when the pelvis first moves is the flexion contracture.

supine position and the hips flexed to 90 degrees, the hips should abduct to 75 degrees. In this patient, there is abduction to only 40 degrees on the left and 60 degrees on the right. The decrease in the amount of hip abduction with

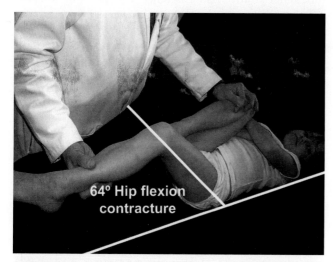

FIGURE 4-23. The Thomas test is performed by flexing the opposite hip and knee into the knee–chest position. This flattens the lumbar spine, correcting the anterior pelvic tilt; the other lower extremity should remain on the table with the hip extended. If the other hip remains flexed, the angle between the thigh and the tabletop measures the flexion contracture of the hip.

the knees extended compared to that with the knees flexed, represents the contribution of the medial hamstrings to the adduction contracture (Phelps-Baker test). Limited abduction, particularly if asymmetric and associated with flexion contracture, may indicate hip subluxation or dislocation. The patient is then placed in the lateral decubitus position, with the lower hip flexed against the chest, flattening the lumbar spine and leveling the pelvis. The higher hip is then adducted with the knee flexed and with the knee extended. The hip will typically adduct to 30 degrees, and any loss of adduction represents an abduction contracture (Ober test) (10). The increase in the abduction contracture with the knee in extension, compared to that with the knee in flexion, demonstrates the contribution of the tensor fascia to the abduction contracture. A patient with spastic cerebral palsy will typically develop an adduction contracture of the hip, whereas a patient with poliomyelitis will often develop an abduction contracture secondary to a tight tensor fasciae latae.

The patient is then placed in the prone position, and is noted to have symmetric hip internal rotation to 90 degrees and external rotation to 70 degrees. Patients with spastic cerebral palsy often have increased anteversion of the proximal femur, which causes an increase in internal rotation and a decrease in external rotation of the hips. In contrast, patients with developmental coxa vara, or slipped capital femoral epiphysis, typically have a retroversion deformity of the femoral neck, which causes an increase in external rotation and a decrease in internal rotation of the hips. With the patient in the prone position, the knee is flexed to 130 degrees, and the clinician notes that the hip spontaneously flexes, causing the buttocks to rise off the table, indicating a contracture of the rectus femoris component of the quadriceps muscle (Ely test) (Fig. 4-25).

The patient is again placed in the supine position, the knees are taken through a full range of motion, and any flexion contractures are recorded. The feet are then examined to determine if there is an equinus or equinovarus contracture. It is important to supinate the hindfoot to lock the subtalar joint when examining for equinus contracture of the ankle, because one can get a false impression that there is adequate ankle dorsiflexion as a result of hypermobility in the subtalar and tarsal joints. In this patient, when the ankle is dorsiflexed, there is a 20-degree plantar flexion contracture, but, when gradual pressure is applied to the foot and ankle, 20 degrees of dorsiflexion is eventually achieved. Performing the test slowly helps to distinguish between the dynamic component of the contracture and the actual static contracture of the Achilles tendon. The decrease in the amount of dorsiflexion achieved with the knee extended, compared to that with the knee flexed, represents the contribution of the gastrocnemius muscle to the equinus contracture (Silverskiöld test) (11).

When the patient is standing, the clinician notes that there is a varus deformity of the hindfoot. In this case, it is beneficial to determine if the hindfoot varus deformity represents a primary deformity of the hindfoot, or if it is caused by a pronated first metatarsal. The patient is asked to stand with his back facing the clinician, and the amount of hindfoot varus is noted. The patient is then asked to stand with the foot on a 1- to 2-cm block, and the first and second metatarsal heads are allowed to fall off the block onto the floor. The amount of correction of the hindfoot

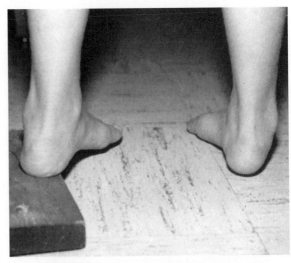

FIGURE 4-26. The patient has bilateral pes cavus deformities, and the clinician observes the amount of hindfoot varus with the patient standing. The patient then stands on a 1- to 2-cm block, and the first and second metatarsal heads are allowed to pronate and fall off the block onto the floor. The amount of correction of the hindfoot varus deformity on the Coleman block test represents the forefoot contribution to the hindfoot varus deformity. (From ref. 13, with permission.)

deformity, when the patient stands on the block, represents the forefoot contribution to the hindfoot varus deformity (Coleman block test) (12) (Fig. 4-26). The peripheral pulses and reflexes in the upper and lower extremities are tested, including the Babinski reflex. Patients with spastic cerebral palsy will typically have an increased stretch reflex of the "clasp-knife type." They will usually have hyperreflexia, clonus, and a positive Babinski reflex. Patients with athetosis will typically have purposeless-type movement patterns, particularly involving the upper extremities. If the athetosis is of the tension type, tension can be "shaken out" of the limb by the clinician. If there is dystonia, the clinician notes distorted posturing of the limbs and trunk without evidence of any contractures. If the patient has rigidity, it can be the "lead-pipe type," with continuous resistance to passive motion, or it can be the "cog-wheel type," with discontinuous resistance to passive motion. If the patient has ataxia, there is a loss of balance, with decreased coordination of the limbs causing a wide-based gait pattern (4).

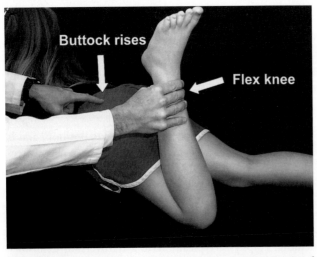

FIGURE 4-25. The Ely test is designed to detect a contracture of the rectus femoris component of the quadriceps muscle. With the patient prone, the clinician gently flexes the knee to 130 degrees. If there is simultaneous flexion of the hip, causing the buttocks to rise off the table, there is a rectus femoris contracture.

A 7-year-old Boy Is Referred for Evaluation of Right-sided Thigh Pain with a Limp That Has Persisted for 4 Months Despite Decreasing His Activities

The patient profile is reviewed with the patient and parents or legal guardian to verify exactly when the symptoms began. Four months earlier, he played baseball all day with his friends, and the next morning, he complained of right thigh pain. Later that afternoon he was playing in the yard, and his parents noted that he was limping on the right side. It is unusual to sustain a groin muscle injury at this age, and symptoms from a groin muscle injury will typically improve in 2 to 4 weeks. The patient is asked about activities that aggravate the symptoms and activities that improve the symptoms. The pain and limp are directly related to activities, and are worse when he plays hard with his friends, and are relieved when he rests. The birth and developmental history are discussed with the parents or legal guardian, although in this case one would expect an unremarkable birth and developmental history, with independent walking by the appropriate time. If the patient is black, he may have sickle cell disease, with a bone infarct involving the femoral head or another bone in the lower extremity. A patient with Legg-Calvé-Perthes disease may be of short stature, and a patient with osteochondrodysplasia will often be of short stature, and may have a family history of the disorder. The insidious onset of pain and a limp is a common presentation for a patient with a bone cyst or tumor involving the femur or tibia. Patients with an osteoid osteoma involving the proximal femur, although typically older, will often complain of night pain that is relieved by aspirin or antiinflammatory medication.

The physical examination of a patient complaining of thigh pain and a limp can begin by asking the patient to walk in the hallway. A patient with Legg-Calvé-Perthes disease, or a bone cyst involving the femur, will often have an antalgic or painful type of limp during gait. This is characterized by a decreased time in the stance phase of the gait cycle, with swaying of the trunk over the painful hip, to decrease the joint reactive forces (Trendelenburg gait). The Trendelenburg gait pattern is an important clinical observation, because it leads the clinician to suspect a problem with the hip, rather than in the knee, leg, or foot. After observation of the patient's gait pattern, an examination of the back and upper extremities is followed by an examination of the lower limbs. During the examination, the clinician compares the symptomatic side with the uninvolved side, looking for any asymmetry. A patient with synovitis involving the hip will typically have a loss of internal rotation, abduction, and extension of the involved hip. This patient has a loss of 40 degrees of internal rotation, 20 degrees of abduction, and 15 degrees of extension, compared with the uninvolved side. The loss of internal rotation is usually the most pronounced, and this is best demonstrated by examining the patient in the prone position with the hips in extension. In this position, with the knees flexed to 90 degrees, the hips are simultaneously internally rotated, and any asymmetry is noted (Fig. 4-7).

The patient is then examined in the supine position, and each hip is flexed to 90 degrees, and gently internally and externally rotated through a range of motion. The clinician notes the range of internal and external rotation of each hip, and observes for any involuntary muscle guarding on the

right side. Guarding indicates that the hip is irritable or inflamed; if present, it is a very important observation, because it indicates that the problem most likely involves the hip. The guarding is typically more pronounced as the clinician takes the hips toward the maximum of internal and external rotation. If there is a limited range of motion without any guarding it may indicate a bony deformity, such as a femoral neck retroversion deformity, which is seen in patients with developmental coxa vara. Because the history and physical examination have isolated the problem to the hip, anteroposterior and frog pelvis radiographs are recommended.

A 5-year-old Boy Is Referred for Evaluation of a Flatfoot Deformity (Pes Planus) That the Parents First Noted When He Began Walking at 13 Months of Age

The patient profile is reviewed with the patient and parents or legal guardian to verify that the pes planus deformity was in fact first noted at 13 months of age. The time that the deformity was first noted might be important, because a rigid pes planus deformity, such as that seen in patients with congenital vertical talus, is typically noted at birth. A rigid pes planus deformity that is seen in patients with tarsal coalition is often not noted until the child is 10 to 12 years of age, when the cartilaginous bar begins to ossify and limits the range of motion of the foot. A flexible pes planus deformity collapses with weightbearing, so it is not unusual that it was first noted by the parents or grandparents when the child first began to walk. A 5-year-old boy with a flexible flatfoot deformity will not usually have any pain associated with the deformity. In fact, a 5-year-old boy usually will not even notice that he has a deformity. This is verified by asking the child if he notices anything different about his feet, compared with his friends, and if he has any pain or limitation of activities because of his feet. It is also valuable to ask the parents or legal guardian if their concern is mainly cosmetic or if they believe that the child is having difficulty with pain, function, or keeping up with his friends. The family history may be relevant, because flexible flatfeet can be familial, and, if the deformity is present in other family members, it is helpful to know if they had or have any functional limitations. Patients who have a tarsal coalition (peroneal spastic flatfoot) are older, and will typically have pain aggravated by activities, and limited subtalar motion that may predispose them to frequent ankle sprains.

The physical examination of a 5-year-old boy with a pes planus deformity begins by asking him to walk in the hallway. He walks with a symmetric heel-toe gait pattern, with a foot-progression angle of 25 degrees of external rotation (Fig. 4-5). This is not surprising, because a patient with a pes planus deformity also has a tendency to toe-out, whereas a patient with a pes cavus deformity has a tendency to toe-in. Before focusing on the feet, a general physical examination of the back, upper extremities, and lower extremities is performed. A flexible pes planus deformity is the most common type of flatfoot deformity in childhood. It is most likely caused by excessive laxity of the ligaments and joint capsules, allowing the tarsal arch to collapse with weightbearing. The key is to differentiate this benign condition from the more serious types of flatfoot deformities, such as congenital vertical talus or tarsal coalition. When standing, patients with a flexible pes planus deformity have a collapsed medial longitudinal arch with a pronated foot and a valgus heel. The arch returns when the patient is sitting, because the weightbearing force that caused the collapse of the arch is relieved. The arch is also recreated by dorsiflexing the great toe, or by asking the child to stand on his tiptoes (Fig. 4-27). The clinician uses these simple tests to document that the patient has a flexible pes planus deformity, a benign condition that does not require any treatment, rather than rigid deformity, which often benefits from treatment.

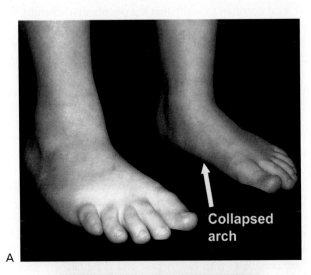

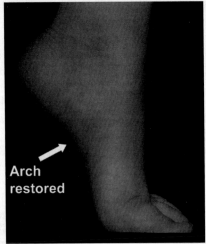

FIGURE 4-27. A: This patient has bilateral flexible pes planus deformities with a collapsed medial longitudinal arch, pronated feet, and valgus heels. **B:** The arch returns when the patient stands on his tiptoes, demonstrating that the pes planus is flexible.

A 6-year-old Boy Is Referred for Evaluation of Acute Pain and Swelling Involving the Left Elbow after Falling from the Monkey Bars at School

This child was apparently in excellent health until earlier in the day, when he fell from the monkey bars and immediately developed pain and swelling about the elbow. The parents called their pediatrician, who recommended that they go directly to the emergency room (ER) at the hospital, and the ER physician is requesting an orthopaedic consultation. In this situation, the patient and family are anxious about the injury, apprehensive about going to the ER, and frightened that the examination or treatment may be painful. The patient is typically found lying on a gurney in the ER, with the elbow in a temporary splint. Knowledge of the mechanism of injury is important for the clinician to assess the magnitude of the trauma that caused the injury and the likelihood of associated complications. The patient remembers that the monkey bars were about 4 ft off the ground, and that he was playing with his friends when he fell, landing on the outstretched arm. A fall on an outstretched arm is the same mechanism of injury that can cause a fracture of the distal humerus, an elbow dislocation, a forearm fracture, a fracture of the distal radius, or any combination of these injuries. If the fall was from a height of 2 ft, the clinician might suspect a contusion or minimally displaced fracture, whereas if the fall was from 20 ft, it could cause a displaced fracture with an associated neurovascular injury. The past history may be helpful, because if the patient has had multiple fractures associated with a disorder such as osteogenesis imperfecta, he may have a pathologic fracture, which is usually minimally displaced and not associated with other injuries. The past history may reveal a kidney problem with renal osteodystrophy, which would increase the likelihood of a pathologic fracture. He has been in excellent health, and does not complain of any numbness or tingling in the hand, and there is no reason to believe that the injury could have been nonaccidental.

The clinician asks if the boy would like to remove the splint himself or if he would prefer to have someone else do it for him. He is asked if he would prefer to be checked while lying down or if he would prefer to be seated. He is also reassured that his parents or legal guardian can stay with him during the examination. Once the patient and family realize that they have the power to make these simple yet important decisions, they become less apprehensive about the entire setting in the ER. When the splint has been removed and the patient is comfortable, the physical examination begins by examination of the uninjured upper extremity, so the patient learns what is involved with the examination. This also allows the clinician to understand what the normal side looks like, and to assess the child's level of apprehension. The injured arm is then observed, and marked swelling and ecchymosis are noted over the distal humerus. These findings are more consistent with a fracture of the distal humerus, or a fracture-dislocation of the elbow, than with a simple contusion. When examining the injured side, the clinician gently palpates the elbow and the distal humerus, and, with the help of the patient, locates the point of maximum tenderness. In most cases, the point of maximum tenderness will be the location of the fracture or contusion.

If the patient has a fracture of the distal humerus, the immediate concern is not the fracture, but whether there is an associated injury to the soft tissues, particularly the arteries and nerves. As a result, a neurocirculatory examination of the hands is performed to compare pulses, capillary fill, pain, light touch, strength, and range of motion of the fingers, between the injured and the uninjured sides. A distal humeral fracture or an elbow dislocation can interfere with the circulation to the hand, either by directly injuring the brachial artery at the elbow or by causing swelling in the compartments of the forearm, which can interfere with capillary blood flow. If the artery is lacerated or trapped in the fracture site, there may be no pulses and the hand may be cool and white. If there is swelling within a compartment that is interfering with capillary blood flow, it may lead to muscle ischemia, and although the pulses and circulation to the hand may appear normal, an early compartment syndrome may be developing. In this case, a high index of suspicion and the finding of pain out of proportion to the mechanism of injury, or pain with passive motion of the fingers, may be the only signs of an impending compartment syndrome.

The results of the neurocirculatory examination may be within normal limits initially, but may change during the next few hours. A compartment syndrome occurs when there is swelling within a closed space, and after an elbow injury; the compartment that most often develops excessive swelling is the volar compartment of the forearm. Swelling in a compartment causes increased pressure that interferes with capillary flow, resulting in muscle ischemia. An early compartment syndrome may be first detected by noticing that the patient is experiencing pain that seems to be out of proportion to the physical findings. Another early sign of a compartment syndrome is pain to passive stretching of the ischemic muscles. If the flexor muscles in the forearm are ischemic, the patient may complain of pain when the fingers are passively extended. As soon as the swelling in the compartment reaches the level of the systolic blood pressure, it will obliterate the pulse at the wrist. However, once a compartment syndrome has reached this stage, the muscles in the forearm may already be necrotic. When the necrotic muscles scar and develop fibrosis, a contracture develops, causing a flexion deformity of the wrist and fingers, termed a "Volkmann ischemic contracture." A Volkmann con-

tracture can markedly interfere with hand function, so it is important to diagnose a compartment syndrome early and avoid this devastating complication.

A distal humeral fracture or an elbow dislocation may injure a nerve, either by direct contusion or by stretching from traction and angulation at the injury site. A complete neurologic examination of the hand is important to document any nerve injuries before embarking on treatment. It is always less stressful for an apprehensive child to begin by examining the uninjured extremity. To evaluate the sensory component of any nerve, it is accurate and nonthreatening to test two-point discrimination using a paper clip to compare the injured side with the noninjured side. The radial nerve is tested by asking the patient to extend his fingers (motor), and checking the sensation in the dorsal web space between the thumb and the index finger (sensory). The median nerve is tested by asking the patient to flex the long and ring fingers (motor), and checking the sensation on the volar aspect of the index finger (sensory). The ulnar nerve is tested by asking the patient to spread his fingers apart (motor), and checking the sensation on the volar aspect of the little finger (sensory). The anterior interosseous nerve is tested by holding the index finger in extension at the metacarpophalangeal and proximal interphalangeal joints, and asking the patient to flex the tip of the finger (motor). The anterior interosseous nerve does not have a sensory component, so an injury to this nerve may not be detected, unless the clinician tests the motor component of the nerve. If the patient and family or legal guardian are extremely anxious, it is possible for the physical examination to be compromised. If that occurs, it is important to document the problem with the examination in the medical record. After the examination is completed, anteroposterior and lateral radiographs centered at the point of maximum tenderness, including a joint above and below, will usually show the fracture or dislocation.

A 9-year-old Boy Is Referred for Evaluation Because He Is Having Pain in His Left Heel That Is Aggravated by Playing Soccer

The history reveals that the patient has been in good health until 1 month earlier, when he began to experience left heel pain. The pain is worse in the evenings after he has played soccer during the day. The patient is a healthy, active boy who is very involved in sports, including soccer, basketball, and baseball. The pain is relieved by rest, and seems to improve when he is not participating in soccer. When asked whether it hurts while he is playing soccer or after he has played, he acknowledges that the pain usually does not bother him while playing, but begins afterwards. The parents have noted swelling in the past, but there is no swelling at the present time. The history is consistent with a calcaneal apophysitis, also termed "Sever disease," but the differential diagnosis also includes tumor, bone cyst, or juvenile rheumatoid arthritis. On further questioning, he denies any morning pain or stiffness, such as one might see in patients with juvenile rheumatoid arthritis. Some children with calcaneal apophysitis will have heel pain in the morning when they first get out of bed.

On physical examination, the feet appear symmetric and no swelling is detected. The pain is located in the heel, right over the calcaneal apophysis, and is aggravated by squeezing the posterior aspect of the calcaneus. There is no pain at the insertion of the Achilles tendon, as would be seen in a patient with Achilles tendonitis, and there is no pain at the origin of the plantar fascia, as would be seen in a patient with plantar fasciitis. Achilles tendonitis and plantar fasciitis, although common in adults, are not frequently seen in children. Calcaneal apophysitis (Sever disease) is an overuse syndrome, and the symptoms should subside with activity modification. If the pain is unilateral or persists despite activity modification, anteroposterior and lateral radiographs may help with the differential diagnosis.

THE ORTHOPAEDIC EXAMINATION FROM 10 TO 18 YEARS OF AGE

A 13-year-old Girl Is Referred for Evaluation of Scoliosis

The pertinent findings in the patient profile are reviewed with the patient and parents or legal guardian. The scoliosis was first detected 4 months earlier, on a routine annual checkup by the family pediatrician. The patient states that she occasionally gets pain in the lower back after sitting for long periods of time, and that otherwise she is in excellent health. She denies any problems with bowel or bladder function, and states that she is active in sports, including soccer and tennis. The family history reveals that she has two maternal cousins with scoliosis, one of whom required operative correction of the deformity. She has a 16-year-old brother and a 9-year-old sister who are in good health, without evidence of scoliosis. There is no family history of anyone with muscular dystrophy or a neuromuscular disorder, and no one in the family died prematurely. She has not yet begun the menses, and her mother states that she has grown 2 in. in the last 6 months. She is 5 ft 2 in. tall, and her mother is 5 ft 6 in. tall.

The physical examination begins with the patient standing; the spine is observed from the back. The clinician looks for any asymmetry in the height of the shoulders, the prominence of the scapular spines, the surface shape of the rib cage, or the contour of the waist. The skin is observed for any café-au-lait marks or freckling in the axilla that may indicate neurofibromatosis. If the patient is tall and has long, prominent fingers (arachnodactyly), it may indicate Marfan syndrome. A plumb bob is suspended from the spi-

nous process of the seventh cervical vertebra, and the clinician notes if it falls over the gluteal cleft. If the spine is compensated and the patient is standing erect, the head should be centered directly over the pelvis and the plumb bob should fall over the gluteal cleft. If the spine is decompensated to the right or left, the distance from the plumb bob to the gluteal cleft is recorded in centimeters. The clinician observes the posterior iliac dimples in stance to determine if they are symmetric and level, indicating equal limb lengths. The clinician's hands are placed on the iliac crests to determine if the pelvis is level, or if there is a limb-length discrepancy. If the patient has a limb-length discrepancy, a compensatory postural scoliosis deformity may develop that is convex toward the shorter limb. If there is a limb-length discrepancy with a compensatory lumbar scoliosis, the waist may be more accentuated on the concave side, which the patient often interprets as the "hip sticking out." Scoliosis that occurs because of a limb-length discrepancy is a postural scoliosis that should correct when the limb-length discrepancy is corrected. This can be accomplished by placing an appropriately sized wooden block under the foot of the short leg to equalize the limb lengths. The spinous processes are palpated to determine if there is any focal tenderness, and the patient is asked to arch her back, to determine if it causes any discomfort. Patients who have spondylolysis or spondylolisthesis will often have discomfort when they hyperextend the lumbar spine.

The patient is then asked to place the hands together in front of her, as if she were diving into a pool, and to bend forward at the waist, as if she were touching her toes. This is termed the "Adams forward-bending test," and is one of the most sensitive clinical tests for detecting a scoliosis deformity (Fig. 4-28). As the patient bends forward, the

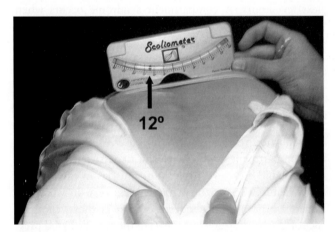

FIGURE 4-28. The Adams forward-bending test is conducted by asking the patient to place the hands together in front of her, as if she were diving into a pool, and to bend forward at the waist, as if she were touching her toes. As the patient bends forward, the clinician observes the spine to determine if it is supple, and if it flexes symmetrically. Once the patient has bent forward so that the spine is parallel to the floor, the clinician measures the rib prominence in degrees using a scoliometer.

clinician observes the spine to determine if it is supple and flexes symmetrically. If the patient bends to one side rather than straight ahead, the clinician should take note, because this may indicate tight hamstring muscles that may be associated with spondylolisthesis, disk herniation, or tumor. As the patient bends forward, if the spine flexes excessively in the thoracic area (thoracic kyphosis), but not in the lumbar area, it may indicate Scheuermann disease. Once the patient has bent forward, the clinician looks for any asymmetry of the trunk, notes any rib or lumbar prominence, and measures the prominence using a scoliometer (14) (Fig. 4-28). The rib prominence reflects the rotational component of the scoliosis deformity that occurs in the axial plane. The most common type of scoliosis deformity is a convex right thoracic curve, in which the vertebrae rotate into the convexity of the curve, twisting the rib cage, so that the ribs are more prominent posteriorly on the patient's right side. The ribs are also more prominent anteriorly on the patient's left side, which may cause some breast asymmetry. While the patient is in the forward-bending position, the clinician asks her to bend from side to side to assess the flexibility of the scoliosis deformity.

Scoliosis is seen in association with neuromuscular disorders, such as muscular dystrophy or cerebral palsy, and is also seen is association with spinal cord anomalies, such as syringomyelia or tethered spinal cord. As a result, a neurologic examination of the patient is essential to rule out an occult neuromuscular or neurologic cause of the scoliosis deformity. With the patient standing, the Romberg sign is tested for by asking the patient to stand with the feet placed closely together. The patient is then asked to close her eyes, and the clinician looks for any sway or instability. The patient with balance problems or cerebellar ataxia will sway or move her feet to maintain balance. This test may be important because scoliosis is commonly seen in patients with Friedreich ataxia. Lower extremity strength and reflexes, including the Babinski reflex, are tested to rule out any occult neurologic problems. With the patient in the supine position, a straight-leg-raising test is performed to look for hamstring tightness or radiculopathy. If the previous examination suggested a limb-length discrepancy, the lower extremity lengths can be measured from the anterior superior iliac spine to the medial malleolus using a tape measure. While measuring the lower extremity lengths, it is important that the hips are in a neutral position, because abduction of one hip and adduction of the other hip will affect the measurements. The abdominal reflexes are tested by gently stroking the side of the abdomen; the umbilicus should deviate toward the stimulus. Any asymmetry of the abdominal reflexes is documented, because this may reflect an underlying spinal cord problem. In patients with adolescent idiopathic scoliosis, it is important to assess their maturity, because the risk of progression of the scoliosis deformity is higher in younger patients and in patients with larger curves. If a scoliosis deformity is suspected on the physical examination, appropriate radiographs are indicated.

A 14-year-old Boy Is Referred for Evaluation of Persistent Right Knee Pain That Causes Him to Limp

The history reveals that the pain and limp developed spontaneously 4 months earlier, and that the patient has otherwise been in good health. There is no history of injury, and he does not recall any swelling in the knee. In describing the pain, he points to the anterior aspect of the right knee and to the inner thigh. He states that the pain is worse with activity, and the parents state that the limp is usually worse toward the end of the day. The birth and developmental history are unremarkable, and there is no family history of any leg problems or arthritis. The personal and social history reveals that he has always been overweight, but in the last year, his weight has increased markedly.

On physical examination, the patient is obese (greater than the 95th percentile for weight), and, on observation of his gait pattern, he is seen to ambulate with a limp (antalgic or painful gait) on the right. When he walks, he leans his head and trunk over his right lower extremity during the stance phase. This shifting of his weight over the right lower extremity in stance is done to decrease the pain in the extremity, and is termed a Trendelenburg gait pattern. He has a shortened stance phase on the right, and his foot-progression angle is 10 degrees of external rotation on the left and 30 degrees of external rotation on the right (Fig. 4-5). With the patient standing, the spine is observed from the back, and any asymmetry is noted. The clinician's hands are placed on the iliac crests, and the right iliac crest is noted to be 1 cm lower than the left, indicating a limb-length discrepancy, with the right shorter than the left. With the examiner's hands still on the iliac crests, the patient is asked to stand on the left lower extremity and lift the right foot off the floor. When the patient stands on the left leg, the right iliac crest rises up 1 cm, indicating that the abductor muscles of the left hip are functioning satisfactorily. In contrast, when the patient stands on the right leg, the left iliac crest drops 1 cm, indicating insufficiency of the abductor muscles on the right (positive Trendelenburg test) (Fig. 4-18). In single-limb support, contraction of the abductor muscles markedly increases the compressive forces between the femoral head and the acetabulum, so patients with hip pain will often limp, rather than experience increased discomfort from contracting the abductor muscles.

In the supine position, the knee has a full range of motion from 0 to 135 degrees. To look for an effusion the suprapatellar pouch and lateral aspect of the knee are milked, while observing for a fluid wave on the medial aspect. If there was a large effusion, the patella would float above its articulation with the femoral trochlea, and when the clinician pushed the patella toward the femur a ballottable patella would be appreciated. The patient points to the anterior aspect of the knee and the inner thigh when describing the pain, yet the knee is nontender to palpation and stable to stress, and the remainder of the knee examination is unremarkable. Because the same nerves that supply the knee (obturator, sciatic, and femoral) also supply the hip, it is not unusual for a patient with hip pathology to perceive that the pain is coming from the knee. As a result, it is important to examine both the knees and the hips in a patient complaining of knee pain.

Examination of the patient's hips reveals flexion to 130 degrees on the left and 120 degrees on the right. Abduction is to 70 degrees on the left and 50 degrees on the right. Internal rotation is to 30 degrees on the left and 0 degrees on the right. External rotation is to 70 degrees on the left and 85 degrees on the right. When the left hip is flexed it remains in neutral rotation, but when the right hip is flexed it simultaneously also goes into abduction and external rotation. These physical findings indicate a retroversion deformity of the right femoral neck, with an increase in external rotation and a decrease in internal rotation of the right hip. An overweight adolescent boy with this type of deformity involving the hip has a high probability of having a slipped capital femoral epiphysis, so rather than obtaining radiographs of the knee, anteroposterior and frog-lateral pelvis radiographs are recommended.

A 14-year-old Girl Is Referred for Evaluation of Right Knee Pain and Giving Way That Is Aggravated by Playing Soccer and Basketball

The history reveals that the patient was in good health until 6 months earlier, when she began noting right knee pain after soccer practice. She states that the knee felt better between the soccer and basketball seasons, but that the pain recurred when she began playing basketball. The pain is also aggravated by sitting with the knee flexed for prolonged periods of time, such as while riding in the back seat of a car or at the movie theater. Patients with anterior knee pain or patellofemoral pain syndrome will often have pain when they have to sit still with the knee flexed for a prolonged period of time. This finding has been termed a positive "movie sign." Two months earlier, while playing basketball, the knee gave out, causing the patient to fall to the floor. She developed swelling after the injury, and the swelling resolved over the next few days.

On physical examination, the patient is asked to point to the area of maximum tenderness. An adolescent can usually point exactly to the spot that is bothering her, and she points to both the medial and lateral sides of the patella in describing her pain. She has tenderness to palpation on the undersurface of the patella, which can be elicited by gently pushing the patella laterally with the knee in extension to palpate the lateral facet, and pushing it medially to palpate the me-

dial facet. If the anterior knee pain is caused by a problem with the patellofemoral joint, it can be identified by performing a patellar inhibition test. This test is performed with the patient relaxed in the supine position with the knee in extension. The patient is asked to do a straight-leg raise while the clinician holds the patella, preventing it from ascending along the femoral sulcus. This maneuver increases the pressure between the patella and the femoral sulcus, causing discomfort in patients who have a disorder involving the patellofemoral joint (Fig. 4-29).

A patient with anterior knee pain may have the miserable malalignment syndrome, with internal femoral torsion in conjunction with external tibial torsion. The internal femoral torsion is associated with squinting patellae, in which the kneecaps are pointing inward when the patient is standing, despite the fact that the feet are pointing straight ahead. The internal femoral and external tibial torsional deformities cause an increase in the Q-angle. The Q-angle is the angle formed between a line connecting the anterior superior iliac spine with the center of the patella and a line connecting the tibial tubercle with the center of the patella, and this patient's Q-angle is 12 degrees (Fig. 4-30). The Q-angle should be measured with the knee in 30 degrees of flexion so that the patella is in contact with the femoral sulcus. Patients with an increased Q-angle may develop anterior knee pain as a result of abnormal tracking of the patella in the femoral sulcus. This maltracking can be detected by observing the patella as the patient extends the knee. With the patient sitting and the knees flexed to 90 degrees over the front of the table, the patient is asked to gradually extend the knee. The patella is observed to remain in the femoral sulcus as it ascends along the axis of the

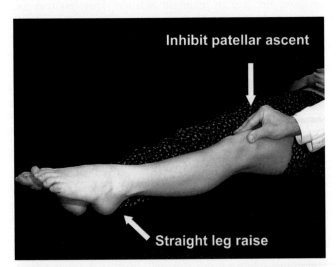

FIGURE 4-29. The patellar inhibition test is performed with the patient supine and the knee in extension. The clinician holds the patella, inhibiting it from ascending, while the patient performs a straight-leg raise. This maneuver increases the forces in the patellofemoral joint. If the patient experiences discomfort, it often indicates a patellofemoral joint disorder.

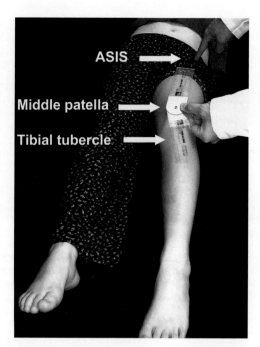

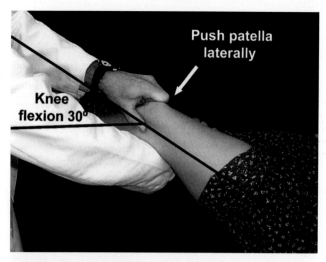

FIGURE 4-31. The patellar apprehension test is performed with the patient supine and the knee flexed to 30 degrees. The clinician gently pushes the patella laterally, and, if the patient experiences discomfort or apprehension, it is a positive test, often indicating patellofemoral instability.

FIGURE 4-30. The Q-angle is the angle formed between a line connecting the anterior superior iliac spine (*ASIS*) with the center of the patella and a line connecting the tibial tubercle with the center of the patella. The Q-angle is measured with the knee in 30 degrees of flexion, so that the patella is in contact with the femoral sulcus.

femur with knee extension, but as the knee reaches full extension, the patella deviates laterally like an upside-down J (positive J-sign). Patients with patellofemoral joint instability may be identified by performing a "patellar apprehension test." This test is performed with the patient in the supine position and the knee flexed to 30 degrees. The clinician gently pushes the patella laterally, subluxating it from the patellofemoral joint, and observes if the patient experiences any discomfort. Patients with patellofemoral joint instability often have discomfort with this maneuver, and some are so apprehensive that they contract their quadriceps, preventing the clinician from performing the test (Fig. 4-31). Another problem often seen in patients with anterior knee pain is a pes planus deformity of the foot. The pes planus deformity causes the tibia to rotate inward, decreasing the Q-angle. A decreased Q-angle is also associated with an increased incidence of patellofemoral pain.

Patients with anterior knee pain do not typically have any pain in the back of the knee. If the patient complains of pain in the back of the knee, particularly if it is associated with swelling, it may indicate a Baker cyst. A Baker cyst is a ganglion that develops between the semimembranosus tendon and the medial head of the gastrocnemius muscle. The cyst usually communicates with the knee joint, and will often develop swelling that is aggravated by activities and relieved by rest.

Patients with anterior knee pain will typically have a full range of motion from 0 to 135 degrees. The straight-leg-raising test is often limited to 60 degrees because of decreased flexibility of the hamstring muscles. There is usually no evidence of an effusion or any swelling about the knee. The knee is palpated to determine if there are specific areas of tenderness. Pain located over the tibial tubercle, at the insertion of the patellar tendon, is seen in patients with Osgood-Schlatter disease. Pain located at the inferior pole of the patella is typical for patients with Sinding-Larsen-Johansson disease (15). Pain elicited by direct palpation over the articular surface of the femoral condyle, with the knee flexed, may be seen in patients with osteochondritis dissecans. The pain can be reproduced by flexing the knee to 90 degrees, internally rotating the tibia, then gradually extending the knee. As the knee approaches 30 degrees of flexion, the patient with an osteochondritis dissecans lesion, located on the medial femoral condyle, will experience pain that is relieved by externally rotating the tibia (positive Wilson test [16]).

Pain that is located directly over the joint line is often seen in a patient with a torn meniscus. A torn meniscus can be evaluated by flexing the knee to 135 degrees, and, while applying a valgus stress, gradually extending the knee and externally rotating the tibia. Pain elicited with this maneuver (often associated with a palpable clunk) is often secondary to a torn meniscus (positive McMurray test). With the patient in the prone position, pressure can be applied to the heel, loading the knee in compression, while the tibia is internally and externally rotated on the femur. Patients with a torn meniscus will often experience pain with this maneuver when the torn meniscus is trapped between the tibia and the femur (positive Apley test). To further evaluate the status of the meniscus, the patient is then asked to relax the knee while the leg is held in full extension. The examiner rapidly pulls up on the foot, then drops it several inches, causing the knee to hyperextend, flex, then hyperextend again. Most patients will tolerate this test without any difficulty, but if the patient has a torn meniscus, this test may be uncomfortable, causing a reflex contraction of the hamstring muscles that prevents the knee from hyperextending (positive bounce test).

Although the patient with anterior knee pain will not typically have any ligamentous instability, these important knee stabilizers are examined. With the patient in the supine position and the knees flexed to 90 degrees, the clinician looks for a posterior sag of the tibia, which is often seen in patients with a posterior cruciate ligament-deficient knee. A torn posterior cruciate ligament can be elicited by the quadriceps active test (17). This test is performed with the patient in the supine position and the knee flexed to 90 degrees. The patient is asked to slide her foot down the table, while the examiner prevents the foot from moving. The force of the quadriceps muscle will pull the tibia anteriorly, reducing the posterior subluxation that is seen in a patient with a posterior cruciate ligament-deficient knee (Fig. 4-32). The anterior drawer test, to evaluate the anterior cruciate ligament, is also performed with the patient supine and the knee flexed to 90 degrees. As the tibia is pulled forward at the knee, the examiner feels a solid stop after 3 to 4 mm of translation of the tibia on the femur, indicating an intact anterior cruciate ligament. A more sensitive test to detect an anterior cruciate ligament-deficient knee is the Lachman test. This test is performed with the patient in

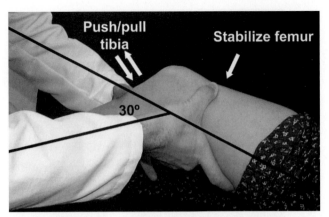

FIGURE 4-33. The Lachman test is performed with the patient supine and the knee flexed to 30 degrees. To test the left knee, the femoral condyles are held with the clinician's right hand, while the tibia is pulled anteriorly with the clinician's left hand. Anterior subluxation greater than 5 mm, without a solid end point, indicates anterior cruciate ligament insufficiency.

the supine position and the knee flexed to 30 degrees. The femoral condyles are held in one hand, while the tibia is pulled anteriorly and pushed posteriorly with the other hand. Subluxation greater than 5 mm, without a solid end point, indicates anterior cruciate ligament insufficiency (Fig. 4-33). The anterior cruciate ligament-deficient knee can also be detected using the pivot-shift test. This test is performed with the patient in the supine position and the knee in extension. A valgus and internal rotation force is applied to the leg, causing the tibia to subluxate anteriorly in an anterior cruciate ligament-deficient knee. As the knee is flexed, when the iliotibial band crosses the axis of the knee joint, the tibia rapidly shifts or reduces to its normal position, and a clunk is seen and felt by the clinician. This pivot shift of the tibia indicates an anterior cruciate ligament-deficient knee.

The medial and lateral collateral ligaments are located just under the skin, so an injury to one of these structures is usually associated with pain to palpation over the ligament. By gently palpating the uninjured side and comparing it with the injured side, the clinician can often pinpoint the location of the injury. The medial and lateral collateral ligaments are tested with the knee in 30 degrees of flexion, because varus or valgus laxity can be masked by the intact cruciate ligaments with the knee in extension. The medial joint line is palpated with a finger while the examiner applies a valgus stress to the knee, and the lateral joint line is similarly palpated while the examiner applies a varus stress to the knee. The amount of joint line widening is recorded in millimeters, and 0 to 5 mm of widening with a solid end point is considered a normal amount of ligamentous laxity. Medial and lateral collateral ligament sprains are classified according to the amount of widening or opening of the joint space on the clinical examination. A grade I sprain

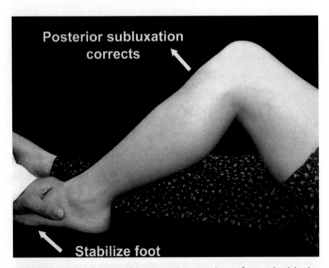

FIGURE 4-32. The quadriceps active test is performed with the patient supine and the knee flexed to 90 degrees. In a patient with a posterior cruciate ligament-deficient knee, the tibia is subluxated posteriorly in this position. The patient is asked to slide her foot down the table while the examiner prevents the foot from moving. The force of the quadriceps muscle pulls the tibia anteriorly, reducing the posterior subluxation of the tibia.

opens 0 to 5 mm, a grade II sprain opens 5 to 10 mm, and a grade III sprain opens more than 10 mm.

A 13-year-old Girl Is Referred for Evaluation of Right Shoulder Pain That Is Aggravated by Swimming

The history reveals that the patient has been a competitive swimmer since she was 6 years old, and that she was in good health until 3 months earlier. She was swimming lengths in practice when she began noting pain in the front of the right shoulder. The pain is relieved by rest, and is particularly aggravated by swimming freestyle. The remainder of the history reveals that she has always been athletic, and has no other medical problems. A swimmer or gymnast who is having difficulty with shoulder pain will usually have an overuse syndrome caused by extensive or improper training. In this situation, it is important to discuss the type of training or workouts that the patient is doing, in view of the fact that they are causing shoulder pain. Often, a training error is discovered that, when corrected, will relieve the symptoms.

On physical examination, inspection of the shoulder reveals that there is no muscle wasting, swelling, or deformity. She is tender to deep palpation over the supraspinatus tendon and the anterior aspect of the acromion. A patient who has an imbalance of the rotator cuff muscles will often have impingement with tendonitis involving the supraspinatus tendon. Range of motion of the shoulder reveals elevation to 180 degrees, external rotation with the arm at the side to 70 degrees, and internal rotation to the point where the thumbs will touch the spinous process of the fifth thoracic vertebra. In this patient, internal rotation is to the spinous process of T4 on the left and T9 on the right. This limited internal rotation indicates tight posterior structures, a common finding in patients who do a great deal of overhead athletics. The tight posterior structures can also be identified by evaluating passive crossed-arm adduction. The arm is positioned in 90 degrees of forward elevation and decreased adduction of the right shoulder, compared with the left, is secondary to tight posterior structures. Muscle strength of the shoulder in flexion, abduction, and internal and external rotation are tested, and the muscles are graded from 0 to 5, according to the scale of the Medical Research Council (18) (Table 4-4). An imbalance of the rotator cuff is often seen in patients with weakness of the periscapular muscles, including the rhomboids, serratus anterior, subscapularis, and trapezius muscles. As a result, it is important to also examine these muscles to determine if there is any associated weakness that may be contributing to the rotator cuff imbalance.

A swimmer or gymnast with shoulder pain may have ligamentous laxity with multidirectional instability and rotator cuff tendonitis with impingement. There are several tests that the clinician can use to detect instability and im-

TABLE 4-4. GRADING OF MUSCLE STRENGTH USING THE MEDICAL RESEARCH COUNCIL RATING SYSTEM

Grade	Rating	Muscle Strength	Assessment
0	Zero	No palpable contraction	Nothing
1	Trace	Muscle contracts, but no movement of the bone	Trace
2	Poor	Muscle moves the bone, but not against gravity	With gravity eliminated
3	Fair	Muscle moves the bone through a full range of motion against gravity	Against gravity
4	Good	Muscle moves the bone against resistance	Near normal
5	Excellent	Normal strength against full resistance	Normal

(From ref. 18, with permission.)

pingement. Ligamentous laxity and instability can be evaluated by palpating the amount of glenohumeral translation. With the patient seated, the clinician evaluates the amount of glenohumeral translation by stabilizing the scapula and clavicle with one hand while pushing and pulling the proximal humerus in an anterior and posterior direction with the other hand. The amount of glenohumeral translation is measured in millimeters, and compared with the uninjured shoulder (Fig. 4-34). This test is essentially a shoulder "drawer sign." Another maneuver that the clinician can use to evaluate for ligamentous laxity is the "sulcus sign." With

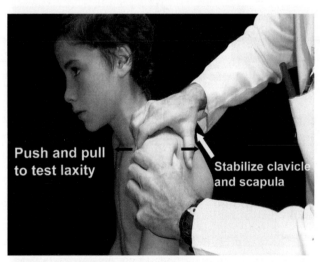

Push and pull to test laxity

Stabilize clavicle and scapula

FIGURE 4-34. Ligamentous laxity of the left shoulder is evaluated with the patient seated, by holding the scapula and clavicle with the right hand while pushing the humeral head anteriorly and pulling it posteriorly with the left hand. The amount of glenohumeral translation is measured in millimeters, and compared with the uninjured shoulder. This test is a shoulder "drawer sign."

the patient standing and relaxed, the clinician applies a longitudinal inferior traction force on the upper extremity while palpating the distance between the humeral head and the acromion. Excessive laxity of the superior glenohumeral ligament will allow the humeral head to subluxate inferiorly (Fig. 4-35).

The apprehension tests to evaluate for anterior instability can be performed with the patient sitting and the clinician standing behind the patient. If the left shoulder is being examined, the clinician abducts the shoulder to 90 degrees, then gradually increases the amount of external rotation using the left hand. The right hand of the clinician is placed over the humeral head, and the clinician gently pushes the humeral head forward with the right thumb, but has the fingers strategically placed anteriorly to control any sudden instability. Patients with anterior instability of the shoulder will experience discomfort or apprehension with this test (Fig. 4-36). Combining the external rotation with controlled anterior translation creates an impending feeling of anterior instability, termed an "apprehension sign." This test has also been referred to as the "crank test." This apprehension is relieved when the clinician pushes posteriorly on the humeral head, reducing it in the glenoid. If the apprehension is relieved with this maneuver, it is termed a positive "relocation test." The apprehension test and the relocation test can also be performed in the supine position, with the shoulder placed in 90 degrees of abduction and external rotation. The apprehension test, when performed in the supine position, is termed the "fulcrum test," because the table is used as a fulcrum to support the scapula. The

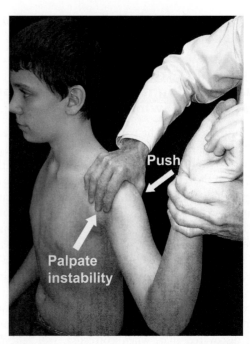

FIGURE 4-36. The apprehension test of the left shoulder is performed with the shoulder abducted to 90 degrees and externally rotated by the clinician's left hand. The clinician gently pushes the humeral head forward with the right thumb, while the fingers are strategically placed anteriorly in front of the humeral head, to prevent any sudden instability. Discomfort or apprehension with this maneuver indicates anterior instability of the shoulder.

supine relocation test is performed by abducting the shoulder to 90 degrees and externally rotating the arm up to the point where the patient experiences apprehension. The amount of external rotation is noted; the clinician then pushes the humeral head posteriorly, and the patient immediately experiences a loss of apprehension with increased external rotation of the shoulder (19) (Fig. 4-37). Posterior instability of the shoulder is typically a subluxation, rather than a dislocation, and can often be demonstrated by the patient. Because the posterior subluxation is usually asymptomatic, a posterior apprehension sign is typically absent. Posterior instability can be evaluated with the Jahnke test. This test is performed by flexing the arm forward to 90 degrees of elevation in neutral rotation, and posteriorly stressing the arm to subluxate the humeral head posteriorly. The arm is then gradually brought toward the coronal plane, while the clinician gently pushes the humeral head anteriorly, and a palpable clunk is felt as the humeral head reduces from its subluxated position (Fig. 4-38).

A swimmer with shoulder pain may have tendonitis involving the rotator cuff muscles, particularly the supraspinatus tendon. To determine if the patient has tendonitis, the clinician can perform several impingement tests. If the patient has tendonitis involving the supraspinatus tendon, forcible elevation of the arm to 180 degrees will cause the inflamed tendon to impinge against the anterior inferior

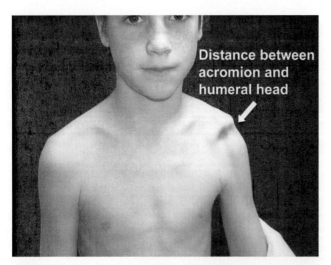

FIGURE 4-35. Ligamentous laxity of the shoulder can also be evaluated with the patient standing with his arms at his sides. The clinician applies a longitudinal inferior traction force to both upper extremities while palpating the distance between the humeral head and the acromion. Excessive laxity of the superior glenohumeral ligament will allow the left humeral head to subluxate inferiorly, compared with the right side. This increased laxity is termed a positive "sulcus sign."

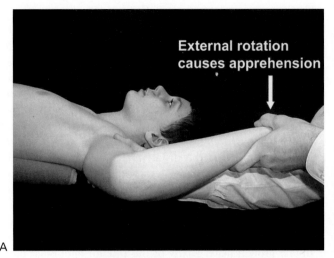

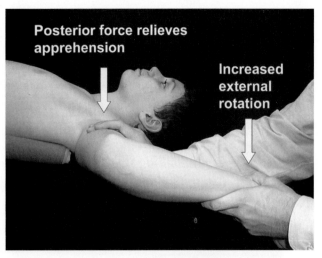

A   B

FIGURE 4-37. A: The apprehension test of the shoulder can also be performed in the supine position with the shoulder elevated to 90 degrees, then externally rotated up to the point where the patient experiences discomfort or apprehension. **B:** In the supine relocation test, after the shoulder is placed in this position, the clinician stabilizes the humeral head by pushing it posteriorly with the right hand. If the patient has increased external rotation, with a loss of apprehension as the shoulder relocates, it reflects a positive relocation test.

acromion and coracoacromial ligament, causing discomfort for the patient. This discomfort or grimacing facial expression is termed a positive Neer impingement sign (Fig. 4-39). Another method to detect shoulder impingement is to flex the shoulder forward to 90 degrees of elevation in neutral rotation, with the elbow flexed to 90 degrees. In this position, forcible internal rotation will cause discomfort or grimacing facial expression, as the supraspinatus tendon im-

pinges against the coracoacromial ligament. This maneuver is termed a positive Hawkins sign (Fig. 4-40). This test is also a good method to evaluate for tightness of the posterior capsule.

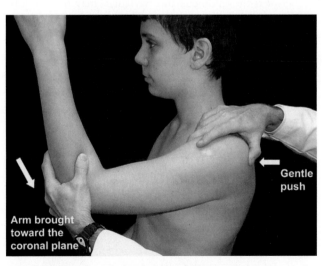

FIGURE 4-38. The Jahnke test, developed to evaluate posterior instability, is performed by flexing the patient's arm forward to 90 degrees of elevation in neutral rotation, and applying a posteriorly directed force to the arm to subluxate the humeral head posteriorly. The elevated arm is then gradually brought toward the coronal plane, while the clinician's thumb gently pushes the humeral head anteriorly. A palpable "clunk" is felt as the humeral head reduces from its subluxated position.

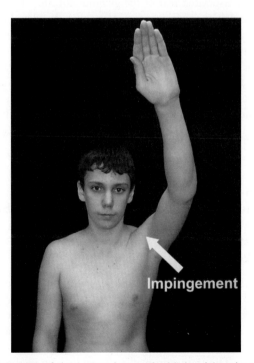

FIGURE 4-39. If the patient has tendonitis involving the supraspinatus tendon, forcible elevation of the arm to 180 degrees will cause discomfort when the inflamed tendon impinges against the anterior inferior acromion and coracoacromial ligament. This discomfort or grimacing facial expression is termed a positive Neer impingement sign.

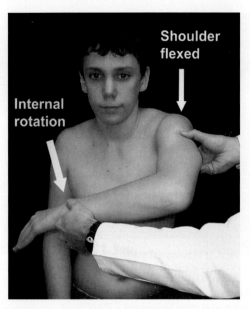

FIGURE 4-40. The Hawkins test is another maneuver that was developed to detect shoulder impingement. This test is performed with the shoulder flexed forward to 90 degrees. If internal rotation in this position causes discomfort, it indicates impingement between the inflamed supraspinatus tendon and the anterior inferior acromion and the coracoacromial ligament.

A patient with shoulder pain that is aggravated by swimming or gymnastics may have multidirectional instability, with an associated tear of the glenoid labrum. The labrum surrounds the glenoid cavity, deepening the glenohumeral joint, and the humeral head rests against the labrum. If there is a tear of the superior labrum, it is termed a "SLAP lesion," for superior labrum anterior and posterior. If the labral tear involves the anteroinferior labrum, it is termed a "Bankart lesion." If the attachment of the labrum to the glenoid is torn, it causes increased shoulder instability because the capsular attachment to the glenoid has been disrupted, further aggravating the symptoms.

A 15-year-old Boy Is Referred for Evaluation of Pain and Swelling of the Right Ankle That Developed after He Twisted His Foot while Playing Basketball

The history reveals that the patient was jumping for a rebound in a basketball game 2 days earlier and twisted his right foot when he landed on an opponent's foot. He developed pain and swelling over the lateral aspect of the ankle immediately after the injury, and was unable to continue playing. The trainer immediately applied ice to the ankle, but he continues to have pain and swelling that are aggravated by walking. He has always been athletic and in good health, but he has had two similar injuries of the right ankle

in the past. One occurred the previous year while playing basketball, and the other occurred 18 months earlier while playing tennis. There is no family history of frequent ankle sprains, and the remainder of the history is unremarkable.

On physical examination, there is marked swelling noted over the lateral malleolus, with ecchymosis over the lateral side of the foot. The patient is exquisitely tender to palpation over the anterior talofibular ligament and the calcaneofibular ligament, but he is not tender over the anterior tibiofibular ligament or the distal fibular growth plate. This pattern of tenderness indicates an injury to the ligaments, a sprained ankle, rather than a fracture of the distal fibular growth plate. In a younger patient, the ligaments are stronger than the growth plate, so the clinician would expect the area of maximum tenderness to be located over the distal fibular growth plate. Laxity of the anterior talofibular ligament can be detected by performing an anterior drawer test. This test is performed by applying anterior traction to the calcaneus with one hand, while holding the tibia in a fixed position with the other hand, and comparing the amount of anterior subluxation of the talus in the ankle joint between the injured and uninjured sides (Fig. 4-41). Laxity of the calcaneofibular ligament can be detected by performing a talar-tilt test, and comparing the injured side with the uninjured side. The talar-tilt test is performed by stabilizing the tibia with one hand while applying a varus stress to the calcaneus with the other hand, and feeling for asymmetry between the injured and uninjured sides.

In a patient with a sprained ankle, it is important to evaluate the range of motion of the ankle, subtalar, tarsal, and tarsometatarsal joints, because limited subtalar or tarsal motion may predispose the patient to frequent ankle sprains. A tarsal coalition between the talus and calcaneus, or between the calcaneus and navicular, may markedly restrict subtalar or tarsal motion. This loss of motion in the

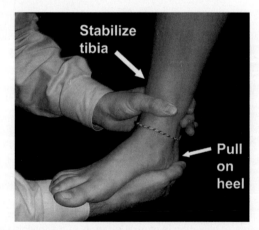

FIGURE 4-41. The anterior drawer test is performed by pulling the calcaneus forward with one hand, while stabilizing the tibia with the other hand. The amount of anterior subluxation is measured in millimeters, and compared with the other side.

subtalar or tarsal joints transmits forces to the ankle during athletic activities, increasing the risk that the patient may sustain an ankle sprain.

A sprained ankle typically occurs after a supination- or inversion-type injury to the ankle. As a result, the injury involves the ligaments on the lateral side of the ankle, and the medial side is not injured. If there is associated pain and swelling over the medial malleolus or the deltoid ligament, it may indicate a rotational type of injury pattern, which is often seen in fractures involving the ankle. This question can be answered by obtaining appropriate radiographs of the ankle.

References

The Orthopaedic Examination from Birth to 4 Years of Age

1. Aronsson DD, Goldberg MJ, Kling TF, et al. Developmental dysplasia of the hip. *Pediatrics* 1994;94:201.
2. Yngve D. Foot-progression angle in clubfeet. *J Pediatr Orthop* 1990;10:467.
3. Staheli LT, Corbett M, Wyss C, et al. Lower-extremity rotational problems in children: normal values to guide management. *J Bone Joint Surg Am* 1985;67:39.
4. Bleck EE. *Orthopaedic management in cerebral palsy.* Philadelphia: JB Lippincott, 1987.
5. Illingworth RS. *The development of the infant and young child: normal and abnormal,* 9th ed. New York: Churchill Livingstone, 1987.
6. Salenius P, Vankka E. The development of the tibiofemoral angle in children. *J Bone Joint Surg Am* 1975;57:259.
7. Nathan PA, Kenniston RC. Crossed polydactyly. *J Bone Joint Surg Am* 1975;57:847.

The Orthopaedic Examination from 4 to 10 Years of Age

8. Sutherland DH, Olshen R, Cooper L, et al. The development of mature gait. *J Bone Joint Surg Am* 1980;62:336.
9. Staheli LT. The prone hip extension test. *Clin Orthop* 1977;123:12.
10. Ober FR. The role of the iliotibial band and fascia: a factor in the causation of low back disorders and sciatica. *J Bone Joint Surg Am* 1936;18:105.
11. Silverskiöld N. Reduction of the uncrossed two joint muscles of the one-to-one muscle in spastic conditions. *Acta Chirurg Scand* 1923;56:315.
12. Coleman SS, Chesnut WJ. A simple test for hindfoot flexibility in the cavovarus foot. *Clin Orthop* 1977;123:60.
13. Sullivan JA. The child's foot. In: Morrissy RT, Weinstein SL, eds. *Lovell and Winter's pediatric orthopaedics,* 4th ed. Philadelphia: Lippincott-Raven, 1996;2:1077.

The Orthopaedic Examination from 10 to 18 Years of Age

14. Bunnell WP. An objective criterion for scoliosis screening. *J Bone Joint Surg Am* 1984;66:1381.
15. Medlar RC, Lyne ED. Sinding-Larsen-Johansson disease: its etiology and natural history. *J Bone Joint Surg Am* 1978;60:1113.
16. Wilson JN. A new diagnostic sign in osteochondritis dissecans of the knee. *J Bone Joint Surg Am* 1967;49:477.
17. Diduch D, Scuderi G, Scott WN. Knee injuries. In: Scuderi GR, McCann PD, Bruno PJ, eds. *Sports medicine: principles of primary care.* St. Louis: Mosby, 1997:336.
18. Medical Research Council. *Aids to the examination of the peripheral nervous system.* Memorandum 45. London: Her Majesty's Stationery Office, 1943.
19. Hawkins RJ, Bokor DJ. Clinical evaluation of shoulder problems. In: Rockwood CA, Matsen FA, eds. *The shoulder.* Philadelphia: WB Saunders, 1998:164.

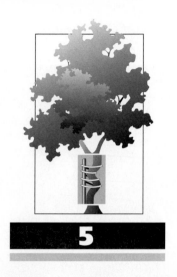

5

NORMAL GAIT AND ASSESSMENT OF GAIT DISORDERS

JON R. DAVIDS

The evolutionary forces that engendered life's emergence from the primordial slime, and subsequent domination of the local environment, greatly favored organisms with the ability to move from one spot to another. Locomotion evolved from reptilian slithering to advanced quadrupedal and bipedal gait. Quadrupedal locomotion is greatly favored in the animal kingdom, because it promotes stability and speed (1). The center of mass of a quadruped is located between the front and hindlimbs, which form a stable base of support. Speed is enhanced by the use of the trunk musculature to augment stride length and power. Ventral flexion of the trunk allows the animal to bring the flexed hind-limbs forward beyond the planted forelimbs. After weight has been transferred to the hindlimbs, the hips, shoulders, and trunk extend in synchrony to advance the forelimbs forward to complete a single cycle (1).

Bipedal gait sacrifices stability and speed to free the upper extremities for prehensile functions, imparting a tremendous evolutionary advantage. An upright position requires the center of mass to be balanced above the base of support, which is an inherently less stable and energy-efficient alignment (2–6). The diminished ability to use the trunk musculature to advance the swing limb limits stride length and power, compromising the speed of ambulation.

The early human fascination with normal gait and its deviations is revealed in the primitive cave paintings that illustrate hunters pursuing their prey. The modern era of motion analysis began with artists and mathematicians who were primarily interested in anatomy, aesthetics, and body segment motion (2,7,8). Eadward Muybridge, a British

J. R. Davids: Department of Orthopaedic Surgery, Duke University Medical Center, Durham, North Carolina 27710; Motion Analysis Laboratory, Shriners Hospital, Greenville, South Carolina 29605.

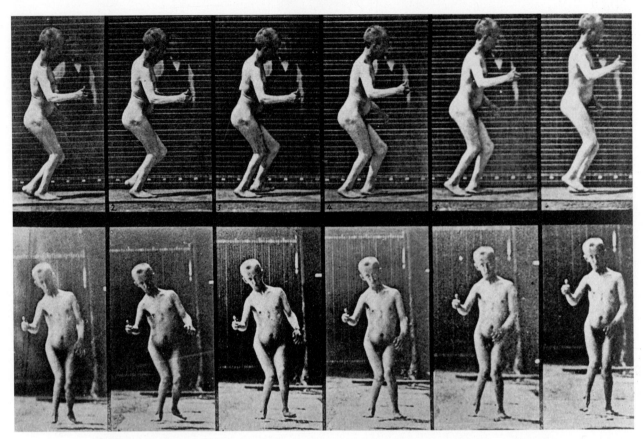

FIGURE 5-1. Muybridge's study of a young man with Little's disease, published in 1887. The subject exhibits many of the common gait deviations seen in children with cerebral palsy. (From ref. 9, with permission.)

photographer working in California, was the first to photograph fast motion (9). In 1872, his technique, which was the forerunner of modern motion pictures, was initially financed by Leland Stanford, who sought to win a wager by proving that a trotting horse, at some point in its stride, had all four feet off the ground at the same time. Muybridge's work was later supported by the University of Pennsylvania, where he created elegant studies of animal and human locomotion (Fig. 5-1). This extensive body of work has been collected into three volumes, and can still be found in the art section of large bookstores (9).

Etienne-Jules Marey was the first to develop a method of graphic notation derived from recording devices attached to the animal or person being studied (2,7,9,10). His "experimental shoe," described in 1873, is the direct forerunner of the electrical foot switch developed in the 1950s. In 1894, Braune and Fischer performed the first systematic study of human gait (10). Their subjects were Prussian soldiers who were placed into rubberized suits with electrical tubes attached to define the body segments (Fig. 5-2). It took 8 h to dress each volunteer, primarily because of concerns about potential electrocution. The mathematical analysis of the data was performed by hand and took several months to

complete. Their analysis, however, was as mechanically sophisticated as that currently performed by computer-driven quantitative motion analysis systems (10). Shortly after World War II, Dr. Verne T. Inman, an orthopaedist and functional anatomist, and defense industry-based colleagues in engineering and physiology became involved in lower limb prosthetics research (3,6). This collaboration led to the development of the first modern motion analysis laboratory. Inman's work was advanced, and the value of motion analysis was disseminated by two of his students and orthopaedic residents, Jacqueline Perry and David H. Sutherland. There are now approximately 70 clinical motion analysis laboratories in North America.

Quantitative motion analysis has had a significant impact on virtually all fields within orthopaedics, primarily by facilitating the objective analysis of an individual's functional deficits of movement. Quantitative motion analysis before and after an intervention allows assessment of the outcome in technical and functional domains not previously possible in clinical orthopaedics. Although some investigators may be discouraged by the cost and labor intensity of performing quantitative motion analysis, the central role of outcome studies in the ongoing reform of health care services in

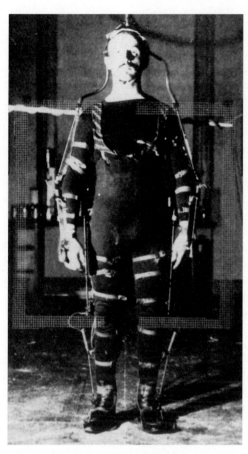

FIGURE 5-2. Rubberized suit with electrical tubes attached to various body segments, used by Braune and Fisher to study human gait in 1894. (From ref. 10, with permission.)

has been used to evaluate the impact of orthotic design on gait and joint loading in three planes, as well as to assess the surgical treatment of calcaneus gait by anterior tibial tendon transfer to the os calcis and Achilles tenodesis (59–65). For children with Duchenne muscular dystrophy, the pathomechanics of the deterioration of their gait have been elucidated, with implications for the timing and nature of surgical intervention (66,67). Children with congenital and acquired limb deficiencies have been studied to evaluate various reconstructive procedures, such as posteromedial release and Van Nes rotationplasty, and to assess prosthesis design (68–77).

Adult orthopaedics has also proven to be fertile ground for the application of quantitative motion analysis. The issues of adult joint disease examined include the energy costs of various arthrodeses, prediction of the efficacy of high tibial osteotomy, and functional recovery after knee and hip arthroplasty (78–84). In sports medicine, the various adaptations and their significance in gait of anterior cruciate ligament deficiency, and the biomechanics of throwing, swimming, running, and cycling have been assessed by motion analysis (85–92). Quantitative motion analysis has also been applied to adults with stroke, closed head injury, acquired limb deficiency, and spinal cord injury (26,93–100).

Using the results of quantitative motion analysis, this chapter defines and describes normal gait, running gait, and the maturation of gait. The most common gait deviations seen in the practice of pediatric orthopaedics are delineated. A technique of observational gait analysis is described, and the technology and technique of quantitative motion analysis are considered, primarily to facilitate a critical review of clinical studies that employ quantitative motion analysis.

NORMAL GAIT

The primary goal of gait is to provide a smooth, energy-efficient transfer of the body through space (2,3,5,8,11, 101,102). Normal gait is an extremely complex process that is built on the manipulation of selective synergistic motor patterns (i.e., "hard wired" spinal cord reflexes) and incorporation of learned sequential motor patterns (1,103,104). The remarkable similarity of gait between individuals is thought to be a consequence of the underlying demand for energy-efficient locomotion (3,6). Mechanically, this phenomenon is observed by considering the excursion of the body's center of gravity, located anterior to the second sacral vertebra, during gait. Although the body grossly appears to be walking a straight path, the center of gravity actually follows a sinusoidal course in the coronal and sagittal planes (Fig. 5-3). The maximum vertical displacement of the body's center of gravity occurs at the point of minimal horizontal displacement, which is a relatively energy-efficient pattern (1,3). In the sagittal plane, the body's center of gravity is at its highest point (i.e., minimum

North America suggests that the application of this technique will play a crucial part in the redefinition of the clinical practice of orthopaedics in the future.

In pediatric orthopaedics, quantitative motion analysis has advanced treatment concepts in cerebral palsy, myelodysplasia, muscle disease, and limb deficiency. The study of patients with cerebral palsy has revealed several principles: the separation of primary gait abnormalities due to the underlying neurologic lesion from secondary or compensatory gait deviations; the value of reducing the energy expenditure associated with pathologic gait by interventions aimed at reestablishing normal mechanical parameters; recognition of the significance of muscles that cross two joints; and the significance of skeletal malalignment, particularly in the transverse plane, in compromising the biomechanical ability of muscles to generate the forces required to stabilize motor limb segments (1,11,12). Quantitative motion analysis has identified common gait deviations at the hip, knee, and ankle (1,12–33). The efficacy of orthoses, tendon releases, tendon transfers, dorsal rhizotomy, and botox injections have been studied with motion analysis (34–58).

In cases of myelodysplasia, quantitative motion analysis

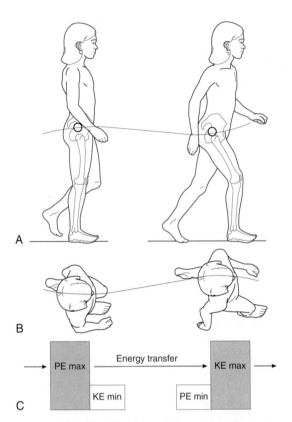

FIGURE 5-3. The excursion of the body's center of gravity follows a sinusoidal path in the sagittal (**A**) and coronal planes (**B**). Notice that the maximal excursion in one plane occurs in synchrony with minimal excursion in the other plane. **C:** Kinetic energy is maximal in double support periods (**left**), and potential energy is maximal in single-limb support periods (**right**). (Adapted from refs. 1 and 3, with permission.)

velocity, maximum potential energy) in midstance, and at its lowest point (i.e., maximum velocity, maximum kinetic energy) in terminal stance, when the two limbs are farthest apart (105,106). The transformation of potential to kinetic energy, and the use of the kinetic energy to accelerate the body and create potential energy, is a cyclic process occurring throughout gait. This form of energy transfer is effective but costly, with only 30 to 50% of the potential energy recovered as kinetic energy (1,101). Gait is therefore most efficient when the magnitude of the energy transferred is minimized. This is accomplished by minimizing the excursion of the center of gravity, one of three significant mechanisms of energy conservation (discussed below), which are best appreciated by applying basic mechanical principles to the analysis of normal gait.

Dynamic mechanical modeling of gait considers the motions that occur at joints and body segments (i.e., kinematics) and the forces that produce the motion (i.e., kinetics). Kinematic data describe gait and its deviations, including sagittal, coronal, and transverse joint angles, velocities, and accelerations (107,108). Kinetic data address the causes of motion and movement abnormalities, including the ground reaction forces, joint moments, and joint powers (107,108). A joint moment is the product of the force generated by a muscle and the distance of the muscle from the joint's estimated center of rotation (11,106,109,110). The ground reaction forces, in conjunction with gravitational and inertial forces, produce an external moment about the joints, and the moments generated by the muscles, ligaments, and joint capsules that cross the joint are called internal moments. Joint power is the product of a net joint moment and the joint's angular velocity (11,106,109,110). Power generation occurs when a muscle contracts concentrically (i.e., shortens), to produce a joint motion in the same direction that the muscle pulls (107). Power absorption occurs when the joint motion is opposite to the direction of the muscle pull, and the muscle exhibits an eccentric (i.e., lengthening) contraction (107).

This mechanical model recognizes three major mechanisms by which the body conserves energy during gait (1,12). The first mechanism involves minimizing the excursion of the center of gravity (2,3,5,6,29,101). This is accomplished by synchronized pelvic, hip, knee, and ankle motions. Multilevel lower extremity joint and segment motions are so well coordinated with and across planes, that pelvis and trunk deviations during normal gait usually cannot be appreciated by observational gait analysis. For this reason, it is helpful to consider the lower extremities as the body's locomotor segment, and the pelvis and trunk as the passenger segment (101). The efficacy of this mechanism is illustrated by the analysis of above-knee amputee gait, in which the energy cost is approximately double that for nonamputee gait (97,111). The second mechanism uses internal moments generated by passive structures (such as ligaments and joint capsules), instead of active internal moments (generated by muscle contractions), to counterbalance applied external moments and achieve joint stability during the gait cycle (1,8,11,12,105–107,112–115).

Because of proper positioning of the ankle in midstance, which is controlled by eccentric contraction of the soleus, the ground reaction force falls in front of the knee, generating an external extension moment in which stability at the knee is achieved by the internal flexion moment generated by the knee ligaments and joint capsules. In children with cerebral palsy, incompetence of the ankle plantar flexors after overlengthening of the heel cord leads to poor control of ankle position in midstance, posterior displacement of the ground reaction force at the knee, and creation of an external flexion moment. With time, this overwhelms the stabilizing internal knee extension moment generated by the quadriceps, resulting in a progressive crouch gait pattern, which is extremely energy inefficient (28,29). A similar coupling occurs at the hip, where the ground reaction force falls behind the joint center to generate an external extension moment, which is stabilized by the internal flexion moment generated by the anterior hip ligaments (101). The final mechanism involves the efficient transfer of energy between body segments (1,12). Early work suggests that two-joint muscles, such as the rectus femoris, which can generate power when serving as a hip flexor, while simultaneously absorbing power in its role as a knee extensor during rapid walking, serve a central role in the efficient transfer of energy between nonadjacent segments (77,116). The physiologic confirmation of this mechanism is under investigation (117). Current investigations of normal and pathologic gait mechanisms include dynamic mechanical modeling of muscle length and calculation of joint stiffness (17,118).

THE GAIT CYCLE

A single gait cycle, also called "stride," functionally defines the events occurring between two sequential floor contacts by the same limb. The gait cycle is logically divided into two phases, stance and swing, respectively defined by the presence or absence of floor contact for the limb being considered. Normal walking allows each limb to accomplish three tasks during each gait cycle: weight acceptance, single-limb support, and limb advancement (101) (Fig. 5-4). Pathologic deviations of gait compromise the achievement of these tasks and increase the energy cost of ambulation. The events of gait are temporally described as occurring at specific percentages of the gait cycle. Stance phase constitutes the first 60% of the gait cycle, and contains two periods of "double support," when both limbs are in contact with the floor. The first period occurs immediately after the

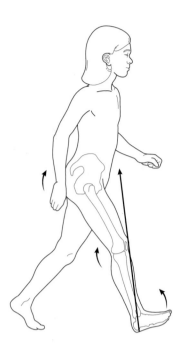

FIGURE 5-5. Initial contact. The *long arrow* represents the ground reaction force. Its position relative to each joint determines the external moment. The *smaller arrows* represent the net internal moments that are generated by the muscles and other soft tissue structures crossing each joint.

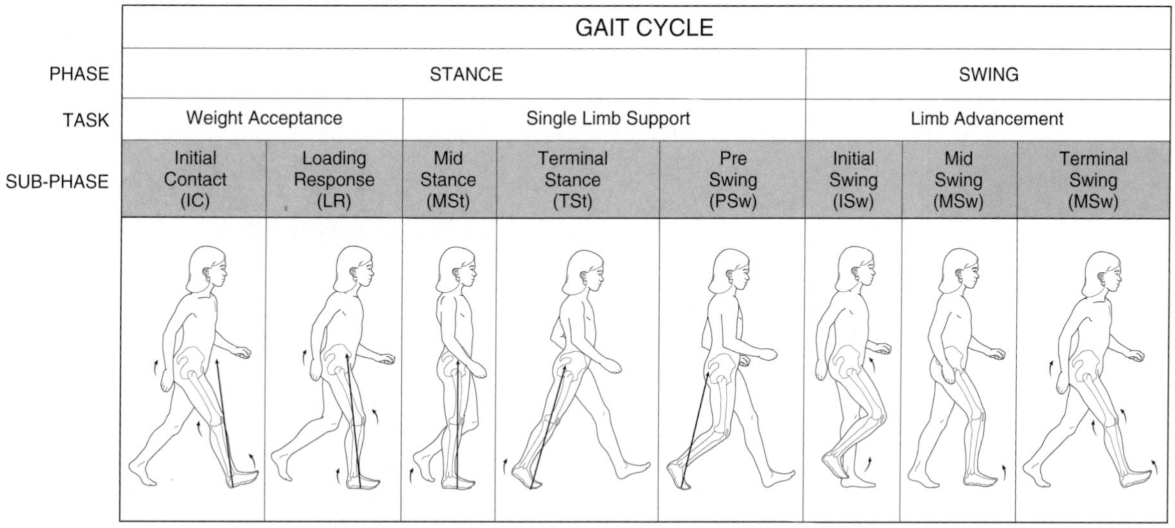

initiation of stance phase, and the second just before the end of stance. Clinically, stance phase is further divided into five subphases, each of which has a functional objective: initial contact, loading response, midstance, terminal stance, and preswing (Figs. 5-5 through 5-9; Table 5-1).

GAIT CYCLE								
PHASE	STANCE					SWING		
TASK	Weight Acceptance		Single Limb Support			Limb Advancement		
SUB-PHASE	Initial Contact (IC)	Loading Response (LR)	Mid Stance (MSt)	Terminal Stance (TSt)	Pre Swing (PSw)	Initial Swing (ISw)	Mid Swing (MSw)	Terminal Swing (MSw)

FIGURE 5-4. The division of the gait cycle into phases, tasks, and subphases facilitates the analysis of normal and pathologic gaits.

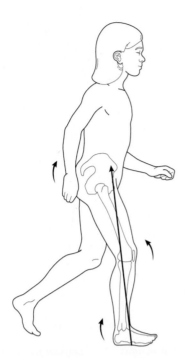

FIGURE 5-6. Loading response. Shock absorption by the quadriceps and controlled ankle plantar flexion are the central events. The ankle plantar flexion sets up the first, or heel, rocker. *Long arrow,* ground reaction force; *curved arrows,* net internal moments generated by muscles crossing each joint.

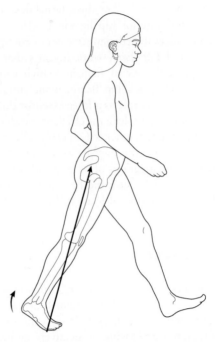

FIGURE 5-8. Terminal stance. Heel rise occurs as the body advances and the ankle plantar flexors resist the large external dorsiflexor moment. (This constitutes the third, or forefoot, rocker.) *Long arrow,* ground reaction force; *curved arrow,* internal plantar flexion moment.

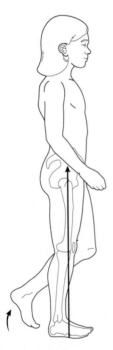

FIGURE 5-7. Midstance. After the ground reaction force (*long arrow*) falls in front of the knee, generating an external extension moment, and behind the hip, generating an external extension moment, internal muscle-generated moments are no longer necessary for joint stability. This is one of the energy-efficient mechanisms often lost in pathologic gait deviations. Tibial advancement over the foot constitutes the second, or ankle, rocker, and is controlled by an internal ankle plantar flexion moment (*small arrow*).

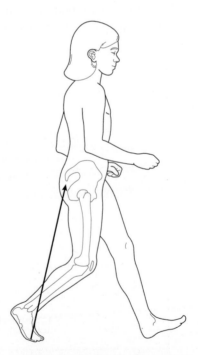

FIGURE 5-9. Preswing. "Passive" ankle plantar flexion, knee flexion (i.e., no internal muscle moments), and active hip flexion occur as the limb is unloaded. *Long arrow,* ground reaction force.

TABLE 5-1. STANCE PHASE OF THE GAIT CYCLE

Initial Contact (see Fig. 5-5)
  Interval: 0% of the gait cycle
  Task: weight acceptance
  Critical events: the ankle is positioned so the heel strikes first
    as the foot comes in contact with the floor
  Kinematics
    Ankle: 0 degrees
    Knee: 0 degrees
    Hip: 25 degrees flexion
  Kinetics
    Ankle: external plantar flexion moment, which is balanced
      by internal dorsiflexion moment by tibialis anterior
    Knee: external extension moment; hamstring activity
      decelerates the advancing limb
    Hip: external flexion moment, controlled by hamstring
      extension moment, which also contributes to
      deceleration

Loading Response (see Fig. 5-6)
  Interval: 0–10% of the gait cycle
  Task: weight acceptance; shock is adsorbed, primarily by the
    quadriceps, as forward moment is preserved
  Critical events: controlled ankle plantar flexion and knee
    flexion; hip stability
  Kinematics
    Ankle: 10 degrees plantar flexion
    Knee: 15 degrees flexion
    Hip: 25 degrees flexion
  Kinetics
    Ankle: external plantar flexion moment; internal
      dorsiflexion moment by tibialis anterior decelerates and
      stabilizes the foot and advances the tibia anterior to the
      ground reaction force vector
    Knee: external flexion moment; internal extension moment
      by quadriceps stabilizes the knee in flexion and absorbs
      the shock of floor contact
    Hip: diminishing external flexion moment as the body
      advances; activity of the hip extensors and abductors
      stabilizes the hip and pelvis

Midstance (see Fig. 5-7)
  Interval: 10–30% of the gait cycle
  Task: single-limb support; the body progresses over the foot
    in a controlled manner; forward momentum is generated
    by the contralateral swing limb
  Critical events: controlled tibial advancement
  Kinematics
    Ankle: 5 degrees dorsiflexion
    Knee: 0 degrees
    Hip: 0 degrees
  Kinetics
    Ankle external dorsiflexion moment; internal plantar

flexion moment by the soleus decelerates ankle
  dorsiflexion, stabilizes the tibia, and controls the position
  of the ground reaction force vector at the knee and hip
  Knee: external moment changes from flexion to extension
    as the ground reaction force vector moves anteriorly;
    internal muscle moments are no longer necessary for
    joint stability after the vector passes in front of the knee
  Hip: external moment changes from flexion to extension as
    the ground reaction force vector moves posteriorly;
    internal extension moment generated by the gluteus
    maximus is no longer required; the pelvis is stabilized in
    the coronal plane by action of the gluteus medius (i.e.,
    internal abduction moment)

Terminal Stance (see Fig. 5-8)
  Interval: 30–50% of the gait cycle
  Task: single-limb support; the body passes in front of the
    foot, and forward progression is accelerated by kinetic
    energy generated primarily by the ankle plantar flexors
  Critical events: heel rise
  Kinematics
    Ankle: 10 degrees dorsiflexion
    Knee: 0 degrees
    Hip: 20 degrees extension
  Kinetics
    Ankle: maximum external dorsiflexion moment is opposed
      by internal plantar flexion moment from the
      gastrocnemius, leading to heel rise as the body advances
      forward; this muscle is the principal source of power,
      accelerating the limb as it enters the swing phase
    Knee: external extension moment is diminishing, but no
      internal muscle moments are required to maintain
      stability
    Hip: maximal external extension moment is attained as the
      body advances

Preswing (see Fig. 5-9)
  Interval: 50–60% of the gait cycle
  Task: swing-limb advancement; the principal objective is
    preparation and positioning of the limb for swing
  Critical events: passive knee flexion
  Kinematics
    Ankle: 20 degrees plantar flexion
    Knee: 40 degrees flexion
    Hip: 0 degrees
  Kinetics
    Ankle: passive plantar flexion as the limb is unloaded
    Knee: passive flexion as the limb is unloaded; the rectus
      femoris, a biarticular muscle, may assist in energy
      transfer between the knee and hip in this subphase
    Hip: passive flexion as the limb is unloaded

The swing phase constitutes the remaining 40% of the gait cycle, and begins at the point where the limb is unloaded and the foot comes off the ground. The limb is advanced from behind the body to in front of the body, reaching out to take the next step. Foot clearance and correct positioning for the initiation of the subsequent stance phase are critical components of swing-limb advancement (101). The velocity of gait can be altered by changing the stride length (i.e., distance covered by a single gait cycle) or the cadence (i.e., number of gait cycles per unit time) (109,116,119). Changes in cadence are primarily accomplished by altering the duration of swing phase (1). A period of variable acceleration (i.e., initial swing), a transitional period (i.e., midswing), and a final period of deceleration and limb positioning (i.e., terminal swing) are the recognized subphases of swing. Kinetic analysis of the joints in swing phase is much simpler, because there is no external moment generated by the ground reaction force. External moments may be generated by gravitational and inertial forces, and are usually dominated by the internal muscle–generated moments (107) (Figs. 5-10 through 5-12; Table 5-2).

In addition to analysis by phase, task, and subphase, the functional assessment of gait is facilitated by considering the kinematics and kinetics of anatomic areas, such as joints and body segments, throughout the gait cycle.

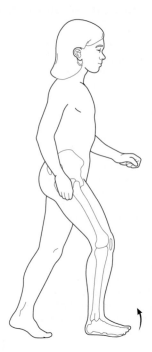

FIGURE 5-11. Midswing. Gravitational and inertial external moments dominate at the hip and knee. The ankle position for clearance is determined by an internal dorsiflexion moment (*curved arrow*).

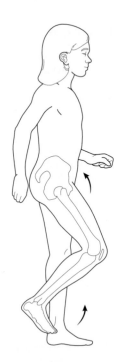

FIGURE 5-10. Initial swing. Hip flexion, knee flexion, and ankle dorsiflexion contribute to limb clearance. *Curved arrows,* internal hip flexion and ankle dorsiflexion moments.

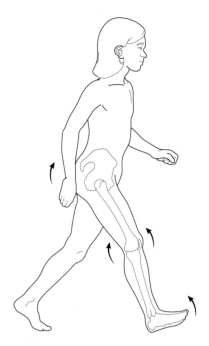

FIGURE 5-12. Terminal swing. Internal muscle moments at the hip, knee (i.e., simultaneous flexion and extension moments), and ankle decelerate the limb, and position it correctly for the initiation of the subsequent stance phase. *Curved arrows,* internal moments generated by the muscles crossing each joint.

TABLE 5-2. SWING PHASE OF THE GAIT CYCLE

Initial Swing (see Fig. 5-10)
  Interval: 60–75% of the gait cycle
  Task: swing-limb advancement; variable acceleration is
    possible
  Critical events: foot clearance
  Kinematics
    Ankle: 10 degrees plantar flexion
    Knee: 60 degrees flexion
    Hip: 15 degrees flexion
  Kinetics
    Ankle: the pretibial musculature generates a dorsiflexion
      moment; diminished plantar flexion alignment
      contributes to foot clearance
    Knee: at a normal cadence, increased knee flexion is
      determined by external flexion moments generated by
      inertial and gravitational forces; at a slower cadence, an
      internal flexion moment, generated by the lateral
      hamstrings, may be present (63,100); at a faster cadence,
      the rectus femoris contributes to limb acceleration by
      generating an extension moment at the knee (21,110)
    Hip: the flexors and adductors generate an internal flexion
      moment, which contributes to limb advancement and
      acceleration
Midswing (see Fig. 5-11)
  Interval: 75–90% of the gait cycle
  Task: swing-limb advancement
  Critical events: vertical alignment of the tibia; foot clearance
  Kinematics
    Ankle: 0 degrees
    Knee: 25 degrees flexion
    Hip: 25 degrees flexion

  Kinetics
    Ankle: internal dorsiflexion moment from the tibialis
      anterior supports the ankle and prevents footdrop
    Knee: external moment from inertial forces begin to
      extend the knee
    Hip: external moment from inertial forces causes further
      hip flexion

Terminal Swing (see Fig. 5-12)
  Interval: 90–100% of the gait cycle
  Task: swing-limb advancement, achievement of maximal step
    length, position the foot for initial contact, and
    deceleration of swing limb
  Critical events: knee extension to neutral
  Kinematics
    Ankle: 0 degrees
    Knee: 0 degrees
    Hip: 25 degrees flexion
  Kinetics
    Ankle: internal dorsiflexion moment maintains the foot in
      the proper position for initial contact
    Knee: internal extension moment by the quadriceps
      extends the knee for stance; internal flexion moment by
      the hamstrings decelerates and stabilizes the advancing
      swing limb
    Hip: internal extension moment by the hamstrings
      contributes to deceleration

Ankle

Stance Phase

Ankle function during stance phase is best considered in terms of three rockers (120,121) (Fig. 5-13). The first, or heel, rocker begins at initial contact, and extends through the loading response. Correct ankle position at initial contact ensures that the heel strikes the floor first, creating an external plantar flexion moment. The 10 degrees of plantar flexion seen in the loading response lowers the foot to the floor, and is resisted by the internal moment generated by the ankle dorsiflexor muscles. The second, or ankle, rocker occurs during midstance, and the external moment favors dorsiflexion. The 5 degrees of dorsiflexion is resisted by the internal moment generated by the ankle plantar flexor muscles. This deceleration of ankle dorsiflexion controls tibial advancement, and contributes to stance stability by ensuring that the ground reaction force is anterior to the knee and posterior to the hip, creating an external extension moment at each joint. This promotes joint stability through ligaments (and other soft tissue structures), and without muscle action, which is energy-efficient. The third, or forefoot, rocker occurs during terminal stance, as the body advances over the stance limb. The greatest external moment of the

gait cycle, favoring ankle dorsiflexion, occurs at this point (101,107,112, 115,122). The ankle plantar flexors meet the challenge, generating the greatest internal muscle moment occurring at any joint at any time in the gait cycle. The net joint moment favors ankle plantar flexion, and accelerates the advancing limb. Minimal ankle movement at this point causes the heel to rise as the forefoot dorsiflexes through the metatarsophalangeal joints, maintaining momentum and efficiently transferring energy between body segments (11,101,115). Heel rise should occur just before the opposite limb enters weight acceptance at initial contact.

Before quantitative analysis and mechanical modeling, heel rise was imprecisely perceived as active ankle plantar flexion and referred to as "push-off," which implies propulsion, but is misleading. Although the ankle plantar flexors are active, they are resisting the external dorsiflexion moment, effectively stabilizing the ankle joint and promoting controlled tibial advancement over the forefoot. A child with a calcaneal gait pattern (e.g., low lumbar-level myelodysplasia) loses heel rise and has uncontrolled tibial advancement over the foot, which leads to instability and poor energy transfer proximally during terminal stance. Twenty degrees of ankle plantar flexion does occur during preswing, as the body weight is transferred to the other limb. This

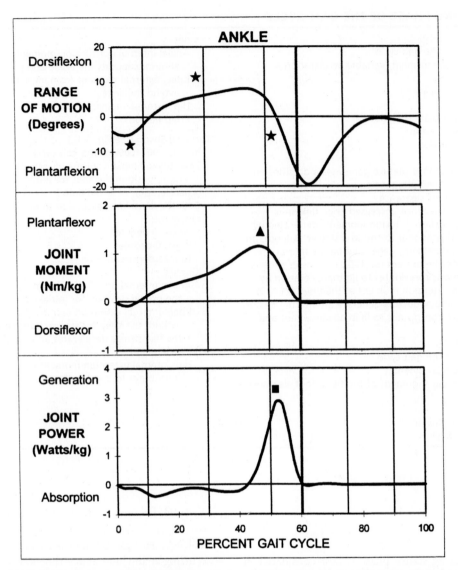

FIGURE 5-13. Normal motion, moments, and powers of the ankle. Motion is in the sagittal plane. Notice the three rockers (★) that occur during stance phase. The joint moment curve describes the net internal muscle moment, generated in response to the external moments from the ground reaction force, gravity, and inertia. The internal plantar flexion moment generated at the end of the terminal stance (TSt) subphase (▲) is the greatest muscle moment occurring at any joint at any time in the gait cycle. The TSt power generation (■) reflects the crucial role of the ankle plantar flexors in accelerating the limb as it enters the swing phase (i.e., energy transfer). (From refs. 8, 101, 107, and 122, with permission.)

plantar flexion takes place during a period of unloading, in response to external moments generated by inertia and gravity forces, not as a result of active internal muscle moments.

Swing Phase

Active ankle dorsiflexion begins during initial swing to assist in early swing-limb clearance. The internal dorsiflexion moment in midswing resists inertia and gravity forces to pro-

mote clearance. In terminal swing, the internal muscle moments position the ankle for initial contact, so the heel strikes the floor first, generating the first, or heel, rocker.

Knee

Stance Phase

The knee exhibits a single flexion wave during stance phase (Fig. 5-14). Full extension at initial contact provides stabil-

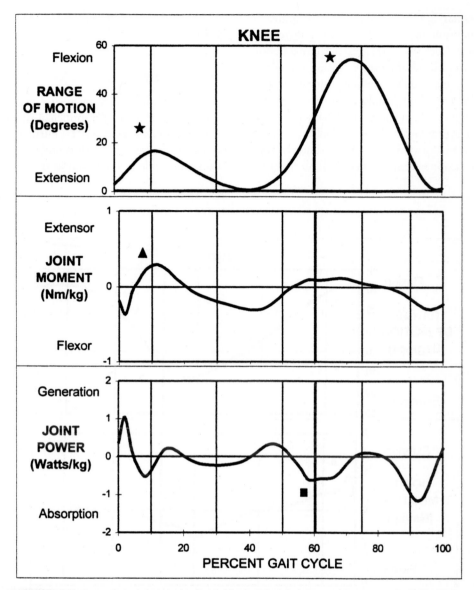

FIGURE 5-14. Normal motion, moments, and powers of the knee. Sagittal plane motion of the knee is characterized by two flexion waves (★). Stance-phase knee flexion (during loading response [LR] subphase) reflects shock absorption, and the swing-phase flexion wave promotes limb clearance. Note that 40 degrees of knee flexion occurs before the extremity enters swing phase. The quadriceps are the primary shock absorbers at the knee, generating the internal muscle extension moment seen during the LR subphase (▲). Power absorption occurs during LR and terminal stance (■). The relatively low level of power generation and absorption reflects the transfer of energy across the knee (between body segments above and below) by two joint muscles, such as the rectus femoris, biceps femoris, and gastrocnemius. (From refs. 8, 101, 107, and 122, with permission.)

ity for weight acceptance and contributes to optimal foot position. Flexion at the knee in the loading response is the principal means of shock absorption, and is a consequence of the external flexion moment generated by the ground reaction force (123). The alignment of this applied force behind the knee is controlled by the heel rocker. Although knee flexion promotes shock absorption, it must not compromise knee stability. Competent quadriceps function to generate an internal knee extension moment to prevent ex-

cessive knee flexion and instability (25). The knee extends in midstance to promote stability and advancement. The ankle rocker correctly aligns the ground reaction force, so that an external knee extension moment is generated, promoting energy-efficient knee stability. The phenomena whereby the position of the foot and ankle in stance phase determines the relative position of the ground reaction force to the knee joint center is known as the ankle plantar flexion–knee extension couple. As implied by the name, increasing ankle plantar flexion is associated with a greater external knee extension moment. Conversely, increasing ankle dorsiflexion is associated with a greater external flexion moment at the knee. Maximum knee extension is attained in terminal stance, maintaining stability during forward progression. As the stance limb is unloaded in preswing, the knee flexes, driven primarily by the external flexion moment from the ground reaction force, which falls behind the knee as the body advances forward (11). Approximately two-thirds of the knee flexion necessary for swing-limb clearance

occurs in the preswing subphase before the foot leaves the floor.

Swing Phase

A second flexion wave of greater peak magnitude occurs during swing phase. The principal function of this flexion wave is limb clearance (101). Further knee flexion occurs during initial swing, which is crucial for foot clearance because the ankle is in equinus at this point (124). After the

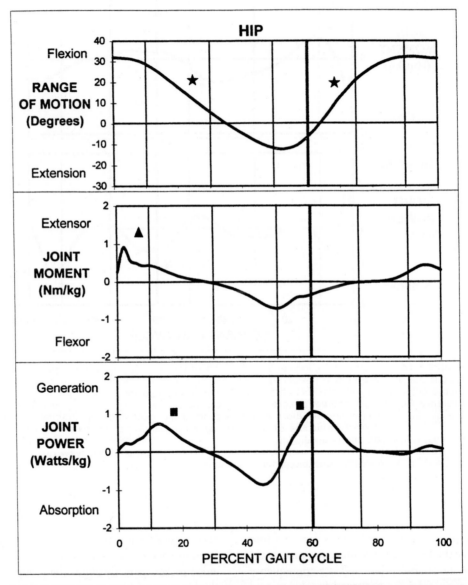

FIGURE 5-15. Normal motion, moments, and powers of the hip. Sagittal plane motion of the hip is characterized by an extension wave in stance phase and a flexion wave in swing phase (★). The extensor moment generated by the hamstrings in the loading response subphase (▲) is the second-greatest internal muscle moment in the gait cycle. The two periods of power generation (■) serve to accelerate the limb in the stance and swing phases. (From refs. 8, 101, 107, and 122, with permission.)

tibia has attained a vertical alignment, clearance has been achieved, and the primary function at the knee becomes limb advancement and stride length (101). The knee therefore extends, primarily because of an external moment derived from the forces of inertia and gravity. Optimal stride length is achieved by further knee extension in terminal stance. Internal (i.e., muscle) and external (i.e., gravitational and inertial) moments contribute to knee extension and limb positioning for the initial contact subphase. An internal flexion moment, generated by the hamstrings, decelerates the advancing limb before beginning the stance phase.

Hip

Stance Phase

The hip exhibits a single extension wave during stance phase (Fig. 5-15). At initial contact, the hip is flexed to promote limb position. During the loading response subphase, the ground reaction force falls in front of the hip joint, generating the second-highest external moment of the entire gait cycle (101,107). The internal muscle extension moment, generated by the hamstrings, stabilizes the hip. In the coronal plane, the weight of the contralateral swing limb causes the ground reaction force to fall medial to the stance-limb hip, creating an adduction moment that is resisted by the internal muscle moment of the gluteus medius (125,126). In midstance, the hip is extending as the body advances. After the ground reaction force falls at or behind the hip joint, an external extension moment is generated, and hip stability is provided by the anterior ligaments—an energy-efficient mechanism. In the coronal plane, the hip adduction moment persists. As the limb is unloaded in the pre-swing subphase, the hip begins to flex. In the coronal plane, the external adduction moment diminishes as the contralateral limb begins weight acceptance.

Swing Phase

The hip exhibits a single flexion wave in swing phase. During the initial swing subphase, internal muscle flexion moments may contribute to hip flexion. The remaining flexion in swing phase is a consequence of inertial and gravitational external moments (106,107). The hip flexion contributes to limb clearance early in swing and limb positioning, for weight acceptance after the terminal swing subphase.

Pelvis/Trunk/Upper Extremities

As noted earlier, it is helpful to consider the pelvis and trunk as the passenger segment during gait. This is most appropriate given the limitations of observational gait analysis. However, appreciation of pelvic and trunk motion during normal gait is possible with qualitative gait analysis. Motion of these segments is clearly coupled to the lower extremities, and is characterized by minimal (i.e., between 0 and 5 degrees) excursion or dynamic range.

In the "sagittal plane," the pelvis and trunk are both tilted slightly anterior throughout the gait cycle. In the "coronal plane," trunk obliquity is inversely coupled to pelvic obliquity, which is directly coupled to hip ab/adduction. When the right hemipelvis is up, the right hip is adducted and the trunk is shifted down to the right. In the "transverse plane," trunk rotation is directly coupled to pelvic rotation, which is inversely coupled to hip rotation. The most significant "cross plane" coupling occurs between the pelvis and the hip. Pelvic external rotation is coupled with hip flexion and adduction (contributing to apparent hip hyperextension in terminal stance), while pelvic internal rotation is coupled to hip extension and abduction.

In the sagittal plane, the upper extremities flex and extend in a reciprocal fashion, relative to each other. The motion of the upper extremity is inversely coupled to the ipsilateral lower extremity, with flexion of the arm occurring as the leg extends during stance phase.

THE RUNNING CYCLE

As the velocity of gait increases, bipedal ambulators progress from walking to running to sprinting. The transitional velocity at which an individual switches from one form of ambulation to the other is not constant; it is a function of multiple factors, including leg length (109). For this reason, children begin to run at lower velocities than adults. Walking is differentiated from running and sprinting by the pattern of ground contact (91,109,119,127). In walking, there is always ground contact with one or both feet, but running and sprinting are characterized by "double float" periods when neither foot is on the ground (Fig. 5-16).

In terms of the gait cycle, walking can be differentiated from running by the duration of the stance phase. In walking, the two periods of double support (i.e., both feet in contact with the floor) ensure that the duration of the stance phase is greater than 50% of the gait cycle (1,109,119). In running, both periods of double support are lost. The toe-off motion occurs before the opposite heel strike, creating two periods of double float (i.e., neither foot in contact with the floor), which constitute portions of the swing phase. In running, the duration of the stance phase constitutes less than 50% of the gait cycle (1,109,119). As the velocity of walking increases, the duration of double support decreases. As the velocity of running/sprinting increases, the duration of double float increases (127).

Running and sprinting are most easily differentiated by the position of the foot at initial contact (109,119,127). In running, the initial contact is made with the heel, as in walking. In sprinting, the initial contact is made with the forefoot, which is advantageous at higher velocities.

Biomechanical analysis of running divides the stance

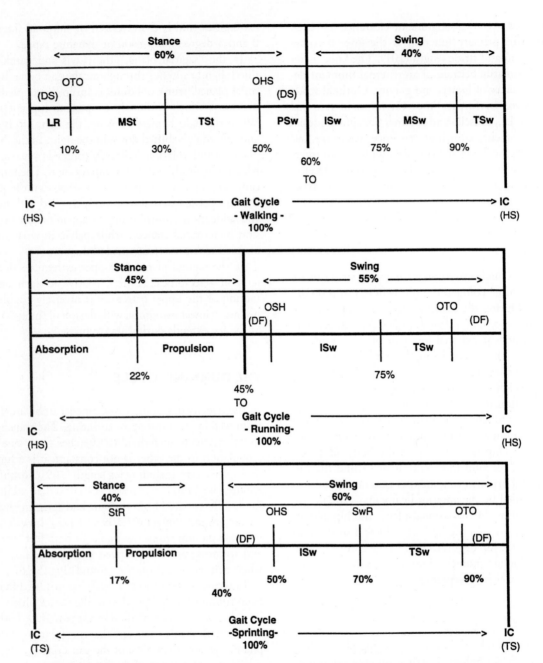

FIGURE 5-16. Comparison of the walking, running, and sprinting gait cycles. In walking, the stance phase constitutes more of the gait cycle than the swing phase. In running, this relation is reversed. In walking, heel strike (HS) and opposite heel strike (OHS) occur before opposite toe-off (OTO) and toe-off (TO), respectively, creating two periods of double support (DS), when both feet are touching the ground. In running, HS and OHS occur after OTO and TO, respectively; both periods of DS are lost, and two additional periods of double float (DF) are created. IC, initial contact; LR, loading response; MSt, midstance; Tst, terminal stance; PSw, preswing; ISw, initial swing; MSw, midswing; TSw, terminal swing; StR, stance phase reversal; SwR, swing phase reversal. (From refs. 1, 109, 119, and 127, with permission.)

phase into two subphases. During the absorption subphase, the hip and knee flex, and the ankle dorsiflexes. Kinetic studies of children running suggest that the knee and ankle are primary and secondary energy absorbers, respectively, during this subphase (109,127). The propulsion subphase is characterized by active hip and knee extension and ankle plantar flexion. Kinetic analysis reveals that the ankle is the primary power generator in running, while the hip is the primary power generator during sprinting (109,127). This period of active ankle plantar flexion occurs during the propulsion subphase of running, and can correctly be called the "push-off period."

MATURATION OF GAIT

The widely recognized developmental milestones of infants, such as rolling over, sitting, crawling, and standing, occur sequentially in conjunction with the physiologic maturation of the neuromuscular system (128). Animal models of spinal cord injury, and the presence of mass flexion and extension reflexes in neonates, suggests the existence of "hard-wired" motor synergies emanating from the spinal cord (103,104). With maturation, these spinal cord reflexes are manipulated to produce and control a reciprocating gait pattern. With further development, complex learned motor activities can be incorporated into the neuronal circuitry (1). With appropriate training, such learned activities can be performed with increasing ease. In all likelihood, the development of a mature gait pattern represents a combination of physiologic maturation of the neuromuscular system and incorporation of complex, learned motor activities (129–133).

Landmark studies by Sutherland et al., employing quantitative gait analysis, have characterized the different stages in the maturation of gait (8,29,131,132). In toddler gait, the upper extremities are held in abduction with elbow extension. Reciprocal arm movement does not occur. The foot and ankle exhibit a toe-strike pattern at initial contact, increased stance-phase dorsiflexion, and increased swing-phase plantar flexion. The knee shows diminished flexion throughout the gait cycle. The hip is externally rotated during the stance and swing phases. The stance phase is characterized by diminished single-limb stance time and a widened base of support in double stance. In the swing phase, circumduction (i.e., hip abduction) is used to clear the externally rotated, extended, and plantar-flexed extremity.

By 2 years of age, significant maturation is exhibited. Reciprocal arm swing is achieved by most children. Heel strike occurs at initial contact, and ankle dorsiflexion facilitates limb clearance during the swing phase. The knee flexion wave also occurs during the stance phase. Rotation at the hip has normalized. The stance phase is characterized by increased single-limb stance time, and the movement during swing phase shows normalized clearance mechanisms.

By 3 years of age, most adult kinematic patterns are present. Subsequent changes in time–distance parameters, such as cadence, velocity, and step length, continue to occur until 7 years of age, when an adult gait pattern is achieved.

Sutherland and coworker's analysis of more than 300 children identified five statistically significant parameters of gait maturity (132):

1. Single-limb stance duration increases with age and maturation.
2. Walking velocity increases with age and limb length.
3. Cadence decreases with age and limb length.
4. Step length increases with age and limb length.
5. The ratio of the interankle distance to the pelvic width decreases with age and maturation.

COMMON GAIT DEVIATIONS

Mechanical modeling of gait assumes mobile body segments powered by internal muscle activity and external applied forces. The pathologic processes that affect gait usually compromise joint mobility and muscle activity by three general mechanisms: deformity, muscle dysfunction, and pain (78,101,134).

In deformity, soft tissue contractures limit joint motion. Fixed contractures create rigid deformity, and elastic contractures lead to dynamic deformity. Ligament laxity causes instability that can contribute to joint deformity. Osseous tissues may be altered by trauma, infection, and vascular compromise. Abnormally applied mechanical forces may affect growth mechanisms, leading to the development of bony deformities that limit joint mobility.

Disorders of the neuromuscular system can cause dynamic muscle weakness that alters gait. Children with lower motor neuron lesions or primary muscle diseases can often compensate for the function deficit. This capacity to substitute depends on the preservation of proprioception and selective control (101,134). Primary compensatory mechanisms include changing the timing of other muscle actions during gait, and use of postural adjustments to substitute for deficient muscle forces. Children with upper motor neuron lesions have the most challenging functional deficits. Their gait deviations are a consequence of spasticity, persistent primitive locomotor patterns (i.e., mass flexion or extension reflexes), poor selective control, and impaired proprioception (1,101).

Pain can contribute to joint deformity and muscle dysfunction. After an injury, the body assumes a natural resting joint position that minimizes intraarticular pressure (101). This mechanism contributes to soft tissue and osseous tissue changes over time. Neurologic control mechanisms exist that protect joint structures from destructive pressures (101). These protective reflexes limit the ability to activate certain muscles after an injury, which over time, cause disuse atrophy, and contributes to a vicious cycle of progressive functional deficits. An antalgic gait reflects the body's efforts to compensate for pain or instability in the stance-phase limb by minimizing the duration and magnitude of loading. It is a gait pattern characterized by diminished single-limb stance time.

Within this framework, gait abnormalities may be seen as primary, if they are the direct result of a mechanical change related to the injury or disease process; secondary, when a primary deviation at another joint causes a pathologic deviation at the reference joint; or compensatory, reflecting an adaptation to an applied pathologic condition. Treatment should be directed toward primary gait deviations that cause functional deficits. Interventions that address secondary or compensatory gait deviations are generally ineffective and should be avoided. It is an error to intervene when a compensatory gait deviation successfully substitutes for a functional deficit. Treatment is appropriate when the compensations are inadequate or when they require excessive energy cost, joint strain, or muscle overuse (12,78,134). This concept may be illustrated by considering the child with Duchenne muscular dystrophy who is ambulatory. The primary functional deficit is weakness, particularly of the muscles about the trunk, hip, and knee. These children favor a toe-toe gait pattern (which, in this case, is a secondary, compensatory deviation), in order to utilize the plantar flexion–knee extension couple to maintain the ground reaction force in front of the knee, effectively substituting for the weak quadriceps during stance phase. Over time, the child will develop diminished ankle range of motion, with myostatic deformity of the gastrocsoleus muscle group. Surgical treatment of the tight heel cord, while the child remains an independent ambulator, will restrict the child's ability to utilize this compensation and greatly limit the child's ability to ambulate independently. In this situation, the secondary deviation (i.e., the toe-toe gait pattern) should be accepted, until the underlying muscle weakness becomes so great that independent ambulation is no longer possible. At this point, correction of the equinus deformity, to facilitate bracing for possible orthotics- and assistive-device–augmented ambulation is appropriate.

Ankle

Excessive Ankle Plantar Flexion

The primary causes of excessive ankle plantar flexion in the stance phase include plantar flexor muscle spasticity, contracture, and impaired proprioception. Compensatory ankle plantar flexion is seen as a substitution pattern for weak quadriceps or for ankle or forefoot pain. Increased ankle plantar flexion in midstance and terminal stance, called "vaulting," may occur as a compensatory mechanism to facilitate swing clearance of a relatively long contralateral limb. The consequences of excessive plantar flexion in stance phase include diminished shock absorption by limiting knee flexion in the loading response subphase, and decreased forward progression of the tibia over the foot and ankle, which interferes with the heel and ankle rockers. The primary causes of excessive ankle plantar flexion in the swing phase include weakness or impaired selective control of the ankle dorsiflexors and plantar flexor spasticity or contracture. Excessive ankle plantar flexion during the swing phase interferes with foot clearance and foot positioning for initial contact.

Excessive ankle plantar flexion is clinically described as an "equinus gait," and is commonly seen in patients with cerebral palsy; muscle diseases, such as Duchenne muscular dystrophy; and posttraumatic conditions, such as anterior compartment nerve injury or compartment syndrome.

Excessive Ankle Dorsiflexion

The most common primary cause of excessive ankle dorsiflexion during the stance phase is weakness of the ankle plantar flexors. This is seen in conditions such as low lumbar-level myelodysplasia, and after overlengthening of the heel cord in children with cerebral palsy. This circumstance is clinically described as a "calcaneous gait." A common secondary cause of excessive ankle dorsiflexion in the stance phase is excessive knee flexion due to hamstring contracture or spasticity, as seen in cerebral palsy. Excessive ankle dorsiflexion may serve as a compensation for forefoot pain, and as a mechanism to shorten the step length of the opposite limb (101,122).

The consequences of excessive ankle dorsiflexion are significant in all of the subphases of stance. In the loading response and midstance subphases, exaggeration of the heel and ankle rockers increases the demand on the quadriceps (i.e., knee extensors) and diminishes limb stability. The crouch gait in cerebral palsy is a consequence of this deviation. In the terminal stance and preswing subphases, heel rise is compromised, which places the ankle plantarflexor muscles at a mechanical disadvantage with respect to power generation, and diminishes the step length of the opposite limb. This decreases the subsequent shock absorption demands of the loading response. Excessive ankle dorsiflexion during the swing phase is unusual, and interferes with the foot position for initial contact.

Knee

Inadequate Flexion/Excessive Extension

Primary inadequate flexion or excessive extension of the knee in the stance phase is usually caused by quadriceps spasticity or contracture. Hyperextension of the knee in stance phase, called "recurvatum gait," may be a primary consequence of overly aggressive medial and lateral distal hamstring lengthening in children with cerebral palsy. The most common secondary cause of these deviations is increased stance-phase ankle plantar flexion, which in the extreme, also causes knee hyperextension or recurvatum deformity by the plantar flexion–knee extension couple. Inadequate flexion or excessive extension of the knee in the stance phase may also reflect a compensatory deviation for knee or patellofemoral pain, or indicate a weakness of the quadriceps, classically seen in children with polio. The consequences of the deviation in the stance phase are decreased shock absorption ability, decreased forward progression of the tibia, and potential injury to the posterior knee joint structures.

A common primary cause of inadequate flexion or excessive extension of the knee in the swing phase is quadriceps spasticity or contracture, as seen in the stiff knee gait pattern in children with cerebral palsy. Hip flexor weakness is a secondary cause of this deviation in swing phase (30). During the terminal-swing subphase, inadequate flexion or excessive extension of the knee may occur as a compensatory mechanism for knee pain or quadriceps weakness. The principal consequence of this deviation in initial and midswing subphases is impaired foot clearance. Suboptimal positioning of the limb for initial contact and loading response is the principal consequence of this deviation in terminal swing.

Excessive Flexion/Inadequate Extension

The primary causes of excessive flexion or inadequate extension of the knee in the stance phase include hamstring spasticity or contracture, as seen in cerebral palsy patients, and quadriceps weakness, as seen in patients with polio. The jump gait and crouch gait deviations seen in children with cerebral palsy are characterized by increased knee flexion in stance phase (30). Secondary causes are related to increased ankle dorsiflexion in the stance phase, usually a consequence of ankle plantar flexor weakness, as seen in low lumbar-level myelodysplasia, or after excessive lengthening of the heel cord in cerebral palsy patients. This deviation is rarely used as a compensatory mechanism, because it is energy-inefficient. The consequences of excessive flexion or inadequate extension of the knee in the stance phase are increased demands on the quadriceps, increased joint reaction forces at the knee and patellofemoral joint, diminished limb stability, and decreased step length of the contralateral limb.

The primary causes of excessive flexion or inadequate extension of the knee in the swing phase are hamstring spasticity or contracture and persistence of primitive locomotor reflex patterns (i.e., inability to extend the knee while flexing the hip), as seen in patients with cerebral palsy (101). Increased knee flexion in the initial and midswing subphases may be a compensatory mechanism to facilitate limb clearance in the face of ankle plantar flexion or diminished hip flexion, which, clinically, is termed a "steppage gait" pattern. Similarly, this deviation during terminal swing allows forefoot strike at initial contact, which would be a compensatory mechanism for a child with heel pain. The consequences of excessive flexion or inadequate extension of the knee in swing phase are diminished step length and impaired positioning of the foot for heel strike at initial contact.

Excessive Varus/Valgus

Primary (or true) excessive varus or valgus dynamic gait deviations are generally related to underlying coronal plane skeletal malalignment. Common examples in pediatric orthopaedics include the stance-phase varus thrust seen in children with rickets and infantile tibia vara. A stance-phase valgus thrust may be seen with other metabolic bone disease (like renal osteodystrophy), longitudinal deficiency of the fibula (with associated lateral femoral condylar hypoplasia), and congenital or obligatory dislocation of the patella.

Secondary (or apparent) excessive varus or valgus dynamic gait deviations at the knee are a consequence of the combination of sagittal plane deviations and transverse plane malalignment or deviations. Increased knee flexion associated with external rotation (e.g., in compensation for internal tibial torsion, or dynamic at the pelvis or hip) will appear as varus on observational gait analysis. Increased knee flexion associated with internal rotation (e.g., as seen with femoral anteversion, or dynamic at the pelvis or hip) will appear as valgus. Quantitative gait analysis is often necessary to accurately characterize these deviations.

Hip

Inadequate Extension/Excessive Flexion

The primary causes of inadequate extension or excessive flexion of the hip in the stance phase include hip flexor spasticity or contracture, as seen in cerebral palsy patients; hamstring or hip extensor weakness, as seen in those with myelodysplasia; iliotibial band contracture, as seen in children with Duchenne muscular dystrophy; and hip joint pain. The most common secondary cause of this deviation in the stance phase is excessive ankle dorsiflexion, as seen in low lumbar-level myelodysplasia patients, and in the crouch gait pattern of patients with cerebral palsy.

The consequences of inadequate extension or excessive flexion of the hip in stance phase are related to the associated anterior pelvic tilt and the result of forward trunk lean. Children have the flexibility to compensate for this hip deformity by increasing their lumbar lordosis (101,122). This places increased strain across the lumbar spine over time. Incomplete compensation for forward trunk lean moves the ground reaction force anteriorly, increasing the external extension moment at the knee and dorsiflexion moment at the ankle.

The most common primary cause of this deviation in the swing phase is hip flexor spasticity or contracture. Compensatory increased hip flexion during the swing phase is used to facilitate limb clearance in the face of inappropriate ankle plantar flexion or knee extension. The main consequence of this deviation in swing phase is increased energy cost.

Excessive Adduction

The primary causes of excessive adduction of the hip during the stance phase are adductor muscle spasticity or contracture and ipsilateral abductor muscle weakness. Secondary causes include contralateral hip abductor muscle contracture and scoliosis with pelvic obliquity. The consequences of this deviation in the stance phase are a decreased base of support in the coronal plane and diminished limb stability.

Excessive adduction of the hip is seen as a primary deviation in the swing phase caused by adductor muscle spasticity or contracture. A common secondary cause is limb-length inequality. A significantly short contralateral limb causes pelvic obliquity in the stance phase, effectively adducting the reference limb in swing phase. Compensatory hip adduction in the swing phase occurs when the hip adductors substitute for weak hip flexors to assist with limb clearance (101,122). The principal consequence of excessive hip adduction in swing phase is a relative increase in the limb length, which can cause problems with clearance. The scissor gait deviation, seen in children with cerebral palsy, may appear to be due to excessive hip adduction during swing phase. However, quantitative gait analysis has shown this deviation to most commonly be a consequence of increased hip flexion and internal rotation (because of increased femoral anteversion or dynamic rotational deviation).

A child who exhibits contralateral pelvic drop when asked to stand on one leg (a sign of ipsilateral hip abductor muscle weakness), is said to have a positive Trendelenburg sign. Contralateral pelvic drop during the stance phase of the reference limb is called a "Trendelenburg gait" or "uncompensated gluteus medius gait" pattern. A common compensation for this inefficient gait deviation is lateral trunk lean over the stance limb, which effectively moves the body's center of mass closer to the stance-phase hip joint, and diminishes the demand on the gluteus medius muscle, the principal hip abductor. This deviation is called the "abductor lurch" or "compensated gluteus medius gait" pattern.

Excessive Abduction

The primary cause of excessive abduction of the hip during the stance phase is abductor muscle contracture. Secondary causes are limb-length inequality, in which the ipsilateral limb is significantly short, and scoliosis with pelvic obliquity. Excessive abduction of the hip in the stance phase may also be a compensatory mechanism for a relatively long limb. The consequences in the stance phase are to increase the base of support in the coronal plane, and to decrease the relative length of the stance limb.

The primary cause of excessive abduction of the hip in the swing phase is ipsilateral abductor muscle contracture. Compensatory excessive hip abduction in swing is seen as a substitution pattern for weak hip flexors (5,101,122). This deviation is also used, in combination with increased pelvic rotation and upward pelvic obliquity, as a means to clear a long limb (i.e., absolute length, or relatively long, due to inadequate knee flexion or ankle dorsiflexion). This complex deviation is called "circumduction." The principal consequence of excessive hip abduction in the swing phase is to decrease the functional length of the ipsilateral limb.

GAIT ANALYSIS

Observational Gait Analysis

A systematic method of observational gait analysis promotes a comprehensive assessment of gait deviations and functional deficits and avoids the common pitfall of focusing exclusively on the most striking component of a complex multilevel problem. The technique described has three phases: preparation, observation, and interpretation.

The preparation begins with determination or confirmation of the underlying diagnosis by taking a clinical history. It is essential to determine the principal gait problems as perceived by the child, the parents, and the referring physician or therapist. A physical examination should assess the active and passive range of motion of the hips, knees, ankles, and subtalar joints. A thorough neurologic evaluation should include muscle strength, selective control, spasticity (i.e., response to fast stretch), contracture (dynamic versus fixed or myostatic), presence or persistence of primitive mass reflexes, sensation, and proprioception.

The observation phase begins with a global assessment of the child's gait, focusing on velocity, cadence, step length, stability, and effort. This is followed by serial horizontal analyses, beginning at the ankle and proceeding to the hip, of each anatomic area relative to the eight subphases of the gait cycle: initial contact, loading response, midstance, terminal stance, preswing, initial swing, midswing, and terminal swing. Analysis of one limb is completed at each joint before analysis of the opposite limb. Sagittal-plane analysis is performed from the right and left sides as the child walks by the observer. Coronal-plane analysis is performed with the child walking toward and away from the observer. The observations are entered, as they are made, on a standardized form (Fig. 5-17).

Interpretation begins with horizontal summation, by anatomic area, of the data collected. This approach can identify the gait deviations at each joint. Vertical summation of the data can identify the functional deficits with respect to gait tasks and the subphases of the gait cycle. A review of the gait deviations and functional deficits helps to determine the primary deviations, secondary deviations, and compensatory deviations. Appropriate interventions can be determined and implemented at this point.

Quantitative Gait Analysis

Technologic advances, many of which have occurred as spin-offs from the defense industry between the 1960s and 1990s, have greatly enhanced the ability to objectively quantify the movements associated with normal gait, and to catalogue common deviations associated with pathologic gait.

NAME _____ Side: Right / Left		Weight Acceptance		Single Limb Support			Swing Limb Advancement			Gait Deviations (By Anatomic Area)
Anatomic Area	**Deviation**	IC	LR	MSt	TSt	PSw	ISw	MSw	TSw	
ANKLE	↑ Dorsiflexion									
	Neutral									
	↑ Plantar Flexion									
	Varus									
	Valgus									
KNEE	↑ Flexion									
	Neutral									
	↑ Extension									
	Varus									
	Valgus									
HIP	↑ Flexion									
	Neutral									
	↑ Extension									
	Adduction									
	Abduction									
FUNCTIONAL DEFICITS (By Gait Tasks)										

FIGURE 5-17. Standardized form used when performing observational gait analysis. IC, initial contact; LR, loading response; MSt, midstance; Tst, terminal stance; PSw, preswing; ISw, initial swing; MSw, midswing; TSw, terminal swing. (From ref. 122, with permission.)

Quantitative gait analysis, as applied to pediatric orthopaedics, is performed in a motion analysis laboratory equipped to study children of all sizes. These laboratories perform analyses in several domains, depending on the nature of the child's gait deviations and the clinical questions being asked.

Kinematic analysis describes gait deviations by determining the magnitude and timing of limb segment motion with joint angles, velocities, and accelerations. Stride analysis may be considered as a subset of kinematic analysis, documenting parameters, such as velocity, cadence, step and stride lengths, and duration of the subphases of the gait cycle. Kinematic data are presented graphically as a waveform for a particular joint or limb segment in a particular plane or dimension.

Kinetic analysis explains gait deviations by determining the magnitude and location of the mechanical forces acting around the joints. Kinetic data are also presented graphi-

cally, and include both moment analysis, which describes the net internal or external forces acting around the joint, and power analysis, which in most situations correlates with the type of muscle activity (i.e., eccentric versus concentric) occurring about the joint.

Dynamic electromyography (EMG) assesses the timing and magnitude of skeletal muscle activity occurring during the gait cycle. Energetics evaluates the energy expenditure associated with walking, and determines the physiologic efficiency of gait.

Kinematic Analysis

Biomechanical analysis of limb movement in gait reduces the skeletal segments to rigid bodies moving through space, which are interconnected by frictionless joints. There are two main types of automated video systems used to generate kinematic data (101,110). The first and most widely used technique consists of video cameras that generate digital data by tracking passive, retroreflective markers fixed to body landmarks based on surface anatomy. A central computer analyzes these data to determine the three-dimensional coordinates of each marker throughout the gait cycle. To generate accurate, reproducible data, all cameras must record data simultaneously, and the image space must be calibrated frequently. Each marker must be traced throughout the duration of the gait cycle by at least two cameras to enable three-dimensional calculations. When attempting to study both limbs simultaneously, five or six cameras are required.

This first technique has several limitations. First, it assumes that surface anatomy, which determines marker placement, is consistently related to the underlying osseous anatomy. It also considers the marker position to be stable throughout the gait cycle. The margin of error is acceptable when calculating limb-segment movement. However, more sophisticated kinetic analysis requires determination of the joint centers from the surface anatomy, which remains a controversial and less widely accepted practice. Current research is directed at validation and improvement of this technique. Second, the cameras require a minimum distance of 5 to 7 cm between markers for recognition (101,110). This can make it difficult to analyze small anatomic areas, such as the foot and ankle of a child. Third, any event that blocks the marker from the camera, such as a swinging hand, an assistive device, or the overlap of two markers in the camera field, causes the computer to lose track of the marker. This is called "marker dropout," and can only be corrected by manual sorting of the marker trajectories, which can be labor intensive. Sampling rates are generally limited to 50 to 60 images per second (2,8). This precludes the study of most athletic activities beyond running, like throwing, batting, and swinging a golf club.

The second type of automated video system uses active markers to designate anatomic sites. Each marker is a light-emitting diode that is activated sequentially by a central computer. A computer-controlled optical detector tracks the markers in a similar sequence. This technique facilitates data differentiation, and has fewer problems with marker spacing and dropout (101,110). Problems with this system include background reflections of the markers from the floor and walls, and electronic interference when simultaneously recording EMG during the gait cycle. As a result, this second technique is less widely used in clinical motion analysis laboratories.

Gait can be characterized by temporal and distance parameters. Velocity is the distance per unit time; cadence is the steps per unit time; stride length is the distance between two sequential initial contacts by the same limb; step length is the distance between the initial contact by each foot;

and single-limb stance time is the period during which the opposite limb is in the swing phase with no floor contact. Compensations for diminished velocity include increased cadence and, when possible, increased stride length (108,135). In children, changes in temporal and distance parameters with age are primarily a function of increasing limb length (101,131–133). Adults have a wide range of safe and comfortable walking velocities, influenced primarily by voluntary variability (136). Age has no significant effect until the person is older than 60 years of age (101).

Stride analysis can be performed by several techniques. The indirect method uses kinematic data. A single foot or ankle marker is tracked with respect to time and distance over a predetermined gait cycle sequence.

Direct techniques measure the foot contact with the floor. This is accomplished with a foot switch system, which consists of individual pressure sensors that are placed beneath the heel and the metatarsal heads (29,32,101, 110,137). Time and distance parameters can be determined directly from the activation patterns of the different sensors. Insertable insole pressure sensors enable analysis of more complex patterns of foot pressure distribution.

Kinetic Analysis

As the body advances forward over the stance-phase limb, a three-dimensional ground reaction force, which is equal in magnitude and opposite in direction to the force being experienced by the stance-phase limb, is generated (i.e., Newton's third law). The magnitude of the vertical, horizontal, and axial components of the ground reaction force can be determined by a force platform (101,107,110,123, 138,139). This device is a rigid plate mounted on four piezoelectric or strain gauge transducers. With each corner having a transducer sensitive to applied loads in three dimensions, the vertical force and horizontal shear forces (i.e., mediolateral and progressional) can be measured directly. Summation of this data allows the examiner to calculate the center of pressure, which is the point on the foot about which the ground reaction force has zero moment, and to calculate its progression (101,110,139).

By combining the position of the ground reaction force with the position of the joint centers, which are derived from the kinematic data, the external joint moments can be calculated (107). These moments reflect the demands applied to the joints by body-segment position, gravity, and inertia. The external moments determine the requirements for the internal moments generated by the muscles and other soft tissue structures. Further kinetic analysis combines the position of the ground reaction force with the joint angular velocity, which is derived from the kinematic data, to determine joint powers (107).

To obtain accurate data, the child must walk across the force platform in a spontaneous, natural fashion. Deliberately stepping onto the platform, an action called "targeting," compromises the data collected, and is avoided by mounting the platform flush with the floor and camouflaging it with a thin "skin" that matches the rest of the floor. The foot of the reference limb must strike the platform completely, while the opposite foot remains clear. Children who use assistive devices, such as walkers or crutches, cannot be studied with a standard force platform, because only a portion of their body weight is supported by the stance-phase limb.

Dynamic Electromyography

EMG documents the electrical activity associated with skeletal muscle contraction on a visual record (29,101, 140–142). Dynamic EMG uses surface or internal electrodes to record these myoelectric potentials. Surface electrodes are pairs of metal pads that are placed directly on the skin overlying the muscle to be studied. They are easy to apply and cause no pain or discomfort. Unfortunately, they pick up signals from other muscles in the same area, which can interfere with the signal from the muscle being studied. This phenomenon is called "muscle cross talk" and limits the use of surface electrodes to superficial muscles, such as the gluteus maximus, or muscle groups, such as the medial or lateral hamstrings (110,143). Internal electrodes are 50-mm–diameter wires, which are introduced through the skin with a 27-gauge needle and embedded in the muscle belly. The principal advantage of the internal electrode is its ability to record the activity of a specific muscle without interference from surrounding muscles (137). It is ideal for studying deeper or smaller muscles, such as the iliacus or posterior tibialis (26,110). The disadvantages associated with the use of fine-wire electrodes include pain on insertion, difficulty of accurate placement, and wire movement with muscle contraction (110,142,144). Moreover, the temporal parameters of gait in children with cerebral palsy can change after insertion of fine-wire electrodes (145).

Controversies encumber the interpretation of EMG data, particularly with respect to the determination of muscle force. The raw EMG signal is quantified by computer-based digital sampling, rectification (i.e., transposition of the negative signals to the positive side of the graphic display to avoid the positive and negative signals cancelling each other out in subsequent data processing), and integration (i.e., summing of the digitized, rectified EMG signals over time) (101,110). The signal is then normalized to a selected reference value, usually that generated by a maximal-effort manual muscle test (106,144). Other investigators have noticed improved reproducibility when the selected reference value is the peak EMG activity generated by the muscle during a representative gait cycle (101,106). The former technique is difficult to apply in children with cerebral palsy who have

poor selective control. The latter technique fails to differentiate between weak and strong muscular activity (101).

The use of dynamic EMG to determine the timing of muscle activity is widely accepted, even though the determination of actual on and off is subjective, with the minimum significant signal arbitrarily defined as being greater than or equal to 5% of the maximal manual muscle test (137, 141–143). There is poor consensus concerning the relation of muscle force to the EMG signal, with linear and nonlinear correlations having been reported (34,106,101, 110) Potentially significant confounders include the type of muscle contraction (i.e., concentric versus eccentric versus isometric), the speed of the contraction, the joint position (i.e., affecting the resting muscle length and the muscle's moment arm), and electromechanical delay (101). It is most accurate to consider dynamic EMG to be a measure of the timing of muscle activation, and not a direct measure of muscle force generation when attempting to relate the activity of a particular muscle to a particular gait deviation.

Energetics

Measurement of the energy required for walking provides a comprehensive parameter of gait performance and a means of quantifying the physiologic cost of various gait deviations (1,110,111,146–148). Total body calorimetry, which is a measurement of the body's heat and work production, is the most accurate technique of energy use assessment, but is not clinically practical.

Indirect calorimetry assumes that anaerobic metabolism contributes little to energy production during steady-state ambulation at a self-determined walking velocity (111,136, 148). In this model, the energy needs of gait are completely met by the aerobic metabolism of inspired oxygen (O_2). The magnitude of O_2 consumed reflects the energy requirements for walking. Indirect calorimetry uses open spirometry to measure O_2 consumption (148).

While ambulating, the child inspires ambient air and expires air into a closed capture system. Analysis and comparison of the O_2 content of the ambient and expired air determines the child's O_2 consumption over time. The O_2 consumption is reported as the O_2 rate, expressed in milliliters per kilogram minute, and is a reflection of the intensity of the effort required to ambulate (111,148).

When comparing gait patterns, the most valuable parameter is the O_2 cost, which is a measure of the physiologic efficiency of gait. In general, children are studied at their self-determined walking speed, which represents the most energy-efficient compromise between progression and stability. The O_2 cost is defined as the O_2 rate divided by the walking velocity, and is expressed as milliliters per kilogram meter. The O_2 cost describes the amount of energy needed to walk a standard distance (111,148). Children with cerebral palsy tend to have O_2 rates similar to healthy normal children, indicating a common range of energy used for walking (102,146,147). However, the self-selected walking velocity is significantly less for the children with cerebral palsy. As a result, their relatively energy-inefficient gait is best described by the O_2 cost, which is greater than the controls (146,147). Energetics analysis has traditionally been performed with a metabolic cart. The facemask worn by the child is directly connected to the cart, which is wheeled alongside the child as he or she walks. More recently, technologic advances have supported the development of a lightweight, telemetric device, which is easily carried by the child in a neoprene fanny pack (149). Such devices should have a less disruptive effect on the subject's gait. In addition, they should facilitate the collection of energetics data outside of the hospital setting, during more relevant community-based activities.

Given the cost and inconvenience of performing quantitative energetics analysis in children with disabilities, some investigators have attempted to utilize the heart rate as a substitute for O_2 rate. Based on a linear relationship between heart rate and O_2 rate, these investigators developed the physiologic cost index (PCI, walking minus resting heart rates, divided by walking velocity) as a measure of gait efficiency (146,147,150). Subsequent investigators have found increased intrasubject variability and poor correlation when comparing the PCI to O_2 cost (151).

Clinical and Research Applications

Although quantitative motion analysis has been practiced in pediatric orthopaedics for over 20 years, its role remains controversial (152). Improved technology has made data collection faster and more accurate. Improved processing has allowed clinical data to be available almost immediately after a study has been performed. Improved graphics have made data output formats more user-friendly. Clinical experience, with the application of quantitative motion analysis for children with cerebral palsy, has improved understanding of pathologic gait (e.g., the functional significance of skeletal malalignment) (1,12,19), resulted in the abandonment of certain procedures (e.g., aggressive adductor muscle release and anterior branch obturator neurectomy for apparent scissoring gait) (31,49,57,153), led to the development of other procedures to address previously poorly understood gait deviations (e.g., rectus femoris transfer and intrapelvic fractional lengthening of the psoas) (38, 45–47,55,56), and provided a rationale for the selection of certain procedures over others (e.g., performing muscle lengthenings at the myotendinous junction, instead of at the level of the tendon, in order to preserve power generation) (17,20,51,58,154).

The role of quantitative motion analysis in biomechanical and clinical research has been widely accepted. Teaching gait analysis techniques to a variety of health care profession-

als utilizing quantitative motion analysis data and principles, although not widely appreciated, has also proven to be very effective. Despite these benefits, widespread acceptance and use of quantitative motion analysis in preoperative decision-making by pediatric orthopaedists have not occurred. Critics argue that the application of quantitative motion analysis is too expensive, and that the testing circumstances (i.e., in the artificial setting of the motion laboratory) have little to do with day to day functional activities. Resistance to the application of this technology is due, in part, to the fact that the data are complex and requires significant experience to interpret. In addition, there are misconceptions about what the data can, and cannot, do. Quantitative motion analysis is a diagnostic tool that complements, but does not replace, clinical judgment. In the same way that technologic advances in dynamic functional assessment have changed the way clinical medicine is practiced in fields such as cardiology, so too should quantitative motion analysis improve the pediatric orthopaedist's ability to diagnose complex gait disorders, and to critically analyze the outcomes of various treatment options. Continued refinement of this technology in the research arena, and earlier exposure to the data in the literature and in residency training programs, should facilitate its ultimate acceptance by clinicians.

ACKNOWLEDGMENTS

The author wishes to recognize the contributions of David H. Sutherland, M.D., Jacqueline Perry, M.D., and James R. Gage, M.D., to the field of motion analysis, and to refer interested readers to ref. 1, 29, 101, and 132.

References

1. Gage JR. *Clinics in developmental medicine*, no. 121. Oxford: MacKeith, 1991.

Normal Gait

2. Hoffinger SA. Gait analysis in pediatric rehabilitation. *Phys Med Rehabil Clin North Am* 1991;2:817.
3. Inman VT, Ralston H, Todd F. *Human walking*. Baltimore: Williams & Wilkins, 1981.
4. Mann RA, Hagy JL, White V, et al. The initiation of gait. *J Bone Joint Surg Am* 1979;61:232.
5. Perry J. Mechanics of walking. *Phys Ther* 1967;47:778.
6. Saunders JBdeCM, Inman VT, Eberhart HD. The major determinants in normal and pathologic gait. *J Bone Joint Surg Am* 1953;35:543.
7. Steindler A. A historical review of the studies and investigations made in relation to human gait. *J Bone Joint Surg Am* 1953; 35:540.
8. Sutherland DH, Valencia FG. Pediatric gait. In: Drennan JC, ed. *The child's foot and ankle*. New York: Raven, 1992:19.
9. Muybridge E. *Complete human and animal locomotion*. New York: Dover, 1980.

10. Braune W, Fischer D. *The human gait*. Berlin: Springer-Verlag, 1987.

11. Gage JR. An overview of normal walking. *Instr Course Lect* 1990;39:291.

12. Gage JR. Gait analysis: an essential tool in the treatment of cerebral palsy. *Clin Orthop* 1993;288:126.

13. Abel MF, Damiano DL. Strategies for increasing walking speed in diplegic cerebral palsy. *J Pediatr Orthop* 1996;16:753.

14. Barto PS, Supinski RS, Skinner SR. Dynamic EMG findings in varus hindfoot deformity and spastic cerebral palsy. *Dev Med Child Neurol* 1984;26:88.

15. Damiano DL, Abel MF. Functional outcomes of strength training in spastic cerebral palsy. *Arch Phys Med Rehabil* 1998;79:119.

16. Davids JR, Bagley AM, Bryan M. Kinematic and kinetic analysis of running in children with cerebral palsy. *Dev Med Child Neurol* 1998;40:528.

17. Delp SL, Arnold AS, Speers RA, et al. Hamstrings and psoas lengths during normal and crouch gait: implications for muscle-tendon surgery. *J Orthop Res* 1996;14:144.

18. DeLuca PA. Gait analysis in the treatment of the ambulatory child with cerebral palsy. *Clin Orthop* 1991;264:65.

19. Gage JR, DeLuca PA, Renshaw TS. Gait analysis: principles and applications. Emphasis on its use in cerebral palsy. *J Bone Joint Surg Am* 1995;77:1607.

20. Gage JR. The clinical use of kinetics for evaluation of pathologic gait in cerebral palsy. *Instr Course Lect* 1995;44:507.

21. Hicks R, Durinick N, Gage JR. Differentiation of idiopathic toe-walking and cerebral palsy. *J Pediatr Orthop* 988;8:160.

22. Kalen V, Adler N, Bleck EE. Electromyography of idiopathic toe walking. *J Pediatr Orthop* 1986;6:31.

23. Norlin R, Odenrick P. Development of gait in spastic children with cerebral palsy. *J Pediatr Orthop* 1986;6:674.

24. Perry J, Hoffer MM, Giovan P, et al. Gait analysis of the triceps surae in cerebral palsy. *J Bone Joint Surg Am* 1974;56:511.

25. Perry J, Antonelli D, Ford W. Analysis of knee-joint forces during flexed-knee stance. *J Bone Joint Surg Am* 1975;57: 961.

26. Perry J. Determinants of muscle function in the spastic lower extremity. *Clin Orthop* 1993;288:10.

27. Skinner SR, Lester DK. Gait electromyographic evaluation of the long-toe flexors in children with spastic cerebral palsy. *Clin Orthop* 1986;207:70.

28. Sutherland DH, Cooper L. The pathomechanics of progressive crouch gait in spastic diplegia. *Orthop Clin North Am* 1978;9:143.

29. Sutherland DH. *Gait disorders in childhood and adolescence*. Baltimore: Williams & Wilkins, 1984.

30. Sutherland DH, Davids JR. Common gait abnormalities of the knee in cerebral palsy. *Clin Orthop* 1993;288:139.

31. Tylkowski CM, Simon SR, Mansour JM. Internal rotation gait in spastic cerebral palsy. In: Nelson JP, ed. *The hip*. St. Louis: CV Mosby, 1982:89.

32. Wills CA, Hoffer MM, Perry J. A comparison of foot-switch and EMG analysis of varus deformities of the feet of children with cerebral palsy. *Dev Med Child Neurol* 1988;30:227.

33. Winters TF, Gage JR, Hicks R. Gait patterns in spastic hemiplegia. *J Bone Joint Surg Am* 1987;69:437.

34. Boscarino LF, Ounpuu S, Davis RB, et al. Effects of selective dorsal rhizotomy on gait in children with cerebral palsy. *J Pediatr Orthop* 1993;13:174.

35. Bowen TR, Miller F, Castagno P, et al. A method of dynamic foot-pressure measurement for the evaluation of pediatric orthopaedic foot deformities. *J Pediatr Orthop* 1998;18:789.

36. Brodke DS, Skinner SR, Lamoreux LW, et al. Effects of ankle-foot orthoses on the gait of children. *J Pediatr Orthop* 1989;9:702.

37. Cahan LD, Adams JM, Perry J, et al. Instrumented gait analysis after selective dorsal rhizotomy. *Dev Med Child Neurol* 1990;32:1037.

38. Chambers H, Laver A, Kaufman K, et al. Prediction of outcome after rectus femoris surgery in cerebral palsy: the role of cocontraction of the rectus femoris and vastus lateralis. *J Pediatr Orthop* 1998;18:703.

39. Corry IS, Cosgrove AP, Duffy CM, et al. Botulinum toxin A compared with stretching casts in the treatment of spastic equinus: a randomized prospective trial. *J Pediatr Orthop* 1998;18:304.

40. Cosgrove HP, Corry IS, Graham HK. Botulinum toxin in the management of the lower limb in cerebral palsy. *Dev Med Child Neurol* 1994;36:386.

41. DeLuca PA, Davis RB III, Ounpuu S, et al. Alterations in surgical decision making in patients with cerebral palsy based on three-dimensional gait analysis. *J Pediatr Orthop* 1997;17:608.

42. DeLuca PA, Ounpuu S, Davis RB, et al. Effect of hamstring and psoas lengthening on pelvic tilt in patients with spastic diplegic cerebral palsy. *J Pediatr Orthop* 1998;18:712.

43. Etnyre B, Chambers CS, Scarborough NH, et al. Preoperative and postoperative assessment of surgical intervention for equinus gait in children with cerebral palsy. *J Pediatr Orthop* 1993;13:24.

44. Hoffer MM. Ten year follow-up of split anterior tibial tendon transfer in cerebral palsied patients with spastic equinovarus deformity. *J Pediatr Orthop* 1985;5:432.

45. Miller F, Cardoso Dias R, Lipton GE, et al. The effect of rectus EMG patterns on the outcome of rectus femoris transfers. *J Pediatr Orthop* 1997;17:603.

46. Ounpuu S, Muik E, Davis RB, et al. Rectus femoris surgery in children with cerebral palsy. Part I: the effect of rectus femoris transfer location on knee motion. *J Pediatr Orthop* 1993;13:325.

47. Ounpuu S, Muik E, Davis RB, et al. Rectus femoris surgery in children with cerebral palsy. Part II: a comparison between the effect of transfer and release of the distal rectus femoris on knee motion. *J Pediatr Orthop* 1993;13:331.

48. Ounpuu S, Bell KJ, Davis RB III, et al. An evaluation of the posterior leaf spring orthosis using joint kinematics and kinetics. *J Pediatr Orthop* 1996;16:378.

49. Perry J, Hoffer MM, Antonelli D, et al. Electromyography before and after surgery for hip deformity in children with cerebral palsy. *J Bone Joint Surg Am* 1976;58:201.

50. Perry J, Hoffer MM. Preoperative and postoperative dynamic electromyography as an aid in planning tendon transfers in children with cerebral palsy. *J Bone Joint Surg Am* 1977;59:531.

51. Segal LS, Sienko TSE, Mazur JM, et al. Calcaneal gait in spastic diplegia after heelcord lengthening: a study with gait analysis. *J Pediatr Orthop* 1989;9:697.

52. Sienko TS, Aiona MD, Buckon CE, et al. Does gait continue to improve 2 years after selective dorsal rhizotomy? *J Pediatr Orthop* 1997;17:387.

53. Stefko RM, deSwart RJ, Dodgin DA, et al. Kinematic and kinetic analysis of distal derotational osteotomy of the leg in children with cerebral palsy. *J Pediatr Orthop* 1998;18:81.

54. Subramanian N, Vaughn CL, Peter JC, et al. Gait before and after rhizotomy in children with cerebral palsy spasticity. *J Neurosurg* 1998;88:1014.

55. Sutherland DH, Santi M, Abel MF. Treatment of stiff-knee gait in cerebral palsy: a comparison by gait analysis of distal rectus femoris transfer versus proximal rectus release. *J Pediatr Orthop* 1990;10:433.

56. Sutherland DH, Zilberfarb JL, Kaufman KR, et al. Psoas release

at the pelvic brim in ambulatory patients with cerebral palsy: operative technique and functional outcome. *J Pediatr Orthop* 1997;17:563.

57. Thometz J, Simons S, Rosenthal R. The effect on gait of lengthening of the medial hamstrings in cerebral palsy. *J Bone Joint Surg Am* 1989;71:345.

58. Yngve DA, Chambers C. Vulpius and Z-lengthening. *J Pediatr Orthop* 1996;16:759.

59. Banta JV, Sutherland DH, Wyatt MP. Anterior tibial transfer to the os calcis with Achilles tenodesis for the calcaneal deformity in myelomeningocele. *J Pediatr Orthop* 1981;1:125.

60. Cudderford TJ, Freeling RP, Thomas SS, et al. Energy consumption in children with myelomeningocoele: a comparison between reciprocating gait orthosis and hip-knee-ankle-foot orthosis ambulators. *Dev Med Child Neurol* 1997;39:239.

61. Duffy CM, Hill AE, Cosgrove AP, et al. Three-dimensional gait analysis in spina bifida. *J Pediatr Orthop* 1996;16:786.

62. Hullin MG, Robb JE, Loudon IR. Ankle-foot orthosis function in low-level myelomeningocele. *J Pediatr Orthop* 1992;12:518.

63. Lim R, Dias L, Vankoski S, et al. Valgus knee stress in lumbosacral myelomeningocoele: a gait-analysis evaluation. *J Pediatr Orthop* 1998;428.

64. Thomson JD, Ounpuu S, Davis RB III, et al. The effects of ankle-foot orthoses on the ankle and knee in persons with myelomeningocele: an evaluation using three-dimensional gait analysis. *J Pediatr Orthop* 1998;18:27.

65. Vankoski C, Moore C, Statler KD, et al. The influence of forearm crutches on pelvic and hip kinematics in children with myelomeningocoele: don't throw away the crutches. *Dev Med Child Neur* 1997;39:614.

66. Hsu JD, Furumasu J. Gait and posture changes in the Duchenne muscular dystrophy child. *Clin Orthop* 1993;288:122.

67. Sutherland DH, Olsen R, Cooper LB, et al. The pathomechanics of gait in Duchenne muscular dystrophy. *Dev Med Child Neurol* 1981;23:3.

68. Asperheim MS, Moore C, Carroll NC, et al. Evaluation of residual clubfoot deformities using gait analysis. *J Pediatr Orthop* 1995;43:49.

69. Davids JR, Meyer LC. Proximal tibiofibular bifurcation synostosis for the management of longitudinal deficiency of the tibia. *J Pediatr Orthop* 1998;18:110.

70. Engsberg JR, Lee AG, Tedford KG, et al. Normative ground reaction force data for able-bodied and below-knee-amputee children during walking. *J Pediatr Orthop* 1993;13:169.

71. Fowler E, Zernicke R, Setoguchi Y, et al. Energy expenditure during walking by children who have proximal femoral focal deficiency. *J Bone Joint Surg Am* 1996;78A:1857.

72. Karol LA, Concha MC, Johnston CE II. Gait analysis and muscle strength in children with surgically treated clubfeet. *J Pediatr Orthop* 1997;17:790.

73. Karol LA, Haideri NF, Halliday SE, et al. Gait analysis and muscle strength in children with congenital pseudarthrosis of the tibia: the effect of treatment. *J Pediatr Orthop* 1998;18:381.

74. Kaufman KR, Miller LS, Sutherland DH. Gait asymmetry in patients with limb-length inequality. *J Pediatr Orthop* 1996;16:144.

75. Lewallen R, Kyck G, Quanbury A, et al. Gait kinematics in below-knee child amputees: a force plate analysis. *J Pediatr Orthop* 1986;6:291.

76. Liu XC, Fabry G, Molenaers G, et al. Kinematic and kinetic asymmetry in patients with leg-length discrepancy. *J Pediatr Orthop* 1998;18:187.

77. Steenhoff JRM, Daanen HAM, Taminiav AHM. Functional analysis of patients who have had a modified Van Nes rotationplasty. *J Bone Joint Surg Am* 1993;75:1451.

78. Andriacchi TP. Evaluation of surgical procedures and/or joint implants with gait analysis. *Instr Course Lect* 1990;39:343.

79. Berman AT, Zarro VJ, Bosacco SJ, et al. Quantitative gait analysis after unilateral or bilateral total knee replacement. *J Bone Joint Surg Am* 1987;69:1340.

80. Kroll MA, Otis JC, Sculco TP, et al. The relationship of stride characteristics to pain before and after total knee arthroplasty. *Clin Orthop* 1989;239:191.

81. Long WT, Dorr LD, Healy B, et al. Functional recovery of noncemented total hip arthroplasty. *Clin Orthop* 1993;288:73.

82. Prodromos C, Andriacchi T, Galante J. A relationship between gait and clinical changes following high tibial osteotomy. *J Bone Joint Surg Am* 1985;67:1188.

83. Skinner HB. Pathokinesiology and total joint arthroplasty. *Clin Orthop* 1993;288:78.

84. Waters RL, Barnes G, Husserl T, et al. Comparable energy expenditure following arthrodesis of the hip and ankle. *J Bone Joint Surg Am* 1988;70:1032.

85. Andriacchi TP, Birac D. Functional testing in the anterior cruciate ligament-deficient knee. *Clin Orthop* 1993;288:40.

86. Berchuck M, Andriacchi TP, Bach BR, et al. Gait adaptations by patients who have a deficient anterior cruciate ligament. *J Bone Joint Surg Am* 1990;72:871.

87. Glousman R. Electromyographic analysis and its role in the athletic shoulder. *Clin Orthop* 1993;288:27.

88. Limbird TJ, Shiavi R, Frazer M, et al. EMG profiles of knee joint musculature during walking: changes induced by anterior cruciate ligament deficiency. *J Orthop Res* 1988;6:630.

89. Pink M, Jobe FW, Perry J, et al. The normal shoulder during the butterfly swim stroke: an electromyographic and cinematographic analysis of twelve muscles. *Clin Orthop* 1993;288:48.

90. Pink M, Jobe FW, Perry J, et al. The painful shoulder during the butterfly stroke: an electromyographic and cinematographic analysis of twelve muscles. *Clin Orthop* 1993;288:60.

91. Schwab GH, Moynes DR, Jobe FW, et al. Lower extremity electromyographic analysis of running gait. *Clin Orthop* 1983;176:166.

92. Tibone JE, Antich TJ. Electromyographic analysis of the anterior cruciate ligament-deficient knee. *Clin Orthop* 1993;288:35.

93. Kozin SH, Keenan MAE. Using dynamic electromyography to guide surgical treatment of the spastic upper extremity in the brain-injured patient. *Clin Orthop* 1993;288:109.

94. Perry J, Waters RL, Perrin T. Electromyographic analysis of equinovarus following stroke. *Clin Orthop* 1978;131:47.

95. Pinzur MS. Dynamic electromyography in functional surgery for upper limb spasticity. *Clin Orthop* 1993;288:118.

96. Water RL, Yakura JS, Adkins RH. Gait performance after spinal cord injury. *Clin Orthop* 1993;288:87.

97. Waters RL, Perry J, Antonelli D, et al. The energy cost of walking of amputees—influence of level of amputation. *J Bone Joint Surg Am* 1976;58:42.

98. Waters RL, Garland DE, Perry J, et al. Stiff-legged gain in hemiplegia: surgical correction. *J Bone Joint Surg Am* 1979;61:927.

99. Waters RL, Lunsford BR. Energy cost of paraplegic ambulation. *J Bone Joint Surg Am* 1985;67:1245.

100. Waters RL, Campbell J, Perry J. Energy cost of three-point crutch ambulation in fracture patients. *J Orthop Trauma* 1987;1:170.

101. Perry J. *Gait analysis: normal and pathologic function.* Thorofare, NJ: Slack, 1992.

102. Waters RL, Hislop HJ, Thomas L, et al. Energy cost of walking in normal children and teenagers. *Dev Med Child Neurol* 1983;25:184.

103. Grillner S. Neurobiological bases of rhythmic motor acts in vertebrates. *Science* 1985;228:143.

104. Joseph J. Neurological control of locomotion. *Dev Med Child Neurol* 1985;27:822.
105. Winter DA. Biomechanical motor patterns in normal walking. *J Motor Behav* 1983;15:302.
106. Winter DA. *The biomechanics and control of human gait.* Waterloo: University of Waterloo Press, 1987.
107. Ounpuu MS, Gage JR, Davis RB. Three-dimensional lower extremity joint kinetics in normal pediatric gait. *J Pediatr Orthop* 1991;11:341.
108. Winter DA. Kinematic and kinetic patterns in human gait: variability and compensating effects. *Human Movement Sci* 1984;3:51.
109. Ounpuu S. The biomechanics of running: a kinematic and kinetic analysis. *Instr Course Lect* 1990;39:305.
110. Sutherland DH, Kaufman KR. Motion analysis: lower extremity. In: Nickel VL, Botte MJ, eds. *Orthopaedic rehabilitation.* 2nd ed. New York: Churchill Livingstone, 1992:223.
111. Waters RL, Lunsford BR. Energy expenditure of normal and pathologic gait: application to orthotic prescription. In: Bunch WH, ed. *Atlas of orthotics.* St. Louis: CV Mosby, 1985:151.
112. Simon SR, Mann R, Hagy JL, et al. Role of the posterior of calf muscles in normal gait. *J Bone Joint Surg Am* 1978;60:465.
113. Skinner SR, Antonelli D, Perry J, Lester DK. Functional demands on the stance limb in walking. *Orthopaedics* 1985;8:355.
114. Sutherland DH. An electromyographic study of the plantar flexors of the ankle in normal walking on the level. *J Bone Joint Surg Am* 1966;48:66.
115. Sutherland DH, Cooper L, Daniel D. The role of ankle plantar flexors in normal walking. *J Bone Joint Surg Am* 1980;62:354.
116. Winter DA. Energy generation and absorption at the ankle and knee during fast, natural, and slow cadence. *Clin Orthop* 1983;175:147.
117. Lieber RL. *Skeletal muscle structure and function.* Baltimore: Williams & Wilkins, 1992.
118. Davis RB, DeLuca PA. Gait characterization via dynamic joint stiffness. *Gait Posture* 1996;4:224.

The Gait Cycle

119. Mann RA, Hagy J. Biomechanics of walking, running, and sprinting. *Am J Sports Med* 1980;8:345.
120. Katoh Y, Chao EYS, Laughman RK, et al. Biomechanical analysis of foot function during gait and clinical applications. *Clin Orthop* 1983;177:23.
121. Perry J. Anatomy and biomechanics of the hindfoot. *Clin Orthop* 1983;177:9.
122. Pathokinesiology Department, Physical Therapy Department. *Observational gait analysis handbook.* Downey: The Professional Staff Association of Rancho Los Amigos Medical Center, 1989.
123. Chao EY, Laughman RK, Schneider E, et al. Normative data of knee joint motion and ground reaction forces in adult level walking. *J Biomechanics* 1983;16:219.
124. Mansour JM, Audu ML. Passive elastic moment at the knee and its influence on human gait. *J Biomech* 1986;19:369.
125. Lyons K, Perry J, Gronley JK, et al. Timing and relative intensity of hip extensor and abductor muscle action during level and stair ambulation: am EMG study. *Phys Ther* 1983;63:1597.
126. Pare EB, Stern JT, Schwartz JM. Functional differentiation within the tensor fasciae latae. *J Bone Joint Surg Am* 1981;63:1457.
127. Novacheck TF. Walking, running, and sprinting: a three-dimensional analysis of kinematics and kinetics. *Instr Course Lect* 1995;44:497.

Maturation of Gait

128. Devivo DC. A clinical approach to neurologic disease. In: Rudolph A, Hoffman J, Rudolph C, eds. *Rudolph's pediatrics.* 20th ed. Norwalk: Appleton & Lange, 1996:1853.
129. Beck RJ, Andriacchi TP, Kuo KN, et al. Changes in the gait patterns of growing children. *J Bone Joint Surg* 1981;63:1452.
130. Statham L, Murray MP. Early walking patterns of normal children. *Clin Orthop* 1971;79:8.
131. Sutherland DH, Olsen R, Cooper L, et al. The development of mature gait. *J Bone Joint Surg Am* 1980;62:336.
132. Sutherland DH, Olsen RA, Biden EN, Wyatt MP. *The development of mature walking.* London: MacKeith, 1988.
133. Todd FN, Lamoreux LW, Skinner SR, et al. Variations in the gait of normal children. *J Bone Joint Surg Am* 1989;71:196.

Common Gait Deviations

134. Perry J. Pathologic gait. *Instr Course Lect* 1990:39;325.

Gait Analysis

135. Andriacchi TP, Ogle JA, Galante JO. Walking speed as a basis for normal and abnormal gait measurements. *J Biomech* 1977;10:261.
136. Waters RL, Lunsford BR, Perry J, et al. Energy-speed relation of walking: standard tables. *J Orthop Res* 1988;6:215.
137. Kadaba MP, Wooten ME, Gainey J. Repeatability of phasic muscle activity: performance of surface and intramuscular wire electrodes in gait analysis. *J Orthop Res* 1985;3:350.
138. Soames RW. Foot pressure patterns during gait. *J Biomed Eng* 1985;7:120.
139. Takegami Y. Wave pattern of ground reaction force of growing children. *J Pediatr Orthop* 1992;12:522.
140. Basmajian JV, DeLuca CJ. *Muscles alive: their functions revealed by electromyography.* 5th ed. Baltimore: Williams & Wilkins, 1985.
141. Shiavi R, Green N, McFadyen B, et al. Normative childhood EMG gait patterns. *J Orthop Res* 1987;5:283.
142. Wootten ME, Kadaba MP, Cochran GV. Dynamic electromyography. II. Normal patterns during gait. *J Orthop Res* 1990;8:259.
143. Perry J, Easterdays CS, Antonelli D. Surface versus intramuscular electrodes for electromyography of superficial and deep muscles. *Phys Ther* 1981;61:7.
144. Perry J, Ireland ML, Gronley J, et al. Predictive value of manual muscle testing and gait analysis in normal ankles by dynamic electromyography. *Foot Ankle* 1986;6:254.
145. Young CC, Rose SE, Biden EN, et al. The effect of surface and internal electrodes on the gait of children with cerebral palsy, spastic diplegic type. *J Orthop Res* 1989;7:732.
146. Butler P, Engelbrecht M, Major RE, et al. Physiological cost index of walking for normal children and its use as an indicator of physical handicap. *Dev Med Child Neurol* 1984;26:607.
147. Rose J, Gamble JG, Medeiros J, et al. Energy cost of walking in normal children and in those with cerebral palsy: comparison of heart rate and oxygen uptake. *J Pediatr Orthop* 1989;9:276.
148. Waters RL. Energy expenditure. In: Perry J, ed. *Gait analysis: normal and pathologic function.* Thorofare, NJ: Slack, 1992:443.
149. Corry IS, Duffy CM, Cosgrove AP, et al. Measurement of oxygen consumption in disabled children by the Cosmed K2 portable telemetry system. *Dev Med Child Neurol* 1996;38:585.
150. Rose J, Gamble JG, Lee J, et al. The energy expenditure index: a method to quantitate and compare walking energy expenditure for children and adolescents. *J Pediatr Orthop* 1991;11:571.
151. Bowen TR, Lennon N, Castagno P, et al. Variability of energy-

consumption measures in children with cerebral palsy. *J Pediatr Orthop* 1998;18:738.

152. Morton R. New surgical interventions for cerebral palsy and the place of gait analysis. *Dev Med Child Neurol* 1999;41: 424.

153. Scott AC, Chambers C, Cain TE. Adductor transfers in cerebral palsy: Long-term results studied by gait analysis. *J Pediatr Orthop* 1996;16:741.

154. Rose SA, DeLuca PA, Davis RB III, et al. Kinematic and kinetic evaluation of the ankle after lengthening of the gastrocnemius fascia in children with cerebral palsy. *J Pediatr Orthop* 1993; 13:727.

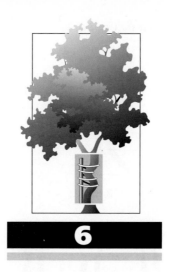

6

GENETIC ASPECTS OF ORTHOPAEDIC CONDITIONS

WILLIAM G. COLE

Many orthopaedic conditions are associated with genetic anomalies that produce congenital, developmental, metabolic, immunologic, and neoplastic disorders. Identification of the genes responsible for many of these conditions has resulted in more precise diagnoses and yielded insights into

the pathogenesis, classification, prognosis, and treatment of the disorders. Further advances are likely to influence the orthopaedic care of families with genetic disorders of the musculoskeletal system. This chapter summarizes the principles of genetics as they apply to orthopaedic conditions, and highlights the advances in knowledge in this field. The information provided, however, will need to be updated periodically, because genetic knowledge is rapidly advancing. The World Wide Web site http://www3.ncbi.nlm.nih.gov:80/Omim/ provides easy access to chronological ac-

W. G. Cole: University of Toronto; Division of Orthopaedics, The Hospital for Sick Children, Toronto, Ontario M5G 1X8, Canada.

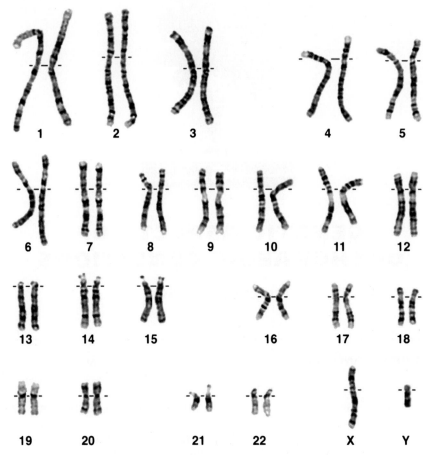

FIGURE 6-1. Normal 46,XY karyotype.

counts of advances in each genetic disorder, as well as access to specialized disease-related databases and other genetic information.

MOLECULAR BASIS OF INHERITANCE

Chromosomes

Chromosomes are rod-shaped organelles in the nucleus. The chromosomes contain genes, which are the DNA units of genetic information. They are linearly arranged along the chromosomes, and each gene occupies a particular position or locus.

The karyotype of a cell refers to its complement of chromosomes (1). Human somatic cells contain 23 pairs of chromosomes, referred to as euploidy (Fig. 6-1). Twenty-two of them are autosomes that occur in males and females. The remaining pair, the sex chromosomes, are designated XX in females and XY in males. The members of a pair of autosomes and a pair of X chromosomes contain matching genetic information.

During the metaphase of mitosis, the chromosomes consist of two chromatids joined at the centromere, which is the primary constriction of the chromosome. The centromere divides the chromosome into the short p arm and the long q arm. Cytogenetic techniques divide the arms into banded regions that are used to indicate the sites of chromosomal rearrangements and the loci of genes. For example, the *COL1A1* gene for one of the type I collagen protein chains is located on chromosome 17 at locus q21.3-22. The latter notation indicates that the gene is located on the q arm of chromosome 17 at the band 21.3-22 (Fig. 6-2).

Somatic cells divide during growth, development, and repair by the process of mitosis. The daughter cells contain the identical genetic profiles of the parent cells. Germline cells undergo meiosis during gametogenesis. In this process, the diploid number of 46 chromosomes is reduced to the haploid number of 23, including one of each of the autosomes and either an X or a Y chromosome. The random assortment of each of the chromosome pairs during meiosis is central to the mendelian inheritance pattern of single-gene disorders and some forms of chromosomal rearrangements.

Gene Structure

About 100,000 genes are present in the human genome of about 7 billion base pairs of DNA. Genes are made up of

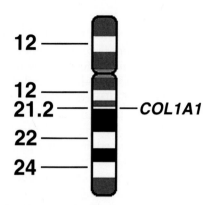

FIGURE 6-2. Diagram of chromosome 17 showing its banded structure and the location of the *COL1A1* gene encoding the pro-α1(I) chain of type I collagen.

linearly aligned nucleotides. Each unit or nucleotide of DNA consists of a deoxyribose sugar, a purine or pyrimidine base, and a phosphate group. There are two purine bases, adenine (A) and guanine (G), and two pyrimidines, thymine (T) and cytosine (C). The nucleotides form long polynucleotide chains.

DNA forms a double-stranded structure, called the double helix, in which the component polynucleotide chains run in opposite directions and contain complementary sequences. Central to the Watson and Crick model of the DNA double helix are the complementary sequences of the chains, which are held together by hydrogen bonding between complementary pairs of nucleotide bases. An A of one chain pairs with a T of the other, and a G of one chain pairs with a C of the other.

A typical gene is illustrated in Figure 6-3. The coding sequence is divided into exons that are separated by noncoding introns or intervening sequences. The exons contain codons that encode specific amino acids. Each codon contains three nucleotides. Exons often delimit functional domains within the protein. The 5′, or upstream, end of the gene contains promotor sequences that regulate the expression of the gene. The promotor immediately precedes the start site of transcription of messenger RNA (mRNA).

Transcription and RNA Processing

During transcription, an exact RNA copy of the gene, called pre-mRNA, is synthesized from the start site of transcription to the 3′ untranslated region. The pre-mRNA undergoes several modifications to form mRNA, which is transported from the nucleus to the cytoplasm and ribosomes. After the introns are spliced out, the remaining exons form a continuous coding sequence. The coding region is flanked by a 5′ untranslated region that contains sequences essential for ribosomal binding and translation. The 3′ untranslated region contains sequences that are important for mRNA stability. The polyadenylation signal contains sequences that result in the addition of a polyA nucleotide tail, a polyadenosine sequence that characterizes most mRNAs.

Translation

Translation of the DNA code, copied by the mRNA to the amino acid code of the corresponding protein, is achieved on the ribosomes. The key to the genetic code is the codon, which is a group of three bases. Because each codon contains three of the four nucleotide bases, there are 64 possible triplet combinations. In humans, there are only 20 relevant amino acids, and most of them are encoded by more than one codon. Three of the codons are called stop or nonsense codons, because they designate the site of termination of translation.

The first codon of the coding sequence of mRNA encodes the amino acid methionine. This codon establishes the translational reading frame, ensuring that the correct amino acids are added sequentially to the growing polypeptide chain. Addition of the appropriate amino acids is achieved by specific transfer RNAs (tRNAs) for each amino acid. They contain the anticodon sequences that recognize the complementary codon sequences of the mRNA. As an amino acid is added to the carboxyl end of the polypeptide

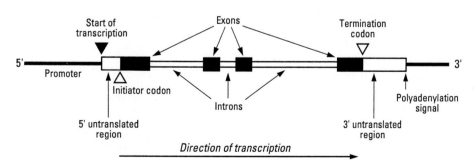

FIGURE 6-3. General structure of a typical human gene, showing the main functional domains. (From ref. 1, with permission.)

chain, the mRNA slides exactly one codon length along the ribosome, and brings the next codon into line for interaction with its specific tRNA. The proteins are synthesized from the amino terminus to the carboxyl terminus, which corresponds to translation of the mRNA from 5′ to 3′. Translation ceases at the first stop codon. The completed polypeptide is released from the ribosome.

Posttranslational Modification and Protein Assembly

Many proteins undergo numerous posttranslational modifications in the rough endoplasmic reticulum, Golgi apparatus, and outside the cell. For example, the core proteins of collagen and glycosaminoglycans undergo extensive enzymatic modification. Many proteins are produced with terminal extensions that are removed to convert the preproproteins into functional proteins. The functional proteins are assembled into complex polymers.

MOLECULAR BASIS OF MUTATIONS

A mutation is any permanent change in the sequence or arrangement of DNA. It can occur in somatic cells, as observed in many cancers, but, when it occurs in germline cells, the mutation can be transmitted to subsequent generations. Permanent changes in DNA sequences are rarely deleterious, but add to the genetic diversity among individuals. Loci that have many alternative forms, called alleles, are polymorphic.

Mutations occur on various scales, from genome mutations that involve misaggregation of chromosomes, to chromosome mutations that involve chromosome rearrangements and specific gene mutations.

Point Mutations

Point mutations are the most common mutations. These nucleotide substitutions can result in several molecular outcomes (1):

- missense mutations that alter the amino acid sequence
- nonsense mutations that introduce a premature termination codon
- alteration of promotor sequences
- mRNA splicing mutations that result in exon loss

Although point mutations are often considered to occur randomly, there are mutational hot spots in the genome, commonly at CG dinucleotides, and mutations tend to recur at such sites. Transitions, which exchange one pyrimidine for the other or one purine for the other, are more common than transversions, which exchange a purine for a pyrimidine, or vice versa. Transitions and transversions are responsible for most of the mutations of the type I collagen genes in osteogenesis imperfecta and of the type II collagen gene in the spondyloepiphyseal dysplasias.

Advanced paternal age is a frequent factor in cases of sporadic point mutations, and is referred to as the paternal age effect on new mutations (2,3). It is common in achondroplasia. Germline mosaicism for the new mutation also occurs in achondroplasia and other skeletal dysplasias. It accounts for the birth of affected siblings from clinically normal parents (4). The paternal age effect and germline mosaicism are explained by differences in gametogenesis in males and females. Spermatogonia go through a few mitotic divisions before embarking on the meiotic divisions that lead to mature sperm (5). Some of the products of the mitotic divisions are returned to the "cell bank" to replenish the supply of spermatogonia. Mutations that occur during DNA replication can accumulate, providing a basis for the paternal age effect and for germline mosaicism.

Missense Mutations

A missense mutation occurs when a single nucleotide substitution alters the sense of a codon and a different amino acid is added to the elongating polypeptide. Mutations of this kind are common in many structural proteins, such as the collagens in osteogenesis imperfecta and in some of the chondrodysplasias.

Nonsense Mutations

Nonsense mutations occur when a single nucleotide substitution converts a codon for an amino acid to a termination codon. The introduction of a termination codon into the sequence results in the premature termination of translation and a truncated protein. Such proteins are rarely functional, because they lack the carboxyl-terminal domains that are usually required for the formation of the secondary and higher orders of protein structure. The mRNAs containing a premature translational termination codon are often retained within the nucleus. Because the mutant allele is essentially functionless, it produces a state of haploid insufficiency. This type of mutation produces the common mild form of osteogenesis imperfecta.

Promotor Mutations

Point mutations within the promotor may alter the transcription of the gene. They have been identified in the β-globin gene and in the factor IX gene in hemophilia B. Few other mutations of this type have been identified in humans.

Mutations of the 3′ untranslated region may result in altered transcription or instability of mRNA, reducing the production of the relevant protein. Such mutations have been identified in the β-globin gene, but not in the genes that produce musculoskeletal diseases.

mRNA Splicing Mutations

Mutations of mRNA splicing are common in large genes that contain numerous exons and introns. Commonly, the point mutations occur in the consensus sequences at the exon–intron boundaries. The adjoining exon is usually spliced out, resulting in a shortened protein chain. If the exon normally starts and finishes with complete codons, the normal translational reading frame is retained, and the amino acid sequence is normal beyond the spliced-out exon. The resulting protein functions abnormally, because it is shorter than normal, and because it lacks the functional domain encoded by the lost exon. If the exon contains split codons at its ends, the translational reading frame beyond the spliced-out exon is abnormal and the amino acid sequence is incorrect. A frequently encountered premature translational termination codon results in the synthesis of a truncated protein.

Abnormal splicing can also occur because of point mutations that create a new or cryptic splice site. The consequences of such mutations are often complex, because splicing may remove part of an exon and include intron sequences. Lethal forms of osteogenesis imperfecta and spondyloepiphyseal dysplasia frequently result from such mutations of the type I and type II collagen genes, respectively.

Deletions and Insertions

Small and large deletions and insertions produce major changes in gene structure and in the transcript. These genetic variations result from several types of molecular alterations:

- frameshift mutations caused by incomplete codon gain or loss
- complete codon deletions or insertions
- gene deletions and duplications
- insertion of duplicated elements

A protein of abnormal length and sequence may be produced. The protein may be partially functional, as observed with the shortened forms of dystrophin produced by deletions in the *DMD* gene in patients with the Becker form of muscular dystrophy (6).

Detection of Mutations

Genetic mutations are identified by specifying the locus that is the cause of the disease, and defining the range of mutations in the disease.

Identification of the disease locus involves several approaches. In some diseases, candidate genes are selected and tested for their association with the disease. For example, the type I collagen genes were the candidate genes in osteogenesis imperfecta, because the type I collagen is found in all of the major tissues affected by the disease, and because protein anomalies were directly identified in these tissues. The candidate gene can be directly studied for mutations in affected individuals. Alternatively, linkage analysis is used to determine whether genetic markers or polymorphisms in, or flanking, the candidate gene are coinherited with the disease phenotype in families.

Knowledge concerning the disease locus is often lacking, and a list of candidate genes cannot be prepared. The chromosome, and region of the chromosome containing the disease gene, may be revealed by cytogenetic analysis. Translocations may disrupt a gene, producing the disease, and a microdeletion may indicate loss of contiguous genes. Linkage and gene-mapping studies can then focus on these regions. Similar conditions in the mouse or other species in which the disease locus has been determined can be used as a guide for analysis of the corresponding part of the human genome. However, no leads may be forthcoming, necessitating a general genome search to identify the disease gene.

The general genome studies rely on access to families, preferably of at least three generations, in which the members have been carefully evaluated for the disease. Blood is collected from each member. DNA is extracted for analysis of polymorphic DNA markers, which are distributed throughout the genome, particularly in regions containing the highest concentrations of genes. Linkage of a DNA marker to a disease locus is a statistical exercise. After a linked gene marker has been identified, additional studies are required to identify the disease locus. Candidate genes are sought in the region. Such an approach was used successfully to identify the Marfan locus, which was at the same site as the fibrillin-1 gene (7). A similar approach successfully identified the fibroblast growth factor receptor 3 (*FGFR3*) gene as the achondroplasia locus (8). However, there may not be any candidate genes known in the region of the genome linked to the disease phenotype. This problem is rapidly being overcome by the identification of known and unknown genes in the DNA sequences being generated from the Human Genome Project. Consequently, the most important aspect of mutational analysis is to identify the region of the genome containing the disease gene of interest.

Mutations can be identified in the disease gene or in its products. Protein analysis may be used to verify that an individual is affected, but it is infrequently used to define the abnormal amino acid sequence, because that is more easily deduced from the abnormal DNA sequence. A popular method of identifying mutations is to prepare mRNA from cells that express the gene. The mRNA, with its compact protein-coding sequence, is converted to complementary DNA (cDNA). The cDNA is amplified millions of times by the polymerase chain reaction (PCR), which is one of the most widely used techniques in molecular biology. The amplified PCR products are screened for mutations, such that only a portion of the cDNA needs to be sequenced.

If mRNA and cDNA are not available, genomic DNA is used for mutational analysis. It is much more difficult to localize the mutation with genomic DNA, because genes contain more noncoding than coding sequences. However,

PCR is used to amplify all exons and exon–intron boundaries for mutational screening, and for DNA sequencing of abnormal fragments.

Coinheritance of the putative gene mutation and the disease phenotype provides indirect evidence that the mutation gives rise to the disease. Direct evidence of disease causation is sought using cells that express the disease gene, such as skin fibroblasts in patients with Marfan syndrome or osteogenesis imperfecta. If the cells that normally express the disease gene, e.g., chondrocytes or osteoblasts, are not available, then the disease genes can be transfected into other types of cells. An alternative means of establishing the importance of the disease gene is to produce mice bearing a mutant disease gene (transgenic mice) or mice lacking the disease gene (knock-out mice).

CHROMOSOME DISORDERS

Chromosome disorders are more frequent than all of the single-gene disorders together (9). They occur in about 0.7% of live births, in 2% of all pregnancies of women older than 35 years of age, and in 50% of all spontaneous first-trimester abortions. They are being recognized with increasing frequency because of improvements in cytogenetic techniques. Chromosome abnormalities of number or structure can involve autosomes or sex chromosomes.

Abnormalities of Autosomal Chromosome Number

Incidence

An abnormal chromosome number, called aneuploidy, occurs in about 4% of pregnancies. Most aneuploid patients are trisomic; they have three, instead of the normal pair, of a particular chromosome. Monosomy, which is the loss of one member of a pair, occurs less commonly. The most common trisomies of an entire autosome compatible with postnatal survival are trisomy 21 (i.e., Down syndrome), trisomy 18, and trisomy 13. They all produce growth retardation, mental retardation, and multiple congenital anomalies. It is likely that the additional dosage of the specific genes on the extra chromosome is responsible for the abnormal phenotype (10).

Down Syndrome

About 1 child in 800 is born with Down syndrome, and the frequency is higher among pregnancies of mothers older than 35 years.

The specific karyotype has little effect on the phenotype, but is important for counseling. In 95% of patients, trisomy 21 results from meiotic nondisjunction of the chromosome 21 pair (Fig. 6-4). The recurrence risk increases with maternal age, particularly in women older than 30 years of age. Nondisjunction usually occurs during maternal meiosis I, and occasionally during paternal meiosis I. The cause of nondisjunction is uncertain.

About 4% of patients have 46 chromosomes, one of which is a translocation between chromosome 21q and the long arm of chromosome 14 or 22. The resulting karyotype for a robertsonian translocation between chromosome 14 and 21 is 46,XX or XY, -14, $+t(14q21q)$, with a loss of chromosome 14, designated -14, and a new hybrid 14q21q chromosome, designated $+t(14q21q)$. This karyotype produces a trisomy 21 state. The translocation forms of Down syndrome are not related to maternal age, but there is a high recurrence risk, particularly when the mother is a carrier of the translocation. A carrier involving chromosomes 14 and 21 has only 45 chromosomes, because one of each of these chromosomes is missing, and is replaced by the translocation chromosome t(14q21q). Down syndrome is produced when the fetus inherits a normal chromosome 21 from one parent and an unbalanced complement of chromosomes, including a normal chromosome 21 and the translocation chromosome, from the other parent. The unbalanced chromosome complement appears in 15% of the progeny of carrier mothers, which is less than the expected proportion, and it rarely appears in the progeny of carrier fathers.

Rarely, Down syndrome is produced by the inheritance of a translocation chromosome t(21q21q), made up of two chromosome 21 long arms from one parent and a normal chromosome 21 from the other parent. Carriers of this translocation chromosome usually only have children with Down syndrome.

About 1% of cases of Down syndrome are mosaic for the trisomy state. There is wide variability in the severity of the phenotype, probably because of the variable proportion of trisomic and euploid cells. Germline mosaicism may account for the higher-than-expected recurrence risk in young mothers.

Abnormalities of Autosomal Chromosome Structure

Structural anomalies occur less frequently than anomalies of chromosome number. They are balanced if the chromosome set has the normal complement of DNA, or unbalanced if there is additional or missing DNA.

Unbalanced rearrangements alter the amount of genetic information, and commonly produce abnormal phenotypes. Duplication of part of a chromosome produces a partial trisomy, and deletion leads to a partial monosomy. Increasingly, small deletions and insertions are detected by cytogenetic techniques. The phenotypes of some of the deletion syndromes can be readily explained by the loss of contiguous genes. For example, in the Langer-Giedion syn-

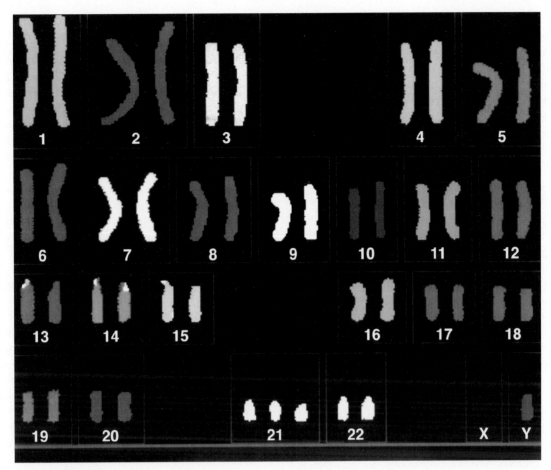

FIGURE 6-4. Karyotype in Down syndrome attributable to meiotic nondisjunction of the chromosome 21 pair. There are three copies of chromosome 21.

drome, deletion of chromosome 8q24.11–q24.13 produces mental retardation, dysmorphism, and osteochondromas. The osteochondromas occur because the deletion includes the *EXT1* locus, which is abnormal in some patients with autosomal dominant multiple exostoses.

Balanced rearrangements do not usually have a phenotypic effect, because all of the genetic information is present, although it is arranged differently. Occasionally, such rearrangements do disrupt a gene at the site of chromosome break. Balanced rearrangements increase the risk of unbalanced rearrangements in progeny.

Abnormalities of Sex Chromosomes

Sex chromosome aneuploidy produces syndromes that are associated with abnormally tall and short statures. The 47,XXY chromosome constitution, called Klinefelter syndrome, and the 47,XYY constitution produce abnormally tall stature in males. Trisomy X (47,XXX) is the female counterpart of Klinefelter syndrome, producing tall stature, and 45,X and its variants (e.g., Turner syndrome) are associated with short stature.

SINGLE-GENE DISORDERS

In contrast to the chromosomal disorders, single-gene defects are not detectable by current cytogenetic methods. Single-gene defects alter one or both copies of a gene. Alternative forms of a gene are called alleles. Many genes have only one allele, and others have many alleles that contain nonpathologic changes of DNA sequence. These loci are polymorphic. Mutant alleles contain changes in DNA sequence that can produce single-gene disorders.

The genetic constitution at one or more loci is the genotype. The detectable expression of the genotype is called the phenotype. Single-gene disorders are produced by a specific allele at a single locus of one or both members of a chromosome pair. If the alleles are identical, the individual is homozygous for that trait; if they are dissimilar, the individual is heterozygous; and if they have two different mutant alleles, the individual is a compound heterozygote. Males are hemizygous for X-linked genes, because they only have one X chromosome.

Patterns of transmission of single-gene defects are determined by pedigree analysis. They may involve genes on autosomes (i.e., autosomal inheritance) or genes on the X chromosome (i.e., X-linked inheritance) (11). The phenotypes are dominant if the disease is expressed when only one chromosome carries a mutant allele, and recessive if both chromosomes need to carry the mutant allele. For many genetic diseases, there is little detailed knowledge of the critical factors that link the genotype and the phenotype. Many other genetic and environmental factors modify the expression of the genotype; some affected individuals show minimal or no clinical anomalies, but others show severe changes.

"Penetrance" is the probability that a gene defect will have any phenotypic expression at all. In pedigrees, particularly autosomal dominant pedigrees, some affected individuals fail to express the genotype. The penetrance of a gene can be defined as the proportion of individuals with the appropriate genotype who express it.

Variable expressivity refers to different severities of the phenotype among individuals who have the same genotype. Many autosomal dominant disorders show variable expressivity. For example, patients with Marfan syndrome may have few or all of the classic features of the condition.

Another form of variable expressivity is called anticipation, which refers to the apparent worsening of the disease in successive generations. This is a feature of pedigrees of myotonic dystrophy, Huntington disease, and fragile X mental retardation, and it is caused by variable and unstable expansions of DNA. Myotonic dystrophy, for example, is caused by the unstable expansion of a CTG trinucleotide repeat located in the 3′ untranslated region of a gene on chromosome 19 that encodes a protein kinase (12).

Variable expressivity can also be a function of the age of onset of the phenotype. Some single-gene disorders, such as achondroplasia, are evident at birth, and are therefore congenital. Others, such as pseudoachondroplasia, are not apparent at birth, but become so after the patient is 2 to 3 years of age, when growth retardation and dysmorphism appear.

Many single-gene defects give rise to the diverse phenotypic effects referred to as pleiotropy. For many diseases, there is no obvious causative link between their diverse manifestations. It is likely, however, that links will be established as more knowledge is obtained about the molecular pathology of the single-gene disorders. For example, the pleiotropic musculoskeletal, ocular, and cardiovascular manifestations of Marfan syndrome are causally linked by fibrillin-1, the microfibrillar protein at fault in this syndrome, which is distributed throughout all of the affected tissues (7).

In contrast to the considerable heterogeneity that exists in the phenotypic expression within and between the single-gene disorders, the underlying molecular changes in their mutant loci are similar, reflecting the limited number of ways in which a single gene can be altered.

Autosomal Dominant Disorders

About half of the known single-gene defects are autosomal dominant traits. Affected individuals are heterozygous for the mutation; they have one normal and one mutant allele of the gene. However, the product of the normal allele is unable to compensate for the abnormality produced by the mutant allele. Matings of two heterozygous individuals can produce homozygous autosomal dominant traits. The homozygotes are usually much more severely affected, often with perinatal death, than heterozygotes.

Many autosomal dominant disorders have major musculoskeletal anomalies. They include many of the chondrodysplasias, osteogenesis imperfecta, Marfan syndrome, Ehlers-Danlos syndrome, acrocephalosyndactyly syndromes, absent tibial syndromes, Charcot-Marie-Tooth disease types IA and IB, and neurofibromatosis 1.

In typical families, the autosomal dominant trait is transmitted from generation to generation by affected individuals who transmit the mutant gene to about half of their offspring (Fig. 6-5). Males and females are equally affected, and unaffected individuals do not carry or transmit the mutant gene. Typical multigeneration autosomal dominant pedigrees (Fig. 6-5) are common in families with neurofibromatosis, osteogenesis imperfecta type I, and Marfan syndrome. However, there is wide variability of penetrance and expression of the genotype in such families. For example, in families with the common type I form of osteogenesis imperfecta, some members have gray-blue scleras and severe osteoporosis with multiple fractures, whereas others have gray-blue scleras, a characteristic feature of the disease, without clinical evidence of bone fragility. Similar variability is observed in families with neurofibromatosis 1 and Marfan syndrome, when the clinical manifestations are correlated with the inheritance of the mutant allele. Many of the individuals shown to carry the mutant allele lack the major

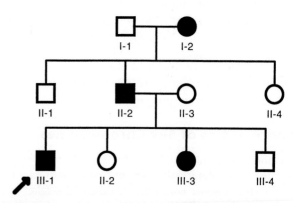

FIGURE 6-5. Typical autosomal dominant pedigree. Each individual is identified by a generation number and the position within each generation. Males are indicated by *squares* and females by *circles. Filled symbols* indicate clinically affected individuals. The proband (*arrow*) is the family member through whom the family history was ascertained.

clinical features required for a firm clinical diagnosis, and are unaware that they have the disease. The latter observation applies particularly to young people, who are likely to develop more obvious features with age.

Atypical autosomal dominant pedigrees occur with new dominant mutations. About half of the individuals with osteogenesis imperfecta or Marfan syndrome, and most individuals with achondroplasia, have new autosomal dominant mutations. The mutation occurs in the ovum, or in the sperm involved in the formation of the fertilized ovum, for the first affected individual in the family. New dominant mutations are often associated with increased paternal age, presumably as a result of an increased level of mutagenesis during spermatogenesis in older men. The affected individuals transmit the trait to half of their offspring, which is typical of an autosomal dominant inheritance pattern.

Some families with osteogenesis imperfecta and Marfan syndrome show an apparently autosomal recessive form of inheritance, with clinically normal parents and multiple affected offspring. In most instances, genetic testing has shown that one parent is mosaic for the dominant mutation, and transmits the trait to multiple children. Presumably, a spontaneous mutation occurs early in the embryogenesis of the mosaic parent, and some of the somatic cells and gametes carry the mutation. Mosaic parents may show some minor clinical features of the disease. Genetic testing of dermal fibroblasts, hair follicles, and leukocytes reveals the proportion of cells carrying the mutant allele. The sperm can be similarly tested. Rapid progress is being made in identifying mutant genes in autosomal dominant disorders that produce musculoskeletal anomalies. Several disorders illustrate important principles, and are discussed in the following sections.

Osteogenesis Imperfecta

Many of the principal features of autosomal dominant diseases are illustrated by recent findings in osteogenesis imperfecta. The majority of cases are inherited as autosomal dominant traits, or occur from new autosomal dominant mutations. The mutations usually involve one of the two genes that encode the chains of type I collagen, the principal collagen of the tissues affected by the disease. The *COL1A1* gene on chromosome 17 encodes the pro-α1(I) chain, and the *COL1A2* gene on chromosome 7 encodes the pro-α2(I) chain. Each type I collagen molecule contains two α1(I) chains and one α2(I) chain.

Although osteogenesis imperfecta is clinically and genetically heterogeneous, the genetic patterns are relatively simple (13,14). The common type IA form, with gray-blue scleras, osteoporosis, mild bone fragility, normal teeth, ligament laxity, and premature deafness, is caused by mutations of the *COL1A1* gene, in which the mutant allele is functionless. The mutant allele usually produces an mRNA containing a premature stop codon that would be expected to pro-

duce a truncated and functionless α1(I) collagen chain. However, the nucleus retains most of the mutant mRNA, and the cytoplasm contains predominantly normal α1(I) mRNA, although in half of the normal amounts. The type I collagen produced by the osteogenesis imperfecta type IA cells is normal, but the amount produced is about half of the normal amount. Each family has been shown to have its own private mutation, leading to premature stop codons at different sites of the mRNA. Despite this genetic heterogeneity, there is a final common pathway of type I collagen deficiency that accounts for this type of osteogenesis imperfecta. Nonetheless, because the severity of the disease varies between and within families, it is likely that modifying genes and epigenetic factors also play a role in the pathogenesis of the disease.

The more severe forms of osteogenesis imperfecta are usually caused by autosomal dominant mutations of the *COL1A1* or *COL1A2* gene, which result in the production of a mixture of normal and mutant collagen chains and type I collagen molecules. A registry of type I collagen mutations is available at http://www.le.ac.uk/genetics/collagen/. The most common mutation involves the substitution of a glycine residue in one of the 338 glycine-X-Y triplets, the mandatory repetitive triplet sequence required for triple helix formation. Proline is often in the X position and hydroxyproline in the Y position of the triplets. Abnormal helix formation occurs after substitution of glycine, the smallest amino acid, with the larger amino acids, alanine, valine, cysteine, arginine, aspartic acid, and glutamic acid. Collagen α chains carrying these substitutions are able to combine with normal chains to produce type I collagen molecules. In cases of *COL1A1* mutations, half of the α1(I) chains are expected to be mutant and half are expected to be normal. Because type I collagen molecules contain two α1(I) chains, it is expected that about 25% of the molecules will be normal and 75% will contain one or two mutant α1(I) chains. The particular α1(I) chain composition of the type I collagen molecules enhances the impact of the heterozygous *COL1A1* mutation.

Similarly, with *COL1A2* mutations, about half of the α2(I) chains will be normal and half will be mutant. Because type I collagen molecules contain only one α2(I) chain, about half of the molecules will be normal and half will contain the mutant α2(I) chain. The mutant molecules, whether containing the mutant α1(I) or α2(I) chain, are more susceptible to degradation and are poorly secreted. Once secreted, they interfere with the formation of the extracellular matrix of bone and other type I collagen-containing tissues. These mutations act in a dominant-negative fashion, because the mutant collagen chains impair the function of the normal α chains.

Most affected families also have their own private mutations, as shown for the perinatal lethal forms of osteogenesis. There are a few examples of unrelated families with the same mutation. Variability in the severity of the disease has also been observed in such families, indicating that modifying genes and epigenetic factors contribute to the pathogenesis of the dominant negative forms of osteogenesis imperfecta.

Little is known about the factors that are important in determining the clinical severity of the disease resulting from dominant negative mutations of the type I collagen genes. However, most of the perinatal lethal cases result from mutations that involve the carboxyl-terminal half of the collagen chains. Substitutions of glycine by cysteine yield a gradient of severity, with lethal cases at the carboxyl terminus, moderately severe cases in the middle, and milder cases at the amino terminus of the α chains.

Mosaic cases giving rise to an apparently autosomal recessive form of inheritance are common. As a result, the empiric risk of recurrence in a family with a sporadic form of osteogenesis imperfecta is about 6%. The risk can be better assessed by genetic testing of the parents, but it is still only a rough estimate, because the proportion of affected gametes is usually unknown. Intrauterine DNA testing for osteogenesis imperfecta is available at specialized centers.

Spondyloepiphyseal Dysplasia

The chondrodysplasias are a diverse group of genetically determined diseases that affect the structure and function of cartilage. Spranger grouped the disorders with similar features into families (15). One family consists of a heterogeneous group of spondyloepiphyseal dysplasias. The severity of these disorders varies markedly among the lethal forms of achondrogenesis type II and hypochondrogenesis, the severely dwarfing forms of spondyloepiphyseal dysplasia congenita and Kniest syndrome, the marfanoid form of Stickler syndrome or hereditary arthroophthalmopathy, and mild forms with premature osteoarthritis. Heterozygous mutations of type II collagen, the principal collagen of cartilage, or type XI collagen, a minor collagen of cartilage, are found in this family of spondyloepiphyseal dysplasias. The general categories of mutations found in osteogenesis imperfecta are also found in this family of dysplasias.

Some patients with Stickler syndrome have null mutations of the *COL2A1* gene on chromosome 12 that encode the pro-α1(II) chains of type II procollagen (16). The types of *COL2A1* mutations observed in these patients are similar to those found in the *COL1A1* gene in patients with osteogenesis imperfecta type IA. In both of these diseases, the mutant alleles of the respective genes are functionless and lead to the production of normal collagen, although in about half of the normal amounts. Other individuals with Stickler syndrome have mutations of the *COL11A1* gene on chromosome 1p21, which encodes the α1(XI) chain, or of the *COL11A2* gene on chromosome 6p21.3, which encodes the α2(XI) chain of type XI collagen.

The other members of this family of spondyloepiphyseal dysplasias are caused by heterozygous mutations that alter the structure of the triple helical domain of type II collagen (14,16). Unlike the marfanoid habitus of individuals with Stickler syndrome, these individuals are often severely dwarfed. The dominant negative effects of the mutations are severe, because type II collagen molecules contain three α1(II) chains. About 12.5% of the molecules contain three normal chains, and 87.5% of them contain one, two, or three mutant chains. As in osteogenesis imperfecta, the mutant molecules are poorly secreted, are more susceptible to degradation, and impair normal formation of the extracellular matrix.

Achondroplasia

Achondroplasia is the most common form of short-limb dwarfism. It is inherited as an autosomal dominant trait with complete penetrance. About 87% of cases are caused by new mutations. There is a considerable reduction in the effective reproductive fitness of patients with achondroplasia.

Patients with achondroplasia have less phenotypic heterogeneity than occurs in other skeletal dysplasias, such as osteogenesis imperfecta and the type II collagen family of spondyloepiphyseal dysplasias. The clinical and radiographic features are remarkably constant, and the growth plates are histologically normal, despite the severe retardation of longitudinal growth. The similarity of phenotype between unrelated patients can be explained by the molecular defects in achondroplasia.

The gene for achondroplasia was assigned to chromosome 4 at locus p16.3 by linkage analysis, and mutations were identified in the gene for fibroblast growth factor receptor 3 (*FGFR3*) (7,17–19). Transcripts of this gene are most abundant in the nervous system, and may account for the megaloencephaly of some patients. Outside the nervous system, the highest levels are found in the cartilage anlage of all bones and in the resting chondrocytes of the growth plates (20). All patients have missense mutations that change glycine residue 380 to arginine, or, less often, that change a nearby amino acid residue (17,21). The codon for amino acid residue 380 includes a CG dinucleotide, which is a "hot spot" for mutations. These mutations are expected to alter the structure of the transmembrane domain of the receptor, and to produce similar functional abnormalities, accounting for the relatively invariant phenotype of achondroplasia.

Hypochondroplasia, which has a milder phenotype than achondroplasia, is caused by mutations of other regions of the *FGFR3* gene. Thanatophoric dwarfism, a lethal chondrodysplasia that shares some phenotypic features with achondroplasia, is also caused by mutations of *FGFR3* (22).

Homozygous achondroplasia, which arises from achondroplasia matings, is extremely severe and often lethal. The same mutations as those observed in heterozygous cases of achondroplasia have been detected in homozygous achondroplasia.

Neurofibromatosis 1

Also known as von Recklinghausen disease, neurofibromatosis 1 shows complete penetrance in that all individuals who carry the mutation express the mutation. However, expression is highly variable, and some individuals within affected families have extremely severe disease and others may have café-au-lait spots as their only manifestation of neurofibromatosis 1.

The gene responsible for this disease, *NF1*, is located on chromosome 17 at locus q11.2 (23). It is a very large gene that encodes a protein called neurofibromin. It is a guanine triphosphatase-activating protein that acts as a tumor-suppressor gene (24,25). The protein is most abundant in the nervous system.

The mutations of *NF1* include deletions, insertions, missense mutations, and nonsense mutations (26). About 80% of these mutations potentially encode a truncated protein because of premature termination of translation. The disease expression is probably the result of haploid insufficiency, because the truncated proteins are likely to be functionless. The normal allele produces a reduced amount of normal neurofibromin that is insufficient for normal development and function of the tissues that express the *NF1* gene.

Patients with affected mothers often have more severe disease than patients with affected fathers (27). This phenomenon probably reflects genomic imprinting, which is a poorly understood process that alters the relative expression of the paternally and maternally derived genes.

In a few cases, the mutation is transmitted from a clinically unaffected father in whom some of the sperm contains a mutant *NF1* allele. This process is an example of gonadal or germline mosaicism.

In about 50% of patients, the disease arises from a new mutation that is not inherited from either parent. The spontaneous mutation rate is about 1 in 10,000 gametes, which is one of the highest levels in humans. This high rate presumably reflects the large size of the gene and its resulting susceptibility to deletions, insertions, point mutations, and major rearrangements. In most cases, the new mutation occurs in the paternally derived gene. This finding suggests that the mutation may occur during mitotic division, which takes place in male gametogenesis but not in female gametogenesis. Because there is little or no evidence of the accumulation of mutations, reflected by the absence of a paternal age effect, the mutations may accumulate in cells that are not involved in the process of replenishment of the germ cell bank.

In neurofibromatosis 1, malignant tumors are homozygous for *NF1* gene anomalies, and benign tumors are still heterozygous for *NF1* anomalies. The malignant process arises by somatic mutation of the normal *NF1* allele, and

results in homozygous loss of the tumor-suppressor activity of the gene (24,28).

Autosomal Recessive Disorders

Autosomal recessive disorders account for about one-third of the single-gene defects (1). Affected individuals are homozygous, having inherited a mutant allele from each parent (Fig. 6-6). The clinically normal parents are heterozygotes, also called carriers. Carrier frequency varies considerably, but, for common autosomal recessive disorders such as cystic fibrosis, it affects about 1 in 45 individuals. The mutant alleles in a population occur much more frequently in carriers than in affected individuals. For example, about 98% of the cystic fibrosis alleles are present in asymptomatic carriers, and only 2% are present in homozygous patients.

Males and females are equally likely to be affected. Autosomal recessive traits are more frequent in consanguineous marriages, particularly if the mutant gene is rare.

Many autosomal recessive diseases produce inborn errors of metabolism, a term introduced by Garrod (29). They result from deficiencies of specific enzymes that lead to a block in a normal metabolic pathway, with accumulation of the substrate and a deficiency of the product. Because most enzymes are normally present in vast excess, a major reduction in their activity is required before a metabolic pathway is blocked. As a result, carriers rarely express inborn errors of metabolism, because the activity of the enzyme produced by the normal allele is sufficient to ensure normal metabolic activity. In the homozygous state, the activity of the specific enzyme is often reduced to about 5% or less of normal values. Reductions of this magnitude are usually required before a metabolic pathway is blocked.

The consequences of an enzyme deficiency result from the accumulation of its substrate, the deficiency of its product, or both. Substrates may be readily diffusible, and are found in excessive amounts in all body fluids and in all

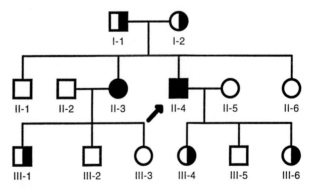

FIGURE 6-6. Typical autosomal recessive pedigree. Homozygous affected individuals are indicated by *filled symbols.* Asymptomatic carriers, who are heterozygotes, are indicated by *half-filled symbols.* The proband is indicated by the *arrow.*

tissues. An example is phenylalanine, which accumulates in phenylketonuria, the classic example of an autosomal recessive disease. In diseases of this kind, the widespread accumulation of the substrate may result in pathologic changes in tissues that are not normally involved in the particular metabolic pathway. Damage to the developing nervous system in phenylketonuria results from this mechanism. Most of the inborn errors of amino acid metabolism produce types of changes similar to those observed in phenylketonuria. Homocystinuria is one of the few inborn errors of amino acid metabolism that produces musculoskeletal anomalies. Affected individuals have a marfanoid appearance.

Nondiffusible substrates accumulate within the cells that are normally involved in the metabolic process. Cell function deteriorates, eventually producing cell death, as the substrate progressively accumulates intracellularly. Diseases caused by this abnormality are often referred to as storage diseases, because the affected tissues progressively enlarge. Typical examples include lysosomal storage diseases, such as Gaucher disease, and the mucopolysaccharidoses. The lysosomal enzymes are responsible for the degradation of macromolecules, such as the mucopolysaccharides of the extracellular matrix. Deficiencies of the lysosomal enzymes involved in the degradative cascade of the mucopolysaccharides produce a heterogeneous group of diseases, some of which manifest severe skeletal anomalies. This group includes Hurler, Scheie, Sanfilippo A to D, Morquio A and B, Maroteaux-Lamy, and Sly syndromes.

Similar clinical phenotypes, such as Sanfilippo A to D syndromes, can occur with different enzyme deficiencies, a phenomenon referred to as "locus heterogeneity." Partial and complete deficiencies of the enzymes can also alter the severity of the phenotype, which is referred to as "clinical heterogeneity." These syndromes may also show wide variation in clinical severity as a result of allelic heterogeneity, in which different defects occur in the same gene.

The clinical manifestations of some enzyme deficiencies are caused by a deficiency of the normal product, rather than an accumulation of the substrate. For example, some forms of congenital hypothyroidism result from enzyme defects in the synthesis of thyroxine.

Autosomal recessive diseases are also produced by other mechanisms, including defects in receptor proteins, membrane transport, and cell organelles. Cystic fibrosis is caused by mutations of a protein called cystic fibrosis transmembrane conductance regulator. Disorders of peroxisomes, which are subcellular organelles, produce a variety of diseases, including rhizomelic chondrodysplasia punctata.

X-linked Disorders

X-linked disorders are readily identified by their characteristic patterns of inheritance (Fig. 6-7). Males are unaffected or affected, because they have only one X chromosome, and

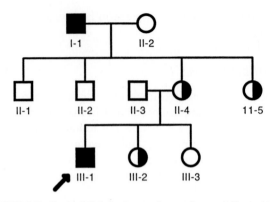

FIGURE 6-7. Typical X-linked recessive pedigree. Affected hemizygous males are indicated by *filled squares*. Asymptomatic carrier females are indicated by *half-filled circles*.

are therefore hemizygous for X-linked genes. Females are homozygous unaffected, homozygous affected, or heterozygous, because they have a pair of X chromosomes.

Heterozygous females show variable expression of X-linked disorders, because of the normal random inactivation of one of the X chromosomes in their somatic cells. The random inactivation of the X chromosome is called the Lyon hypothesis, which accounts for the similar levels of expression of one allele in males and a pair of alleles in females. This process is also referred to as "dosage compensation"; the level of expression of one dose of an X-linked gene in a male is equivalent to that of two doses of an X-linked gene in a female.

At the 16- to 64-cell stage of embryogenesis, random inactivation of the paternal or maternal X chromosome occurs in each somatic cell. The descendants of each cell have the same inactive X chromosome. As a result, the somatic cells of females are mosaic, with some cells expressing one X chromosome and the remainder expressing the other. The inactive X chromosome is condensed, and, with the exception of the pseudoautosomal region, its genes are not expressed. Because heterozygous females have various proportions of cells expressing either X-linked allele, there is marked variability in the expression and clinical phenotypes. Some females appear normal, whereas others, referred to as manifesting heterozygotes, have the typical phenotype displayed by hemizygous males.

X-linked disorders are classified as dominant, recessive, and atypical forms of inheritance.

X-linked Dominant Disorders

Classification and Incidence. An X-linked phenotype is classified as dominant if it is expressed in heterozygous females. A characteristic feature of such pedigrees is that all of the daughters and none of the sons of affected males are affected. The affected females transmit the mutation in a manner similar to an autosomal dominant trait, because they have a pair of X chromosomes. As a result, affected females transmit the mutation to half of their children, regardless of gender. Affected females are usually less severely affected than affected males, because of random inactivation of one of the X chromosomes. The expression depends on the proportion of cells that express the normal or mutant allele.

Typical X-linked dominant disorders with musculoskeletal manifestations include X-linked hypophosphatemic rickets and Rett's syndrome. Rett's syndrome is lethal in males at birth, but heterozygous affected females are severely mentally retarded.

Hypophosphatemic Rickets. This disorder is also called vitamin D-resistant rickets. It resembles metaphyseal chondrodysplasia-type Schmid, which results from mutations of type X collagen. This collagen is specific to the hypertrophic zone of the growth plate. These disorders are differentiated by the low serum inorganic phosphorus levels in children with hypophosphatemic rickets.

The males always express the disease, because they are hemizygous, with only one X chromosome. Variable expression occurs in heterozygous females, because of random inactivation of the paternal and maternal X chromosomes (30). Mutations of the *PHEX* gene (phosphate-regulating gene with homologies to endopeptidases on the X chromosome) cause the disease.

X-linked Recessive Disorders

Classification and Incidence. An X-linked phenotype is classified as recessive if it is expressed in all males, but only in homozygous females. The latter situation is rare, because expression in females is usually limited to the manifesting heterozygotes in whom the normal X chromosome has by chance been inactivated in most somatic cells.

The X-linked gene causing the disorder is transmitted from an affected male through all his daughters. Consequently, a daughter's sons have a 50% chance of inheriting the gene. Males do not transmit the gene directly to their sons.

Typical X-linked recessive disorders include hemophilia A, which produces a deficiency of factor VIII, and Duchenne muscular dystrophy, which produces a deficiency of dystrophin.

Duchenne Muscular Dystrophy. In males, this X-linked recessive disorder is lethal in the late teenage years. It is caused by mutations of the large *DMD* gene that encodes the protein dystrophin, a normal component of the muscle membrane. About one-third of cases are new mutations, and the remainder are inherited from carrier females. Most of the mutations are deletions (6). Affected males infrequently reproduce, and the disease is transmitted by carrier females who are usually clinically unaffected. Some muta-

tions produce Becker muscular dystrophy, which has a milder phenotype.

Atypical X-linked Disorders

Classification. The inheritance pattern of an X-linked disorder may not fall into the typical dominant or recessive pattern. Fragile X syndrome is an example of a disorder with an atypical X-linked inheritance pattern.

Fragile X Syndrome. After Down syndrome, fragile X syndrome is the most common cause of mental retardation in males. Females can be affected, although the phenotype is usually milder, and is characterized by learning disabilities or mild mental retardation. Postpubertal males have a marfanoid appearance, macroorchidism, and mental retardation. They also have lax joints, resembling milder forms of Ehlers-Danlos syndrome.

The name for fragile X syndrome came from a characteristic cytogenetic anomaly. The chromatin in the fragile site at position Xq27.3 fails to condense during mitosis. The molecular defect is attributable to an amplification of a region containing a variable CGG trinucleotide repeat in the 5′ untranslated region of the *FMR1* gene (31). Expression of the *FMR1* gene is deficient in affected males, although normal individuals, carrier females, and males with the premutation all show normal expression (32). Allele sizes vary from 6 to 54 repeats in normal individuals, from 52 to 200 repeats in individuals with premutations, and from 200 to more than 1000 repeats in affected individuals (31). Expansion of premutations to full mutations occurs only after passage through the female germline. Males can pass on the premutation for this condition to their daughters, but it is only after female gametogenesis that sufficient trinucleotide expansion occurs to silence the *FMR1* gene, and give rise to the clinical manifestations found in grandsons of the premutation males (33).

Huntington disease and myotonic dystrophy are caused by unstable expansion of trinucleotide repeats in other genes. They, like fragile X syndrome, also have a parental sex bias in the transmission of the mutation, with respect to the age of onset or clinical expression (34).

Other Patterns of Single-gene Inheritance

Most single-gene disorders are inherited in accordance with mendelian principles. However, alternative modes of inheritance have been identified in humans. For example, some neuromuscular and ocular diseases are caused by mutations of mitochondrial, rather than nuclear, DNA. They are inherited from the mother, because mitochondria are transmitted in the ovum, but not in sperm. As a result, women transmit their mitochondrial DNA to all of their children, but men do not transmit their mitochondrial DNA to any of their children.

Other patterns include mosaicism, genomic imprinting, and uniparental disomy.

Mosaicism

All somatic cells are usually considered to contain identical nuclear DNA derived from a single zygote. However, mutations can produce cell clones that are genetically different from the original zygote (34). Such individuals are said to be mosaic. Mosaicism can be somatic, gonadal, or both.

Somatic Mosaicism. Mutations that occur early in embryogenesis may produce somatic and gonadal mosaicism; later in embryogenesis or in postnatal life, mutations are limited to producing somatic mosaicism. Some unusual clinical manifestations and inheritance patterns have been observed. Asymmetrical Marfan syndrome affects one side of the body, and segmental neurofibromatosis 1 affects one segment of the body. These mutations appear to arise early in embryogenesis, and produce somatic and gonadal mosaicism, with transmission of the typical disease to offspring. Many mutations, however, occur later in embryogenesis and are limited to somatic cells.

McCune-Albright Syndrome. This syndrome is a sporadic disease that produces polyostotic fibrous dysplasia, café-au-lait spots, sexual precocity, and other dysfunctional endocrinopathies. Activating missense mutations in the gene for the α-subunit of Gs, the G protein that stimulates cyclic adenosine monophosphate formation, have been identified in these patients (35). The mutations are found in variable abundance in different affected endocrine and nonendocrine cells, including osteoblast precursors, consistent with the mosaic distribution of abnormal cells generated by somatic cell mutation early in embryogenesis. However, because the mutations are not transmitted to offspring, presumably they occur after cells are committed to form gametes.

Other examples of sporadic segmental and symmetrical disorders that probably arise by a similar mechanism of somatic mosaicism include Proteus syndrome, other hemihypertrophy and local gigantism syndromes, and Ollier disease.

Malignant Tumors. Somatic mosaicism also plays a major role in the cascade of genetic events leading to the development of malignant neoplasms (36,37). Using retinoblastoma, which can be associated with osteosarcomas, as a model, the inherited types can be explained by a germline mutation of the *RB1* gene, followed by a somatic mutation of the remaining normal allele in a given cell. In the sporadic form, the two mutations are somatic in origin, affecting both copies of the normal allele of the *RB1* gene in the same cells. A similar mechanism applies to the development of

malignant tumors in individuals with neurofibromatosis 1. However, more complex arrangements occur, with combinations of somatic mutations and chromosomal rearrangements. The chromosomal rearrangements in tumors, such as the t(11;12)(q24;q12) translocation in Ewing sarcoma, alter the structure or regulation of cellular oncogenes or tumor-suppressor genes (37). Mutations involving the tumor-suppressor gene *P53* are common in many malignant tumors.

Germline Mosaicism. Germline mosaicism has been observed in autosomal dominant diseases, such as osteogenesis imperfecta and Marfan syndrome, and in X-linked disorders. In affected families, multiple affected children can be shown by genetic testing to be heterozygous for the mutation, although the parents are clinically normal. Such pedigrees were previously considered to show autosomal recessive inheritance of the trait, with the resulting prediction that 25% of offspring would be homozygous for the mutation, and clinically affected. The predicted recurrence risk may be greater, depending on the proportion of germline cells that contain the mutant gene. If there is only one affected child, the prediction of recurrence risk is difficult. If neither parent is mosaic for the mutation, the recurrence risk is equal to the spontaneous occurrence rate of the disease in that ethnic group, which is usually low. However, the recurrence rate is significantly higher if either parent has germline mosaicism. In the absence of genetic testing of germline cells, the empiric recurrence risk of autosomal dominant or X-linked disorders for phenotypically normal parents, is about 6%. The affected heterozygous children will transmit the mutation to half of their offspring.

Genomic Imprinting

Genomic imprinting refers to the concept that certain genes are marked, or imprinted, in such a way that they are expressed differently when they are inherited from the mother than when they are inherited from the father (34). The process of imprinting often involves differences in DNA methylation that alter the transcriptional regulation of the paternally derived and the maternally derived genes.

Genomic imprinting is an important process in many human diseases, including familial cancers, chromosomal deletion syndromes, and single-gene disorders such as retinoblastoma, neurofibromatosis 1, Beckwith-Wiedemann syndrome, Huntington disease, and myotonic dystrophy. More severe forms of myotonic dystrophy and neurofibromatosis 1 occur when the mutant gene is inherited from the mother. More severe forms of Huntington disease and autosomal dominant spinocerebellar ataxia occur when the mutant gene is inherited from the father.

Beckwith-Wiedemann syndrome is a generalized overgrowth syndrome. Hemihypertrophy, Wilms tumors, and other tumors are common in affected individuals. Cytogenetic duplication of band p15 of chromosome 11 occurs in these patients, and it is paternal in origin (38). There is increased expression of the insulin-like growth factor type 2 gene (*IGF2*), which maps to this band. The maternal *IGF2* allele is normally repressed, but is activated in some maternally inherited forms of the syndrome. These women carry chromosomal rearrangements involving chromosome 11 at locus p15, which appear to activate the *IGF2* gene. The syndrome results from increased expression of *IGF2* by paternal duplication or maternal activation of the gene.

The chromosome deletion disorders, Prader-Willi and Angelman syndromes, highlight further the importance of genomic imprinting and the parental origin of genetic material (34,36). Prader-Willi syndrome produces hypotonia, obesity with hyperphagia, hypogonadism, mental retardation, short stature, and small hands and feet. Angelman syndrome is clinically distinct. Affected individuals have a happy disposition, mental retardation, repetitive ataxic movements, abnormal facies with a large mouth and protruding tongue, and an unusual type of seizure. Despite their clinical dissimilarity, these syndromes share the same cytogenetic deletion of chromosome 15 (15q11q13). In Prader-Willi syndrome, the deletion is inherited from the father, and in Angelman syndrome, it is inherited from the mother.

Uniparental Disomy

Individuals with uniparental disomy have cells that contain two chromosomes of a particular type that have been inherited from only one parent (34,36). Isodisomy exists when one chromosome is duplicated, and heterodisomy exists when both homologs have been inherited from one parent. Examples include patients with Prader-Willi syndrome lacking cytogenetic anomalies, in whom both copies of chromosome 15 had been inherited from the mother. Conversely, some cases of Angelman syndrome lacking cytogenetic anomalies result from the inheritance of both copies of chromosome 15 from the father. Some of these individuals carry two identical copies of the same chromosome 15, and have uniparental isodisomy, and others carry two different copies of chromosome 15 from one parent and have uniparental heterodisomy. These findings suggest that the lack of the q11-13 region of the paternal chromosome 15 leads to Prader-Willi syndrome, and that the lack of the equivalent region of the maternal chromosome 15 produces Angelman syndrome. These observations also indicate that both parental chromosome contributions serve necessary and complementary functions in normal growth and development.

Uniparental disomy has been observed in a few patients with cystic fibrosis who had unexplained short stature at birth. It is unclear whether there is a higher frequency of uniparental disomy in patients with intrauterine growth retardation syndromes, such as Russell-Silver syndrome, which is also associated with limb-length discrepancy.

Uniparental disomy can involve the X and Y chromosomes. For example, a boy with hemophilia A inherited both sex chromosomes from his father, with no contribution of sex chromosomes from his mother. Although such events occur rarely, they add to the difficulties of predicting recurrence risks.

MULTIFACTORIAL DISORDERS

Many diseases of orthopaedic importance show multifactorial inheritance (39). Neural tube defects, congenital talipes equinovarus, and developmental dislocation of the hip are examples of multifactorial disorders that involve a combination of multiple genetic and environmental factors. Little is known about the genetic or environmental factors involved in the pathogenesis of clubfeet or developmental dislocation of the hip. However, folic acid intake during pregnancy appears to be an important nutritional factor in the pathogenesis of neural tube defects.

Many of the multifactorial disorders behave as multifactorial threshold traits (39). There appears to be an underlying continuous variation in liability to each multifactorial disease that has to exceed a threshold before the abnormal phenotype appears.

Several additional principles have emerged from studies of the multifactorial inheritance of diseases (1). The disorders are familial, but do not show the inheritance patterns typical of single-gene defect disorders. The risk to first-degree relatives is about the square root of the population risk, but the risk is much lower for second-degree relatives. For example, the risk of congenital talipes equinovarus in the general population is about 0.001, but it is 25 times higher in first-degree relatives, only 5 times higher in second-degree relatives, and only twice as common in third-degree relatives. If the disorder is more common in one sex, the recurrence risk is higher for relatives of the less susceptible sex. The recurrence risk is higher when there is more than one affected family member, and when the malformation is more severe. The recurrence risk is also increased when the parents are consanguineous.

Genetic counseling about multifactorial disorders involves the provision of empiric risk, which is the recurrence risk observed in similar families. It may not be accurate for a given family. Progress in defining the genes at fault can be expected to improve the risk estimates. Preventative measures, such as taking folic acid during the periconception period, may diminish the risk of neural tube defects. The pregnancy can also be monitored using α-fetoprotein levels in maternal serum and amniotic fluid, and by ultrasonography of the fetus.

TERATOLOGIC DISORDERS

Principles of Teratology

The effects of known teratogens on the fetus are determined by the timing of exposure and dosage (40,41). During blastocyst formation, teratogens usually result in fetal death and spontaneous abortion. During the period of organogenesis, 18 to 60 days after conception, the fetus is most vulnerable to the effects of teratogens. Easily recognizable structural defects are the usual result. Later in pregnancy, teratogens may produce no anomaly or subtle changes.

Most teratogens act by interfering with metabolic processes. They may act on cell membranes or the metabolic machinery of cells. The final common pathway of these various levels of action is cell death or a failure of replication, migration, or fusion of cells. These changes often involve specific organs, but can produce more general changes in the fetus.

Exposure of the father to teratogens does not appear to play a significant role in the development of birth defects. Most agents that interfere with the DNA of sperm produce sterility, rather than teratogenic effects in the fetus.

Current methods for detecting potential teratogens are inadequate. Interspecies differences in sensitivity are common. For example, thalidomide is teratogenic in rabbits, but not in rats and mice. Many agents known to be teratogenic in animals, such as glucocorticoids in rats, do not produce any detectable anomalies in humans.

Most known teratogenic agents in humans have been identified from clinical observations of unexpected outbreaks of malformations. In most instances, however, unexpected clusters of cases result from natural fluctuations in the frequency of specific birth defects, as shown by birth defect registers. Epidemiologists associated with birth defects registers play an important role in assessing whether apparent outbreaks are potentially important.

Teratogenic Agents

The selected items in the following list are teratogenic agents in humans (41):

drugs and environmental chemicals
androgens
aminopterin
chlorobiphenyls
Warfarin (Coumadin)
cyclophosphamide
diethylstilbestrol
D-penicillamine
goitrogens and antithyroid drugs
isoretinoin
methyl mercury
phenytoin
tetracyclines
thalidomide
valproic acid
infections
cytomegalovirus
rubella

syphilis
toxoplasmosis
maternal metabolic imbalance
alcoholism
diabetes mellitus
phenylketonuria
virilizing tumors
ionizing radiation

There is continuing concern about the possible adverse effects of drugs and other environmental factors on the developing fetus. However, relatively few agents have proven to be teratogenic.

Thalidomide

Lenz (42) in Germany and McBride (43) in Australia reported an increased frequency of limb-deficient babies born to mothers who used thalidomide as a sedative during pregnancy. The agent was shown from clinical studies to produce its major effects during the period of limb formation.

Warfarin

Teratogenic effects occur from exposure of the fetus to warfarin from 6 to 9 weeks of gestation. Stippling of the epiphyses is one of the characteristic changes. Exposure during the second and third trimesters produces severe neural anomalies.

Retinoic Acid

Retinoic acid has been used in the treatment of severe cystic acne. Recipient females are often of childbearing age and are at risk from the potent teratogenic effects of this agent. It produces craniofacial, cardiac, thymic, and central nervous system defects. Megadoses of vitamin A are also teratogenic. Vitamin A, retinoic acid, and its analogs should be avoided during pregnancy. If women of childbearing age use these agents, unplanned pregnancies should be avoided by contraception.

Alcohol

Alcohol is the most common teratogen to which a pregnancy is likely to be exposed (11,35). Regular intake of two alcoholic drinks each day during pregnancy results in a slightly reduced birth weight. Chronic intake of eight to ten drinks each day is likely to produce babies with low birth weights, craniofacial anomalies, mental retardation, incoordination, short stature, and increased frequency of congenital heart disease. A gradient of severity of these effects is seen with intermediate levels of alcohol intake. Alcohol should be avoided during pregnancy.

Radiation

Pregnant women should avoid unnecessary exposure to radiographs and isotopes. Doses in excess of 1 Gy should be avoided, and doses in excess of 10 Gy produce microcephaly, growth retardation, and mental retardation. Women of childbearing age should not be exposed to unnecessary radiation, if they may be, or are known to be, pregnant.

Infections

Syphilis was the first known infectious teratogen. Its deleterious effects on the fetus can be prevented by routine testing of pregnant women, and treatment when necessary. The virus that causes acquired immunodeficiency syndrome has emerged as a major teratogen. Rubella embryopathy is preventable by vaccination of young girls. When the fetus is exposed to the virus in the first trimester, blindness, deafness, cataracts, microphthalmos, congenital heart disease, limb deficiencies, and mental retardation occur. Cytomegalovirus infection and toxoplasmosis also produce birth defects.

Diabetes Mellitus

Abnormal embryogenesis occurs more often in babies of diabetic mothers, particularly if their diabetes is poorly controlled in the first trimester of the pregnancy. For example, cardiac malformations occur three to four times more often in babies of diabetic mothers than of normal mothers, and anencephaly and myelomeningocele occur in 1 to 10% of babies born to diabetic mothers. Caudal regression syndrome, with sacral hypoplasia and fusion of the legs, is a rare disorder, but it is more common in babies of diabetic mothers.

GENETIC COUNSELING AND PRENATAL DIAGNOSIS

Genetic counseling aims to provide sufficient information for an individual or couple to make an informed decision about future pregnancies, and to assist them in coming to terms with the issues they face (44).

Indications for Genetic Counseling

Anyone who suspects that there may be an increased risk of producing a child with a birth defect should receive formal genetic counseling. Appropriate genetic counseling requires diagnostic precision and knowledge of the recurrence risk, the burden of the disorder, and the reproductive options. There are several indications for genetic counseling (28,44):

- couples who have a stillbirth or multiple miscarriages
- a child with a birth defect

- mental retardation
- a family history of any of the above problems
- relatives with known genetic diseases, such as muscular dystrophy
- exposure to radiation, drugs, or infections during pregnancy
- advanced maternal age
- consanguinity
- chromosomal translocations

Diagnostic Precision

The most important element in counseling is establishing the correct diagnosis. A precise diagnosis cannot be made for about half of the children who present with mental retardation or dysmorphic features. However, there is a large amount of empiric data that can be used for counseling in this group.

Estimation of Recurrence Risk

After diagnostic evaluation, an estimate of the recurrence risk is made. This is a numeric estimate of the likelihood of a particular disorder occurring in subsequent children, such as a 1 in 4 risk of an autosomal recessive disorder and a 1 in 2 risk of an autosomal dominant disorder. The recurrence risk for multifactorial disorders, after a single affected child, is about 3 to 5%.

Many families do not have a grasp of probabilities and need a careful discussion to give meaning to any risk estimate. For example, a 1 in 4 risk applies to each pregnancy, but many families believe that they can have three more children without worry, if they already have one abnormal child.

Another aspect of risk is the background level of risk for major birth defects. About 1 in 25 children are born with a major defect. In this setting, risks of 1 in 2 and 1 in 4 are high, and risks of 1 in 100 are low.

Burden of Genetic Diseases

The burden of genetic diseases is important in genetic counseling. Clinodactyly is a common autosomal dominant condition with a high recurrence risk of 1 in 2, although it has minimal or no burden to those who have it. Clubfeet and congenital dislocation of the hip are multifactorial diseases with lower risks of recurrence. The potential burden of these conditions is minimized by early diagnosis and treatment. In contrast, the burden of additional children with Duchenne muscular dystrophy, severe osteogenesis imperfecta, or severe chondrodysplasia is considerable, because there are no curative treatments available.

There may be disparities between the doctor's concept of burden and the family's concept. Some families are prepared to accept a 1 in 4 risk of a perinatally lethal disorder, knowing that the child will die at, or soon after birth, or be normal. Other families may not be willing to accept the burden of recurrent deformities such as clubfeet, despite the lower risk and the availability of treatment.

Neonatal and Prenatal Diagnosis

General neonatal screening programs for inborn errors of metabolism, such as phenylketonuria and hypothyroidism, have been highly successful. The severe consequences of these diseases have been prevented by early diagnosis and treatment.

Prenatal diagnosis is used more selectively, but is being offered to an increasing number of families, as the number of diseases that can be detected in early pregnancy increases. The most common indication is a maternal age of 35 years or older. The indications for prenatal diagnosis are shown in the following list:

- advanced maternal age (older than 35 years)
- known chromosomal anomaly in one parent or in a previous pregnancy
- previous neural tube defect, high serum level of α-fetoprotein, or neural tube defect suspected from ultrasound results
- family history of disorders detectable by biochemical or DNA technology, including Duchenne and Becker muscular dystrophy, myotonic dystrophy, hemoglobinopathies, hemophilia A or B, Huntington disease, cystic fibrosis, and other rare detectable genetic diseases

In most instances, prenatal diagnosis does not reveal an abnormality, providing reassurance to the parents. The availability of prenatal diagnosis increases the number of families willing to have children, instead of refraining from having them, because of a fear of birth defects.

Serum α-Fetoprotein Screening

α-Fetoprotein is a fetal protein produced by the yolk sac and liver. It reaches a peak in fetal serum at about 13 weeks of gestation and decreases thereafter. Amniotic levels are high in the fetus with a lesion that is not covered by skin, such as open spina bifida, anencephaly, and exomphalos. The protein leaks into the amniotic fluid and into the maternal circulation. An increased maternal serum level of α-fetoprotein is not diagnostic of open spina bifida, but is an indication for further investigation. Abnormally high levels also occur in cases of fetal death, cystic hygroma, polycystic kidneys, and Turner syndrome.

Ultrasound Screening

Real-time ultrasonography is used to visualize the fetus and fetal movements. Ultrasonography is commonly undertaken to determine gestational age. However, more extensive studies by experienced ultrasonographers are required when examining for fetal abnormalities in at-risk pregnancies. Such examinations are increasingly undertaken as screening investigations in all pregnancies.

Amniocentesis and Chorionic Villus Sampling

Ultrasound-guided amniocentesis is a relatively safe procedure when undertaken at 16 weeks of gestation. The risk of fetal loss is about 0.5 to 1%. The amniotic fluid is most often used for determination of α-fetoprotein levels. The amniotic cells are used for karyotype analysis for the determination of enzyme levels in cases of inborn errors of metabolism, and for DNA diagnosis using direct detection of a previously defined mutation, or indirect detection using polymorphisms. Chorionic villus sampling can be undertaken between 9 and 11 weeks of gestation, and allows earlier diagnosis of many genetic diseases, and first-trimester termination. The risk of fetal loss is about 4%.

Prenatal Counseling

Families at risk for genetic diseases and birth defects should seek counseling before the mother becomes pregnant. This approach ensures that there is sufficient time to establish the diagnosis, recurrence risk, burden of the disorder, reproductive alternatives, and suitability for prenatal diagnosis. These options may be limited when counseling is sought during the pregnancy. Parents must be fully informed about the risks of investigational procedures and anticipated delays in receiving test results. They must be given all test results and appropriate explanations of their significance. Parents require much support at this difficult time, and are responsible for the decision to terminate a pregnancy.

TREATMENT OF GENETIC DISEASES

Early treatment of phenylketonuria and hypothyroidism has effectively prevented mental retardation and other consequences of these diseases. However, they are the exceptions, because treatment is not available for most genetic diseases, and, when available, it is relatively ineffective. Table 6-1 lists the various levels at which intervention is possible.

Most methods of treatment, such as metabolic manipulations and protein replacement, occur beyond the level of the gene. However, bone marrow transplantation has been used successfully to cure or ameliorate diseases such as congenital immune deficiencies, infantile malignant osteopetrosis, thalassemia, lysosomal storage diseases, infantile agranulocytosis, and chronic granulomatous disease. The normal genes of the transplanted cells produce the protein, usually an enzyme, which corrects the metabolic defect. The stem cells within the donor marrow continue to replicate, providing a continuing source of the normal protein. As

TABLE 6-1. LEVELS OF TREATMENT OF GENETIC DISEASES

Level of Intervention	Treatment Strategy
Mutant gene	Modification of somatic genotype
	Modulation of gene expression
Mutant messenger RNA	Modulation of mutant messenger RNA expression
Mutant protein	Protein replacement or stimulation of residual function
Metabolic or biochemical dysfunction	Specific metabolic manipulation
Clinical phenotype	Nonspecific medical or surgical intervention
The family	Genetic counseling, carrier detection, and pre-symptomatic diagnosis

(From ref. 45, with permission.)

transplantation technology improves, it is likely that specific subsets of stem cells within the bone marrow, peripheral blood, or other tissues will be used to target specific organs. For example, stem cells that can develop into osteoblasts, fibroblasts, or chondrocytes may be used as a form of cell therapy to correct genetic defects of the appropriate connective tissues. Growth factors will be needed to direct the cell differentiation pathways. An alternative approach to cell therapy is to use embryonic stem cells, which are pluripotential. Despite the great potential of this treatment, many ethical and practical issues need to be resolved before embryonic stem cells can be used in clinical practice.

Somatic gene therapy is in its infancy, but is likely to become available for many genetic diseases. Gene transfer is used to replace a gene that is nonfunctional, such as the *DMD* gene in boys with Duchenne muscular dystrophy. For other diseases, the adverse effects of the mutant allele are blocked by specific gene therapy directed to the mutant sequence. Therapy of the latter kind is most applicable to diseases in which many affected individuals share the same mutation. Designing gene therapy is more difficult for diseases in which most individuals have their own mutations, as occurs in osteogenesis imperfecta.

There are many challenges to achieving safe and effective somatic gene therapy. One of the challenges is to target the therapy to specific cells. Transplantation of modified autologous bone marrow cells is likely to be suitable for hematologic diseases and for some bone diseases. Specific cell surface receptor-mediated gene transfer is likely to be more suitable for other diseases, as in transferring a replacement gene into the skeletal and cardiac muscle cells of young children with Duchenne muscular dystrophy.

Less-dramatic solutions are likely to be applicable in patients with autosomal dominant disorders that give rise to haploid insufficiency. In such patients, the protein produced is qualitatively normal, but is reduced in amount because only the normal allele is functional. In this situation, the amount of normal protein produced from the normal allele can be increased by specific pharmacologic modulation of gene expression. Therapy of this kind is potentially curative for half of all patients with osteogenesis imperfecta and Marfan syndrome.

References

Molecular Basis of Inheritance

1. Thompson MW, McInnes RR, Willard HF. *Genetics in medicine,* 5th ed. Toronto: WB Saunders, 1991.
2. Penrose LS. Parental age in achondroplasia and mongolism. *Am J Hum Genet* 1957;9:167.
3. Stoll C, Roth M-P, Bigel P. A reexamination of parental age effect on the occurrence of new mutations for achondroplasia. In: Papadatos CJ, Bartsocas CS, eds. *Skeletal dysplasias.* New York: Alan R. Liss, 1982:419.
4. Bowen P. Achondroplasia in two sisters with normal parents. *Birth Defects* 1974;10:31.
5. Clermont Y. Renewal of spermatogonia in man. *Am J Anat* 1966; 118:509.
6. Gillard EF, Chamberlain JS, Murphy EG, et al. Molecular and phenotypic analysis of patients with deletions within the deletion-rich region of the Duchenne muscular dystrophy (DMD) gene. *Am J Hum Genet* 1989;45:507.
7. Dietz HC, Cutting GR, Pyeritz RE, et al. Marfan syndrome caused by a recurrent de novo missense mutation in the fibrillin-1 gene. *Nature* 1991;352:337.
8. Shiang R, Thompson LM, Zhu Y-Z, et al. Mutations in the transmembrane domain of FGFR3 cause the most common genetic form of dwarfism, achondroplasia. *Cell* 1994;78:335.

Chromosome Disorders

9. Borgaonkar DS. *Chromosomal variation in man: a catalog of chromosomal variants and anomalies,* 5th ed. New York: Alan R. Liss, 1989.
10. Epstein CJ. *The consequences of chromosome imbalance: principles, mechanisms and models.* New York: Cambridge University Press, 1986.

Single-gene Disorders

11. McKusick VA. *Mendelian inheritance in man: catalogs of autosomal dominant, autosomal recessive, and X-linked phenotypes,* 9th ed. Baltimore: The Johns Hopkins University Press, 1990.
12. Redman JB, Fenwick SK, Fu TH, et al. Relationship between parental trinucleotide GCT repeat length and severity of myotonic dystrophy in offspring. *JAMA* 1993;269:1960.

13. Byers PH, Wallis GA, Willing MC. Osteogenesis imperfecta: translation of mutation to phenotype. *J Med Genet* 1991;28:433.

14. Cole WG. Collagen genes: mutations affecting collagen structure and expression. *Prog Nucleic Acid Res Mol Biol* 1994;47:29.

15. Spranger J. Bone dysplasia "families." *Pathol Immunopathol Res* 1988;7:76.

16. Spranger J, Winterpacht A, Zabel B. The type II collagenopathies: a spectrum of chondrodysplasias. *Eur J Pediatr* 1994;153:56.

17. Francomano CA, Ortiz de Luna RI, Hefferon TW, et al. Localization of the achondroplasia gene to the distal 2.5 Mb of human chromosome 4p. *Hum Mol Genet* 1994;3:787.

18. Le Merrer M, Rousseau F, Legeai-Mallet L, et al. A gene for achondroplasia: hypochondroplasia maps to chromosome 4p. *Nat Genet* 1994;6:314.23.

19. Velinov M, Slaugenhaupt SA, Stoilov I, et al. The gene for achondroplasia maps to the telomeric region of chromosome 4p. *Nat Genet* 1994;6:318.

20. Peters K, Ornitz D, Werner SM, et al. Unique expression pattern of the FGF receptor 3 gene during mouse organogenesis. *Dev Biol* 1993;155:423.

21. Superti-Furga A, Eich G, Bucher HU, et al. A glycine 375-to-cysteine substitution in the transmembrane domain of the fibroblast growth factor receptor-3 in a newborn with achondroplasia. *Eur J Pediatr* 1995;154:215.

22. Aterman K, Welch JP, Taylor PG. Presumed homozygous achondroplasia: a review and report of a further case. *Pathol Res Pract* 1983;178:27.

23. Goldgar DE, Green P, Parry DM, et al. Multipoint linkage analysis in neurofibromatosis type 1: an international collaboration. *Am J Hum Genet* 1989;44:6.

24. Legius E, Marchuk DA, Collins FS, et al. Somatic deletion of the neurofibromatosis type 1 gene in a neurofibrosarcoma supports a tumour suppressor gene hypothesis. *Nat Genet* 1993;3:122.

25. Nakafuku M, Nagamine M, Ohtoshi A, et al. Suppression of oncogenic Ras by mutant neurofibromatosis type 1 genes with single amino acid substitutions. *Proc Natl Acad Sci USA* 1993;90:6706.

26. Weiming X, Yu Q, Lizhi L, et al. Molecular analysis of neurofibromatosis type 1 mutations. *Hum Mutat* 1992;1:474.

27. Miller M, Hall JG. Possible maternal effect of severity of neurofibromatosis. *Lancet* 1978;11:1071.

28. Shannon KM, O'Connell P, Martin GA, et al. Loss of the normal NF1 allele from the bone marrow of children with type 1 neurofibromatosis and malignant myeloid disorders. *N Engl J Med* 1994;330:597.

29. Harper PS. *Practical genetic counselling*, 2nd ed. Bristol, England: Wright, 1984.

30. Glorieux F, Scriver CR. Loss of a PTH sensitive component of phosphate transport in X-linked hypophosphatemia. *Science* 1972;175:997.

31. Fu Y, Kuhl DP, Pizzuti A, et al. Variation of the CGG repeat at the fragile X site results in genetic instability: resolution of the Sherman paradox. *Cell* 1991;67:1047.

32. Pieretti M, Zhang F, Fu Y, et al. Absence of expression of the FMR-1 gene in fragile X syndrome. *Cell* 1991;66:817.

33. Driscoll DJ. Genomic imprinting in humans. *Mol Genet Med* 1994;4:37.

34. Austin KD, Hall JG. Nontraditional inheritance. *Pediatr Clin North Am* 1992;39:335.

35. Shenker A, Weinstein LS, Sweet DE, et al. An activating Gs α mutation is present in fibrous dysplasia of bone in the McCune-Albright syndrome. *J Clin Endocrinol Metab* 1994:79:750.

36. Cohen MM, Rosenblum-Vos LS, Prabhakar G. Human cytogenetics: a current overview. *Am J Dis Child* 1993;147:1159.

37. Delattre O, Zucman J, Melot T, et al. The Ewing family of tumors: a subgroup of small round-cell tumors defined by specific chimeric transcripts. *N Engl J Med* 1994;331:294.

38. Weksberg R, Shen DR, Fei YL, et al. Disruption of insulin-like growth factor 2 imprinting in Beckwith-Wiedemann syndrome. *Nat. Genet* 1993;5:143.

Multifactorial Disorders

39. Carter CO. Genetics of common single malformations. *Br Med Bull* 1976;32:21.

Teratologic Disorders

40. Danks DM, Rogers JG. Birth defects. In: Robinson MJ, ed. *Practical paediatrics*, 2nd ed. London: Churchill Livingstone, 1990:19.

41. Shepard TH. *Catalog of teratologic agents*, 6th ed. Baltimore: The Johns Hopkins University Press, 1989.

42. Lenz W. Thalidomide embryopathy in Germany, 1959–1961. *Prog Clin Biol Res* 1985;163C:77.

43. McBride WG. Thalidomide embryopathy. *Teratology* 1977;16:79.

Genetic Counseling and Prenatal Diagnosis

44. Rogers JG. Genetic counselling. In: Robinson MJ, ed. *Practical paediatrics*, 2nd ed. London: Churchill Livingstone, 1990:55.

Treatment of Genetic Diseases

45. Valle D. Genetic disease: an overview of current therapy. *Hosp Pract* 1987;22:167.

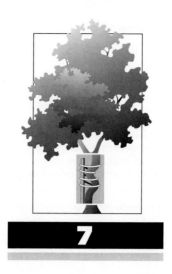

7

METABOLIC AND ENDOCRINE ABNORMALITIES

DAVID J. ZALESKE

Metabolic bone disease includes systemic disorders of calcium and phosphorus that affect osseous tissue. The immature skeleton forms bone through turnover, which is affected by all the disorders considered to be metabolic bone disease, and bone is formed at the interface between vascular tissue and proliferating cartilage, which can be affected by genetic and endocrine disturbances that interfere with growth (1–3).

The advances in molecular biology tend to blur traditional disciplines (4,5). Pediatric patients with metabolic and endocrine abnormalities are usually under the care of pediatric endocrinologists, nephrologists, or gastroenterologists, in addition to a primary pediatrician. The pediatric orthopaedic surgeon is presented with children with alterations in morphology. He or she may have to participate in the diagnosis and needs to understand the basic science for an intelligent approach to treatment. This chapter describes the physiology and pathophysiology of the formation of bone and cartilage in the immature skeleton as the basis for pediatric orthopaedic care. Certain aspects of the clinical entities described are most completely understood when the reader also refers to information in Chapter 1, "Embryology and Development of the Musculoskeletal System"; Chapter 6, "Genetic Aspects of Orthopaedic Conditions"; Chapter 8, "The Skeletal Dysplasias"; and Chapter 9, "Syndromes of Orthopaedic Importance."

REVIEW OF FACTORS IN SKELETAL DEVELOPMENT

Genetic, metabolic, endocrine, and physical factors interact to produce the shape of the immature skeleton (4,5). Em-

D. J. Zaleske: Department of Orthopaedics, Harvard Medical School, Boston, Massachusetts 02115; Pediatric Orthopaedics Unit, Massachusetts General Hospital, Boston, Massachusetts 02114.

TABLE 7-1. GROWTH FACTORS

Factors	Effects
TGF-β superfamily	
TGF-β1 (CIF-A)	Upregulate bone and cartilage components of types I, II, III, V, VI, and X collagen, fibronectin,
TGF-β2 (CIF-B)	osteopontin, osteonectin, thromospondin, proteoglycans, alkaline phosphatase
BMP-2 through BMP-7	Downregulate metalloproteinases, osteoclasts
BMP-3 (osteogenin)	Indefinite effect on chondrocytes
BMP-1 (OP-1)	Osteoclasts lead to or promote up regulation of TGF-β
FGF	
Acidic (aFGF) and basic (bFGF)	Upregulate endothelial cell and chondrocyte replication and neovascularization
Insulin-like growth factors	
Somatomedins	In skeletal growth, mediate many growth-promoting effects of growth hormone
	Upregulate the incorporation of sulfate into proteoglycan
PDGF	
A and B chains	Potent mitogen for cells of connective origin
	TGF-β leads to or promotes up regulation of PDGF-B, which leads to or promotes up-regulation of protooncogenes MYC and FOS

BMP, bone morphogenetic protein; *CIF,* cartilage-inducing factor; *FGF,* fibroblast growth factor; *OP,* osteogenic protein; *PDGF,* platelet-derived growth factor; *TGF,* transforming growth factor.

bryology has been discussed extensively in Chapter 1. A brief review here of this topic is intended to add the perspective that factors active in morphogenesis are important in postnatal skeletal growth, homeostasis, and repair (6). During the embryonic period (i.e., from 1 week after conception to the end of the second month of gestation), morphogenesis occurs (7). An interactive cascade of events (i.e., epigenesis) produces shape. The molecular basis of this complex process is being elucidated (8,9). Activation of genes involved in specifying shape may in turn control the synthesis and release of morphogens, such as the growth factors (Table 7-1), the spatial distribution of which defines body plan (4,9–11). At 8 weeks of gestation, vascular invasion occurs at the midshaft of the humerus, in association with endochondral bone formation; this marks the end of the embryonic period and the beginning of the fetal period.

Primary centers of ossification appear rapidly at other sites. In long bones, chondrocyte hypertrophy and death, followed by osseous replacement, advance toward both ends, leaving the cartilaginous growth plates or physes, which continue to function as endochondral bone generators until adolescence. Bone formation in the cartilaginous epiphyses occurs in the secondary centers of ossification, many of which do not appear until after birth. The timing of endochondral bone formation in various anatomic sites can be useful in establishing biologic or bone age (12).

The fine structures of bone and cartilage have certain similarities. Both have well-defined cell populations and a characteristic extracellular matrix, and collagen is an important constituent of the matrices of both of these tissues (13–15) (Table 7-2). Class 1 collagens (i.e., types I, II, III, V, and XI) are the banded, fiber-forming collagens. The fibrillar collagens consist of three parallel protein chains, called α-chains, organized into triple helices. The α-chains

differ in their primary amino acid sequences, total amino acid compositions, and degrees of glycosylation (13,14). In bone, the matrix is mostly type I collagen, organized to allow nucleation and growth of hydroxyapatite crystals at a finite number of sites (16). The type I collagen consists of two α1(I)-chains and one α2(I)-chain. Type II collagen is the major collagen of cartilage matrix. It consists of three identical α1(II)-chains.

Class 2 collagens (i.e., types IX and XII) do not form aggregates alone, but rather bind to the other collagens in forming fibrils. Class 3 collagens (i.e., types IV, VI, VII, and X) form fibrous structures separate from the banded collagen fibers. Class 4 includes types VIII and XIII, the function of which is still being investigated.

Several noncollagenous proteins are not so abundant as collagen, but they may be important in the regulation of mineralization (17–19). These proteins are proteoglycans, phosphoproteins, and osteocalcin, which binds calcium through an α-carboxyglutamic acid moiety.

The cell types of osseous tissue are osteoblasts, osteocytes, and osteoclasts. It appears that osteoblasts are derived from mesenchymal osteoprogenitor cells. Osteoblasts are large, active cells that elaborate the matrix for bone formation. Osteoblasts that become surrounded by matrix, and eventually become ossified bone, persist in the form of osteocytes. Osteoclasts are multinucleated cells, originating from hematopoietic tissues, which are responsible for bone resorption (20). Bone is a dynamic tissue, and its turnover results from a fairly close coupling of resorption and formation. The net effect of these processes in the normal immature skeleton is an increase in mass throughout growth. Bone tissue remodeling or turnover is a complex phenomenon mediated by the variety of metabolic and endocrine factors that are being presented in this chapter. Turnover is important, not

TABLE 7-2. COLLAGEN TYPES

Types of Collagen	Tissues
Class 1: fiber-forming collagens	
Type 1 $\alpha1(I)_2\alpha2(I)$	Skin, tendon, ligament, bone, cornea
Gene for $\alpha1(I)$ = *COL1A1* on chromosome 17	
Gene for $\alpha2(I)$ = *COL1A2* on chromosome 7	
Type II $\alpha1(II)_3$	Cartilage, nucleus pulposus
Gene for $\alpha1(II)$ = *COL2A1* on chromosome 12	
Type III $\alpha1(III)_3$	Skin and a variety of connective tissues with type 1
Type V $\alpha1(V)\alpha2(V)\alpha3(V)$	Fetal and vascular tissues
Type XI	Cartilage
Class 2: fibril-associated collagens	
Type IX	Cartilage
Type XII	Ligament, tendon, perichondrium, periosteum
Class 3: independent fiber systems	
Type IV	Basement membranes
Type VI	In cartilaginous and noncartilaginous connective tissues
Type VII	Anchoring fibrils
Type X	Hypertrophic chondrocytes during endochondral ossification
Class 4: unknown fiber forms and functions	
Type VIII	
Type XIII	

only in skeletal homeostasis but in fracture healing and bone graft incorporation (6,10,21,22).

There are three types of cartilage in the body: hyaline (e.g., articular cartilage, growth plates), fibrocartilage (i.e., menisci), and elastic cartilage (i.e., ear cartilage). All cartilages have an extracellular matrix consisting of collagen and proteoglycan; the matrix is particularly well defined in hyaline cartilage. Proteoglycan occurs in several macromolecular forms consisting of long-chain sugar polymers (i.e., chondroitin sulfates and keratin sulfate) attached to a core protein. Large numbers of proteoglycans form hydrophilic, highly electronegative aggregates along a filament of hyaluronic acid, and are crucial to the structure of the cartilaginous mass. Collagen and proteoglycan are synthesized by chondrocytes.

Different types of cartilage have different compositions. Articular cartilage is aneural, alymphatic, and avascular. The property of resisting vascular invasion is important to the function of physeal cartilage. Growth plates or physes are specialized hyaline cartilaginous structures responsible for bone growth (23). In long bones, a physis becomes radiographically distinct at either end with the appearance of the secondary center of ossification. In round and flat bones, the growth plate is a roughly spherical structure and therefore is never visualized as a distinct radiolucency. The growth characteristics of physeal regions are endowed during the embryonic period, but are subject to a variety of postnatal modifications, including metabolic factors and physical force (7).

A longitudinal section of a growth plate reveals several zones (23). On the epiphyseal side of the growth plate is the resting zone, which appears to participate in storing lipids and other materials. The proliferative zone contains the dividing cells of the growth plate. In the hypertrophic zone, the flattened cells of the proliferative zone enlarge and become spherical to ellipsoid. On the metaphyseal side is the zone of provisional calcification and formation of the primary spongiosa. The blood supply to the growth plate is dual, with epiphyseal vessels supporting the zone of growth and metaphyseal vessels supporting ossification. In the lower hypertrophic zone, matrix vesicles, membrane-bound particles that contain calcific materials, are formed by the chondrocytes and are deposited in the longitudinal septa, presumably as a prerequisite for bone formation (24,25). Neutral protease and pyrophosphatase activity located in this region decrease the concentration of inhibitors of calcification and allow ossification to proceed (26). A mini–growth plate beneath the articular cartilage serves to enlarge the epiphysis during growth, but rather than ossifying at maturity, it remains cartilaginous and may be subject to stimulation even after maturity.

Cartilage proliferation and growth plate function throughout the body are subject to control by several humoral and local factors (11,27,28). Most notable are growth hormone and the somatomedins (Table 7-1). Early experimental studies showed that growth was at least partially regulated by growth hormone by demonstrating that administration of pituitary extracts to hypophysectomized rats caused a significant proliferative response in growth plates (29). Subsequent experiments demonstrated that the relation between administration of growth hormone and the phenomenon of epiphyseal growth was indirect and that it was mediated by somatomedins, materials synthesized in the liver in response to the administration of the pituitary preparation (2).

Somatomedins are a group of short-chain polypeptides that affect DNA synthesis in the growth plate chondrocytes and enhance amino acid transport, RNA synthesis, and synthesis of proteoglycan and collagen (11). Sensitivity to somatomedins is reduced in cartilage from older persons and in cartilage from early embryonic tissues, so that it is postulated that these materials are less important for growth in early development. The growth plate chondrocytes also demonstrate sensitivity to basic fibroblast growth factor (30,31).

Numerous other factors are important in growth plate regulation. Nutrition and insulin regulate growth plate function. Protein in the diet exerts a positive control over the somatomedins. Excess glucocorticoids appear to inhibit growth, partly by an inhibitory effect on protein synthesis in cartilage, but also by interference with somatomedin production and action. Estrogens decrease somatomedin production; androgens increase growth, but not through the somatomedin system. Similarly, increased thyroxin causes increased growth, but it is not clear whether this effect is mediated through growth hormone and somatomedins (32,33).

The regulation of bone formation is equal in complexity to that of cartilage proliferation. In the immature skeleton, under conditions of normal physiology, the two are linked at the physis, and many of the humoral factors discussed have an effect on osseous, as well as cartilaginous, tissue (17,22,34–38). Bone formation is also controlled by the serum concentration of ions, such as calcium and phosphate, which contribute to the mineral phase; by the hormones (e.g., parathyroid hormone, calcitonin) that regulate these ions; and by a variety of other factors, such as prostaglandin E_2, osteoclast-activating factor, and forms of transforming growth factor-β (19,39–41).

Excess glucocorticoids inhibit bone formation in a complex manner. Glucocorticoid excess is associated with a decrease in calcium and phosphate levels and an inhibition of matrix synthesis (42). Insulin is associated with an increase in bone formation (18). Although *in vitro*, direct, anabolic effects on bone have been demonstrated, *in vivo* effects may be mediated by interaction with somatomedins and nutrition. Conversely, defects in early fracture healing have been documented in experimental diabetes (43). Thyroid hormones are necessary for normal turnover of bone. Thyroid hormone increases osteoclastic bone resorption, but, as indicated previously, it is also associated with increased growth, possibly mediated through the somatomedins.

Androgens and estrogens affect skeletal growth and net bone formation. Testosterone has been shown to cause an increase in growth plate activity, but estrogens appear to be inhibitory in their action. Estrogen is important in growth plate closure in both genders (44,45). The action on bone

is far less clear. In the growing skeleton, testosterone seems to increase skeletal mass (possibly on the basis of androgen-induced increase in muscle mass), whereas estrogen appears to stabilize the skeleton (or at least has an antiosteoporotic effect in postmenopausal women).

Prostaglandin E_2 is a potent stimulator of bone resorption (39). Perhaps because of the combination of bone resorption and formation, bone synthesis may also be stimulated in the immature skeleton. Cyanotic infants treated with prostaglandin E_2 to maintain patency of the ductus arteriosus have been observed to have increased periosteal bone formation (43,46). Osteoclast-activating factor is elaborated by lymphocytes and may have a role in the formation of hematopoietic marrow (19).

The physiology of parathyroid hormone (PTH), vitamin D, and calcitonin are fully discussed later in this chapter. At this point, it is sufficient to indicate that calcium levels are normally maintained constant by the body; phosphate levels vary more with intake, but are also defended. Vitamin D exists in a variety of forms. It stimulates the transport of calcium and phosphate across the intestine and can also stimulate bone resorption. PTH, in response to low serum calcium, stimulates osteoclastic resorption of bone, mediated through osteoblasts (20). PTH increases the renal tubular reabsorption of calcium and decreases that of phosphate. Calcitonin has the reverse effect, promoting the movement of calcium and phosphate into bone. However, at least in humans, its importance does not seem to be as great as that of PTH.

Physical factors are important in regulating bone formation (47,48). Two laws define the effect of load on proliferating cartilage and bone (49). The Hueter-Volkmann principle states that growth plates exhibit increased growth in response to tension and decreased growth in response to compression (50). Wolff's law states that osseous tissue remodels in response to the stress placed across it (51). An example of compressive inhibition of growth, according to the Hueter-Volkmann principle, is the decreased growth anticipated from the concavity of the kyphotic spine in untreated Scheuermann disease. An example of bone remodeling, according to Wolff's law, is the arrangement of the trabeculae in the femoral neck. The basis of these laws at the level of the cell is gradually being elucidated (52,53). Experimental data link mechanical force to a class of cell receptors, called integrins, which transduce the force to changes in the cytoskeleton and, presumably, ultimately to the genome (54).

Although all the factors described previously play a role in the development and function of the skeletal system, genetic determinants expressed through the biology of the cell, even in postnatal life, may be the critical unifying factor. The concentrations of the enzymes necessary for normal differentiation of the skeleton, the number and availability of hormone receptors on chondrocytes and bone cells, the production of hormones, the transport systems for calcium and phosphate, and the synthetic systems for vitamin D may be genetically determined, and, in normal populations, may ultimately dictate such variations in the size, thickness, and shape of bones. In people whose skeletal morphology falls outside the normal range and who are regarded as displaying metabolic bone disease, genetic errors may be significant factors in the development of the often stereotypical syndrome, either as a primary cause or as an accessory cause. In the pediatric population, in whom acquired disorders are less common, genetic causes should not be overlooked.

The following sections contain discussions of pathologic states and specific disorders often grouped as metabolic bone diseases. They are classified according to whether the primary abnormality is mainly in the mineral phase, in the organic phase, in the endocrine system, or in an indeterminate site.

MINERAL PHASE

Excluding the rachitic syndromes, the bone diseases of children in which disorders of calcium and phosphorus metabolism play a significant role are for the most part either genetic (e.g., pseudohypoparathyroidism, hypophosphatasia, hyperphosphatasia) or iatrogenic (e.g., corticosteroid-induced osteopenia, anticonvulsant rickets, and others). True metabolic bone diseases as seen in adults are rare in children, and disorders such as hyperparathyroidism and milk alkali syndrome are so infrequently seen in the pediatric population that they are rarely mentioned. A discussion of metabolic bone disease in children is mostly confined to the subjects of rickets and renal osteodystrophy (1). To appreciate the aberrations seen in these two still-prevalent disorders, a brief review of calcium and phosphorus balance and homeostasis is essential.

Calcium and Phosphorus Homeostasis

With the exception of the small but important amount of protein-bound and ionic calcium in the serum and extracellular space, most of the body's calcium is stored in the bones and is held in the form of hydroxyapatite, a salt with the generic formula $Ca_{10}(PO_4)_6(OH)_2$, which is composed of very tiny crystals embedded in the collagen fibers of the cortical and cancellous bone (55–58). The small size of the crystals ($5 \times 10 \times 20$ nm) provides an enormous surface area, and this factor, combined with the reactivity of the crystal surface and the hydration shell that surrounds it, allows a vast and rapid exchange process with the extracellular fluid. This process converts the mechanically solid structure of bone to a highly interactive reservoir for calcium, phosphorus, and a number of other ions (57,59). In disorders such as rickets and renal osteodystrophy, the depleted extracellular compartment of calcium can be replenished

from the bone compartment, although at the expense of the strength and integrity of the skeleton.

In analyzing the homeostatic mechanisms that control the metabolism of calcium and phosphorus, three truths become evident. These principles underlie all internal shifts, and it is necessary to understand them fully to comprehend the causes and mechanisms of the rachitic syndromes.

First, a principle of inorganic chemistry states that the salt, $CaHPO_4$, is not freely soluble in water. At the pH of body fluids, calcium and phosphate concentrations in the serum exceed the critical solubility product, and are presumed to be held in solution by an elaborate inhibitor system. This metastable state allows the deposition of hydroxyapatite during bone formation, with minimal expenditure of energy, and simultaneously makes the body potentially susceptible to ectopic calcification and ossification as a result of increments in either or both of these materials.

Second, a principle of physiology states that the irritability, conductivity, and contractility of smooth and skeletal muscle, and the irritability and conductivity of nervous tissue, are inversely proportional to the calcium ion concentration. The equation for cardiac muscle is the reverse: a direct proportionality. Calcium is also an intracellular messenger, and it may be fundamental to biologic function in differential cellular organelle function (24,60,61). The concentration of calcium in each of these compartments is a fine balance, and, under certain circumstances, an exquisite one, and minimal decreases in ionic calcium concentration can lead to tetany, convulsions, or diastolic death. Conversely, increases in the concentration of calcium can lead to muscle weakness, somnolence, and ventricular fibrillation. It is obviously important for the body to guard the concentration of ionized calcium, and many of the mechanisms to be described are designed to protect against such disasters (62,63).

Third, a principle of biochemistry states that diffusion of calcium across a cellular barrier cannot take place without a transport system. The discoveries of the components of this transport system have constituted some of the major scientific accomplishments of the twentieth century, and have greatly altered our approaches to the treatment of the rachitic syndromes.

The transport of calcium across a gut cell occurs during absorption of calcium from the lumen of the gastrointestinal tract, across the renal tubular cell to the peritubular space in the process of tubular reabsorption of calcium, or across a bone cell in the process of crystal lysis, which occurs during bone resorption (57,59,62,64,65). Although some evidence suggests that the mechanisms for these three processes differ somewhat, they all involve the action of the active form of vitamin D and PTH, and are inhibited by an increase in the concentration of cytosol phosphate (59,66–68). The principal and best-defined model is transport across the gut cell.

The gut cell at the site of absorption of calcium (i.e., distal duodenum and proximal jejunum) has a surface recep-

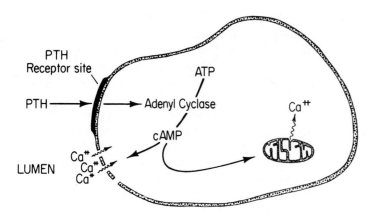

FIGURE 7-1. Action of parathyroid hormone (PTH) in calcium transport in the gut cell. Circulating PTH binds to the receptor site on the cell membrane and activates an adenyl cyclase system that induces the synthesis of cyclic adenosine monophosphate (cAMP) from adenosine triphosphate (ATP). cAMP acts to render the cell membrane more permeable to calcium ions and to induce the mitochondria to release calcium. Both of these actions fill the cytosol with ionized calcium (Ca^{++}). *ECF*, extracellular fluid.

tor for PTH. The circulating level of PTH is increased in response to a decrease in the serum ionized calcium. The circulating hormone binds to the receptor and activates an intracellular mechanism in which adenosine triphosphate is converted to cyclic adenosine monophosphate (cAMP) by the action of adenyl cyclase (Fig. 7-1). cAMP has two effects. It renders the cell membrane more permeable to ionic calcium, presumably by altering the charge on the membrane, and it induces the mitochondria, which are intracellular storehouses for calcium, to release their calcium. Both actions markedly increase the intracellular concentration of calcium, but do not promote transport to the extracellular space.

At this point, the active form of vitamin D, 1,25-dihydroxyvitamin D_3, or calcitriol, acts intranuclearly to enhance the transcription from DNA of a messenger RNA that codes for the synthesis of calcium transport factor or binding protein (69). This low-molecular-weight protein is capable of binding and transporting calcium across the cell into the pericellular space and the extracellular fluid (70–74) (Fig. 7-2). PTH and vitamin D work independently, but not completely so. Increased concentrations of

PTH are partly responsible for the increased rate of synthesis of 1,25-dihydroxyvitamin D from 25-hydroxyvitamin D. The active form of vitamin D is essential to the system, but the role of PTH is less important (48,66,75,76). This explains why the vitamin D-deficient state is more serious than hypoparathyroidism.

Phosphate does play a role in the calcium transport system. Increases in the cytosol concentration of phosphate, such as those that occur with chronic renal failure, turn off the system and act at the level of the renal tubule to decrease the synthesis of the potent vitamin D (77). Presumably as a protective action against exceeding the critical solubility product for calcium acid phosphate (first principle), high levels of phosphate prevent absorption of phosphate from the gastrointestinal tract, prevent reabsorption of calcium from the renal tubules, and probably prevent lysis of bone crystal. High levels of phosphate do not protect against the osteoclastic resorption of the skeleton associated with excessive concentrations of PTH.

A review of the process by which the ingested or synthesized provitamins D are converted into the active material necessary for transport of calcium can aid in the understand-

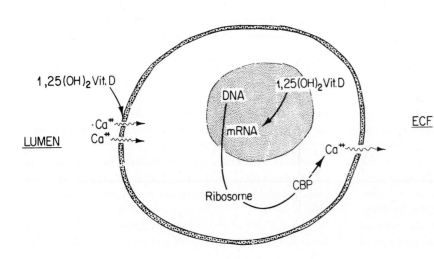

FIGURE 7-2. Actions of vitamin D on intracellular transport of calcium by the gut cell. The active hormone derived from ingested or synthesized vitamin D, 1,25-dihydroxyvitamin D [*1,25(OH)₂Vit.D*], acts intranuclearly to enhance transcription of messenger RNA (*mRNA*) for the synthesis of a calcium-binding protein (*CBP*), a low-molecular-weight protein that is material in the transport of calcium ion across the cell membrane. As for most sterols, 1,25-dihydroxyvitamin D exerts a *nonspecific* effect on the cell membrane to render it more permeable for the transport of the ionized calcium (Ca^{++}). *ECF*, extracellular fluid.

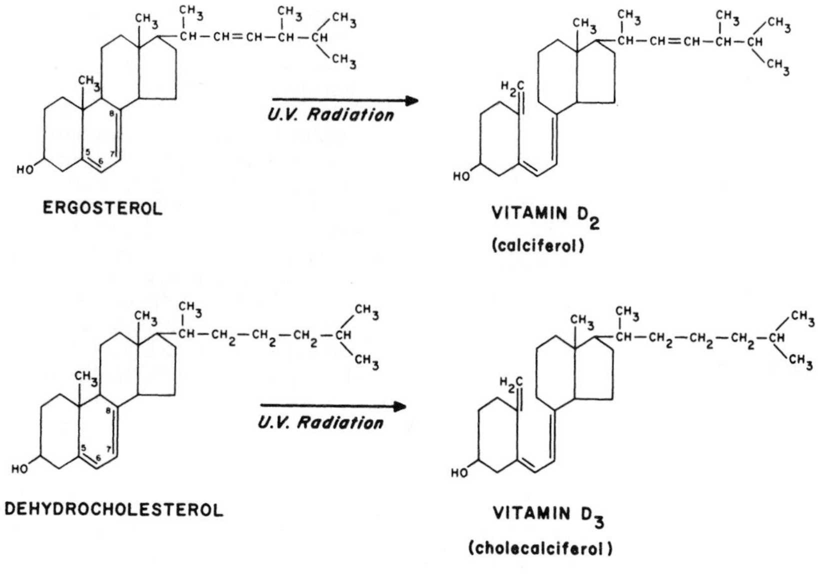

FIGURE 7-3. Provitamins ergosterol and 7-dehydrocholesterol are stored in the skin and activated by ultraviolet (*U.V.*) radiation to vitamins D_2 and D_3, respectively, by opening a bond in the first ring.

ing of calcium homeostasis and the development of the rachitic syndromes (69). The provitamins D consist of ergosterol ingested in the form of animal fats and 7-dehydrocholesterol synthesized in the liver (55,65) (Fig. 7-3). Both sterols are metabolically inactive, are transported in the serum by a special transport protein, and are stored in the skin (75). In the presence of ultraviolet light at a wavelength of about 315 nm, a chemical conversion occurs with the opening of a bond on the first ring. The structures are activated to form calciferol (i.e., vitamin D_2) and cholecalciferol (i.e., vitamin D_3) (55,78) (Fig. 7-3). The compounds are then transported to the liver, in which, in the presence of an appropriate hydrolase, they are converted to the first polar metabolite, 25-hydroxyvitamin D (Fig. 7-4). In experimental circumstances, the latter material has been found to be more active than the parent compounds, and acts considerably more rapidly (79–83).

The final and most critical conversion occurs in the kidney. In the presence of specific hydrolases and a number of biochemical cofactors, the 25-hydroxyvitamin D is converted to either 24,25-dihydroxyvitamin D or 1,25-dihydroxyvitamin D. The former acts as a balance hormone, probably with only limited action on gut, kidney, and bone. The latter serves as the potent transport promoter for the three cellular sites (48,84,85) (Fig. 7-5). The generic name of 1,25-dihydroxyvitamin D_3 is calcitriol. The conditions that seem to dictate which of the two polar metabolites is synthesized have been established. The data suggest that a low serum calcium level and a high PTH level favor conversion to the 1,25 analog, and a high serum calcium level, a higher serum phosphate level, and a low PTH level favor formation of the less-potent 24,25-dihydroxyvitamin D (47,48,86–88) (Fig 7-5). The protective action of the level of serum phosphate on the calcium-absorptive mechanisms is essential. A high concentration of phosphate appears to shunt the 25-hydroxyvitamin D into the less active 24,25-dihydroxy form and away from the more active 1,25-dihydroxy form.

In understanding calcium homeostasis, it is important to review some aspects of PTH metabolism and action. PTH is elaborated by the normal glands, almost entirely in response to the serum concentration of ionized calcium (59,62). Magnesium plays a role in release of the hormone, but the synthetic response is directed by a negative feedback system with calcium only (59,89,90). The lower the serum level,

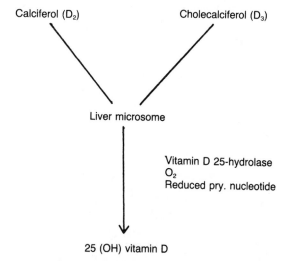

FIGURE 7-4. The first conversion of vitamin D takes place in the liver, where a specific enzyme, vitamin D 25-hydrolase, acts on the molecules to form 25-hydroxyvitamin D, a more active form of the sterol.

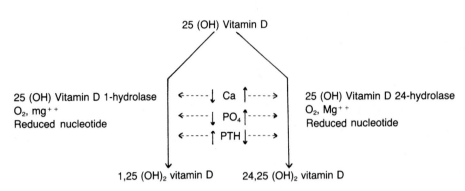

FIGURE 7-5. The second conversion of vitamin D takes place in the kidney, where at least two pathways have been described. The *maintenance* pathway (when the need is minimal, as defined by a normal calcium and phosphorus and a low parathyroid hormone [*PTH*]) occurs in the presence of a specific enzyme (25-hydroxyvitamin D 24-hydrolase) and results in the less-active 24,25-dihydroxyvitamin D. If calcium transport is required, as signaled by the presence of low serum calcium and phosphorus levels and a high PTH level, the body converts the 25-hydroxyvitamin D to the much more active form, 1,25-dihydroxyvitamin D.

the more PTH is synthesized and elaborated. PTH acts with 1,25-dihydroxyvitamin D to facilitate cellular calcium transport in absorption from the gut, reabsorption from the renal tubule, and lysis of hydroxyapatite crystal (59,66,90). PTH acts independently of vitamin D to activate the osteoclast population to resorb bone; this action, and the three others mentioned, tend to flood the extracellular space and serum with ionized calcium, correcting the deficit that initiated the demand (68,90). Such activity puts the patient at risk of exceeding the critical solubility product for calcium and phosphate. Another action of PTH (also probably independent of vitamin D) is to diminish markedly the tubular reabsorption of phosphate. This causes a phosphate diabetes and eliminates, at least partially, the threat posed by the increased concentration of ionized calcium (63,77,90).

In considering the actual handling of calcium and phosphorus by the intact mammalian system, it should be apparent that there are three sites of cell-mediated transport, particularly for calcium—the gut cell, the renal tubule, and bone—and that the transport taking place at these sites is mediated by the synergistic action of at least two hormones exogenous to the cell: PTH and 1,25-dihydroxyvitamin D. Both hormones are at least partially controlled by negative feedback to the concentrations of calcium. Both also appear to be inhibited at the level of the cell by hyperphosphatemia. Two other actions of PTH, which are independent of vitamin D and uninhibited by hyperphosphatemia, are osteoclastic resorption of bone and decreased tubular reabsorption of phosphate.

Because of the tight control exerted by the calcium transport system on calcium absorption from the gastrointestinal tract, it is difficult to define a minimum daily requirement for balance (62,78,91). Most people on a well-balanced diet ingest approximately 1.0 g of calcium per day, but, if a person does not eat or drink dairy products regularly, this value may decrease considerably (Fig. 7-6). If a person is in neutral balance for calcium, less than 200 mg of the ingested 1.0 g is absorbed; the remainder passes out in the feces.

In addition to vitamin D and PTH, additional factors

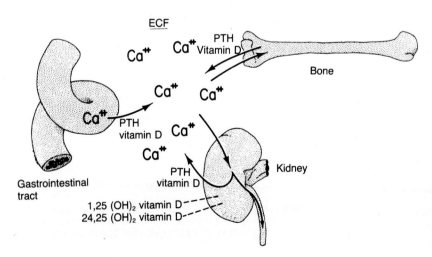

FIGURE 7-6. Calcium kinetics in the normocalcemic state. The synergistic actions of vitamin D and parathyroid hormone (*PTH*) appear to be necessary for the transport of calcium ions across the gut wall. Depending on the need for increased transport, 25-hydroxyvitamin D is converted to 24,25- or 1,25-dihydroxyvitamin D. *ECF*, extracellular fluid.

operating in the gastrointestinal tract significantly affect the absorption of calcium. The first factor is pH (92). All calcium salts are more soluble in acid media, and the ingested ionized calcium is no exception. Loss of the normal contribution of acid from the stomach reduces the solubility of the calcium salts and decreases the absorption of the ionized cation. The second factor is also a function of solubility; $CaHPO_4$ is not freely soluble at the pH of body solutions, even in the acidic medium of the upper gastrointestinal tract. A diet rich in phosphate may decrease the absorption of calcium by binding the cation to HPO_4^{2-} and precipitating most of the ingested calcium as insoluble material (57,93).

Ionic calcium can be chelated by some organic materials with a high affinity for the element. Although these materials may remain soluble, they cannot be absorbed (93). The materials that bind calcium in this manner include phytate, oxalate, and citrate, and excesses of these substances in the diet may markedly reduce the absorption of calcium (57,93–95). Calcium, in the presence of a free fatty acid, forms an insoluble soap that cannot be absorbed (93,96). Disorders of the biliary or enteric tracts, associated with steatorrhea, are likely to reduce the absorption of calcium, because it forms an insoluble compound, and because ingested fat-soluble vitamin D is less likely to be absorbed under these circumstances (97).

Absorption of phosphorus occurs somewhat lower in the gastrointestinal tract than that of calcium, and probably requires some cellular action (57,62,98) (Fig. 7-7). The action, however, is not selective, and there is not much control exerted by the endogenous or exogenous systems, because most of the phosphorus presenting to the cell in the ionized form (mostly as $H_2PO_4^-$ or HPO_4^{2-}) is absorbed. Approximately 2 g of phosphorus is ingested daily by people on a normal diet; more than three-fourths of this amount is absorbed and eventually excreted in the urine. The only additional conditions in the gastrointestinal tract that exert

any influence on the absorption of phosphate are high concentrations of calcium and the presence of beryllium, an unusual enteric constituent, or aluminum, which is much more common because of the use of $Al(OH)_3$ in many antacid preparations (57,62,98). Aluminum phosphate is a relatively insoluble material, and its formation markedly reduces the rate of absorption of phosphate.

A balance diagram for calcium is shown in Fig. 7-6. The absorption of calcium from the gastrointestinal tract, reabsorption of calcium from the renal tubule, and bone–blood exchange are the three major components of the calcium control system. All are under control of the potent 1,25-dihydroxyvitamin D and PTH synergistic transport system. If calcium concentrations diminish (e.g., in a deficiency state for calcium or vitamin D), the response in the intact normal person is brisk and highly effective (Fig. 7-8). The decreased serum calcium level stimulates the production of PTH, which activates the synthesis of 1,25-dihydroxyvitamin D. Together, the two agents act to increase calcium absorption from the gut, tubular reabsorption of filtered calcium in the kidney, and resorption of bone. (Bone resorption occurs by lysis of the crystalline apatite and by osteoclastic resorption.) Any excess phosphate that appears as a result of the breakdown of bone is, under the influence of excess PTH, rapidly excreted by the kidney by means of a marked decrease in tubular reabsorption of phosphate. In this manner, short-term calcium deficits, even if profound, may be rapidly corrected by a highly effective balance system.

The system in humans that counteracts hypercalcemia is not nearly as efficient as the system that responds to hypocalcemia (Fig. 7-9). The principal mechanism of control is to turn off PTH action and vitamin D metabolism, but there is also a mechanism for decreasing serum calcium, which, at least in humans, is not very effective. The hormone calcitonin mediates this direct mechanism. In avian species, calcitonin is very potent in this role. In mammals,

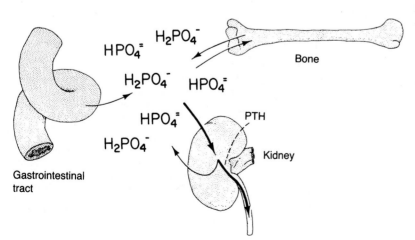

FIGURE 7-7. Diagrammatic representation of phosphate kinetics. Phosphate (*PO₄*) is absorbed lower in the gastrointestinal tract than calcium, and is freely transported across the gut cell to enter the extracellular space, in which it represents a major buffer system. Transport into and out of the bone is passive and related to the kinetics of the formation and breakdown of hydroxyapatite crystals. Tubular reabsorption of phosphate, however, is highly variable, with reabsorption ranging from almost 100% to less than 50%. The principal factor in decreasing tubular reabsorption of phosphate is parathyroid hormone (*PTH*).

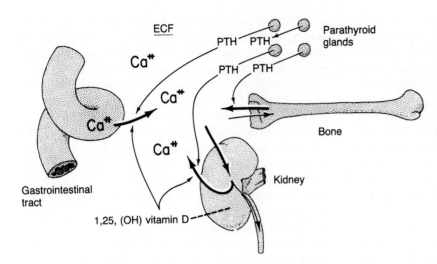

FIGURE 7-8. Calcium kinetics in the hypocalcemic state. A reduced concentration of calcium ion in the extracellular fluid (*ECF*) signals the parathyroid glands to release more of the potent hormone, which then acts at the level of the gut cell, renal tubule, and bone to increase transport of calcium and rapidly replenish the body fluids with calcium. An increase in parathyroid hormone (*PTH*) favors the synthesis of 1,25-dihydroxyvitamin D in the kidney and acts to promote phosphate diuresis by markedly diminishing the tubular reabsorption of phosphate.

calcitonin elicits only a limited response. Moreover, the autogenous calcitonin secreted by the C-cells of the thyroid gland is not adequate to counteract a significant calcium overload, acutely or chronically (59,63,99). If exogenous calcitonin is added (even from a different species), it may be effective in reducing hypercalcemia. This effect suggests that the calcitonin receptors, particularly on the bone cell, are operative, but that the autogenous supply or release under control of the response feedback loop is inadequate. The major action of either endogenous or exogenous calcitonin is at the level of bone. Numerous studies have demonstrated that calcitonin decreases the number of osteoclasts and the activity of the remaining osteoclasts (67,99,100). This action reduces the rate of bone breakdown. Such a reduction in bone breakdown seems to be precisely what is desired in Paget disease, and calcitonin has been used

extensively in the treatment of this disease. The actions of calcitonin on the enteric tract and the renal cell remain far less well defined.

Rickets and Osteomalacia

The earliest reports describing the syndrome of rickets appeared in the English literature around 1650, suggesting that the disease is an ancient one (101,102). The history of discovery of the causes of the disorder is a fascinating saga of medical detective work and should be reviewed by the interested reader (1,57,62).

Although there are numerous etiologic pathways, all the disease states grouped under the term "rickets" have as their pathogenic mechanism a relative decrease in calcium, phosphorus, or both, which is of such magnitude that it interferes

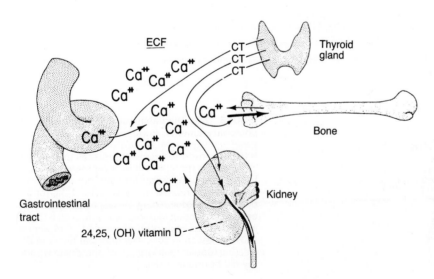

FIGURE 7-9. Calcium kinetics in the hypercalcemic state. Increased concentrations of calcium in the extracellular fluid (*ECF*) can cause release of calcitonin (*CT*) from the C-cells of the thyroid gland (the ultimobranchial body in avian species), which acts to diminish calcium concentration principally by stabilizing the osteoclast and decreasing its action on the bone. Hypercalcemia and a low concentration of parathyroid hormone act independently to diminish the synthesis of 1,25-dihydroxyvitamin D and decrease transport of calcium in the gut cell, tubule, and bone. The mechanism is not effective in humans.

with the processes of epiphyseal growth and normal mineralization of the skeleton of the growing child. The counterpart of these disorders in the adult, osteomalacia, lacks the factor of growth abnormality, but the effects on the bones are identical. When rickets or osteomalacia occurs in patients with chronic renal failure, it has additional features that affect the skeleton; it is then known as renal osteodystrophy.

Despite the rather extensive list of possible causes of rickets and osteomalacia, the clinical presentation, histologic abnormality, radiographic changes, and at least some of the chemical abnormalities are virtually identical. All patients with rickets show a striking similarity to one another, and the disease, regardless of cause, is stereotypical in presentation.

Clinical Manifestations of Rickets

Children with rickets are described as apathetic and irritable, often with a short attention span and seeming indifference. They are content to sit for long periods of time, and, as has been noted frequently in earlier texts, often assume a Buddha posture (103,104). The height of children with rickets is often under the third percentile, although their weight may be normal or higher than that of age-matched normal cohorts (105,106).

In younger children with florid disease, a rather remarkable constellation of characteristic signs may be demonstrated. Children with rickets show flattening of the skull, prominence of the frontal bones (i.e., frontal bossing), enlargement of the cartilaginous components of the suture lines (i.e., caput quadratum or hot-cross-bun skull), delayed dentition, enamel defects, and frequent and severe carious lesions in the teeth (107). Examination of the chest is likely to show enlargement of the costal cartilages (i.e., rachitic rosary), indentation of the lower ribs where the diaphragm inserts (i.e., Harrison's groove), and occasionally a pectus carinatum (103,107,108). Children often have respiratory infections, and, in earlier days, pneumonia was a common cause of morbidity and mortality.

The spine is commonly affected in the rachitic child, most characteristically with a long, smooth dorsal kyphosis, known as the rachitic cat back; occasionally, slight to moderate scoliosis of limited progression is seen. Abdominal distension is common (i.e., rachitic pot belly), and diarrhea and constipation have been described.

Children with florid rickets may have weak musculature of the abdomen (contributing to the pot-belly appearance) and of the extremities, which sometimes appear flaccid (109–111). Abductor weakness and a lurching gait are prominent features in some children who are walkers, and the onset of walking is often delayed.

The extremities are most profoundly affected in rickets, and cause the child to be brought to the orthopaedist. Ligamentous laxity is common. The long bones are often somewhat shortened and deformed, usually with bowing abnormalities in the lower extremities and varus deformities of the humeri and forearms. Because of the cupping and flaring of the epiphyseometaphyseal regions, the elbows, wrists, knees, and ankles appear enlarged on physical examination. Fractures are frequent. Slipped capital femoral epiphyses are rarely seen in vitamin D-deficient or vitamin D-resistant rickets, but are commonly seen in renal osteodystrophy (112–115). Mehls and colleagues believe that epiphyseal slippage in renal osteodystrophy results more from the associated hyperparathyroidism and metaphyseal resorption and failure than from the widening of the growth plate (115). This, together with the increasing availability of chronic dialysis while awaiting renal transplantation, increases the population at risk for epiphyseal slippage at the proximal femur and at other anatomic locations (116).

These changes are characteristic of children with severe and florid disease, usually caused by vitamin D deficiency. The changes are rarely seen in the United States today, but may be prevalent in other areas of the world (117–121). The findings usually are subtle and vague (122). The child with rickets is irritable and inattentive. He or she is short, has slightly thickened wrists or ankles, and possibly has bowing of one or both tibias. The diagnostic challenge is much greater with these limited findings.

Histologic Changes in Rickets

The osseous and epiphyseal changes in the rachitic skeleton are striking (107,123–126). The cortices are thinned and often show areas of increased resorption (107,127). The quantity of medullary bone is decreased, and the trabeculae are thin and irregularly shaped. The feature that most significantly helps to establish the diagnosis is the presence of a layer of unmineralized bone (osteoid seam) surrounding a mineralized segment (127–131) (Fig. 7-10). This failure to mineralize newly formed bone appears most prominently in the spicules of the medulla and can be highlighted by appropriate staining techniques (130). Although the finding is not pathognomonic (i.e., it also occurs in hyperparathyroidism, fibrous dysplasia, and some bone tumors), wide osteoid seams are characteristic of rickets and osteomalacia. Bone morphometricians can often establish the diagnosis with certainty on the basis of a properly studied iliac crest biopsy (114,127,128,132). Extensive focal collections of osteoid may be seen in specific locations of the skeleton that correspond to the Looser lines; this finding is pathognomonic of the disease (57,107).

Histologic alterations in the epiphyseal plate seen in rickets are equally striking and are diagnostic. With the exception of hypophosphatasia and, to a lesser extent, the milder forms of metaphyseal dysostosis (Schmid type), no other syndrome produces changes remotely resembling rickets. The resting and proliferative zones of the rachitic physeal plate are relatively normal in appearance, although some

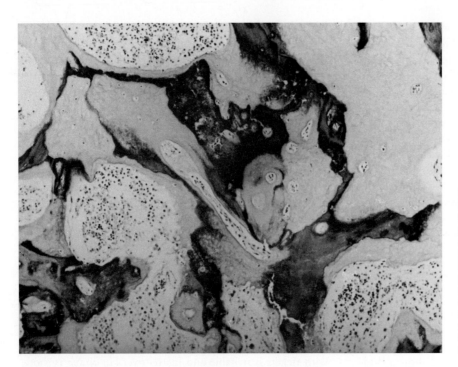

FIGURE 7-10. Histologic appearance of trabecular bone in a patient with rickets. The trabeculae are smaller than normal, but the striking feature is the presence of large masses of unmineralized osteoid surrounding central portions of irregularly mineralized bone. These osteoid seams are not pathognomonic, but when they are as wide as shown in this figure, they are diagnostic of rickets and osteomalacia. The darker-staining central portions of the bone are mineralized, and the lighter outer portions are osteoid. (von Kossa stain; 350× original magnification.)

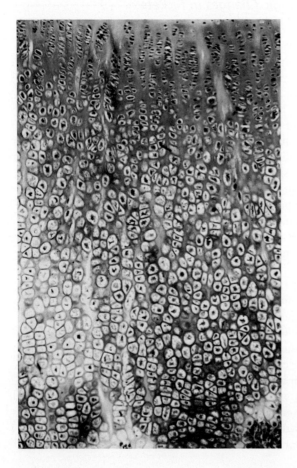

FIGURE 7-11. Histologic appearance of the epiphyseal plate in rickets. The resting and proliferative zones are relatively normal, but there is an extensive and pathognomonic alteration in the maturation zone, which shows a loss of columnization, a marked increase in the axial height of the zone, and a profligate profusion of the cells. The zone of provisional calcification is poorly calcified and irregular. (Safranin-O, fast green, iron hematoxylin stain; 100× original magnification.)

researchers have described a shortening of the columns in the region of the proliferative zone. The maturation zone, however, shows a gross distortion (Fig. 7-11). The normally orderly columnation is usurped by a disorderly increase in the hypertrophic zone, with only a small amount of intervening matrix (107,123,124). The plate is enlarged in its width, presumably because of the softening of the structure, with limited resistance to the mechanical forces acting on it, and, more characteristically, in its axial height, by as much as 5 to 15 times normal (107,123,133).

The zone of provisional calcification seen in patients with rickets is poorly defined, with only a few of the defective bars between the almost nonexistent columns of chondrocytes showing the deposition of mineral (125). Tongues of viable cartilage, without evidence of active endochondral replacement, descend far into the metaphyseal regions (134,135). The blood supply of the physes is altered. The zone of primary spongiosa shows only limited bone formation. The few spicules of bone that form are poorly mineralized or nonmineralized and have wide osteoid seams (107).

Radiographic Changes in Rickets

When the clinician has knowledge of the altered histology, it is simple to define the radiographic changes observed in children with rickets (136,137). The decreased bone mass of the skeletal system can be translated into osteopenia, with thin cortices and smaller trabeculae (62,138–140). However, the irregular mineralization of bone, which causes the histologic finding of osteoid seams, creates an indistinct image on radiographs, and the cortical and trabecular markings are often described as fuzzy or coarse and irregular (140–142). The appearance of the physis or growth plate, however, is the most remarkable feature and is virtually pathognomonic (138) (Figs. 7-12 and 7-13). The normally curvilinear, or almost transverse, well-defined line on radiography often shows irregular cupping and widening. In-

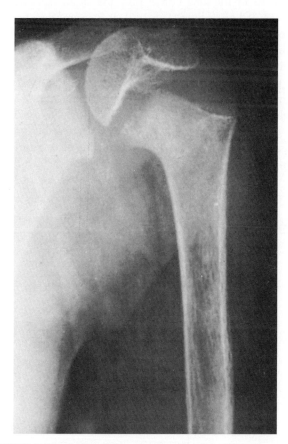

FIGURE 7-12. Radiographic appearance of rachitic changes in the humerus of an 11-year-old girl with florid vitamin D-resistant rickets. Notice the thin and indistinct cortices and the fuzzy, poorly defined trabeculae. The axial height of the epiphyseal plate is markedly increased, and the zone of provisional calcification is almost completely absent.

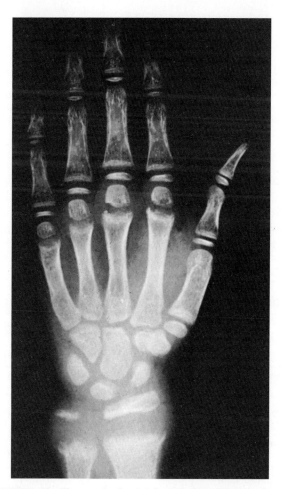

FIGURE 7-13. Changes in the epiphyseal plates of the wrist and hand are seen in this radiograph of an 8-year-old child with florid rickets. The distal radial and ulnar epiphyseal lines are markedly increased in axial height and show cupping; the zone of provisional calcification is absent. The changes in the slower-growing physes of the more distally placed bones are less marked, emphasizing the fact that rickets is a disease of the growing skeleton (in contrast to osteomalacia), and if the physeal regions grow slowly, the findings are much less prominent.

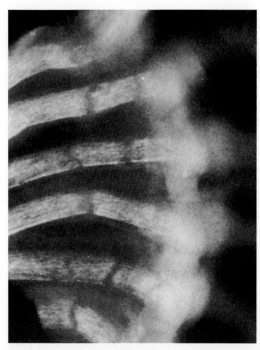

FIGURE 7-14. Looser lines seen in the rib cage of a child with florid rickets. These transverse radiolucent lines, which resemble incomplete fractures, are localized accumulations of osteoid of unknown cause. They are pathognomonic for rickets and osteomalacia.

the remainder of the bones, giving a washed-out appearance to the juxtaepiphyseal region (107,139,140,143).

In children with rickets, the most significant finding among the bone changes is the Looser lines, also known as umbauzonen or Milkman pseudofractures (Fig. 7-14). These localized collections of osteoid appear as ribbon-like linear radiolucent lines, transverse to the long axis of the bone, often not extending completely across the bone and preferring the concave sides of the long bones, medial femoral neck, ischial and pubic rami, ribs, clavicles, and axillary borders of the scapulas. Although not true fractures, the Looser lines represent areas of weakening of the bone and may become complete transverse fractures, sometimes with only minor trauma (144). Looser lines occur in 20% of patients with rickets of all types, but are more common in the vitamin D-resistant and renal osteodystrophic groups (143).

Radiographic changes in patients with florid rickets are extensive and virtually unmistakable. However, in mild cases, there may be minimal or no changes, which makes the diagnosis more difficult. Bone scanning is sometimes helpful, because there may be patchy increased activity over the shafts of the long bones, ribs, and skull, especially at the sites of Looser lines (145,146). It is appropriate first to order laboratory tests for calcium, phosphorus, and alkaline phosphatase in suspected metabolic bone disease. After obtaining the history and performing a physical examination, the physician customarily orders radiographs and analysis of the serum calcium, phosphorus, and alkaline phosphatase levels. Although changes may be subtle, this approach usually detects an abnormality (Table 7-3) that establishes the diagnosis or merits proceeding with further testing and obtaining appropriate consultation.

variably, the axial height of the line is markedly increased (1,62,138). The zone of provisional calcification, which is ordinarily a thin, dense, white line on the radiograph, appears indistinct or is absent (136,140). The primary spongiosa of the metaphysis is often even more osteopenic than

TABLE 7-3. CHEMICAL FINDINGS IN VARIOUS FORMS OF RICKETS

Type of Rickets	Serum						Urine		Miscellaneous Serum and Urine Values
	Ca^{2+}	P	Alk Phos	PTH	25(OH) Vit D	1,25(OH)₂ Vit D	% TRP	Ca^{2+}	
Vitamin D-deficient rickets	↓ or →	↓	↑	↑	↓	↓	↑	↓	
Dietary phosphate deficiency	→	↓	↑	→	→	→	→	→	
Gastrointestinal rickets	↓	↓	↑	↑	↓	↓ or →	↓	↓	↓ Absorption from gastrointestinal tract
Vitamin D-resistant rickets									Amino acids, sugar, water, base in urine
Phosphate diabetes	→	↓↓		→	→	→	↓↓	→	
Reduced 1,25-dihydroxyvitamin D production	↓	↓	↑	↑	→	↓↓	↓	↓	
End-organ insensitivity	↓	↓	↑	↑	↑ or →	↑ or →	↓	↓	
Renal tubular acidosis	↓	↓	↑	↑	↑ or →	↑ or →	↓	↑	Na ↓, K ↓, Cl ↑; acidosis alkaline urine
Renal osteodystrophy	↓	↑	↑	↑↑	↓↓	↓↓	?	↓↓	BUN ↑

↑, increased; ↓, decreased; →, unchanged or normal; *Alk Phos*, alkaline phosphatase; *BUN*, blood urea nitrogen; *Ca*, calcium; *Cl*, chloride; *K*, potassium; *Na*, sodium; *P*, phosphate; *PTH*, parathyroid hormone; *TRP*, tubular reabsorption of phosphate; *Vit D*, vitamin D forms.

TABLE 7-4. CAUSES OF RICKETS AND OSTEOMALACIA

Deficiency diseases
  Vitamin D deficiency
  Chelators in the diet
  Phosphorus deficiency

Gastrointestinal disorders
  Gastric rickets
  Hepatobiliary disease
  Enteric disorders

Vitamin D-resistant rickets (acquired or genetic)
  Phosphate diabetes
  Decrease in 1,25-dihydroxyvitamin D production
  End-organ insensitivity
  Renal tubular acidosis

Unusual forms of rickets
  Rickets with fibrous dysplasia
  Rickets with neurofibromatosis
  Rickets with soft tissue and bone tumors
  Rickets with anticonvulsant medication

Renal osteodystrophy

Causes of Rickets

Numerous factors are involved in the pathogenesis of rickets (Table 7-4). The symptoms, physical findings, and radiographic alterations rarely provide clues to the cause of the disease, with the exception of renal osteodystrophy. Most patients present for evaluation with a remarkably stereotypical pattern.

In general, changes associated with nutritional rickets appear earlier and are milder that those seen with vitamin D-resistant disease (122). Changes occurring with gastrointestinal disease often are consistent with the stigmata of those disorders. Patients with chronic renal disease have findings consistent with severe secondary hyperparathyroidism and may radiographically display ectopic calcification, ossification, and occasionally osteosclerosis. To understand the manifestations of the different types of rickets and how to differentiate them and how to plan treatment, it is essential to consider their pathogenesis.

Deficiency rickets primarily include vitamin D-deficient rickets, possibly chronic calcium deficiency (147), phosphate deficiency (107) (a rare cause), and the presence of chelators in the diet (57,62,128,148,149). All forms are rare in the United States, except in children subjected to highly atypical diets (150–152) or in infants born prematurely (48,131,153–156). The model for the pathogenesis of deficiency rickets (except rickets resulting from primary hypophosphatemia) is shown in Fig. 7-15 (62). The patient's intake of vitamin D is inadequate, and an insufficient quantity of 1,25-dihydroxyvitamin D is synthesized by the kidney. The result is diminished absorption of calcium from the gastrointestinal tract and resultant hypocalcemia, which promotes the release of PTH. Release of PTH partially restores the serum calcium to normal, but causes a marked

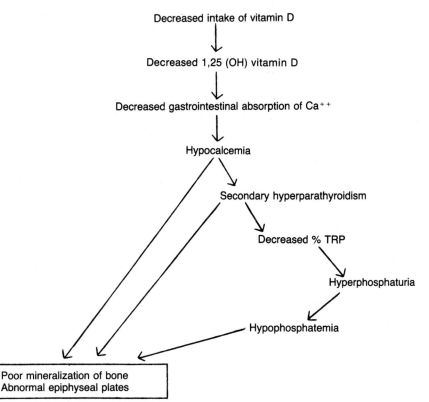

FIGURE 7-15. Mechanism of development of vitamin D-deficient rickets. A diminished intake of vitamin D causes a decreased synthesis of the potent 1,25-dihydroxyvitamin D, which causes a reduction in the absorption of calcium from the gastrointestinal tract. This progression leads to hypocalcemia, which causes a secondary hyperparathyroidism, and a reduced tubular reabsorption of phosphate (*TRP*), which decreases the serum phosphate. The reduced concentrations of calcium and phosphorus and the secondary hyperparathyroidism cause the clinical, histologic, and radiographic manifestations of rickets and osteomalacia.

decrease in phosphate reabsorption in the kidney. The combination of low serum calcium, mild secondary hyperparathyroidism, and hypophosphatemia produces the syndrome of classic or vitamin D-deficient rickets. Children with this disorder usually show low to low-normal serum calcium levels, low serum levels of phosphorus, elevated levels of serum alkaline phosphatase, elevated PTH levels, low concentrations of 25-hydroxyvitamin D and 1,25-dihydroxyvitamin D, diminished levels of urinary calcium, and markedly diminished tubular reabsorption of phosphate (Table 7-3) (1,57,62,157–159).

Gastrointestinal Rickets. Gastrointestinal causes of rickets are more common in most settings in the United States today than those associated with deficiency states. Gastric rickets, an unusual sequel to ulcer surgery and the dumping syndrome, is rare in children, but hepatic and small bowel problems are considerably more common, and probably account for most of the acquired forms of the disease seen in pediatric practice (160–162). The hepatic causes are principally disorders in which there is an obstructive jaundice or a significant interference with the production of bile salts (163,164). Without the emulsification action of these salts, fat accumulates in the feces and causes a significant interference with the absorption of fat-soluble vitamin D and, if free fatty acids are present, with the precipitation of the ingested calcium ions as insoluble soaps (165,166). In addition, if sufficient hepatic damage is present, synthesis of 25-hydroxyvitamin D is reduced (55,167,168).

In the enteric forms of rickets, injury to the gut wall, caused by such disorders as the malabsorption syndrome (164,169), gluten-sensitive enteropathy (170,171), Crohn's disease, chronic ulcerative colitis, sarcoidosis, and tuberculosis, and by surgical bypass procedures (62,98,164, 172,173), decreases the rate of absorption of both vitamin D and calcium. If the factors of steatorrhea and rapid transit are added, there may be a profound decrease in the extracellular compartment of calcium and the development of mild to moderately severe rickets (157,174). The mechanism by which these disorders produce rickets is not unlike that shown in Fig. 7-15 for classic vitamin D-deficiency disease, except that the causes of the decrease in gastrointestinal absorption of calcium are those just cited. Beyond that level, the disorder progresses in a manner similar to that shown in the illustration. Chemically, the patients are found to be hypocalcemic, hypophosphatemic, hyperphosphatasic, and hypocalciuric, and they demonstrate elevated levels of PTH and variable concentrations of 25-hydroxyvitamin D and 1,25-dihydroxyvitamin D (depending on the amount of interference with the absorption of the vitamin) (175). These patients commonly have test results that show altered hepatic function and diminished absorptive capacity by the gut wall, and abnormalities are discovered on endoscopic and imaging studies designed to elucidate the nature of the disease process in the small bowel (Table 7-4).

Vitamin D-resistant Rickets. Vitamin D-resistant rickets may be acquired or genetic in origin, and have a rather wide distribution of patterns, many of which are eponymically and, less commonly, biochemically distinct (1,57, 62,96,108,152,176–188). Historically, patients with these diseases were first differentiated on the basis of their resistance to the ordinary treatment doses of vitamin D, and were found to have abnormal urinary excretory patterns for phosphate, sugar, amino acids, water, fixed base, bicarbonate, and some unusual materials, such as ketone bodies (i.e., Lowe syndrome) and glycine (i.e., superglycine syndrome) (186,189,190). Others were found to have deposition of crystals of cystine in the liver, bone marrow, and anterior chamber of the eye (i.e., Lignac-Fanconi syndrome) (177,191), or the presence of pure renal tubular acidosis (Butler-Albright syndrome) (192–195). Although it is historically correct and sometimes valuable to categorize vitamin D–resistant rickets in this way, there are only four basic pathogenic mechanisms operative, and all the syndromes result from one (or sometimes two) of these mechanisms (196,197). Grouping the syndromes according to pathogenic mechanisms is a much sounder system, because it better directs the plan of treatment.

There are four types of vitamin D-resistant rickets: phosphate diabetes (i.e., failure of the reabsorptive mechanism for phosphate); failure of production of 1,25-dihydroxyvitamin D (i.e., vitamin D-dependent rickets); end-organ insensitivity to 1,25-dihydroxyvitamin D; and renal tubular acidosis.

In patients with phosphate diabetes, the defect principally lies in the renal tubule and is characterized by a failure to resorb phosphate filtered by the glomerulus (108, 128,197). Although there may be other resorptive defects for glucose (1,183,185,190), amino acids (182, 183,198), or even water and fixed base (1,199) and an impairment of vitamin D synthesis in some cases (197), the main cause of rachitic disease is probably hyperphosphaturia and profound hypophosphatemia (197,200). After examining the mechanism for vitamin D-deficient rickets (Fig. 7-15), it should be apparent that children with phosphate diabetes rickets absorb vitamin D normally, make an adequate amount of 1,25-dihydroxyvitamin D, absorb calcium normally from the gastrointestinal tract, and have no mild secondary hyperparathyroidism. However, they become rachitic because of a vast decrease in phosphate available for mineralization of the skeleton (201). The same mechanism is operative in the rare patient who develops a dietary hypophosphatemia. The chemical findings in this group of patients are unique in that the calcium, PTH, 25-hydroxyvitamin D, and 1,25-dihydroxyvitamin D levels are often normal or only slightly decreased, but the serum level of inorganic phosphate is markedly reduced and the rate of tubular reabsorption of phosphate is often less than 50% (1,108,202) (Table 7-3). Treatment of this group of patients with excessive amounts of vitamin D is of little value, and, to achieve even a partial cure, fairly large doses of neutral phosphate must be added to the diet often (203–207).

Patients who synthesize inadequate amounts of the potent 1,25-dihydroxyvitamin D are similarly resistant to standard doses of the vitamin, because they are less able to convert 25-hydroxyvitamin D to 1,25-dihydroxyvitamin D (208,209) (Fig. 7-15). Biochemically, they show all the manifestations of the vitamin D-deficient group, except that their 25-hydroxyvitamin D levels may be normal, but their concentrations of 1,25-dihydroxyvitamin D are remarkably diminished (208) (Table 7-3). Treatment of this group is best achieved by the addition of exogenous 1,25-dihydroxyvitamin D, which, if the syndrome has been diagnosed correctly, should be curative (209–212).

Patients who have end-organ insensitivity are similar to patients in the second group, because they ingest adequate amounts of vitamin D, but, instead of a block to synthesis, they produce both polar metabolites, 25-hydroxyvitamin D and 1,25-dihydroxyvitamin D, in ample quantities. The problem appears to lie with the gut cell, which displays a relative insensitivity to autogenous 1,25-dihydroxyvitamin D (142,213). Despite adequate amounts of the active D vitamins, the gut cell is unable to synthesize the transport system, and the movement of calcium is sharply reduced. These patients develop hypocalcemia, secondary hyperparathyroidism, hypophosphatemia, reduced urinary calcium, and reduced tubular reabsorption of phosphate, but the values for 25-hydroxyvitamin D and 1,25-dihydroxyvitamin D are normal or, in many cases, elevated (213) (Table 7-3). Management of patients with end-organ insensitivity is difficult. In some patients, the insensitivity is relatively mild, and can be overcome by increased amounts of exogenous 1,25-dihydroxyvitamin D (still less than the level of toxicity) (213). In other patients, calcium infusions may present a temporary solution, but obviously have limited application in long-term management (214).

The fourth form of vitamin D-resistant rickets, renal tubular acidosis, is a misnomer, because it is not directly related to vitamin D, but is due to an acquired or genetic error in renal handling of fixed base and bicarbonate (192,195,215–217). In one form, the kidney is unable to establish a hydrogen ion gradient, and therefore must excrete fixed base, including sodium and calcium (193). In another form, the failure of the tubule to resorb bicarbonate causes a loss of fixed base as a cation (193). Regardless of cause, the patient develops renal tubular acidosis, characterized chemically by a hyperchloremic, hyponatremic, and hypokalemic acidosis with an alkaline urine (193–195, 218–220) (Table 7-3). In many patients with a broader lesion, resorption of phosphate is also impaired, heightening the degree of metabolic bone disease. In some patients, because of the increased movement of calcium through the collecting system at an alkaline pH (and failure of citrate production), renal calcinosis can be severe and can lead to renal failure (1,62,92,218,221).

Because of the pathogenesis of these syndromes, the use of vitamin D in other than low doses is usually contraindicated. The treatment of choice is correction of the metabolic abnormality by alkalinization. For most patients, this rectifies the metabolic disturbance (219,222).

Unusual Forms of Rickets. Several unusual forms of rickets deserve attention. Three are certain types of vitamin D-resistant rickets and are defined in terms of the disease state and the associated syndrome. For example, severe rickets may be a concomitant finding in patients with neurofibromatosis (1,223,224) or fibrous dysplasia (225–229). Rickets may also occur in certain patients with benign or even low-grade malignant soft tissue tumors or, less frequently, with bone tumors of the fibrous series (230–233). Production of an antivitamin D factor or a phosphaturic agent by the lesion has been postulated, primarily on the basis of the almost immediate reversal of the metabolic and radiographic alteration with resection of the tumor (234) (and the prompt return of the metabolic problem with recurrence of the lesion). A report partially characterizing such a factor has been made (235). The occurrence of hypercalcemia in association with malignancy is discussed in a later section. Its cause has been linked in some cases to the systemic release of an agent related to PTH, parathyroid-related protein. A section describing parathyroid-related protein and its role in metabolic bone disease is included at the end of this section on the entities with pathophysiology primarily in the mineral phase.

Another unusual form is rickets associated with anticonvulsant medication. Patients who receive almost any anticonvulsant medication may develop mild chemical (and occasionally osseous) rickets (111,138,236–242). Although the disorder is reversible with administration of vitamin D, it represents a major problem, partly because it is difficult to diagnose by standard means and, more important, because the irritability of the central nervous system is inversely proportional to calcium ion concentration (i.e., second principle) (243,244). As the concentration of calcium decreases in relation to the use of anticonvulsant medication, the patient may not respond to medication, and may experience more convulsions. The biochemical defect in these patients appears to result from a mild injury to the hepatic cell, which alters the microsomal enzyme system sufficiently to decrease the concentration of 25-hydroxyvitamin D (201,240,242,245). Diagnosis is based on the findings of classic vitamin D deficiency in a child who is receiving anticonvulsant medication. The concentrations of 25-hydroxyvitamin D are usually sharply reduced. The goal of treatment is to increase vitamin D and, if possible, to reduce the levels of the anticonvulsant drugs (246). The relation between the administration of anticonvulsant medication and the occurrence of rickets, in an otherwise healthy population, may not be a simple one (247).

Renal Osteodystrophy

The constellation of clinical problems associated with chronic renal failure affect most of the organ systems and produce moderate to severe impairment of these systems. The skeletal system shares in these disabilities to an extraordinary degree. It is affected by the problems associated with the chronic debilitating illness itself (e.g., osteoporosis, osteomyelitis, gout, and disturbances in calcium and phosphorus homeostasis) and the problems associated with attempts at management (e.g., corticosteroid-induced osteoporosis, osteonecrosis, dialysis osteomalacia, arthropathy). This constellation of problems is subsumed under the term "renal osteodystrophy" (248,249).

In the years that preceded the period of aggressive therapy of chronic renal disease, the prognosis for survival of patients with renal failure was so poor that the osseous manifestations were considered a medical curiosity, worthy only of emergency treatment for fractures and other acute changes, but of little importance to the overall picture. This pattern has changed radically. With dialysis systems and renal transplantation, patients with chronic renal disease can live considerably longer, and can be expected to participate in activities that require a competent skeleton. Management of the whole patient now demands careful attention to the problems of the skeletal system and a thorough understanding of their pathogenesis (250,251).

Pathophysiology.   The pathophysiologic events that lead to the syndrome of renal osteodystrophy are illustrated in Fig. 7-16. Damage to the glomerulus causes retention of phosphate, producing hyperphosphatemia (57,252). Concomitant tubular injury leads to a reduction in the production of 1,25-dihydroxyvitamin D (1,55,253–256). Hyperphosphatemic suppression of 1,25-dihydroxyvitamin D synthesis and reduced tubular mass conspire to offer only a small fraction of the potent principle to the gut cell (257). The

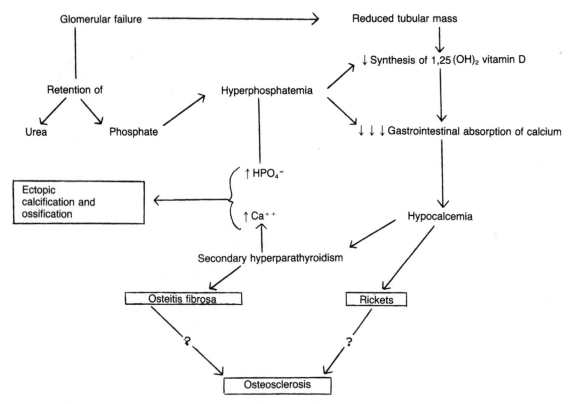

FIGURE 7-16. Mechanism of development of the chemical and bony changes in renal osteodystrophy. Reduced renal function and glomerular failure cause retention of urea and phosphate, leading to hyperphosphatemia, which, along with a reduction in tubular mass, causes a profound reduction in the synthesis of 1,25-dihydroxyvitamin D. This condition, plus the direct effect of increased concentrations of phosphate in the serum, reduces the gastrointestinal absorption of calcium and causes a profound hypocalcemia and severe secondary hyperparathyroidism. These changes produce the clinical syndromes of rickets and osteitis fibrosa. For unknown reasons, 20% of patients with this combination of chemical abnormalities also have an osteosclerosis. Because the phosphate concentration is chronically increased, an occasional increment in the serum calcium level can lead to rapid ectopic calcification and ossification in the conjunctivae, skin, blood vessels, and periarticular regions.

increased concentration of phosphate in the cytosol reduces the absorption of calcium to virtually zero. Balance studies have shown that more calcium is excreted in the feces than is ingested in the diet, suggesting intestinal secretion of the mineral. All these factors conspire to produce a profound hypocalcemia (253,258–264).

If it were not for the acidosis characteristic of chronic renal disease, which makes more soluble the small quantity of available calcium salts, the level of calcium in the serum would lead to severe neural, motor, and cardiac disorders in many patients. The negative feedback system that causes elaboration of PTH in response to decreases in serum calcium is unimpaired by chronic renal failure, and, within a short period of time, marked secondary hyperparathyroidism occurs, usually in the form of a clear-cell hyperplasia of all four glands (1,198,256,265,266). The increased elaboration of PTH is ineffective in increasing gastrointestinal absorption or renal tubular reabsorption, because of the absence of vitamin D and the presence of increased phosphate. The principal action of the increased PTH is on the skeleton (107). The syndrome that occurs includes rickets (associated with the reduced concentration of calcium in the body fluids) and osteitis fibrosa, a severe lysis of the skeleton from overproduction of PTH (107,256,267).

For reasons not fully understood, 20% of patients with renal osteodystrophy also show osteosclerosis, most frequently in the spine, but sometimes affecting the long bones as well, which is characterized histologically by an increase in the numbers of trabeculae, rather than an increased mineral accretion in the osteoid of the rachitic bone or repair of the destructive lesions associated with chronic hyperparathyroidism (268–272).

Patients with chronic renal disease are hyperphosphatemic, and even when there is reduced pH, which shifts the solubility product, they depend on a decreased serum calcium to avoid precipitation of the relatively insoluble $CaHPO_4$. If for any reason, such as spontaneous improvement, dietary indiscretions, or dialysis factors, calcium increases to near-normal levels, then calcium salts may be precipitated in a variety of ectopic sites. The principal findings in this unfortunate group of patients depend on the sites of deposition of the salts, but calcification or ossification of the corneas and conjunctivae (red eyes of renal failure) (273–277), skin, muscular coats of the major arteries and arterioles (249,278–281), and periarticular soft tissues is the typical pattern encountered (276,280).

The four pathophysiologic entities—rickets-osteomalacia, osteitis fibrosa (secondary hyperparathyroidism), osteosclerosis, and ectopic calcification/ossification—constitute the syndrome of renal osteodystrophy (282). Frequently associated with this syndrome are the side effects of treatment (e.g., dialysis, steroid treatment), infections, and pathologic fractures.

The pediatric patient with renal osteodystrophy is almost always shorter than his or her peers, and is slow in reaching milestones and exhibiting age-related phenomena, such as appearance of secondary centers of ossification or signs of sexual maturation (283). Older terms for the disorder, such as renal infantilism or renal nanism, are reflections of this retardation, which is considerably more marked in these patients than in patients with rickets of other causes.

Clinical Manifestations. The patient with chronic renal failure may show all the features of rickets and exhibit bone tenderness and skeletal fragility (107,256,263,283,284). Fractures occur frequently with minor trauma and are very disabling. The presence of calcification in the conjunctivae and skin can produce significant irritation and itching. The periarticular calcification and ossification can cause severe limitation and pain in one or several joints (Fig. 7-17). The gait is disturbed, sometimes because of rickets-associated ligamentous laxity and muscular weakness, and because of slipped femoral epiphyses that can occur from alterations in the mechanics and physiology of the proximal femurs (112,113,115,130) (Fig. 7-18). Slippage of epiphyses at other anatomic sites has been described (115,116). The profound hyperparathyroidism seen in renal osteodystrophy and the consequent resorption of metaphyseal regions, combined with the chronicity of this entity because of modern medical management, provide the basis for the common occurrence of slipped epiphyses (115). Although hyperparathyroidism does exist with vitamin D-deficient or vitamin D-resistant rickets, it is less profound in patients with these entities than in patients with renal osteodystrophy. Moreover, the time for medical correction of these conditions is

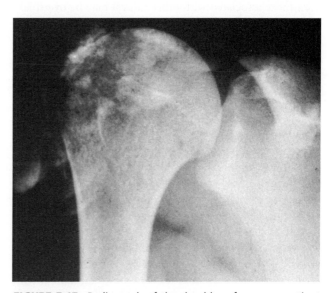

FIGURE 7-17. Radiograph of the shoulder of a young patient with renal osteodystrophy shows extensive calcification in the deltoid muscle, which has caused severe limitation of movement. Because of the radiographic projection, most of the calcification projects over the humeral head.

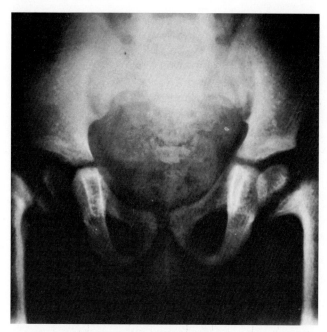

FIGURE 7-18. Renal osteodystrophic changes on a radiograph of the pelvis of a 12-year-old child. Notice the bony changes, suggestive of osteomalacia, and the marked abnormalities of the epiphyseal line, with increased axial height, cupping, and loss of sharp definition of the zone of provisional calcification. Epiphysiolysis also is present. This finding is not commonly seen with vitamin D-deficient or vitamin D-resistant rickets, but occurs frequently with renal osteodystrophy.

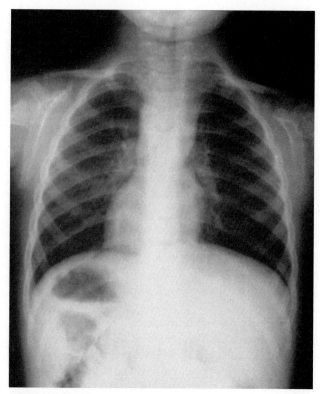

FIGURE 7-19. The radiographic changes of hyperparathyroidism are seen in this patient with renal osteodystrophy. Notice the resorption at the distal ends of the clavicles.

relatively short, and slipped epiphyses are rarely seen in vitamin D-deficient or vitamin D-resistant rickets.

The radiographic changes seen in renal dystrophy are also unique in that the findings of rickets (indistinguishable from those associated with other causes) may be overshadowed by the changes of osteitis fibrosa (268,269,272, 283–287). "Salt-and-pepper" skull, absence of the lamina dura on dental films, loss of the cortical outline of the outer centimeter of the clavicles (288,289), subperiosteal resorption of the ulnas (290) and terminal tufts of the distal phalanges (291–293), and rarefaction and subperiosteal resorption of the medial proximal tibias may dominate the picture (293,294) (Fig. 7-19).

In severe and long-standing cases of renal osteodystrophy, brown tumors, large oval or round rarefactions with indistinct margins, which sometimes thin and expand the cortex and provide the sites of pathologic fractures, may be present in the pelvis or long bones (Fig. 7-20). These may suggest to the unwary examiner the presence of a primary bone tumor or metastatic disease, such as lymphoma or leukemia (107). Areas of sclerosis are occasionally seen next to the areas of rarefaction. This is most common in the spine, in which the alternating areas look like the stripes of a rugby jersey, but a similar pattern is seen occasionally in the long bones. Ectopic calcification and ossification are frequently noted on routine radiographs and, particularly

in the pediatric age group, are helpful in establishing the diagnosis.

The biochemical alterations in patients with chronic renal disease and osteodystrophy clearly reflect the general state of the disturbances in both renal and osseous physiology. Blood urea nitrogen (BUN), creatinine, and uric acid levels are elevated, and acidosis and hypoalbuminemia usually are detected. The calcium concentration is almost invariably low (usually less than 8.0 mg per dL), and the serum inorganic phosphate level is elevated (greater than 5 mg per dL). The alkaline phosphatase and PTH levels are increased commensurate with the extent of the disease. Concentrations of 25-hydroxyvitamin D and 1,25-dihydroxyvitamin D are always diminished, and urinary calcium is low, although fecal calcium is increased (Table 7-3).

Management

The orthopaedist's role in the diagnosis and treatment of the many disorders associated with rickets and renal osteodystrophy has shifted considerably with the understanding of the basic science of these entities. Pediatric orthopaedic surgeons and pediatricians continue to be the principal diagnosticians dealing with children who have findings suggestive of rachitic disease. The various forms of rickets should

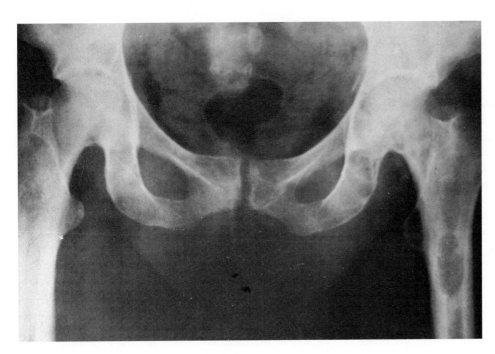

FIGURE 7-20. Radiograph of the pelvis of a patient with renal osteodystrophy shows the marked changes of secondary hyperparathyroidism. Several brown tumors are seen in the femoral shafts and ischial rami. These appear as expanded destructive lesions, resembling primary or metastatic bone tumors.

continue to be important elements of the differential diagnosis in children who present for evaluation with a bowed extremity, repeated fractures, abnormalities of the spine, gait disturbances, diminished height, and failure to thrive. Radiography, radionuclide imaging, and measurements of BUN, creatinine, calcium, phosphorus, alkaline phosphatase, 25-hydroxyvitamin D, 1,25-dihydroxyvitamin D, PTH, and a variety of urinary measurements, also including calcium, are invaluable aids in establishing the diagnosis of rickets and in categorizing according to precise cause. The physician begins with a history and physical examination. Radiographs of the knee, including the most active growth plates in the body, the distal femoral and proximal tibial physes, are useful as a screen. Serum calcium, phosphorus, and alkaline phosphatase levels are customarily measured as part of this initial evaluation. Additional radiographic studies, and the chemical studies suggested in Table 7-3, may then be pursued to a diagnosis. If the pediatric orthopaedist is making the diagnosis, communication with the primary pediatrician is then appropriate, after which further consultation may be obtained with specialists in pediatric nephrology or gastroenterology.

Determination of the change in skeletal morphology associated with metabolic bone disease is guided by general principles, and is designed specifically to address the pathophysiology of the subcategory of illness and the needs of the individual patient. Management of the underlying metabolic disturbance is always the necessary first step, because it alone may be curative, the general health status of the individual depends on it, and orthopaedic intervention without it will prove disappointing. However, will manage-

ment of the metabolic disturbance alone be sufficient to address the skeletal abnormality? Generally, the extent of remodeling that is likely to occur depends on the growth remaining after correction of the abnormal physiology. There are no definitive data about the change in morphology with bracing. Because of the wider experience with children's fractures, remodeling in this setting tends to be appreciated under the heading of clinical judgment. The problem in metabolic bone disease in childhood is more complicated. The underlying pathophysiology may be improved, but not actually rendered normal; growth, the basis for remodeling, may itself be abnormal; and the biomechanical properties of the bone may be particularly adversely affected when the child is most ill, making fixation difficult if operative intervention is undertaken. Every clinical situation requires individual analysis.

In its various forms, rickets tends to manifest in infancy or early childhood. The pediatrician, pediatric endocrinologist, nephrologist, or gastroenterologist addresses the altered physiology with the use of agents such as vitamin D, 1,25-dihydroxyvitamin D, calcium infusions, neutral phosphate solutions, and other dietary and pharmacologic interventions. It is usually possible to achieve a cure in many rickets patients, with expectations of normal growth and lifestyle (250). In fractures and rickets in very low birth weight infants, improved enteral intake is the major intervention, with orthopaedic intervention largely a matter of occasional splinting and observation (295). Similarly, deficiency rickets, gastrointestinal rickets, and vitamin D-resistant rickets in infancy or early childhood usually respond to the correction of the metabolic abnormality. However, remodeling of skeletal deformity, even in childhood rickets, is not necessarily universal, and intervention may be required, particularly in vitamin D-resistant rickets (206,296). Fractures in childhood require appropriate management. Vigilance for uncommon subsequent physeal disturbances is still appropriate. In the multiple-handicapped patient during adolescence, the existence of vitamin D deficiency as the basis of underlying fractures needs to be considered (297).

Angular and rotatory deformities of the lower extremities in metabolic bone disease need to be interpreted from a perspective of natural history. Salenius and Vankka (298) described the physiologic development of the tibiofemoral angle, starting at 15 degrees of varus at birth, becoming neutral at 18 months of age, then proceeding to valgus of approximately 10 degrees, and achieving physiologic valgus at 7 years of age. This general progression is associated with an internal tibial torsion that also tends to change to an external torsion during early childhood (299). The extant alignment at the time of occurrence of the metabolic bone disease is usually accentuated (300). Rickets occurring within the first year of life usually leads to a pronounced genu varum and internal tibial torsion. With correction of the metabolic abnormality, return to the pattern described by Salenius and Vankka is anticipated. If this is not the case, coordination of care between the pediatric orthopaedic surgeon and the physician making the metabolic adjustments is important to ensure that metabolic response is appropriate. After that is ascertained, the issue of bracing arises.

The use of bracing, presumably using the Hueter-Volkmann principle intelligently, to change the morphology of the skeleton usually generates some controversy. For physiologic alignment changes, there is little need to brace, and what in the past had been interpreted as a response to brace treatment is generally regarded as the progress of normal development (298,299). For metabolic problems, the pediatric orthopaedist can observe for some relatively arbitrary period. If the malalignment fails to improve in the face of metabolic correction, bracing to counteract the deformity should be considered. Although uncommon in rickets, refractory cases may require surgery (301). Full-length standing radiographs in anteroposterior and lateral planes are essential to establish the deviations in the mechanical axis (302). The sites of the deviations can be established, and the plan for osteotomy or osteotomies can be devised with tracings. In early childhood rickets, fixation that does not affect the growth plates is particularly important [➥6.1–6.6]. Plates have been advocated (301). Before using plates, the osseous tissue quality must be corrected by metabolic intervention, or there is a tendency for the screws to lose purchase. Intramedullary fixation is generally easier to use when there are multiple deviations in the mechanical axis necessitating multiple osteotomies and/or the quality of the osseous tissue cannot be rendered normal, such as in osteogenesis imperfecta and some types of rickets [➥4.11,6.7] (303).

Management of renal osteodystrophy is more complicated and involves management of the primary disorder by dialysis or renal transplantation and control of the calcium and phosphate levels by appropriate drug treatment and infusions (155,304). Occasionally, parathyroidectomy is necessary to control the hyperparathyroidism, particularly in patients with tertiary hyperparathyroidism (304,305). Administration of vitamin D must be carried out with considerable care to avoid the complications of ectopic ossification and calcification (256). Intravenous infusion of 1,25-dihydroxyvitamin D has been advocated in some refractory cases of osteitis fibrosa (306).

As with rickets, the orthopaedic manifestations include fractures, growth disturbances, and angular malalignments. Only some of these resolve with improvement in metabolic status (251). Site-specific fracture management is important. The incidence of fractures should decrease with correction of the metabolic disturbances. Slipped epiphyses are common in renal osteodystrophy at the proximal femur, distal femur, distal tibia, and forearm (115,116,251). Correction of the metabolic status is always the first step to restore the overall physiologic status of the patient and improve the quality of the bone. At sites other than the proximal femur, some period of observation is logical for the remodeling considerations discussed previously, and subsequent corrective osteotomy is performed if remodeling is not occurring. Slipped capital femoral epiphysis in renal osteodystrophy is perhaps more controversial. Although some of the general principles governing idiopathic slipped capital femoral epiphyses also apply, the questions of fixation and bilaterality have led to different approaches (307). Because these slips in renal osteodystrophy can occur in patients younger than 10 years of age, methods of fixation that might allow growth, rather than promoting growth plate closure, at least merit consideration (308). In adolescence, after correction of metabolism, fixation to promote growth plate closure can be performed [➥3.14] (251,309). Concerns have been noted that with metabolic bone problems fixation to achieve growth plate closure may be difficult. Presumably, the purchase of a screw on the weakened bone of the secondary center of ossification and the metaphysis can be overcome by the distractive force of the growth plate. The use of a bone peg to transgress the growth plate and promote ossification has been advocated in such situations, but it is not the only approach (310).

The mechanism of growth disturbance is not completely defined. In addition to the overall physiologic status of the patient, disturbance in the growth factor control of physes has been implicated. Somatomedin disturbance and disturbance in the bone morphogenetic proteins and osteogenic proteins may also occur (311). Because the major production site of one of the osteogenic proteins is the kidneys, renal failure could interfere with its production. The problem of growth disturbance in renal osteodystrophy, even after treatment with transplantation, has yet to be solved.

Because renal osteodystrophy tends to occur in later

childhood, and because there is a physiologic valgus at that point in development, genu valgum is frequently encountered and may persist even after metabolic abnormalities are corrected (251). The principles applied in genu varum can be applied in this condition. Observation during the period of medical management is prudent. Failure to improve over months, in the face of medical improvement, should prompt consideration of bracing. Persistence is appropriately treated surgically. The deviations in the mechanical axis are established with full-length radiographs (302). Valgus occurring through the distal femur is common in renal osteodystrophy and may be treated with stapling toward the end of growth. The amount of overgrowth from the lateral aspect of the growth plate required for correction may be determined from the Green-Anderson growth charts (300). Stapling of the medial aspect of the growth plate may then be performed at the time indicated. If this option cannot be enacted because of insufficient growth remaining, metaphyseal osteotomies may be required using either staple or blade plate fixation (303). An alternative approach is to perform a gradual angular correction with an external fixator (312).

Hypophosphatasia

In some classification systems, hypophosphatasia is included with deficiency states of calcium and vitamin D, renal tubular disorders, and renal glomerular disorders (renal osteodystrophy) as a cause of rickets. Although there are some clinical and roentgenographic similarities, hypophosphatasia has a different pathophysiology from that of rickets. The link should be noted, but the distinction of hypophosphatasia from rickets and osteomalacia must also be made.

Hypophosphatasia was described as early as 1929, but it was subsequently differentiated from the rachitic syndromes by Rathbun in 1948 (313,314). It has since been documented as resulting from a genetic error in the synthesis of alkaline phosphatase by bone, leukocytes, intestinal mucosa, and kidney (314,315). Hypophosphatasia is transmitted as an autosomal recessive trait (316,317). Asymptomatic heterozygotes may also be readily identified by a decrease in serum and leukocyte alkaline phosphatase and, as in patients with clinical disease, by the presence of large concentrations of phosphoethanolamine in the urine.

Patients affected with hypophosphatasia usually show changes early in life (314,316,318). The principal findings in individuals with the fully developed syndrome are growth retardation, failure to thrive, irritability, fever, vomiting, constipation, and signs of increased intracranial pressure (316). Craniosynostosis is a common finding in infants, and the cranial bones may be poorly ossified. Suture lines may be enlarged and bear a close resemblance to craniotabes. As in rickets, dentition may be markedly delayed, and the teeth show extensive caries (319). Examination of the extremities and thorax is likely to show enlargement of the metaphyseal areas adjacent to the joints, bowing, and knock-knee de-

formities, prominent costochondral junctions, and kyphosis. Milder forms of the disorder, in which the onset of symptoms is delayed, have been described and may not be present until adolescent or adult life (317,320,321). Manifestations include fractures after minor trauma, poor fracture healing with laboratory study abnormalities, and the radiographic appearance of osteomalacia (322).

Radiographic studies of the patient affected with hypophosphatasia show generalized osteopenia, most marked in the calvarium and metaphyseal regions of the long bones (323). The bones may be bowed, and the epiphyseometaphyseal areas may show a peculiar cupped or wedge-shaped deformity, principally affecting the center of the physis and irregular notches at the margins (323) (Fig. 7-21). This is similar to the radiographic appearance of rickets. The epiphyseal centers are somewhat delayed in appearance, but normal in outline. Histologic studies show large quantities of unmineralized osteoid in the bones, particularly in regions of active growth and in the region of the synostotic sutures (316). As in rickets, the epiphyseal cartilages are irregular, with lengthening of the columns and diminished vascular invasion and mineralization (314,320).

The cause of hypophosphatasia is believed to be a decreased production of alkaline phosphatase, presumably because of an error in DNA coding by the cells that ordinarily produce the enzyme (316,324). Because the enzyme is necessary for the maturation of the primary spongiosa of the developing epiphyseal plate, the deformities that develop in affected patients are mostly evident in the skeleton, in which they mimic the change of rickets. Synthesis of bone is probably unimpaired, but, because of the relative absence of alkaline phosphatase, the mineralization process is inadequate, and large quantities of osteoid are produced. Diagnosis is based on the finding of a uniformly low concentration of serum alkaline phosphatase, with usually normal values for calcium, 25-hydroxyvitamin D, 1,25-dihydroxyvitamin D, and PTH (313,316,320,321,325). Some severely affected children may have marked hypercalcemia of unknown cause, which is thought to be caused by hypersensitivity to vitamin D (325). An unusual feature of the disease is the increased serum concentration and excessive urinary excretion of phosphoethanolamine (314,325–327). The significance of this finding, which is not specific to hypophosphatasia, is still unexplained (328).

Children or adults with mild forms of hypophosphatasia are often shorter in stature than their peers, but have limited symptoms or signs (317,322). Those with florid disease at birth present major problems in management. Increased intracranial pressure, hypercalcemia, renal failure, and overwhelming infections may cause considerable threat to life. The mortality for the infantile form of hypophosphatasia is high, ranging from 50 to 70% (318). If the child survives, considerable skeletal deformity and disability occur. Fractures are common in these patients and have been shown to heal very slowly (322,329).

There is no definitive therapy. In theory, diseases with

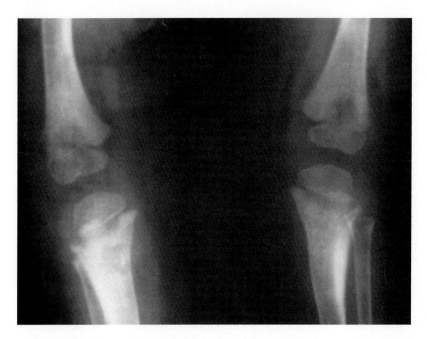

FIGURE 7-21. The central cup- or wedge-shaped ossification defects of the physes are particularly prominent at the distal femurs in a patient with hypophosphatasia.

an enzyme deficiency as the underlying cause may ultimately be treated by introduction of the appropriate gene into a stem cell population, but practical application is still in the future. Vitamin D in large doses has provided some benefit that was reversed with withdrawal of the medication (325). Pathologic fracture in hypophosphatasia (as in metabolic and endocrine entities with bone of poor mechanical quality) may be a difficult problem for the orthopaedist. In the pediatric patient with the severe form of hypophosphatasia, the dilemmas bear a resemblance to those encountered in osteogenesis imperfecta. Intramedullary fixation can be undertaken in an attempt to avoid growth plate injury. In the adult patient, intramedullary fixation and bone grafting may be indicated (322,330).

Parathyroid Disorders

Primary disorders of calcium homeostasis, except for rickets and renal osteodystrophy, are not common in children. Although it is unlikely that the pediatric orthopaedist will be the first practitioner to see patients with parathyroid disorders, it is worthwhile for him or her to be aware of several such entities.

Hyperparathyroidism. An increased level of PTH in renal failure has been discussed previously. In chronic renal failure, the hyperparathyroidism is secondary or tertiary. Secondary hyperparathyroidism is compensatory for the hypocalcemia, and remains reversible with correction of the underlying renal failure. Tertiary hyperparathyroidism is also compensatory originally, but because of the long-standing stimulation of the parathyroid glands, becomes autono-

mous, even with correction of the renal failure. In primary hyperparathyroidism, autonomous hyperfunction of the glands occurs not as a compensation for any antecedent stimulus, and hypercalcemia itself is the basis for the presenting symptoms (331–333). In the clinical situation, because of the diffuse effects of the disturbance in calcium homeostasis, the symptoms at first are bewildering. If the mnemonic device, "stones, bones, and abdominal groans," is remembered, the bewildering complaints become explicable on the basis of hypercalcemia. The critical solubility product of calcium and phosphorus is exceeded; precipitation in the urinary tract leads to renal calculi and colic. The induced osteoclastic resorption of bone causes skeletal pain. Smooth muscle action in the gut is inhibited by hypercalcemia. Abdominal pain, constipation, and weight loss follow. The irritability and conductivity of nervous tissue are decreased by hypercalcemia. Aberrations of mental status and, ultimately, lethargy and obtundation ensue. Hypertension is frequently present.

The radiographic features of primary hyperparathyroidism are similar to those of secondary hyperparathyroidism. There is generalized osteopenia and cortical thinning. Resorption is particularly severe at the terminal tufts of the distal phalanges and the distal clavicles (Fig. 7-19).

The classic laboratory findings in patients with hyperparathyroidism are elevated serum calcium, decreased serum phosphorus, and elevated alkaline phosphatase (333). Unfortunately, these values can be normal, despite an elevated PTH. Further testing may be required in difficult situations to establish the diagnosis. These tests include a urinary clearance study to clarify a decreased percentage of tubular reabsorption of phosphate, measurement of urinary cAMP, and assaying directly for serum PTH.

Treatment is directed toward correcting the underlying cause of hyperparathyroidism. For adenomas and hyperplasia, treatment is usually surgical (334). Preliminary metabolic management may be required. Although fractures can occur and need to be managed by customary principles, there should be pediatric endocrinologic management of the hypercalcemia (335,336).

Hypoparathyroidism. The manifestations of hypoparathyroidism are recognized more easily by the disturbance of calcium homeostasis than by the skeletal changes (337). The principles of calcium homeostasis discussed previously logically explain the symptoms and signs that are seen. Irritability of nervous and muscle tissue is high because the serum calcium is low (338). Tetany, paresthesias, and alteration in mental status may be seen. If hypocalcemia occurs early in development, mental retardation may result. If it occurs later, mood changes may be seen. The Chvostek and Trousseau signs are used to elicit the tetany and spasm.

Radiographic findings in patients with hypoparathyroidism include increased density of the long bones and skull. Soft tissue calcifications, including the basal ganglia, may also be seen.

Laboratory changes include a decrease in total and serum ionized calcium and elevated serum phosphorus. As with all calcium measurements, hypocalcemia must be interpreted with the serum albumin, because decreased albumin necessarily leads to decreased bound serum calcium and total serum calcium.

Treatment for hypoparathyroidism is endocrine-related, rather than orthopaedic (339). The principal treatment agent is vitamin D. Vitamin D and PTH work synergistically to facilitate the transport of calcium across the gut, by the renal tubule, and from the bone. Vitamin D is capable of exerting its effect at each of these sites. Considerably higher than physiologic (i.e., pharmacologic) doses of vitamin D are required. Management must be carried out very carefully to avoid vitamin D toxicity.

Albright Hereditary Osteodystrophy. In 1942, Albright et al. described a syndrome of short stature, short metacarpals, and rounded facies, and termed it "pseudohypoparathyroidism" (PHP) because of the associated hypocalcemia and hyperphosphatemia that were unresponsive to parathormone (340). A similar syndrome was subsequently described in which affected patients demonstrated all the clinical stigmata of PHP but showed no chemical alterations. This disorder, also genetic and presumably a variant, was termed "pseudopseudohypoparathyroidism" (PPHP). The hypocalcemia was demonstrated to be a variable expression in the same entity, so both PHP and PPHP are now included under Albright hereditary osteodystrophy (AHO).

AHO is more an endocrine than an orthopaedic entity (341). Skeletal changes are present, however, and the disorder represents an unusual but important form of metabolic bone disease that is associated with end-organ insensitivity.

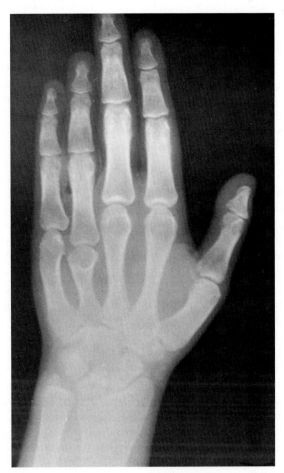

FIGURE 7-22. Radiograph of the hand of a patient with pseudohypoparathyroidism. Notice the shortened fourth and fifth metacarpals.

In addition to the characteristics of AHO already mentioned, mental retardation and central nervous system irritability and tetany are also present. Radiographs may reveal soft tissue calcifications that are especially common in the basal ganglia. Hand films demonstrate shortening of the fourth and fifth metacarpals (Fig. 7-22). Brachydactyly can be seen as part of many syndromes (342). In AHO, workup is usually pursued by genetics and pediatric endocrine services. Biochemical findings include a low serum calcium and a high serum inorganic phosphorus concentration in PHP, and these may require metabolic management.

The phenotype of AHO with PHP became regarded as a genetic disorder in which production of PTH was normal, but the cells that serve as the target for the hormone were unresponsive (341,343–346). Several different types of defects were felt to cause the lack of response. A sex-linked dominant mode of transmission with variable penetrance was one type. Heterogeneity existed even beyond the PHP/PPHP presentations, and other modes of transmission were suggested.

Because of advances in the molecular biology of development, mechanisms are gradually being established linking developmental genes (Chapters 1 and 6), growth factors, and autocrine, paracrine, and endocrine factors (347–349). Perhaps the most important issue for a pediatric orthopaedic surgeon to appreciate in AHO is how these factors interact; it is also important to contrast this entity with fibrous dysplasia. This necessitates an introduction and short review of G proteins. G (guanine nucleotide-binding) proteins are on–off switches in cellular signaling (350). They consist of three polypeptide subunits (α, β, and γ) that are noncovalently associated. In the off position, guanosine diphosphate is tightly bound to the α-subunit. When a hormone binds with its cellular receptor, the G protein is activated by displacing guanosine diphosphate and replacing it with guanosine triphosphate. A variety of second messengers can in turn be activated. The G protein that mediates the activation of adenyl cyclase is termed G_s. In AHO, there is a germline mutation in $G\alpha_s$ (*GNAS1*) that leads to loss of function. It is this loss of function of the G protein that causes the end-organ resistance to parathormone (351). At least in some patients with the AHO phenotype, the genetic defect has been localized to chromosome 2q37. Genes important in skeletal and neural development may lie in this region (352). The pediatric orthopaedic surgeon should be aware of this correlation among several factors, which is now being linked back to the genome. Although the pediatric orthopaedic surgeon is usually not directly involved in patients with AHO, this entity can now be contrasted with fibrous dysplasia, which will be discussed later in the chapter.

Hypercalcemia

In addition to the hypercalcemia associated with hyperparathyroid states, there are several other causes of hypercalcemia in childhood (353,354). These causes are relatively rare and are more frequently based on endocrine disorders than on metabolic bone disease. These entities are often of considerable importance; therefore, despite their rarity in orthopaedic practice, a brief review is necessary.

Hypervitaminosis D can cause a profound and occasionally life-threatening hypercalcemia. Vitamin D and the potent 1-hydroxyvitamin D and 1,25-dihydroxyvitamin D are used in the treatment of rickets, osteomalacia, and hypoparathyroidism. Despite the clear need of the patient, it is possible to overdose with these drugs, especially with potent analogs, and the resultant hypercalcemia causes a situation similar to that described in the section on primary hyperparathyroidism. Treatment consists of decreasing the serum calcium. Vitamin D administration should be stopped, and the patient should be promptly treated by diuresis, which is usually accomplished by administration of large volumes of saline and furosemide. Replacement of urinary losses of water, sodium, and potassium is often necessary, and these should be carefully monitored. Although sodium phosphate

infusions were advocated at one time, they are now contraindicated, because a reconsideration of the calcium homeostasis mechanism clearly indicates that such an infusion is likely to cause precipitation of calcium acid phosphate. Administration of oral phosphate in a nonabsorbable preparation binds calcium in the intestinal lumen and decreases absorption. Glucocorticoids can diminish calcium absorption and decrease tubular reabsorption.

Hypercalcemia can be seen in association with some neoplasms, although more frequently in adults than in children (355,356). The mechanisms postulated are multiple. Direct invasion of bone by massive metastases can produce hypercalcemia. Some tumors tend to produce agents that act in a manner similar to PTH or prostaglandins and cause significant increases in the resorption of bone, and sometimes profound hypercalcemia (39). The discovery of parathyroid-related protein occurred because of its role in the hypercalcemia of malignancy. Its role in the physiology of cartilage regulation has been demonstrated to be essential, and this will be described in detail in the following section.

Treatment of the hypercalcemia of malignancy begins as just described for hypervitaminosis D. In some cases of malignant disease, treatment with mithramycin, a chemotherapeutic agent that interferes with osteoclastic resorption, may be justified.

Hypercalcemia arising during periods of immobilization has been reported, more often in adults than in children (357–361). Disuse osteoporosis is not an unusual consequence of immobilization, but it is almost never associated with hypercalcemia. Children placed on prolonged bed rest, in traction or casts, can rarely develop a florid hypercalcemia, with lethargy, obtundation, abdominal symptoms, and urinary calculi (361). However, hypercalcemia must be considered in the differential diagnosis in immobilization situations. Treatment is as described for hypervitaminosis D.

Idiopathic hypercalcemia of childhood is a rare condition, seen more often in Great Britain than in the United States. The disorder is not clearly a single entity, and most recently it has been considered to be a series of heterogeneous syndromes. One of the more common syndromes, Williams syndrome, is characterized by a peculiar elfin facies with a small mandible and upturned nose (362). Cardiovascular anomalies, such as supravalvular aortic stenosis, have been reported, in addition to mental retardation. The multiple anomalies suggest an *in utero* mesenchymal defect, but the relationship of the abnormality in calcium handling to the other defects is not clear. Williams syndrome should be distinguished from the idiopathic hypercalcemia that was first described in Great Britain and thought to be due to hypervitaminosis D secondary to overzealous supplementation.

Parathyroid-related Protein

The hypercalcemia of malignancy has been studied. A circulating peptide was detected that seemed to be mediating this phenomenon. PTH was a logical candidate. However, this peptide shared homology with PTH, yet was distinct from it. It was named "parathyroid-related protein" (PTHrP). Subsequently, it was shown that PTH and PTHrP, although distinct, shared the same cellular receptor. Under physiologic conditions, PTH is a circulating hormone and PTHrP exerts its effect locally in autocrine or paracrine fashion. In the growth plate, PTHrP is part of a negative feedback loop that slows the conversion of chondrocytes from the small cell to the hypertrophic phenotype. In certain malignancies, PTHrP may be released into the circulation. The shared PTH/PTHrP receptors are activated. The result is hypercalcemia through the mechanism described for hyperparathyroidism, yet the PTH levels are not elevated.

Further work then demonstrated that the Jansen-type chondrodysplasia results from a continually active PTH/PTHrP receptor. This abnormal receptor mediates a too-rapid conversion from small to hypertrophic chondrocyte in the growth plates, with resultant short stature. Because the receptor is continually on, a hypercalcemia results from the systemic effects on bone and kidney, as in hyperparathyroidism (363,364).

The Schmid-type chondrodysplasia has the radiographic appearance of rickets. This dysplasia results from an abnormality in type X collagen, the collagen associated with endochondral ossification at the lower hypertrophic zone of the growth plate (365).

The molecular bases of these two types of metaphyseal chondrodysplasias are included here to illustrate the correlations that may now be drawn among embryology (Chapter 1), molecular genetics (Chapter 6), metabolic and endocrine abnormalities (Chapter 7), and clinical genetics (Chapters 8 and 9). The signals that regulate embryonic cartilage and bone formation are recapitulated during growth and in fracture repair (6).

Heavy Metal Intoxication

Heavy metal poisoning is usually not considered among the metabolic bone diseases of children. Indeed, the manifestations of lead intoxication, which is the most common variety of metal poisoning, are more frequently neurologic and gastrointestinal than osseous (366). However, the pediatric orthopaedist may be presented with certain radiographic findings that should be recognized (367).

Lead can be stored in the metaphyses, where bone is being rapidly laid down by growth plates. The radiographic appearance is characteristically broad bands of markedly increased radiodensity located in the metaphyseal area, adjacent to the epiphyseal plates (Fig. 7-23). Normally, the metaphyseal region in growing children may appear slightly more dense than in adults, because the zone of provisional calcification and the primary spongiosa on the metaphyseal side of the growth plate contain calcified cartilage. Calcified cartilage has more mineral than bone, and is more radio-

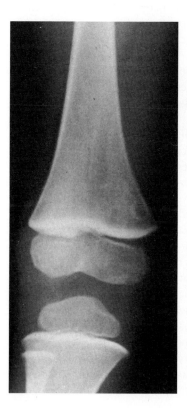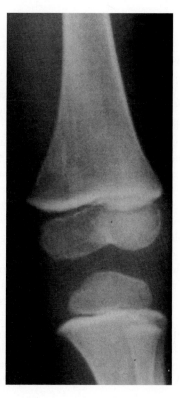

FIGURE 7-23. Radiograph of the knee of a patient with lead poisoning. Notice the broad, radiodense metaphyseal lines. Lead has accumulated at the site of bone formation.

dense. The radiodensity in most cases of lead intoxication is far beyond the normal range. In a few cases, the radiographs are negative or equivocal. Lead lines in the gums and hematologic and chemical findings establish the diagnosis (343).

ORGANIC PHASE

Although differentiation of the mineral phase from the organic phase of bone metabolism is simplistic and neglects interactions between the two phases, the classification is useful for discussing physiology and differentiating clinical syndromes. Mineral homeostasis was discussed earlier in this chapter. The diseases of the organic phase are introduced by a brief review of the cellular and organic aspects of bone physiology.

Bone Physiology

Bone is a specialized form of connective tissue with several important roles. It is rigid, provides form, and contributes to structural stability. Bone is the primary body store for calcium and phosphorus and also serves as an envelope for the blood-forming marrow elements. When injured, bone normally heals with its native tissue rather than scar. In the child, the modeling process accounts for growth and continued reshaping of the bones (368). In the adult, although the shape of the bones in general remains unchanged, the tissue undergoes continued internal remodeling, in which bone cells are responsible for continued resorption and formation, resulting in the replacement of old bone by new bone (369,370).

Bone is a composite material. Based on dry weight, 77% is inorganic, primarily hydroxyapatite. The remaining 23% is organic, and almost 90% of this is in the form of collagen. The remaining noncollagenous organic material consists of phospholipids, other glycoproteins, and proteoglycans. The collagen molecules within the fibers are highly ordered, with the fibrillar arrangement consisting of a three-fourths stagger (16). There is an 8% overlap that produces hole zones essential to the deposition of hydroxyapatite crystals and the linkage to the noncollagenous proteins within and in juxtaposition to the collagen fibers. The biomechanical properties of bone in part result from the organic and inorganic components. Bone is anisotropic; the collagen molecules and fibrils, haversian systems, and trabeculae are not randomly oriented. Their orientation ensures that the biomechanical properties of the materials composing the tissue are maximized.

The collagen molecule is a macromolecule made up of three polypeptide chains, each of about 1,000 amino acids, arranged in a triple helix (371–373). One-third of the amino acids are glycine, and 20 to 30% are proline or hydroxyproline. Many different types of collagen have been described (13,371,372,374) (Table 7-2; refer also to Chapter 6). Type I collagen, the most common, is found in bone, tendon, and skin. Type II collagen is the predominant form in cartilage.

The individual chains of collagen are synthesized in the rough endoplasmic reticulum, and assembled into a triple helix intracellularly before extrusion. Several posttranslational changes occur, including hydroxylation of some of the proline and lysine residues and glycosylation of some of the hydroxylysine residues. The hydroxyproline residues make the triple helix more heat-stable, and the hydroxylysine residues are important in the development of crosslinks. After translocation to the extracellular space, portions of the amino- and carboxy-terminal nonhelical portions of the procollagen molecule are cleaved, and the collagen molecules aggregate to form fibrils in which additional reactions occur to produce stable intramolecular and intermolecular cross-links. Interspersed around the collagen molecules are the other noncollagenous proteins.

After collagen production, additional events occur that render the bone matrix (osteoid) mineralizable. Under appropriate conditions, including the presence of adequate amounts of calcium and phosphorus and the production of alkaline phosphatase by the cells, the hydroxyapatite crystals are deposited within the collagen fiber. Many aspects of the mineralization process are still being investigated (13,25, 375–377). Some investigators have suggested that the process is due primarily to physicochemical phenomena that occur as a result of the specific nature of collagen and noncollagenous organic structure. Others have suggested that mineralization begins as an energy-dependent intracellular process that requires the presence of one or more vitamin D metabolites. Proteoglycans also may play a significant role in the process (378).

The process is not completed with the end of mineralization. Because of incompletely understood signals, bone as an organ responds to stress, according to Wolff's law. After mineralization, bone may undergo partial resorption with subsequent new formation, possibly in a different location, for the purpose of producing bone that is more appropriately oriented to resist stress. This action depends on combined osteoclastic and osteoblastic activity (20). Its mediation at the cellular level may occur by mechanical transduction across the cell membrane and through the cytoskeleton, with an effect on the genome (54).

Advances in knowledge of collagen biochemistry, physiology of mineralization, and cellular processes responsible for bone cell differentiation and function have led to a better understanding of many metabolic bone diseases. Defects in the mineralization process are numerous and may lead to the rachitic diseases discussed previously. There are many sites for disturbances in collagen production; some of these defects have been identified in diseases such as osteogenesis imperfecta, the Ehlers-Danlos syndromes (EDS), and some skeletal dysplasias (14). Problems with bone cell differentiation, function, or both have been found in osteopetrosis and idiopathic juvenile osteoporosis. As additional metabolic and biochemical abnormalities are identified in these diseases, greater insight will be gained regarding pathogenesis, and more effective forms of treatment will evolve.

Osteogenesis Imperfecta

The molecular genetics of osteogenesis imperfecta is covered in Chapter 6. The discussion here focuses on the clinical aspects of this condition.

Osteogenesis imperfecta has traditionally been categorized as a heritable disorder of connective tissue, affecting both the bone and the soft tissue; studies have also revealed a number of metabolic abnormalities (379). The disease was probably first described by Malebranche (380) in 1674, and since then it has been discussed under at least 40 different names or eponyms, some of the more common of which are Lobstein disease (381), Vrolik disease (382), van der Hoeve disease, fragilitas ossium, osteomalacia congenita, and osteoporosis fetalis (383–386). Advances in collagen biochemistry and electron microscopy, and recent genetic, epidemiologic, and dental studies, support the concept that osteogenesis imperfecta is a series of syndromes representing classes of molecular defects, each with a reasonably well-defined clinical pattern (385,387,388). Most types of osteogenesis imperfecta have been linked to mutations in type I collagen (14).

Clinical Manifestations

The nature and severity of the clinical features depend on the type of osteogenesis imperfecta (14,385,389,390). General features include the characteristic fragility of bone, short stature, scoliosis, defective dentinogenesis of deciduous or permanent teeth or both, middle ear deafness, laxity of ligaments, and blue sclerae and tympanic membranes. Many patients have misshapen skulls with wide intertemporal measurements and small, triangular faces. The bones are gracile and diffusely osteopenic, with thin cortices and an attenuated trabecular pattern. The long bones have narrow diaphyses, and bowing and fractures are common. The fracture-healing process is undisturbed in terms of sequence of events, but the new bone has the same deficient biomechanical characteristics. Fractures may occur at any age, and the age of occurrence is one basis for classification. In the milder forms of osteogenesis imperfecta, the incidence of fractures decreases with age.

The pelvis in osteogenesis imperfecta may have a trefoil shape, and protrusio acetabuli is common, presumably because of repeated fractures. A softened base of the skull may lead to platybasia and potential neurologic sequelae. Dentinogenesis imperfecta results in soft, translucent, and brownish teeth. The teeth are affected in a nonuniform manner; the primary and secondary teeth may be involved

to a greater or lesser degree. The osteopenic vertebrae may fracture easily, resulting in a flattened or biconcave shape. The laxity of the ligaments results in hypermobile joints and an increased incidence of joint dislocation. Inguinal, umbilical, and diaphragmatic hernias are common. The skin is thin, translucent, and easily distendible. Although increased vascular fragility is common, major arterial or aortic aneurysms are rarely encountered. The differential diagnosis includes juvenile osteoporosis, nonaccidental injury (391), and, rarely, a malignancy such as leukemia. The severity of involvement ranges from a crushed stillborn fetus, in the most severe cases, to an infant with multiple or unusual fractures (392) or severe postnatal deformities, to an almost symptom-free adult (393). The adult, on careful clinical evaluation, reveals a history of occasional fracture and mild osteopenia, and family history may be contributory.

The issue of discerning nonaccidental injury from osteogenesis imperfecta can arise. Because a given, single fracture may occur in nonaccidental injury or osteogenesis imperfecta, it is inadvisable to exclude osteogenesis imperfecta by the radiographic pattern alone (391). Conversely, multiple fractures at different stages of healing, posterior rib fractures, and metaphyseal corner fractures are highly specific for nonaccidental injury (394,395). The history is extremely helpful. Fractures from child abuse occur most frequently in children younger than 3 years of age (394). If the physician is caring for a patient who is not yet ambulatory and has multiple fractures, interpreting the data as osteogenesis imperfecta would imply a severe type, which is usually diagnosed with fractures at birth. It is possible for a child with a mild form of osteogenesis imperfecta to become ambulatory and sustain a fracture with relatively mild trauma. A positive family history, signs such as abnormal dentition or blue sclerae, or a systemic osteopenia revealed by radiography might be helpful in this situation.

Culture of dermal fibroblasts for characterization of the type I collagen may be part of the workup, but the molecular basis for the entire spectrum of osteogenesis imperfecta has not been established (14). The matching of a child's type I collagen with a previously described molecular abnormality may establish the diagnosis of osteogenesis imperfecta, but not matching does not necessarily exclude osteogenesis imperfecta in problem situations. The combination of history, physical examination, and radiographic pattern still remains of paramount significance. Fractures and rickets can occur in very low birth weight infants, but the setting of a birth weight less than 1,500 g, hospitalization, biochemical abnormalities, and subsequent resolution with development are key features of this syndrome (295). Fractures can occur as noted in primary hyperparathyroidism, but there are biochemical abnormalities in this setting (335,336). A patient with Menkes kinky-hair syndrome can present with metaphyseal corner fractures, but the presentation is more likely in the setting of a newborn boy (X-linked recessive trait) with failure to thrive and the sparse, kinky hair that gives the syndrome its name (396). "Overdiagnosis of child abuse is a tragedy, but an incorrect diagnosis of osteogenesis imperfecta may put a child's life at risk" (394).

The inheritance of osteogenesis imperfecta was thought to be autosomal dominant. The fact that there was considerable variability of phenotypic expression in different members of a kindred led to the concept of variable penetrance and expressivity (386). Investigations of multiple kindreds led some authors to conclude that there was a high rate of spontaneous mutation, but others emphasize the need for a careful history, physical examination, and metabolic studies and collagen typing to detect subclinical involvement in some patients in a pedigree.

Classification

It is not surprising that numerous classifications have been proposed for osteogenesis imperfecta. Looser used the terms congenita and tarda to differentiate what he believed were different forms of the disease, based on when the first fractures occurred, applying congenita only to intrauterine fractures (384). Seedorff used this definition of congenita, but divided tarda into gravis (i.e., fractures occurring at birth or within the first year of life) and levis (fractures occurring after 1 year) (397). Bauze et al. used deformity of the femurs as a guide to distinguish clinical types (389).

The classification most widely accepted is the Sillence classification. The Sillence classification of osteogenesis imperfecta takes into account multiple features of this entity to provide some order to the wide heterogeneity (385,388). This classification provides the framework to which much of the molecular biology is being added (14). Sillence proposed a numeric classification, types I to IV, with several modifiers. Types I and IV were felt to be transmitted by an autosomal dominant mode and types II and III by an autosomal recessive mode. Dental findings were used to further subtype (i.e., A indicates without and B indicates with dentinogenesis imperfecta). Sillence also recognized several pedigrees that seemed to have an X-linked inheritance pattern, although these are not included in the classification that he proposed (Table 7-5).

Type I osteogenesis imperfecta is the common mild form. The molecular basis for this is a 50% reduction in the production of type I collagen (14). Overall morphology may be normal or nearly so, with fractures occurring in later childhood and decreasing toward adolescence. Type II is lethal in the perinatal period, with many of the mutations being mutations in glycine residues of type I collagen. Type III osteogenesis imperfecta is the severe form, with fractures present at birth. The molecular basis for this type of osteogenesis imperfecta has not been as fully characterized as it has been for the other types. Types II and III are not difficult to diagnose clinically, but correlation of these clinical entities with molecular defects expands our knowledge of bone physiology, and ultimately may provide more effective

TABLE 7-5. OSTEOGENESIS IMPERFECTA CLASSIFICATION

Type	Inheritance	Clinical Features
I	Autosomal dominant	Bone fragility, blue sclerae, onset of fractures after birth (most preschool age). Type A, without dentinogenesis imperfecta; type B, with dentinogenesis imperfecta
II	Autosomal recessive	Lethal in perinatal period, dark blue sclerae, concertina femurs, beaded ribs
III	Autosomal recessive	Fractures at birth, progressive deformity, normal sclerae and hearing
IV	Autosomal dominant	Bone fragility, normal sclerae, normal hearing. Type A, without dentinogenesis imperfecta; type B, with dentinogenesis imperfecta

(From refs. 385 and 388, with permission.)

forms of treatment. Type IV is a moderately severe form of osteogenesis imperfecta, with glycine point mutations in type I collagen. Clinically, this type has great variation, overlapping types I and III, and it may represent a heterogeneous group of patients who do not readily fit into the other categories. A molecular characterization of this group aids in establishing the diagnosis of osteogenesis imperfecta and typing it in problematic situations.

Orthopaedic management for type I osteogenesis imperfecta is customary fracture management. Management for types III and IV includes adaptive equipment, rehabilitation, intramedullary rodding, and scoliosis management. This approach also points to another problem. The Sillence classification, which has been and remains the most helpful classification for the geneticist in ordering the many features of this entity, may be less helpful for the pediatric orthopaedist consulted in the perinatal period and confronted by concerned parents with questions about musculoskeletal prognosis.

Shapiro has advanced a congenita/tarda classification to try to address this issue (398). In this classification scheme, congenita implies fractures occurring *in utero* or at birth. The congenita group is further subdivided into A (i.e., crumpled femurs and ribs) and B (i.e., normal bone contours, but with fractures). The tarda group is also divided into A (i.e., fractures before walking) and B (i.e., fractures after walking). At follow-up, the congenita A group had a high mortality rate (94%). The congenita B mortality rate was only 8%; 59% were in wheelchairs and 33% were ambulatory. In the tarda A group, 33% were in wheelchairs and 67% were ambulatory. In the tarda B group, 100% were ambulatory. Most intramedullary rodding was performed in the congenita B and tarda A groups.

The problems of the Sillence classification for the pediatric orthopaedist do not obviate its usefulness and general acceptance, and it will be the classification used for the remainder of the discussion.

The radiographic features of osteogenesis imperfecta patients are variable, depending on the disease type, but they must be interpreted with history and physical examination to establish the type (385,388,399) (Figs. 7-24 through 7-27). Findings may or may not be obvious at birth, depending on the type. In almost every case, some degree of generalized osteopenia can be detected. In type II and, to a certain extent, in type III, the femurs have a crumpled "concertina" appearance. A similar deformity, presumably caused by previous fractures, may or may not be seen early in type I. Later in childhood in type I, the long bones appear slender and gracile, with thin cortices and deformities resulting from multiple fractures. In type III in later childhood, the bones are often short, and children may have disproportionate short stature. The head is misshapen, and the skull exhibits wormian bones. The vertebrae may show evidence of multiple fractures, with resultant platyspondylia and sometimes severe scoliosis. In severe cases, the metaphyses may appear cystic, a finding occasionally present at birth but more often developing during infancy or childhood.

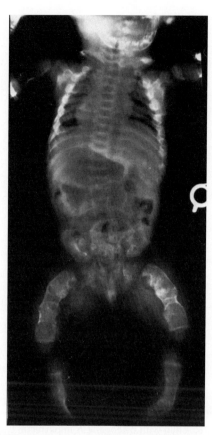

FIGURE 7-25. Child with osteogenesis imperfecta, type II. Notice the concertina-like appearance of the femurs and the beading of the ribs.

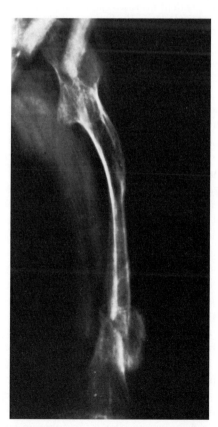

FIGURE 7-24. Radiograph of a patient with osteogenesis imperfecta, type I. The patient had blue sclerae. Fractures began soon after birth, with resulting deformity.

The histologic changes in the bones of patients with osteogenesis imperfecta have been the subject of considerable investigation, and researchers vary in their description of them, in part reflecting the heterogeneity of the entity. Toward the more severe end of the spectrum of osteogenesis imperfecta, fairly uniform agreement exists with regard to the nature of the bone, which often appears woven and only occasionally exhibits a lamellar pattern. The cortices are thin, with poorly developed haversian systems, and the trabeculae in the metaphyses are markedly attenuated. Several investigators have observed a hypercellularity, with increased numbers of osteocytes per unit area or volume of bone (400). No change has been noted in the osteoclast population. The collagen fibers of the cornea and skin share in the disturbance and have a looser arrangement and thinner fibers. Histologic study of the epiphyseal and articular cartilages have failed to show an abnormality. Ultrastructural studies confirm the more random arrangement of the collagen fibers of the bone (and other sites) and the thinner fiber diameters. The osteoblasts contain excessive concentrations of glycogen. In type II osteogenesis imperfecta, chondrogenesis at the growth plates is normal, with the skeletal dysmorphology arising from abnormal endochondral ossifi-

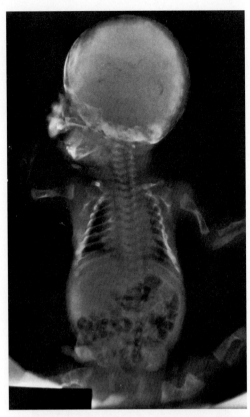

FIGURE 7-26. Child with osteogenesis imperfecta, type III. Fractures were present at birth; progressive deformity occurred with further development.

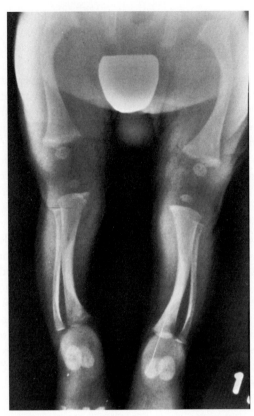

FIGURE 7-27. Patient with osteogenesis imperfecta, type IV. The patient had normal sclerae. The femurs and tibias are bowed. The type IV phenotype, when severe, can overlap with that of type III.

cation on the metaphyseal side of the physis, failure of the ring of LaCroix, and multiple fractures with axial and angular distortion (401).

The techniques of molecular biology demonstrated abnormalities in type I collagen as the basis for at least some types of osteogenesis imperfecta (14). Elucidation of this cause required much classic investigative work to provide the pertinent information on which to build the molecular search. Biochemical studies of osteogenesis imperfecta patients have shown the calcium, phosphorus, magnesium, vitamin D, and PTH levels to be within normal limits. Subsequent research began to reveal abnormalities in collagen (402,403). In normal bones, the collagen is almost entirely type I, although, in fetal tissues and in very young infants, some of the collagen is in the form of type III or V. This finding diminishes with age; in most older children, only type I collagen can be recognized. In lethal osteogenesis imperfecta, a considerable increase in the concentration of types III and V and a marked variation in cross-linking were found (404). Changes in the various types of osteogenesis imperfecta were documented, including an increase in collagen hydroxylysine residues in bone, a decrease in hydroxylysinonorleucine in skin collagen, and abnormalities of α1-

and α2-polypeptides of type I collagen in cultured skin fibroblasts (387,405–407). With an improved classification system of the heterogeneity in osteogenesis and expanding techniques in molecular biology, increasingly precise abnormalities in type I collagen are being correlated with the clinical syndromes and with entities such as the Ehlers-Danlos syndromes and skeletal dysplasias (14,408).

Not all the clinical manifestations nor all the subtypes of osteogenesis imperfecta may be linked directly to collagen abnormalities, and other metabolic disturbances may at least be contributory (400,409,410). Increased sweating, heat intolerance, increased body temperature, and resting tachycardia and tachypnea have been described. Although this finding suggested the possibility of hyperthyroidism, increased serum thyroxine levels have been an inconsistent finding. Hyperthermia during anesthesia has been reported, and occasionally a patient manifests true malignant hyperthermia. The serum inorganic pyrophosphate concentrations can be increased, and studies of leukocyte metabolism suggest an uncoupling of oxidative phosphorylation. Platelet function studies have demonstrated defects in adhesion and clot retraction.

Management

Treatment depends on the type of osteogenesis imperfecta. Type I osteogenesis, at least in its milder forms, may have little impact on the patient, and the role of the pediatric orthopaedic surgeon may be limited to conventional fracture care. Type II, lethal perinatal osteogenesis imperfecta, has some degree of variability. In the most severe cases, the very early death occurs before pediatric orthopaedic intervention. Types III and IV represent the greatest challenges.

Several systemic treatment modalities have been attempted. Investigators have used calcium, vitamin C, vitamin D, fluoride, calcitonin, diphosphonates, and magnesium without benefit (411). An early report on the efficacy of (3-amino-1-hydroxypropylidene)-1,1-bisphosphonate (pamidronate) was made (412). Subsequent reports in the basic science and clinical literature further support the use of this bisphosphonate in severe cases of osteogenesis imperfecta (413,414). Pamidronate does not cure osteogenesis imperfecta. It inhibits osteoclastic resorption, but the abnormality in the type I collagen remains.

The theoretical possibilities of molecular treatments for specific types of osteogenesis imperfecta loom on the horizon (14). Stimulating production of type I collagen in type I osteogenesis imperfecta or correcting the point mutations in certain cases of types II or IV should, in theory, cure the disease, but achieving this outcome in practice remains a goal for the future. Other strategies include bone marrow transplantation to replace abnormal stem cells with normal stem cells and suppression of mutant collagen gene expression (415).

Orthopaedic management of even the severe types III and IV osteogenesis imperfecta can be important in fracture prevention, fracture management, and function (416–421). As with any heterogeneous condition, controversies about the efficacy of any specific treatment abound. It does seem worthwhile to proceed with an aggressive program of exercises, standing with bracing, working to develop ambulatory potential, and proceeding with appropriate seating, including wheelchair locomotion, if required (422).

The treatment for fractures in osteogenesis imperfecta is sometimes difficult, because of the patient's ligamentous laxity, structural abnormalities of the bones, and frequency of multiple fractures with even minor or no trauma. Fractures heal readily, often with exuberant callus, but the callus formed in response to the fracture is identical in structure to the rest of the skeleton; it is plastic and easily deformed by forces associated with weight-bearing or simply the action of muscles across the fracture site. As a result, uncontrollable deformities or shortening often occur during or after the treatment phase, which contribute to the crippling and disability experienced by patients with severe forms of the disease.

Closed treatment methods are often used. Use of light-weight polypropylene splints or braces may prove helpful in getting the child to bear weight quickly to avoid the compounding problems of immobilization. Devices such as a parapodium may help a child to acquire an upright posture. Vacuum pants have been described for use in this situation (423). If management by closed means proves difficult, treatment with internal fixation may be enacted. Intramedullary fixation is superior to plates and screws, which tend to dislodge from the weakened bones.

The issue of the optimal age for operation has attracted different opinions. Ryoppy et al. advocated proceeding as early as 6 weeks of age (424). Their criteria for this decision were recurrent fractures with appropriate care, progressive deformation, a cycle of immobilization leading to further weakening, and humanitarian reasons. Solid devices were used to anticipate a change to elongating devices. It was thought that this approach decreased the incidence of refracture and aided function. The insertion of solid rods percutaneously after closed osteoclasis has been reported (424–426).

The alternative, which has been elected more frequently, has been to accept deformity or to treat deformity with closed methods as soon as possible in the course of early fracture management, get the child to the approximate age of 5 years, and proceed with corrective osteotomies of larger bones. The method of multiple corrective osteotomies with intramedullary fixation for the lower and upper extremities has been accepted for managing recurrent fractures with deformity and maintaining function (427–429). Such procedures have been done with solid rods, using exchanges as the child grew [→4.11]. The introduction of the elongating Bailey-Dubow rod seemed to provide a solution, but also generated problems, such as disconnection of the T-piece from the rods. Crimping the T-piece seems to provide an effective, although incomplete, solution. Nevertheless, use of the Bailey-Dubow rods seems to be a method of intramedullary fixation that diminishes the rate of reoperation and has a complication rate similar to that of use of nonelongating rods (430–432) (Fig. 7-28). Other alternatives include closed osteoclasis with subsequent management using pneumatic splints or casting (433).

Fractures in the more mild types of osteogenesis imperfecta may present some problems with different options for solution. In the very mild forms, customary fracture management may apply. In more severe forms, recurrent fracture and subsequent bowing may be seen, especially at the femurs or tibias. There is no absolute rule on which to base intervention with intramedullary rodding in these situations. The risk-benefit analysis should consider recurrent fracture (i.e., two to three fractures being an arbitrary but practical limit before surgery) and deformity versus possible injury to the blood supply and physeal regions of the growing ends of long bones.

One of the most difficult disorders to treat in osteogenesis imperfecta, and in other disorders with osteopenia,

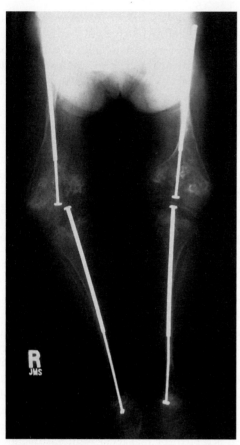

FIGURE 7-28. Radiograph of a patient with osteogenesis imperfecta, type III, after insertion of Bailey-Dubow rods.

is scoliosis. The curves tend to advance relentlessly, and bracing is ineffective in controlling the progression of the deformity. Internal fixation is considerably hampered by the poor quality of the bone. Newer methods of segmental instrumentation are changing the approach to scoliosis in

osteogenesis imperfecta and other diseases with osteopenia (434) [➥2.5, 2.9]. Curves may be fused early (at 40 degrees) to halt the relentless progression (434,435). This should help to maintain function and prevent respiratory complications.

Idiopathic Juvenile Osteoporosis

It is important to clarify any confusion regarding the terminology of metabolic bone disease. Osteopenia is a nonspecific term, indicating only a reduction in bone mass as determined by radiographic study or by special techniques, such as computed tomographic analysis or absorption photometry. Within this category, there are four diagnostic groups, based on the pathology and special studies of tissue, such as histology and bone morphometric analysis. These groups are osteoporosis, in which the bone is normal in appearance and structure but reduced in amount; osteomalacia, in which the bone matrix is laid down normally but is not properly mineralized; osteitis fibrosa, in which the bone is resorbed rapidly as a result of excessive PTH; and malignant disease, in which the bone is replaced and at times actively resorbed by local deposits of malignant cells. When radiographic examination reveals decreased bone mass, it is essential to view the process initially as osteopenia, rather than to make a more specific diagnosis such as osteoporosis, and to seek to define its cause among the various syndromes within the four broad categories defined.

Idiopathic juvenile osteoporosis is a rare, self-limited disorder of unknown cause, which affects previously healthy children (436,437). Since it was first described, at least 45 patients have been reported, but much remains to be learned about its cause and pathophysiology (438–442). Although one series has been reported in which several patients had symptoms before 5 years of age, the age of onset of symp-

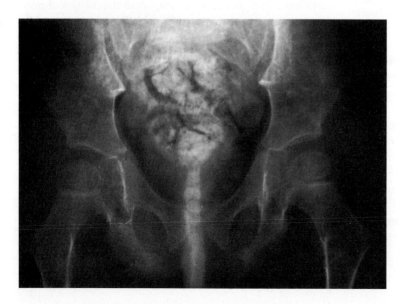

FIGURE 7-29. Child with juvenile osteoporosis. The osteoporosis affects the pelvis and the femurs.

toms is usually between 8 and 14 years, and resolution usually occurs spontaneously within 2 to 4 years after onset or after puberty. Idiopathic juvenile osteoporosis must be differentiated from other osteopenic conditions affecting children, especially from osteogenesis imperfecta, hematologic malignancies, thyrotoxicosis, and Cushing disease. The diagnosis of idiopathic juvenile osteoporosis is made by the positive identification of features of this disease, and by ruling out other diseases with similar manifestations.

Idiopathic juvenile osteoporosis is initially characterized by bone and joint pain, followed by an arrest of growth, varying degrees of osteopenia, vertebral body collapse, and metaphyseal fractures (Figs. 7-29 and 7-30). The disease may be limited to the spine. When long bones are involved, bone loss is generalized, but usually more marked at the metaphyses. The diaphyses, affected to a lesser degree, are not as thin and narrow as in osteogenesis imperfecta. Prolonged disuse may exaggerate and enhance this situation.

The pathophysiology of idiopathic juvenile osteoporosis is obscure (443–445). Symptoms usually resolve after puberty, which suggests that the disease is endocrine in origin. Biochemical measurements of these patients are difficult to interpret, because of the extraordinarily rapid alterations in metabolism that occur just before puberty. Serum calcium

and phosphorus levels are normal. Alkaline phosphatase and urinary hydroxyproline levels are normal or slightly above normal. Metabolic studies have shown these patients to be in a negative calcium balance initially and in a positive calcium balance during recovery. Intestinal calcium absorption is abnormally low, and hypercalciuria may exist. Normal 25-hydroxyvitamin D levels with very low 1,25-dihydroxyvitamin D levels have been reported (446). Few data regarding PTH levels are available.

Microradiographic and histomorphometric studies of bone biopsies of patients with idiopathic juvenile osteoporosis have been confusing (437). Increased resorbing surfaces have been demonstrated with microradiographic techniques, but the rates of formation were not evaluated. A normal osteoclast population with a decrease in the number of osteoblasts has been reported, suggesting a defect in bone formation. Other evidence suggests increased resorption and increased formation or a combined high turnover state. One serious problem with these studies is that of sampling error. The osteopenic changes are most marked in the metaphyseal regions, but the biopsies are obtained from the iliac crests.

Because the cause and pathophysiology of idiopathic juvenile osteoporosis are poorly understood, it is not surprising that effective treatment remains ill defined. It is not clear whether any of these regimens can favorably alter the natural history. A greater awareness of idiopathic juvenile osteoporosis, using careful metabolic studies before and after treatment, should help to elucidate the pathophysiology of this rare but interesting disease.

The pediatric orthopaedic surgeon sees patients with idiopathic juvenile osteoporosis for the spinal deformity (i.e., kyphosis) and pain, which may be present, especially at the outset of the disease (447). He or she must be aware of the stage of workup for the patient, so that the differential diagnosis has been excluded and idiopathic juvenile osteoporosis has been established. In this setting, antikyphotic bracing has been recommended (448). It is initiated at 23 hours per day for approximately 1 year, then weaned down, consistent with maintaining a normal kyphosis with relief of symptoms. Because this is a relatively small group of patients with a tendency to improve, the efficacy of bracing might be questioned, but residual deformity without bracing has been noted (448).

Although osteoporosis secondary to disuse is not idiopathic, it is mentioned for two reasons. First, the lack of stress across osseous tissue can affect the balance between absorption and formation, causing a net decrease in bone mass (Fig. 7-31). Although the precise link between mechanical force and cell physiology is unknown, such a link may play a role in the development of osteoporoses of unknown cause (52,54). Second, disuse atrophy has practical consequences in pediatric orthopaedics. After prolonged cast immobilization, children often show some degree of osteoporosis with resultant weakening of the skeleton. This

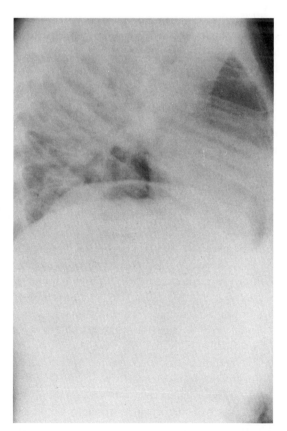

FIGURE 7-30. Juvenile osteoporosis. This lateral radiograph of the spine shows the typical biconcave appearance of the vertebrae.

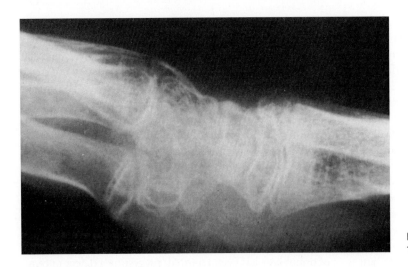

FIGURE 7-31. Disuse atrophy of the wrist and distal forearm after cast immobilization.

phenomenon is accentuated in children with neuromuscular diseases. A gradual return to activity is important in fracture rehabilitation in patients with neuromuscular diseases, including functional polypropylene bracing, to avoid vicious cycles of increased fragility followed by recurrent fracture after removal of the immobilizing devices.

Osteopetrosis

Osteopetrosis is an unusual disorder of the skeletal system in which, because of a failure of osteoclastic and chondroclastic resorption, the bones become exceedingly dense. The marrow spaces and foraminal openings are encroached on by the unresorbed masses of dense bone, and these features, plus the fragility of the pathologic bone, dominate the clinical picture (449,450). Three clinically distinct forms of osteopetrosis are now recognized (451). The infantile-malignant form is transmitted as an autosomal recessive type and is fatal within the first several years of life without treatment. An intermediate form, also transmitted as an autosomal recessive type, appears within the first decade of life and does not follow a malignant course. The patient with the autosomal dominant type has a normal life expectancy but many orthopaedic problems. The autosomal dominant form was first described by Albers-Schonberg (i.e., Albers-Schonberg disease) (452). Other names applied to both forms of the disease are marble bone disease and osteosclerosis fragilis generalisata (453–455). Although generally considered a primary disorder of bone metabolism, with diminished bone resorption due to an osteoclast defect, studies indicate that osteopetrosis may more appropriately be considered an immune disorder resulting from a thymic defect that leads to the osteoclast abnormality (456).

The autosomal recessive malignant form of osteopetrosis is manifested in infancy with thick, poorly remodeled dense bones and poor development of the medullary canal (457). The child generally shows a failure to thrive, myelophthisic anemia and thrombocytopenia, hepatosplenomegaly, lymphadenopathy, spontaneous bruising, abnormal bleeding, and multiple fractures. Because of the abnormal bone modeling process, the neural foramina in the skull become small, causing neural encroachment and optic, oculomotor, and facial palsies. There are no reports of any person with untreated autosomal recessive malignant osteopetrosis surviving for more than 20 years; death usually occurs from overwhelming infection or hemorrhage.

The autosomal recessive intermediate form of osteopetrosis tends to be diagnosed in later childhood after a fracture (451). In retrospect, some of the features noted in the malignant form, such as anemia, dental anomalies, or disproportion (short limb/short stature), can be identified in milder presentations in this condition.

Radiographically, the bones are overly dense in osteopetrosis patients (Figs. 7-32 and 7-33). There may be transverse bands in the metaphyseal regions and longitudinal striations in the shafts. The metaphyseal regions, particularly in the proximal humerus and distal femur, may develop a flask-shaped configuration. The pelvis may appear as a bone within a bone, and the sclerotic vertebrae may have a rugby jersey appearance.

The autosomal dominant form of osteopetrosis is much more benign, and the general health and life span of the patient are usually unaffected. Mild anemia may be present; facial palsies and deafness can occur, but are not necessarily features of this form of osteopetrosis. Fractures and subsequent deformities such as coxa vara are common.

The histology of the osteopetrotic bone shows that, in addition to thickened trabeculae and cortices, tongues of cartilage bars persist at the sites of endochondral bone formation, and may project far into the metaphysis and even

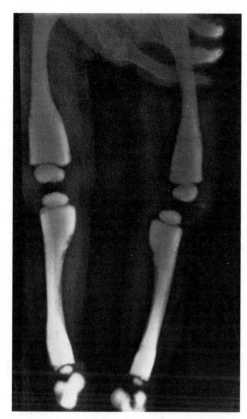

FIGURE 7-32. Patient with osteopetrosis and generalized increased density of the bones.

calcified, and their central portions undergo osseous metaplasia. The bone is relatively hypocellular, with a paucity of osteoblasts and an almost complete absence of osteoclasts. The subperiosteal new bone is in part nonlamellar, suggesting that intramembranous bone formation is also abnormal, but it is less well defined than the abnormality in endochondral bone formation. Kinetic data for calcium in osteopetrotic rats and humans have shown a low accretion rate and a dramatically reduced resorption rate (459–463). These observations suggest a defect in bone cell differentiation and function, the most obvious of which involves the osteoclast (464).

The classic experiments of Walker demonstrated that osteopetrosis in mice was reversible with parabiosis or marrow transplantation (463,465,466). Several studies in osteopetrotic rodents and humans have revealed the role of a thymic defect in this disease. Osteopetrotic mice of the *op* strain have been found to have precocious thymic atrophy. Milhaud and co-workers have found that the cell mitogens concanavalin A and phytohemagglutinin have little effect on tritiated thymidine incorporation in thymic cells from osteopetrotic rats, and several other immune defects have been demonstrated in these rodent models (467,468). In some strains, parenteral administration of bone marrow or transplantation of thymic tissue from normal littermates appears to correct the bone abnormalities, but in other strains, splenic or thymic lymphocytes alone may cure the disease (465,469).

Systemic treatment is an issue in the autosomal recessive malignant form. High-dose 1,25-dihydroxyvitamin D₃ coupled with a low-calcium diet has been used because of its ability to simulate osteoclasts and bone resorption (451). The autosomal recessive malignant form of osteopetrosis

into the diaphysis (457,458). The persistence of cartilage bars, normally resorbed by osteoclastic action in the zone of primary spongiosa, is a characteristic of both rickets and osteopetrosis, but, in osteopetrosis, the cartilage bars are

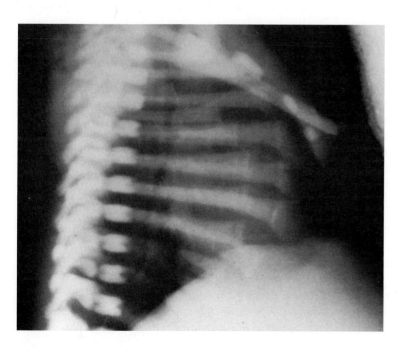

FIGURE 7-33. Patient with osteopetrosis. The increased bone density is also present in the vertebrae. In some patients, an alternating pattern of density is seen, producing a rugby jersey spine.

has been treated successfully by allogeneic bone marrow transplantation from human leukocyte antigen–identical siblings, or by marrow ablation with cyclophosphamide and total body irradiation, or busulfan followed by marrow transplantation from a human leukocyte antigen–mismatched donor (470–475). Treatment of osteopetrosis with recombinant human interferon-γ was reported more recently (476). These studies represent significant progress in the treatment of this disease and also provide further insight into the origin of the osteoclast (477).

The pediatric orthopaedic concerns about osteopetrosis are numerous (451). Transverse fractures with minimal displacement occur in the infantile malignant form and may be difficult to recognize. Without immobilization, abundant callus can occur in the healing phase. Fractures in the intermediate recessive and dominant forms are common and require conventional treatment. Although healing does occur, time to healing can be prolonged (450). Coxa vara and long-bone deformity can result during the course of treatment of multiple fractures. Both are amenable to corrective osteotomy (450,451). Intramedullary fixation is desirable, but can be difficult because of the hardness of the bone and compromise of the marrow space. Osteomyelitis is common because of the diminished vascularity and immune response. This problem is most common in the mandible, but it also can be seen in the long bones. Back pain is frequently encountered in the benign dominant form of osteopetrosis and responds to rest, bracing, and antiinflammatory medication.

Periosteal Reaction and Soft Tissue Calcification and Ossification

Numerous metabolic, inflammatory, traumatic, neoplastic, and idiopathic disorders of the infant's or child's skeleton may produce symptoms of localized or diffuse periosteal new bone formation on radiographic study (478,479). Unlike that of adults, the child's periosteum is easily stimulated to form new bone, and depending on the nature of the process, new bone formation may be diffuse and may cause considerable disability. Three of these disorders—hypervitaminosis A, Caffey disease, and scurvy—are discussed in this chapter in detail, but a brief history and a chronologic differential for the various syndromes are first provided.

The salient features of periosteal reaction, or cortical thickening in infancy or early childhood, are listed in Table 7-6. Physiologic periosteal reaction of the newborn is most prominent from 1 to 6 months of life. This is usually an incidental finding on radiographs obtained for other reasons. The periosteal reaction is thin, even, and symmetric, occurring along the femur, tibia, and humerus on both sides. Periosteal reaction can be seen in Menkes kinky-hair syndrome, an X-linked recessive disorder producing defective copper absorption (396). Although the radiographic

pattern with metaphyseal spurs and adjacent periosteal reaction may suggest abuse or healing rickets, the typical child is a male neonate with profound failure to thrive and progressive central nervous system degeneration, in addition to the characteristic kinky hair for which the entity is named.

In Engelmann-Camurati disease, which is autosomal dominant in transmission, the progressive cortical thickening of long bones is customarily seen at 4 to 6 years of age, in association with a waddling gait resulting from progressive neuromuscular degeneration (480).

Infection can occur at any age; in bacterial osteomyelitis, the periosteal reaction is usually associated with lytic and blastic metaphyseal changes. Congenital syphilis rarely is manifested in children younger than 3 months of age. Severe spirochetal infection may lead to fetal loss; survivors may develop early or late childhood lesions in rather protean manifestations. However, during infancy, a periosteal reaction resulting from syphilis usually occurs with metaphyseal lesions (481).

A periosteal reaction resulting from trauma can occur at any age; the features that differentiate accidental trauma from nonaccidental trauma were discussed previously. Periosteal new bone can be associated with burns (482). Metabolic conditions can cause periosteal reaction in a variety of settings. Hypervitaminosis A and scurvy usually appear no earlier than 9 months of age.

The neoplastic conditions that can result in the periosteal reaction in early childhood are leukemia, neuroblastoma, and retinoblastoma. Diffuse periosteal reaction associated with leukemia most often appears in children older than 2 years of age. Neuroblastoma and retinoblastoma can have similar radiographic appearances and may be seen earlier.

Although the peak occurrence of Caffey disease is at 6 weeks to 6 months of age, it can occur before 6 weeks. Periosteal new bone formation before 6 weeks is consistent with infection, trauma, or Caffey disease (391,394,395).

Caffey Disease

Infantile cortical hyperostosis, or Caffey disease, is a disorder of unknown cause affecting the skeleton and contiguous myofascial tissues (483–486). It is characterized by a febrile illness with hyperirritability, swelling of soft tissues, and cortical thickening of bone (487). The bones of the jaw and forearm are the most common sites, but occasionally the lesion is diffuse. The average age of onset is usually younger than 9 weeks of age, and several cases in which the disease began *in utero* have been described.

The child with Caffey disease may be febrile. The sedimentation rate and serum alkaline phosphatase are often elevated, but cultures and serologic studies fail to show an infectious agent. Radiographs reveal a periosteal reaction involving any bone except the vertebrae and phalanges. Caf-

TABLE 7-6. CAUSES OF PERIOSTEAL REACTION AND CORTICAL THICKENING IN INFANCY AND EARLY CHILDHOOD

Entity	Peak Age at Detection	Characteristics
Physiologic periosteal reaction of newborn	1–6 mo	Thin, even periosteal reaction symmetric along femora, tibiae, humeri
Congenital or genetic		
Menkes kinky-hair syndrome	Newborn	Failure to thrive; X-linked defective copper absorption; boys; sparse; kinky hair; central nervous system degeneration, metaphyseal fractures, and periosteal reaction confused with abuse and rickets
Engelmann-Camurati disease	4–6 yr	Autosomal dominant; progressive midshaft thickening of long bones; waddling gait; normal laboratory findings, except slight elevation of alkaline phosphatase
Infective		
Osteomyelitis	Any age	Classic bacterial osteomyelitis with lytic or blastic changes at metaphysis and periosteal reaction as disease progresses; elevated erythrocyte sedimentation rate (ESR); viral and fungal types exist; *Salmonella* osteomyelitis in sickle cell disease may begin at diaphysis; ESR not elevated
Congenital syphilis	>3 mo (severe spirochetal infection can cause fetal loss)	Many manifestations possible; osteochondritis with metaphyseal lytic lesions; diaphyseal osteitis; periostitis; positive serology for syphilis
Inflammatory		
Juvenile chronic arthritis	5–10 yr	Periarticular reaction at phalanges, metacarpals, and metatarsals
Traumatic		
Accidental or nonaccidental injury	Any age	Accidental injury should result in local reaction consistent with age-appropriate activities (i.e., single tibial reaction 7–10 d after injury in a child who is walking); nonaccidental injury can result in multiple areas of periosteal reaction inconsistent with age-appropriate activities
Burns	Weeks to months after burn	Usually a local response, but can have elements of hypertrophic osteoarthropathy
Metabolic		
Hypertrophic osteoarthropathy	Any age	Usually associated with physiologic abnormality in pulmonary, cardiac, or gastrointestinal system; tibial, fibular, radial, ulnar diaphyseal and metaphyseal involvement; clubbing
Hypervitaminosis A	>9 mo	Periosteal reaction in long bones, typically ulnas and metatarsals; epiphyseal and metaphyseal ossification abnormalities and physeal lesions possible; elevation of serum vitamin A level
	>9 mo	Epiphyseal and metaphyseal changes most prominent around knees, with associated subperiosteal hemorrhages; abnormal vitamin C levels in serum or blood
Hyperphosphatemia	Associated with tumoral calcinosis; second and third decades of life, but reported in childhood and infancy	Periostitis in tubular bones; calcified soft tissue masses; elevated serum phosphorus level
Healing phase of rickets	After treatment of rickets	Periosteal reaction adjacent to healing growth plates
In prostaglandin-induced hyperostosis	After weeks of prostaglandin E₁ administration to maintain ductus patency in congenital heart disease	Symmetric, diffuse periosteal reaction in long bones and ribs; elevated alkaline phosphatase level
Neoplastic		
Acute leukemia	2–5 yr	Diffuse osteopenia, metaphyseal rarefactions; commonly, symmetric periosteal reaction in long bones
Metastatic neuroblastoma, retinoblastoma	Similar to leukemia, with presentations <2 yr	Similar to leukemia
Idiopathic		
Caffey disease	6 wk–6 mo	Mandibular involvement, asymmetric involvement of clavicle, scapula, ribs, or tubular bones without associated lytic lesions; elevated alkaline phosphatase level and ESR

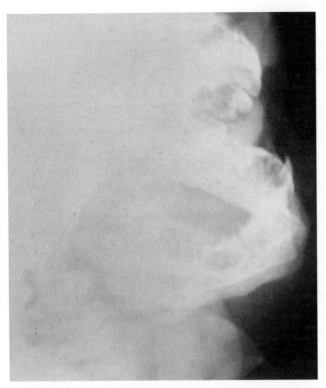

FIGURE 7-34. This oblique view of the mandible of a patient with Caffey disease demonstrates the characteristic periosteal reaction.

fey makes the point that involvement of a single bone, with the exception of the mandible, suggests trauma (484). Mandibular involvement is characteristic (Fig. 7-34). In the extremities, the ulna is most frequently involved (Fig. 7-35).

Pathologic study of the involved tissue in patients with Caffey disease has failed to define a specific alteration, although hyperplasia of collagen fibers and fibrinoid degeneration have been seen. A case report described the absence

of cortical bone at the diaphyses, which were entirely cancellous (487). Most patients recover spontaneously, but, for some, the disease becomes sufficiently severe to require short periods of corticosteroids to reduce the morbidity. Occasionally, a patient develops a chronic syndrome that persists into late childhood. The possibility of coexistent infection needs to be considered (488).

Hypervitaminosis A

Overdosage with vitamin A can be acute or chronic (489–491). Vitamin A is a necessary constituent in the synthesis of visual pigments, but it is also required in appropriate amounts for membrane stability. Excess or deficiency may lead to rupture of lysosomal membranes. Vitamin A participates in the biology of the epithelium, and, in excess, it causes a proliferation of basal cells and hyperkeratinization. Acute hypervitamin A intoxication causes intracranial pressure, vomiting, and lethargy. Several weeks or months of chronic overingestion (if the child survives) leads to a syndrome characterized by pruritus, skin lesions, failure to thrive, and muscle and bone tenderness. Radiographs in this later phase show the periosteal reaction in many of the long bones. Epiphyseal and metaphyseal ossification abnormalities occur with central physeal arrests. Hypercalcemia may be present, and serum vitamin A levels are elevated. Histologic study of the bones shows an increase in resorptive surfaces, suggesting that the combination of resorption and formation has been accelerated to a hypermetabolic state.

Scurvy

Scurvy, the pathologic state associated with a deficiency of vitamin C, is perhaps the best-understood metabolic disease, and is certainly the most preventable (492). All the clinical and pathologic manifestations of scurvy are based on the now well-defined role of ascorbic acid in the synthesis of

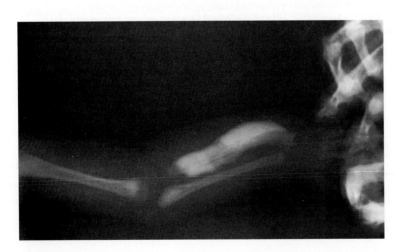

FIGURE 7-35. The ulna is the most frequently involved bone in the extremities of patients with Caffey disease.

collagen. In the course of collagen synthesis, a necessary step is the hydroxylation of the amino acids proline and lysine to hydroxyproline and hydroxylysine, both active participants in the intramolecular and intermolecular cross-links that stabilize collagen. The hydroxylation step takes place early in the synthetic process and requires ferrous iron, oxygen, α-ketoglutarate, and ascorbic acid. In the absence of ascorbate (neither humans nor guinea pigs can synthesize vitamin C), this step cannot occur, and the collagen that is synthesized is defective. If the mother's intake of vitamin C is adequate during pregnancy, the infant usually does not manifest the disease for several months (i.e., late onset), even if there is dietary insufficiency. Breast-feeding by a mother who has an adequate supply of vitamin C is usually sufficient to prevent scurvy.

The pathologic process that results from inadequate intake of vitamin C is characterized by production of collagen fibers of poor quality; all the body's systems are affected. Blood vessels become excessively permeable and rupture readily, normal bone formation is reduced, and bone that forms is lacking in tensile strength and is defective in structural arrangement.

Clinically, children with scurvy appear undernourished, apathetic, and irritable. They show generalized weakness, poor wound healing, petechial hemorrhages, ecchymoses, and bone pain that often leads to pseudoparalysis.

Radiographic findings in the skeleton of patients with scurvy may be seen in any of the long bones, but are most prominent around the knees (Fig. 7-36). Bone density is diminished, and the cortices are markedly thinned. An area of marked radiolucency, which causes the zone of provisional calcification at the physeometaphyseal junction to stand out in bold relief (i.e., white line of Fraenkel), is observed in the metaphysis. Brittleness of the zone of provisional calcification may lead to fractures and marginal spurs (i.e., Pelken sign). A zone of radiolucency forms beneath this zone, and separation may occur. The epiphyseal nucleus is also markedly radiolucent, but the calcification front of the cartilage is unaffected, producing an appearance of ringed epiphyses (i.e., Wimberger sign). Subperiosteal hemorrhages occur, lifting the periosteum and causing pain and pseudoparalysis. These areas calcify with treatment and have the appearance of periosteal new bone.

Laboratory studies may help to differentiate scurvy from other possible entities, most notably sepsis. A fasting serum vitamin C level can be determined if scurvy is being considered. This can be difficult to interpret. Ascorbic acid concentration in the buffy coat of blood is believed to be a better measure. A nonspecific aminoaciduria also exists in scurvy. Treatment is replacement of the deficient ascorbic acid. Minimal daily requirements are 30 mg for infants and 50 mg for adults. Therapeutic dosages may be 200 mg or higher.

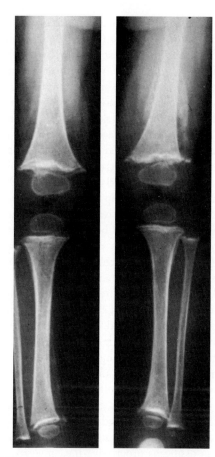

FIGURE 7-36. Patient with scurvy, early in treatment. The subperiosteal hemorrhage, especially on the left femur, has begun to ossify. The white lines of Fraenkel can still be seen at the distal femurs.

Calcification of Soft Tissues

Calcification or ossification in the soft tissues can represent diagnostic and therapeutic problems. Cutaneous calcification may be secondary to injury, to disturbance in calcium and phosphorus metabolism, as described previously, or to unknown factors. Depending on distribution, cutaneous calcification may be termed "calcinosis universalis" or "calcinosis cutis circumscripta" (493). True ossification or cutaneous osteomatosis has been reported, although rarely in the pediatric age group (491). If these entities are caused by a metabolic disturbance, treatment is directed toward rectifying the underlying problem. For idiopathic types of soft tissue calcification, such as that associated with collagen vascular diseases, no specific treatment exists, and removal of symptomatic deposits may be indicated.

Tumoral calcinosis consists of lobulated, calcified soft tissue masses adjacent to joints (494–496). Although it usually is seen in the second and third decades of life, it can be seen in infants and children. The serum phosphorus level is sometimes elevated. A defect in phosphorus transport or metabolism has been implicated, but not established as the cause of the tumoral calcinosis (497). The differential diagnosis includes collagen vascular diseases, hyperparathyroidism, and hypervitaminosis D, which must be excluded by history, physical examination, and laboratory data. Excision of the lesions surgically has not been entirely satisfactory, because of the possibilities of skin ulceration or recurrence (495,498). Treatment of tumoral calcinosis in adults has been successfully accomplished medically with phosphorus deprivation (496,499). Reports of tumoral calcinosis in children (495,498) and infants (494,500) have been made. The best treatment in this age group remains open to some judgment. Use of phosphorus deprivation in the immature skeleton, at least in theory, would be rachitogenic; hence, excision of symptomatic lesions may be the logical course (494,498,500). However, successful medical treatment with aluminum hydroxide antacid administration to bind phosphate and dietary phosphate restriction for 6 months has been reported for a 6-year-old child (495). An initial medical approach appears justified, even for a patient who is skeletally immature. A pediatric orthopaedist and a pediatric nephrologist or gastroenterologist make a logical team to balance the ongoing calcium and phosphorus needs of the skeleton with a restriction sufficient to affect the lesions favorably. If these somewhat conflicting goals cannot be met, excision may be indicated (494,498,500).

Ossification in the deeper soft tissues may represent fibrodysplasia ossificans progressiva (i.e., myositis ossificans progressiva) or myositis ossificans circumscripta or traumatica. Fibrodysplasia ossificans is a genetic condition (501,502). Digital abnormalities are present at birth, the most common being underdevelopment of the great toes and short, abnormal first metatarsals. Hearing loss, premature baldness, and mental retardation also can be clinical features of this entity. There is an abnormal modulation of pluripotential fibroblasts into osteoblasts. A bone morphogenetic protein (BMP) may mediate this process (503). Because of the knowledge of limb development at the molecular level, abnormal expression of BMP would be an attractive candidate to explain heterotopic ossification and brachydactyly (504). At present, there is no satisfactory treatment. Excision alone does not halt progressive ossification and limitation of the range of motion of joints. The effect of adjunctive metabolic treatments is difficult to assess. Respiratory failure with chest wall constriction may be terminal. The characterization of a BMP antagonist may provide a more effective treatment for this difficult entity (504).

In myositis ossificans circumscripta, there is usually either a clear history of trauma or an associated condition, such as neurologic or thermal injury, in which case the entity is usually termed "myositis ossificans traumatica" (482, 505,506). In spontaneous myositis ossificans circumscripta without a clear history of trauma or an associated condition, the entity may be called "pseudomalignant myositis" (507). Spontaneous myositis ossificans circumscripta is uncom-

mon, but has been reported in early childhood (508). The history of the patient with myositis ossificans traumatica usually facilitates the radiographic distinction from malignant processes. The ossification is more mature at the surface peripheral to the underlying bone, with an intervening space without osseous tissue. Although the periosteum as a source of the ossification has been considered, pluripotential fibroblasts modulating into osteoblasts may also be the source of myositis ossificans traumatica.

In myositis ossificans traumatica, spontaneous resolution can occur with only observation. When there is limitation of joint range of motion (particularly in association with conditions such as burns and head injuries), resection of a traumatically induced myositis may be undertaken during the quiescent phase when it is clear that it is no longer growing or resolving spontaneously (482,505). Adjunctive regimens such as radiation (509) are not indicated in children, but antiinflammatory programs have been used (506). Occasionally, the distinction of pseudomalignant myositis from malignant conditions may prove difficult, necessitating biopsy, and this is best coordinated with the pathologist to review all features of the case in interpreting the histologic findings.

Connective Tissue Syndromes

Marfan Syndrome

Marfan syndrome is a genetic disorder of connective tissue, and, like osteogenesis imperfecta and EDS, it has some degree of heterogeneity. The mode of inheritance is thought to be autosomal dominant transmission (379,510). Common findings are in the skeletal, ocular, and cardiovascular systems. The skeleton shows arachnodactyly (i.e., abnormally long and slender digits), dolichostenomelia (i.e., long, narrow limbs), pectus deformities, and scoliosis. In the cardiovascular system, aortic regurgitation, aortic dilatation, aneurysms, and mitral valve prolapse can occur. Ocular findings are myopia and superior displacement of the lens (compare with homocystinuria, in which the lens displacement is inferior).

Marfan syndrome has been classified into four more or less distinct types: asthenic, nonasthenic, contractural, and hypermobile. Cardiac manifestations are particularly pronounced in the asthenic type. In contractural Marfan syndrome, the joints have a decreased range of motion. In the hypermobile type, joint motion is increased (compare with EDS, type III).

Marfan syndrome has been linked to a fibrillin gene on chromosome 15, as has ectopia lentis; congenital contractural arachnodactyly has been linked to a fibrillin gene on chromosome 5 (511). These findings make possible the diagnosis of Marfan syndrome on the basis of genetic linkage and analysis. However, the diagnosis is still established by a combination of findings in two of the three affected systems (i.e., ocular, cardiac, and musculoskeletal) and a

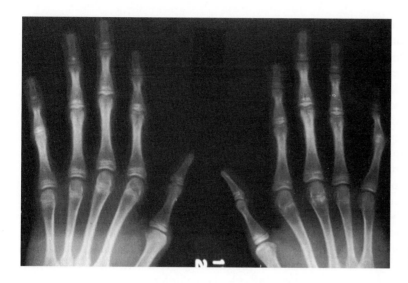

FIGURE 7-37. Hands showing arachnodactyly. Notice the long, thin metacarpals and phalanges.

positive family history (510). Although genetic analysis usually establishes the diagnosis, the pediatric orthopaedist frequently participates in this process at some point relative to the musculoskeletal findings. The ratio of upper segment (i.e., head to pubic symphysis) to lower segment (i.e., pubic symphysis to plantar surface) is calculated. In the normal mature skeleton, this ratio is 0.93. (Tables are required to calculate the normal ratio at various points during growth.) Because of the dolichostenomelia, in Marfan syndrome this ratio is decreased to approximately 0.85 or less (512). Steinberg (513) described the thumb sign. The thumb is grasped in a clenched fist. In Marfan syndrome, because of the arachnodactyly, the thumb protrudes past the ulnar border of the hand. Similarly, when the thumb and index finger are wrapped around the opposite wrist, there is overlap. Arachnodactyly alone does not make a diagnosis of Marfan syndrome.

Although the radiographic findings in patients with Marfan syndrome are fairly typical for this disorder, no single sign is pathognomonic, because of variable expressivity in this syndrome and considerable overlap with the normal population. Arachnodactyly can easily be defined by radiographic examination because of the long, slender phalanges, metatarsals, and metacarpals, and the increased ratio of length to width of the second to fifth metacarpals (Fig. 7-37). The lengths of the second to fifth metacarpals are divided by the widths of the respective diaphyses. The ratios are averaged. Positive arachnodactyly is defined as a ratio greater than 8.8 in males and greater than 9.4 in females (514). These findings may also be seen in minimally affected individuals who have no other manifestations of the disease.

Scoliosis may be present and is relatively indistinguishable from that in other patients, but in some patients, the vertebral height is notably increased (Fig. 7-38). Bone density is normal compared with the osteopenia seen in homo-

cystinuria. The curve pattern frequently is either single right thoracic or double right thoracic and left lumbar (515). The thoracic curve is most commonly lordoscoliotic. The thoracolumbar junction is prone to kyphosis, probably related to the underlying ligamentous laxity (516).

It is important for the orthopaedist who sees undiag-

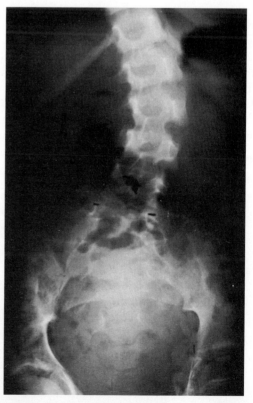

FIGURE 7-38. Patient with Marfan syndrome. Scoliosis is obvious. The bone quality is normal, unlike the osteopenia seen in homocystinuria.

nosed patients with the Marfan phenotype to consider it when treating sprains and other injuries associated with the altered ligamentous structure or scoliosis. The potential for serious ocular abnormalities and life-threatening cardiac abnormalities exists in association with the musculoskeletal problems. The potential cardiac problems are aortic and mitral valvular disease, aortic aneurysm, and conduction defects that can cause sudden death. After the diagnosis of Marfan syndrome has been considered and workup pursued, an electrocardiogram and an echocardiogram are customarily obtained. If the echocardiogram reveals positive findings, the cardiology service should participate in the patient's care. Scoliosis should be treated aggressively [➡2.9]. The treatment guidelines follow those for idiopathic scoliosis. Curves greater than 50 degrees require surgery (517). The cardiac status is important at this juncture. Valvular disease requires antibiotic prophylaxis, with specific recommendations varying among cardiology services.

Ehlers-Danlos Syndrome

Ehlers-Danlos syndrome (EDS) once was considered to be a single genetically induced entity characterized by hyperextensibility of the skin, joint hypermobility, easy bruisability, soft tissue and bony fragility, calcification of soft tissues, and various degrees of osteopenia. The syndrome was thought to result from a single error, but to have variable expressivity. It has now been clearly established, however, that EDS is a family of disorders embracing a large variety of defects in collagen metabolism (13). At least 13 types of EDS have been identified, and the groups are now considered to be the most common heritable disorder of connective tissue (14). The genetic basis for types I, II, and III does not seem to reflect a difference in the type I or III collagens, which are in skin and ligaments. Presumably, the mechanism underlying these types must involve other collagens or noncol-

lagenous proteins in the matrix. Type VII EDS has abnormalities in type I collagen similar to the abnormality found in type IV osteogenesis imperfecta, but the two syndromes are distinct (14). Type VII EDS has multiple joint dislocations but no clinical bone fragility, whereas type IV osteogenesis imperfecta has joint hypermobility, but no instability, and the bone fragility characteristic of osteogenesis imperfecta.

The orthopaedic manifestations of EDS vary with the type, but may also be considered collectively (518,519). This has practical significance for the pediatric orthopaedic surgeon because, like individuals with Marfan syndrome, these patients may present to the pediatric orthopaedist without a previous diagnosis. Consideration of the diagnosis of EDS may then prompt further consultation, such as with the genetics and dermatology services, leading to a diagnosis, subtyping, and a clearer definition of the associated conditions. The general orthopaedic conditions include joint hypermobility, joint instability (520,521), arthralgias, and scoliosis. Scoliosis is particularly common in types III and VI EDS. As in Marfan syndrome, treatment generally proceeds according to guidelines for idiopathic scoliosis, with an awareness of associated conditions and a particularly cautious monitoring of the response to bracing.

In EDS type I, the gravis variety, joint hypermobility, and skin hyperextensibility dominate the picture. The skin, although hyperextensible, is not lax and returns to its original configuration. Areas of recurrent bruising can be recognized by the accumulation of pigment (Fig. 7-39). Subcutaneous calcified nodules may be present in these regions and may be seen on radiographs. EDS type I is transmitted as an autosomal dominant trait.

In EDS type II, or the mitis variety, the manifestations are similar to those in EDS type I, but milder. Transmission is also as an autosomal dominant trait.

In EDS type III, also known as benign familial hypermo-

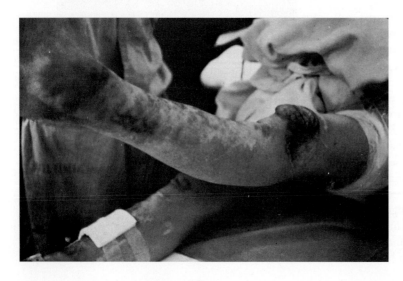

FIGURE 7-39. Patient with Ehlers-Danlos syndrome, type I. The knees and pretibial regions have been subjected to recurrent injury and have accumulated heme pigmentation. (Courtesy of Michael G. Ehrlich, M.D., Providence, RI.)

bility, joint hypermobility is present, but scar formation is normal, unlike the situation in EDS types I and II. The inheritance pattern is autosomal dominant. There is not a clinical laboratory test to establish a diagnosis of EDS type III, which is made on the basis of history (including family history) and physical examination. It is worthwhile for the orthopaedist to consider this diagnosis in a patient with instability of multiple joints. In such a setting, successful surgical reconstruction may be difficult, and ultimately, fusion may be required (519). Cardiac evaluation for the possibility of a floppy mitral valve may be desirable.

EDS type IV is the vascular or ecchymotic type and can be further subtyped. It results from abnormalities in type III collagen, the type required for vascular integrity. Autosomal dominant and recessive modes of transmission have been described. The clinical findings are thin skin, usually normal joint mobility, and visceral rupture.

In EDS type V, the skin hyperextensibility is similar to that in EDS type II, but with less marked joint mobility and skin fragility. Its transmission is considered to be X-linked.

EDS type VI is the most clearly biochemically characterized syndrome. Patients with this ocular-scoliotic type show a relative decrease in concentrations of lysine hydroxylase and therefore deficient concentrations of hydroxylysine in the collagen (522). Because lysine hydroxylation is a post-translational modification of the collagen necessary for normal cross-links, the collagen fibers are loosely organized and more soluble. As with most enzymatically based genetic diseases, transmission occurs as an autosomal recessive trait. Ocular fragility and scoliosis are present.

EDS type VII, arthrochalasis multiplex congenita, is notable for extreme joint laxity. Three subtypes with abnormalities in type I collagen metabolism have been identified (14). Developmental dysplasia of the hip is common (521). Autosomal dominant and recessive modes of transmission exist.

In EDS type VIII, the usual stigmata are present, but progressive periodontal disease is a distinguishing feature. The biochemical defect is unknown. Inheritance is as an autosomal dominant trait.

Homocystinuria

Cysteine (SH CH$_2$ CH [NH$_2$] COOH) is not an essential amino acid; it is synthesized from methionine and serine. Cystine or dicysteine is the disulfide resulting from the oxidation of two cysteine moieties. The homolog homocysteine (SH CH$_2$ CH$_2$ CH [NH$_2$] COOH) contains an additional methyl group compared with cysteine. Homocystine is the disulfide from two homocysteine groups. Homocysteine is an intermediary metabolite in the production of cysteine from methionine. There are three enzymatic steps in this pathway for which defects have been described that lead to

the accumulation of homocysteine and homocystine in the blood and homocystine in the urine (523,524).

Type I homocystinuria has a phenotype similar to that of Marfan syndrome (525). Patients with homocystinuria are tall with long limbs and may have arachnodactyly and scoliosis. Dislocation of the lens in common, but, unlike that seen in Marfan syndrome, the displacement is inferior. Osteoporosis is a marked feature of type I homocystinuria, but in Marfan syndrome, bone quality is normal. Vertebral osteoporosis may be present in homocystinuria, producing biconcavity and flattening of vertebral bodies. Florid arachnodactyly and scoliosis are more common in Marfan syndrome, in which the vertebral bodies are normal or excessively tall. Widening of the epiphyses and metaphyses of long bones is more typically seen in homocystinuria. Mental retardation is not a feature of Marfan syndrome. Mental retardation does occur in approximately half of all patients with homocystinuria (526). Another notable feature of type I homocystinuria is an abnormality in clotting, which leads to venous and arterial thromboembolic episodes (527).

The biochemical defect in type I homocystinuria is thought to be a deficiency of cystathionine synthetase, which normally catalyzes the chemical union of homocysteine and serine to form cystathionine. The enzyme uses pyridoxine (vitamin B$_6$) as a cofactor. Blood levels of methionine are increased in patients with this metabolic error. Screening of marfanoid patients for homocystine in the urine with the cyanide nitroprusside test can differentiate type I homocystinuria from the phenotypically similar Marfan syndrome.

Types II and III homocystinuria are biochemically distinct, because the errors cause blocks at other points. Blood levels of methionine are normal. The other stigmata, such as skeletal changes and thromboses, are absent.

Treatment for homocystinuria depends on the type. In type I, the typical course is methionine restriction and pyridoxine supplementation. This may also have the beneficial effect of preventing thromboses (527). For types II and III, methionine restriction is harmful. Treatment with cofactors also varies for the other types. Vitamin B$_{12}$ is suggested in the management of type II, and folic acid for type III.

As with all inborn errors of metabolism, homocystinuria may reveal other physiologic aspects. Hyperhomocysteinemia has been determined to be an independent risk factor for vascular disease (528). It may have a role in the generation of neural tube defects (529). The role of folate, B$_6$, and B$_{12}$ in treating hyperhomocysteinemia and its sequelae is evolving.

ENDOCRINOPATHIES

Although the spectrum of disorders of the endocrine glands can manifest symptoms in several ways, alterations in rate of growth and skeletal morphology are common in children.

The pediatrician usually detects the problem, then consults the orthopaedist; it is essential that he or she be aware of the nature and significance of these disorders. Although skeletal growth has been discussed extensively in Chapters 1 and 2, some salient features of the growth process are particularly germane to endocrine physiology and are reviewed briefly here.

Several parameters are useful in assessing growth: height, sitting height, arm span, head circumference, and body weight (530,531). These factors must be interpreted in relation to chronologic and biologic age. Because of difficulties in interpretation, investigators have advocated increasingly sophisticated means of assessment (532,533). Nevertheless, these factors are appropriate in the primary study of the patient. All parameters must be interpreted according to cross-sectional distributions in the general population, or, if possible, longitudinally in the individual over time. The latter approach is especially useful in determining whether a borderline value is actually pathologic for a given patient.

Examples of different growth patterns are shown in Figs. 7-40 through 7-43. The child whose curve continues to fall below the normal percentiles is much more likely to have

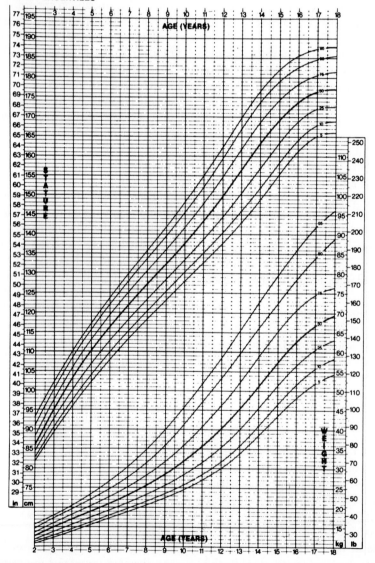

FIGURE 7-40. Normal growth chart for boys, 2 to 18 years of age. (Adapted from ref. 534, with permission.)

a hormonal problem than the child whose curve stays constantly in a low percentile. Placement in the third percentile and below in absolute height raises suspicion, and, when combined with a commensurate decrease in growth velocity, such an abnormality warrants further investigation.

Several features of morphometry and growth can be assessed in a crude manner without consulting the available standard charts. The first of these is the ratio or percentage of sitting height relative to total height. At birth, the ratio should approximate 70%. (This value also can be expressed as a ratio of upper segment [i.e., head to pubic symphysis]

to lower segment [i.e., pubic symphysis to plantar surface] and should equal 1.69.) By 3 years of age, the sitting height should constitute 57% of total height, and, in adolescence, the value should be 52%. As a rough approximation, 25 cm of growth can be expected in the first year of life, 10 cm in the second year, 6 cm in the third and fourth years, and 5 cm annually thereafter, with a spurt at the beginning of adolescence. The velocity of growth throughout childhood has been the subject of extensive analytic study and is a far more sensitive indicator than absolute stature in the detection of a problem (Fig. 7-43).

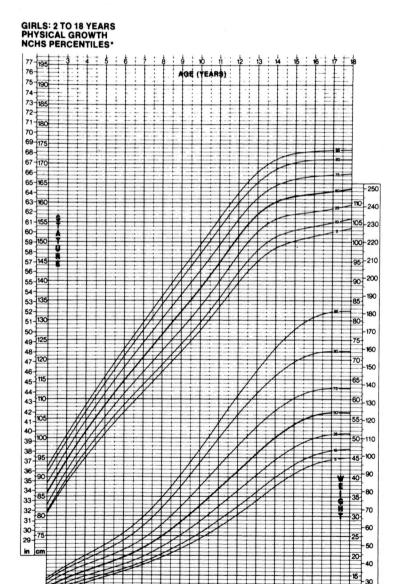

FIGURE 7-41. Normal growth chart for girls, 2 to 18 years of age. (Adapted from ref. 534, with permission.)

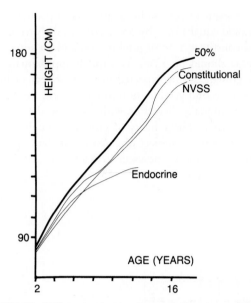

FIGURE 7-42. Different patterns of growth disturbance. The normal fiftieth percentile serves as a reference. In the endocrine disturbance, a progressive deceleration in growth occurs. In constitutional growth delay, growth starts normally, decreases during the first few years of life, and finally regains its earlier percentile level. In normal variant short stature (NVSS), growth remains at a constant but low (third or less) percentile.

Correlating these parameters relative to some index of maturity is obviously an important issue, and Tanner and associates have devoted a great deal of thought to this (530,531). Because any stage of development is a combination of anatomic and physiologic changes, and this combi-

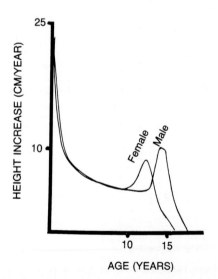

FIGURE 7-43. Growth velocity curves. Plotted in this manner, changes in growth rates frequently can be detected early. (Adapted from ref. 531, with permission.)

nation may be different for each person, any single parameter for a person compared with standard parameters may not accurately reflect that person's maturity. A combination of physical and radiographic criteria may have to be invoked. For most orthopaedic applications, radiographs of the left wrist and hand are the customary index of bone age in children 2 years of age and older, but the orthopaedist must be aware that there are limitations to this method (12,533). These include interobserver variability in determining the bone age, variation in the correlation of growth with bone age among different genetic populations, and a relatively large standard deviation in the correlation within a population during the growth spurt.

The initial diagnostic approach for patients suspected of having an endocrine-related growth problem should include a careful history of the pattern of growth, a family history, and a history of associated gastrointestinal, renal, and neurologic signs or symptoms. Endocrine disturbances should be evaluated. Menarchial history is important in girls. In addition to a general physical examination, the growth patterns described previously must be measured accurately. Breast development and the age of appearance and the extent of development of axillary and pubic hair and gonads should be assessed. Routine laboratory studies should include complete blood count, urinalysis, and glucose, BUN, creatinine, electrolytes, calcium, phosphorus, and alkaline phosphatase levels, and left wrist and hand radiographs should be obtained for the determination of bone age. Additional laboratory studies may be necessary in the pursuit of specific entities.

Normal Variant Short Stature

By definition, normal variant short stature (NVSS) involves a current and predicted height below the third percentile, a birth weight greater than 2.5 kg, no apparent organic cause for growth retardation, and a normal serum growth hormone level (when tested with pharmacologic provocation) (535). NVSS has tentatively been further classified, but the significance of this has yet to be established. Practically speaking, the majority of short-statured persons (85%) fall into this category, for which no specific cause can be established. A slightly different category of short stature is described by the term "constitutional growth delay." In this situation, there is normal early growth, then a deceleration during the first 2 years, and subsequent reestablishment of a normal pattern. As with NVSS, no metabolic or endocrine abnormality can be established. This growth pattern is clear in retrospect, but causes concern at the time of presentation; workup is recommended to rule out other problems. The differential diagnosis includes conditions (discussed in subsequent sections) that cause short stature.

Treatment is usually a matter of explanation and reassurance. One report suggested a role for growth hormone as therapy for a subgroup of this population; the use of growth hormone is still evolving (535,536). The role of nutrition as a cause of NVSS has yet to be evaluated fully, and improving dietary intake of proteins and other important constituents remains part of the management (537).

Growth Hormone Deficiency and Hypopituitarism

Deficiency of growth hormone leads to progressive inhibition of linear growth and maturation (538,539). Birth weight and height are usually normal in children with this disorder. Typically, the deviations begin to become evident after the first year of life. Deficiency of growth hormone may or may not be associated with other deficiencies of hypothalamic-releasing factors or other pituitary hormones, including, from the anterior portion, human growth hormone, adrenocorticotropin (ACTH), thyroid-stimulating hormone (TSH), follicle-stimulating hormone, prolactin or lactogenic hormone, luteinizing hormone, or testicular interstitial cell-stimulating hormone; from the middle portion, melanocyte-stimulating hormone; and from the posterior portion, antidiuretic hormone and oxytocin (540,541). The clinical manifestations of growth hormone deficiency can be narrow, affecting only growth, or diffuse, with a broad range of additional abnormalities. Deficiencies of ACTH and TSH can be recognized by appropriate biochemical tests, but deficiencies of gonadotropins usually cannot be diagnosed until the age at which puberty would otherwise be expected. The basic clinical manifestation is progressive retardation in growth and maturation (Fig. 7-44).

When growth hormone deficiency is suspected on clinical grounds, laboratory testing is essential (542). The studies available are one-time assay tests, with results varying according to stress and alterations in response to chemical and pharmacologic manipulation. The first major investigative effort is an exercise test in which growth hormone levels are measured by radioimmunoassay during walking. Resting values are usually less than 5 ng per mL; minimum peak values are in the 7 to 12 ng per mL range. If the exercise test result is normal, the production of growth hormone is considered adequate. If it is abnormal, a pharmacologic stress test can be performed. Several protocols have been advanced, including insulin-induced hypoglycemia, arginine infusion, and an L-dopa–propranolol test (543). If the increase in growth hormone is still inadequate and thyroid function is normal, growth hormone deficiency has been confirmed.

The underlying cause of growth hormone deficiency may be idiopathic, previous head injury, psychosocial problems, including malnutrition and neglect, and intracranial tumor (544,545). It is particularly important to rule out the presence of a craniopharyngioma by thorough neurologic examination, visual field studies and funduscopic examination,

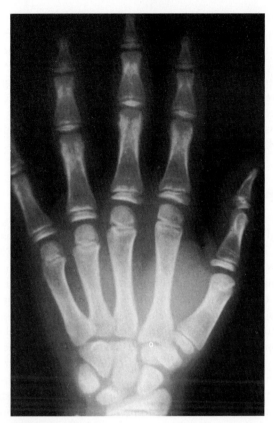

FIGURE 7-44. Patient with panhypopituitarism. The patient had retarded height and maturation. The bone age was 11 years; the chronologic age was 20 years.

skull radiography, and computed tomography or magnetic resonance imaging.

The differential diagnosis of growth hormone–deficient short stature includes several entities. In NVSS, the patient continues to grow at a constant but low level, but, in constitutional growth delay, there is a return to a higher growth curve without intervention. Although delayed puberty may be difficult to distinguish from growth hormone deficiency, maturity milestones, once established, continue to appear at a normal rate. A growth hormone assay may be helpful in making these differential diagnoses. At times, children with one of the gastrointestinal or renal diseases mentioned in previous sections may present for evaluation because of growth retardation, but the general initial workup will reveal the presence of such disease. Disorders associated with chromosomal abnormalities should be considered. Turner syndrome usually has many other stigmata, but an XO/XX mosaic may be more difficult to differentiate. Hypothyroidism and gonadal dysfunction also must be included in the differential diagnosis.

Treatment for growth hormone deficiency must start with the exclusion and correction of the psychosocial causes of the deficiency, because in these cases, response to administration of growth hormone will be suboptimal. In other cases, human growth hormone administration is the treatment of choice (536,546). If growth hormone deficiency is associated with other hormonal deficiencies, replacement treatment for these factors must be included in the therapeutic regimen. The response to growth hormone in these selected cases is usually dramatic. Unfortunately, a few patients develop antibodies to the hormone, and its value is markedly diminished.

Hypothyroidism

The manifestations of a deficiency in thyroid hormone depend on age. In the newborn period, hypothyroidism manifests itself as cretinism; the infant is described as sluggish and shows increasingly short stature and developmental delay, immature facies, a broad flat nasal bridge, and coarse hair. The child often manifests constipation, severe feeding problems, persistence of jaundice, a protruding tongue, and a protuberant abdomen with an umbilical hernia. Mental development is retarded, and if recognition and treatment are delayed, irreparable nervous system damage may occur.

In the older child, manifestations usually more closely resemble those seen in adults with hypothyroidism. Changes in facial appearance are less commonly seen. Retardation of growth is characteristic, and radiographically, the secondary centers of ossification appear late and show a peculiar fragmentation that may be misinterpreted as evidence of osteonecrosis (547). Lethargy, changes in personality, and poor school performance may be the presenting features. Slipped capital femoral epiphyses may be seen (548) **[➡3.14]**. In untreated cases, slippage may not be seen until the child is older; because it can also occur during the treatment for hypothyroidism as the bone age advances, vigilance is important at this time (549) (Fig. 7-45). In some children

with mild hypothyroidism, retarded linear growth and delayed skeletal maturation may be the only manifestations.

Specific laboratory studies for hypothyroidism include measurement of thyroid hormones and TSH. Additional thyroid studies may be necessary to define the precise locus of the hypothyroidism. Normal values must be interpreted in terms of age. In the case of growth retardation, a growth hormone assay must also be performed. However, the serum growth hormone level usually does not increase, even in response to the provocative tests, until the hypothyroidism has been corrected. Bone age is typically delayed to a more severe degree than in other endocrinopathies affecting maturation. Delay in the appearance of secondary centers involves all epiphyses. For congenital hypothyroidism, a knee film is more useful than a wrist film (Fig. 7-46). The distal femoral secondary center of ossification, which should be present at term, is absent. Occasionally, irregularities in ossification give a stippled appearance to the secondary centers. In the proximal femur, this may impart a Perthes-like radiographic appearance, but both proximal femurs are symmetrically involved (Fig. 7-47). One study found a group of Perthes patients to be generally euthyroid but to have a moderate elevation of free thyroxine, suggesting a disturbance in chondrocyte maturation in this disease (550).

Treatment for hypothyroidism is replacement with an appropriate dosage of thyroid hormone, a therapy that requires careful fine-tuning to avoid acceleration in bone maturation and premature closure of epiphyseal plates. Even with appropriate treatment, evidence indicates that juvenile acquired hypothyroidism results in a permanent height deficit relative to the duration of hypothyroidism before treatment (547).

Gonadal Abnormalities and Sex Steroids

Some of the effects of sex steroids on growth and turnover were discussed in the early part of this chapter. The manner

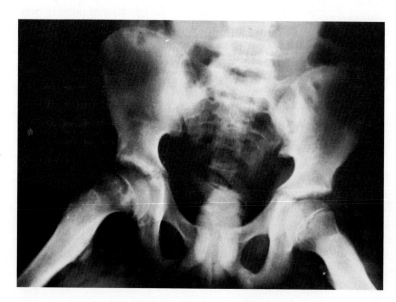

FIGURE 7-45. Slipped capital femoral epiphysis in a boy being treated for hypothyroidism. The patient's chronologic age was 13 years, 11 months, and his bone age was 12 years, 6 months.

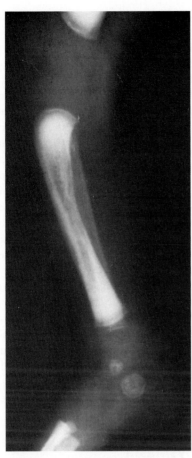

FIGURE 7-46. Child with congenital hypothyroidism at term. The distal femoral secondary center should be ossified, but is absent.

by which these hormones act is still not completely clear, but according to theory, specific receptors for these steroids are on the membrane or in the cytoplasm of the target cells (551,552). No receptors for androgens or estrogens have been identified in chondrocytes from the epiphyseal plate, in contrast to specific receptors for somatomedins (30).

Despite the absence of specific binding sites, two major effects of sex steroids on the skeleton have been identified: promotion of maturation and an increase in the rate of growth. The typical early finding in syndromes associated with sexual precocity is accelerated growth. At first, the child is taller than his or her peer population, according to chronologic age. Later, the acceleration of maturation predominates, and if untreated, the patient ultimately suffers a growth impairment compared with his or her peer group. As an example, an increased concentration of testosterone in childhood results in virilization and initially increased epiphyseal growth. With advancing time, the plate closes prematurely, and ultimately, the child is shorter in stature than his peers. Conversely, in humans and animals, early castration initially slows the rate of growth, but materially increases the length of time until epiphyseal closure; the eunuch is often taller than the average child. Estrogens also promote maturational changes in the epiphysis, but cell proliferation and matrix production are often retarded, so that the person with an abundance of estrogen may be considerably shorter.

Sex steroids are also produced by the adrenal cortex. They may be especially important for girls, because they are converted to testosterone activity and may initiate the adolescent growth spurt.

It is evident from the foregoing facts that the syndromes associated with precocious puberty and adrenal hyperplasia

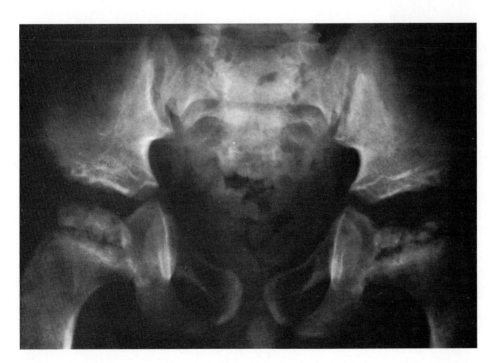

FIGURE 7-47. Patient with later-onset hypothyroidism. A Perthes-like pattern can be seen in the femoral epiphyses, but both are at a similar stage of fragmentation.

must be considered in the differential diagnosis of disturbances of growth or premature skeletal maturation, and the abnormalities associated with decreased gonadal function, such as Turner syndrome or Prader-Willi syndrome, must be considered in the differential diagnosis of delayed skeletal maturation.

Glucocorticoid-related Abnormalities

The abnormalities in the skeleton associated with alterations in adrenal glucocorticoid production are encountered considerably less frequently in children than in adults. However, Cushing syndrome occurs (Fig. 7-48), and the musculoskeletal abnormalities of Addison disease have also been reported (540,553). Iatrogenic problems secondary to the administration of steroids for asthma, neoplasms, immuno-

suppression, and other diseases are more common in childhood.

Although no definite receptor for glucocorticoids has been found in epiphyseal chondrocytes, the effects of these agents on the growing skeleton are profound. Proteoglycan and collagen synthesis are sharply decreased, and chondrocyte differentiation in the zone of growth is impaired. An excess of glucocorticoids may exert an effect through suppression of growth hormone synthesis or somatomedin production. Corticoids also inhibit calcium absorption; however, based on this factor alone, rickets must be rare.

Of greatest concern is the action of glucocorticoids on the skeleton itself, because sustained high doses produce profound and usually irreversible osteopenia, even after the drug is discontinued. However, a study in adults demonstrated that 1,25-dihydroxyvitamin D_3 and calcium, used prophylactically, prevented corticosteroid bone loss in the lumbar spine (554). Children on corticosteroids may exhibit fairly severe osteoporosis, often with compression fractures of the vertebrae. The possibility of osteonecrosis occurring in 6 to 25% of children receiving prolonged therapy with high doses of corticosteroids is significant; it is a major cause of disability. Unfortunately, there is no absolutely safe dosage of glucocorticoids for children. These agents should be used when absolutely necessary and at the lowest possible dosage consistent with clinical well-being.

Fibrous Dysplasia

Fibrous dysplasia (i.e., osteitis fibrosa cystica disseminata) results from a somatic mutation that produces sites in one, several, or occasionally many bones in which the normal medullary mix of osseous and marrow elements is replaced by what appears to be benign neoplastic fibrous tissue (555–557).

Traditionally, fibrous dysplasia has been a difficult entity to classify. It can be classified under neoplasms and is discussed partially in that Chapter 14 of this text. The intriguing, but previously unexplained, association with multiple endocrine problems has always earned a place for this entity in a metabolic chapter. In affected areas of the skeleton, there is both decreased formation and increased absorption of bone. The fibrous tissue undergoes ossification by a form of intramembranous bone formation, without apparent conversion of the fibroblasts to osteoblasts; the bone produced consists of small, irregular, purposeless, and often poorly mineralized trabeculae. The disease process is most active during growth, showing considerable activity on bone scan and causing internal scalloping of the cortices, weakening of the bone, and pathologic fracture. It often persists into adult life. Fibrous dysplasia may be associated with significant endocrine disturbances, which can dominate the picture (558).

The clinical manifestations of fibrous dysplasia may vary greatly (555). The lesions may be isolated (i.e., monostotic),

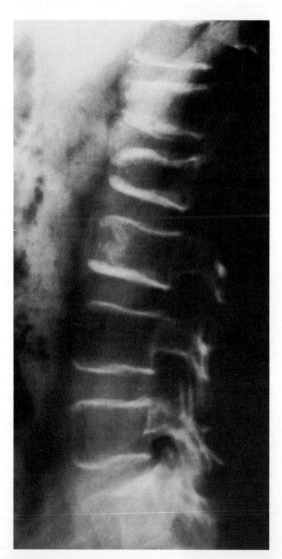

FIGURE 7-48. Cushing syndrome in an adolescent. There is marked steroid-induced osteoporosis.

or found in several bones on one side of the skeleton, or scattered throughout the skeleton (i.e., polyostotic). Solitary lesions are rarely accompanied by endocrine problems and usually are of no concern to the patient unless fracture occurs. At the opposite end of the spectrum are the cases in which the lesions are polyostotic and widely disseminated. The patient may display multiple sites of skeletal involvement, with severe distortion of the normal bony configuration and facial appearance as a result of asymmetric enlargement of the facial bones (i.e., hemihypertrophy cranii). Patients with florid disease suffer frequent fractures, particularly at such sites as the pelvic rami and necks of femurs. Lesions in the necks of femurs may cause progressive coxa vara, leading to the shepherd's crook deformity.

Radiologic findings in patients with fibrous dysplasia vary somewhat, depending on the bone involved and the site, but the bone usually is expanded at the site. The cortices are thinned but intact and scalloped from within. The area of the lesion shows few trabecular markings; instead, the fibrous tissue and small bony spicules (below the resolution of the x-ray beam) project a ground-glass consistency. In florid cases of fibrous dysplasia, deformities and other sequelae of old fractures are evident. Skin abnormalities are frequently seen in the more florid types of polyostotic fibrous dysplasia. These lesions are macular and light brown (cafe au lait spots). They often have an irregular border ("coast of Maine"), unlike similar lesions with a smooth border ("coast of California") seen in neurofibromatosis.

The McCune-Albright syndrome (MAS) includes polyostotic fibrous dysplasia, cafe au lait spots, precocious puberty, and hyperfunction of multiple endocrine glands. This entity, like Albright hereditary osteodystrophy (AHO), has been linked to an abnormality in G protein function. As discussed in the section on AHO, G proteins are trimers

of three different protein subunits (α, β, and γ) that link many different cell membrane receptors, such as hormone receptors, to their effector molecules, such as enzymes or ion channels (350,559,560). The G protein that couples receptors to adenyl cyclase activity is designated G_s. Mutations in the α-subunit of G_s (*GNAS1*) have been shown to cause both AHO and MAS. However, the mutation in AHO is a germline loss of function, whereas the mutation in MAS is a somatic gain of function with sporadic distribution. Activating mutations of G_s protein have also been demonstrated in monostotic fibrous lesions of bone (561). Furthermore, in an animal model, the activating mutation of the G_s protein also induced higher expression of interleukin-6, which may be responsible for the increased bone resorption in this disease (562). Therefore, there is an evolving molecular explanation for the various manifestations of fibrous dysplasia.

The natural history of fibrous dysplasia is variable (556). If multiple lesions become obvious during early childhood, the skeletal deformity may become severe. Localized lesions that manifest in adolescence are less likely to cause problems.

Treatment for fibrous dysplasia has been surgical intervention at the site at which the lesion has caused, or is likely to cause, pathologic fracture. Deformity at the proximal femur may be particularly difficult to treat (Fig. 7-49). Generous osteotomies may be required in this location to move the femoral neck out of the considerable varus. As in other diseases with bone of poor quality, intramedullary fixation is preferable to plates and screws alone, which tend to dislodge from such bone (563,564). The issue of the best graft or bone-inducing agent or synthetic in this condition has been debated. Bone grafting in fibrous dysplasia is challenging. Autografts tend to be replaced with fibrous tissue, reflecting the increased resorption seen in this condition. One study

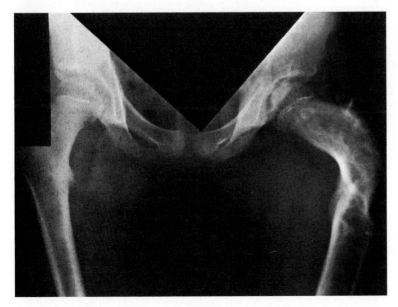

FIGURE 7-49. A patient with fibrous dysplasia has a shepherd's crook deformity of the left hip.

has indicated that valgus osteotomy alone is as effective as osteotomy and autogenous bone grafting (565) [➡**4.5**]. In general, allografted bone is more slowly revascularized than autografted bone (566–569). The persistence of an allograft on a clinical radiograph may not correlate with increased biomechanical strength. Nevertheless, the use of allografts applied to fibrous dysplasia raises interesting possibilities (570). Fibular strut allografts have been used successfully in combination with sliding compression screws (571).

The advent of agents that are effective in inhibiting absorption, particularly the bisphosphonates, has opened the possibility of medical management of several conditions with diminished bone strength seen in pediatric orthopaedics. Studies in the literature for osteogenesis imperfecta were cited in that section. These agents may have wider application, including use in fibrous dysplasia. The safety and efficacy of the various agents will need to be established by protocols. Pediatric orthopaedic surgeons will need to interact with pediatric endocrinologists at their institutions as these treatments bring basic science to clinical application and increase optimism for favorably affecting an extremely difficult condition.

References

1. Mankin HJ. Metabolic bone disease. *J Bone Joint Surg Am* 1994; 76:760.
2. Phillips LS, Vassilopoulos-Sellin R. Somatomedins. *N Engl J Med* 1980;302:371, 438.
3. Zaleske DJ. Cartilage and bone development. In: Cannon WD Jr, ed. *Instructional course lectures.* Rosemont, IL: American Academy of Orthopaedic Surgeons, 1998:461.
4. Erlebacher A, Filvaroff EH, Gitelman SE, et al. Toward a molecular understanding of skeletal development. *Cell* 1995;80:371.
5. Zaleske DJ. Overview of musculoskeletal development. In: Buckwalter JA, Ehrlich MG, Sandell LJ, et al, eds. *Skeletal growth and development.* Rosemont, IL: American Academy of Orthopaedic Surgeons, 1998:5.

Review of Factors in Skeletal Development

6. Vortkamp A, Pathi S, Peretti GM, et al. Recapitulation of signals regulating embryonic bone formation during postnatal growth and in fracture repair. *Mech Dev* 1998;71:65.
7. Sledge CB, Zaleske DJ. Developmental anatomy of joints. In: Resnick D, Niwayama G, eds. *Diagnosis of bone and joint disorders,* 2nd ed. Philadelphia: WB Saunders, 1988:604.
8. Tabin CJ. Retinoids, homeoboxes, and growth factors: toward molecular models for limb development. *Cell* 1991;66:199.
9. Johnson RL, Tabin CJ. Molecular models for vertebrate limb development. *Cell* 1997;90:979.
10. Sandberg MM, Aro HT, Vuorio EI. Gene expression during bone repair. *Clin Orthop* 1993;289:292.
11. Trippel SB. Basic science of the growth plate. *Curr Opin Orthop* 1990;1:279.
12. Greulich WW, Pyle SI. *Radiographic atlas of skeletal development of the hand and wrist,* 2nd ed. Stanford: Stanford University Press, 1959.
13. Burgeson RE, Nimni ME. Collagen types: molecular structure and tissue distribution. *Clin Orthop* 1992;282:250.
14. Cole WG. Etiology and pathogenesis of heritable connective tissue diseases. *J Pediatr Orthop* 1993;13:392.
15. Hiltunen A, Aro HT, Vuorio E. Regulation of extracellular matrix genes during fracture healing in mice. *Clin Orthop* 1993; 297:23.
16. Glimcher MJ, Krane SM. The organization and structure of bone and the mechanism of calcification. In: Ramachandran GN, Gould BS, eds. *Treatise on collagen.* New York: Academic, 1968:67.
17. Canalis E. Effect of growth factors on bone cell replication and differentiation. *Clin Orthop* 1985;193:246.
18. Canalis EM, Dietrich JW, Maina DM, et al. Hormonal control of bone collagen synthesis in vitro: effects of insulin and glucagon. *Endocrinology* 1977;100:668.
19. Raisz LG, Kream BE. Regulation of bone formation. *N Engl J Med* 1983;309:29, 83.
20. Vaes G. Cellular biology and biochemical mechanism of bone resorption: a review of recent developments on the formation, activation, and mode of action of osteoclasts. *Clin Orthop* 1988; 231:239.
21. Friedlaender GE. Current concepts review. Bone grafts. *J Bone Joint Surg Am* 1987;69:786.
22. Einhorn TA. The cell and molecular biology of fracture healing. *Clin Orthop* 1998;355S:7.
23. Brighton CT. Longitudinal bone growth: the growth plate and its dysfunctions. In: Griffin PP, ed. *Instructional Course Lectures XXXVI.* Park Ridge, IL: American Academy of Orthopaedic Surgeons, 1987:3.
24. Wuthier RE. A review of the primary mechanism of endochondral calcification with special emphasis on the role of cells, mitochondria and matrix vesicles. *Clin Orthop* 1982;169:219.
25. Reinholt FP, Hjerpe A, Jansson K, et al. Stereological studies on the epiphyseal growth plate in low phosphate, vitamin D-deficiency rickets with special reference to the distribution of matrix vesicles. *Calcif Tissue Int* 1984;36:95.
26. Ehrlich MG, Armstrong AL, Neuman RG, et al. Patterns of proteoglycan degradation by a neutral protease from human growth-plate epiphyseal cartilage. *J Bone Joint Surg Am* 1982; 64:1350.
27. Goddard AD, Covello R, Luoh S-M, et al. Mutations of the growth hormone receptor in children with idiopathic short stature. *N Engl J Med* 1995;333:1093.
28. Wilsman NJ, Farnum CE, Leiferman EM, et al. Differential growth by growth plates as a function of multiple parameters of chondrocytic kinetics. *J Orthop Res* 1996;14:927.
29. Daughaday WH, Reeder C. Synchronous activation of DNA synthesis in hypophysectomized rat cartilage by growth hormone. *J Lab Clin Med* 1968;68:357.
30. Trippel SB, Van Wyk JJ, Mankin HJ. Localization of somatomedin-C binding to bovine growth-plate chondrocytes in situ. *J Bone Joint Surg Am* 1986;68:897.
31. Trippel SB, Chernausek SD, Van Wyk JJ, et al. Demonstration of type I and type II somatomedin receptors on bovine growth plate chondrocytes. *J Orthop Res* 1988;6:817.
32. Froesch ER, Zapf J, Audhya TK, et al. Non-suppressible insulin-like activity and thyroid hormones: major pituitary-dependent sulfation factors for chick embryo cartilage. *Proc Natl Acad Sci USA* 1976;73:2904.
33. Burch WM, Van Wyk JJ. Triiodothyronine stimulates cartilage growth and maturation by different mechanisms. *Am J Physiol* 1987;252:E176.
34. Ibbotson KJ, Twardzik DR, D'Souza SM, et al. Stimulation of bone resorption *in vitro* by synthetic transforming growth factor-alpha. *Science* 1985;228:1007.
35. Rosier RN. Orthopaedic basic science: update. *Orthopedics* 1987;10:1793.

36. Sporn M, Roberts AB, Wakefield LM, et al. Transforming growth factor-beta: biological function and chemical structure. *Science* 1986;233:532.

37. Urist MR, DeLange RJ, Finerman GAM. Bone cell differentiation and growth factors. *Science* 1983;220:680.

38. Sadowski H, Shuai K, Darnell JE Jr, et al. A common nuclear signal transduction pathway activated by growth factor and cytokine receptors. *Science* 1993;261:1739.

39. Bennett A, Harvey W. Prostaglandins in orthopaedics. *J Bone Joint Surg Br* 1981;63:152.

40. Centrella M, McCarthy TL, Canalis E. Transforming growth factor-beta and remodeling of bone. *J Bone Joint Surg Am* 1991;73:1418.

41. Glowacki J. Angiogenesis in fracture repair. *Clin Orthop* 1998;355S:82.

42. Tam CS, Wilson DR, Hitchman AJ, et al. Protective effect of vitamin D_2 on bone apposition from the inhibitory action of hydrocortisone in rats. *Calcif Tissue Int* 1981;33:167.

43. Drvaric DM, Parks WJ, Wyly JB, et al. Prostaglandin-induced hyperostosis. *Clin Orthop* 1989;246:300.

44. Smith EP, Boyd J, Frank GR, et al. Estrogen resistance by a mutation in the estrogen-receptor gene in a man. *N Engl J Med* 1994;331:1056.

45. Federman DD. Life without estrogen. *N Engl J Med* 1994;331:1088.

46. Ueda K, Saito A, Nakano H, et al. Cortical hyperostosis following long-term administration of prostaglandin E in infants with cyanotic congenital heart disease. *J Pediatr* 1980;97:834.

47. DeLuca HF. Parathyroid hormone as a trophic hormone for 1,25-dihydroxy vitamin D_3, the metabolically active form of vitamin D. *N Engl J Med* 1972;287:250.

48. Cheeney RW. Current clinical applications of vitamin D metabolite research. *Clin Orthop* 1981;161:285.

49. Moss ML. The design of bones. In: Owen R, Goodfellow J, Bullough P, eds. *Scientific foundations of orthopaedics and traumatology*. Philadelphia: WB Saunders, 1980:59.

50. Hueter C. Anatomische Studien an den Extremitatengelenken Neugebornener und Erwachsener. *Virchows Arch* 1862;25:572.

51. Wolff J. *Das Gesetz der Transformation de Knochen*. Berlin: Hirschwald, 1892.

52. Brighton CT, Strafford B, Gross SB, et al. The proliferative and synthetic response of isolated calvarial bone cells of rats to cyclic biaxial mechanical strain. *J Bone Joint Surg Am* 1991;73:320.

53. Greco F, DePalma L, Speddia N, et al. Growth plate cartilage metabolic response to mechanical stress. *J Pediatr Orthop* 1989;9:520.

54. Wang N, Butler JP, Ingber DE. Mechanotransduction across the cell surface and through the cytoskeleton. *Science* 1993;260:1124.

Mineral Phase

55. Avioli LV, Haddad JG. Progress in endocrinology and metabolism. Vitamin D: current concepts. *Metab Clin Exp* 1973;22:507.

56. Hoffman WS. *The biochemistry of clinical medicine*, 4th ed. Chicago: Year Book, 1970.

57. Morgan B. *Osteomalacia, renal osteodystrophy, and osteoporosis*. Springfield, IL: Charles C Thomas, 1973.

58. Widdowson EM, McCance RA. The metabolism of calcium, phosphorus, magnesium and strontium. *Pediatr Clin North Am* 1965;12:595.

59. Raisz LG. Bone metabolism and calcium regulation. In: Avioli LV, Krane SM, eds. *Metabolic bone disease*. New York: Academic, 1978.

60. Iannotti JP, Brighton CT, Stambough JL, et al. Calcium flux and endogenous calcium content in isolated mammalian growth-plate chondrocytes, hyaline-cartilage chondrocytes, and hepatocytes. *J Bone Joint Surg Am* 1985;67:113.

61. Rasmussen H. The calcium messenger system. *N Engl J Med* 1986;314:1094.

62. Fourman P, Royer P. *Calcium metabolism and bone*, 2nd ed. Philadelphia: FA Davis, 1968.

63. Rasmussen H. Ionic and hormonal control of calcium homeostasis. *Am J Med* 1971;50:567.

64. Borle AB. Membrane transfer of calcium. *Clin Orthop* 1967;52:267.

65. DeLuca HF. Vitamin D: new horizons. *Clin Orthop* 1971;78:423.

66. Arnaud C, Fischer J, Rasmussen H. The role of the parathyroids in the phosphaturia of vitamin D deficiency. *J Clin Invest* 1964;43:1256.

67. Arnaud C, Tsao HS, Littledike T. Calcium homeostasis, parathyroid hormone and calcitonin: preliminary report. *Mayo Clin Proc* 1970;45:125.

68. Harrison HE, Harrison HC. The interaction of vitamin D and parathyroid hormone on calcium, phosphorus and magnesium homeostasis in the rat. *Metab Clin Exp* 1964;13:952.

69. Kanis JA. Vitamin D metabolism and its clinical application. *J Bone Joint Surg Br* 1982;64:542.

70. Drescher D, DeLuca HF. Vitamin D stimulated calcium binding protein from rat intestinal mucosa: purification and some properties. *Biochemistry* 1971;10:2302.

71. Fullmer CS, Wasserman RH. Bovine intestinal calcium-binding proteins (CaBP): purification and some properties. *Fed Proc* 1972;31:693.

72. MacGregor RR, Hamilton JW, Cohn DV. The induction of calcium-binding protein biosynthesis in intestine by vitamin D_3. *Biochim Biophys Acta* 1970;222:482.

73. Taylor AM. Intestinal vitamin D-induced calcium-binding protein: time course of immunocytological localization following 1,25-dihydroxyvitamin D_3. *J Histochem Cytochem* 1983;31:426.

74. Taylor AM, Wasserman RH. Vitamin D-induced calcium binding protein: comparative aspects in kidney and intestine. *Am J Physiol* 1972;223:110.

75. Harmeyer J, DeLuca HF. Calcium-binding protein and calcium absorption after vitamin D administration. *Arch Biochem Biophys* 1969;133:247.

76. Norman AW. Evidence for a new kidney-produced hormone 1,25-dihydroxy-cholecalciferol, the proposed biologically active form of vitamin D. *Am J Clin Nutr* 1971;24:1346.

77. Bijovet OLM. Kidney function in calcium and phosphate metabolism. In: Avioli LV, Krane SM, eds. *Metabolic bone disease*. New York: Academic, 1977:49.

78. Beal VA. Calcium and phosphorus in infancy. *J Am Diet Assoc* 1968;53:450.

79. Blunt JW, DeLuca HF. The synthesis of 25-hydroxycholecalciferol: a biologically active metabolite of vitamin D_3. *Biochemistry* 1969;8:671.

80. Blunt JW, DeLuca HF, Schnoes HK. 25-Hydroxycholecalciferol: a biologically active metabolite of vitamin D_3. *Biochemistry* 1968;7:3317.

81. Blunt JW, Tanaka Y, DeLuca HF. The biological activity of 25-hydroxycholecalciferol: a metabolite of vitamin D_3. *Proc Natl Acad Sci USA* 1968;61:1503.

82. Jones G, Schnoes HK, DeLuca HF. Isolation and identification of 1,25 dihydroxy vitamin D_2. *Biochemistry* 1975;14:1250.

83. Lund J, DeLuca HF. Biologically active metabolite of vitamin D from bone, liver and blood serum. *J Lipid Res* 1966;7:739.

84. Holick MF, Schnoes HK, DeLuca HF, et al. Isolation and iden-

tification of 24,25-hydroxycholecalciferol, a metabolite of D_3 made in the kidney. *Biochemistry* 1972;11:4251.

85. Holick MF, Schnoes HK, DeLuca HF, et al. Isolation and identification of 1,24-dihydroxycholecalciferol: a metabolite of vitamin D active in intestine. *Biochemistry* 1971;10:2799.

86. Boyle IT, Gray RW, DeLuca HF. Regulation by calcium of *in vivo* synthesis of 1,25-dihydroxycholecalciferol and 21,25-dihydroxycholecalciferol. *Proc Natl Acad Sci USA* 1971;68:2131.

87. Fraser DR, Kodicek E. Regulation of 25-hydroxycholecalciferol-1-hydrolase activity in kidney by parathyroid hormone. *Nature* 1973;241:163.

88. Rasmussen H, Wong M, Bikle D, et al. Hormonal control of 25-hydroxycholecalciferol to 1,25-dihydroxycholecalciferol. *J Clin Invest* 1972;51:2502.

89. Albright F, Reifenstein EC. *The parathyroid glands and metabolic bone disease.* Baltimore: Williams & Wilkins, 1948.

90. Arnaud CD, Tenenhouse AM, Rasmussen H. Parathyroid hormone. *Annu Rev Physiol* 1967;29:349.

91. *Food and Nutrition Board recommended dietary allowances*, 7th ed. Washington: National Academy of Sciences, National Research Council, 1968; publication no 1694.

92. Huth EJ, Webster GD Jr, Elkinton JR. Renal excretion of hydrogen ion in renal tubular acidosis. III. An attempt to detect latent cases in a family: comments on nosology, genetics, and etiology of primary disease. *Am J Med* 1960;29:586

93. Avioli LV. Intestinal absorption of calcium. *Arch Intern Med* 1972;129:345.

94. Bruce HM, Callow RK. Cereals and rickets: the role of inositalhexaphosphoric acid. *Biochem J* 1934;28:517.

95. Wills MR, Phillips JB, Day RC, et al. Phytic acid and nutritional rickets in immigrants. *Lancet* 1972;1:771.

96. DeToni G. Renal rickets with phospho-gluco-amino renal diabetes. *Ann Paediatr* 1956;187:42.

97. Tryfus H. Hepatic rickets. *Ann Paediatr* 1959;192:81.

98. Moore JH, Tyler C. Studies on the intestinal absorption and excretion of calcium and phosphorus in the pig. 2. The intestinal absorption and excretion of radioactive calcium and phosphorus. *Br J Nutr* 1955;9:81.

99. Minkin C, Talmage RV. A study in secretion and function of thyrocalcitonin in normal rats. In: Talmage RV, Balanger LF, eds. *Parathyroid hormone and thyrocalcitonin (calcitonin).* Amsterdam: Excerpta Medica, 1968:339.

100. Austen LA, Heath H. Calcitonin: physiology and pathophysiology. *N Engl J Med* 1981;304:269.

Rickets and Osteomalacia

101. Glisson R. *De rachitide sive marbo puerili qui vulgo The Rickets Dicitur Tracttatus. Adscitis in operis societatem Georgio Bate et Ahasuero Regemortero.* London: G Du-Gardi, 1650.

102. Whistler D. *Disputatio Medica Inauguralis de Morbo puerili Anglorum quem patrio idiomate indigenae vocant the rickets.* London: Wilhemi, Christiani, Boxii, 1645.

103. Smith R. The pathophysiology and management of rickets. *Orthop Clin North Am* 1972;3:601.

104. Smith R, Stern G. Muscular weakness in osteomalacia and hyperparathyroidism. *J Neurol Sci* 1969;8:511.

105. Streeter GL. Developmental horizons in human embryos. IV. A review of the histogenesis of cartilage and bone. *Contrib Embryol* 1949;33:149.

106. Olin A, Creasman C, Shapiro F. Free physeal transplantation in the rabbit: an experimental approach to focal lesions. *J Bone Joint Surg Am* 1984;66:7.

107. Jaffe HL. *Metabolic, degenerative, and inflammatory diseases of bones and joints.* Philadelphia: Lea & Febiger, 1972:381.

108. Parfitt AM. Hypophosphatemic vitamin D-refractory rickets and osteomalacia. *Orthop Clin North Am* 1972;3:653.

109. Schott GD, Wills MR. Muscle weakness in osteomalacia. *Lancet* 1976;1:626.

110. Skaria J, Katiyar BC, Srivastava TP, et al. Myopathy and neuropathy associated with osteomalacia. *Acta Neurol Scand* 1975;51:37.

111. Villareale ME, Chiroff RT, Bergstrom WH, et al. Bone changes induced by diphenylhydantoin in chicks on a controlled vitamin D intake. *J Bone Joint Surg Am* 1978;60:911.

112. Floman Y, Yosipovitch Z, Licht A, et al. Bilateral slipped upper femoral epiphysis: a rare manifestation of renal osteodystrophy. Case report with discussion of its pathogenesis. *Isr J Med Sci* 1975;11:15.

113. Goldman AB, Lane JM, Salvati E. Slipped capital femoral epiphyses complicating renal osteodystrophy: a report of three cases. *Radiology* 1978;126:33.

114. Martin W, Riddervold HO. Epiphysiolysis in rickets. *Va Med Mon* 1980;107:566.

115. Mehls O, Ritz E, Krempien B, et al. Slipped epiphyses in renal osteodystrophy. *Arch Dis Child* 1975;50:545.

116. Tebor GB, Ehrlich MG, Herrin J. Slippage of the distal tibial epiphysis. *J Pediatr Orthop* 1983;3:211.

117. Goel KM, Sweet EM, Logan RW, et al. Florid and subclinical rickets among immigrant children in Glasgow. *Lancet* 1976;1:1141.

118. Laditan AA, Adeniyi A. Rickets in Nigerian children: response to vitamin D. *J Trop Med Hyg* 1975;78:206.

119. Miller CG, Chutkin W. Vitamin D-deficiency rickets in Jamaican children. *Arch Dis Child* 1976;51:214.

120. Ohara-May J, Widdowson EM. Diets and living conditions of Asian boys in Coventry with and without signs of rickets. *Br J Nutr* 1976;36:23.

121. Salimpour R. Rickets in Tehran: study of 200 cases. *Arch Dis Child* 1975;50:63.

122. Rudolf M, Arulanatham K, Greenstein RM. Unsuspected nutritional rickets. *Pediatrics* 1980;66:72.

123. Dodds GS, Cameron HC. Studies on experimental rickets in rats. IV. The relation of rickets to growth, with special reference to the bones. *Am J Pathol* 1943;19:169.

124. Dodds GS, Cameron HC. Studies on experimental rickets in rats. III. The behavior and rate of cartilage remnants in the rachitic metaphysis. *Am J Pathol* 1939;15:723.

125. Dodds GS, Cameron HC. Studies on experimental rickets in rats. II. The healing process in the head of the tibia and other bones. *Am J Pathol* 1938;14:273.

126. Dodds GS, Cameron HC. Studies on experimental rickets in rats. I. Structural modifications of the epiphyseal cartilages in the tibia and other bones. *Am J Anat* 1934;55:135.

127. Frost HM. *Bone dynamics in osteoporosis and osteomalacia.* Springfield, IL: Charles C Thomas, 1966.

128. Arnstein AR, Frame B, Frost HM. Recent progress in osteomalacia and rickets. *Ann Intern Med* 1967;67:1296.

129. Jaworski ZFG. Pathophysiology, diagnosis, and treatment of osteomalacia. *Orthop Clin North Am* 1972;3:623.

130. Marie PJ, Pettifor JM, Ross FP, et al. Histological osteomalacia due to dietary deficiency in children. *N Engl J Med* 1982;307:584.

131. Oppenheimer SJ, Snodgrass GJ. Neonatal rickets: histopathology and quantitative bone changes. *Arch Dis Child* 1980;55:945.

132. Ramser JR, Villaneuva AR, Frost HM. Cortical bone dynamics in osteomalacia, measured by tetracycline bone labeling. *Clin Orthop* 1966;49:89.

133. Park EA. Observations on the pathology of rickets with particu-

lar reference to the changes at the cartilage shaft junctions of the growing bones. *Bull NY Acad Med* 1939;14:495.

134. Huffer WE, Lacey DL. Studies on the pathogenesis of avian rickets. II. Necrosis of perforating epiphyseal vessels during recovery from rickets caused by vitamin D_3 deficiency. *Am J Pathol* 1982;109:302.

135. Lacey DL, Huffer WE. Studies on the pathogenesis of avian rickets. I. Changes in epiphyseal and metaphyseal vessels in hypocalcemic and hypophosphatemic rickets. *Am J Pathol* 1982; 109:288.

136. Pitt MJ. Rachitic and osteomalacia syndromes. *Radiol Clin North Am* 1981;19:581.

137. Swischuk LE, Hayden CK. Rickets: a roentgenographic scheme for diagnosis. *Pediatr Radiol* 1979;8:203.

138. Caffey J. *Pediatric x-ray diagnosis*, 5th ed. Chicago: Year Book, 1967.

139. Reynolds WA, Karo JJ. Radiologic diagnosis of metabolic bone disease. *Orthop Clin North Am* 1972;3:521.

140. Steinbach HG, Noetzli M. Roentgen appearance of the skeleton in osteomalacia and rickets. *AJR* 1964;91:955.

141. Feist JH. The biologic basis of radiologic findings in bone disease: recognition and interpretation of abnormal bone architecture. *Radiol Clin North Am* 1970;8:183.

142. Stamp TCB, Baker LR. Recessive hypophosphatemic rickets and possible etiology of the vitamin D–resistant syndrome. *Arch Dis Child* 1976;51:360.

143. Steinbach HL, Kolb FO, Gilfillan R. Mechanism of production of pseudofractures in osteomalacia (Milkman's syndrome). *Radiology* 1954;62:388.

144. Hodkinson HM. Fracture of the femur as a presentation of osteomalacia. *Gerontol Clin* 1971;13:189.

145. Paul PD, Lloyd DJ, Smith FW. The role of bone scanning in neonatal rickets. *Pediatr Radiol* 1983;13:89.

146. Singh BN, Spies SM, Mehta SP, et al. Unusual bone scan presentation in osteomalacia: symmetrical uptake. A suggestive sign. *Clin Nucl Med* 1978;3:292.

147. Pettifor JM, Ross P, Wang J, et al. Rickets in children of rural origin in South Africa: is low dietary calcium a factor? *J Pediatr* 1978;92:320.

148. Sognen E. Calcium-binding substances and intestinal absorption. *Acta Pharmacol Toxicol* 1964;21[Suppl 1]:1.

149. Winnacker JL, Yeager H, Saunders RB, et al. Rickets in children receiving anticonvulsant drugs: biochemical and hormonal markers. *Am J Dis Child* 1977;131:286.

150. Backrach S, Fisher J, Parks JS. An outbreak of vitamin D-deficiency rickets in a susceptible population. *Pediatrics* 1979;64: 871.

151. Dwyer JT, Dietz WH, Hass G, et al. Risk of nutritional rickets among vegetarian children. *Am J Dis Child* 1979;133:134.

152. Harrison HE, Harrison HC. Rickets then and now. *J Pediatr* 1975;87:1144.

153. Callenback JC, Sheehan MB, Abramson SJ, et al. Etiologic factors in rickets of very low birthweight infants. *J Pediatr* 1981; 98:800.

154. Bosley AR, Verrier-Jones ER, Campbell MJ. Aetiological factors in rickets of prematurity. *Arch Dis Child* 1980;55:683.

155. Crutchlow WP, David DS, Whitsell J. Multiple skeletal complications in a case of chronic renal failure treated by kidney homotransplantation. *Am J Med* 1971;50:390.

156. Glass EJ, Hume R, Hendry GMA, et al. Plasma alkaline phosphatase activity in rickets of prematurity. *Arch Dis Child* 1982; 57:373.

157. Garabedian M, Vainsel M, Mallet E, et al. Circulating vitamin D-metabolite concentrations in children with nutritional rickets. *J Pediatr* 1983;103:381.

158. Arnaud SB, Stickler GB, Haworth JC. Serum 25-hydroxy-vitamin D in infantile rickets. *Pediatrics* 1976;57:221.

159. Raghuramulu N, Reddy V. Serum 25-hydroxy vitamin D levels in malnourished children with rickets. *Arch Dis Child* 1980;55: 285.

160. Clark CG, Crooks J, Dawson AA. Disordered calcium metabolism after Polya partial gastrectomy. *Lancet* 1964;1:734.

161. Deller DJ, Begley MD. Calcium metabolism and the bones after partial gastrectomy. I. Clinical features and radiology of the bones. *Aust Ann Med* 1963;12:282.

162. Eddy RL. Metabolic bone disease after gastrectomy. *Am J Med* 1971;50:442.

163. Atkinson M, Nordin BEC, Sherlock S. Malabsorption and bone disease in prolonged obstructive jaundice. *Q J Med* 1956;25: 299.

164. Nordin BEC. Effect of malabsorption syndrome on calcium metabolism. *Proc R Soc Lond* 1961;54:497.

165. Kooh SW, Jones G, Reilly BJ, et al. Pathogenesis of rickets in chronic hepatobiliary disease in children. *J Pediatr* 1979;94: 870.

166. Long RG, Wills MR. Hepatic dystrophy. *Br J Hosp Med* 1978; 20:312.

167. Daum F, Rosen JF, Roginsky M, et al. 25-Hydroxycholecalciferol in the management of rickets associated with extrahepatic biliary atresia. *J Pediatr* 1976;88:1041.

168. Heubi JE, Tsang RC, Steichen JJ, et al. 1,25-Dihydroxy-vitamin D_3 in childhood hepatic osteodystrophy. *J Pediatr* 1979;94:977.

169. Thompson GR, Lewis B, Booth CC. Absorption of vitamin D_3-^{3}H in control subjects and patients with intestinal malabsorption. *J Clin Invest* 1966;45:94.

170. Mann JG, Brown WR, Kern F. The subtle and variable expressions of gluten-induced enteropathy (adult celiac disease, nontropical sprue). *Am J Med* 1970;48:357.

171. Moss AJ, Waterhouse C, Terry R. Gluten-sensitive enteropathy with osteomalacia without steatorrhea. *N Engl J Med* 1965;272: 825.

172. Clayton BE, Cotton DA. A study of malabsorption after resection of the entire jejunum and the proximal half of the ileum. *Gut* 1961;2:18.

173. Zerwekh JE, Glass K, Jowsey J, et al. A unique form of osteomalacia associated with end-organ refractoriness to 1,25-dihydroxyvitamin D and apparent defective synthesis of 25-hydroxyvitamin D. *J Clin Endocrinol Metab* 1979;49:171.

174. Franck WA, Hoffman GS, Davis JS, et al. Osteomalacia and weakness complicating jejunoileal bypass. *J Rheumatol* 1979;6: 51.

175. Hepner GW, Jowsey J, Arnaud C, et al. Osteomalacia and celiac disease: response to 25-hydroxyvitamin D. *Am J Med* 1965;65: 1015.

176. Albright F, Butler AM, Bloomberg E. Rickets resistant to vitamin D therapy. *Am J Dis Child* 1937;54:529.

177. Baar HS, Bickel H. Cystine storage disease with aminoaciduria and dwarfism. Part 8. Morbid anatomy, histology, and pathogenesis of Lignac-Fanconi disease. *Acta Paediatr Scand Suppl* 1952;90:171.

178. Burnett CH, Dent CE, Harper C, et al. Vitamin D–resistant rickets: analysis of twenty-four pedigrees with hereditary and sporadic cases. *Am J Med* 1964;36:222.

179. Butler AM, Wilson JL, Farber S. Dehydration and acidosis with calcification at renal tubules. *J Pediatr* 1936;8:489.

180. Dent CE. Rickets and osteomalacia from renal tubule defects. *J Bone Joint Surg Br* 1952;34:266.

181. DeToni G. Remarks on the relations between renal rickets (renal dwarfism) and renal diabetes. *Acta Paediatr Scand* 1933;16:479.

182. Fanconi G. Der fruhinfantile nephrotisch-glykosurische Zwerg-

wuchs mit hypophosphatamishcer Rachitis. *Jahrb Kinderheilkd* 1936;147:299.

183. Fraser DR, Salter RB. The diagnosis and management of the various types of rickets. *Pediatr Clin North Am* 1958;26:417.

184. Harrison HE, Harrison HC. The effect of acidosis upon the renal tubular absorption of phosphate. *Am J Physiol* 1941;134:781.

185. Lightwood R, Payne WW, Black JA. Infantile renal acidosis. *Pediatrics* 1953;12:628.

186. Lowe CU, Terrey M, MacLachlan EA. Organic aciduria, decreased from renal ammonia production, hydrophthalmos, and mental retardation. *Am J Dis Child* 1952;83:164.

187. Perry W, Stamp TC. Hereditary hypophosphatemic rickets with autosomal recessive inheritance and severe osteosclerosis. *J Bone Joint Surg Br* 1978;60:430.

188. Yong JM. Cause of raised serum alkaline phosphatase after partial gastrectomy and in other malabsorption states. *Lancet* 1966;1:1132.

189. Chutorian A, Rowland LP. Lowe's syndrome. *Neurology* 1966;16:115.

190. Dent CE, Harris H. Hereditary forms of rickets and osteomalacia. *J Bone Joint Surg Br* 1956;38:204.

191. Bickel H, Baar HS, Astley R, et al. Cystine storage disease with aminoaciduria and dwarfism. *Acta Paediatr Scand Suppl* 1952;90:1.

192. Morris RC. Renal tubular acidosis: mechanisms, classification, and implication. *N Engl J Med* 1969;281:1405.

193. Morris RC, Sebastian A, McSherry E. Renal acidosis. *Kidney Int* 1972;1:322.

194. Relman AS, Levinsky NG. Kidney disease: acquired tubular disorders with special reference to disturbances of concentration and dilution and of acid-base regulation. *Annu Rev Med* 1961;12:932.

195. Seldin DW, Wilson JD. Renal tubular acidosis. In: Stanbury JB, Wyngaarden JB, Fredrickson DS, eds. *The metabolic basis of inherited disease*, 2nd ed. New York: McGraw-Hill, 1966:1230.

196. Habener JF, Mahaffey JE. Osteomalacia and disorders of vitamin D metabolism. *Annu Rev Med* 1978;29:327.

197. Isogna KL, Broadus AD, Gertner JM. Impaired phosphorus conservation and 1,25-dihydroxyvitamin D generation during phosphorus deprivation in familial hypophosphatemic rickets. *J Clin Invest* 1983;71:1562.

198. Harrison HE. The varieties of rickets and osteomalacia associated with hypophosphatemia. *Clin Orthop* 1957;9:61.

199. Morris RC, Sebastian A. Renal tubular acidosis and Fanconi syndrome. In: Stanbury JB, Wyngaarden JB, Fredrickson DS, et al., eds. *The metabolic basis of inherited disease*, 5th ed. New York: McGraw-Hill, 1983:1808.

200. Walton J. Familial hypophosphatemic rickets: a delineation of its subdivisions and pathogenesis. *Clin Pediatr* 1976;15:1007.

201. Hahn TJ, Scharp CR, Halstead LR, et al. Parathyroid hormone status and renal responsiveness in familial hypophosphatemic rickets. *J Clin Endocrinol Metab* 1975;41:926.

202. Dancaster CP, Jackson WPU. Familial vitamin D–resistant rickets. *Arch Dis Child* 1957;34:383.

203. Chan JC, Bartter FC. Hypophosphatemic rickets: effect of 1,alpha,25-hydroxyvitamin D_3 on growth and mineral metabolism. *Pediatrics* 1979;64:448.

204. Evans GA, Arulanantham K, Gage J. Primary hypophosphatemic rickets: effect of phosphate and vitamin D on growth and surgical treatment. *J Bone Joint Surg Am* 1980;62:1130.

205. Frame B, Smith RW Jr, Fleming JL, et al. Oral phosphates in vitamin D-refractory rickets and osteomalacia. *Am J Dis Child* 1963;106:147.

206. Loeffler RD, Sherman FC. The effect of treatment on growth

and deformity in hypophosphatemic vitamin D–resistant rickets. *Clin Orthop* 1982;162:4.

207. Mason RS, Rohl RG, Lissner D, et al. Vitamin D metabolism in hypophosphatemic rickets. *Am J Dis Child* 1982;136:909.

208. Scriver CR, Reade TM, DeLuca HF, et al. Serum 1,25-dihydroxy vitamin D levels in normal subjects and in patients with hereditary rickets or bone disease. *N Engl J Med* 1978;299:976.

209. Tsuchiya Y, Matsuo N, Cho H, et al. Vitamin D and vitamin dependency. *Contrib Nephrol* 1980;22:80.

210. Balsan S, Garabedian M. 1,25-Dihydroxyvitamin D_3 and 1,alpha-hydroxy vitamin D_3 in children: biologic and therapeutic effects in nutritional rickets and different types of vitamin D resistance. *Pediatr Res* 1975;9:586.

211. Delvin EE, Glorieux FH, Marie PJ, et al. Vitamin D dependency: replacement therapy with calcitriol. *J Pediatr* 1981;99:26.

212. Etches P, Pickering D, Smith R. Cystinotic rickets with vitamin D metabolites. *Arch Dis Child* 1977;52:661.

213. Brooks MH, Bell NH, Love L, et al. Vitamin D-dependent rickets, type II: resistance of target organs to 1,25-dihydroxy-vitamin D. *N Engl J Med* 1978;298:996.

214. Colombo JP, Donath A. The effect of calcium infusions on renal handling of amino acids in hypophosphatemic vitamin D–resistant rickets. *Acta Paediatr Scand* 1975;64:703.

215. Elkinton JR. Renal acidosis. *Am J Med* 1960;28:165.

216. Elkinton JR, Huth EJ, Webster GD Jr, et al. The renal excretion of hydrogen ion in renal tubular acidosis. I. Quantitative assessment of the response to ammonium chloride as an acid load. *Am J Med* 1960;29:554.

217. Relman AS. Renal acidosis and renal excretion of acid in health and disease. *Adv Intern Med* 1964;12:295.

218. Baines GH, Barclay JA, Cooke WT. Nephrocalcinosis associated with hyperchloremia and low plasma bicarbonate. *Q J Med* 1945;14:113.

219. Mautalen C, Montoreano R, LaBarrere C. Early skeletal effect of alkali therapy upon the osteomalacia of renal tubular acidosis. *J Clin Endocrinol Metab* 1976;42:875.

220. Schreiner GE, Smith LH, Kye LH. Renal hyperchloremic acidosis: familial occurrence of nephrocalcinosis with hyperchloremia and low serum bicarbonate. *Am J Med* 1953;15:122.

221. Cooke RE, Kleeman CR. Distal tubular dysfunction with renal calcification. *Yale J Biol Med* 1950;23:199.

222. Cunningham J, Fraher LJ, Clemens TL, et al. Chronic acidosis with metabolic bone disease: effect of alkali on bone morphology and vitamin D metabolism. *Am J Med* 1982;73:199.

223. Salassa RM, Jowsey J, Arnaud CD. Hypophosphatemic osteomalacia associated with "nonendocrine" tumors. *N Engl J Med* 1970;283:65.

224. Swann GF. Pathogenesis of bone lesions in neurofibromatosis. *Br J Radiol* 1954;27:623.

225. Dent CE, Gertner JM. Hypophosphatemic osteomalacia in fibrous dysplasia. *Q J Med* 1976;45:411.

226. Halvorsen S, Aas K. Renal tubular defects in fibrous dysplasia of the bones: report of two cases. *Acta Paediatr Scand* 1961;50:297.

227. Kunin AS. Polyostotic fibrous dysplasia with hypophosphatemia: a metabolic study. *Metab Clin Exp* 1962;11:978.

228. McArthur RG, Hayles AG, Lambert PW. Albright's syndrome with rickets. *Mayo Clin Proc* 1979;54:313.

229. Tanaka T, Swann S. A case of McCune-Albright syndrome with hyperthyroidism and vitamin D–resistant rickets. *Helv Paediatr Acta* 1977;32:263.

230. Asnes RS, Berdon WE, Bassett VA. Hypophosphatemic rickets in an adolescent cured by excision of a non-ossifying fibroma. *Clin Pediatr* 1981;20:646.

231. Daniels RA, Weisenfeld I. Tumorous phosphaturic osteomala-

cia: report of a case associated with multiple hemangiomas of bone. *Am J Med* 1967;67:155.

232. Moncrieff MW, Brenton DP, Arthur LJ. Case of tumor rickets. *Arch Dis Child* 1978;53:740.

233. Pollack JA, Schiller AL, Crawford JD. Rickets and myopathy cured by removal of a nonossifying fibroma of bone. *Pediatrics* 1973;52:364.

234. Parker MS, Klein I, Haussler MR, et al. Tumor-induced osteomalacia: evidence of a surgically correctable alteration in vitamin D metabolism. *JAMA* 1981;245:492.

235. Cai Q, Hodgson SF, Kao PC, et al. Brief report. Inhibition of renal phosphate transport by a tumor product in a patient with oncogenic osteomalacia. *N Engl J Med* 1994;330:1645.

236. Aponte CJ, Petrelli MP. Anticonvulsants and vitamin D metabolism. *JAMA* 1973;225:1248.

237. Borgstedt AP, Bryson MF, Young LW, et al. Long-term administration of anti-epileptic drugs and the development of rickets. *J Pediatr* 1972;81:9.

238. Christiansen C, Kristensen M, Rodbro P. Latent osteomalacia in epileptic patients on anticonvulsants. *Br Med J* 1972;3:738.

239. Crosley CJ, Chee C, Berman PH. Rickets associated with long-term anticonvulsant therapy in a pediatric outpatient population. *Pediatrics* 1975;56:52.

240. Dent CE, Richens A, Rowe DJF, et al. Osteomalacia with long-term anticonvulsant therapy in epilepsy. *Br Med J* 1970;4:69.

241. Frame B. Hypocalcemia and osteomalacia associated with anticonvulsant therapy. *Ann Intern Med* 1971;74:294.

242. Morijiri Y, Sato T. Factors causing rickets in institutionalized handicapped children on anticonvulsant therapy. *Arch Dis Child* 1981;56:446.

243. Liakakos D, Papadopoulos Z, Vlachos P, et al. Serum alkaline phosphatase and urinary hydroxyproline values in children receiving phenobarbital with and without vitamin D. *J Pediatr* 1975;87:291.

244. Winters RW, Graham JB, Williams TF, et al. A genetic study of familial hypophosphatasia and vitamin D–resistant rickets with a review of the literature. *Medicine* 1958;37:97.

245. Gascon-Barre M, Cote MG. Influence of phenobarbital and diphenylhydantoin on the healing of rickets in the rat. *Calcif Tissue Res* 1978;25:93.

246. Hoikka V, Savolainen K, Karjalainen P, et al. Treatment of osteomalacia in institutionalized epileptic patients on long-term anticonvulsant therapy. *Ann Clin Res* 1982;14:72.

247. Timperlake RW, Cook SD, Thomas KA, et al. Effects of anticonvulsant drug therapy on bone mineral density in a pediatric population. *J Pediatr Orthop* 1988;8:467.

248. Liu SH, Chu HI. Studies of calcium and phosphorus with special reference to pathogenesis and effects of dihydrotachysterol (AT10) and iron. *Medicine* 1943;22:103.

249. Mallick NP, Berlyne GM. Arterial calcification after vitamin D therapy in hyperphosphatemic renal failure. *Lancet* 1968;2:1316.

250. Blockey NJ, Murphy AV, Mocan H. Management of rachitic deformities in children with chronic renal failure. *J Bone Joint Surg Br* 1986;68:791.

251. Oppenheim WL, Salusky IB, Kaplan D, et al. Renal osteodystrophy in children. In: Castells S, Finberg L, eds. *Metabolic bone disease in children*. New York: Marcel Dekker, 1990:197.

252. Goldman R, Basset SH, Duncan GB. Phosphorus excretion in renal failure. *J Clin Invest* 1954;33:1623.

253. Brickman AS, Coburn JW, Norman AW. Action of 1,25-dihydroxycholecalciferol, a potent kidney-produced metabolite of vitamin D$_3$ in uremic man. *N Engl J Med* 1972;287:891.

254. DeLuca HF. The biochemical basis of renal osteodystrophy and post-menopausal osteoporosis: a view from the vitamin D system. *Curr Med Res Opin* 1981;7:279.

255. Mason RS, Lissner D, Wilkinson M, et al. Vitamin D metabolites and their relationship to azotemic osteodystrophy. *Clin Endocrinol* 1980;13:375.

256. Parfitt AM. Renal osteodystrophy. *Orthop Clin North Am* 1972;3:681.

257. Ritz E, Malluche HJ, Krempien B, et al. Pathogenesis of renal osteodystrophy: roles of phosphate and skeletal resistance to PTH. *Adv Exp Med Biol* 1978;103:423.

258. Brautbar N, Kleemna CR. Disordered divalent ion metabolism in kidney disease: comments on pathogenesis and treatment. *Adv Nephrol* 1979;8:179.

259. Coburn JW, Popovtzer MM, Massry SG, et al. The physicochemical state and renal handling of divalent ions in chronic renal failure. *Arch Intern Med* 1969;124:302.

260. Juttman JR, Hagenouw-Taal JC, Lameyer LD, et al. Intestinal calcium absorption, serum phosphate, and parathyroid hormone in patients with chronic renal failure and osteodystrophy before and during hemodialysis. *Calcif Tissue Res* 1978;26:119.

261. Kessner DM, Epstein FH. Effect of renal insufficiency on gastrointestinal transport of calcium. *Am J Physiol* 1965;209:141.

262. Kleeman CR, Massry SG, Coburn JW, et al. Calcium and phosphorus metabolism and bone disease in uremia. *Clin Orthop* 1970;68:210.

263. Stanbury SW. Bone disease in uremia. *Am J Med* 1968;44:714.

264. Stanbury SW, Lamb GA. Metabolic studies of renal osteodystrophy. I. Calcium, phosphorus, and nitrogen metabolism in rickets, osteomalacia, and hyperparathyroidism complicating uremia and in the osteomalacia of the adult Fanconi syndrome. *Medicine* 1962;41:1.

265. Berson SA, Yalow RS. Parathyroid hormone in plasma in adenomatous hyperparathyroidism, uremia, and bronchogenic carcinoma. *Science* 1966;154:907.

266. Stanbury SW, Lamb GA. Parathyroid function in chronic renal failure: a statistical survey of the plasma biochemistry in azotaemic renal osteodystrophy. *Q J Med* 1966;35:1.

267. Brown DJ, Dawborn JK, Thomas DP, et al. Assessment of osteodystrophy in patients with chronic renal failure. *Aust NZ J Med* 1982;12:250.

268. Greenfield GB. Roentgen appearance of bone and soft-tissue changes in chronic renal disease. *AJR* 1972;116:749.

269. Craven JD. Renal glomerular osteodystrophy. *Clin Radiol* 1964;15:210.

270. Kaye M, Pritchard JE, Halpenny GW, et al. Bone disease in chronic renal failure with particular reference to osteosclerosis. *Medicine* 1960;39:157.

271. Lalli AF, Lapides J. Osteosclerosis occurring in renal disease. *AJR* 1963;93:924.

272. Weller M, Edeiken J, Hodes PJ. Renal osteodystrophy. *AJR* 1968;104:354.

273. Abrams JD. Corneal and other findings in patients on intermittent dialysis for renal failure. *Proc R Soc Lond* 1966;59:533.

274. Berlyne GM. Microcrystalline conjunctival calcification in renal failure: a useful sign. *Lancet* 1968;2:366.

275. Berlyne GM, Shaw AG. Red eyes in renal failure. *Lancet* 1967;1:4.

276. Platt R, Owen TK. Renal dwarfism associated with calcification of arteries and skin. *Lancet* 1934;2:135.

277. Putkonen T, Wangel GA. Renal hyperparathyroidism with metastatic calcification of the skin. *Dermatologica* 1959;118:127.

278. Andersen DH, Schlesinger ER. Renal hyperparathyroidism with calcification of the arteries in infancy. *Am J Dis Child* 1942;63:102.

279. Friedman SA, Novack S, Thomson GE. Arterial calcification and gangrene in uremia. *N Engl J Med* 1969;280:1392.

280. Parfitt AM. Soft-tissue calcification in uremia. *Arch Intern Med* 1969;124:544.

281. Rosen H, Friedman SA, Raizner AE, et al. Azotemic arteriopathy. *Am Heart J* 1972;84:250.

282. Norman ME, Mazur AT, Borden S, et al. Early diagnosis of juvenile renal osteodystrophy. *J Pediatr* 1980;97:226.

283. Hsu AC, Kooh SW, Fraser D, et al. Renal osteodystrophy in children with chronic renal failure: an unexpectedly common and incapacitating complication. *Pediatrics* 1982;70:742.

284. David DS. Calcium metabolism in renal failure. *Am J Med* 1975;58:48.

285. Andersen J, Neilsen HJ. Renal osteodystrophy in non-dialysed patients with chronic renal failure. *Acta Radiol* 1980;21:803.

286. Debnam JW, Bates ML, Kopelman RC, et al. Radiological/pathological correlations in uremic bone disease. *Radiology* 1977;125:653.

287. Eastwood JB. Renal osteodystrophy: a radiological review. *CRC Crit Rev Diagn Imaging* 1977;9:77.

288. Anton HC. Thinning of the clavicular cortex in adults under the age of 45 in osteomalacia and hyperparathyroidism. *Clin Radiol* 1979;30:307.

289. Bonavita JA, Dalinka MK. Shoulder erosions in renal osteodystrophy. *Skeletal Radiol* 1980;5:105.

290. Kricun ME, Resnick D. Elbow abnormalities in renal osteodystrophy. *AJR* 1983;140:577.

291. Resnick D, Deftos LJ, Partemore JG. Renal osteodystrophy: magnification radiography of target sites of absorption. *AJR* 1981;136:711.

292. Sundaram M, Joyce PF, Shields JB, et al. Terminal phalangeal tufts: earliest site of renal osteodystrophy findings in hemodialysis patients. *AJR* 1981;136:363.

293. Sundaram M, Wolverson MK, Heiberg E, et al. Erosive azotemic osteodystrophy. *AJR* 1981;136:363.

294. Kricun ME, Resnick D. Patellofemoral abnormalities in renal osteodystrophy. *Radiology* 1982;143:667.

295. Koo WWK, Sherman R, Succop P, et al. Fractures and rickets in very low birth weight infants: conservative management and outcome. *J Pediatr Orthop* 1989;9:326.

296. Stamp WG, Whitesides TE, Field MH, et al. Treatment of vitamin D–resistant rickets: a long-term evaluation of its effectiveness. *J Bone Joint Surg Am* 1964;46:965.

297. Lee JJK, Lyne ED, Kleerekoper M, et al. Disorders of bone metabolism in severely handicapped children and young adults. *Clin Orthop* 1989;245:297.

298. Salenius P, Vankka E. The development of the tibio-femoral angle in children. *J Bone Joint Surg Am* 1975;57:259.

299. Staheli LT, Corbett M, Wyss C, et al. Lower-extremity rotational problems in children. *J Bone Joint Surg Am* 1985;67:39.

300. Kling TF Jr. Angular deformities of the lower limbs in children. *Orthop Clin North Am* 1987;18:513.

301. Rubinovitch M, Said SE, Glorieux FH, et al. Principles and results of corrective lower limb osteotomies for patients with vitamin D–resistant hypophosphatemic rickets. *Clin Orthop* 1988;237:264.

302. Paley D, Tetsworth K. Mechanical axis deviation of the lower limbs. *Clin Orthop* 1992;280:65.

303. Ferris B, Walker C, Jackson A, et al. The orthopaedic management of hypophosphataemic rickets. *J Pediatr Orthop* 1991;11:367.

304. Felts HJ, Whitley JE, Anderson DD, et al. Medical and surgical treatment of azotemic osteodystrophy. *Ann Intern Med* 1965;62:1272.

305. Esselstyn CB Jr, Popowniak KL. Parathyroid surgery in treatment of renal osteodystrophy and tertiary hyperparathyroidism. *Surg Clin North Am* 1971;51:1211.

306. Andress DL, Norris KC, Coburn JW, et al. Intravenous calcitriol in the treatment of refractory osteitis fibrosa of chronic renal failure. *N Engl J Med* 1989;321:274.

307. Crawford AH. Current concepts review. Slipped capital femoral epiphysis. *J Bone Joint Surg Am* 1988;70:1422.

308. Hagglund G, Bylander B, Hansson LI, et al. Bone growth after fixing slipped femoral epiphyses: brief report. *J Bone Joint Surg Br* 1988;70:845.

309. Nixon JR, Douglas JF. Bilateral slipping of the upper femoral epiphysis in end-stage renal failure. *J Bone Joint Surg Br* 1980;62:18.

310. Crawford AH. Correspondence. *J Bone Joint Surg Am* 1990;72:632.

311. Alper J. Boning up: newly isolated proteins heal bad breaks. *Science* 1994;263:324.

312. Stanitski DF. Treatment of deformity secondary to metabolic bone disease with Ilizarov technique. *Clin Orthop* 1994;301:38.

313. Huhne R, Schonfeld H. Eine eigenartige Wachtumsstorung im Kindeslater. *Monatsschr Kinderheilkd* 1929;42:267.

314. Rathbun JC. Hypophosphatasia. *Am J Dis Child* 1948;75:822.

315. Sobel EH, Clark LC, Fox RP, et al. Rickets: deficiency of "alkaline" phosphatase activity and premature loss of teeth in childhood. *Pediatrics* 1953;11:309.

316. McCane RA, Fairweathr DVI, Barrett AM, et al. Genetic, clinical, biochemical, and pathological features of hypophosphatasia. *Q J Med* 1956;25:523.

317. Whyte MP, Teitelbaum SI, Murphy WA. Adult hypophosphatasia: clinical, laboratory, and genetic investigation of a large kindred with review of the literature. *Medicine* 1979;58:329.

318. Fraser D, Yendt ER, Christie FHE. Metabolic abnormalities in hypophosphatasia. *Lancet* 1955;1:286.

319. Pimstone B, Eissenberg E, Silverman S. Hypophosphatasia: genetic and dental studies. *Ann Intern Med* 1966;65:722.

320. Bartter FC. Hypophosphatasia. In: Stanbury JB, Wyngaarden JB, Fredrickson DS, eds. *The metabolic basis of inherited disease*, 2nd ed. New York: McGraw-Hill, 1966.

321. Bethune JD, Dent CD. Hypophosphatasia in the adult. *Am J Med* 1960;28:615.

322. Anderton JM. Orthopaedic problems in adult hypophosphatasia: a report of two cases. *J Bone Joint Surg Br* 1979;61:82.

323. Currarino G, Neuhauser EBD, Reyersback GC, et al. Hyposphosphatasia. *AJR* 1957;78:392.

324. Kretchmer N, Stone M, Bauer C. Hereditary enzymatic effects as illustrated by hypophosphatasia. *Ann NY Acad Sci* 1958;75:279.

325. Fraser D. Hypophosphatasia. *Am J Med* 1957;22:730.

326. Goyer RA. Ethanolamine phosphate excretion in a family with hypophosphatasia. *Arch Dis Child* 1963;38:205.

327. McCane RA, Morrison AB, Dent CD. The excretion of phosphoethanolamine in hypophosphatasia. *Lancet* 1955;1:131.

328. Licata AA, Radfar N, Bartter FC. The urinary excretion of phosphoethanolamine in diseases other than hypophosphatasia. *Am J Med* 1978;64:133.

329. Jacobson DP, McClain EJ. Hypophosphatasia in monozygotic twins: a case report. *J Bone Joint Surg Am* 1967;49:377.

330. Coe JD, Murphy WA, Whyte MP. Management of femoral fractures and pseudofractures in adult hypophosphatasia. *J Bone Joint Surg Am* 1986;68:981.

331. Arnaud SB, Goldsmith RS, Stickler GB, et al. Serum parathyroid hormone and blood minerals: interrelationships in normal children. *Pediatr Res* 1973;7:485.

332. Bergman L, Hagberg S. Primary hyperparathyroidism in a child investigated by determination of ultrafiltrable calcium. *Am J Dis Child* 1972;123:174.

333. Bjernulf A, Hall K, Sjogren I, et al. Primary hyperparathyroidism in children. *Acta Paediatr Scand* 1970;59:249.

334. Cutler RE, Reiss E, Ackerman LV. Familial hyperparathyroidism. *N Engl J Med* 1964;270:859.

335. Randall C, Lauchlan SC. Parathyroid hyperplasia in an infant. *Am J Dis Child* 1963;105:364.

336. Stuart C, Aceto T Jr, Kuhn JP, et al. Intrauterine hyperparathyroidism: postmortem findings in two cases. *Am J Dis Child* 1979;133:67.

337. Bronsky D, Kiamko RT, Waldstein S. Familial idiopathic hyperparathyroidism. *Am J Med* 1974;57:34.

338. Whyte MP, Weldon W. Idiopathic hypoparathyroidism presenting with seizures during infancy: X-linked recessive inheritance in a large Missouri kindred. *J Pediatr* 1981;99:608.

339. Avioli LV. The therapeutic approach to hypoparathyroidism. *Am J Dis Child* 1974;57:34.

340. Albright F, Burnett C, Smith P, et al. Pseudohypoparathyroidism: an example of "Seabright-Bantam syndrome." Report of three cases. *Endocrinology* 1942;30:922.

341. Weinberg AG, Stone RT. Autosomal dominant inheritance in Albright's hereditary osteodystrophy. *J Pediatr* 1971;79:997.

342. Temtamy SA, McKusick VA. Brachydactyly as part of syndromes. In: Bergsma D, ed. *The genetics of hand malformations.* New York: Alan R. Liss, 1978:227.

343. Drezner M, Neelon FA, Lebovitz HE. Pseudohypoparathyroidism type II. A possible defect in the reception of the cyclic AMP signal. *N Engl J Med* 1973;289:1056.

344. Farfel Z, Brickman AS, Kaslow HR, et al. Defect of receptor-cyclase coupling protein in pseudohypoparathyroidism. *N Engl J Med* 1980;303:237.

345. Glass EJ, Barr DGD. Transient neonatal hyperparathyroidism secondary to maternal pseudohypoparathyroidism. *Arch Dis Child* 1981;56:555.

346. Marcus R, Wilber JF, Aurbach GD. Parathyroid hormone-sensitive adenyl cyclase from the renal cortex of a patient with pseudohypoparathyroidism. *J Clin Endocrinol Metab* 1971;33:537.

347. Cohn MJ, Izpisua-Belmonte JC, Abud H, et al. Fibroblast growth factors induce additional limb development from the flank of chick embryos. *Cell* 1995;80:739.

348. Zou H, Niswander L. Requirement for BMP signaling in interdigital apoptosis and scale formation. *Science* 1996;272:738.

349. Muragaki Y, Mundlos S, Upton J, et al. Altered growth and branching patterns in synpolydactyly caused by mutations in HOXD13. *Science* 1996;272:548.

350. Lefkowitz RJ. G proteins in medicine. *N Engl J Med* 1995;332:186.

351. Ringel MD, Schwindinger WF, Levine MA. Clinical implications of genetic defects in G proteins: the molecular basis of McCune-Albright syndrome and Albright hereditary osteodystrophy. *Medicine* 1996;75:171.

352. Wilson LC, Leverton K, Luttikhuis O, et al. Brachydactyly and mental retardation: an Albright hereditary osteodystrophy-like syndrome localized to 2q37. *Am J Hum Genet* 1995;56:400.

353. David NJ, Verner JV, Engel FL. The diagnostic spectrum of hypercalcemia. *Am J Med* 1962;33:88.

354. Forbes GB, Cafarelli C, Manning J. Vitamin D and infantile hypercalcemia. *Pediatrics* 1968;42:203.

355. Muggia F, Heineman HO. Hypercalcemia associated with neoplastic disease. *Ann Intern Med* 1970;73:281.

356. Powell D, Singer FR, Murray TM, et al. Nonparathyroid humoral hypercalcemia in patients with neoplastic diseases. *N Engl J Med* 1973;289:176.

357. Hyman LR, Boner G, Thomas JC, et al. Immobilization hypercalcemia. *Am J Dis Child* 1972;124:723.

358. King LR, Knowles HC, McLaurin RL. Calcium, phosphorus, and magnesium metabolism following head injury. *Ann Surg* 1973;177:126.

359. Lawrence GD, Loeffler RG, Martin LG, et al. Immobilization hypercalcemia. *J Bone Joint Surg Am* 1973;55:87.

360. Millard FJC, Nassim JR, Woollen JW. Urinary calcium excretion after immobilization and spinal fusion in adolescents. *Arch Dis Child* 1970;45:399.

361. Pezeshki C, Brooker AF Jr. Immobilization hypercalcemia. *J Bone Joint Surg Am* 1977;59:971.

362. Williams JCP, Baratt-Boyes BG, Lowe JB. Supravalvular aortic stenosis. *Circulation* 1961;24:1311.

363. Schipani E, Kruse K, Juppner H. A constitutively active mutant PTH-PTHrP receptor in Jansen-type metaphyseal chondrodysplasia. *Science* 1995;268:98.

364. Lanske B, Karaplis AC, Lee K, et al. PTH/PTHrP receptor in early development and Indian Hedgehog-regulated bone growth. *Science* 1996;273:663.

365. Warman ML, Abbott M, Apte SS, et al. A type X collagen mutation causes Schmid metaphyseal chondrodysplasia. *Nat Genet* 1993;5:79.

366. Chisholm JJ Jr. Increased lead absorption and lead poisoning. In: Behrman RE, Vaughan VC III, eds. *Nelson's textbook of pediatrics,* 12th ed. Philadelphia: WB Saunders, 1983:1684.

367. Kumar S, Shahabuddin S, Haboubi N, et al. Angiogenesis factor from human myocardial infarcts. *Lancet* 1983;2:364.

Organic Phase

368. Cruess RL. Physiology of bone formation and resorption. In: Cruess RL, ed. *The musculoskeletal system.* New York: Churchill Livingstone, 1982:219.

369. Frost HM. *Mathematical elements of lamellar bone remodeling.* Springfield, IL: Charles C Thomas, 1964.

370. Rasmussen H, Bordier P. The cellular basis of metabolic bone disease. *N Engl J Med* 1973;289:25.

371. Hollister DW, Byers PH, Holbrook KA. Genetic disorders of collagen metabolism. *Adv Hum Genet* 1982;12:1.

372. Gordon MK, Gerecke DR, Nishimura I, et al. A new dimension in the extracellular matrix. In: Glimcher MJ, Lian JB, eds. *The chemistry and biology of mineralized tissues: proceedings of the third international conference.* New York: Gordon and Breach, 1988:179.

373. Dunker AK, Zaleske DJ. Stereochemical considerations for constructing alpha-helical protein bundles with particular application to membrane proteins. *Biochem J* 1977;163:45.

374. Lane JM, Suda M, von der Mark K, et al. Immunofluorescent localization of structural collagen types in endochondral fracture repair. *J Orthop Res* 1986;4:318.

375. Hay ED. Embryonic induction and tissue interaction. *Excerpta Med Int Congr Ser* 1977;432:126.

376. Boskey AL. Current concepts of the physiology and biochemistry of calcification. *Clin Orthop* 1981;157:225

377. Boskey AL. Mineral-matrix interactions in bone and cartilage. *Clin Orthop* 1992;281:244.

378. Buckwalter JA. Proteoglycan structure in calcifying cartilage. *Clin Orthop* 1983;172:207.

Osteogenesis Imperfecta

379. McKusick VA. *Heritable disorders of connective tissues,* 4th ed. St. Louis: Mosby, 1972.

380. Malebranche N. *Traite de la recherche de la verite.* Paris: Chez Andre Pralard, 1674.

381. Lobstein JF. De la fragilite des os, ou de l'osteopsathyrose. In: Levrault FG, ed. *Traite de l'anatomie pathologique,* vol 2. Paris: L.T. Cellot, 1833.

382. Vrolik W. *Tabulae ad illustradam embryogenesin hominis et mammalium, tam naturalem quam abnormen.* Amsterdam: GMP Londonck, 1949.

383. Castells S, Colbert C, Chakrabarti C, et al. Therapy of osteogenesis imperfecta with synthetic salmon calcitonin. *J Pediatr* 1979;95:807.

384. Looser E. Zur Kenntnis der Osteogenesis imperfecta congenita et tarda. *Mitt Grenzbiet Med Chir* 1906;15:161.

385. Sillence DO. Osteogenesis imperfecta: an expanding panorama of variance. *Clin Orthop* 1981;159:11.

386. Wynne-Davis R, Gormley J. Clinical and genetic patterns in osteogenesis imperfecta. *Clin Orthop* 1981;159:26.

387. Francis MJO, Bauze RJ, Smith R. Osteogenesis imperfecta: a new classification. *Birth Defects* 1985;11:99.

388. Sillence DO, Senn A, Danks DM. Genetic heterogeneity in osteogenesis imperfecta. *J Med Genet* 1979;16:101.

389. Bauze RJ, Smith R, Francis MJO. A new look at osteogenesis imperfecta. *J Bone Joint Surg Br* 1975;57:2.

390. Minch CM, Kruse RW. Osteogenesis imperfecta: a review of basic science and diagnosis. *Orthopedics* 1998;21:558.

391. Dent JA, Paterson CR. Fractures in early childhood: osteogenesis imperfecta or child abuse. *J Pediatr Orthop* 1991;11:184.

392. DiCesare PE, Sew-Hoy A, Krom W. Bilateral isolated olecranon fractures in an infant as presentation of osteogenesis imperfecta. *Orthopedics* 1992;15:741.

393. Rao S, Patel A, Schildhauer T. Osteogenesis imperfecta as a differential diagnosis of pathologic burst fractures of the spine. *Clin Orthop* 1993;289:113.

394. Carty HML. Fractures caused by child abuse. *J Bone Joint Surg Br* 1993;75:849.

395. Kleinman PK, Blackbourne BD, Marks SC, et al. Radiologic contributions to the investigation and prosecution of cases of fatal infant abuse. *N Engl J Med* 1989;320:507.

396. Kozlowki K, McCrossin R. Early osseous abnormalities in Menkes' kinky hair syndrome. *Pediatr Radiol* 1980;8:191.

397. Seedorff KS. *Osteogenesis imperfecta: a study of clinical features and heredity based on 55 Danish families comprising 180 affected persons.* Copenhagen: Ejnar Munksgaard, 1949.

398. Shapiro F. Consequences of an osteogenesis imperfecta diagnosis for survival and ambulation. *J Pediatr Orthop* 1985;5:456.

399. Duffrin H, Sundaram M. Radiologic case study: osteogenesis imperfecta. *Orthopedics* 1987;10:1304.

400. Cropp GJ, Meyers DN. Physiological evidence of hypermetabolism in osteogenesis imperfecta. *Pediatrics* 1972;49:375.

401. Marion MJ, Gannon FH, Fallon MD, et al. Skeletal dysplasia in perinatal lethal osteogenesis imperfecta. *Clin Orthop* 1993;293:327.

402. Smith R, Francis MJO, Bauze RJ. Osteogenesis imperfecta: a clinical and biochemical study of a generalized connective tissue disorder. *Q J Med* 1975;44:555.

403. Trelstad RL, Rubin D, Gross J. Osteogenesis imperfecta congenita: evidence for a generalized molecular disorder of collagen. *Lab Invest* 1977;36:501.

404. Pope FM, Nicholls AC, Eggleton C, et al. Osteogenesis imperfecta (lethal) bones contain types III and V collagen. *J Clin Pathol* 1980;33:534.

405. Barsh GS, David KE, Byers PH. Type I osteogenesis imperfecta: a nonfunctional allele for pro alpha (I) chains for type I procollagen. *Proc Natl Acad Sci USA* 1982;79:3838.

406. Peltonen L, Palotie A, Prockop DJ. A defect in the structure of type I procollagen in a patient who had osteogenesis imperfecta: excessive mannose in the COOH-terminal peptide. *Proc Natl Acad Sci USA* 1980;77:6179.

407. Pettinen RP, Lichtenstein JR, Martin GR, et al. Abnormal collagen metabolism in cultured cells in osteogenesis imperfecta. *Proc Natl Acad Sci USA* 1975;72:586.

408. Eyre DR, Upton M, Shapiro F, et al. Non-expression of cartilage type II collagen in a case of human achondrogenesis (Langer-Saldino variant). *Trans Orthop Res Soc* 1986;11:459.

409. Delvin EE, Glorieux FH, Lopez E. *In vitro* sulfate turnover in osteogenesis imperfecta congenita and tarda. *Am J Med Genet* 1979;4:349.

410. Turkainen J. Altered glycosaminoglycan production in cultured osteogenesis imperfecta skin fibroblasts. *Biochem J* 1983;213:171.

411. Cowell HR, Ray S. Talipes equinovarus and syndrome identification. *Contemp Orthop* 1984;9:51.

412. Huaux JP, Lokietek W. Is APD a promising drug in the treatment of severe osteogenesis imperfecta? *J Pediatr Orthop* 1988;8:71.

413. Acito AJ, Kasra M, Lee JM, et al. Effects of intermittent administration of pamidronate on the mechanical properties of canine cortical and trabecular bone. *J Orthop Res* 1994;12:742.

414. Glorieux FH, Bishop NJ, Plotkin H, et al. Cyclic administration of pamidronate in children with severe osteogenesis imperfecta. *N Engl J Med* 1998;339:947.

415. Marini JC. Osteogenesis imperfecta: managing brittle bones [editorial]. *N Engl J Med* 1998;339:986.

416. Cole NL, Goldberg MH, Loftus M, et al. Surgical management of patients with osteogenesis imperfecta. *J Oral Maxillofac Surg* 1982;40:578.

417. King JD, Bobechko WP. Osteogenesis imperfecta: an orthopaedic description and surgical review. *J Bone Joint Surg Br* 1971;53:72.

418. Miller EA. Observation on the surgical management of osteogenesis imperfecta. *Clin Orthop* 1981;159:154.

419. Morefield WG, Miller GR. Aftermath of osteogenesis imperfecta: a disease in adulthood. *J Bone Joint Surg Am* 1980;62:113.

420. Quisling RW, Moore GR, Jahrsdoefer RA. Osteogenesis imperfecta. *Arch Otolaryngol* 1979;105:207.

421. Roberts JM, Solomons CC. Management of pregnancy in osteogenesis imperfecta. *Obstet Gynecol* 1975;45:168.

422. Gerber LH, Binder H, Weintrob J, et al. Rehabilitation of children and infants with osteogenesis imperfecta. *Clin Orthop* 1990;251:254.

423. Letts M, Monson R, Weber K. The prevention of recurrent fractures of the lower extremities in severe osteogenesis imperfecta using vacuum pants: a preliminary report in four patients. *J Pediatr Orthop* 1988;8:454.

424. Ryoppy S, Alberty A, Kaitila I. Early semiclosed intramedullary stabilization in osteogenesis imperfecta. *J Pediatr Orthop* 1987;7:139.

425. Sijbrandij S. Percutaneous nailing in the management of osteogenesis imperfecta. *Int Orthop* 1990;14:195.

426. Middleton RWD, Frost RB. Percutaneous intramedullary rod interchange in osteogenesis imperfecta. *J Bone Joint Surg Br* 1987;69:429.

427. Tiley F, Albright JA. Osteogenesis imperfecta: treatment by multiple osteotomy and intramedullary rod insertion. *J Bone Joint Surg Am* 1973;55:701.

428. Williams PF. Fragmentation and rodding in osteogenesis imperfecta. *J Bone Joint Surg Br* 1965;47:23.

429. Sofield HA, Millar EA. Fragmentation, realignment, and intramedullary rod fixation of deformities of the long bones in children: a ten-year appraisal. *J Bone Joint Surg Am* 1959;41:1371.

430. Nicholas RW, James P. Telescoping intramedullary stabilization of the lower extremities for severe osteogenesis imperfecta. *J Pediatr Orthop* 1990;10:219.

431. Gamble JG, Strudwick WJ, Rinsky LA, et al. Complications of intramedullary rods in osteogenesis imperfecta: Bailey-Dubow rods versus nonelongating rods. *J Pediatr Orthop* 1988;8:645.

432. Porat S, Heller E, Seidman DS, et al. Functional results of operation in osteogenesis imperfecta: elongating and nonelongating rods. *J Pediatr Orthop* 1991;11:200.

433. Morel G, Houghton GR. Pneumatic trouser splints in the treatment of severe osteogenesis imperfecta. *Acta Orthop Scand* 1982;53:547.

434. Herring JA. Indications, patient selection, and evaluation in pediatric orthopedics. In: Luque ER, ed. *Segmental spinal instrumentation*. Thorofare, NJ: Slack, 1984:64.

435. Lubicky JP. The spine in osteogenesis imperfecta. In: Weinstein SL, ed. *The pediatric spine*. New York: Raven, 1994:943.

436. Brenton DP, Dent CE. Idiopathic osteoporosis. In: Bickel H, Stern J, eds. *Inborn errors of calcium and bone metabolism*. Baltimore: University Park, 1976.

437. Cloutier MD, Hayles AB, Riggs BL, et al. Juvenile osteoporosis: report of a case including a description of some metabolic and microradiographic studies. *Pediatrics* 1967;40:649.

438. Dent CE. Idiopathic juvenile osteoporosis. *Birth Defects* 1969; 5:134.

439. Jowsey J. *Metabolic diseases of bone*. Philadelphia: WB Saunders, 1977.

440. Jowsey J, Johnson KA. Juvenile osteoporosis: bone findings in seven patients. *J Pediatr* 1972;81:511.

441. Kooh SW, Cumming WA, Fraser D, et al. *Transient childhood osteoporosis of unknown cause*. Amsterdam: Excerpta Medica, 1973.

442. Teotia M, Teotia S, Singh RK. Idiopathic juvenile osteoporosis. *Am J Dis Child* 1979;133:894.

443. Evans RA, Dunstan CR, Hills E. Bone metabolism in idiopathic juvenile osteoporosis: a case report. *Calcif Tissue Int* 1983;35: 5.

444. Gallagher CJ, Riggs BL, Eisman J. Intestinal calcium absorption and serum vitamin D metabolites in normal subjects and osteoporotic patients. *J Clin Invest* 1979;64:729.

445. Harris WH, Heaney RP. Skeletal renewal and metabolic bone disease. *N Engl J Med* 1969;280:193.

446. Marder HK, Tsang RC, Hug G, et al. Calcitriol deficiency in idiopathic juvenile osteoporosis in the young. *J Bone Joint Surg Br* 1980;62:417.

447. Greene WB. Idiopathic juvenile osteoporosis. In: Weinstein SL, ed. *The pediatric spine*. New York: Raven, 1994:933.

448. Jones ET, Hensinger RN. Spinal deformity in idiopathic juvenile osteoporosis. *Spine* 1981;6:1.

Osteopetrosis

449. Manzke E, Gruber HE, Hines RW, et al. Skeletal remodeling and bone-related hormones in two adults with increased bone mass. *Metab Clin Exp* 1982;31:25.

450. Milgram JW, Jasty M. Osteopetrosis. *J Bone Joint Surg Am* 1982;64:912.

451. Shapiro F. Osteopetrosis: current clinical considerations. *Clin Orthop* 1993;294:34.

452. Albers-Schonberg H. Eine Bisher Nicht Beschriebene Allgemeinerkrankung Skelettes Im Rontgenbild. *Forschr Geb Rontgenstr* 1907;11:261.

453. Beighton P, Hamersma H. The orthopaedic implications of the sclerosing bone dysplasias. *S Afr Med J* 1980;11:600.

454. Hasenhuttl K. Osteopetrosis: review of the literature on comparative studies on a case with a 24-year follow-up. *J Bone Joint Surg Am* 1962;44:359.

455. Hinkel CL, Beiler DD. Osteopetrosis in adults. *AJR* 1955;74: 46.

456. Milhaud G, Labat ML. Osteopetrosis reconsidered as a curable immune disorder. *Biomedicine* 1979;30:71.

457. Shapiro F, Glimcher MJ, Holtrop ME, et al. Human osteopetrosis: a histological, ultrastructural, and biochemical study. *J Bone Joint Surg Am* 1980;62:384.

458. Kramer B, Yuska H, Steiner MM. Marble bones. II. Chemical analysis of bone. *Am J Dis Child* 1939;57:1044.

459. Brown DM. Pathogenesis of osteopetrosis: a comparison of human and animal spectra. *Pediatr Res* 1971;5:181.

460. Dent CE, Smellie JM, Watson L. Studies in osteopetrosis. *Arch Dis Child* 1965;40:7.

461. Pearce L. Hereditary osteopetrosis of the rabbit. III. Pathological observations: skeletal abnormalities. *J Exp Med* 1950;92:591.

462. Pinchus JB, Gittleman IF, Kramer B. Juvenile osteopetrosis: metabolic studies in two cases and further observations on the composition of the bones in this disease. *Am J Dis Child* 1947; 73:458.

463. Walker DG. Experimental osteopetrosis. *Clin Orthop* 1973;97: 158.

464. Marks SC. Pathogenesis of osteopetrosis in the rat: reduced bone resorption due to reduced osteoclast function. *Am J Anat* 1973;138:165.

465. Walker DG. Bone resorption restored in osteopetrotic mice by transplants of normal bone marrow and spleen cells. *Science* 1975;190:784.

466. Walker DG. Osteopetrosis cured by temporary parabiosis. *Science* 1973;180:875.

467. Marks SC, Walker DG. The hematogenous origin of osteoclasts: experimental evidence from osteopetrotic (microphthalmic) mice treated with spleen cells from beige mouse donors. *Am J Anat* 1981;161:1.

468. Milhaud G, Labat ML, Parant M, et al. Immunologic defect and its correction in the osteopetrotic mutant rat. *Proc Natl Acad Sci USA* 1977;74:339.

469. Hofer M, Hirschel B, Kirschner P, et al. Brief report. Disseminated osteomyelitis from *Mycobacterium ulcerans* after a snakebite. *N Engl J Med* 1993;328:1007.

470. Ballet JJ, Griscelli C. Lymphoid cell transplantation in human osteopetrosis. In: Horton JE, Tarpley TM, Davis WF, eds. *Mechanisms of localized bone loss: proceedings of the first scientific evaluation workshop on localized bone loss*. Washington: Information Retrieval, 1978:399.

471. Ballet JJ, Griscelli C, Coutris C, et al. Bone marrow transplantation in osteopetrosis. *Lancet* 1977;2:1137.

472. Coccia BF, Krivit W, Cervenka J. Successful bone marrow transplantation for infantile osteopetrosis. *N Engl J Med* 1980;302: 701.

473. Kaplan FS, August CS, Fallon MD, et al. Successful treatment of infantile malignant osteopetrosis by bone-marrow transplantation. *J Bone Joint Surg Am* 1988;70:617.

474. Sieff CA, Levinsky RJ, Rogers DW, et al. Allogeneic bone-marrow transplantation in infantile malignant osteopetrosis. *Lancet* 1983;1:437.

475. Sorell M, Kapoor N, Kirkperuch C. Marrow transplantation for juvenile osteopetrosis. *Am J Med* 1981;70:1280.

476. Key LL Jr, Rodgriguiz RM, Willi SM, et al. Long-term treatment of osteopetrosis with recombinant human interferon gamma. *N Engl J Med* 1995;332:1594.

477. Whyte MP. Chipping away at marble-bone disease. *N Engl J Med* 1995;332:1639.

478. Aegerter E, Kirkpatrick J. *Orthopaedic diseases*. Philadelphia: WB Saunders, 1975:440.

479. Talab YA, Mallouh A. Hyperostosis with hyperphosphatemia: a case report and review of the literature. *J Pediatr Orthop* 1988; 8:338.

480. Naveh Y, Kaftori JK, Alan V, et al. Progressive diaphyseal dysplasia: genetics and clinical and radiographic manifestations. *Pediatrics* 1984;74:399.

481. Resnick D, Niwayama G. Osteomyelitis, septic arthritis, and soft tissue infection: the organisms. In: Resnick D, Niwayama G, eds. *Diagnosis of bone and joint disorders*, 2nd ed. Philadelphia: WB Saunders, 1988:2647.

482. Evans EB. Musculoskeletal changes complicating burns. In: Epps CH Jr, ed. *Complications in orthopaedic surgery*, 2nd ed. Philadelphia: Lippincott-Raven, 1986:1307.

483. Caffey J. *Pediatric x-ray diagnosis.* Chicago: Year Book, 1972.

484. Caffey J. Infantile cortical hyperostosis: a review of the clinical and radiographic features. *Proc R Soc Lond* 1957;50:347.

485. Staheli LT, Church CC, Ward BH. Infantile cortical hyperostosis (Caffey's disease). *JAMA* 1968;203:96.

486. Bernstein RM, Zaleske DJ. Familial aspects of Caffey's disease: a report of a family and review of the English literature. *Am J Orthop* 1995;24:777.

487. Pazzaglia UE, Byers P, Beluffi G, et al. Pathology of infantile cortical hyperostosis (Caffey's disease). *J Bone Joint Surg Am* 1985;67:1417.

488. Blasier RB, Aronson DD. Infantile cortical hyperostosis with osteomyelitis of the humerus. *J Pediatr Orthop* 1985;5:222.

489. Frame B, Jackson CE, Reynolds WA, et al. Hypercalcemia and skeletal effects in chronic hypervitaminosis and skeletal effects in chronic hypervitaminosis A. *Ann Intern Med* 1974;80:44.

490. Gamble JG, Ip SC. Hypervitaminosis A in a child from megadosing. *J Pediatr Orthop* 1985;5:219.

491. Lim MO, Mukherjee AB, Hansen JW. Dysplastic cutaneous osteomatosis. *Arch Dermatol* 1981;117:797.

492. Banks SW. Bone changes in acute and chronic scurvy: an experimental study. *J Bone Joint Surg Am* 1943;25:553.

493. Hurwitz S. *Clinical pediatric dermatology.* Philadelphia: WB Saunders, 1981:185.

494. Heydemann JS, McCarthy RE. Tumoral calcinosis in a child. *J Pediatr Orthop* 1988;8:474.

495. Gregosiewicz A, Warda E. Tumoral calcinosis: successful medical treatment. *J Bone Joint Surg Am* 1989;71:1244.

496. Mozaffarian G, Lafferty FW, Pearson OH. Treatment of tumoral calcinosis with phosphorus deprivation. *Ann Intern Med* 1972;741:745.

497. Mitnick PD, Goldfarb S, Slatopolsky E, et al. Calcium and phosphorus metabolism in tumoral calcinosis. *Ann Intern Med* 1980;92:482.

498. Aprin H, Sinha A. Tumoral calcinosis: report of a case in a one-year-old child. *Clin Orthop* 1984;185:83.

499. Kirk TS, Simon MA. Tumoral calcinosis: report of a case with successful medical management. *J Bone Joint Surg Am* 1981;63:1167.

500. Rodriguez-Peralto JL, Lopez-Barea F, Torres A, et al. Tumoral calcinosis in two infants. *Clin Orthop* 1989;242:272.

501. Cohen RB, Hahn GV, Tabas JA, et al. The natural history of heterotopic ossification in patients who have fibrodysplasia ossificans progressiva. *J Bone Joint Surg Am* 1993;75:215.

502. Kaplan FS, Tabas JA, Gannon F, et al. The histopathology of fibrodysplasia ossificans progressiva. *J Bone Joint Surg Am* 1993;75:220.

503. Kaplan FS, Hahn GV, Zasloff MA. Heterotopic ossification: two rare forms and what they can teach us. *J Am Acad Orthop Surg* 1994;2:288.

504. Brunet LJ, McMahon JA, McMahon AP, et al. Noggin, cartilage morphogenesis, and joint formation in the mammalian skeleton. *Science* 1998;280:1455.

505. Garland DE, Hanscom DA, Keenan MA, et al. Resection of heterotopic ossification in the adult with head trauma. *J Bone Joint Surg Am* 1985;67:1261.

506. Mital MA, Garber JE, Stinson JT. Ectopic bone formation in children and adolescents with head injuries: its management. *J Pediatr Orthop* 1987;7:83.

507. Ogilvie-Harris DJ, Fornasier VL. Pseudomalignant myositis ossificans: heterotopic new-bone formation without a history of trauma. *J Bone Joint Surg Am* 1980;62:1274.

508. Pazzaglia UE, Beluffi G, Colombo A, et al. Myositis ossificans in the newborn. *J Bone Joint Surg Am* 1986;68:456.

509. Ayers DC, Evarts CM, Parkinson JR. The prevention of heterotopic ossification in high risk patients by low-dose radiation therapy after total hip arthroplasty. *J Bone Joint Surg Am* 1986;68:1423.

510. Pyeritz RE, McKusick VA. The Marfan syndrome: diagnosis and management. *N Engl J Med* 1979;300:772.

511. Tsipouras P, Del Mastro R, Sarfarazi M, et al. Genetic linkage of the Marfan syndrome, ectopia lentis, and congenital contractural arachnodactyly to the fibrillin genes on chromosomes 15 and 5. *N Engl J Med* 1992;326:905.

512. Keech MR, Wendt VE, Reed RC, et al. Family studies of the Marfan syndrome. *J Chronic Dis* 1966;19:57.

513. Steinberg I. A simple screening test for the Marfan syndrome. *AJR* 1966;97:118.

514. Parrish JG. Heritable disorders of connective tissue. *Proc R Soc Med* 1960;53:515.

515. Moe JH, Winter RB, Bradford DS, et al. Scoliosis in Marfan's syndrome. In: *Scoliosis and other spinal deformities.* Philadelphia: WB Saunders, 1978:315.

516. Amis J, Herring JA. Iatrogenic kyphosis: a complication of Harrington instrumentation in Marfan's syndrome. *J Bone Joint Surg Am* 1984;66:460.

517. Robins PR, Moe JH, Winter RB. Scoliosis in Marfan's syndrome. *J Bone Joint Surg Am* 1975;57:358.

518. Beighton P, Horan F. Orthopaedic aspects of the Ehlers-Danlos syndrome. *J Bone Joint Surg Br* 1969;51:444.

519. Ainsworth SR, Aulicino PL. A survey of patients with Ehlers-Danlos syndrome. *Clin Orthop* 1993;286:250.

520. Rames RD, Strecker WB. Recurrent elbow dislocations in a patient with Ehlers-Danlos syndrome. *Orthopedics* 1991;14:705.

521. Badelon O, Bensahel H, Csukonyi Z, et al. Congenital dislocation of the hip in Ehlers-Danlos syndrome. *Clin Orthop* 1990;255:138.

522. Pinnell SR, Krane SM, Kenzora JE, et al. A heritable disorder of connective tissue: hydroxylysine-deficient collagen disease. *N Engl J Med* 1972;386:1013.

523. Finkelstein JD. Methionine metabolism in mammals: the biochemical basis for homocystinuria. *Metab Clin Exp* 1974;23:387.

524. Gaull G, Sturman JA, Schaffner F. Homocystinuria due to cystathionine synthase deficiency: enzymatic and ultrastructural studies. *J Pediatr* 1974;84:381.

525. Brenton DP, Dow CJ, James JIP, et al. Homocystinuria and Marfan's syndrome. *J Bone Joint Surg Br* 1972;54:277.

526. Brill PW, Mitty JA, Gaull GE. Homocystinuria due to cystathionine synthetase deficiency: clinical roentgenologic correlations. *AJR* 1974;121:45.

527. Boers GHJ, Smals AGH, Trijbels FJM, et al. Heterozygosity for homocystinuria in premature peripheral and cerebral occlusive arterial disease. *N Engl J Med* 1985;313:709

528. Clarke R, Daly L, Robinson K, et al. Hyperhomocystinemia: an independent risk factor for vascular disease. *N Engl J Med* 1991;324:1149.

529. Steegers-Theunissen RPM, Boers GHJ, Trijbels FJM, et al. Neural-tube defects and derangement of homocysteine metabolism. *N Engl J Med* 1991;324:199.

Endocrinopathies

530. Tanner JM, Goldstein H, Whitehouse RH. Standards for children's height at ages 2 to 9 years allowing for height of parents. *Arch Dis Child* 1970;45:755

531. Tanner JM, Whitehouse RH, Takaishi M. Standards from birth to maturity for height, weight, height velocity, and weight velocity: British children, 1965. *Arch Dis Child* 1966;41:454–471.

532. Bunch WH, Dvonch VM. Pitfalls in the assessment of skeletal

immaturity: an anthropologic case study. *J Pediatr Orthop* 1983; 3:220.

533. Tanner JM, Whitehouse RH, Marshall WA, et al. *Assessment of skeletal maturity and prediction of adult height (TW2 method)*. London: Academic, 1975.

534. Hamill PV, Drizd TA, Johnson CL, et al. Physical growth: National Center for Health Statistics percentiles. *Am J Clin Nutr* 1979;32:607.

535. Rudman D, Kutner MH, Blackston RD, et al. Children with normal variant short stature: treatment with human growth hormone for six months. *N Engl J Med* 1981;305:123.

536. Vance ML, Mauras N. Growth hormone therapy in adults and children. *N Engl J Med* 1999;341:1206.

537. Crawford JD. Meat, potatoes, and growth hormone. *N Engl J Med* 1981;305:163.

538. Marshall WA. *Human growth hormone and its disorders*. London: Academic, 1977.

539. Raisz LG, Kream B. Hormonal control of skeletal growth. *Annu Rev Physiol* 1981;43:225.

540. Jennings AS, Liddle TW, Orth DN. Results of treating childhood Cushing's disease with pituitary irradiation. *N Engl J Med* 1977;297:957.

541. Root AW, Bongiovanni AM, Eberlai WR. Diagnosis and management of growth retardation with special reference to the problem of hypopituitarism. *J Pediatr* 1971;78:737.

542. Lin T, Tucci JR. Provocation tests of growth hormone release. *Ann Intern Med* 1974;80:464.

543. Chaknakjian ZH, Marks JF, Fink CW. Effect of levodopa (L-dopa) on serum growth hormone in children with short stature. *Pediatr Res* 1973;7:71.

544. Powell GF, Brasil JA, Blizzard RM. Functional deprivation and growth retardation simulating idiopathic hypopituitarism. I. Clinical evaluation of the syndrome. *N Engl J Med* 1967;276:1271.

545. Powell GF, Brasil JA, Ruiti S, et al. Emotional deprivation and growth retardation simulating idiopathic hypopituitarism. II. Endocrinologic evaluation of the syndrome. *N Engl J Med* 1967;276:1279.

546. Soyka LF, Bode HH, Crawford JD, et al. Effectiveness of long term human growth therapy for short stature in children with human growth hormone deficiency. *J Clin Endocrinol Metab* 1970;30:1.

547. Rivkees S, Bode HH, Crawford JD. Long-term growth in juvenile acquired hypothyroidism: the failure to achieve normal adult stature. *N Engl J Med* 1988;318:599.

548. Wells D, King JD, Roe TF, et al. Review of slipped capital femoral epiphysis associated with endocrine disease. *J Pediatr Orthop* 1993;13:610.

549. Zubrow AB, Lane JW, Parks JS. Slipped capital femoral epiphysis occurring during treatment for hypothyroidism. *J Bone Joint Surg Am* 1978;60:256.

550. Neidel J, Boddenberg B, Zander D, et al. Thyroid function in Legg-Calve-Perthes disease: cross-sectional and longitudinal study. *J Pediatr Orthop* 1993;13:592.

551. Kan K, Cruess RL, Posner B, et al. Receptor proteins for steroid and peptide hormones at the epiphyseal line. *Trans Orthop Res Soc* 1981;6:110.

552. Simpson JL. *Disorders of sexual differentiation: etiology and clinical delineation*. New York: Academic, 1976.

553. Zaleske DJ, Bode HH, Benz R, et al. Association of sciatica-like pain and Addison's disease: a case report. *J Bone Joint Surg Am* 1984;66:297.

554. Sambrook P, Birmingham J, Kelly P, et al. Prevention of corticosteroid osteoporosis: a comparison of calcium, calcitriol, and calcitonin. *N Engl J Med* 1993;328:1747.

555. Danon M, Crawford JD. The McCune-Albright syndrome. *Ergeb Inn Med Kinderheilkd* 1987;55:81.

556. Harris WH, Dudley HR, Barry RJ. The natural history of fibrous dysplasia. *J Bone Joint Surg Am* 1962;44:207.

557. Henry A. Monostotic fibrous dysplasia. *J Bone Joint Surg Br* 1969;51:300.

558. Albin J, Wu R. Abnormal hypothalamic-pituitary function in polyostotic fibrous dysplasia. *Clin Endocrinol* 1981;14:435.

559. Spiegel AM. The molecular basis of disorders caused by defects in G proteins. *Horm Res* 1997;47:89.

560. Schnabel P, Bohm M. Mutations of signal-transducing G proteins in human disease. *J Mol Med* 1995;73:221.

561. Alman BA, Greel DA, Wolfe HJ. Activating mutations of Gs protein in monostotic fibrous lesions of bone. *J Orthop Res* 1996;14:311.

562. Motomura T, Kasayama S, Takagi M, et al. Increased interleukin-6 production in mouse osteoblastic MC3T3-E1 cells expressing activating mutant of the stimulatory G protein. *J Bone Miner Res* 1998;13:1084.

563. Andrisano A, Soncini G, Calderoni PP, et al. Critical review of infantile fibrous dysplasia: surgical treatment. *J Pediatr Orthop* 1991;11:478.

564. Connolly JF. Shepherd's crook deformities of polyostotic dysplasia treated by osteotomy and Zickel nail fixation. *Clin Orthop* 1977;123:22.

565. Guille JT, Kumar SJ, MacEwen GD. Fibrous dysplasia of the proximal part of the femur. *J Bone Joint Surg Am* 1998;80:648.

566. de Boer HH. The history of bone grafts. *Clin Orthop* 1988;226:292.

567. Virolainen P, Vuorio E, Aro HT. Gene expression at graft-host interfaces of cortical bone allografts and autografts. *Clin Orthop* 1993;297:144.

568. Hopp SG, Dahners LE, Gilbert JA. A study of the mechanical strength of long bone defects treated with various bone autograft substitutes: an experimental investigation in the rabbit. *J Orthop Res* 1989;7:579.

569. Pelker RR, McKay J Jr, Troiano N, et al. Allograft incorporation: a biomechanical evaluation in a rat model. *J Orthop Res* 1989;7:585.

570. Jofe MH, Gebhardt MC, Tomford WW, et al. Reconstruction for defects of the proximal part of the femur using allograft arthroplasty. *J Bone Joint Surg Am* 1988;70:507.

571. Shih HN, Chen YJ, Huang TJ, et al. Treatment of fibrous dysplasia involving the proximal femur. *Orthopedics* 1998;21:1263.

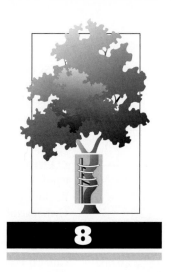

THE SKELETAL DYSPLASIAS

PAUL D. SPONSELLER

P. D. Sponseller: Orthopaedic Surgery, Johns Hopkins Medical Institutions; Department of Orthopaedic Surgery, Johns Hopkins Hospital, Baltimore, Maryland 21287.

GENERAL PRINCIPLES

Terminology

The skeletal dysplasias are a heterogeneous group including over 200 conditions recognized to date. In common, they are disorders of the growth and remodeling of bone and its cartilaginous precursor. The pathogenesis of many of these conditions is slowly being worked out, teaching us little by little about the growth of the skeleton. In the preface to his classic text, *Heritable Disorders of Connective Tissue*, McKusick quoted, "Nature is nowhere more openly to display her secret mysteries than in cases where she shows traces of her workings apart from the beaten path . . ." (1). It may even be true that there is a mutation and a disorder representing nearly each step of skeletal development. Most disorders result in short stature, defined as height more than two standard deviations below the mean for the population at a given age. The term "dwarfing condition" is used to refer to disproportionately short stature. The disproportion is commonly referred to as "short-trunk" or "short-limb." The short-limb types are further subdivided into categories based on which segment of the limb is short. "Rhizomelic" refers to shortening of the root (proximal) portion of the limb; "mesomelic," to the middle segment, and "acromelic," to the distal segment. Achondroplasia is a classic example of rhizomelic involvement, with the femora and especially the humeri being most affected by shortening. Some of these disorders are named after the appearance of the skeleton (diastrophic means "to grow twisted," camptomelic means "bent limbs," and chondrodysplasia punctata refers to stippled cartilage). Eponyms are used to name others, such as Kneist, Morquio, and McKusick.

Classification

Classification of skeletal dysplasias has traditionally been done according to the pattern of bone involvement, as in the International Classification of Osteochondrodysplasias (2) (Table 8-1). The newer trend, however, is to group them according to the specific causative protein, enzyme, or gene defect, in cases in which this is known (Table 8-2). A schematic representation of the effects of the known mutations on cartilage development is shown in Figure 8-1. It is also

TABLE 8-1. INTERNATIONAL CLASSIFICATION OF SKELETAL DYSPLASIAS, 1992 (A PARTIAL LIST)

Defects of the tubular and flat bones and/or the axial skeleton
  Achondroplasia group
    Achondroplasia
    Hypochondroplasia
    Thanatophoric dysplasia
  Metatropic dysplasia
  Atelosteogenesis/diastrophic dysplasia group
  Osteogenesis imperfecta
  Kneist-Stickler group
  Spondyloepiphyseal dysplasia congenita group
  Other Spondyloepi-(metaphyseal) dysplasia group
    Storage disorders
    Mucopolysaccharidoses
    Mucolipidoses
    Multiple epiphyseal dysplasia (MED)
    Metaphyseal dysplasia
    Dysplasias with defective mineralization
    Hypophosphatasia
    Hypophosphatemic rickets
    Neonatal hypoparathyroidism
    Dysplasias with increased bone density

Disorganized development of cartilaginous and fibrous components of the skeleton
  Multiple cartilaginous exostoses
  Dysplasia epiphysealis hemimelica
  Enchondromatosis
  Fibrous Dysplasia

Idiopathic osteolyses

TABLE 8-2. CLASSIFICATION OF DYSPLASIAS BASED ON ETIOLOGY

FGFR3 group (local regulator of cartilage growth)
Achondroplasia
  Hypochondroplasia
  Thanatophoric dysplasia

COL1A group (structural osseous protein)
Osteogenesis imperfecta

COL2A1 group (structural cartilage protein)
Spondyloepiphyseal dysplasia (SED)
  Kneist dysplasia
  Stickler dysplasia
  Strudwick dysplasia
  SED tarda

Diastrophic dysplasia sulfate transport-defective sulfate
  transport enzyme group
    Diastrophic dysplasia
    Achondrogenesis
Collagen oligomeric matrix protein group (structural
  cartilage protein)
    Multiple epiphyseal dysplasia
    Pseudoachondroplasia
Storage disorders
  Mucopolysaccharidoses
  Mucolipidoses

useful for the orthopaedic surgeon to mentally classify the dysplasias into those that are free from spinal deformity (for instance, hypochondroplasia and multiple epiphyseal dysplasia [MED] rarely have significant spinal abnormalities) versus those for which it is a frequent problem (such as spondyloepiphyseal dysplasia, diastrophic dysplasia, and metatropic dysplasia). Which disorders are free from epiphyseal involvement, and therefore from risk of degenerative joint disease down the road? Achondroplasia and hypochondroplasia, cleidocranial dysplasia, and diaphyseal aplasia rarely present these problems in adulthood, but spondyloepiphyseal dysplasia, multiple epiphyseal dysplasia, diastrophic dysplasia, and others commonly do.

Prenatal Diagnosis

With the increasing availability of prenatal screening, more patients with skeletal dysplasia are being diagnosed before birth. When ultrasound shows a fetus with shortening of the skeleton, femur length is the best biometric parameter to distinguish among the five most common possible conditions. Fetuses with femur length below 40% of the mean for gestational age most commonly had achondrogenesis; those with femur length between 40 and 60% most commonly had thanatophoric dysplasia or osteogenesis imper-

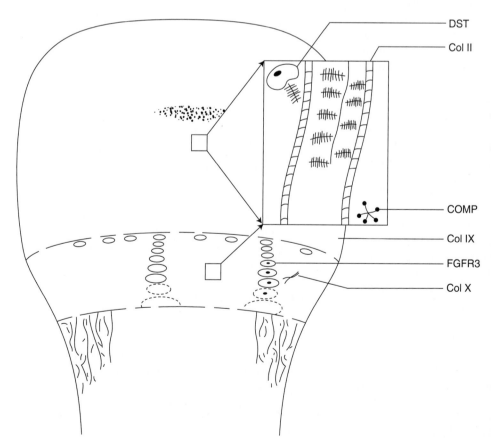

FIGURE 8-1. Schematic illustration of the sites and effects of the known cartilage defects in the skeletal dysplasias. Section of cartilage matrix of physis and epiphysis is simplified and enlarged; genetic abnormalities often affect both regions. *DST*, diatrophic sulfate transporter, deficiency of which leads to undersulfation of proteoglycans in epiphysis and physis of diastrophic dysplasia and achondrogenesis types 1B and 2; *Col II*, type II collagen, which is defective in Kneist dysplasia and spondyloepiphyseal dysplasia; *COMP*, cartilage oligomeric matrix protein, abnormal pseudoachondroplasia, and some forms of multiple epiphyseal dysplasia; *Col IX*, type IX collagen, which is closely linked to type II collagen, and is abnormal in some forms of multiple epiphyseal dysplasia; *FGFR3*, fibroblast growth factor receptor 3, which inhibits chondrocyte proliferation in achondroplasia, hypochondroplasia, and thanatophoric dysplasia; *Col X*, type X collagen, which is synthesized only by the hypertrophic cells of the growth plate, and is abnormal in Schmid-type metaphyseal chondrodysplasia.

fecta type II; and those with femur length over 80% most commonly had achondroplasia or osteogenesis imperfecta type III (3). Further testing may be performed, if indicated, by chorionic villous sampling and mutation analysis.

Evaluation

In evaluating a patient with short stature or abnormal bone development for skeletal dysplasia, several aspects of the medical history should be investigated for diagnosis and for coordination of care. Respiratory difficulty in infancy may occur as a result of restrictive problems in the syndromes with a small thorax, neurologic problems such as foramen magnum stenosis in achondroplasia, or upper airway obstruction in various conditions. A history of heart disease suggests the possibilities of chondroectodermal dysplasia, which may be associated with congenital heart malformations, or storage disorders such as Hurler or Morquio syndromes, in which cardiac dysfunction may be acquired. History of immune deficiency or malabsorption is common in cartilage-hair hypoplasia. Retinal detachment may occur with Kneist syndrome or spondyloepiphyseal dysplasia. Pertinent family history of short stature or dysmorphism should be sought, as well as any prior skeletal surgery the patient has had. Birth length, head circumference, and weight should be recorded. Unusual facial characteristics, cleft palate, and extremity malformations should be noted. Height percentile for age should be determined using standard charts. Measurement of the upper:lower segment ratio may be helpful in distinguishing disproportion early. This can be done by measuring the distance from the superior pubic ramus to the sole of the plantigrade foot, and subtracting it from the overall length. The normal ratio is 1.6 at birth (given that extremities develop later than the trunk), and diminishes to 0.93 in adults and teens. A thorough neurologic examination is needed because of the frequent incidence of spinal compromise—at the upper cervical level in spondyloepiphyseal dysplasia, diastrophic dysplasia, Larsen syndrome, metatropic dysplasia, or at any level in achondroplasia.

A skeletal survey should be ordered if one is not available: lateral film of head and neck, anteroposterior views of the entire spine, pelvis, arms, hands, and legs. Flexion–extension films of the cervical spine should be ordered if instability is suspected to be caused by delay in reaching milestones, or loss of strength or endurance. In many syndromes, such as spondyloepiphyseal dysplasia, in which cervical instability is common, these films should be ordered as a matter of course.

Laboratory tests may include calcium, phosphate, alkaline phosphatase, and protein, to rule out metabolic disorders such as hypophosphatemia or hypophosphatasia. The urine should be screened for storage products (under the guidance of a geneticist), if a progressive disorder is found. Serum thyroxine should be measured if the fontanels in an infant are bulging and bone development is delayed, to rule out hypothyroidism. DNA testing for mutation analysis is not currently done in the clinical setting for skeletal dysplasias. When treating a child with a skeletal dysplasia, a geneticist should be consulted to help establish a diagnosis and, therefore, a prognosis, and to deal with medical problems. The geneticist sometimes functions as a primary physician for a patient with a genetic disorder, because a geneticist has the best overview of the medical issues facing the patient.

Treatment

The orthopaedic surgeon caring for the person with skeletal dysplasia should focus on several aspects: prevention of future limitations; treatment of current deformity, and treatment of pain. The patient's parents should be counseled about the mode of inheritance and risk of recurrence, so that they can make future family plans appropriately. In most cases, it is advisable to see these patients on a routine basis for surveillance, so that skeletal problems can be detected at the optimum time for treatment. Weight management is a continuing challenge for many, and reasonable attention should be paid to this.

If surgery becomes necessary on a person with skeletal dysplasia, special considerations apply. Anesthesia management is more difficult if the dysplasia involves oropharyngeal malformations, limited neck mobility cervical instability, or stenosis (4). Cervical instability is so common in the skeletal dysplasias that the surgeon should make a point of mentally ruling it out by knowledge of the patient, knowledge of the condition, and whether cervical instability is associated with it, or else by obtaining special radiographs in flexion and extension (5,6). Restrictive airway problems accompany some dysplasias, and laryngotracheomalacia affects many young diastrophic children. Skeletal distortion may make deep venous access challenging, and, in some cases, a general surgeon should be consulted in advance for this. Intraoperative positioning must accommodate both small stature and any contractures that are present. Postoperative planning must be done in advance, because most of these patients have decreased ability to accommodate postoperative immobilization, stiffness, or functional restrictions. In some situations, postoperative placement in a rehabilitative setting may be most helpful to the patient and family. The organization, Little People of America, may be a significant resource for information and support.*

ACHONDROPLASIA

Overview and Etiology

Achondroplasia is the most common form of skeletal dysplasia, although even it is uncommon, with an incidence of

---

* P.O. Box 9897, Washington DC, 20016.

approximately 1 in 30,000 to 1 in 50,000 (7,8). It is the only form of skeletal dysplasia that most physicians come in contact with. The name of the condition itself is not strictly accurate, since cartilage does develop both at the physes and at other locations. Whatever the origin of the term, bone that is formed from endochondral means is most underdeveloped in length, resulting in disproportionate short stature. The etiology of achondroplasia has recently been determined to be a mutation in the gene for fibroblast growth factor receptor-3 (*FGFR3*), which is present in cartilage (9–12).

Achondroplasia is transmitted as an autosomal dominant condition, and that information should be used to counsel the family and affected patient. However, looking backward, at least 80% of patients with achondroplasia have the disorder as the result of a spontaneous mutation (13). The risk of having a child with achondroplasia increases with increasing paternal age.

Etiology

The cause of achondroplasia is a point mutation in the gene for fibroblast growth factor receptor-3 (12). The gene for this receptor is on the short arm of chromosome 4. The mutation is always at the same nucleotide (1138), which is part of the transmembrane domain of this receptor. This is said to be the single most mutable nucleotide in humans. It causes a change in a single amino acid, from arginine to glycine. Fibroblast growth factor receptor is expressed in physeal cartilage and in the central nervous system. FGFR3 seems to limit endochondral bone formation in the proliferative zone of the physis, and this is a mutation that actually increases that inhibition (a so-called "gain-of-function" mutation). As discussed later in this chapter, this same receptor is also the site of different mutations, causing hypochondroplasia and thanatophoric dysplasia.

Histologically, the growth plates of persons with achondroplasia show a reduced hypertrophic cell zone and large collagen fibrils (14). However, intramembranous and periosteal ossification processes are normal (15).

Clinical Features

The appearance of a person with achondroplasia has numerous features that are uniform and predictable. Facial appearance is characterized by frontal bossing and midface hypoplasia (8,16). This hypoplasia develops because of the endochondral origin of the facial bones (16). The trunk length is within the lower range of normal, whereas the extremities are much shorter than normal (17), in a pattern which is termed "rhizomelic" (Fig. 8-2). The term "rhizo-" means "root." The proximal segments (roots) of the extremities—the humeri and femora—are the most foreshortened. The fingertips usually reach only to the top of the greater trochanters, and this leads to difficulties in personal care

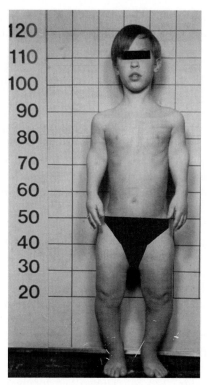

FIGURE 8-2. A 10-year-old boy with achondroplasia. Note pronounced shortening of proximal limb segments (rhizomelic pattern). The humeri are most affected. The elbows have a mild flexion contracture. There is mild genu varum.

(16). The digits of the hand have extra space between the third and the fourth rays, so that the digits are separated into three groups, including the thumb—the "trident hand." There is usually a flexion contracture of the elbows, and the radial heads may be subluxated. Neither of these features causes functional impairment. Kyphosis at the thoracolumbar junction is common, especially in infancy. The condition usually improves with increasing patient age (18). Lumbar lordosis increases. Ligamentous laxity is common at the knees and ankles. The knees are most commonly in varus alignment, but may be in excessive valgus. The ankles usually have varus alignment, as well. Internal tibial torsion is common. The joints are otherwise not directly affected by this condition to any significant degree. The limbs generally have a muscular appearance. Intelligence is normal. Life expectancy is not significantly diminished in this condition.

Growth and Development

Growth curves are available for children with achondroplasia (17). The stature of children with achondroplasia is diminished proportionately throughout childhood, but the proportion declines during the adolescent growth spurt (19). The predicted adult height is 132 cm for men, and 122 cm women (13). When the growth pattern of specific long bones is studied, it is found that the growth of the femur deviates from the population mean even more during the growth spurt, and the fibula overgrows the tibia (8). This latter fact is considered to explain the phenomenon of genu varum, which is seen in many children with achondroplasia.

Hydrocephalus was originally thought to be a cause of much of the macrocephaly seen in children with achondroplasia, but, although three-fourths of patients have ventriculomegaly, only a small subset have clinically important hydrocephalus (20). Charts of head circumference are available for children with achondroplasia to assist in following these features (21). Ventriculoperitoneal shunt surgery is indicated only for patients with rapidly progressive head enlargement or signs of increased intracranial pressure. Mental development is normal. but motor development is delayed (22). Muscle tone is low in the trunk and extremities in infancy. The most evident cause for this delay is neural compression at the foramen magnum. This occurs most likely because of asynchronous growth between the neural elements and the skull base, which is formed by endochondral bone (9). The foramen magnum is small for age in all infants with achondroplasia, although there is some "biologic variability" (23,24). Diminished foramen magnum measurements have been correlated with respiratory dysfunction and delayed motor development (20) (Fig. 8-3). Signs most predictive of severe stenosis of the foramen magnum requiring surgery are presence of clonus or hyperreflexia, and central hypopnea, as seen on sleep study. Developmental milestones are met later by children with achondroplasia than average-stature children. As an example, the mean age at which children with achondroplasia walk alone is 17 months. Normative tables for standard

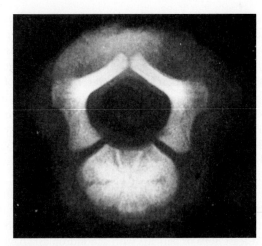

FIGURE 8-4. This specimen radiograph shows the obliquely oriented neurocentral synchondroses that contribute, by endochondral ossification, to both dimensions of the spinal canal. Because this process is impaired in achondroplasia, stenosis results.

milestones are available (22) and allow parents to detect complications. Development of spinal stenosis is explained by the formation of the spinal canal through endochondral ossification at the neurocentral synchondroses (Fig. 8-4). These obliquely oriented growth plates contribute to both the length of the pedicles and the distance between them. These dimensions are decreased at all levels of the achondroplastic spine. It remains a mystery why the dimensions are most diminished in the distal lumbar spine.

Radiographic Characteristics

The radiographic alterations involve regions in which the growth and development occur primarily through processes of endochondral ossification. Thus, in the skull, the facial bones, skull base, and foramen magnum are underdeveloped, whereas the cranial bones are normal in size and shape (8). There are growth curves available for the foramen magnum, which demonstrate that the dimensions of this aperture, as measured by computed tomography (CT), are reduced at birth in achondroplasia, accelerate in early childhood, but never quite reach normal (24). The spine displays central and foraminal stenosis, which becomes worse at progressively caudal levels (25,26). Although stenosis may occur at any level, it is most common in the lumbar spine. This is evident on plain films as a constant or diminishing distance between pedicles, from the first to the fifth lumbar levels on the anteroposterior view (Fig. 8-5), compared with the average-statured population, in whom 60% have increasing interpedicular distance at more caudal levels, and 40% have a constant distance. There is also decreased space between the vertebral body and the lamina on the lateral view. The stenosis of the spinal canal is best seen on CT, which graphically illustrates the tapering of the spinal

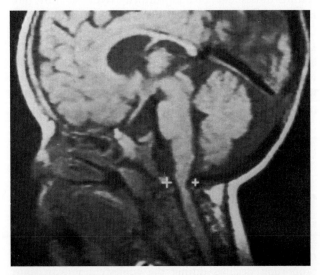

FIGURE 8-3. Magnetic resonance image of a child with achondroplasia shows stenosis at the foramen magnum. (Courtesy of George Bassett, M.D.)

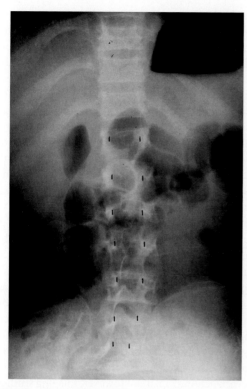

FIGURE 8-5. This anteroposterior view of the entire spine shows the progressive narrowing of the interpedicular distance at more caudal levels of the lumbar spine. This is the opposite of the normal pattern.

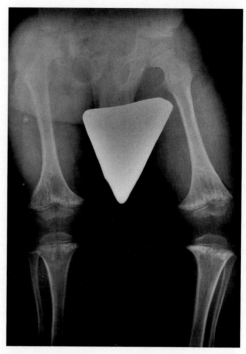

FIGURE 8-7. Radiograph of the lower extremities in a six-year-old with achondroplasia. The distal femoral physes have a pronounced inverted-"V" shape, and the knee is in varus. The acetabular roofs are horizontal.

canal to a slit-like space at the lumbosacral junction (Fig. 8-6). The vertebral bodies have a scalloped appearance (13). If thoracolumbar kyphosis fails to resolve, the apical vertebrae develop a progressively round or wedge shape. Lumbar lordosis increases, and the sacrum may even become horizontal. Significant scoliosis is rare. A point to remember is that cervical instability, although so common in many forms

of skeletal dysplasia, is not usually seen in this, the most common type of dysplasia.

The iliac wings have a squared appearance. The metaphyses of all long bones are flared in appearance. The diaphyses of all long bones are thick, despite being short, owing to subperiosteal bone apposition. Angulation at both the distal femoral and the proximal tibial metaphyses contributes to abnormal knee alignment (Fig. 8-7). The growth of the fibula is typically greater than that of the tibia, which also

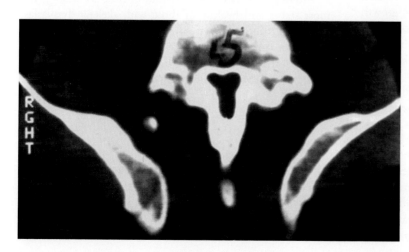

FIGURE 8-6. Computed tomogram of the fifth lumbar vertebra in achondroplasia, showing the slit-like spinal canal.

contributes to the varus in some cases. The shape of the distal femoral physis is an exaggeration of the normal inverted "V" in the midline, and the sites of major muscle insertions (such as the tibial tubercle and the greater trochanter) are more prominent than usual. The metacarpals and metatarsals are all of almost equal length. In 50% of individuals with achondroplasia, there is increased space between the third and fourth metacarpals, which is the basis for the appearance of the "trident" hand (13). The epiphyses throughout the skeleton are virtually normal in appearance and development, and consequently degenerative joint changes are rare.

General Medical Treatment

Infants with achondroplasia should be closely monitored in the first 2 years of life for signs of foramen magnum stenosis. These may include severe developmental delay, sleep apnea, persistent hypotonia, or spasticity. Sleep studies may be used, if this is suspected, to evaluate brain stem functions (27). If the diagnosis of foramen magnum stenosis is made, and the clinical picture persists, decompression of the brain stem should be undertaken by an experienced neurosurgeon. This consists of enlargement of the foramen magnum and sometimes laminectomy of the atlas. The clinical response is usually gratifying (23).

People with achondroplasia have a continuous challenge identifying and maintaining ideal body weight. Obesity is more common than in the general population, but standard curves of weight-for-height or weight-for-age used in the general population are not applicable to persons with achondroplasia. It is recommended that these individuals be followed using triceps skinfold thickness or weight/height squared, a measure that is less sensitive to short stature. Weight control measures should be instituted when these values exceed the 95% range for the general population (28).

Persons with achondroplasia are not deficient in growth hormone. Growth hormone has been used with only limited success in this disorder (11,29,30). The most noticeable results seem to be in those patients with the lowest growth velocities. Early data from the National Cooperative Growth Study has shown that treated children with achondroplasia gain a mean 0.3 standard deviations in height after 2 years of treatment, but the ability to maintain this over time is not known (11), nor is the effect on final height. One study (30) showed a significant increase in the growth rate during the first year of treatment, with a slower increase the second year, as well as variation in the response between patients. Clinically its use has not been widespread, to date.

A number of ear, nose, and throat problems occur as a result of underdevelopment of the midfacial skeletal structure. Maxillary hypoplasia leads to dental crowding and malocclusion, which may require orthodontic attention (31). The eustachian tubes may not function normally, and

this may lead to recurrent otitis media. Given that this may result in hearing loss, the physician should have a high index of suspicion, and early hearing screening should be performed in all children with achondroplasia (31). In one study, 60% of all achondroplastic children screened had hearing loss (32). Other causes of hearing deficit include ossicular chain abnormalities and neurologic causes, resulting from brain stem compression. Obstructive sleep apnea is found in three-fourths of children with achondroplasia when studied in the sleep laboratory (27,33). Treatment, if necessary, begins with adenotonsillectomy, and may progress to include more advanced procedures to enlarge the airway.

Respiratory complications are a greater risk in people with achondroplasia, due not only to upper airway obstruction, but also to decreased respiratory drive and decreased pulmonary function. Early correction of brain stem compression by decompression of critical foramen magnum stenosis may help preserve ventilatory potential. Spirometry shows that patients with achondroplasia also have decreased vital capacity (approximately 70% of predicted for height), although this is rarely a clinically limiting factor (34,35).

Enlargement of head circumference is the norm in individuals with achondroplasia. However, imaging studies have shown that the cerebrospinal fluid dynamics are variable. Examples of true megaloencephaly, dilated ventricles without hydrocephalus, and communicating and noncommunicating forms of hydrocephalus have been identified. It is thought that intracranial venous pressure increases as a result of jugular foraminal stenosis, causing arrested hydrocephalus without elevated intracranial cerebrospinal pressure. Treatment is not required. However, there are occasional patients who do appear to have clinical hydrocephalus, and it is recommended that head circumference should be measured throughout infancy and plotted against norms published for achondroplastic individuals (21). Those with progressive head enlargement should be seen by a neurosurgeon familiar with skeletal dysplasia, and they may benefit from treatment with a ventriculoperitoneal shunt.

Although patients with achondroplasia are among the most stable and healthy of those with skeletal dysplasias, nevertheless mortality rates are elevated in all age groups. The most common causes are sudden death in young infants, central nervous system events and respiratory problems in older children and young adults, and cardiovascular problems in older adults (28).

Orthopaedic Treatment

The major orthopaedic problems seen in children with achondroplasia include angular deformities of the knees, thoracolumbar kyphosis, and spinal stenosis. The former two are related to the pathogenetic factors of ligamentous laxity and muscular hypotonia. Genu varum is more common than valgus. Genu valgus almost never becomes severe or requires treatment. Varus may progress in some patients and appear to cause pain and difficulty walking. The fibula is long compared with the tibia, and it has been proposed that this differential growth between the long bones may be a cause of the deformity (15). However, the deformity involves the distal femur, as well as the proximal tibia. Often incomplete ossification of the epiphyses makes it impossible on plain films to determine the joint line, and to calculate the contributions of the tibia and the femur to the deformity. An arthrogram may be helpful in such cases. Along with the varus, there is often tibial torsion. Decision making about treatment is clouded by the fact that there are no natural history studies to suggest what degree of varus in young children is likely to progress, and what degree of varus, if any, is likely to cause degenerative problems in adulthood. The clinician should rely on the patient or parents for a history of walking difficulty or knee pain. Pain originating from the knee joint should be differentiated from the leg pain of spinal stenosis. In spinal stenosis, the aching is more diffuse and is relieved by decreasing the lumbar lordosis by flexing the lumbar spine, or "hunching over."

Treatment of genu varum, if it is severe, usually involves surgery. There is no evidence that bracing children with achondroplasia is effective. Their short thighs make it difficult to exert mechanical pressure unless the brace is extended to the waist. Lax ligaments make it difficult to transmit any force to the growth plates themselves. It does not seem wise to subject these children to unproven therapies, in light of all of the other medical problems they face. Tibial osteotomy may be done in any of several ways [➡6.1–6.4]: opening or closing, with internal or external fixation (36,37). Usually, a decision for surgery is not made until age 4 at the earliest. In skeletally immature patients, the osteotomy should be performed below the tibial tubercle. If internal tibial torsion exceeds 10 to 20 degrees, this should be corrected at the same time. Fibular shortening alone has been advocated as a treatment for young children with genu varum (15), but no long-term studies are available. Severe degenerative arthritis of the knee is not seen in adults with achondroplasia with any frequency.

Limb-lengthening for achondroplasia remains controversial, but is gradually gaining greater acceptance by patients and physicians. In contrast to most other skeletal dysplasias, conditions are favorable for extensive lengthening, in that the joints are normal and the musculotendinous units and nerves have excellent tolerance for stretch. Lengthening of 40 to 50% per segment has been reproducibly achieved for the femur and the tibia (38,39), with lengthening indices of between 30 and 40 days per centimeter. Care must be taken to minimize the complications of angular deformity and joint stiffness. The expected benefits of limb lengthening include increased function in the average-height world, improved self-image, and possibly a decrease in the lumbar

lordosis. The latter is purported to occur if the hip flexors are lengthened and an extension osteotomy is performed at the time of femoral lengthening (40). This combination of steps has been claimed to produce a relative pull of the pelvis into extension. However, most of these claims have not yet been clinically validated. The improved function has not been conclusively documented using standard outcome measures. This is important information to have, because lengthening may have an effect on muscle strength and joint status. Because most achondroplasts would need approximately 25 to 30 cm of additional height to enter the range of average stature, some do not quite achieve this goal. If the lower extremities are lengthened significantly, the humeri should be lengthened also to facilitate personal care. Six segments of major lengthening is a major time commitment, even when opposite limbs are lengthened at the same time. The total time required for such an undertaking may exceed 2 years, during a patient's critical years of adolescence or young adulthood. The effects on the lumbar spine require prospective study. The long-term effects of lengthening in this population also require study. In helping patients to come to a decision about whether limb-lengthening is personally appropriate, several discussions should be held with the involved family members to ensure that all the implications of the treatment plan have been discussed and that the information has been understood. Discussions with knowledgeable counselors, as well as with others with achondroplasia who have undergone lengthening, can be of help. In the proper setting, patients may be gratified with the results of lengthening.

Kyphosis

Kyphosis is present in most infants with achondroplasia, presumably due to low muscle tone, ligamentous laxity, and a large cranium. The kyphosis is noncongenital and is centered at the twelfth thoracic or first lumbar vertebrae. These vertebrae become wedge-shaped anteriorly, although this is a reversible phenomenon (Fig. 8-8). Most improve by the second or third year of life after walking begins and muscle strength increases (8,18,41,42). However, between 10 and 15% of patients retain kyphosis (Fig. 8-9), which can increase the risk of symptomatic stenosis through pressure on the conus, as well as the secondary lumbar lordosis that it induces. Therefore, treatment may be indicated at several phases of life: in infancy, to prevent development of kyphosis; in childhood, to assist in correction of those that do not correct with time; and in adulthood, to correct surgically those kyphoses that contribute to symptomatic spinal stenosis. Pauli et al. reported favorable results from early intervention (18). They recommend prevention of unsupported sitting, as well as keeping children from sitting up over 60 degrees, even with support, while kyphosis was present. We dispute the efficacy of this latter recommendation, because the drive to sit is irrepressible, and it seems to be more appropriate to provide earlier support, in the form of a firm-

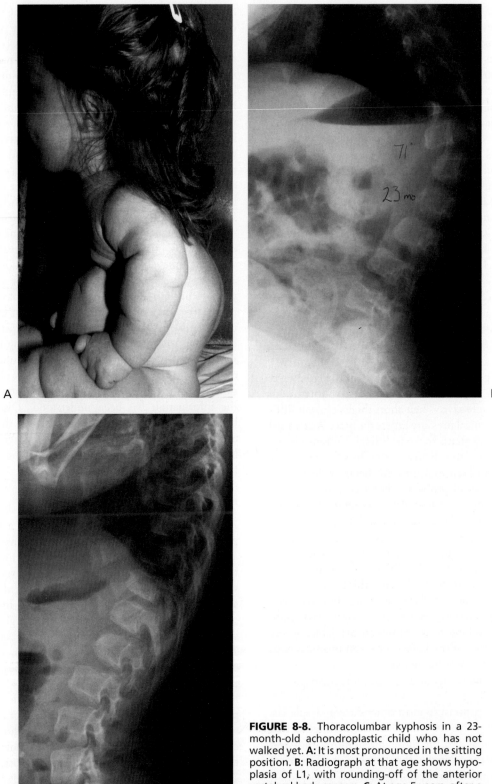

FIGURE 8-8. Thoracolumbar kyphosis in a 23-month-old achondroplastic child who has not walked yet. **A:** It is most pronounced in the sitting position. **B:** Radiograph at that age shows hypoplasia of L1, with rounding-off of the anterior vertebral body corners. **C:** At age 5 years, after a period of brace treatment, the shape of L1, as well as the overall kyphosis, has improved.

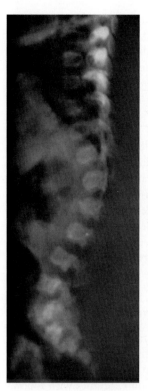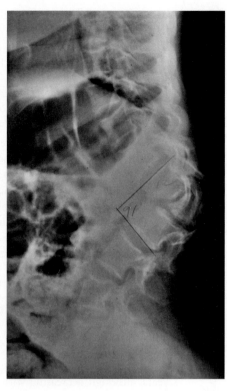

A,B

FIGURE 8-9. Thoracolumbar kyphosis has progressed in this patient, who had no medical follow-up between age 6 months (**A**) and 12 years (**B**). Although the latter figure resembles a congenital kyphosis, the former does not support it, and suggests that it was instead caused by compression over time.

backed chair, when sitting begins. Bracing is indicated if the kyphosis is accompanied by significant and progressive vertebral wedging, if it does not reduce below 30 degrees on prone hyperextension radiographs, or if it does not resolve by the age of 3 years. We prefer the use of a modified Knight brace; a double-upright thoracolumbosacral orthosis that has an adjustable posterior pad under the apex of the kyphosis and that does not constrain the thorax laterally. This should be worn full-time during waking hours until resolution of the vertebral wedging occurs, and a lateral film, taken while the patient is out of the brace, shows no significant kyphosis; then it should be gradually weaned. For children who fail treatment with a brace, we have had some success with a hyperextension cast incorporating the thighs, changed until elimination of the kyphosis in cast is achieved, and worn for several months, until the same end-point is achieved. This has the advantage of not being removable, and, consequently, a more sustained corrective force is applied to the spine. For patients in whom this therapy also fails, two options exist: prophylactic posterior fusion during childhood, or observation, with stabilization or correction of kyphosis only in those requiring decompression for spinal stenosis. Although there are no data directly comparing the two approaches, the former may be preferable for those with severe kyphosis because of the difficulty and risk of correcting a large kyphosis at an older age in these patients (43).

Stenosis

Spinal stenosis is the most common serious problem in individuals with achondroplasia. Most present with symptoms of neurogenic claudication. However, a small number develop muscle weakness alone, some of which is detected only on routine physical examination, thus emphasizing the importance of periodic neurologic screening. The neurologic deficit may involve upper or lower motor neuron signs, or both. Symptomatic stenosis usually develops in the third decade, although it has been noted as early as age 11 years. Diagnosis is best made by myelography performed through a cervical puncture with CT. This is, in many cases, more sensitive and specific than magnetic resonance imaging (MRI), to evaluate the site of block in a canal that is diffusely narrow. Spinal decompression is usually indicated as soon as the diagnosis has been confirmed. This decompression should extend from several levels above the myelographic block, down to the second sacral vertebra (44,45). The laminectomy should be done by a surgeon experienced in this procedure and should involve minimal use of instruments, such as rongeurs or probes, inside the canal. The laminae to be removed should be thinned with a high-speed bur. The dura often adheres to the lamina, and the incidence of dural tearing is high. The nerve roots, which are relatively long, often protrude through any hole in the dura. Careful foraminotomy should be done if there are signs of root stenosis.

HYPOCHONDROPLASIA

Etiology and Pathogenesis

Hypochondroplasia is an autosomal dominant disorder that has phenotypic and genotypic similarities to achondroplasia, but the two disorders are distinct, nevertheless. There are no known instances of achondroplasia and hypochondroplasia existing in the same family, except by marriage. The mutation causing most cases of hypochondroplasia has been found to be in the gene for fibroblast growth factor receptor-3 on the short arm of the fourth chromosome, just as in achondroplasia and thanatophoric dysplasia (9,46,47). In all these conditions, the mutation results in increased activation of factors that slow cell growth (48). In the case of hypochondroplasia, the mutation arises in a different portion of the gene (the tyrosine kinase domain, in contrast to the transmembrane domain in achondroplasia). However, there is more heterogeneity in this condition than in achondroplasia: between 30 and 40% of patients with hypochondroplasia have mutations in a different gene, instead. As mentioned earlier, almost all patients with achondroplasia have a uniform mutation in the same gene. This finding probably accounts for the clinical variability seen in hypochondroplasia. There does not appear to be an increased paternal age in fathers of children with hypochondroplasia.

Clinical Features

This is one of the most subtle of the skeletal dysplasias. The clinical abnormalities in hypochondroplasia are rather mild, and may go unnoticed until the pubertal growth spurt in some cases. The eventual height ranges from 118 to 160 cm (13,49). Head circumference is normal and frontal bossing is mild to absent. Because of the absence of obvious midface hypoplasia, these patients do not have a distinctive appearance. The limbs are not short in a rhizomelic pattern, but rather in a mesomelic one. Body proportions are closer to normal. The trident hand characteristic of achondroplasia is not seen in hypochondroplasia. Thoracolumbar kyphosis is also not a feature of this condition. Varus angulation of the knees is mild, and may resolve with growth. Joint laxity is mild. Spinal stenosis has been reported in about one-third of patients (13), but it is usually mild and does not require surgical treatment. Mental retardation has been reported in some of these patients.

Radiographic Features

Radiographic findings, as with clinical findings, are generally subtle. Hall and Spranger have proposed primary and secondary radiographic criteria (13,50). The primary criteria are narrowing of the lumbar pedicles, square iliac crests, short, broad femoral necks, mild metaphyseal flaring, and brachydactyly. Secondary criteria are shortening of the lum-

bar pedicles, mild posterior scalloping of the vertebral bodies, and elongation of the distal fibula and ulnar styloid. The pelvis has sciatic notches that are normally wide, in contrast to the narrowed notches seen in achondroplasia (51).

Differential Diagnosis

Although generally a mild skeletal dysplasia, hypochondroplasia has more variation than achondroplasia in its severity. In its more extreme form, it may resemble achondroplasia. Conversely, it may be mistaken for constitutionally short stature. It may also resemble Schmid metaphyseal dysplasia, in its mild short stature and mild genu varum. Dyschondrosteosis also produces mild short stature, but it is distinguished by Madelung deformity and triangular carpal bones.

Treatment—General and Orthopaedic

People with hypochondroplasia rarely have serious medical problems. The response to growth hormone administration in pharmacologic doses has been shown to persist up to 4 years, although decreasing with time. Studies with follow-up to maturity are still needed, but this treatment remains an option (30,52,53). Genetic counseling should be given about pattern of transmission for this autosomal dominant condition. If a female patient becomes pregnant, extra vigilance should be exercised for possible disproportion during childbirth.

Limb-lengthening is usually as successful as it is in achondroplasia in achieving significant gains without undue risks, because the joints are sound and the muscles tolerate lengthening (54). Because these patients are generally about 20 cm taller than patients with achondroplasia, limb-lengthening may place them within the normal range of stature. This is a personal decision for patients, who may benefit from talking to others who have considered it or undergone it. Long-term follow-up is still needed to determine the effects on the joints.

METATROPIC DYSPLASIA

The term "metatropic dwarfism" comes from the Greek word metatropos, or "changing form," because patients with this condition appear to have short-limb dwarfism early in life, but later develop a short-trunk pattern as spinal length is lost to the development of kyphosis and scoliosis. The condition has been likened to Morquio syndrome, due to the enlarged appearance of the metaphyses and the contractures (55).

It is a rare condition, which may be inherited in an autosomal dominant or recessive manner. The cause of this dysplasia has not been elucidated. However, histologic abnor-

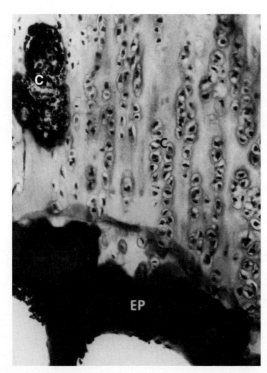

FIGURE 8-10. Histology of the growth plate in metatropic dysplasia, showing relatively normal columns of proliferating chondrocytes (*C*), but absence of the hypertrophic or degenerating zones, as well as a "seal," or bony end plate (*EP*), over the metaphysis. (From ref. 56, with permission.)

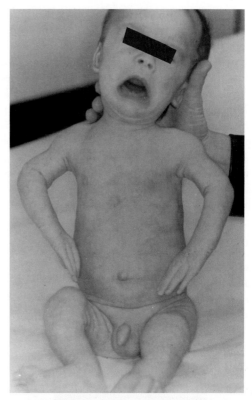

A

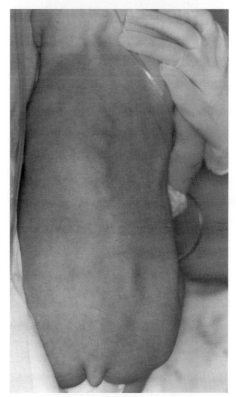

B

FIGURE 8-11. A 1-year-old infant with metatropic dysplasia, illustrating knee-flexion contractures, "bulky" metaphyses (**A**), and a coccygeal tail (**B**).

malities of the growth plate have been studied and appear to be characteristic, as shown in the study published by a group led by Boden (56). The physis shows relatively normal columns of proliferating chondrocytes. However, there is an abrupt arrest of further development, with absence of a zone of hypertrophic or degenerating chondrocytes. Instead, there is a mineralized seal of bone over the metaphyseal end of the growth plate (Fig. 8-10). The perichondral ring remains intact, and circumferential growth was preserved. This uncoupling of endochondral and perichondral growth appears to account for the characteristic "knobby" metaphyses. Further understanding of the defect in this disorder will undoubtedly shed light on the normal maturation of the physis.

Clinical Features

One of the most characteristic features of this condition is the presence of the "coccygeal tail," a cartilaginous prolongation of the coccyx that is not present in other dysplasias (Fig. 8-11). It is usually a few centimeters long and arises from the gluteal fold. The facial appearance is not determined by the condition, although there may be a high arched palate. The sternum may display a pectus carinatum, and the limbs have flexion contractures of up to 30 to 40 degrees from infancy, and may have ligamentous laxity. They appear relatively short with respect to the trunk. The metaphyses are enlarged, which, when combined with underdeveloped musculature, gives a bulky appearance to the limbs. Ventriculomegaly or hydrocephalus has been reported in up to 25% of patients (57). Upper cervical spine instability develops in some patients. Scoliosis develops in early childhood and is progressive (58,59). Inguinal hernias are common. Some restrictive lung disease is usually present, which may cause death in infancy for the one-third of patients who are afflicted by the autosomal recessive form of the disease. However, others survive into adulthood, and adult height varies from 110 to 120 cm.

Radiographic Features

Prenatal sonographic diagnosis may be possible in the first or second trimester, with finding of significant dwarfism, narrow thorax, and the enlarged metaphyses (60,61). Odontoid hypoplasia frequently exists in patients with this condi-

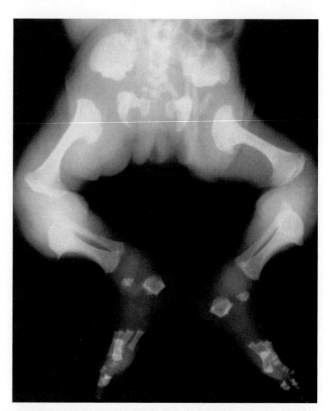

FIGURE 8-13. Newborn with metatropic dysplasia. The diaphyses are short and the metaphyses are broad, flared, and their appearance has been likened to dumbbells. The iliac wings are flared, and the acetabulae deep. (Courtesy of George S. Bassett, M.D.)

tion, as in many patients with skeletal dysplasia. In infancy, the vertebrae are markedly flattened throughout the spine, but normal in width. Kyphosis and scoliosis are almost always seen. The ribs are short and flared, with cupping at the costochondral junctions (Fig. 8-12).

The epiphyses and metaphyses are enlarged, giving the long bones an appearance that has been likened to that of a barbell (Fig. 8-13). The epiphyses have delayed and irregular ossification. Protrusio acetabuli has been reported. Genu varum of mild to moderate degree usually develops. Degenerative changes of major joints often occurs in adulthood.

Treatment/Orthopaedic Considerations

Respiratory problems often dominate infancy, and may be fatal. They result from the small thorax, and may also, in part, result from cervical instability. These children need to be observed on a follow-up basis at a center where pediatric pulmonary expertise is available. The neck should be imaged early with lateral flexion–extension radiographs. Because cervical quadriplegia has been reported from falls, fusion is recommended if the translation is greater than about 8 mm, or neurologic compromise is present. If a patient has atlan-

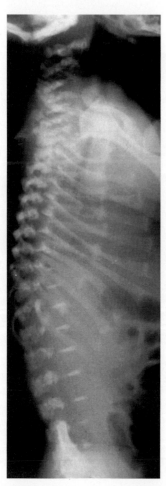

FIGURE 8-12. Newborn with metatropic dysplasia. Note platyspondyly with delayed vertebral ossification, and flared ribs. (Courtesy of Judy Hall, Vancouver, British Columbia.)

toaxial instability between 5 and 8 mm but is neurologically intact, MRI should be obtained in flexion and extension. Fusion should be recommended if cord compromise is seen [➥2.17].

The patients should be examined early for spinal curvature. There is no documentation of the efficacy of brace treatment for this condition. It may be tried in small curves (under 45 degrees) in young patients or those who need support to sit, but I do not recommend it for large curves, even if the patients are young and still actively growing. Spinal fusion for scoliosis may be advisable in patients with more severe curves. Deciding exactly when to intervene is more of an informed judgment than a science. This author recommends observation and accepting a larger curve threshold for surgery in younger patients (under age 10) to document medical health, and to have a chance of bone size adequate for instrumentation. However, progressive sharp angular kyphosis with paraparesis may occur in metatropic dysplasia, and should be treated early with fusion if, in the surgeon's estimation, neurologic compromise is a risk. When surgery is undertaken, anterior as well as posterior fusion is recommended if the patient is able to tolerate it, because of the high rate of pseudarthrosis in this condition (5). Given that the curves are often rigid, obtain only the amount of correction that can be achieved safely. Halo-cast immobilization is an option if patient size, stenosis, or poor bone density make instrumentation inadvisable.

CHONDROECTODERMAL DYSPLASIA

Disproportionately short stature and abnormalities in the mouth, teeth, limbs, and heart characterize this uncommon skeletal dysplasia, also known as Ellis–van Creveld syndrome (62). It is transmitted as an autosomal recessive condition, and is therefore more common in closely knit populations, most notably in the Pennsylvania Amish community. The basic defect is not known, but the chromosomal defect has been localized to the short arm of the fourth chromosome (63,64).

Clinical Features

About one-third of patients with this syndrome die in the neonatal period (the most severely affected age group). The cardiac defects are present in about one-half of patients, and most commonly consist of atrial septal defects or single atrium. As the name of this disorder would suggest, the teeth are also abnormal, both appearing and being lost early. The nails are hypoplastic. Urologic features include hypospadias and epispadias. The skeletal features are shortening of the middle and distal parts of the extremities (acromesomelic) in combination with a normal spine (65). This distal shortening is the opposite of that seen in achondroplasia (66–68). The chest is narrow. The ligaments are lax, and there is often sig-

nificant genu valgum. Rotational abnormalities often accompany this, such as external rotation of the femur and internal rotation of the tibia. The combination of these findings can give the limb an appearance of a flexion contracture, whereas in fact the problem is really valgus. Postaxial polydactyly is quite common, usually in the hands, and much less commonly in the feet.

Radiographic Features

The ribs are short and the chest is narrow. Bilateral knee valgus is usually relatively symmetric. It is partially due to uneven growth of the proximal tibial epiphysis, with the lateral side being underdeveloped (Fig. 8-14). An exostosis may arise medially from the proximal tibial metaphysis. The acetabulae have spike formation at the medial and lateral edges. The capital femoral epiphyses ossify early, and the greater trochanteric apophyses are pronounced. The wrists display fusion of the capitate and the hamate, and sometimes other bones. The carpal bones have delayed maturation but the phalanges are accelerated.

Orthopaedic Management

Reconstruction of the poly/syndactyly, performed when the cardiac status is stable, is usually successful. The angular and rotational disturbance of the lower extremities is usually addressed when it becomes clinically significant or rapidly progressing, usually at about 20 degrees of valgus (69). Unfortunately, bracing seems to have little or no effect, and

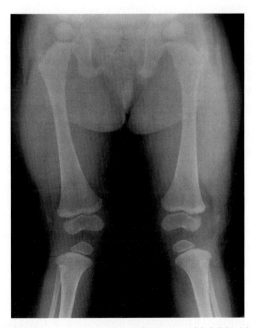

FIGURE 8-14. Lower extremities of a 5-year-old child with chondroectodermal dysplasia, demonstrating the characteristic pronounced hypoplasia of the lateral proximal tibial epiphysis with marked genu valgus. (Courtesy of Michael Ain, M.D.)

surgery remains the mainstay of treatment. Careful preoperative planning is needed, taking into account deformity at all locations from the proximal femur to the ankle and aiming to correct the mechanical axes and the malrotation with as few procedures as possible (70). Usually external fixation is the most expeditious way of handling the correction. If the deformity is one of simple valgus, simple medial hemiepiphyseal stapling may be adequate.

DIASTROPHIC DYSPLASIA

Diastrophic dysplasia (DD) is perhaps the dysplasia with the most numerous, disparate, and severe skeletal abnormalities. The term "diastrophic" comes from a Greek root meaning "distorted," which aptly describes the ears, spine, long bones, and feet. Before the current level of understanding of the skeletal dysplasias was developed, an early authority referred to this condition as "achondroplasia with clubbed feet" (71,72). Certainly the abnormalities are much more extensive than that.

The disorder is autosomal recessive and is extremely rare, except in Finland, where between 1 and 2% of the population are carriers, and there are over 160 people known to be affected due to an apparent founder effect. The defect is on chromosome 5 in the gene that codes for a sulfate transporter protein (aptly named "diastrophic dysplasia sulfate transporter") (73,74). This protein is expressed in virtually all cell types. Decreased content of sulfate in cartilage from patients with DD has been demonstrated (75). It is presumed that a defect in this gene leads to undersulfation of proteoglycan in the cartilage matrix. If one considers proteoglycans to be the "hydraulic jacks" of cartilage at the ultrastructural level, it is understandable that there should be such impairment of performance of physeal, epiphyseal, and articular cartilage throughout the body. Achondrogenesis types 1B and 2 are more serious disorders causing mutations on the same gene.

Histopathology reveals that chondrocytes appear to degenerate prematurely, and collagen is present in excess (76,77). Tracheal cartilage has some of the same abnormalities seen in other cartilage types. This still does not explain some of the focal, specific malformations seen in DD, such as proximal interphalangeal joint fusion in the hands, short first metacarpal causing hitchhiker thumbs, or cervical spina bifida. Further work on the role of this sulfate transporter on skeletal growth and development must be done to explain these curious findings.

Clinical Features

Prominent cheeks and circumoral fullness gave rise to the previously used name "cherub dwarf" (Fig. 8-15). The nasal bridge is flattened. Up to one-half of patients have a cleft palate, which may contribute to aspiration pneumonia (76). The cartilage of the trachea is abnormally soft, and its

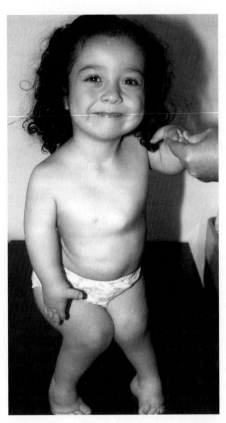

FIGURE 8-15. A 5-year-old girl with diastrophic dysplasia. Note prominent cheeks, circumoral fullness, equinovarus feet, valgus knees with flexion contracture, and abducted or "hitchhiker" thumbs.

diameter may be narrowed. The ear is normal at birth, but develops a peculiar acute swelling of the pinna at 3 to 6 weeks in 80 to 85% of cases. The reason for this event and this timing is not known. The cartilage hardens in a deformed shape—the "cauliflower ear," which is one of the pathognomonic features of this dysplasia.

Patients with diastrophism have a slightly increased (approximately 5%) perinatal mortality as a result of respiratory problems, especially aspiration pneumonia and tracheomalacia.

The skeleton displays abnormalities from the cervical spine down to the feet (78). The posterior arches of the lower cervical spine are often bifid. There are no external clues to this underlying abnormality, which is occult. Cervical kyphosis is seen in one-third to one-half of patients (6,79). This may be present in infancy, and its course is variable. Spontaneous resolution has been reported in a number of patients, even with curves of up to 80 degrees (80,81) (Fig. 8-16A and B). However, others progress, and several reports of quadriparesis from this deformity exist (6,82). Scoliosis develops in at least one-third of patients (79), but many curves do not exceed 50 degrees. Tolo and Kopits state that the scoliosis may be one of two types:

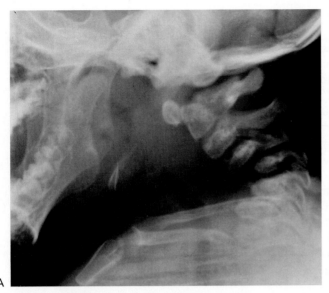
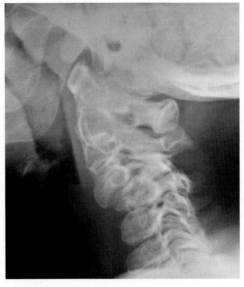

A

B

FIGURE 8-16. Cervical kyphosis, in a 1-year-old child (**A**) with diastrophic dysplasia, is pronounced, with marked deformity of C4. Results of findings on neurologic examination are normal. Four years later, it is markedly improved without any intervention (**B**).

idiopathic-like or sharply angular (83). The sharply angular type is usually characterized by kyphosis at the same level as the scoliosis. Spinal stenosis is not common, in contrast to achondroplasia. Most patients have significant lumbar lordosis, likely to compensate for the hip flexion contractures in diastrophism.

The extremities display rhizomelic shortening. The shoulders may be subluxated, as may the radial heads (possibly because of ulnar shortening). The hands are short, broad, and ulnarly deviated. The hitchhiker thumb is due to a short, proximally placed, often triangular, first metacarpal that may be hypermobile. This finding is seen in up to 95% of diastrophic persons. The proximal interphalangeal joints of the fingers are often fused (symphalangism).

The hips maintain a persistent flexion contracture. The proximal femoral epiphyses progressively deform, and even subluxate in some patients. Epiphyseal flattening and hinge abduction develop in many patients (84). Arthritic changes develop by early to middle adulthood. The knees usually have flexion contractures, which result from a combination of ligamentous contracture and epiphyseal deformation (Fig. 8-17). Excessive valgus is also common. As much as one-fourth of patients have a dislocated patella. Degenerative joint disease of the hips and knees develops in early to mid adulthood.

The feet of diastrophic persons are commonly described as being clubfeet, but many different variations exist. In the large Finnish series of Ryoppy, the most common finding was adduction and valgus (seen in 43%), followed in prevalence by equinovarus in 37%, then by pure equinus. The great toe may be in additional varus, beyond the degree

commonly seen in idiopathic clubfoot. This is analogous to the hitchhiker thumb. The navicular may not be so medially displaced as in typical clubfoot. The foot deformities are very stiff and involve bony malformations, as well as contracture and malalignment. These feet are as difficult to correct as any type of clubfoot.

There is great variation in severity of DD. Height is

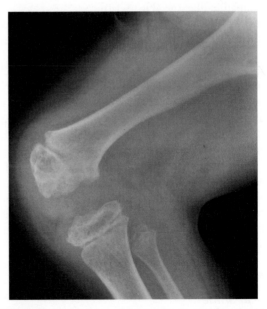

FIGURE 8-17. The joint contracture in diastrophic dysplasia is accompanied by epiphyseal deformity, as this knee radiograph illustrates.

related to overall severity of involvement, with taller people being less severely affected (85,86). These are part of the same spectrum of disorder. Growth curves for persons with DD are available (87). The median adult height is 136 cm for male patients and 129 cm for females (88). Therefore, people with achondroplasia are shorter in stature, and are approximately equal to those with pseudoachondroplasia and spondyloepiphyseal dysplasia congenita. The pubertal growth spurt is diminished or absent, so the overall growth failure is progressive, suggesting that the physes are unable to respond to normal hormonal influences.

The life expectancy of diastrophic persons is not significantly reduced, except for the small number of patients (approximately 8%) who die in infancy from respiratory causes, or during childhood from cervical myelopathy. Patients with severe spinal deformities are more prone to develop respiratory problems. Many patients are able to lead productive work and family lives.

Radiographic Features

Prenatal diagnosis may be made by sonography in the second trimester with demonstration of long-bone measurements at least three standard deviations below normal, as well as clubfeet and adducted thumbs. In infancy, calcification develops in the pinna of the ear, and later in the cranium and the costal cartilages. The vertebrae are poorly ossified. The lower cervical spine may demonstrate kyphosis. MRI may be necessary to judge the severity of this in relation to the spinal cord. Only one case of atlantoaxial instability has been reported in this condition. The interpediculate distances narrow only slightly at descending levels of the lumbar spine, unlike achondroplasia. Scoliosis may occur in the form of either a sharp, angular curve or a gradual, idiopathic-like one (Fig. 8-18).

Images of the hand are characterized by several findings The first metacarpal is small, oval, and proximally placed. Although the proximal interphalangeal joints of the digits are ankylosed, a radiolucent space is present early on, which later fuses. Both the ulna and the fibula are shortened, contributing to the valgus of the knees and the radial head subluxation, which is sometimes seen. The diaphyses of the long bones are short and broad. The epiphyses of both the proximal and the distal femur are delayed in appearance. The capital femoral epiphyses may show signs of osteonecrosis well into childhood. Arthrograms show flattening of both the proximal and the distal femur, accounting for the stiffness observed clinically. The proximal femur is usually in varus, but, even so, hip dysplasia or subluxation may develop progressively with time.

Treatment

Cervical Spine

A neurologic examination should be performed periodically on all children. A lateral cervical radiograph should be per-

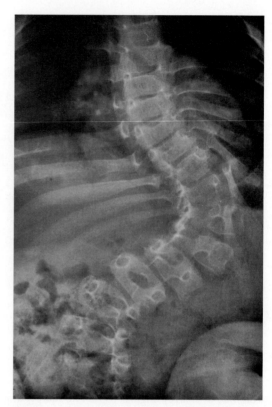

FIGURE 8-18. Significant scoliosis may occur early in diastrophic dysplasia, as in this 6-year-old child.

formed during the first 2 years of life, as well. If cervical kyphosis is noted, the patient should be followed with clinical and radiographic examinations every 6 months. If the kyphosis is nonprogressive, and there is no neurologic deficit, it should only be observed. If the kyphosis progresses, but there is no neurologic deficit, bracing may be employed. Successful control of cervical kyphosis by full-time use of the Milwaukee brace was reported by Bethem et al. (6,13). If the curve continues to progress despite the brace, or a neurologic deficit occurs, posterior fusion should be performed. The surgeon should be cognizant of the bifid lamina during the exposure. Instrumentation is usually technically not possible. If adequate bone graft is not available from the iliac crests, it may be taken from the proximal tibia(s) or other sources. Immobilization by a halo and vest is needed for 2 to 4 months. The pins should be inserted at a lower torque than in adults (4 inch-pounds), and the surgeon may elect to use a slight distractive moment and a slight posterior translation of the head. A pad may be used behind the apex of the kyphosis to help keep it from increasing. If neurologic deficit is present along with the curve, MRI in a neutral position and in extension will help to determine the degree of anterior compression and the type of procedure required. If there is severe anterior cord compression, corpectomy and strut graft may be indicated. Posterior fusion is indicated as well.

Thoracolumbar Spine

Scoliosis affects about one-half of diastrophic patients but often begins early in childhood. The success of bracing in preventing or slowing curve progression has not been documented. It seems reasonable to offer it to patients, if the curve is less than 45 degrees, but to discontinue it for those in whom there is no apparent benefit. Large curves often continue to progress in adulthood (79). Surgery has a role in preventing progression for curves over about 50 degrees [➡2.1–2.5]. Posterior fusion is the mainstay of treatment (83). For younger patients, or those whose associated kyphosis is over 50 degrees, anterior fusion may be added as well. Instrumentation should be used carefully, bearing in mind the short stature, the stiffness of the spine, and the slightly diminished bone density. Small hooks may be used if needed (83). Spinal stenosis is seen much less commonly than in achondroplasia, but it may occur if degenerative changes are superimposed on the baseline canal size. Mild stenosis may be masked in some cases by the patients' relative inactivity.

Hips

Hip flexion contractures and knee flexion contractures should be assessed together. If they are significant (over 40 degrees) release may be considered if an arthrogram shows no epiphyseal flattening and good potential for gaining range of motion. If there is epiphyseal flattening it is probably better to avoid releases, given that recurrence is likely. Hip dysplasia is often progressive because of deformation of the abnormal cartilage under muscle forces and body weight. No long-term series has been done to show the ability of surgery to arrest this process. Therefore, the surgeon should use individual judgment as to whether an acetabular augmentation or femoral osteotomy will help provide good coverage without restricting range of motion or function. Conservative treatment cannot be faulted in this condition.

Degenerative changes in the hip are one of the main reasons for decreasing walking ability in those with diastrophism. Hip joint arthroplasty is an option, usually after the patient reaches the midthirties. Small or custom components are needed. The femur often has an increased anterior bow, probably in compensation for the hip flexion contracture. The isthmus of the femur is only 13 mm on average. Contracture release may be needed along with the arthroplasty, but femoral nerve palsy may follow if it is done extensively. Autograft augmentation of the acetabulum is often necessary. The largest series of hip arthroplasty in this condition is by Peltonen et al., with 15 hips in 10 patients who had a mean age of 37 years (89). Three patients required femoral osteotomy or trochanteric transfer. Two had femoral palsies, which recovered. Hip range of motion was increased slightly.

Knees

The knees in diastrophism usually lack both flexion and extension. Complete correction of knee flexion contractures is prohibited by the shape of the condyles, which may be triangular, creating a bony block to flexion, extension, or both. Residual contracture at maturity may be diminished by distal femoral osteotomy. Patellar subluxation is present in one-fourth of diastrophic persons; correcting these may help improve extensor power.

Feet

Although the classic foot deformity in this condition is equinovarus, other types may be seen, including isolated equinus, forefoot adduction, or valgus. The feet are rigid, and cast treatment is usually futile. A plantigrade foot is the goal of treatment. Surgical treatment should be deferred until the feet are large enough to work on (usually after 1 year), and the neck is safe. If soft tissue release is performed, it should be as extensive as needed to correct the deformity [➡7.1]. Sometimes, this requires release of the posteroinferior tibiofibular ligament to bring the dome of the talus into the mortise. Partial recurrence of deformity is common (72), and salvage procedures include talectomy, talocalcaneal decancellation, or arthrodesis (in the older child).

KNEIST DYSPLASIA

Kneist syndrome is a profoundly affecting skeletal dysplasia characterized by typical facial features, and large, stiff joints with contractures (90,91). It has been likened by some to metatropic dysplasia, because of the enlarged stiff joints, and to spondyloepiphyseal dysplasia, because of the generalized disorder of both spinal and epiphyseal growth. It is now known to be due to a defect in type II collagen, the predominant protein of cartilage. Most mutations are between exons 12 and 24 of the *COL2A1* gene. Although numerous different mutations have been described, their phenotypic similarity results from the fact that they are all in this region, and that they tend to occur at splice sites, resulting in exon skipping, and thus in shorter type II collagen monomers (92,93). These combine with normal-length monomers from both ends to form heterotrimers with the missing segment excluded from the helix (94). This allows the mutation to express autosomal dominant behavior, in that one copy of the mutant allele disrupts the structure of the entire cartilage matrix. Most patients are affected as a result of a new mutation.

Pathologically, the cartilage has been termed "soft and crumbly," with a "Swiss-cheese" appearance (95). Scanning electron microscopy of cartilage demonstrates deficiency and disorganization of cartilage fibrils, and large, open cyst-like spaces.

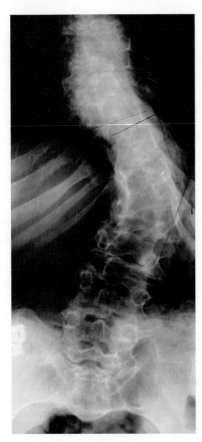

FIGURE 8-19. Scoliosis is common in Kneist dysplasia, but rarely severe enough to require intervention.

Clinical Features

As with many dysplasias, patients with this condition have a somewhat characteristic facial appearance, with prominent eyes and forehead and a depressed midface. Many patients have a cleft palate. The sternum may be depressed, and the trunk is broad, unlike findings with metatropic dysplasia. However, as with that condition, the joints appear enlarged because of broad metaphyses of the long bones, and they are stiff—often lacking both extension and full flexion. This stiffness affects the hands as well as the large joints. Motor development may be delayed because of contractures or myelopathy. Intellectual development, however, is normal. Inguinal and abdominal hernias are also common.

Respiratory impairment may occur because of aspiration, which is made more likely by cleft palate or tracheomalacia. As with many other patients with skeletal dysplasia, otitis media may be a recurrent problem, and may even contribute to hearing impairment. Myopia is common, and retinal detachment and glaucoma may cause severe visual loss, as in Kneist's original patient, who became blind during adolescence (91). Adult height ranges from 106 to 145 cm.

Radiographic Features

There is osteopenia of both spine and extremities, perhaps as a result of disuse. All regions of the spine are affected, from atlantoaxial instability (due to odontoid hypoplasia) to hypoplasia of the cervical vertebrae and flattening of all vertebrae (96). The vertebral bodies have vertical clefts (97). There is kyphosis, and often mild scoliosis (Fig. 8-19), in the thoracolumbar spine. The femoral necks, as with all metaphyses, are short and broad. There are irregular calcifications in the epiphyseal and metaphyseal regions. Valgus deformities often develop in the distal femur or proximal tibia. The epiphyses are flattened and irregular (Fig. 8-20). Degenerative arthritis of the major weightbearing joints develops early, even in the second decade of life.

Orthopaedic Treatment

It is important to rule out cervical instability when the diagnosis is first made, when intubation is planned, or with

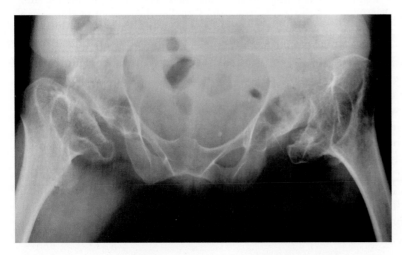

FIGURE 8-20. Like most epiphyses in Kneist dysplasia, the femoral heads are flattened and irregular. Also note the short, broad femoral necks.

any loss of milestones or of strength or coordination (98). Although kyphoscoliosis should be monitored, efficacy of brace treatment has never been studied, and remains doubtful. Surgery for spinal deformity is not often needed. Physical therapy has been recommended to increase joint mobility, but the efficacy of this too has not been proven.

Osteotomies about the hip or the knee may be helpful in certain circumstances. Osteotomy of the proximal femur may help improve joint congruity, if hinge abduction is developing [➥4.5]. An arthrogram in different positions may aid in making this decision. Any flexion deformity can be corrected at the same time by incorporating an extension component into the osteotomy, as long as adequate range of flexion will remain for sitting (at least 80 to 90 degrees). Osteotomy of the distal femur or proximal tibia is indicated if knee valgus is excessive. Equinovarus of the foot may be treated initially with casts, but surgery is often indicated [➥7.1]. If the stiffness of the first metatarsophalangeal joint produces hallux rigidus, traditional measures such as cheilectomy or arthrodesis may help.

SPONDYLOEPIPHYSEAL DYSPLASIA CONGENITA

Spondyloepiphyseal dysplasia congenita is a rare disorder with an estimated prevalence of about 3 to 4 per million population (8). Its key features include significant spinal and epiphyseal involvement, without metaphyseal enlargement or contractures of other joints (99). It is heritable in an autosomal dominant form, but most patients acquire the disease because of a new mutation. The genetic defect has recently been characterized as a defect in type II collagen, the gene for which is located on chromosome 1293. This is the predominant protein of cartilage, and mutations have been observed in the α1 chain, resulting in alteration in length (100). Like many skeletal dysplasias, electron microscopy has demonstrated intracellular inclusions, which are probably due to intracellular retention of procollagen (101).

Clinical Features

The severity of disease is variable. In general, the face is taut, the mouth small, and appearance somewhat characteristic. Cleft palate is common. The trunk and extremities are both shortened, although the extremities are more shortened proximally because of the coxa vara (Fig. 8-21). There is pectus carinatum, in part because the rib growth outpaces the increase in trunk height. There are many similarities to Morquio syndrome but a lack of visceral involvement. Scoliosis and kyphosis usually develop before the teen years. Back pain is common by this time, as well.

The hips are most commonly in varus, but this is variable. The degree of varus has been felt to be the best marker for the severity of the disease (102). If the varus is severe,

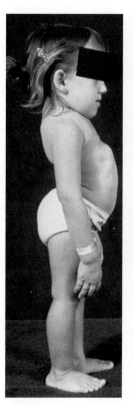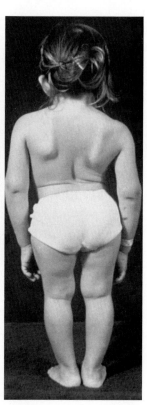

FIGURE 8-21. An 11-year-old child with spondyloepiphyseal dysplasia congenita. Markedly short stature is result of flattening of vertebrae at all levels, scoliosis, increased lumbar lordosis, and hip flexion contractures. Also note pectus carinatum. (Courtesy of George S. Bassett, M.D.)

it is often accompanied by a significant hip flexion contracture. Patients often walk with the trunk and head held back to compensate for this contracture. The knees are often in mild varus, and a combination of external rotation of the femora and internal rotation of the tibiae often coexists.

The most common foot deformity is equinovarus, but this is not nearly as stiff as the involvement with DD. Growth curves are available for this condition (102). Adult height varies from 90 to 125 cm.

Radiographic Features

One of the traits of this condition is that ossification is delayed in almost all regions (103,104). There is often odontoid hypoplasia or os odontoideum. Flattened vertebral ossification centers with posterior wedging give the vertebral appearance, on lateral view, a "pear shape." If scoliosis is present, it is often sharply angulated over a few vertebrae (Fig. 8-22). Disc spaces become narrow and irregular by maturity. Ossification of the pubis is delayed. The proximal femora are in varus with short necks, but the degree of this involvement varies. The proximal femur may not ossify for up to 9 years (102). Often, the varus is progressive (Fig. 8-

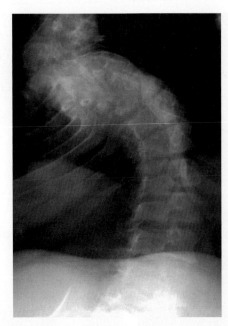

FIGURE 8-22. Scoliosis, with a sharp apex concentrated over a limited number of vertebrae, is characteristic of spondyloepiphyseal dysplasia congenita.

23). There is possible progressive extrusion of the femoral head. This may require an arthrogram to clearly demonstrate it. The distal femoral metaphyses are flared. Genu valgum is more common than genu varum. Early osteoarthritis is likely in the hips, more so than in the knee. The carpals are delayed in ossification, but the tubular bones of the hands are near normal.

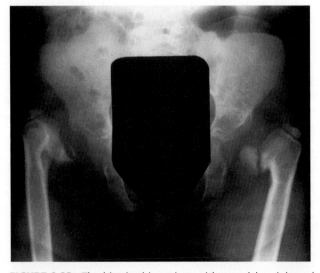

FIGURE 8-23. The hips in this patient with spondyloepiphyseal dysplasia congenita show severe coxa vara, with delayed ossification of the capital femoral epiphyses. (Courtesy of George S. Bassett, M.D.)

Medical Problems

Respiratory problems occur in infants due, in many cases, to a small thorax. The most common disabling problem in this syndrome involves the eyes: retinal detachment is common. It is reported to occur especially during the adolescent growth spurt. Regular ophthalmologic examinations are recommended. Hearing impairment is noted in a minority of patients.

Orthopaedic Problems and Treatment

Orthopaedically, the most potentially serious sequelae can involve neck instability. Os odontoideum, or odontoid hypoplasia, or aplasia may all cause instability and, potentially, myelopathy (Fig. 8-24A–C). Numerous cases have been reported (5). Careful neurologic examination should be done at each clinic visit. Flexion–extension radiographs should be performed about every 3 years if an upper cervical anomaly is identified. If the odontoid is difficult to see, one can use CT or MRI. Stenosis often coexists and makes subluxation more critical. It is recommended to fuse the atlantoaxial interval if instability exceeds 8 mm, or if symptoms develop [➥2.17]. If severe stenosis exists, or if a fixed subluxation cannot be reduced, it may be necessary to perform an atlas decompression and, consequently, fusion to the occiput (105). Bone strength or canal size often make rigid internal fixation impractical or unsafe; in these cases, bone graft and halo-cast immobilization are usually successful. Scoliosis is present in more than one-half of patients with spondyloepiphyseal dysplasia. It may become severe. Curve control with a brace may be attempted if it is less than 40 degrees. However, long-term efficacy has not been demonstrated. Fusion may be necessary if the curve is progressive. Thoracolumbar stenosis is not as severe as in achondroplasia. Instrumentation is not contraindicated but should be used judiciously. If internal stabilization is not judged to be strong, consider use of a halo brace immobilization postoperatively. Correction is usually modest (17% in one series [5]). Anterior surgery should be used if the patient is young (under about age 11) or the curve is rigid (correcting to less than approximately 45 degrees). Kyphosis is also common; use of a Milwaukee brace has been shown to be effective if it can be worn until maturity (5).

Hip osteotomies are indicated if the neck-shaft angle is less than 100 degrees [➥4.4]. Insufficient correction makes recurrence more likely. It is helpful to correct any flexion contracture at the same time if enough flexion will remain. Malrotation should be corrected as well. If a patient is experiencing painful hinge abduction, a valgus osteotomy may improve symptoms. An arthrogram may help in operative planning.

Dislocation may be reconstructed if done early. The surgeon may need a combination of femoral and iliac osteoto-

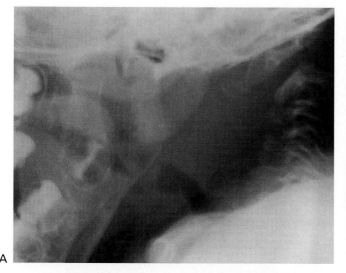

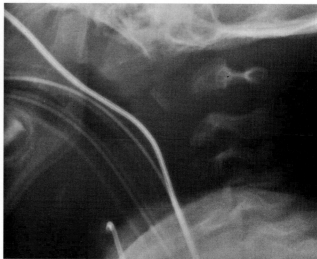

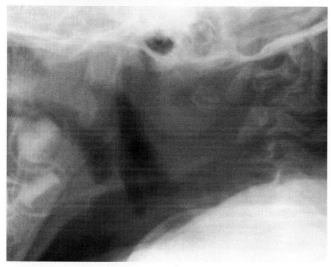

FIGURE 8-24. Atlantoaxial instability is common in spondyloepiphyseal dysplasia congenita. This 2-year-old patient had delayed motor milestones. The upright lateral film (**A**) of the cervical spine demonstrates odontoid hypoplasia with marked atlantoaxial subluxation. Less evident is the stenosis of the ring of the atlas. When supine in a neutral position (**B**), the alignment improved. Following decompression of the atlas and fusion of occiput to C2 (**C**), he gained the ability to walk.

mies. When doing any procedure on the hip, assess the knee alignment at the same time and correct it if necessary. The clinician should also consider the effect that knee angular correction will have on the hip. For instance, correction of severe knee valgus deformity has the same effect on hip congruity as does a varus osteotomy of the proximal femur.

Total joint replacement is a very difficult procedure: the hip is stiff, custom components are often needed, and concomitant osteotomy is sometimes necessary.

Foot deformities can usually be treated according to standard clubfoot principles [➡7.1]. If the foot is stiff, an osteotomy or decancellation of the talus, calcaneus, and/or cuboid may be needed.

SPONDYLOEPIPHYSEAL DYSPLASIA TARDA

Spondyloepiphyseal dysplasia (SED) tarda is distinguished from the congenita form by later age at diagnosis and more mild features. Manifestations first appear in later childhood, or even in adulthood. The spine and only the larger joints are affected. Several genetic patterns of transmission have been reported (106–108). The most common is X-linked, in which male patients are more commonly or more severely affected and female patients may show milder manifestations. A recessive form has also been reported. SED-tarda is one of several conditions (termed the COL2A1 group or the SED family), which may result from a mutation in type II collagen (7,46). The mechanism by which the particular mutation for this condition produces the mildest phenotype in this family will doubtlessly be elucidated in the near future.

Clinical Features

Manifestations first are called to clinical attention at about 4 years old, in the earliest cases. Stature is mildly shortened. The condition may be first diagnosed as bilateral Perthes syndrome (109). Back pain and hip or knee pain may be present in childhood. Joint range of motion is minimally limited, if at all. Varus or valgus deformities are rare. Degenerative changes may occur in the hip or the knee by young adulthood. Adult height may be to 60 in. or more (108).

Radiographic Features

Involvement of shoulders, hips, and knees predominates. The hips manifest varying degrees of coxa magna, flattening, or epiphyseal extrusion, differing markedly even within the same family (Fig. 8-25). A minority of patients present with bilateral coxa vara. Odontoid hypoplasia or os odontoideum may cause atlantoaxial instability. Spinal involvement ranges from mild platyspondyly (Fig. 8-26), with ax-like configuration of the vertebral bodies on the lateral view, to isolated disc-space narrowing. Mild-to-moderate scoliosis develops in a minority of cases.

Orthopaedic Problems and Treatment

The severity of orthopaedic conditions varies widely, even within a family. There are undoubtedly many affected individuals whose problems are so mild that no diagnosis is ever made. One large family was reported in which only 4 of the 31 affected members requested any orthopaedic treatment (110). This is one condition to consider whenever spine, hip, and/or knee pains run in a family, and the radiographs seem to be just a little atypical. Bracing may be recommended if scoliosis exceeds 30 degrees in the skeletally immature patient. Surgery should be offered for the rare patient in whom it exceeds 50 degrees. All patients should be screened for atlantoaxial instability. Fusion should be

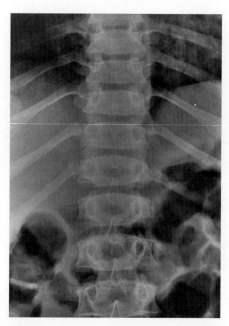

FIGURE 8-26. The spine in this patient with spondyloepiphyseal dysplasia tarda shows typical mild flattening of the vertebral bodies, but no scoliosis.

recommended if the spine is unstable in either flexion or extension, according to criteria given earlier for the congenita form [➥**2.17**]. The role for procedures to increase coverage of the dysplastic, extruded femoral head by the acetabulum during the childhood years is not well documented. However, it may be helpful in the rare young patient with increasing extrusion and persistent pain, in whom the hip contact surface is markedly compromised. If hip pain becomes a problem after the femoral heads are mature or nearly mature, osteotomy may help to increase congruity or decrease hinge abduction. Usually, a valgus or valgus-extension osteotomy is most appropriate, so long as there is reasonable joint space and adequate contact remaining. A preoperative arthrogram is helpful in the younger patient to see the full outline of the articular surface. Osteotomies of knees or ankles are rarely needed. Total joint replacement is often needed for the hips or knees, at an age much younger than the general population.

PSEUDOACHONDROPLASIA

Pseudoachondroplasia was first described in 1959 by Maroteaux and Lamy as a form of spondyloepiphyseal dysplasia (111). It has subsequently been reclassified as being distinct from SED, because of late-onset physical findings and more mild spinal involvement. It involves the metaphyses, as well as the spine and epiphyses. The significant features are ligamentous laxity and "windswept" knees. With a prevalence of approximately four per million, it is one of the more

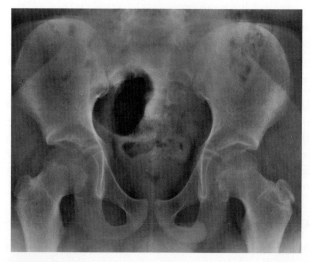

FIGURE 8-25. The pelvis in this patient with spondyloepiphyseal dysplasia tarda shows minimally small, flattened epiphyses.

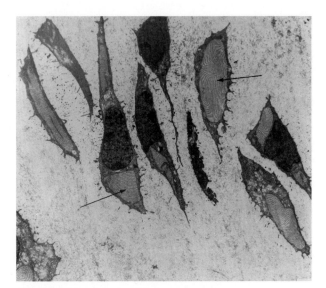

FIGURE 8-27. Abnormal lamellar inclusion bodies in endoplasmic reticulum of growth plate chondrocytes of a patient with pseudoachondroplasia. (From ref. 112, with permission.)

common skeletal dysplasias. Early histologic studies demonstrated that the chondrocytes of persons with pseudoachondroplasia contained lamellar inclusions within the endoplasmic reticulum (58,112). It has since been demonstrated that pseudoachondroplasia results from a mutation in cartilage oligomeric matrix protein (COMP), the same protein that is disordered in MED (113,114). COMP is normally a large extracellular matrix glycoprotein that is found in the territorial matrix surrounding chondrocytes. It is also found in the extracellular matrix of ligament and tendon tissues. A number of different mutations have been found in this gene (113). Some of the mutations involve a GAC trinucleotide repeat within this gene; it has been found that either expansions or deletions in this region may cause the disease. COMP accumulates in the rough endoplasmic reticulum of chondrocytes and tenocytes in persons with this disorder (115) (Fig. 8-27). Normal growth and development occur in mice whose *COMP* gene has been deleted, illustrating that it is accumulation of an abnormal form of COMP, not its absence, which causes pseudoachondroplasia. It is thought that the abnormality of the matrix does not maintain the shape of the cells, and allows them to become flatter (116,117). Three separate families have been reported who have somatic/germline mosaicism, which allows this dominant condition to behave like a recessive disorder, with up to a 50% recurrence risk, even from two normal-statured parents (114).

Clinical Features

Most patients with pseudoachondroplasia are not recognized as having a skeletal dysplasia at birth. The length at birth is a mean of 49 cm, which is within normal limits. Growth tapers soon after this, however, so that the height falls to below the fifth percentile by the age of 2 years (118). The eventual height is the same as that of a person with DD. This pattern of progressive involvement is typical of storage disorders, which is essentially the nature of this condition. Usually, the diagnosis is made by the age of 2 to 4 years old.

Facial features have variously been termed "delicate" or normal (Fig. 8-28). In any event, they are not distinctive enough to be involved in the diagnostic process (119,120). Cervical instability is present in a minority of cases. Increased thoracic kyphosis and lumbar lordosis are often present (116). Mild scoliosis often occurs, but few cases become severe. The pattern of shortening of the extremities is rhizomelic and progresses with time. This finding helps explain why early writers often confused this disorder with achondroplasia. However, the hands are not tridentine. In almost all cases, the hips are dysplastic and the patient exhibits a waddling gait. Knees are most commonly in excessive valgus, or windswept (one in varus, one in valgus), due to lax ligaments, as well as epiphyseal and metaphyseal abnormalities. The joints may have flexion contractures or recurvatum. Adult height is a mean of 119 cm (range 106 to 130 cm) (118). No changes outside the skeletal system

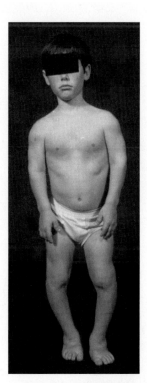

FIGURE 8-28. A 12-year-old patient with pseudoachondroplastic dysplasia. The head and trunk are normal, but there is rhizomelic shortening of the extremities. The hands and feet are short and broad. (Courtesy of George S. Bassett, M.D.)

have been noted as part of the disorder. Patients have normal intelligence, and a normal life expectancy (121).

Radiographic Changes

The vertebral bodies are very flat with anterior indentations, even in early childhood, and this may be one of the earliest ways to make the diagnosis, because affected babies are outwardly normal (Fig. 8-29). This flattening may be discovered if a routine chest radiograph is ordered, for instance. Almost one-half have odontoid hypoplasia or aplasia. Therefore, flexion–extension radiographs are advised at the initial evaluation. These should be repeated at intervals, because the degree of instability may increase with time. In the lumbar spine, the pedicles are not narrower caudally, as in achondroplasia, but are short in the sagittal plane. Sternal deformities may appear (carinatum or excavatum).

The long-bone metaphyses are broad, irregular at the ends, and flared at the edges. The epiphyses are late to ossify and irregular in appearance. There is progressively irregular ossification of epiphyses. Delayed maturation of triradiate cartilage is more common than in any other dysplasia. The pubic rami are delayed in closing, and the greater trochanteric apophysis is delayed also (122). The femoral head is enlarged, and undergoes progressive subluxation (Fig. 8-

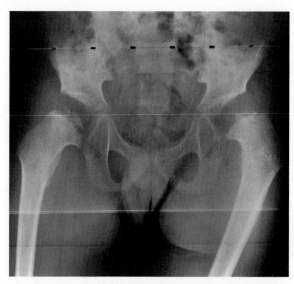

FIGURE 8-30. Deformation and delay in the ossification of the epiphyses are frequently seen in pseudoachondroplasia.

30). The metaphyses all show irregularity and beaking. The height of the epiphysis of the distal femur decreases (Fig. 8-31). An arthrogram may be helpful if operative intervention is planned, to visualize the joint surface and determine the location of the deformity(ies), because epiphyseal ossification is delayed, and this can be difficult to visualize. The tibial plateau may be depressed on one side, and the fibula may be relatively long. Delayed maturation of carpal bones makes predicting bone age or skeletal maturity difficult.

Orthopaedic Problems and Treatment

The cervical spine should be monitored and treated according to guidelines given earlier in this chapter. Myelopathy

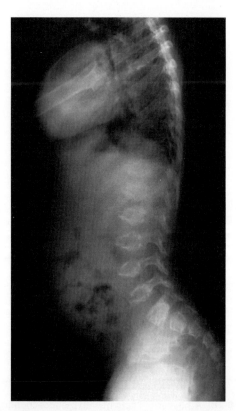

FIGURE 8-29. A 3-year-old child with pseudoachondroplastic dysplasia has platyspondyly with anterior beaking. (Courtesy of George S. Basset, M.D.)

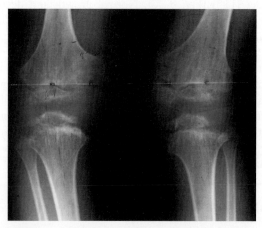

FIGURE 8-31. Epiphyseal flattening and a "windswept" alignment are characteristic of the knees in pseudoachondroplasia.

has been reported in several series. Posterior cervical fusion [➡2.17] may be indicated if translation of the atlas on the axis exceeds approximately 8 mm, or if neurologic signs are present. Many patients, surprisingly, have normal cervical spines.

If scoliosis is present, and is between 25 and 45 degrees in the skeletally immature individual, a trial of brace is warranted. Larger curves (over 50 degrees) may require surgery. Spinal stenosis is not a clinical problem, so the surgeon can use sublaminar fixation, if needed, to supplement other fixation methods [➡2.1–2.5].

Hip subluxation and dislocation may be due to intrinsic cartilage deformation to a hip adduction contracture or to valgus of the knee. It is recommended to try to arrest this process. A femoral osteotomy, as well as an iliac procedure, may be needed. Preoperatively, it is wise to make radiographs with the patient in corrected position, to see whether the hip will be congruous in this position. If it is aspherical or incongruous, one may need an acetabular augmentation to achieve coverage. This is generally a more versatile procedure than a rotational iliac osteotomy in the person with skeletal dysplasia. At the same time, the surgeon should look for and correct flexion and rotation contractures as well.

Valgus or varus deformities about the knee often need correction. It is up to the discretion of the patient and the surgeon when this should be done. The objective of the procedure is to obtain a horizontal joint surface with a well-aligned knee. Both tibial and femoral procedures may be necessary. The risk of recurrence is high, even with a well-done procedure, so it is wise to educate patients about this risk. Early onset of osteoarthritis often occurs—about one-half of adults in one long-term study had undergone at least one arthroplasty (116,121).

MULTIPLE EPIPHYSEAL DYSPLASIA

Multiple epiphyseal dysplasia is one of the most widely known and commonly occurring skeletal dysplasis. It is dominantly inherited. It affects many epiphyses, produces symptoms mainly in those with significant loadbearing, and has few changes in the physes or metaphyses. Historically, it was described as occurring in two separate forms, with eponyms that are still used today: Ribbing's dysplasia, having mild involvement, or Fairbank's dysplasia, a more severe type (123–125). With current understanding of the genetic basis, this may not be an absolute distinction.

Histologically, intracytoplasmic inclusions are seen that are similar to, but not so severe as, those seen in pseudo-achondroplasia. Growth plate organization is still noticeably abnormal, despite the minimal changes seen in the metaphyses. The genetic basis for this disorder is now reasonably well understood. It is a genetically heterogeneous disorder. Mutations have been found in the gene for COMP on chromosome 19, as in pseudoachondroplasia. However, in other cases of MED, abnormalities have been found in the α_2

fibers of collagen type 9 (*COL9A2*). Collagen type 9 is normally a trimer that is found on the surface of type II collagen in cartilage. It may form a macromolecular bridge between type II collagen fibrils and other matrix components—it thus may be important for the adhesive properties of cartilage. A *COL9A2* mutation has been described in one large family, with peripheral joint involvement only (126).

Clinical Features

Patients typically present later in childhood, for one of several reasons. They may be referred for joint pain in the lower extremities, decreased range of motion, gait disturbance, or angular deformities of the knees (127). There may be flexion contractures of knees or elbows. Symptoms may develop as late as adulthood. These patients have minimal short stature, ranging from 145 to 170 cm (57 to 67 in) (124). The face and spine are normal. There is no visceral involvement.

Radiographic Features

Most changes in MED involve the epiphyses; almost all of the ossification centers are delayed in appearance. There are occasional irregularities of streaking in the metaphyses, but they are minor. The appearances of the epiphyses in the immature and in the mature patient are different and characteristic (128). In the growing patient, the epiphyses are fragmented and small in size (Fig. 8-32). The epiphyseal

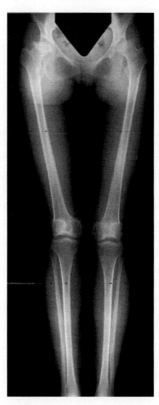

FIGURE 8-32. Multiple epiphyseal dysplasia.

ossification centers eventually coalesce, but the overall shape of the epiphysis is smaller. An arthrogram may be helpful when it is necessary to assess the shape of the joint surface. The more fragmentation there is in the capital femoral epiphysis, the earlier onset of osteoarthritis (129). Coxa vara occurs in some patients. After maturity, there is some degree of flattening of the major load-bearing epiphyses: flattening of the femoral condyles, an ovoid femoral head, decreased sphericity of the humeral head, and squaring of the talus. In adulthood, major joints develop premature osteoarthritis. This is most common and most severe in the hips.

Avascular necrosis may be superimposed on MED. This occurs in about one-half the femoral heads. It can be recognized by appearance of a crescent sign, resorption of bone that had already been formed, and, sometimes, by the presence of metaphyseal cysts (130). MRI at this time may show loss of signal in a portion of the femoral head. A "sagging rope sign" may develop later (121).

Any orthopaedic surgeon who examines children must be able to differentiate MED from Perthes disease (109). Several radiographic clues may be helpful. In MED, abnormalities in the acetabulum are primary, and are more pronounced. The radiographic changes are symmetric and fairly synchronous. It is also helpful to obtain radiographs of the knees, ankles, shoulders, and wrists.

Radiographs of the knees show that the femoral condyles are flattened, and may be in valgus. There may be irregular ossification, just as in the hip. The condyles are somewhat squared on lateral view. Osteochondritis dissecans may be superimposed. Some MED patients also show a double-layered patella on the lateral view (132). This is a complete or partial double radiodensity, which is rarely seen in other conditions. There may be a synovial-lined joint between the two layers of the patella.

The ankles in MED are also in valgus; changes occur more in the talus than in the distal tibia. Upper extremity involvement is less severe; there may be irregularities in the proximal and distal humerus and radius. The humeral head involvement in adulthood has been termed a "hatchet-head" appearance, and results from undergrowth of the head and neck. It occurs in children more severely affected with MED. Radial ray hypoplasia may occur sporadically (133). The carpal ossification centers are delayed in appearing. The hand and wrist involvement may predict stature (134). The spine may be normal, or may have slight end-plate irregularities or ossification defects on the anterior margins of the vertebrae (135).

Orthopaedic Implications

The orthopaedic surgeon may become involved in the care of the patient with MED in either of two periods. There is a small role for realignment procedures in the early, deforming period of the hip if there is progressive subluxation or pain. Pain is more likely to occur in cases in which avascu-

lar necrosis has supervened (130). Although the principle of coverage is the same as that used in Perthes disease, there is often a degree of coxa vara preexisting in hips with MED, which contraindicates use of a femoral osteotomy. Acetabular shelf augmentation is a worthwhile procedure in these instances (136,137).

Not all patients need surgical treatment; however, some can be helped. Significant deformities may be corrected near maturity, either in the femur or tibia, depending on the site of abnormality. Degenerative joint disease is the biggest problem, and it occurs in the second or third decade. It results not so much from malalignment of the joints, but from intrinsic defect in cartilage. It produces stiffness, from an early age, and pain leading to a total joint arthroplasty. Even the shoulder is commonly affected by degeneration, and shoulder arthroplasty may be necessary (138).

CHONDRODYSPLASIA PUNCTATA

This skeletal dysplasia is also known by the synonyms "congenital stippled epiphysis" and "chondrodystrophia calcificans congenita." Key features include multiple punctate calcifications in infancy, which are best visualized on the newborn's radiographs (139). It has been subclassified into three groups: an X-linked dominant type (Conradi-Hünermann syndrome), an autosomal recessive rhizomelic type, which is usually lethal in infancy, and a rare X-linked recessive type. Four others have been described that are even more rare (140). Although the appearance of neonatal epiphyseal calcification is striking, it is not very specific. Wulfsberg has listed various other conditions that may present with the same phenomenon: Zellweger (cerebrohepatorenal) syndrome, gangliosidosis, rubella, trisomy 18 or 21, vitamin K deficiency, hypothyroidism, or fetal alcohol or hydantoin syndromes (140–145). Rhizomelic chondrodysplasia punctata is a peroxisomal deficiency of dihydroxyacetone-phosphate acyltransferase; it is often (but not always) fatal in the first year of life (146,147). The genetic defect and pathogenesis of the Conradi-Hünermann syndrome has not been elucidated. Histologic examination shows perilacunar calcifications throughout the cartilage matrix (148).

Clinical Features

Patients with Conradi-Hünermann syndrome are characterized by hypertelorism, a depressed nasal bridge, and a bifid nasal tip (149–152). In addition, many have alopecia, congenital heart and/or renal malformations, and mental retardation. In rhizomelic chondrodysplasia punctata, findings include microcephaly, a high incidence of congenital cataracts, growth retardation, and a well-formed nasal bridge (153–156). Some have feeding difficulties, and most succumb to respiratory death or seizures in the first year. Diag-

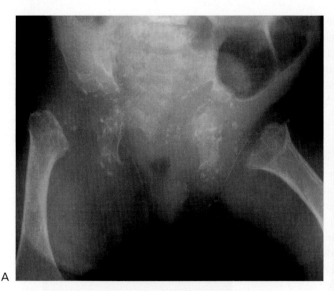

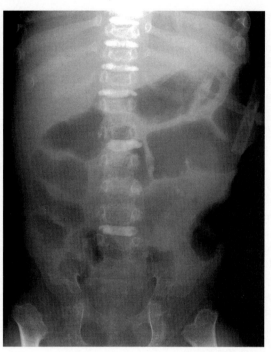

FIGURE 8-33. A: Diffuse punctate epiphyseal calcifications in infancy are a hallmark for which chondrodysplasia punctata was named. **B:** At age 2-1/2 years, the epiphyseal calcifications are mostly resolved, but calcification of the intervertebral discs persists.

nosis may be made by amniocentesis, with measurement of plasmalogen biosynthesis and phytanic acid oxidation.

Skeletal findings in the extremities include limb-length inequality, coxa vara, and clubfoot or other foot deformities (157). Spinal findings include atlantoaxial instability, congenital scoliosis, or kyphosis (158).

Radiographic Features

Skeletal calcifications are visible at birth, but most disappear by 1 year. These involve the epiphyses, carpal bones, and pelvis (159) (Fig. 8-33A and B). Extraskeletal sites include the trachea and larynx. The appearance is of small flecks of calcium, "which appear as if paint had been flecked on by a brush" (160). The ossification centers themselves may be delayed in appearance. Coxa vara may affect one or both hips, or it may be absent (161). The fibula often overgrows the tibia significantly. Spine radiographs may show presence of a hemivertebra or a congenital bar. Calcification of the intervertebral discs may develop (Fig. 8-33B). Odontoid hypoplasia and os odontoideum have been described (158).

Orthopaedic Implications

Because of the risk of cervical instability, each patient should have a lateral cervical radiograph and, if instability appears possible, a flexion–extension view. Scoliosis may occur early due to secondary congenital anomalies. It may require early fusion if progression is documented and the patient, medically, is a candidate. Coxa vara should be treated

if the neck-shaft angle is less than 100 degrees [➥4.4]. Lower limb-length inequality should be monitored and treated appropriately.

METAPHYSEAL CHONDRODYSPLASIAS

The metaphyseal chondrodysplasias are actually a group of disorders characterized by metaphyseal irregularity and deformity but preservation of epiphyseal structure, which, of course, is a contrast to almost all the dysplasias previously described in this chapter (162–164). The name may be a bit misleading, because it refers to the end result: radiographic changes in the metaphyses. Of course, logically, the real defect is in the growth plate itself, resulting in failure of uniform ossification of the cartilage columns, with persistence of cartilage islands, undergrowth, and deformity as the sequelae (165,166). There are many different named disorders that come under the heading of metaphyseal chondrodysplasia. We discuss here the commonest types: McKusick, Schmid and Jansen types, as well as Kozlowski-type spondylometaphyseal dysplasia, which has mild changes in the vertebral bodies.

McKusick-type Metaphyseal Chondrodysplasia

This condition is rather common in the Amish community of Lancaster County, Pennsylvania, as well as in Finland. It also occurs sporadically throughout the world. It is also known by the term "cartilage-hair hypoplasia." It is autosomal recessive and maps to chromosome 9 (167). Although etiology has not been further elucidated at this point, defects in hematopoietic colony development have been found in bone marrow samples of a number of patients, perhaps explaining the hematologic aspects of the disease.

Clinical Findings

The first thing that distinguishes this group of patients is their fine, light, and sometimes sparse hair (Figs. 8-34 and 8-35) . This should serve as a clue to the more important medical problems that this group of patients may have. An alteration in T-cell immunity causes an increased risk of viral infection (especially *varicella zoster,* which may be more severe in these persons). Continued antibiotic prophylaxis in the first 6 months of life has been recommended (168,169). Anemia may develop, and 16% of patients require a blood transfusion (170). Bone marrow transplant has been reported in one infant with severe recurrent infections; it corrected the immune problem, but did not improve skeletal growth (171). Hematologic problems have a tendency to become less severe after childhood. Hirschsprung disease, intestinal malabsorption, and megacolon

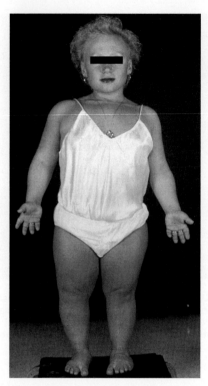

FIGURE 8-35. A 22-two-year-old woman with metaphyseal chondrodysplasia, McKusick type (cartilage-hair hypoplasia). Note disproportionately short stature, fine light hair, and genu varum.

may also develop. There is an increased risk of malignancy, such as lymphoma, sarcoma, and skin cancer. In the largest series reported, 8% of patients had malignancies (168,172). Clearly, then, these patients need medical surveillance into adulthood, more than would most patients with skeletal dysplasia.

Orthopaedically, these patients have generalized ligamentous laxity, but the elbows actually have flexion contractures. There is mild genu varum, which may bring them to see an orthopaedist. Pectus excavatum or carinatum may be observed. The adult height is 106–147 cm (42–58 in.).

Radiographic Features

In the McKusick type of metaphyseal chondrodysplasia (Fig. 8-36), there is more shortening and less varus of the long bones than seen in the Schmid type. The metaphyseal involvement is more evenly distributed, not all on the medial side of the knee. There is distal fibular overgrowth, perhaps because this bone is less inhibited by the forces of weightbearing. Atlantoaxial instability has been reported. The thoracolumbar spine shows some minimal changes, which are not of much clinical importance: columnization (increased height) of the vertebrae and increased lumbar lordosis.

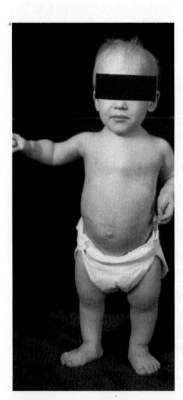
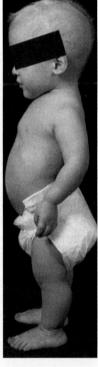

FIGURE 8-34. An 18-month-old child with McKusick-type metaphyseal chondrodysplasia. Notice the characteristic light, sparse hair, disproportionate short stature, pectus excavatum, and varus deformities of the lower extremities. Mild increased lumbar lordosis, flexion contractures of the elbows, and expansion of the wrists are also part of the deformity. (Courtesy of George S. Bassett, M.D.)

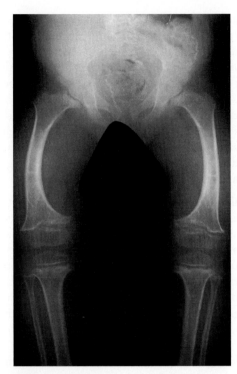

FIGURE 8-36. A 4-year-old patient with McKusick-type metaphyseal chondrodysplasia. Pelvis is normal, apart from silver clips from surgical treatment of megacolon. Mild coxa vara, bowing of the femurs and tibias with metaphyseal expansion, and irregular zones of provisional calcification are evident. (Courtesy of George S. Bassett, M.D.)

Orthopaedic Implications

It is prudent to obtain flexion–extension films for atlantoaxial instability, at least on the first visit. MRI in flexion and extension may be helpful, if the plain films seem equivocal diagnostically. Posterior spine fusion should be performed if there is more than 8 mm of translation, or if any signs of cord compression are present [➡2.17]. Congenital hip dislocation has been reported in 3% of patients, and successful closed reduction may be performed if detected early (168). In some patients (15%), the varus at knee or ankle should be corrected, if severe.

Schmid-type Metaphyseal Chondrodysplasia

The Schmid type is more common than the McKusick type, and is better understood at a genetic level (173). It is autosomal dominant. The defect is in the α_1 chain of type X collagen (174,175). Type X is a highly specialized extracellular matrix component, the synthesis of which is restricted only to hypertrophic chondrocytes in the calcifying zones of the growth plate and in zones of secondary ossification. It is a homotrimer of three α_1 chains, which has been implicated in morphogenetic events of endochondral ossification,

including calcification of hypertrophic cartilage prior to its replacement by bone. Many mutations described involve the C-terminal end, where joining of the three individual chains starts, and prevents the abnormal chains from forming trimeric structures (176). On histologic examination, one sees cartilage islands that extend into the metaphyses. The differential diagnosis for this and other forms of metaphyseal dysplasia, most importantly, includes various types of rickets and hypophosphatasia.

Clinical Features

Patients with the Schmid dysplasia show rather minimal clinical abnormalities. They are normal at birth. The facial appearance is normal. They may present to the orthopaedic surgeon with leg pains, varus knees and ankles, short stature, or a waddling gait. The adult height is minimally shortened, at an average 150 cm (59 inches).

Radiographic Features

The metaphyses of the long bones are widened and flared, and may have cysts. The physes are slightly widened. Weight-bearing may play a role in these changes—they have been reported to improve after rest or cast immobilization, and to recur after resumption of loading (173). There is a varus deformity of the knees. Atlantoaxial instability has been reported, but is rare.

Orthopaedic Implications

The epiphyses are normal, and patients rarely get degenerative changes. The orthopaedic surgeon may be called on to correct bowing of the knees if it becomes severe. Otherwise, there is little need for care in these patients.

Jansen Metaphyseal Dysplasia

This is a rarer type of dysplasia. It is an autosomal dominantly inherited disorder, which has been linked to a defect in the receptor for parathyroid hormone and parathyroid hormone related protein (177). This provides an interesting link between the skeletal dysplasias and the metabolic bone diseases. Patients with Jansen syndrome may have hypercalcemia, and they have more severe metaphyseal changes than the previous two types.

Kozlowski-type (Spondylometaphyseal Dysplasia)

Clinical Features

This uncommon autosomal dominant disorder has spinal, as well as metaphyseal, changes. It is recognized in preschool-age children by the findings of short stature and mildly increased kyphosis. There may be slight limitation of joint movement, a Trendelenburg gait, and early osteoarthritis. Adult height reaches about 150 cm (54 in.).

Radiographic Features

There is mild platyspondyly, in contrast to the three disorders just described. There is a retarded bone age of the carpals and tarsals. The metaphyseal chondrodysplasia is most pronounced in the proximal femur.

DIAPHYSEAL ACLASIA (MULTIPLE OSTEOCARTILAGINOUS EXOSTOSIS)

Although solitary exostoses do not qualify as skeletal dysplasias, it is clear that patients with multiple exostoses have a generalized disturbance of skeletal growth. The condition has been localized to three different chromosomal locations: sites on chromosomes 8, 11, and 19. The specific genes have not been identified. The differing locations of mutation may account for the phenotypic variability of the condition. It is likely that tumor suppressor genes may be involved (7). Most cases are transmitted as autosomal dominant, but a large number of patients acquire it as a spontaneous mutation. The metaphysis of a person with multiple osteochondromas is characterized by thinning of the cortex, innumerable small bumps, and cartilage rests extending into the trabecular bone.

Clinical Features

The condition is not usually noted until age 3 to 4 years, when the first exostoses are noted and other features develop. The features become progressively more pronounced until maturity, at which point bony prominences should cease to grow. Affected persons are at the low end of normal for stature. The metaphyses are circumferentially enlarged throughout the body, not only in regions where there are obvious exostoses. This gives a rather "stocky" appearance, which is then further exaggerated by the appearance of the exostoses. They may cause soreness when they arise under tendons or in an area vulnerable to bumping, such as the proximal humerus. The exostoses tend to steal from the longitudinal growth of the long bones. The categories of problems caused by this condition are fourfold:

1. Localized pressure on tendons and nerves, among other places. Peroneal palsy may arise from a lateral exostosis, and it may occur in such a way as to cause brachial plexus or spinal cord compression.
2. Angular growth of two-bone segments—the arms and forearms. Usually the thinner of these two bones is more inhibited in its growth than the wider one, so it tethers the growth of the latter. Valgus may develop at the wrist, knee, and ankle. The radial head may subluxate or dislocate.
3. Limb length inequality. Often one limb is more involved than the other with exostoses, and it may undergrow as much as 4 cm.
4. Malignant degeneration. Transformation to chondrosarcoma occurs in about 1% of patients after maturity. Such change may be signaled by increased growth of an exostosis, or pain over an exostosis. Bone scans every two years in adulthood have been advocated as one way to detect this change.

Radiographic Features

The metaphyses are very wide, and internal irregularities can be seen. The exostoses may be sessile or pedunculated,

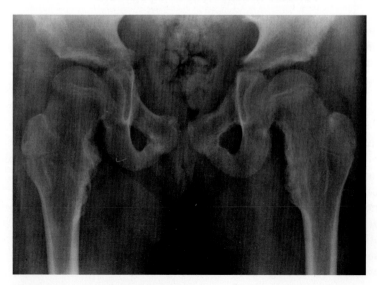

FIGURE 8-37. The hips in diaphyseal aclasia are characterized by broad, irregular femoral necks that are usually in valgus. There are osteochondromas and irregularities in formation of the pelvis also, which can be difficult to monitor over time.

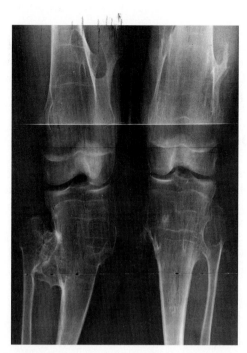

FIGURE 8-38. This figure of the knees in a patient with diaphyseal aclasia best illustrates that this defect is a systemic abnormality of bone formation, rather than a series of discrete tumors. The metaphyses are broad and irregular in the region where the exostoses are located. The knees are developing a valgus alignment, due to the short fibulae, as are the ankles.

and have continuity with the main cortex, like solitary exostoses do. Exostoses on the undersurface of the scapula may be identified on plain films, but are best evaluated by CT. The femoral necks are usually wide and in valgus (Fig. 8-37). Valgus is much more common than varus at the knee (Fig. 8-38), and the distal tibial epiphysis may be triangular if the fibula is pulling the ankle into valgus. Radial head subluxation may occur with ulnar shortening, and the resultant carpal subluxation can readily be identified by wrist films.

Orthopaedic Implications

Monitoring in childhood should mostly be done by clinical examination, because all bones are affected, and the lesions are too numerous to image routinely. Perform a brief neurologic examination, and check joint range of motion. Measure knee, ankle, elbow, and wrist angulation and limb lengths. Remove any exostoses that are causing significant symptoms, but warn the patients that the metaphyseal widening will persist, so the effect on appearance may not match expectations. Removal of lesions impairing radioulnar motion may result in slight increase in range, but not a dramatic improvement. Ulnar lengthening may help avert radial head subluxation. Hemiepiphysiodesis is a minimally invasive way to correct angulation at the wrist, knee, and ankle. If

the patient is near maturity and needs correction, osteotomy may be indicated. Limb-length inequality can be corrected by the standard algorithm, since the growth remains proportionate. Patients should be taught to examine themselves for signs of growth after maturity, because this may signal malignant degeneration. Bone scan may be a helpful adjunct if a problem is suspected.

DYSCHONDROSTEOSIS (LERI-WEILL SYNDROME)

Dyschondrosteosis, which was described by Leri and Weill in 1929 (178), is characterized by mild mesomelic short stature (middle segments are shortest). The growth disturbance of the middle segments is most notable in the distal radius, which usually develops a Madelung deformity (178–180). It is inherited in an autosomal dominant fashion, with about 50% penetrance (179,181). The expression is more severe in female patients than in males. It has been demonstrated to involve a mutation or deletion in the short-stature homeobox-containing gene *SHOX* (182).

Clinical Features

Patients usually present by age 8 years because of short stature, disproportion or deformity of the forearms, or wrist pain or deformity (183). The deformity of the distal forearm, or Madelung deformity, is characterized by a deficiency of growth of the volar–ulnar portion of the radius. The differential diagnosis of this phenomenon includes Turner syndrome, trauma, Ollier disease, or multiple hereditary exostoses. Most patients begin to experience pain in the wrist during adolescence, as well as limitation of pronation and supination. A variation on this theme, seen in some patients with dyschondrosteosis, is shortening of both radius and ulna, together without angulation. The mesomelic shortening also involves the lower extremities, specifically the tibiofibular segments. Here, however, there is not so much angular deformity—only a mild genu varum or ankle valgus usually exists. Short stature is usually, but not always, a feature; adult height ranges from 135 to 170 cm (53 to 66 in.). In one series of patients, deficiency in growth hormone was found, and stature was increased by growth hormone supplementation (184).

Radiographic Features

Madelung deformity is a failure of development of the volar–ulnar part of the distal radial epiphysis. The distal radial epiphysis develops a triangular appearance and a tilt

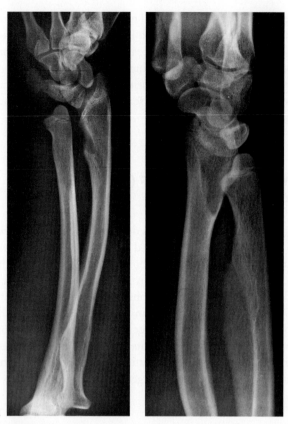

A   B

FIGURE 8-39. A: Madelung deformity in the forearm of a patient with dyschondrosteosis. **B:** The distal radial epiphysis has a markedly triangular epiphysis, and the ulna is dorsally subluxated.

of joint surface (185) (Fig. 8-39A and B). A physeal bar may be seen on CT at the lunate facet (183). The ulna is subluxated or dislocated dorsally. It is as long as, or longer than, the radius, in contrast to other causes of Madelung deformity mentioned in the differential diagnosis (186). The tibia and fibula are short, with the fibula longer than the tibia at the ankle and/or the knee. There may be some degree of genu varum or ankle valgus. Cubitus valgus, hypoplasia of the humeral head, and coxa valga have all been noted, but rarely do all occur in the same patient.

Orthopaedic Implications

Human growth hormone treatment may produce a sustained response, and patients concerned about short stature may be referred to an endocrinologist for discussion of this treatment (184,187). Patients who experience wrist pain may be treated initially by a wrist splint and antiinflammatory agents. If still symptomatic, a reconstruction with a double osteotomy of the distal radius and an ulnar recession, provides good results (188). This has shown improvement in symptoms and clinical appearance, but lunate subluxa-

tion, grip strength, and range of motion were minimally influenced (180). Although it has been described, it is unclear whether bar resection can allow normal growth to occur. Osteotomy of the tibia is occasionally indicated to correct genu varum (179).

CLEIDOCRANIAL DYSPLASIA

Cleidocranial dysplasia is a true skeletal dysplasia, because it affects the growth of many bones in all parts of the skeleton, primarily those of membranous origin. Classic features include a widening of the cranium, as well as dysplasia of the clavicle and the pelvis (189,190). The incidence is estimated at 1:200,000 (191). It is transmitted as an autosomal dominant condition, and the defect is in the *CFBA1* gene, which encodes a transcription factor required for osteoblast differentiation (192–194).

Clinical Features

Although the name suggests that only two bones are affected, there are numerous abnormalities. The patients have mildly to moderately diminished stature, with most female and some male patients below the fifth percentile for age. There is bossing in the frontal parietal and occipital regions. The maxillary region is underdeveloped, giving apparent exophthalmos and maxillary micrognathism. Cleft palate and dental abnormalities are common (195–198).

The clavicles are partially or completely absent (197); complete absence is present only 10% of the time. This causes the shoulders to drop and the neck to appear longer. The classic diagnostic feature is that the shoulders can be approximated, an ability which helped one college wrestler to escape holds (198). The pelvis is narrow. The hips are occasionally unstable at birth. Coxa vara may occur, causing limitation of abduction and a Trendelenburg gait. There is an increased incidence of scoliosis, and often a double thoracic curve. Syringomyelia has been reported in several patients with cleidocranial dysplasia and scoliosis (199–201). It has been recommended to perform MRI in patients with this dysplasia who have progressive scoliosis.

Radiographic Features

Prenatal radiographic diagnosis may be made on the basis of small or absent clavicles (Fig. 8-40). Nomograms are available for clavicular size during gestation (202). If a portion of the clavicle is present, it is usually the medial end. The skull of a newborn with this disorder has the maturation of a 20-week fetus (195). Wormian bones are present in the skull. The anterior fontanel may be open in adulthood (Fig. 8-41). In the vertebral column, spina bifida occulta and spondylolysis are common (203). The pelvis is narrow,

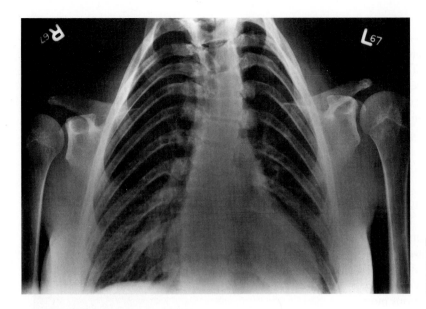

FIGURE 8-40. The clavicles are completely absent in the patient with cleidocranial dysplasia, although in many patients they are merely hypoplastic. There is also a characteristic mild scoliosis and an occult bifid lamina of T2.

and shows widening of the triradiate cartilage, delay in pubic ossification, and progressive deformation of the base of the femoral neck into varus (Fig. 8-42).

Orthopaedic Implications

No treatment is indicated for the clavicles. The coxa vara may be treated by valgus osteotomy if the neck shaft angle is less than 100 degrees (204). If there is acetabular dysplasia, this should be corrected first. Scoliosis should be treated according to usual guidelines. MRI should be performed if the curve is progressive, because of the increased risk of syringomyelia.

Cesarean section is often necessary. Craniofacial surgery may be helpful in correcting the skull defects, and many dental problems may develop. Pregnant women may have cephalopelvic disproportion, especially if the fetus has the same disorder, because of the mother's narrow pelvis and the fetus' enlarged cranium.

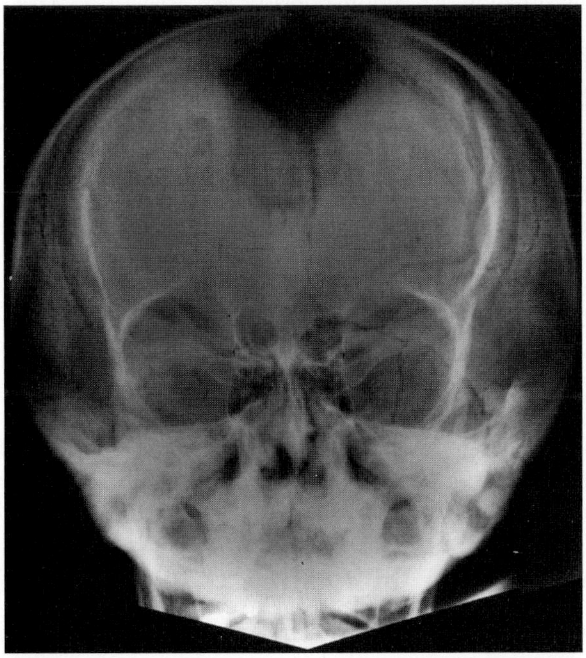

FIGURE 8-41. The skull in this teenager with cleidocranial dysplasia shows an enlarged cranium, widened sutures, and a persistent anterior fontanel.

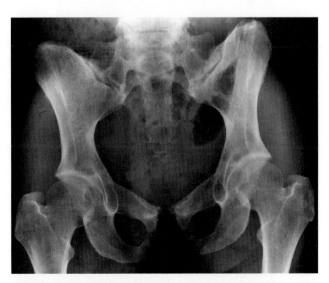

FIGURE 8-42. The pelvis in cleidocranial dysplasia is narrow. The symphysis pubis is widened, the ischiopubic synchondrosis is unossified, and there is mild coxa vara.

LARSEN SYNDROME

This syndrome was first described in 1950, when six cases were described having the unique combination of hypertelorism, multiple joint dislocations, and focal bone deformities (205). It has been reported in both autosomal dominant and recessive patterns. The gene is on chromosome 3 near, but distinct from, *COL7A1* locus 4,207; nothing more is currently known about it.

Clinical Features

The facial appearance involves widely spaced eyes, a depressed nasal bridge, and a prominent forehead. Cleft palate is common. The thumb has a wide distal phalanx and the fingers do not taper distally. Hypotonia has also been reported, but this may result from cervical compression (207). Sudden death has been reported (205,208), most was likely due to exacerbation of this compression. Dislocations most commonly involve the elbows (or radial heads), hips, and knees (Fig. 8-43), followed by the midfoot and shoulders. Characteristic foot deformities involve equinovarus or equinovalgus. Atrial and ventricular septal defects have been reported. Within the range of abnormalities just described, every patient with this syndrome is unique in his or her pattern of associated problems.

Radiographic Features

There does not appear to be a theme to the radiographic findings in this syndrome. Virtually every patient described,

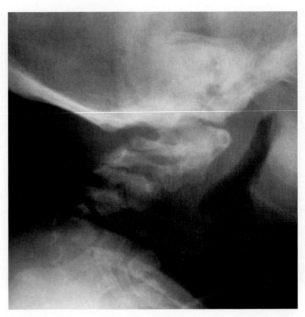

FIGURE 8-44. Cervical kyphosis occurs in many patients with Larsen syndrome, in association with spina bifida occulta of this region. The disorder is usually progressive. (Courtesy of George S. Bassett, M.D.)

however, has some abnormality in some part of the spine. The cervical spine is the most commonly and severely affected. Spina bifida is very common in the cervical spine. Perhaps because of this, the cervical vertebrae may develop a progressive kyphosis (Fig. 8-44). The vertebral bodies in this situation are very hypoplastic, especially C4 and C5. It is not clear whether this vertebral hypoplasia is a result of pressure from the kyphosis, or a separate, coincidental phenomenon that coexists with the posterior element deficiency. The incidence of cervical kyphosis in different series ranges from none to 60% (207,209,210). Other cervical problems that may occur include atlantoaxial or subaxial instability (209) and spondylolisthesis of vertebrae. The thoracic spine may also manifest spina bifida; scoliosis is seen in many, but it is usually mild and rarely requires treatment (209). In the lumbar spine, spondylolysis, kyphosis, scoliosis, and back pain may occur (209). Sacral spina bifida is common, but no neurologic compromise is reported.

One of the characteristic (although not universal) findings in Larsen syndrome is the presence of accessory calcaneal or carpal ossification centers (Fig. 8-45). Shortened metacarpals are also noted.

Orthopaedic Implications

At the beginning of treatment, the orthopaedic surgeon must rule out the cervical kyphosis that may accompany this syndrome, because of the catastrophic complications that have been reported. It may be easy to ascribe any developmental delay to the many other skeletal problems these

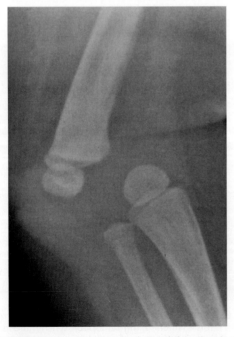

FIGURE 8-43. Congenital anterior knee dislocation is common in Larsen syndrome.

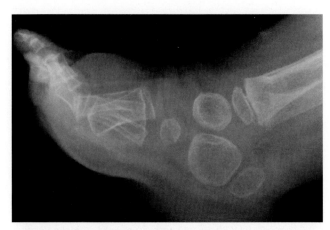

FIGURE 8-45. The feet in Larsen syndrome are usually in equino-varus, and show a characteristic accessory calcaneal ossification center.

children have, when in fact the cervical kyphosis may cause a neurologic basis for it. Because spontaneous improvement has not been reported in this kyphosis, as it has been in DD, it should be fused posteriorly if it exceeds about 35 to 45 degrees. At this level, posterior fusion alone over the involved segments may be successful, and may result in spontaneous correction with growth by acting as a posterior tether. If the kyphosis progresses to the point of myelopathy, an anterior corpectomy and fusion may be needed, and anterior growth will not occur. If enough iliac crest bone is not available for fusion, tibial bone may be used. After surgery, the patient should be in a brace or cast for 4 to 6 months (207). Laryngotracheomalacia may complicate induction of anesthesia.

The lower extremity problems are usually treated in a sequence beginning with the feet and the knees, then the hips. Treatment for clubfeet may be started early, inasmuch as some respond to manipulation and cast treatment with tenotomy. Recurrence is common, and should then be treated with complete subtalar release and shortening osteotomy or decancellation, as necessary. Knees that are hyperextended or subluxatable may be treated with casts as well, but this is unlikely to succeed in cases of complete dislocation. Such cases usually require open reduction with V-Y quadricepsplasty, anterior capsulotomy, and release of the anterior portions of the collateral ligaments. If cruciate deficiency leads to persistent anterior instability, reconstruction using parapatellar fascia is usually successful.

Whether to reduce hip dislocations in this condition remains controversial. Some series report that they are resistant to treatment (209,210), whereas others report some successful results (208,210). A failed treatment of a dislocated hip is less functional than one left untreated. A reasonable approach is to consider treatment of those hips in which the dislocation is not too high and the acetabulum is not too shallow, for patients with otherwise good prospects for activity. The medial approach [➡3.3, 3.4] may be used for infants, but for older children or those with a shallow acetabulum, an anterolateral approach [➡3.2] is preferred, with osteotomy or augmentation. If the hip subluxates easily or has a narrow safe zone, the clinician should not hesitate to perform a femoral shortening and derotation. My preference is to begin cast treatment for the feet and knees together, then to operate on the knees if they are resistant, then the feet if they are resistant. By that time, the surgeon will have a better idea of the patient's potential and can decide on the most appropriate approach to the hips.

PERINATAL LETHAL SKELETAL DYSPLASIAS

With the increasing use of prenatal diagnostic tests, the orthopaedic surgeon may be questioned about some of the lethal dysplasias that would not otherwise be encountered in practice. These are mentioned here to provide passing familiarity. The combined incidence of lethal dysplasias has been estimated at 15 per 100,000 births in one population. The natural history of these conditions should be considered carefully if one is facing a decision to provide respiratory support.

Thanatophoric dysplasia is characterized by disproportionately small limbs, normal trunk length, a protuberant abdomen, and a large head with frontal bossing. The chest is narrow and the lungs hypoplastic. The femora are bowed, and their appearance has been likened to old-style telephone receivers. There is phenotypic resemblance to homozygous achondroplasia, and in fact this condition results from a mutation in the same gene, fibroblast growth factor receptor protein-3. Only a few children with this disorder have been reported to survive past age 2 years, even with full respiratory support.

Achondrogenesis is characterized by a short trunk, large head, distended abdomen, and severely underdeveloped limbs. It has been subclassified into four types. It may be autosomal dominant or recessive. In fact, achondrogenesis type I results from a mutation in the DD sulfate transporter.

Survival beyond birth is very rare. No treatment is available to prolong the life span at present. Atelosteogenesis, of which there are two types, is characterized by dislocations of large joints and in some cases, clubfeet. Midface hypoplasia, micrognathism, and a narrow chest are also seen. At least one of the two types results from a mutation in the DD sulfate transporter.

Short rib–polydactyly syndrome is autosomal recessive and is characterized by polydactyly, which is classically postaxial but may be preaxial, short horizontal ribs, and defects in the kidneys and lungs.

Osteogenesis imperfecta type II is arguably a skeletal dysplasia. Because of the poor prognosis, some of these children have been treated by bone marrow transplants, with reports of prolonged survival.

Conditions that may be, but are not always, lethal in the neonatal period include: achondroplasia (homozygous form), rhizomelic chondrodysplasia punctata, camptomelic dysplasia, and a congenital form of hypophosphatasia.

Appendix 1: Clinical Summaries of Important Skeletal Dysplasias

Achondroplasia
Genetic Transmission: Autosomal dominant, but most patients have *de novo* mutation
Gene Defect: Highly uniform mutation in fibroblast growth factor receptor-3
Key Clinical Features: Stenosis of spine (esp. lumbar) or foramen magnum; thoracolumbar kyphosis; genu varum
Key Treatment Points: Brace thoracolumbar kyphosis if over 2 years old; decompress symptomatic stenosis; C-spine is stable; osteotomies for genu varum if symptomatic

Hypochondroplasia
Genetic Transmission: Autosomal dominant
Genetic Defect: Most in fibroblast growth factor receptor protein-3 (different domain)
Key Clinical Features: Mild short stature; mild spinal stenosis
Key Treatment Implications: May benefit from growth hormone and/or limb lengthening

Metatropic Dysplasia
Genetic Transmission: Autosomal dominant or recessive
Genetic Defect: Unknown
Key Clinical Features: Infant mortality risk; coccygeal tail, enlarged metaphyses, and contractures; kyphoscoliosis
Key Treatment Points: Rule out cervical instability; possible role for spine fusion

Chondroectodermal Dysplasia
Genetic Transmission: Autosomal recessive
Genetic Defect: Unknown
Key Clinical Features: Cardiac defects, teeth and nails abnormal, postaxial polydactyly; genu valgus, external femoral rotation

Diastrophic Dysplasia
Genetic Transmission: Autosomal recessive
Genetic Defect: Diastrophic dysplasia sulfate transporter abnormal in all cartilage
Key Clinical Features: "Hitchhiker" thumbs and "cauliflower" ears; joint contractures, cervical kyphosis; scoliosis; degenerative joint disease, equinovarus feet
Key Treatment Points: Monitor cervical kyphosis, fuse if increasing; correct feet; treat scoliosis, DJD

Kneist Dysplasia
Genetic Transmission: Autosomal dominant
Genetic Defect: Type II collagen, *COL2A1*, usually exons 12–24
Key Clinical Features: Large stiff joints; equinovarus; risk retinal detachment and odontoid hypoplasia

Spondyloepiphyseal Dysplasia Congenita
Genetic Transmission: Autosomal dominant
Genetic Defect: Type II Collagen, *COL2A1*
Key Clinical Features: Severely short stature, C1-2 instability, scoliosis, hip dysplasia, possible equinovarus foot

Spondyloepiphyseal Dysplasia Tarda
Genetic Transmission: X-linked most common
Genetic Defect: Type II collagen (*COL2A1*)
Key Clinical Features: Hip, back, or knee pain develop in later childhood/adolescence; mild scoliosis

Pseudoachondroplasia
Genetic Transmission: Autosomal dominant
Genetic Defect: Cartilage oligomeric matrix protein (COMP)
Key Clinical Features: Ligamentous laxity, windswept knees; size normal at birth, but falls behind

Multiple Epiphyseal Dysplasia
Genetic Transmission: Autosomal dominant
Genetic Defect: Some forms from cartilage oligomeric matrix protein (COMP), other forms from type IX collagen
Key Clinical Features: Near-normal stature; epiphyseal deformation of large joints with symptoms in late childhood or adulthood
Key Treatment Points: Observation versus acetabular coverage in childhood; joint replacement in adulthood

Chondrodysplasia Punctata
Genetic Transmission: Multiple
Genetic Defect: Rhizomelic form from peroxisomal enzyme deficiency; other forms unknown
Key Clinical Features: Neonatal stippling of epiphyses; early mortality (most rhizomelic patients)
Key Treatment Points: Evaluate and treat atlantoaxial instability, congenital scoliosis, coxa vara

Metaphyseal Chondrodysplasias
Mode of Inheritance: McKusick: autosomal recessive; Schmid, Jansen, and Kozlowski: autosomal dominant
Key Clinical Features: Metaphyseal irregularities with normal epiphyses; genu varum, mild short stature, fine sparse hair; immune and GI disorders in McKusick type
Key Treatment Points: Rule out rare atlantoaxial instability; correct genu varum if severe; monitor medical problems in McKusick type

Diaphyseal Aclasia (Multiple Osteocartilaginous Exostosis)
Genetic Transmission: Autosomal dominant
Genetic Mutation: Mutations found on chromosomes 8, 11, and 19
Key Clinical Features: Short stature, impingement on tendons and nerves, angular deformities, limb length inequality, malignant degeneration
Key Treatment Implications: Monitor for growth disturbances, remove symptomatic exostoses, educate about signs of slight malignant degeneration

Dyschondrosteosis (Leri-Weill Syndrome)
Genetic Mutation: Short stature homeobox gene (*SHOX*)
Key Treatment Points: Osteotomies may be indicated to correct forearm deformities

Cleidocranial Dysplasia
Genetic Transmission: Autosomal dominant
Genetic Defect: Defect in human *CBFA1* gene
Key Clinical Features: Widened cranium, clavicles partially or completely absent, unossified pubic rami; hip abnormalities
Key Treatment Issues: Hip surgery for dysplasia or varus; care of dental, cranial, and obstetric problems

Larsen Syndrome
Genetic Transmission: Autosomal dominant or recessive
Genetic Defect: Unknown
Key Clinical Features: Widely spaced eyes, depressed nasal bridge, multiple joint dislocations, cervical kyphosis

References

General Principles

1. Beighton P. *McKusick's heritable disorders of connective tissue*. St. Louis: Mosby–Year Book, 1993.

2. Beighton P, Geidon A, Gorlin R, et al. International classification of osteochondrodysplasias. *Am J Med Genet* 1992;44:223.

3. Goncalves L, Jeanty P. Fetal biometry of skeletal dysplasias: a multicentric study. *J Ultrasound Med* 1994;13:767.

4. Tobias JD. Anesthetic implications of Larsen syndrome. *J Clin Anesth* 1996;8(3):255.

5. Bethem D, Winter RB, Lutter I, et al. Spinal disorders of dwarfism: review of the literature and report of eighty cases. *J Bone Joint Surg Am* 1981;63:1412.

6. Bethem D, Winter RB, Lutter I. Disorders of the spine in diastrophic dwarfism. *J Bone Joint Surg Am* 1981;62:529.

Achondroplasia

7. Dietz FR, Matthews KD. Current concepts review: update on the genetic bases of disorders with orthopaedic manifestations. *J Bone Joint Surg Am* 1996;78:1583.

8. Hall JG. The natural history of achondroplasia. *Basic Life Sci* 1988;48:3.

9. Horton WA. Fibroblast growth factor receptor 3 and the human chondrodysplasias. *Curr Opin Pediatr* 1997;9:437.

10. Muenke M, Schell U. Fibroblast growth factor receptor mutations in human skeletal disorders. *Trends Genet* 1981;11:308.

11. Seino Y, Moriwake T, Tanaka H, et al. Molecular defects in achondroplasia and the effects of growth hormone treatment. *Acta Pediatr* 1999;428(suppl):118.

12. Shiang R, Thompson LM, Zhu Y-Z, et al. Mutations in the transmembrane domain of FGFR3 cause the most common genetic form of dwarfism, achondroplasia. *Cell* 1994;78:335.

13. Wynn-Davies R, Walsh WK, Gormley J. Achondroplasia and hypochondroplasia: clinical variation and spinal stenosis. *J Bone Joint Surg Br* 1981;63:508.

14. Maynard JA, Ippolito EG, Ponseti IV, et al. Histochemistry and ultrastructure of the growth plate in achondroplasia. *J Bone Joint Surg Am* 1981;63:969.

15. Ponseti IV. Skeletal growth in achondroplasia. *J Bone Joint Surg Am* 1970;52:701.

16. Bailey JA. Orthopaedic aspects of achondroplasia. *J Bone Joint Surg Am* 1970;52:1285.

17. Nehme A-ME, Riseborough EJ, Tredwell SJ. Skeletal growth and development of the achondroplastic dwarf. *Clin Orthop* 1976;116:88.

18. Pauli RM, Breed A, Horton VK, et al. Prevention of fixed, angular kyphosis in achondroplasia. *J Pediatr Orthop* 1997;17:726.

19. Scott CI. Achondroplastic and hypochondroplastic dwarfism. *Clin Orthop* 1976;114a:18.

20. Pauli RM, Horton VK, Glinske LP, et al. Prospective assessment of risks for cervicomedullary-junction compression in infants with achondroplasia. *Am J Human Genet* 1995;56:732.

21. Pierre-Kahn A, Hirsch JF, Renier D. Hydrocephalus and achondroplasia: a study of 25 observations. *Childs Brain* 1980;7:205.

22. Todorov AB, Scott CI, Warren AE, et al. Developmental screening tests in achondroplastic children. *Am J Med Genet* 1981;9:19.

23. Hecht JT, Nelson FW, Butler IJ, et al. Computerized tomography of the foramen magnum: achondroplastic values compared to normal standards. *Am J Med Genet* 1985;20:355.

24. Hecht JT, Horton W, Reid CS, et al. Growth of the foramen magnum in achondroplasia. *Am J Med Genet* 1989;32:528.

25. Lutter LD, Lonstein JE, Winter RB, et al. Anatomy of the achondroplastic lumbar canal. *Clin Orthop* 1977;126:139.

26. Lutter LD, Langer LO. Neurological symptoms in achondroplastic. *J Bone Joint Surg Am* 1977;59:87.

27. Waters KA, Everett FM, Sillence DO, et al. Treatment of obstructive sleep apnea in achondroplasia; evaluation of sleep, breathing and somatosensory-evoked potentials. *Am J Med Genet* 1995;59:460.

28. Hecht JA, Francomano C, Horton W, et al. Mortality in achondroplasia. *Am J Hum Genet* 1987;41:454.

29. Horton WA, Hecht JT, Hood OJ, et al. Growth hormone therapy in achondroplasia. *Am J Med Genet* 1992;42:667.

30. Tanaka H, Kubo T, Yamate T, et al. Effect of growth hormone therapy in children with achondroplasia: growth pattern, hypothalamic-pituitary function and genotype. *Eur J Endocrinol* 1998;138:275.

31. Berkowitz RG, Grundfast KM, Scott C, et al. Middle ear disease in childhood achondroplasia. *Ear Nose Throat J* 1991;70:305.

32. Glass L, Shapiro I, Hodge S, et al. Audiological findings of patients with achondroplasia. *J Pediatr Otorhinolaryngol* 1981;11:129.

33. Zucconi M, Weber G, Castronov V, et al. Sleep and upper airway obstruction in children with achondroplasia. *J Pediatr* 1996;129:743.

34. Stokes DC, Pyeritz RE, Wise RA, et al. Spirometry and chest wall dimensions in achondroplasia. *Chest* 1988;93:34.

35. Stokes DC, Woh ME, Wise RA, et al. The lungs and airways in achondroplasia. Do little people have little lungs? *Chest* 1988;98:145.

36. Dietz FR. Spike osteotomy for angular deformities of the long bones in children. *J Bone Joint Surg Am* 1988;70:848.

37. Rab GT. Oblique tibial osteotomy for tibia vara. *J Pediatr Orthop* 1988;8:715.

38. Aldigheri R. Femoral callotasis. *J Pediatr Orthop* 1997;17B:42.

39. Aldigheri R. Distraction osteogenesis for lengthening of the tibia in patients who have limb-length discrepancy of short stature. *J Bone Joint Surg Am* 1999;81:624.

40. Villarrubias JM, Ginebreda I, Jimeno E. Lengthening of the lower limbs and correction of lumbar hyperlordosis in achondroplasia. *Clin Orthop* 190;250:143.

41. Siebens AA, Hungerford DS, Kirgy NA. Curves of the achondroplastic spine: a new hypothesis. *Johns Hopkins Med J* 1978;142:205.

42. Kopits SE. Orthopaedic complications of dwarfism. *Clin Orthop* 1976;114:153.

43. Tolo VT. Surgical treatment of kyphosis In: Nicoletti B, ed. *Achondroplasia: human achondroplasia, a multidisciplinary approach.* New York: Plenum, 1986:257.

44. Pyeritz RE, Sack GH, Udvarhelyi GB. Thoracolumbosacral laminectomy in achondroplasia: long-term results in 22 patients. *Am J Med Genet* 1987;28:433.

45. Uematsu S, Hurko O. The subarachnoid fluid space in achondroplastic spinal stenosis: the surgical implications. In: Nicoletti B, ed. *Achondroplasia: human achondroplasia, a multidisciplinary approach.* New York: Plenum, 1986:275.

Hypochondroplasia

46. Horton WA. Evolution of the bone dysplasia family. *Am J Med Genet* 1996;63:4.

47. Rousseau F, Bonaventure J, Legeai-Mallet L, et al. Clinical and genetic heterogeneity of hypochondroplasia. *J Med Genet* 1996;33:749.

48. Su WC, Kitawaga M, Xue N, et al. Activation of Stat1 by mutant fibroblast growth-factor receptor in thanatophoric dysplasia type II dwarfism. *Nature* 1997;386:288.

49. Beals RK. Hypochondroplasia: a report of five kindreds. *J Bone Joint Surg Am* 1969;51:728.

50. Hall BD, Spranger J. Hypochondroplasia: clinical and radiological aspects in 39 cases. *Radiology* 1979;133:95.

51. Fasanelli S. Hypochondroplasia: radiological diagnosis and differential diagnosis. In: Nicoletti B, ed. *Achondroplasia: human*

achondroplasia, a multidisciplinary approach. New York: Plenum, 1999:163.

52. Oberklaid F, Danks DM, Jansen F, et al. Achondroplasia and hypochondroplasia. Comments on frequency, mutation rate, and radiological features in skull and spine. *J Med Genet* 1979; 16:140.

53. Ramaswami U, Hindmarsh PC, Brook CGD. Growth hormone therapy in hypochondroplasia. *Acta Pediatr* 1999;428(suppl): 116.

54. Yasui N, Kawabata H, Kojimoto H, et al. Lengthening of the lower limbs in patients with achondroplasia and hypochondroplasia. *Clin Orthop* 1997;Nov(344):298.

Metatropic Dysplasia

55. Rimoin DW, Siggers DC, Lachman RS, et al. Metatropic dwarfism, the Kneist syndrome and the pseudoachondroplastic dysplasias. *Clin Orthop* 1982;176:70.

56. Boden SD, Kaplan FS, Fallon MD, et al. Metatropic dwarfism. uncoupling of endochondral and perichondral growth. *J Bone Joint Surg Am* 1987;69:174.

57. Shohat M, Lachman R, Rimoin DL. Odontoid hypoplasia with vertebral subluxation and ventriculomegaly in metatropic dysplasia. *J Pediatr* 1989;114:239.

58. Beck M, Roubecheck M, Rogers JG, et al. Heterogeneity of metatropic dysplasia. *Eur J Pediatr* 1983;140:231.

59. Maroteaux P, Sprange JW, Weidemann HR. Der metatrophische Zwergwuchs. *Arch Kinder* 1966;173: 211.

60. Gordienko IY, Grechanin EY, Sopko NI, et al. Prenatal diagnosis of osteochondrodysplasias in high risk pregnancy. *Am J Med Genet* 1996;63:90.

61. Manouvrier-Hanu S, Devisme L, Zelasko MC, et al. Prenatal diagnosis of metatropic dwarfism. *Prenatal Diag* 1995;15:753.

Chondroectodermal Dysplasia

62. Ellis RWB, van Creveld S. A syndrome characterized by ectodermal dysplasia, polydactyly, chondrodysplasia and congenital morbis cordia. *Arch Dis Child* 1940;15:65.

63. Ide SE, Ortiz de Luna RI, Francomano CA, et al. Exclusion of the MAX1 homeobox gene as the gene for the Ellis van Creveld syndrome in the Amish. *Hum Genet* 1996;98:572.

64. Polymeropoulos MH, Ide SE, Wright M, et al. The gene for the Ellis-van Creven syndrome is located on chromosome 4p16. *Genomics* 1996;35:1.

65. Quereshi F, Jacques SM, Evans MI, et al. Skeletal histopathology in fetuses with chondroectodermal dysplasia (Ellis van Creveld syndrome). *Am J Med Genet* 1996;3:471.

66. Kaitila H, Leisti JT, Rimoin DL. Mesomelic skeletal dysplasias. *Clin Orthop* 1976;114:94.

67. McKusick VA, Egeland JA, Eldridge R. Dwarfism in the Amish. *Johns Hopkins Hosp Bull* 1964;115:125.

68. Pinelli G, Cottefava F, Senes FM, et al. Ellis-van Creveld syndrome: description of four cases: orthopedic aspects. *Ital J Orthop Traumatol* 1990;16:113.

69. Kruse RK, Bowen JR. Oblique tibial osteotomy in the correction of tibial deformity in children. *J Pediatr Orthop* 1989;9: 476.

70. Paley D, Tetsworth K. Mechanical axis deviation of the lower limbs: preoperative planning of uniapical frontal plane angular and bowing deformities of the femur or tibia. *Clin Orthop* 1992; 280:65.

Diastrophic Dysplasia

71. Hollister DW, Lachman RS. Diastrophic dwarfism. *Clin Orthop* 1976;114:61.

72. Ryoeppy S, Poussa M, Merikanto J, et al. Foot deformities in diastrophic dysplasia. An analysis of 102 patients. *J Bone Joint Surg Br* 1992;74:441.

73. Hastbacka J, Kaitila I, Sistonene P, et al. A linkage map spanning the locus for diastrophic dysplasia (DTD). *Genomics* 1991; 11:968.

74. Hastbacka J, De la Chapelle A, Mahtani MM, et al. The diastrophic dysplasia gene encodes a novel sulfate transporter. *Cell* 1664;78:1073.

75. Superti-Furga A, Rossi A, Steinmann B, et al. Achondrodysplasia family produced by mutations in the diastrophic dysplasia sulfate transporter gene: genotype/phenotype correlations. *Am J Med Genet* 1996;63:144.

76. Lamy M, Maroteaux P. Le nanisme diastrophique. *Presse Med* 1990;68:1977.

77. Qureshi F, Jacques SM, Johnson SF, et al. Histopathology of fetal diastrophic dysplasia. *Am J Med Genet* 1995;56:300.

78. Walker BA, Scott CI, Hall JG, et al. Diastrophic dwarfism. *Medicine (Baltimore)* 1972;51:41.

79. Poussa M, Merikano J, Ryoppy S, et al. The spine in diastrophic dysplasia. *Spine* 1991;16:881.

80. Herring JA. The spinal disorders in diastrophic dwarfism. *J Bone Joint Surg Am* 1978;60:177.

81. Remes V, Marttinen E, Poussa M, et al. Cervical kyphosis in diastrophic dysplasia. *Spine* 1999;24:1990.

82. Kash IJ, Sane SM, Samaha FJ. Cervical cord compression in diastrophic dwarfism. *J Pediatr* 1974;84:862.

83. Tolo VT, Kopits SE. Spinal deformity in diastrophic dysplasia. *Orthop Trans* 1983;7:1983.

84. Vaara P, Peltonen J, Poussa M, et al. Development of the hip in diastrophic dysplasia. *J Bone Joint Surg Br* 1998;80:315.

85. Horton WA, Rimoin DL, Lachman RS, et al. The phenotypic variability of diastrophic dysplasia. *J Pediatr* 1978;93:609.

86. Merrill KD. Occipitoatlantal instability in a child with Kneist syndrome. *J Pediatr* 1990;116:596.

87. Horton WA, Hall JG, Scott CL, et al. Growth curves for height for diastrophic dysplasia, spondyloepiphyseal dysplasia congenita and pseudoachondroplasia. *Am J Dis Child* 1982;136: 316.

88. Makitie O, Kaitila I. Growth in diastrophic dysplasia. *J Pediatr* 1991;130:641.

89. Peltonen JL, Hoikka V, Poussa M, et al. Cementless hip arthroplasty in diastrophic dysplasia. *J Arthroplasty* 1992; 7(suppl):369.

Kneist Dysplasia

90. Kneist W. Zur abgrenzung der dysostoses endochondralis von der chondrodystrophie. *Z Kinder* 1952;70:633.

91. Spranger J, Winterpracht A, Zabel B. Kneist dysplasia: Dr. W. Kneist, his patient, the molecular defect. *Am J Med Genet* 1997; 9:79.

92. Cole WG. Abnormal skeletal growth in Kneist dysplasia caused by type II collagen mutations. *Clin Orthop* 1997;341:169.

93. Wilkin DJ, Artz AS, South S, et al. Small deletions in the type II collagen triple helix produce Kneist dysplasia. *Am J Med Genet* 1999;85:105.

94. Poole AR, Pidoux I, Reiner A, et al. Kneist dysplasia is characterized by an apparent abnormal processing of the C-propeptide of type II collagen resulting in imperfect fibril assembly. *J Clin Invest* 1988;81:579.

95. Gilbert-Barnes E, Langer L. O. Kneist dysplasia: radiologic histopathologic and scanning EM findings. *Am J Med Genet* 1996; 63:34.

96. Lachman R, Sillence D, Rimoin D. Diastrophic dysplasia: death of a variant. *Radiology* 1981;140:79.

97. Spranger JW, Maroteaux P. Kneist disease. *Birth Defects* 1974; 10:50.
98. Siggers DC, Rimoin DL, Dorst JP, et al. The Kneist syndrome. *Birth Defects* 1974;10:193.

Spondyloepiphyseal Dysplasia Congenita

99. Cole WG, Hall RK, Rogers JG. The clinical features of spondyloepiphyseal dysplasia congenita resulting from the substitution of glycine 997 by serin in the alpha1(II) chain of type II collagen. *J Med Genet* 1993;30:27.
100. Harrod MJ, Friedman JM, Currarino G, et al. Genetic heterogeneity in spondyloepiphyseal dysplasia congenita. *Am J Med Genet* 1984;18:311.
101. Tiller GE, Weis MA, Polumbo PA, et al. An RNA-splicing mutation in the type II collagen gene in a family with spondyloepiphyseal dysplasia congenita. *Am Hum Genet* 1995;56:388.
102. Wynne-Davies R, Hall C. Two clinical variants of spondyloepiphyseal dysplasia congenita. *J Bone Joint Surg Br* 1982;64:435.
103. Spranger JW, Langer LO Jr. Spondyloepiphyseal dysplasia congenita. *Radiology* 1970;94:313.
104. Williams B, Cranley RE. Morphologic observations on four cases of SED congenita. *Birth Defects* 1974;10:75.
105. LeDoux MS, Naftalis RC, Aronin PA. Stabilization of the cervical spine in spondyloepiphyseal dysplasia congenita. *Neurosurgery* 1991;28:580.

Spondyloepiphyseal Dysplasia Tarda

106. Yang SS, Chen H, Williams P, et al. Spondyloepiphyseal dysplasia congenita: a comparative study of chondrocyte inclusions. *Arch Pathol Lab Med* 1980;104:208.
107. Kaibara N, Takagishi K, Katsuki I. Spondyloepiphyseal dysplasia tarda with progressive arthropathy. *Skeletal Radiol* 1983;10: 13.
108. Pinelli G, Cottefava F, Senes FM. Spondyloepiphyseal dysplasia tarda: linkage with genetic markers from the distal short arm of the X chromosome. *Hum Genet* 1988;81:61.
109. Crossan JF, Wynne-Davies R, Fulford GE. Bilateral failure of the capital femoral epiphysis: bilateral Perthes disease, multiple epiphyseal dysplasia, pseudoachondroplasia, and spondyloepiphyseal dysplasia. *Pediatr Orthop* 1986;8:197.
110. Diamond LS. A family study of spondyloepiphyseal dysplasia. *J Bone Joint Surg Am* 1970;52:1587.

Pseudoachondroplasia

111. Maroteaux P, Lamy M. Les formes pseudoachondroplastique des dysplasies spondyloepisaires. *Presse Med* 1959;67:383.
112. Cooper RR, Ponseti IV, Maynard JA. Pseudoachondroplastic dwarfism. A rough-surfaced endoplasmic reticulum storage disorder. *J Bone Joint Surg Am* 1973;55:475.
113. Deere M, Sanford T, Francomano CA, et al. Identification of nine novel mutations in COMP in patients with pseudoachondroplasia and multiple epiphyseal dysplasia. *Am J Med Genet* 1999;85:486.
114. Ferguson HL, Deere M, Evans R, et al. Mosaicism in pseudoachondroplasia. *Am J Med Genet* 1997;70:287.
115. Stevens JW. Pseudoachondroplastic dysplasia: an Iowa review from human to mouse. *Iowa Orthop J* 1999;19:53.
116. Hecht JT, Montufar-Solis D, Decker G, et al. Retention of COMP and cell death in redifferentiated pseudoachondroplasia chondrocytes. *Matrix Biol* 1998;17:33.
117. Pedrini-Mille A, Maynard JA, Pedrinie VA. Pseudoachondroplasia: biochemical and histochemical studies of cartilage. *J Bone Joint Surg Am* 1984;66:1408.

118. Horton WA, Hall JG, Scott CI, et al. Growth curves for height for diastrophic dysplasia, spondyloepiphyseal dysplasia congenita and pseudoachondroplasia. *Am J Dis Child* 1982;136: 316.
119. Hall JG. Pseudoachondroplasia. *Birth Defects* 1975;11:187.
120. Hall JG, Bailey JA, Dorst JP, et al. Pseudoachondroplastic SED, recessive Maroteaux-Lamy type. *Birth Defects* 1969;5:254.
121. McKeand J, Rotta J, Hecht JT. Natural history study of pseudoachondroplasia. *Am J Med Genet* 1996;63:406.
122. Wynne-Davies R, Hall CM, Young ID. Pseudoachondroplasia: clinical diagnosis at different ages and comparison of autosomal dominant and recessive types. A review of 32 patients. *J Med Genet* 1986;23:425.

Multiple Epiphyseal Dysplasia

123. Fairbank T. Dysplasia epiphysealis multiplex. *Br J Surg* 1947; 34:325.
124. Ribbing S. Studien uber Hereditaire multiple Epiphysenstorungen. *Acta Radiol* 1937;(suppl):34.
125. Stanescu T, Stanescu V, Muriel ME, et al. Multiple epiphyseal dysplasia, Fairbank type: morphologic and biochemical study of cartilage. *Am J Med Genet* 1993;45:501.
126. Van Mourik JB, Hamel BC, Mariman EC. A large family with multiple epiphyseal dysplasia linked to COL9A2 gene. *Am J Med Genet* 1998;77:234.
127. Jacobs PA. Dysplasia epiphysealis multiplex. *Clin Orthop* 1968; 58:117.
128. Schlesinger AE, Poznanski AK, Pudlowski RM, et al. Distal femoral epiphyses: normal standards for thickness and application to bone dysplasias. *Radiology* 1968;159:515.
129. Treble NJ, Jensen FO, Bankier A, et al. Development of the hip in multiple epiphyseal dysplasia. Natural history and susceptibility to premature osteoarthritis. *J Bone Joint Surg Br* 1990; 72.
130. MacKenzie WG, Gassett GS, Mandell GA, et al. Avascular necrosis of the hip in multiple epiphyseal dysplasia. *J Pediatr Orthop* 1989;9:666.
131. Apley AG, Weintroub S. The sagging rope sign in Perthes disease and allied disorders. *J Bone Joint Surg Br* 1981;63:43.
132. Hodkinson HM. Double layered patellae in multiple epiphyseal dysplasia. *J Bone Joint Surg Br* 1962;44:569.
133. Eddy MC, Steiner RD, McAlister WH, et al. Bilateral radial ray hypoplasia with multiple epiphyseal dysplasia. *Am J Med Genet* 1998;77:182.
134. Haga N, Nakamura K, Takikawa K, et al. Stature and severity in multiple epiphyseal dysplasia. *J Pediatr Orthop* 1998;18:394.
135. Spranger J. The epiphyseal dysplasias. *Clin Orthop* 1976;114: 46.
136. Kruse RW, Guille JT, Bowen JR. Shelf arthroplasty in patients who have Legg-Calvé-Perthes disease. *J Bone Joint Surg Am* 1991;73:1338.
137. Willet K, Hudson I, Catterall A. Lateral shelf acetabuloplasty: an operation for older children with Perthes disease. *J Pediatr Orthop* 1992;12:563.
138. Ingram RR. The shoulder in multiple epiphyseal dysplasia. *J Bone Joint Surg Br* 1991;73:277.

Chondrodysplasia Punctata

139. Andersen PE, Justesen P. Chondrodysplasia punctata: report of two cases. *Skeletal Radiol* 1987;16:223.
140. Wulfsberg EA, Curtis J, Jayne CH. Chondrodysplasia punctata: a boy linked with X-linked recessive chondrodysplasia punctata due to an inherited x-y translocation with a current classification of these disorders. *Am J Med Genet* 1992;43:823.

141. Borg SA, Fitzer PM, Young LY. Roentgenologic aspects of adult cretinism. *AJR Am J Roentgenol* 1975;123:820.

142. Hanson JW, Smith DW. The fetal hydantoin syndrome. *J Pediatr* 1975;87:285.

143. Harrod MJ, Sherrod PS. Warfarin embryopathy in siblings. *Obstet Gynecol* 1981;57:673.

144. Pauli RM, Lian JB, Mosher DF, et al. Association of congenital deficiency of multiple vitamin K-dependent coagulation factors and the phenotype of the warfarin embryopathy: clues to the mechanism of teratogenicity of coumarin derivatives. *Am J Med Genet* 1987;41:566.

145. Pike MG, Applegarth DA, Dunn HG, et al. Congenital rubella syndrome associated with calcific epiphyseal stippling and peroxismal dysfunction. *J Pediatr* 1990;116:88.

146. Curry CJR, Magenis RE, Brown M, et al. Inherited chondrodysplasia punctata due to deletion of the terminal short arm of X-chromosome. *N Engl J Med* 1984;311:1010.

147. Wardinsky TD, Pagon RA, Powell BR, et al. Rhizomelic chondrodysplasia punctata and survival beyond one year: a review of the literature and five case reports. *Clin Genet* 1990;38:84.

148. Gilbert EF, Opitz JM, Spranger JW, et al. Chondrodysplasia punctata—rhizomelic form, pathologic and radiographic studies of three infants. *Eur J Pediatr* 1976;123:89.

149. Happle R. X-linked dominant chondrodysplasia punctata. *Hum Genet* 1979;53:65.

150. Manzke H, Christophers E, Wiedmann H-R. Dominant sex-linked inherited chondrodysplasia punctata. *Clin Genet* 1980;17:97.

151. Silengo MC, Luzzatti L, Silverman FN. Clinical and genetic aspects of Conradi-Hunermann disease: a report of three familial cases and review of the literature. *J Pediatr* 1980;97:911.

152. Spranger JW, Opitz JM, Bidder U. Heterogeneity of chondrodysplasia punctata. *Humangenetik* 1971;11:190.

153. Heymans HAS, Oorthuys J, Nelck G, et al. Rhizomelic chondrodysplasia punctata: another peroxismal disorder. *N Engl J Med* 1985;313:187.

154. Hoefler S, Hoefler G, Moser AB, et al. Prenatal diagnosis of rhizomelic chondrodysplasia punctata. *Prenat Diagn* 1988;8:571.

155. Mueller RF, Crowle PM, Jones R, et al. X-linked dominant chondrodysplasia punctata. *Am J Med Genet* 1985;20:137.

156. Rittler M, Menger H, Spranger J. Chondrodysplasia punctata, tibia-metacarpal (TM) type. *Am J Med Genet* 1990;37:200.

157. Burck U. Mesomelic dysplasia with punctate epiphyseal calcifications. *Eur J Pediatr* 1982;138:67.

158. Bethem D. Os odontoideum in chondrodystrophia calcificans congenita. A case report. *J Bone Joint Surg Am* 1982;64:1385.

159. Sheffield LJ, Halliday JL, Danks DM, et al. Clinical, radiologic, and biochemical classification of chondrodysplasia punctata. *Am J Med Genet* 1989;45(suppl A):A64.

160. Fairbank HAT. Dysplasia epiphysealis punctata. Symptoms: stippled epiphyses, chondrodystrophia calcificans congenita Hünermann. *J Bone Joint Surg Br* 1949;31:114.

161. Lawrence JJ, Schlensinger AE, Kozlowski K, et al. Unusual radiographic manifestations of chondrodysplasia punctata. *Skeletal Radiol* 1989;18:15.

Metaphyseal Chondrodysplasias

162. Cooper RR. Metaphyseal dysapostosis: description of an ultrastructural defect in the epiphyseal plate chondrocytes. *J Bone Joint Surg Am* 1973;55:485.

163. Evans R, Caffey J. Metaphyseal dysostosis resembling vitamin D-refractory rickets. *Am J Dis Child* 1958;95:640.

164. Kozlowski K. Metaphyseal and spondylometaphyseal chondrodysplasia. *Clin Orthop* 1976;114:83.

165. Maynard JA, Ippolito EG, Ponseti IV, et al. Histochemistry and ultrastructure of the growth plate in metaphyseal dystosis: further observations on the structure of the cartilage matrix. *J Pediatr Orthop* 1981;1:161.

166. Tiller GE, Polumbo PA, Weis MA, et al. Dominant mutations in the type II collagen gene, COL2A1, produce spondyloepimetaphyseal dysplasia, Strudwick type. *Nat Genet* 1995;11:87.

167. Sulisalo T, van der Burgt I, Rimoin DL, et al. Genetic homogeneity of cartilage-hair hypoplasia. *Hum Genet* 1995;95:157.

168. Makitie O, Kaitila I. Cartilage-hair hypoplasia—clinical manifestations in 108 Finnish patients. *Eur J Pediatr* 1993;152:211.

169. Makitie O, Marttinen E, Kaitila I. Skeletal growth in cartilage-hair hypoplasia: a radiologic study of 82 patients. *Pediatr Radiol* 1992;22:434.

170. Juvonen E, Makitie O, Makipernaa E, et al. Defective in-vitro colony formation of haematopoietic progenitors in patients with cartilage-hair hypoplasia and history of anemia. *Eur J Pediatr* 1995;154:30.

171. Berthet F, Siegrist CA, Ozsahin H, et al. Bone marrow transplantation in cartilage-hair hypoplasia. *Eur J Pediatr* 1996;155:286.

172. van der Burgt I, Haraldsson A, Oosterwijk JC, et al. Cartilage hair hypoplasia. description of seven patients and review of the literature. *Am J Med Genet* 1991;41:371.

173. Wasylenko MJ, Wedge JH, Houston CS. Metaphyseal chondrodysplasia, Schmid type. *J Bone Joint Surg Am* 1980;62:660.

174. Paschalis EP, Jacenko O, Olsen B, et al. Fourier transform infrared microspectroscopic analysis identifies alterations in mineral properties in bones from mice transgenic for type X collagen. *Bone* 1996;19:151.

175. Wallis GA, Rash B, Sykes B, et al. Mutations within the gene encoding the alpha1 (X) chain of type X collagen cause metaphyseal chondrodysplasia type Schmid but not several other forms. *J Med Genet* 1996;33:450.

176. Chan D, Weng YM, Hocking AM, et al. Site-directed mutagenesis of type X collagen. *J Biol Chem* 1996;271:13566.

177. Schipani E, Jensen GS, Pincus J, et al. Constitutive activation of the cyclic adenosine monophosphate signaling pathway by parathyroid hormone receptors mutated at the two loci for Jansen's metaphyseal chondrodysplasia. *Mol Endocrinol* 1997;11:851.

Dyschondrosteosis (Leri-Weill Syndrome)

178. Leri A, Weill J. Une affection congenitale et symmetrique du developpement asseux: la dyschondrosteose. *Bull Med Soc Hosp Paris* 1929;53:1491.

179. Dawe C, Wynne-Davies RW, Fulford GE. Clinical variation in dyschondrosteosis. *J Bone Joint Surg Br* 1982;64:377.

180. Murphy MS, Linscheid RL, Dobyns JH, et al. Radial opening wedge osteotomy in Madelung's deformity. *J Hand Surg* 1996;21A:1035.

181. Mohan V, Gupta RP, Helmi K, et al. Leri-Weill syndrome: a family study. *J Hand Surg Br* 1988;13:16.

182. Shears DJ, Vassal HJ, Goodman FR, et al. Mutation and deletion of the pseudoautosomal gene SHOX causes Leri-Weill dyschondrosteosis. *Nat Genet* 1998;19:70.

183. Cook PA, Yu JS, Wiand W, et al. Madelung deformity in skeletally immature patients: morphologic assessment using radiography, CT and MRI. *J Comput Assist Tomogr* 1996;20:505.

184. Thuestad IJ, Ivarsson SA, Nilsson KO, et al. Growth hormone treatment in Leri-Weill syndrome. *J Pediatr Endocrinol Metab* 1996;9:201.

185. Felman AH, Kirkpatrick JA. Dyschondrosteoses: mesomelic dwarfism of Leri and Weill. *Am J Dis Child* 1999;120:329.

186. Langer LO. Dyschondrosteosis, a heritable bone dysplasia with

characteristic roentgenographic features. *AJR Am J Roentgenol* 1965;95:178.

187. Burren CP, Werther GA. Skeletal dysplasias: response to growth hormone therapy. *J Pediatr Endocrinol Metab* 1996;9:31.

188. Vickers D, Nielsen G. Madelung deformity: surgical prophylaxis (physiolysis) during the late growth period by resection of the dyschondrosteosis lesion. *J Hand Surg Br* 1992;17:401.

Cleidocranial Dysplasia

189. Bick EM, Marie P, Saiton P. The classic: on hereditary cleidocranial dysostosis. *Clin Orthop* 1968;58:5.

190. Marie P, Seinton P. Observation d'hydrocephalie hereditaire par vice de developpement du crane et du cerveau. *Rev Neurol* 1897;5:394.

191. Martinez-Frias ML, Herranz I, Salvador AI. Prevalence of dominant mutations in Spain: effect of changes in maternal age distribution. *Am J Med Genet* 1988;31:645.

192. Geoffroy V, Corral DA, Ahou L, et al. Genomic organization, expression of the human CBFA1 gene, and evidence for an alternative splicing event affecting protein function. *Mamm Genome* 1999;9:54.

193. Lee B, Thirunavukkarasu K, Zhou L, et al. Missense mutations abolishing DNA binding of the osteoblast-specific transcription factor OSF2/CBFA1 in cleidocranial dysplasia. *Nat Genet* 1997;16:307.

194. Otto F, Thornell AP, Crompton T. cfba1, a candidate gene for cleidocranial dysplasia syndrome, is essential for osteoblast differentiation and bone development. *Cell* 1997;89:765.

195. Jensen BL. Somatic development in cleidocranial dysplasia. *Am J Med Genet* 1990;35:69.

196. Jensen BL. Development of the skull in infants with cleidocranial dysplasia. *J Craniofac Genet Dev Biol* 1993;13:89.

197. Miles PW. Cleidocranial dysostosis: a survey of six new cases and 126 from the literature. *J Kansas Med Soc* 1940;41:462.

198. Gupta SK, Sharma OP, Malhotra S, et al. Cleidocranial dysostosis—skeletal abnormalities. *Australas Radiol* 1992;36:238.

199. Dore DD, MacEwen GD, Boulos MI. Cleidocranial dysostosis and syringomyelia: case report and review of the literature. *Clin Orthop* 1987;214:231.

200. Taglialavoro G, Fabris D, Agostini S. A case of progressive scoliosis in a patient with craniocleidopelvic dysostosis. *Ital J Orthop Traumatol* 1999;9:507.

201. Vari R, Puca A, Meglio M. Cleidocranial dysplasia and syringomyelia. *J Neurol Sci* 1996;49:125.

202. Hamner LH, Fabbri EL, Browne PC. Prenatal diagnosis of cleidocranial dysostosis. *Obstet Gynecol* 1994;83:856.

203. Jarvis JL, Keats TE. Cleidocranial dysostosis: a review of 40 new cases. *Am J Radiol* 1974;21:5.

204. Richie MF, Johnston CE II. Management of developmental coxa vara in cleidocranial dysostosis. *Orthopedics* 1989;12:1001.

Larsen Syndrome

205. Larsen LJ, Schottstaedt ER, Bost FC. Multiple congenital dislocations associated with characteristic facial abnormality. *J Pediatr* 1950;37:574.

206. Vujic M, Hallstensson K, Wahlstrom J, et al. Localization of a gene for autosomal dominant Larsen syndrome to chromosome region 3p21.1-14.1 in the proximity of, but distinct from, the COL7A1 locus. *Am J Hum Genet* 1999;57:1104.

207. Johnston CE, Birch JG, Daniels JL. Cervical kyphosis in patients who have Larsen syndrome. *J Bone Joint Surg Am* 1996;78:538.

208. Micheli LJ, Hall JE, Watts HG. Spinal instability in Larsen syndrome: report of three cases. *J Bone Joint Surg Am* 1976;58:562.

209. Bowen JR, Ortega K, Ray S, et al. Spinal deformities in Larsen's syndrome. *Clin Orthop* 1985;197:159.

210. Laville JM, Lakermore P, Limouzy F. Larsen's syndrome: review of the literature and analysis of thirty-eight cases. *J Pediatr Orthop* 1994;14:63.

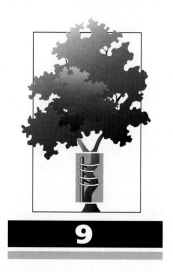

9

SYNDROMES OF ORTHOPAEDIC IMPORTANCE

BENJAMIN A. ALMAN
MICHAEL J. GOLDBERG

B. A. Alman: Department of Surgery, University of Toronto; Department of Orthopaedic Surgery/Developmental Biology, The Hospital for Sick Children, Toronto, Ontario M5G 1X8, Canada.

M. J. Goldberg: Department of Orthopaedics, Tufts University School of Medicine; Department of Orthopaedics, New England Medical Center, Boston, Massachusetts 02111.

The word "syndrome" is derived from a Greek word that means to run together. When several relatively uncommon anomalies occur in the same individual, it may be nothing more than coincidence. However, if they all result from the same cause, or occur in the same pattern in other children, that particular combination of birth defects is called a syndrome. A syndrome should be suspected if a characteristic orthopaedic malformation (e.g., radial clubhand) is encountered, if all four extremities are affected, if limb deformities are symmetric, if there are several associated nonorthopaedic anomalies, or if there is a familiar dysmorphic face (1–4). Children who have syndromes look more like each other than they do their parents.

It is not unusual for an orthopaedist to be the first physician to recognize that a child has features of a syndrome. In such cases, appropriate referrals should be made to a geneticist to assist in syndrome identification, order appropriate confirmatory tests, and arrange for management of the nonorthopaedic manifestations of the syndrome. The evaluation of a child for a syndrome includes a family history, a systems review, and a search for minor dysmorphic features, such as abnormal palm creases or abnormal shape of digits or toes. These may not be of immediate orthopaedic significance, but they are the clues to look further.

Syndromes can be caused by gene defects, environmental abnormalities during fetal development (a teratogen), or both. The relationship between the clinical (phenotypic) features and the cause of a syndrome is not always as simple as one would wish. There can be phenotypic variability, even within a family in which all the members carry the identical gene mutation. Some individuals are minimally affected, whereas others have all of the findings of the syndrome. This may be due to the presence of modifying genes, which may not be inherited in the same way as the gene mutation that causes the syndrome. Teratogenic agents present during fetal development can cause syndromes, such as the fetal alcohol syndrome. These teratogens affect developmental signaling pathways, which are cascades of genes expressed in a controlled fashion, to produce normal fetal development. A genetic defect can sometimes cause the same perturbation in such a pathway as a teratogen. Thus, some syndromes can be caused either by a gene defect or a teratogenic agent. A single gene can be responsible for a number of syndromes. This occurs because the products of different mutations have different cellular functions. Such is the case with the dystrophin gene, which causes both Duchenne and Becker muscular dystrophies.

Information about the etiology of a syndrome is important, because it has implications for the parents as to the risk of recurrence in subsequent pregnancies, and may hold the key to the development of novel treatments. The rapid pace of basic research in developmental biology and genetics makes it difficult for a traditional textbook to contain the most up-to-date information about syndrome etiology. The Internet is becoming an excellent source for such information. One useful site is the On-Line Mendelian Inheritance in Man (OMIM), administered by the National Institutes of Health. This site can be accessed at http//www.ncbi .nlm.nih.gov/Omim/, and can be searched by syndrome name, causative gene, or clinical findings (5).

The care of children with syndromes involves multiple specialists (6). Discussions of the risk of subsequent pregnancies is in the realm of the genetic counselor. For parents, naming the condition often implies that it is then treatable or curable. This, sadly, is not the case. The importance of understanding syndromes is recognizing that associated medical abnormalities may adversely influence orthopaedic outcomes, and may influence surgical timing and management. The orthopaedic surgeon also needs information from the geneticist. Associated conditions may influence the outcome of orthopaedic problems and can affect anesthesia (e.g., cardiac or renal anomalies). Even if parents are not planning subsequent pregnancies, and if there are no plans for their child to undergo surgery in the near future, genetic evaluation is still important for proper syndrome diagnosis. Correct diagnoses are essential for research into syndrome etiology. Patients should be given the opportunity to participate in such research, especially in cases of relatively rare syndromes.

Nomenclature can confuse syndrome identification, because a single syndrome may have several names. Eponyms are not descriptive of the syndrome, nor do they give information about etiology. Classifying syndromes by the causative gene is problematic because some genes cause more than one syndrome, and some syndromes are caused by more than one gene. Furthermore, the gene names are frequently unrelated to clinical findings. A numbering system is used by most computer databases; the most widely used is that of the On-line Mendelian Inheritance in Man (5), but this is only helpful for database searches. The ideal nomenclature system would be descriptive, but also give information about etiology. Unfortunately, such a system has not yet been developed.

NEUROFIBROMATOSIS

There are several forms of neurofibromatosis (NF), the most common of which are type I and type II (NF1 and NF2). Orthopaedic manifestations are common in NF1, which is also called "von Recklinghausen disease," whereas they are rare in NF2, which is also called "central neurofibromatosis" or "familial acoustic neuroma." The clinical findings in NF1 are quite variable, and many of these findings develop over time. Children may exhibit none of the typical findings at birth, but the diagnosis can be made as they grow older and develop the characteristics necessary to confirm a

TABLE 9-1. NEUROFIBROMATOSIS TYPE 1: DIAGNOSTIC CRITERIA

At least two of the following are necessary to establish the diagnosis of NF1:

- At least six café-au-lait spots, larger than 5 mm in diameter for children, and larger than 15 mm for adults
- Two neurofibromas, or a single plexiform neurofibroma
- Freckling in the axillae or inguinal region
- An optic glioma
- At least two Lisch nodules (hamartoma of the iris)
- A distinctive osseous lesion, such as vertebral scalloping, or cortical thinning
- A first-degree relative with NF1

diagnosis of NF1 (7,8). This diagnosis is made by identifying at least two of the clinical findings in Table 9.1.

Cutaneous Markings

Café-au-lait spots are discrete, tan spots (Fig. 9-1). They often appear after 1 year of age, then the numbers and size steadily increase. The spots have a smooth edge, often described as similar to the coast of California, as opposed to the ragged edge of spots associated with fibrous dysplasia, which are described as similar to the coast of Maine. There exists great variation in the number of café-au-lait spots and their shape and size, although six lesions greater than 1 cm in size are required for the diagnostic criteria. Axillary and inguinal freckling is common, and serve as good diagnostic markers, because such freckling is exceptionally rare, except in people with NF. Hyperpigmented nevi are dark brown areas that are sensitive to touch. They typically overlie a deeper plexiform neurofibroma.

Neurofibroma

The two types of neurofibromas are different in their anatomic configuration and in clinical morbidity. The most common is the cutaneous neurofibroma, composed of benign Schwann cells and fibrous connective tissue (Fig. 9-2). They may occur anywhere, but are usually just below the skin. They may not be detectable until 10 years of age, and with puberty there is a rapid increase in their number. When many are grouped together on the skin, it is known as a fibroma molluscum. Plexiform neurofibromas are usually present at birth and are highly infiltrative in the surrounding tissues. The overlying skin is often darkly pigmented. They are highly vascular, and plexiform neurofibromas lead to limb giantism, facial disfigurement, and invasion of the neuroaxis (Figs. 9-3 and 9-4).

Osseous Lesions

There are many skeletal manifestations, but the presence of an unusual scoliosis, nonunion of a long bone, overgrowth of a part, or a congenital pseudarthrosis lesion seen on radiographs should alert the physician to consider a diagnosis of NF (9). There are a variety of radiographic anomalies of bone observed, ranging from a scalloping of the cortex to cystic lesions in long bones that look much like nonossifying fibromas, to permeative bone destruction (Fig. 9-5). These radiographic findings can mimic benign and malignant bone lesions (10–12). Roentgenograms of the pelvis usually show various degrees of coxa valga, and in nearly 20% of patients there is radiographic evidence of protrusio acetabuli (13,14).

Lisch Nodules

Lisch nodules are hamartomas of the iris. They are present in 50% of all 5-year-olds with NF1, and in all adults with NF1. It is unusual for Lisch nodules to be present in individuals without NF1, and their detection can be used to aid in making this diagnosis. However, it may be difficult to

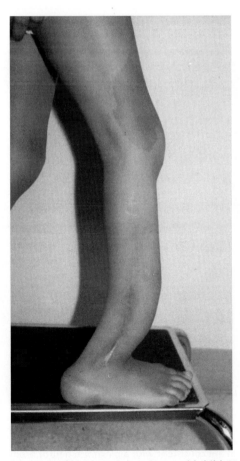

FIGURE 9-1. Neurofibromatosis in a 6-year-old child. Notice the large café-au-lait spot on the thigh and the anterior bowed tibia typical of pseudarthrosis. (From ref. 1, with permission.)

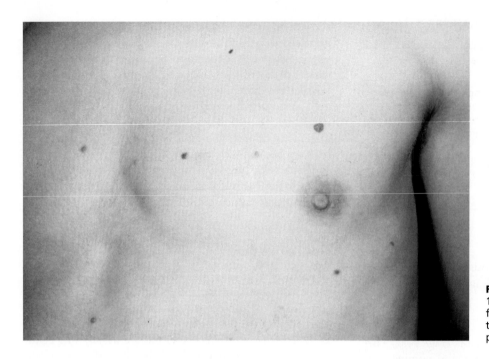

FIGURE 9-2. Neurofibromatosis in a 14-year-old patient. Cutaneous neurofibromas make their appearance with the onset of puberty. (From ref. 1, with permission.)

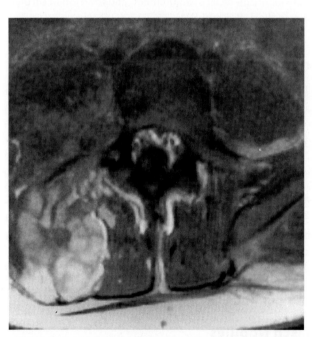

FIGURE 9-3. Neurofibromatosis in a 16-year-old patient. The magnetic resonance image at the level of L4–5 demonstrates a large plexiform neurofibroma that invades the neural axis. It extends from the level of L3 to the sacrum.

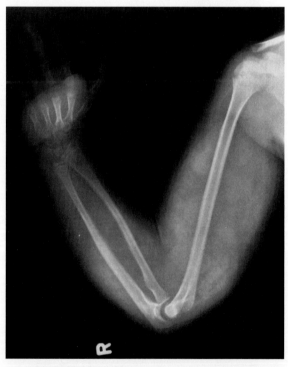

FIGURE 9-4. Neurofibromatosis in a 10-year-old patient. Hypertrophy affects the arm from the shoulder to the fingertips; the major component is soft tissue. Nodular densities throughout the upper arm are consistent with a plexiform neurofibroma. Notice the lack of skeletal overgrowth and some attenuation of the radius and ulna, from external compression by the neurofibroma. (From ref. 1, with permission.)

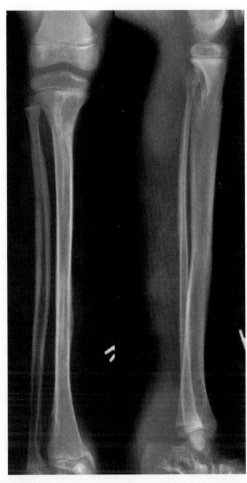

FIGURE 9-5. Neurofibromatosis in a 10-year-old patient. The radiograph shows an array of cystic and scalloped skeletal lesions in the tibia and os calcis of the right leg. Some of the lesions are characteristic of neurofibromatosis. Other lesions, occurring in isolation, can mimic benign fibrous tumors. Scalloped cortical erosion at the upper end of the femur, permeative bone destruction in the region of the os calcis, and metaphyseal cystic lesions are other features. (From ref. 1, with permission.)

detect these lesions, and individuals should be sent to an experienced ophthalmologist to make this diagnosis. The lesions do not cause any visual disturbances. Once the diagnosis is established further, ophthalmologic evaluation is not necessary (15,16).

Etiology

Neurofibromatosis is the most common single-gene disorder in humans, affecting 1 of 3,000 newborns (17–19). NF1 is an autosomal dominant disorder with 100% penetrance, but one-half of the cases are sporadic mutations and are associated with an older-than-average paternal age. The most renowned patient with NF, Joseph Merrick, called the Elephant Man, probably did not have this diagnosis and better fits Proteus syndrome (20). The *NF1* gene is located

on chromosome 17 (21). Its protein product is called neurofibrillin, and it acts as a tumor suppressor (22). There are also other potential genes within the *NF1* gene, located in introns, whose functional significance is unclear.

Neurofibrillin has similarity to the G-protein family of signal transduction proteins. These proteins convey messages from cell surface receptors to cytoplasmic effectors. Neurofibrillin plays such a role in the Ras signaling system, which is involved in the control of cell growth (23). Mutations in the *NF1* gene cause a disruption in its normal regulatory function of Ras signaling. This gives the affected cells an abnormal growth pattern.

Neurofibrillin is expressed at higher levels in the neural crest during development. Cells from the neural crest migrate to become pigmented cells of the skin, parts of the brain, spinal cord, peripheral nerves, and adrenals, thus explaining the common sites of abnormalities in the disorder. The gene defect gives a clue into potential novel therapies, because pharmacologic agents that block Ras signaling could be used to treat the disorder. Disruption of the normal Ras signaling cascade is probably responsible for the malignant potential in this disorder. Only one of the two copies of the *NF1* gene is mutated in affected patients; however, tumors from such individuals have been found to have only a mutated gene because of loss of the normal copy (24–27).

Other Types of Neurofibromatosis

Although patients with other forms of neurofibromatosis rarely present to an orthopaedist, one should be aware of these because musculoskeletal malformations occasionally are present. Patients with NF2 present with acoustic neuromas, central nervous system tumors, and rare peripheral manifestations. There are usually less than six café-au-lait spots, and no peripheral neurofibromata. These patients are very unlikely to present with an orthopaedic deformity. There are two much less common types of neurofibromatosis, type III and type IV (NF3 and NF4), which are more likely to develop a problem requiring orthopaedic intervention. Individuals with NF3 present with some of the characteristics of NF1, but also have acoustic neuromas, which are characteristic of NF2. These individuals often have spinal deformity, especially in the cervical region. NF4 presents with the same clinical findings as in NF1, except that one of the cardinal features of NF1, iris Lisch nodules, is absent (7,8). One reason to distinguish these types from NF1 is that they are probably caused by mutations in a different gene than that which causes NF1 (this has already been demonstrated in NF2), and thus will not be diagnosed using DNA testing for NF1.

Orthopaedic Manifestations

The common orthopaedic manifestations of NF, including scoliosis, limb overgrowth, pseudarthrosis, and radiographic appearances of lesions, enable the initial diagnosis to be made, if the syndrome is kept in mind. Patients with NF often exhibit overgrowth, ranging from a single digit to an entire limb, and from mild anisomelia to massive giantism. Any child with focal giantism, such as macrodactyly, is best thought of as having NF until proven otherwise. When NF is compared with the more symmetric idiopathic hemihypertrophy, there is disproportional overgrowth involving the skin and subcutaneous tissue more than bone (see Fig. 9-4).

Scoliosis is common, and although there is no standard curve pattern, curves tend to fall into two behavioral patterns: a dystrophic curve and an idiopathic curve. Most curves in NF resemble idiopathic scoliosis curves. Their relation to NF is not understood, and their precise incidence debated. These curves can be managed like any other idiopathic curve.

The dystrophic scoliotic curve is a short, sharp, single thoracic curve typically involving four to six segments (Fig. 9-6) (13,28–35). It is associated with distortion of the ribs and vertebrae. The onset is early in childhood, and it is relentlessly progressive. Curves that initially appear to be idiopathic in children under age 7 have almost a 70% chance of becoming dystrophic over time, although there may be subtle clues, for example mild rib penciling, that the curve is really dystrophic. The most important risk factors for progression is an early age of onset, a high Cobb angle, and an apical vertebrae that is severely rotated, scalloped, and located in the middle-to-lower thoracic area (32). The combination of curve progression and vertebral malformation mimics congenital scoliosis in appearance and behavior. Dystrophic curves are refractive to brace treatment. Sagittal plane deformities may occur, including an angular kyphosis (i.e., gibbus) and a scoliosis that has so much rotation that curve progression is more obvious on the lateral than on the anteroposterior roentgenogram (32). In those with angular kyphosis, there is a risk of paraplegia. Dystrophic curves are difficult to stabilize, and it is best to intervene with early surgery involving both anterior and posterior fusion (32,36–38). Kyphotic deformities are often the most difficult to manage surgically, and strut grafts across the kyphosis anteriorly may be necessary. In cases with extremely severe deformity, halo-femoral or halo-gravity traction may be necessary to safely straighten the spine to a more acceptable deformity, without producing neurologic sequelae.

There are several vertebral abnormalities evident on radiographs. These include scalloping of the posterior body, enlargement of the neural foramina, and defective pedicles, occasionally with a completely dislocated vertebral body (39–43). Such findings may mean that there is a dumbbell-shaped neurofibroma in the spinal canal extending out through a neural foramina. In NF patients, the dura behaves like the dura in patients with a connective tissue disorder, and dural ectasia is common, with pseudomeningoceles protruding through the neural foramina. Unlike neurofibromas, dural ectasia is an out-pouching of the dura, without an underlying tumor or overgrowth of spinal elements (Fig. 9-7) (44–47). The incidence of anterolateral meningoceles was underestimated until asymptomatic patients were screened with magnetic resonance imaging (MRI) (9,48). The erosion of the pedicles may lead to spinal instability, especially in the cervical spine. In rare cases, this can even lead to dislocation of the spine (49,50). MRI and computed tomography (CT) scans are helpful preoperatively to delineate the presence of defective vertebrae or dural abnormalities, and may assist in choosing the levels on which to place instrumentation.

Pseudarthrosis of a long bone is typically associated with NF (30). It usually affects the tibia, with a characteristic anterolateral bow obvious in infancy (Fig. 9-8) (51,52). Fracture usually follows, with spontaneous union rare and surgical union a challenge. An anterolateral bowed tibia should be managed with a total-contact orthosis to prevent fracture. Intramedullary rod fixation seems to offer the best results for the initial management of a pseudarthrosis [➥6.11]. The cause of the pseudarthrosis is not known;

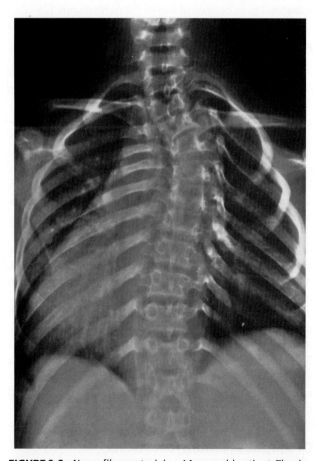

FIGURE 9-6. Neurofibromatosis in a 14-year-old patient. The dystrophic curve is produced by a short-segment scoliosis. Ribboned ribs show cystic irregularities. (From ref. 1, with permission.)

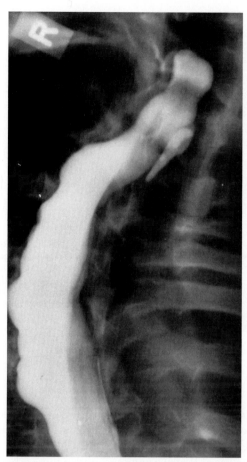

FIGURE 9-7. Myelogram of a young adult with neurofibromatosis and scoliosis with pseudomeningoceles and dural ectasia.

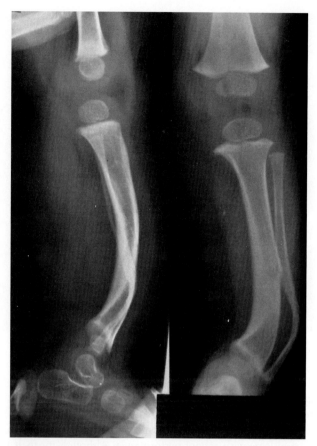

FIGURE 9-8. Neurofibromatosis in a 1-year-old patient. The anterolateral bow of the tibia and fibula warrant concern for impending fracture and pseudarthrosis. (From ref. 1, with permission.)

however, neurofibromas have not been identified at the pseudarthrosis site. The pseudarthrosis process may affect the ulna, radius, femur, or clavicle (53–59). In each of these locations, there is a course similar to that in the tibia, with bone loss and difficulty achieving union (Fig. 9-9). Not all pseudarthroses of the forearm require treatment (60), but if they are symptomatic, options include proximal and distal synostosis to produce a single-bone forearm, or the use of a vascularized fibula graft.

There are a variety of benign and malignant neoplastic processes that affect individuals with NF1. Most neurofibromas do not require treatment, but symptomatic lesions may require excision. Plexiform neurofibromas that become symptomatic are very difficult to manage. Their vascularity and infiltrative nature make complete extirpation almost impossible, with a substantial risk of uncontrollable hemorrhage and neurologic deficit. Although speculative, the use of angiogenesis inhibitors, such as interferon, or some experimental agents based on modulating the affect of the causative gene mutation, may be beneficial (61,62).

The exact incidence of malignancy in NF is controversial, with reported rates ranging from under 1% to over 20%

(63–67). The most common tumor location is in the central nervous system, with lesions such as optic nerve glioma, acoustic neuroma, and astrocytoma (68). There is a risk of malignant degeneration of a neurofibroma to a neurofibrosarcoma. This process can occur in a central or peripheral neurofibroma (69–72). It can be quite difficult to distinguish a malignant from a benign lesion. CT scans show areas of low-enhancing density in neurofibrosarcomas (73), but there are no studies determining the sensitivity and specificity of this finding. Similar patterns can also be visualized using MRI. Routine surveillance for sarcomatous change is impossible due to the large number of neurofibromas. Lesions that increase in size, or that develop new symptoms, should be investigated. There is a propensity for children with neurofibroma to develop other malignancies, such as Wilms tumors or rhabdomyosarcomas.

Hypertension, on the basis of renal artery stenosis or pheochromocytoma, is reported regularly, as is a curious type of metabolic bone disease similar to hypophosphatemic osteomalacia (74,75). Hypertension is a major risk factor for early death (67). Precocious puberty may occur due to

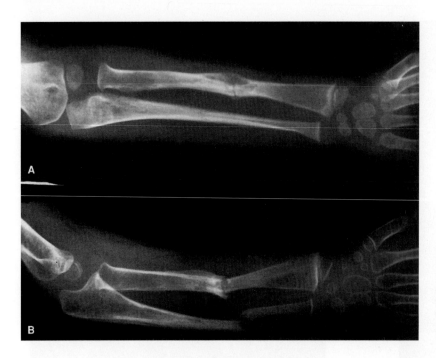

FIGURE 9-9. Neurofibromatosis in a 3-year-old patient. The radiograph shows progressive pseudarthrosis of the radius and ulna after a pathologic fracture. **A:** Fracture through the cystic lesion of the radius and thinning of the mid ulna. **B:** After 10 months of cast immobilization, pseudarthrosis affects the radius and ulna. (From ref. 1, with permission.)

an intracranial lesion (76). Affected children are short, but tend to have large heads. Approximately 50% have an intellectual handicap that varies from frank mental retardation to problems with school performance. Although mean IQ is low, there is quite a broad range of IQ (77). A high incidence of concentration problems may interfere with learning, more than a low IQ (78). The concentration problems can sometimes be managed pharmacologically.

PROTEUS SYNDROME

Proteus syndrome is an overgrowth condition, in which there is a bizarre array of abnormalities that include hemihypertrophy, macrodactyly, and partial giantism of the hands or feet, or both. The key to this diagnosis is worsening of existing features, and the appearance of new ones over time (79–82).

The cause of this syndrome is not known. Although there are case reports of familial occurrence, the vast majority of cases are sporadic (83–85). It is most likely due to a gene that is mutated in a mosaic manner (mutated in the affected tissues, but not the normal tissues), similar to McCune-Albright syndrome (polyostotic fibrous dysplasia). Such a mutation can occur very early in development in a single cell, which will divide to ultimately form various structures throughout the body.

The Proteus syndrome is named after the ancient Greek demigod who could change appearance and assume different shapes. The progressive nature of the deformities seen

in this syndrome can lead to grotesque overgrowth, facial disfigurement, angular malformation, and severe scoliosis (86). Joseph Merrick, called the Elephant Man, is thought to have had this syndrome, rather than NF (87).

The signs of Proteus syndrome overlap those other hamartomatous overgrowth conditions, such as idiopathic hemihypertrophy, Klippel-Trenaunay syndrome, Maffucci syndrome, and neurofibromatosis. However, unlike these other syndromes, the features here are more grotesque and involve multiple tissue types and sites. Proteus can be differentiated from NF1 by the lack of café-au-lait spots and Lisch nodules (88). A rating scale, which assigns points based on clinical findings (macrodactyly, hemihypertrophy, thickening of the skin, lipomas, subcutaneous tumors, verrucae, epidermal nevus, and macrocephaly) may be used to assist in diagnosis (89). However, the finding of worsening overgrowth features over time is usually sufficient to make this diagnosis.

Most children who present with macrodactyly do not have this as part of Proteus syndrome. In these sporadic cases, an isolated digit is involved, or, when multiple digits are involved, these are located adjacent to each other. Macrodactyly affecting nonadjacent toes or fingers or opposite extremities is almost always due to Proteus syndrome. There is a characteristic thickening and deep furrowing of the skin on the palms of the hands and soles of the feet. The array of cutaneous manifestations include hemangiomas and pigmented nevi of various intensities, and subcutaneous lipomas (Fig. 9-10). Varicosities are present, although true arteriovenous malformations are rare. There are cranial hyperostoses, and occasionally exostosis of the hands and feet.

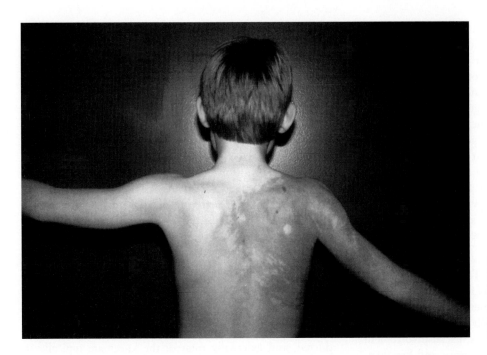

FIGURE 9-10. Proteus syndrome. Notice the cutaneous markings, large hemangioma of the shoulder, and lightly pigmented area on the back. There is some atrophy of the shoulder and arm muscles and a fixed contracture of the elbow.

Macrodactyly seems to correspond to overgrowth along the terminal branches of a peripheral sensory nerve. Digital involvement in the hand favors the sensory distribution of the median nerve (1). The index is the most frequently affected finger, followed by the long finger and the thumb. It is the second toe that is most commonly macrodactylous. The regional sensory nerve is greatly increased in size, taking a tortuous route through the fatty tissue.

There is a wide range of orthopaedic deformities, including focal and regional giantism, scoliosis, and kyphosis (90,91). Rather large vertebral bodies, known as megaspondylodysplasia, are present (92). Angular malformations of the lower extremities, especially genu valgum, are common. Because the genu valgum is often associated with restricted range of motion, joint stiffness, flexion contractures, and joint pain, it is postulated that an intraarticular growth disturbance contributes to the angular malformation. Roentgenographic hip abnormalities, such as acetabular dysplasia, are frequently discovered in asymptomatic patients. Deformities in the hindfoot are frequent and are usually heel valgus, but congenital equinovarus and "Z-foot" deformities have also been described (88,91).

Most of the literature on Proteus syndrome consists of case reports or case series, and there are no data comparing results of different types of treatments.

In addition, recurrences after surgical intervention are very common. This is probably due to an underlying growth advantage in affected tissues which cannot be corrected operatively. Thus, musculoskeletal deformities due to Proteus syndrome are very difficult to manage.

When the foot becomes difficult to fit into a shoe due to macrodactyly, it is best managed by ablation rather than

debulking (93) [➡**7.22**]. Anisomelia is best managed with epiphysiodesis [➡**4.19, 4.20, 6.12, 6.13**], although limb-lengthening may be considered in cases with very large differences [➡**4.15, 4.16, 6.9, 6.10**]. Osteotomies can correct angular malformations, but must be tempered by the chance of a rapid recurrence of deformity after corrective surgery (90,91). In some cases, sudden overgrowth of the operative limb have been reported. There are anecdotal reports of soft tissue procedures to "debulk" overgrown lesions; however, there are no series in the literature reporting results of these procedures, and our experience with them is that the results are only temporary. In rare cases, nerve or spinal cord impingement can occur. Nerve compression can be managed using decompression, but spinal cord compression is difficult, if not impossible, to successfully treat operatively (94,95). Mixed results are obtained from surgical treatment in this disorder, and operative treatment should be reserved for individuals who have exhausted nonsurgical management. Sometimes the operative procedures can be used as a temporizing measure, and patients may need to have repeat procedures performed throughout life.

Functional ability depends on the severity of the limb deformity and the presence of intracranial abnormalities (82,96). The life expectancy is unknown, but many adult patients are reported. Intubation can be difficult due to overgrowth of structures surrounding the trachea.

ARTHROGRYPOSIS

Arthrogryposis is really a physical finding, not a diagnosis, and represents a large group of disorders, all of which have in common joint contractures present at birth. This term is used as a noun to describe specific diseases, and as an adjective, "arthrogrypotic," to refer to rigid joint contractures. There are 65 distinct syndromes coded under the term "arthrogryposis" in the On-Line Mendelian Inheritance in Man (5), illustrating the large variety of etiologies associated with this term. Most of the syndromes have different clinical courses, prognoses, genetics, causes, and pathologic processes, often making it difficult for the orthopaedist to determine management for an individual patient (97,98). A simple way to think about these disorders is to consider them as contracture syndromes, which can be grouped into a few general categories, each of which can be represented by a prototypic disease.

Contracture syndrome groups:

1. Involving all four extremities. This includes arthrogryposis multiplex congenita and Larsen syndrome, with more or less total body involvement.
2. Predominantly or exclusively involves the hands and feet. These are the distal arthrogryposes. Facial involvement can occur with some of these syndromes, and Freeman-Sheldon whistling face is included.
3. Pterygia syndromes in which identifiable skin webs cross the flexion aspects of the knees, elbows, and other joints. Multiple pterygias and popliteal pterygia fit in this group.

CONTRACTURE SYNDROMES INVOLVING ALL FOUR EXTREMITIES

Arthrogryposis Multiplex Congenita

Arthrogryposis multiplex congenita is the best-known of the multiple congenital contracture syndromes (99,100). Although attempts have been made to change the name "arthrogryposis multiplex congenita" to "multiple congenital contractures" or "amyoplasia," the popularity of arthrogryposis remains.

The etiology of arthrogryposis multiplex congenita is unknown. It was initially described in 1841 by Adolf Wilhelm Otto, who referred to his patient as a "human wonder with curved limbs" (101). The disorder is sporadic, with affected individuals having reproduced only normal children. There is, however, an increased incidence of classic arthrogryposis affecting only one of identical twins (102,103). The development of arthrogryposis may be influenced by an adverse intrauterine factor or the twinning process itself. Teratogens have been suggested, but none are proven, despite the multiple animal models that lend support to that theory (100,104–107). Some mothers of children with arthrogryposis have serum antibodies that inhibit fetal acetylcholine receptor function. One possibility is that maternal antibodies to these fetal antigens cause the disorder (108).

Histologic analysis discloses a small muscle mass with fibrosis and fat between the muscle fibers. Myopathic and neuropathic features often are found in the same muscle biopsy specimen. The periarticular soft tissue structures are fibrotic, and in essence, there is a fibrous ankylosis. The number of anterior horn cells in the spinal cord is decreased, without an increase in the number of microglial cells (109–111). The pattern of motor neuron loss in specific spinal cord segments correlates with the peripheral deformities and the affected muscles, suggesting a primary central nervous system disorder as important in the cause (112).

Clinical examination remains best for establishing a diagnosis. The limbs are striking in appearance and position (Fig. 9-11). They are featureless and tubular. Normal skin creases are lacking, but there may be deep dimples over the joints. Muscle mass is reduced, although, in infancy, there is often abundant subcutaneous tissue. Typically, the shoulders are adducted and internally rotated, the elbow more often extended than flexed, and the wrist flexed severely, with ulnar deviation. The fingers are flexed, clutching the thumb. In the lower extremities, the hips are flexed, abducted, and externally rotated; the knees are typically in extension, although flexion is possible; and clubfeet are the rule. Joint motion is restricted. The condition is pain-free, with a firm, inelastic block to movement beyond a very

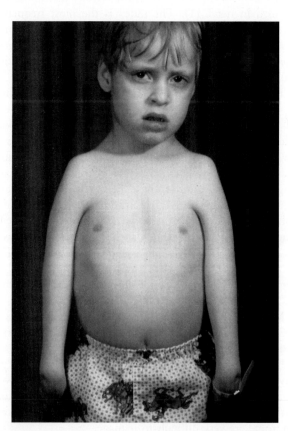

FIGURE 9-11. Arthrogryposis multiplex congenita. The picture shows the classic limb position and fusiform limbs lacking flexion creases.

limited range. In two-thirds of the patients, all four limbs are affected equally, but in one-third, lower-limb deformities predominate, and only on rare occasions do the upper extremities predominate. Deformities tend to be more severe and more rigid distally. The hips may be dislocated unilaterally or bilaterally.

The viscera usually are spared malformations, although gastroschisis has been reported. As a consequence of the general muscle weakness, there is a 15% incidence of inguinal hernia. Major feeding difficulties, due to a stiff jaw and an immobile tongue, are frequently encountered in infancy, and lead to respiratory infections and failure to thrive (113). The face is not particularly dysmorphic. A few subtle features, such as a small jaw, narrowing of the face, and occasionally, limited upward gaze (secondary to ocular muscle involvement), and a frontal midline hemangioma, may help with the diagnosis (see Fig. 9-11).

Radiographs reveal that the joints are normal, and that changes are adaptive and acquired over time as a consequence of fixed position (Fig. 9-12). There is evidence of a loss of subcutaneous fat and tissue. Electromyograms and muscle biopsies are of questionable diagnostic value. They have been used to separate patients with primarily neuro-

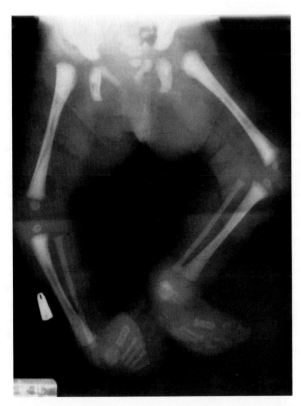

FIGURE 9-12. Arthrogryposis multiplex congenita at birth. Features include club feet, knee flexion deformity, and dislocated right hip. The articular surfaces are normal. Adaptive changes occur as a consequence of the fixed position. (From ref. 1, with permission.)

pathic changes from those with myopathic, but the clinical implications of such distinctions are not clear. A diagnosis of arthrogryposis can be suspected when prenatal ultrasound detects an absence of fetal movement, especially if seen in combination with polyhydramnios (104).

Despite every large medical center having treated patients with arthrogryposis, the natural history and long-term outcomes are not well known (114,115). Some contractures seem to worsen with age, and the joint becomes stiffer. No new joints become involved. At least 25% of affected patients are nonambulators, and many others are limited household walkers (116). As a rule, those with arthrogryposis who are very weak as infants stay weak, and those who appear stronger as infants stay strong. Adult interdependency seems to be related to education and coping skills, more than to the magnitude of joint contractures.

Treatment

Each of the multiple joints involved have their own unique opportunities for orthopaedic intervention, but at times an overview of the total patient must be borne in mind. The overall goals are lower-limb alignment and stability for ambulation, and upper extremity motion for self care (97,117,118). Outcomes seem better if joint surgery is done early, before adaptive intraarticular changes. Osteotomies are usually performed closer to the completion of growth. Early motion, and avoidance of prolonged casing, may increase joint motion, improving function. Many children require long-term bracing or other assistive devices (100).

Joint contractures make the birthing process difficult, and neonatal fractures may result (119). Physical therapy should not be initiated in the newborn until such fractures are ruled out (120). Mobilization of joints may be accomplished by early and frequent range of motion exercises and splinting of the joint in a position of function with a removable orthotic (100,120). There are no studies clearly demonstrating that early mobilization improves these patient outcomes, but such a program may improve passive range of motion, whereas active range of motion does not improve very much (100). In our experience, early mobilization seems to be useful primarily in the upper extremity. Fractures may accompany an overly vigorous range of motion program.

Approximately two-thirds of patients have developmental dysplasia of the hip or frank dislocation (100, 121–123) (see Fig. 9-12). At birth, the hips are flexed and abducted. There is considerable controversy about the management of the hips in these children. Closed reduction is rarely, if ever, successful. Operative reduction of a dislocated hip should be performed if it will improve function or decrease pain. Studies to date have not found pain to be a problem with these hips; however, only relatively short-term follow-up is reported. There is significant variability in function in these individuals due to the underlying severity of the disease, and this variability makes it difficult to determine any change in function from treating the hips. Range of motion of the hips may be important for function, because hip contractures, especially those causing flexion deformity, adversely affect the gait pattern. Operative procedures to locate dislocated hips, therefore, have the potential to worsen function if they produce significant contractures (122,124).

Studies of children with untreated dislocated hips concluded that those with bilateral dislocations frequently had satisfactory range of motion, their hips did not prevent them from walking, although rarely around the community, and pain was uncommon (121,123,124). Those with unilateral dislocations fared less well. More were limited to the household with walkers, and, although scoliosis was present in most patients, it was worse and more frequent in those with unilateral dislocations (100). In both groups, limitation of ambulation results more from the severe involvement of all four extremities than from the dislocated hips (100). These data, and case series suggesting little functional improvement with surgery for bilateral hip dislocations, supports the concept of leaving bilateral dislocated hips alone (100,121,122,124). However, in these studies, hip surgery was delayed until the knees were mobilized, and reductions did not occur until at least 1 year of age. This later age at reduction may be associated with higher rates of contractures, and worse function. Reports of early open reduction of unilateral and bilateral dislocated hips, with a reduced period of immobilization, show improved postoperative range of motion (123,125,126). Hip reduction may not benefit the child who is not an ambulator; however, there is no way to comfortably predict which children will become ambulators at the age early surgical treatment is contemplated. Thus, it seems reasonable to perform early open reduction in most children. Both medial and anterior approaches are advocated for early hip reduction (123,125,126) [➡3.2–3.4]. The key factor may be performing the hip reduction early in life, with minimal immobilization, rather than the specific operative approach utilized. This may be more easily accomplished using a medical approach.

Although the classic description of the knees is that they are hyperextended, most are in flexion (100,127–129) (Fig. 9-12). The precise plane of motion is often difficult to determine, and although physical therapy is recommended, medial lateral instability may result. Hyperextension deformity responds better to physical therapy and splinting than do flexion deformities. If the flexion deformity remains more than 30 degrees, ambulation is precluded because of the associated overall muscle weakness, especially of the quadriceps and gluteus maximus. Sometime before 2 years of age, soft tissue surgery, including posterior capsulotomy, should be performed. The actual procedure needs to be individualized, because each knee has a different degree of deformity. Posterior soft tissue procedures often need to be repeated

later in life, but before nearing skeletal maturity. Supracondylar osteotomies of the femur are recommended toward the end of growth to correct residual deformity (100,128–130). Femoral shortening may need to be added to the osteotomies. Many hyperextension deformities of the knee can be treated without surgery, but quadricepsplasty may be needed in cases with residual lack of motion. Traditional teaching is for correction of the knee deformity, before treating a dislocated hip, to allow stretching out of the muscles, which cross both joints. However, with early operative treatment of the hip, using a short period of immobilization, the hip may be operated upon at the same time as a surgical procedure to correct a hyperextended knee deformity. In this case, the hamstring muscles are relaxed by both procedures, and the knee can be immobilized, flexed in the hip spica cast. The flexed knee cannot be easily managed at the same time as hip surgery, because it is impossible to appropriately immobilize the hip with the knee held extended. Despite good initial nonoperative results in the hyperextended knee, there may be recurrence of the contracture over time, with surgery often needed later in life. An alternative technique of correction of the knee deformity is using an external fixator, with gradual correction (131); however, in most cases, an open procedure to release the contracted structures will be adequate. Late osteoarthritis seems more common in those with persistent hyperextension contracture.

A severe and resistant clubfoot is characteristic (100, 132,133) (Fig. 9-12). It is rare for the arthrogrypotic clubfoot to respond to physical therapy and casts, and surgical intervention is usually necessary. However, as in the knee deformity, there is a wide range of severity. Some feet, therefore, respond better to surgery than others. Surgery for clubfoot is sometimes delayed until 1 year of age or later, as other joints, especially the knees, are attended to first. However, as in management of the hip, performing combined procedures, with minimal immobilization earlier in life, is gaining in popularity. Primary talectomy has been recommended because of the high incidence of failed soft tissue surgery (134,135); however, recent reports show good outcome with circumferential release alone, if performed before 1 year of age (136,137) [➡7.1]. This is probably a better initial approach, because salvage talectomy can always be performed later, if necessary. Positioning of the calcaneus is key to achieving a good result after talectomy (138). Residual deformity in the teenage years can be treated using a triple arthrodesis, or with multiple osteotomies, to maintain motion of the subtalar joints, while producing a plantigrade foot. A vertical talus is an unusual foot deformity in arthrogryposis multiplex congenita, and, if encountered, the physician must think of the distal arthrogryposes or pterygia syndromes.

Most patients do not require upper-extremity surgical procedures. The physician should never think of an individual joint in the upper extremity, but only the whole arm (139,140). Analysis needs to include each hand alone, and how the two hands work together as an effective functional unit, and a functional assessment should be made before deciding on an operation. Because of this, surgical procedures on the upper extremity are usually delayed until the children are old enough to make such an assessment. There are two key goals in treatment of the upper extremities self-help skills, such as feeding and toileting, and mobility skills, such as pushing out of a chair and use of crutches.

The shoulder is usually satisfactory without treatment. For the elbow, it is ideal to achieve flexion to 90 degrees from the fixed extended position. However, when both elbows are involved, surgery to increase flexion should only be done on one side. The fibrotic joint capsule and the weak muscles make the prospect of achieving active elbow flexion unlikely. Passive elbow flexion to a right angle is a prerequisite for considering a tendon transfer for active elbow flexion. Restoration of elbow motion by capsulotomy and triceps-lengthening has had only fair success, diminishing the likelihood for success when an arthrogrypotic muscle is used to motor the joint (141). The triceps brachii and pectoralis have been the most frequently tried. Success is best in children greater than 4 years of age, and who have at least grade four strength of the muscle to be transferred (140,142–144). Distal humeral osteotomy, designed to place the elbow into flexion and correct some of the shoulder internal rotation deformity, may be performed toward the end of the first decade (124,140). It is designed to improve hand-to-mouth function. Care must be taken not to excessively externally rotate the distal humerus. The hand and wrist is usually flexed and ulna deviated, but variations within this pattern exist (145,146). In general, the ulna-side digits are more involved. Proximal interphalangeal flexion deformities rarely respond to physical therapy or surgery. The thumb is flexed and adducted into the palm, and responds better to surgery than do the other digits.

Approximately one-third of patients develop scoliosis (147). There are no comprehensive natural history studies of scoliosis in arthrogryposis, but the curves usually have a C-shaped, neuromuscular pattern and respond poorly to orthoses. Surgery is indicated for progressive curves interfering with balance or function that are generally greater than 50 degrees.

Intelligence is normal, and these children often have a natural ability to learn substitution techniques. There is, however, a strong association between initial feeding difficulties and subsequent language development, which should not be mistaken for retardation (113).

Larsen Syndrome

The essential features of Larsen syndrome are multiple congenital dislocations of large joints, a characteristic flat face, and ligamentous laxity (148) (Fig. 9-13). The cause of the facial flattening is unclear, but it is especially noticeable when observed in profile, and is associated with some hyper-

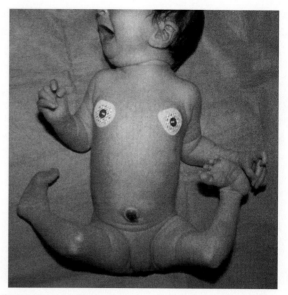

FIGURE 9-13. Larsen syndrome in a 1-week-old patient who has bilateral dislocated knees and clubfeet. (From ref. 1, with permission.)

telorism and a broad forehead. Dislocation of multiple joints appears in a characteristic pattern that includes bilateral dislocated knees, with the tibia anterior on the femur; bilateral dislocated hips; bilateral dislocated elbows; and bilateral clubfeet (149–153). The physician should think of this syndrome whenever dislocated knees are detected. The ligaments are lax or entirely absent. The ligamentous laxity is often so substantial that Larsen syndrome may be confused with Ehlers-Danlos syndrome.

On radiographs, the knees are dislocated, with the tibia anterior to the femur (151). Arthrograms show a small or absent suprapatellar pouch, absent cruciate ligaments, and a misaligned patella (Fig. 9-14). The elbows have complex radial–humeral, ulnar–humeral, and radial–ulnar dislocations. Radial–ulnar synostosis is common and usually associated with ulnar–humeral dislocation (Fig. 9-15B). A spheroid ossicle frequently occurs anterior to the elbow joint; its origin is unknown. There are an increased number of carpal centers (Fig. 9-15A), extra ossification centers in the foot, and a curious double ossification pattern of the calcaneus (Fig. 9-15C). Abnormal cervical spine segmentation, with instability, is typical, and kyphosis a complication often associated with myelopathy. Some cases are inherited in an autosomal dominant manner, aiding in the diagnosis.

Autosomal dominant and recessive inheritance are both reported in Larsen syndrome, although many cases are sporadic (154–156). Autosomal recessive inheritance may have the more severe phenotype. A linkage study of a large kindred from Sweden identified a region on chromosome 3, where the causative gene probably is located (157). The actual causative gene in this region has yet to be identified.

The large number of deformities of the lower extremities

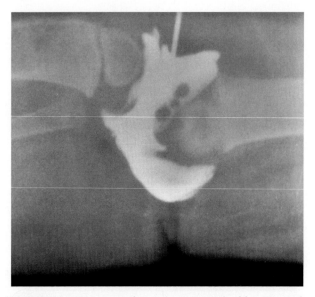

FIGURE 9-14. Larsen syndrome in a 5-month-old patient. The arthrogram of a knee shows anterior dislocation of the tibia on the femur and no suprapatellar pouch.

require treatment to achieve stable, located joints. Knee stability is necessary to achieve ambulation. Reduction almost always requires surgery. The knee may remain unstable after reduction because of the lack of major stabilizing ligaments, such as the anterior cruciate ligament. Long-term orthoses are often needed. Successful anterior cruciate ligament reconstruction has not been reported. The knee is usually reduced before the hips, although simultaneous procedures are possible (151,158). Although most knees do not respond to attempts at manipulation and cast correction, it has been traditional to try this approach initially. Too vigorous manipulations result in distal femoral metaphyseal–physeal fractures. Because manipulation has not been helpful in our hands for true dislocations, we believe that it can be abandoned once a dislocation is confirmed. Surgery may be undertaken as early as 3 to 4 months of age. Cautious restoration of the range of motion (gaining full extension is often a problem), while guarding against redislocation by using a flexion splint or brace may be required after operative reduction.

The hips are dislocated, often despite a rather normal-appearing acetabulum. There is a sensation of good range of motion, although the hip may prove to be irreducible

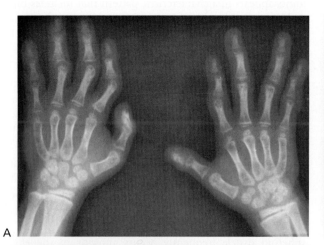

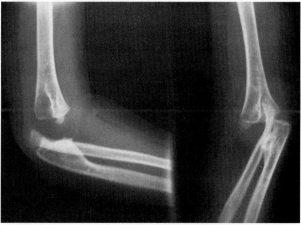

FIGURE 9-15. A 4-year-old patient with Larsen syndrome. Characteristic roentgenograms. **A:** The hands show an increased number of carpal centers and interphalangeal joint subluxations. **B:** The elbow demonstrates total dislocation but full functional ability. (**A** and **B** from ref. 1, with permission.) **C:** The foot has an abnormal os calcis containing two ossification centers.

(153). The evolution of hip management in Larsen syndrome mirrors that in arthrogryposis multiplex congenita, and there is a trend toward earlier treatment. The relative rarity of this syndrome, however, accounts for the lack of good comparative data on how to best manage the hip dislocations. Reduction of the hip is associated with a high redislocation rate and revision surgery (151–153). For this reason, some advocate either leaving bilateral dislocated hips alone, or waiting until after 1 year of age and performing femoral and pelvic osteotomies, along with the open reduction. However, we prefer an approach similar to that in arthrogryposis, with early surgical relocation (usually through a medial approach) [➥3.3, 3.4]. Because the knees are hyperextended when dislocated, and casted flexed after surgical relocation, both knees and hips can be operated on at the same time. Secondary osteotomy of the pelvis and femur can be performed later, if necessary.

The clubfeet can be managed in a cast until the knee deformity is corrected. Some feet can be corrected with serial casting, but long-term results suggest less residual deformity when the foot is treated surgically (151) [➥7.1]. The foot may need to be braced to control ankle instability. Despite the dislocations of the elbow or shoulder, the arms remain functional and rarely require treatment. Crutches or walkers can be used despite the dislocations.

The major concern involving the spine is structural abnormalities of the cervical vertebrae (159,160). This manifestation may occur more frequently than previously recognized, and children should have cervical spine films taken in the first year of life to identify this deformity. Kyphosis is often due to hypoplasia of the vertebral bodies. A combination of cervical kyphosis and forward subluxation may result in quadriplegia and death. Posterior stabilization early (within the first 18 months of life) may avoid the significant problems associated with treatment after myelopathy has occurred, and allow for correction of a kyphotic deformity with growth (161).

Anesthesia complications are common. The mobile infolding arytenoid cartilage creates airway difficulties. The associated tracheomalacia can be especially problematic in the newborn, and may delay surgery for the hips and knees (162). The anesthesiologist should be aware of possible cervical spine instability, and a preoperative lateral film is recommended.

The children have normal intelligence. The prognosis is generally good with aggressive orthopaedic treatment, if the child survives the first year of life. The mortality figures for the first year may be as high as 40%. During the neonatal period, the cartilage-supporting structure of the larynx and trachea is soft, and there may be alarming elasticity of the thoracic cage at the costochondral junction, leading to respiratory failure and death. Cervical spine problems may also contribute to early mortality. Congenital cardiac septal defects and acquired lesions of the mitral valve and aorta,

similar to those found in Marfan syndrome, further complicate medical and anesthesia management (163).

CONTRACTURE SYNDROMES INVOLVING PREDOMINANTLY THE HANDS AND FEET

Distal Arthrogryposis

Children with distal arthrogryposis have characteristic fixed hand contractures and foot deformities, but the major large joints of the arms and legs are spared (164–166). Craniofacial abnormalities are often associated, which has caused distal arthrogryposis to be separated into several eponymic syndromes (e.g., Gordon syndrome), a situation that leads to confusion (167). The cardinal features of distal arthrogryposis are the hand deformity with ulna deviation of the fingers at the metacarpophalangeal joint, flexion deformities at the proximal interphalangeal and metacarpophalangeal joints, and a cup-like palm with a single palmar crease (Fig. 9-16). The thumb is flexed and adducted, with a web at its base (168). Distal arthrogryposis is common, and is sometimes incorrectly called multiple camptodactyly. The inheritance pattern of distal arthrogryposis is autosomal dominant, but there may be considerable variation in families, which leads to missing the diagnosis (167–170).

Linkage analysis shows that the causative gene in some families with distal arthrogryposis is located on chromosome 1 (5). Because there are a variety of subtypes of distal arthrogryposis, it is likely that a number of causative genes will be identified.

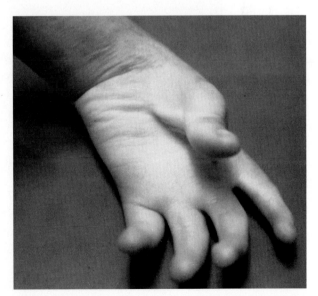

FIGURE 9-16. Distal arthrogryposis. Characteristic hand is the result of ulnar deviation at the metacarpophalangeal (MCP) joints. Notice the deeply cupped palm and webbing of the MCP joint of the thumb.

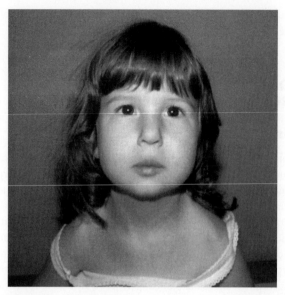

FIGURE 9-17. Freeman-Sheldon syndrome in a 3-year-old patient. Notice the small chin and mouth, long philtrum, puffy cheeks, deeply set eyes, and small chin cleft. (From ref. 1, with permission.)

Although the hand deformity is characteristic and constant, the feet may be clubbed, have stiff metatarsus adductus, and have a vertical talus. The major joints in the upper and lower extremities are otherwise normal, although a minor knee-flexion deformity may be found. Intelligence is normal. The associated craniofacial anomalies are cleft lip or cleft palate, and, in those families, the syndrome of distal arthrogryposis may have an eponymous name, such as Gordon syndrome (171,172). Radiographs show normal bony architecture, and only with persistence of deformities in the hand and feet are articular changes detected. This syndrome can be diagnosed prenatally in the fetus by detecting an unchanged position and lack of motion of the hands in contrast to the normal activity of the large uninvolved joints (173).

Overall, children with distal arthrogryposis have good function. The hands function well because the shoulders, elbows, and wrists are normal. Thumb surgery to lengthen the flexor pollicis longus and rebalance the extensor is the most common surgery. The feet more frequently require surgery. Some clubfeet can be corrected with manipulation and serial casts. Most are treated with circumferential releases [➡7.1]. The outcome of treatment of clubfoot is better in this syndrome than for other arthrogrypotic clubfeet.

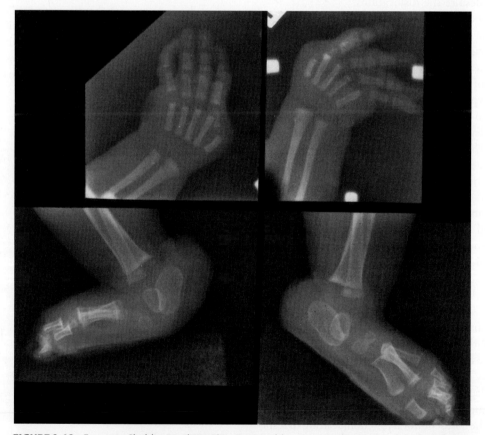

FIGURE 9-18. Freeman-Sheldon syndrome in a 5-year-old patient. Radiographs of the hands demonstrate ulnar deviation at the metacarpophalangeal joint, typical of a distal arthrogryposis syndrome. The feet show bilateral congenital vertical tali. All other joints in this patient were normal. (From ref. 1, with permission.)

Freeman-Sheldon Syndrome

Freeman-Sheldon syndrome is sometimes called "distal arthrogryposis type II," because of the hand and foot deformities similar to distal arthrogryposis. It is recognized by its most characteristic feature, a "whistling face" (Fig. 9-17). The original name, "craniocarpotarsal dystrophy" is misleading, because it does not involve the cranium (174,175). This syndrome is usually sporadic, although there is evidence of autosomal dominant and autosomal recessive inheritance (176–178). The eyes are deeply set. The cheeks are fleshy, and pursed lips simulate whistling. There is a small mouth and a curious H-shaped dimple in the chin.

Scoliosis was not initially recognized as a common feature, but it affects more than one-half of the patients. The onset is in the first decade. It is often severe, with a left thoracic pattern reported regularly. The vertebrae are normally shaped. Although the scoliosis can be managed as in idiopathic scoliosis, the curves are more rigid, and may not respond well to brace treatment (177,179).

The hands demonstrate the classic distal arthrogryposis pattern described earlier (177,179,180). There are other contractures, including flexion deformities of the elbow and knee, decreased shoulder range of motion, decreased neck range of motion, and dislocated hips (181). Operative management principles for the upper extremity are similar to that with distal arthrogryposis. The hands are treated with physical and occupational therapy, but there is less improvement than seen with the other distal arthrogryposis syndromes (182). Most of the other associated contractures can be treated like those in the other arthrogrypotic syndromes.

Clubfoot is the most common foot deformity, with vertical talus being second most common (Fig. 9-18) (177,179,180). The clubfoot and vertical talus deformities are resistant to nonoperative measures.

During infancy, dysphagia and aspiration lead to failure to thrive, and to death. Surgery to permit adequate mouth opening for feeding may be necessary (183). Children who survive the neonatal period do well and have normal intelligence. Anesthesia complications are common; some are the result of abnormalities related to the laryngeal cartilages (183–186). The cause is unknown, but the buccinator muscle is hypoplastic, and electromyograms and muscle biopsies are identical to the peripheral muscle studies in classic arthrogryposis multiplex congenita (187), suggesting some similarity in pathophysiology.

CONTRACTURE SYNDROMES WITH SKIN WEBS

Pterygia Syndrome

"Pterygium" comes from a Greek word meaning "little wing." A pterygium is a web. It can be seen as an isolated malformation in some syndromes, such as the pterygium colli in the neck of patients with Klippel-Feil syndrome.

There are two clinically important pterygia syndromes: multiple pterygium syndrome and popliteal pterygia syndrome (188). Several pterygium syndromes are lethal, with the affected patients not surviving pregnancy or the newborn period (189,190). The web syndromes are separated genetically as autosomal recessive (i.e., lethal pterygium syndrome and multiple pterygium) and autosomal dominant (i.e., popliteal pterygium) (191). However, they often overlap. Lethal pterygium syndrome may be diagnosed prenatally by detecting hydrops and cystic hygroma colli (192).

Multiple pterygia syndrome (i.e., Escobar syndrome) is characterized by a web across every flexion crease in the extremities, most prominently across the popliteal space, the elbow, and in the axilla (193,194) (Fig. 9-19). There also are webs across the neck laterally and anteriorly from sternum to the chin, drawing the facial features down. The fingers are webbed. The webs can be obvious, but if they are not, the affected children can look very much like those with arthrogryposis multiplex congenita. The two features that differentiate this syndrome from classic arthrogryposis

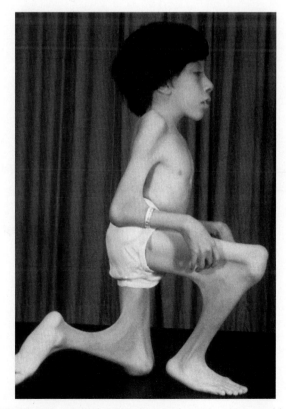

FIGURE 9-19. Multiple pterygium syndrome in a 12-year-old patient. Antecubital webs fix the elbows, and popliteal webs prevent ambulation. The patient had normal intelligence and became a college graduate. (From ref. 1, with permission.)

are vertical talus and congenital spine deformity. The vertical talus is fairly constant in multiple pterygium syndrome and can only be managed surgically. Circumferential release and prolonged protection, as in managing any arthrypotic foot deformity, is necessary. The spine deformity is significant, with multiple segmentation abnormalities and a lordoscoliosis (195) (Figs. 9-20 and 9-21). The lordoscoliosis may be substantial enough to interfere with trunk and chest growth, leading to respiratory death during the first or second year of life (Fig. 9-21). Mobility depends much on the magnitude of the lower extremity webs and the remaining joint motion, with many patients limited to wheelchair for locomotion. The children have normal intelligence, and efforts for their independence should be maximized. Surgery is rarely needed for the upper extremities.

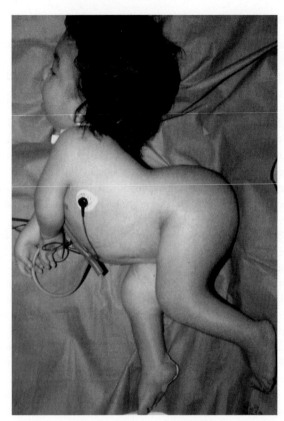

FIGURE 9-21. Multiple pterygium syndrome. Severe limitation of trunk growth was caused by vertebral fusions and lordoscoliosis. Death occurred at 24 months of age because of respiratory failure.

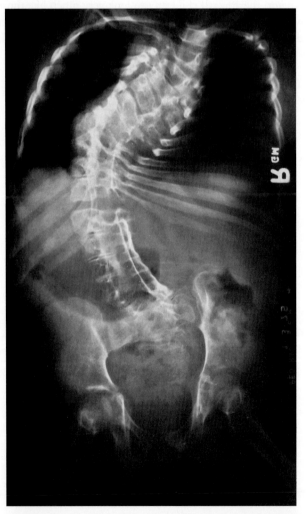

FIGURE 9-20. Multiple pterygium syndrome in a 13-year-old patient. Radiograph shows severe scoliosis, vertebral abnormalities, and an unsegmented bar from T9 to T12 and from L1 to S1, with an apparent gap between the bars. (From ref. 1, with permission.)

Popliteal pterygium syndrome (i.e., fascial-genital-popliteal syndrome) has recognizable features in the face, the genitals, and the knee (196–200). The features include a cleft lip and palate, lip pits, and intraoral adhesions (201,202). A fibrous band crosses the perineum and distorts the genitalia (203). A popliteal web is usually present bilaterally (200). It runs from ischium to calcaneus, resulting in a severe knee-flexion deformity. Tibia hypoplasia may be associated. Within the popliteal web is a superficial fibrous band, over which lies a tent of muscle running from the os calcis to the ischium, and known in the older literature as a "calcaneoischiadicus muscle." The popliteal artery and vein are usually deep, but the sciatic nerve is superficial in the web, just underneath the fibrous band (Fig. 9-22). There is a distinctive foot abnormality in this syndrome: a bifid great toenail and syndactyly of the lesser toes.

Although the original cases of multiple and popliteal pterygium syndromes were clearly defined, there is more phenotypic variation in both than originally thought. For example, mild webs in joints of the upper extremity may be found in patients with popliteal pterygium syndrome. Adaptive changes in the joints occur over time. Radiographically, the

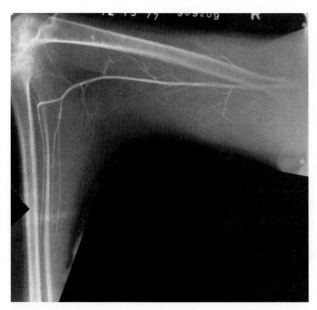

FIGURE 9-22. Popliteal pterygium in a 13-year-old patient. Arteriogram shows that the popliteal artery has been drawn up from its normal position. At the margin of the web is the sciatic nerve. (From ref. 1, with permission.)

patella becomes elongated, and the femoral condyles flattened, as a result of knee flexion deformity.

From a management perspective, the determining factors are the magnitude of scoliosis and the size of the web crossing the knee. The thoracic vertebral dysplasia, thoracic lordosis, and the small chest impairs lung development, resulting in death in the first years of life in those with multiple pterygium syndrome. For the longer-term survivor, management of the spine deformity is identical to those with nonsyndromic congenital scoliosis. Preoperative evaluation of intraspinal contents by MRI and ultrasound of the kidney are indicated.

The knee is the joint that limits mobility in both syndromes and is the joint that most determines future ambulatory potential (200,204–206). Traditionally, treatment of the knee begins with physical therapy, but its effectiveness is doubtful. Early popliteal web surgery is recommended before the onset of adaptive changes in the articular surfaces, and before further vascular shortening. The nerve is usually located just deep to the skin and web, and care must be taken to avoid nerve damage. The web is resected, and Z-plasty of the skin performed. There is a high recurrence rate despite braces. Femoral shortening and extension osteotomy are usually postponed until near or after maturity. However, if almost full knee extension cannot be achieved at surgery, even if during infancy or childhood, femoral shortening should be considered (207). Gradual distraction techniques can be used, but the advantage over traditional techniques has not been demonstrated (208). Posterior soft tissue pro-

cedures can be combined with distraction techniques to gradually extend the knee.

DOWN SYNDROME

Down syndrome is the most common and perhaps the most readily recognizable malformation in humans (209) (Fig. 9-23). Patients have a characteristic facial appearance including upward-slanting eyes, epicanthal folds, and a flattened profile. Examination of the hands reveals a single flexion crease, often referred to as a simian crease. There is also clinodactyly of the small finger. These hand malformations have no clinical significance (210). Milestones are delayed, with most children not walking until 2 to 3 years of age. The classic gait pattern is broad based, toed out, and waddling.

The bones in Down syndrome have subtle malformations. The best-studied changes are in the pelvis, which is characterized by flat acetabula and flared iliac wings (211). These pelvic changes are so characteristic that prior to use of chromosome analysis pelvic radiographs were used to confirm the diagnosis. Short stature is a cardinal feature; the average for male adults is 155 cm (61 in.), and the average for female adults is 145 cm (57 in.) (212). Bone changes can be used in prenatal diagnosis, in which a combination of bone length and maternal lab tests (human chorionic gonadotropin and alpha-fetoprotein levels) may predict the diagnosis, although the positive and negative predictive values are not as good as initially hoped (213). Cytogenetic study, which identifies complete trisomy 21 in 95% of cases, remains the best confirmative test.

Complete trisomies account for 95% of the cases, with 2% mosaics and 3% translocations. The overall risk is 1 per 660 live births, and the incidence is closely related to maternal age. If the mother is younger than 30 years of age, the risk is 1 of 5000 live births, and if the mother is older than 35 years of age, the incidence rises to 1 in 250. The critical region necessary for Down syndrome resides in part of the long arm of chromosome 21. Duplication of a 5-megabase region of chromosome 21 (located at 21q22.2-22.3) causes the classic phenotypic features, such as the characteristic facies, hand anomalies, congenital heart disease, and some aspects of the mental retardation (214). This region probably contains a number of genes whose duplication is necessary to produce the syndrome.

The general features of Down syndrome are well known. There is a characteristic flattened face. Mental retardation is typical, but performance is far better than expected from standard IQ testing. Congenital heart disease occurs in about one-half of patients, and is usually a septal defect (e.g., arteriovenous communis, ventricular septal defect). Duodenal atresia is found regularly. Leukemia occurs in about 1% (1,5). There is a high incidence of endocrinopathies, hypothyroidism in particular. Infections are common, although the precise molecular mechanism is not apparent.

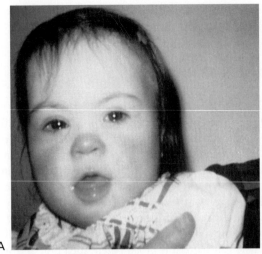
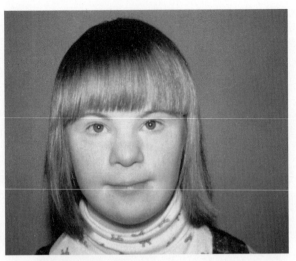

FIGURE 9-23. Down syndrome. The child has the characteristic face, with upward-slanting eyes, epicanthal folds, open mouth of early childhood, and flattened profile. **A:** At 1 year of age. (Courtesy of Murray Feingold, M.D., Boston, MA.) **B:** At 10 years of age. (From ref. 1, with permission.)

The appearance of premature aging is obvious, and there often is an early onset of Alzheimer disease (215).

Approximately 10% of people with Down syndrome show an increased atlantodens interval on lateral spine films (216–220) (Fig. 9-24A). In most, the increased interval is not associated with symptoms (217,221). In addition, there is a broad array of other abnormalities in the upper cervical spine, including instability at occiput and C1 (220, 222–224), odontoid dysplasia (217,225) (Fig.9-24C), laminal defects at C1 (226) (Fig. 9-24B), spondylolisthesis (Fig.

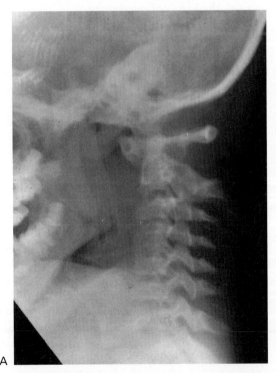
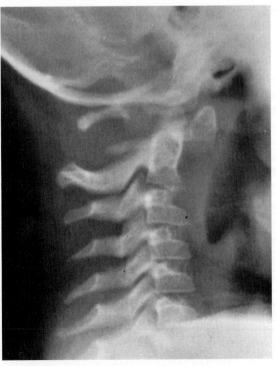

FIGURE 9-24. Cervical spine abnormalities in a patient with Down syndrome. **A:** Atlantodens instability at 8 years of age. **B:** Hypoplastic posterior elements of C1 at 3 years of age.

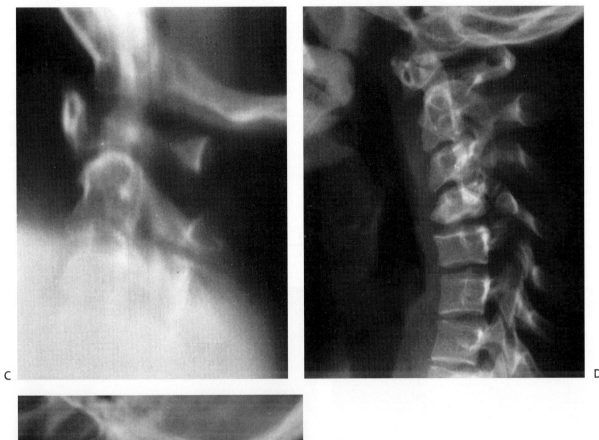

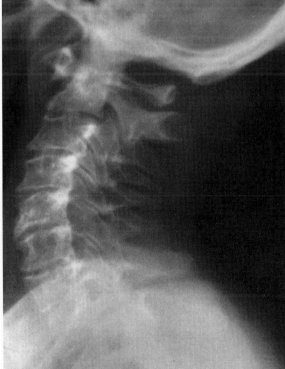

FIGURE 9-24. *(continued)* **C:** Os odontoideum and increased atlantodens interval at 14 years of age. **D:** Midcervical spondylolysis at 16 years of age. **E:** Precocious osteoarthritis of the midcervical spine at 40 years of age. (From ref. 1, with permission.)

9-24D), and precocious arthritis in the midcervical region (227,228) (Fig. 9-24E). These other abnormalities often complicate decision-making about spinal instability. Although routine screening radiographs often disclose these cervical spine abnormalities, radiographs are not reliable in predicting myelopathy (219,221,225,229–232). Thus, their use in the management of the cervical spine in patients with Down syndrome is uncertain. Details of managing the cervical spine in Down syndrome are found in Chapter 21 of this text.

About one-half the patients with Down syndrome have scoliosis, with an idiopathic pattern in most (233). Scoliosis is five times more likely to be detected in a severely retarded institutionalized population than in an ambulatory setting,

which suggests confounding variables of detection and neuromuscular factors. Management is the same as in idiopathic scoliosis. Spondylolisthesis occurs in about 6%, with the lower lumbar spine being most commonly involved. Spondylolisthesis can also occur in the cervical spine.

Congenital dislocated hips are rare, but progressive dysplasia may begin during later childhood. This loss of acetabular containment may lead to an acute or gradual complete dislocation (Fig. 9-25A, B). Although the onset of acetabular dysplasia is in late childhood, it can be progressive even after maturity, leading to adult dislocations (234–236) (Fig. 9-25C, D). Although hip instability and developmental dysplasia are thought to lead to functional disability, interfering with walking, and reducing independent mobility, there are

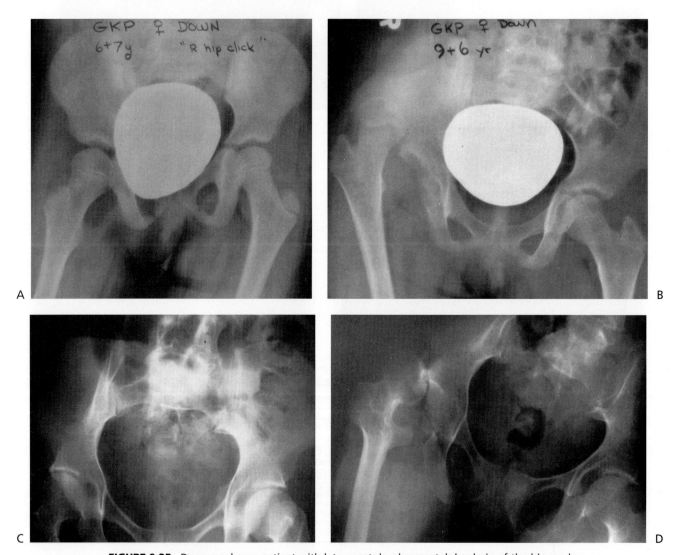

FIGURE 9-25. Down syndrome patient with late-onset developmental dysplasia of the hip, and dislocation. **A:** Standing radiograph of the pelvis at 6.5 years of age. **B:** At 9.5 years of age, the patient suddenly refused to walk because of hip dislocation. (From ref. 1, with permission.) **C:** Pelvic radiograph of a 31-year-old man with Down syndrome. **D:** Three years later, dislocation of right hip occurred. (From ref. 230, with permission.)

no studies showing this to be the case. The etiology of the hip instability is probably multifactorial, with ligamentous laxity, subtle changes in the shape of the pelvis and acetabular alignment, and behavior (some children become habitual dislocators) all contributing. Treatment of the unstable hip is difficult, and the multiple causative factors also contribute to higher treatment failure rates. Both operative and nonoperative treatment are reported. Prolonged bracing after reduction for the hip that acutely dislocates shows success in children under 6 years (237). In cases in which there are repeated dislocations, surgical reconstruction is warranted, especially in children over 6 years. Operative treatment is technically demanding, and requires correction of all the deforming factors. Reconstruction must take into account the abnormal bone alignment, and should include femoral [➥4.1, 4.2, 4.6] and acetabular osteotomies [➥3.5, 3.7, 3.8], as well as imbrication of the redundant capsule. The recurrence rate following hip surgery is high, suggesting that other factors related to the underlying disease, but not necessarily related to the hip anatomy itself, contribute to this high recurrence rate (238–240).

Slipped capital femoral epiphyses are reported in all Down syndrome series, although the precise incidence is unknown (233,241) (Fig. 9-26) [➥3.14]. There appears to be a higher-than-expected risk for avascular necrosis. The reasons are not clear, but the factors include an increased number of acute slips and more late diagnoses. It is tempting to speculate about an association with the hypothyroid

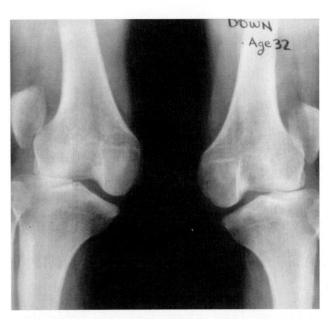

FIGURE 9-27. Down syndrome effects in a 32-year-old patient. The radiograph shows bilateral dislocated patellae and an oblique orientation of the joint line. The patient is fully ambulatory, but before standing, must manually reduce the patellae to the midline. (From ref. 1, with permission.)

state, which is common in Down syndrome. All children with Down syndrome should have thyroid function tests.

The configuration of the knee is that of genu valgum, with a subluxed and dislocated patella (Fig. 9-27). Many individuals will have asymptomatic patellar dislocations, and do not require treatment (242). Symptomatic cases should be initially managed with orthoses and a physiotherapy program. Individuals who continue to be symptomatic can be considered for operative treatment [➥5.1, 5.2]. As in hip dysplasia, operative interventions that correct all of the deformities (bone and soft tissue) have the best success.

The characteristic appearance of the feet in childhood is one of an asymptomatic flexible planovalgus shape, with an increased space between the great and second toes. Because maintaining mobility in adults with Down syndrome is important, foot impairment should be treated. This treatment is shoe-wear modification in many cases, but may require surgery in cases that are symptomatic despite appropriate shoe wear [➥7.4, 7.5, 7.11]. In many, hallux valgus develops in adolescence, and in adulthood bunions may become quite symptomatic. There is no evidence that prophylactic orthotics are beneficial in childhood. Repair of hallux valgus and bunion may be needed in late adolescence or young adulthood. Because of the hindfoot valgus, pronation, and external tibial torsion, the forces that produce bunions are obvious, and fusion of the first metatarsophalangeal joint should be considered, along with osteotomy, to correct hindfoot valgus [➥7.4].

A polyarticular arthropathy occurs in approximately 10%

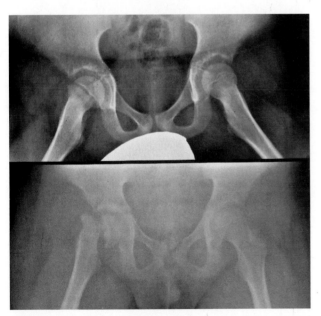

FIGURE 9-26. Effects of Down syndrome in a 12-year-old boy with 4 months of knee pain. The grade I slipped capital femoral epiphysis progressed to a total slip while the patient was undergoing preoperative evaluation and bed rest. (From ref. 1, with permission.)

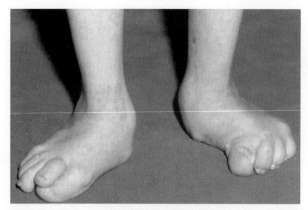

FIGURE 9-28. Polyarthritis of Down syndrome and valgus feet led to significant deformity in a 16-year-old patient. (From ref. 1, with permission.)

of those with Down syndrome (243–245). Whether this is true juvenile rheumatoid arthritis, or a unique inflammatory arthritis due to genetic or immune defects, is unknown; the natural history is not documented. Delayed diagnosis is common. Nonsteroidal antiinflammatory drugs have been the mainstay of treatment. Foot symptoms are exceptionally frequent with the onset of polyarthropathy (Fig. 9-28).

Marked joint hypermobility is evident; the children are able to assume the most intriguing sitting postures. Ligamentous laxity was traditionally thought to be the cause of joint hypermobility and to predispose patients with Down syndrome to orthopaedic pathology. However, ligamentous laxity correlates poorly with joint hypermobility. This suggests that other factors, such as subtle malformations in the shapes of bones and insertion sites of ligaments, play a role in hypermobility (229,246).

The natural history of those with Down syndrome has changed in the last few decades. Longevity has increased because of the aggressive surgical approach to congenital heart disease, chemotherapy for leukemia, and antibiotics for infection. Survival into the sixties is common. Approximately 1 of 5 persons with Down syndrome has a musculoskeletal problem. Many, however, are merely radiographic abnormalities or curious physical findings. These patients often have excellent functional performance despite the abnormalities. There is a paucity of well-documented, long-term orthopaedic studies. Treatment programs should focus on functional performance rather than on radiographic findings.

FETAL ALCOHOL SYNDROME

Fetal alcohol syndrome is a pattern of malformations delineated in children of alcoholic mothers. The full-blown syndrome is usually only seen in children of chronic alcoholics who drink throughout pregnancy. Lesser manifestations of the syndrome, known as fetal alcohol effects, may be related to more moderate alcohol ingestion (247). Although the risk to alcoholic mothers is known, there is substantial difference of opinion about the effects of moderate alcohol use during pregnancy (248–250). Alcohol is the most likely teratogen for a mother to encounter (251). The overall incidence of full-blown fetal alcohol syndrome is 0.33 per 1000 live births (252,253). For an alcoholic mother, there is a 30% risk for fetal alcohol syndrome in her child.

A cardinal clinical feature is disturbed growth; the children have intrauterine growth retardation, small weight, and small length at birth, and these limitations remain despite good nutrition during childhood (254,255) (Fig. 9-29). Their smallness and a loss of fat suggest a search for endocrine dysfunction; the patients often look similar to those who are growth hormone deficient. The second cardinal feature is disturbed central nervous system development. Many children with fetal alcohol syndrome are found in cerebral palsy clinics. The typical child has a small head, a small brain, and delayed motor milestones. Accomplishing fine motor skills is also delayed. Hypotonia is present early but many develop spasticity later. The typical face has three characteristic features: short palpebral fissures (i.e., the eyes

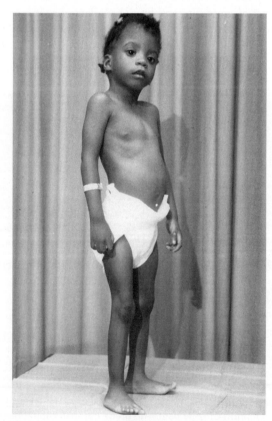

FIGURE 9-29. The 3-year-old patient is small and has the characteristic face of fetal alcohol syndrome. (From ref. 1, with permission.)

appear small), a flat philtrum (i.e., no groove below the nose), and a thin upper lip (256,257) (Fig. 9-29).

Approximately 50% have an orthopaedic abnormality, but most are not disabling (258–260). At birth, the range of motion is restricted, especially of the hands and feet, and occasionally these contractures are fixed. The contractures typically respond well to physical therapy, although residual stiffness in the proximal interphalangeal joints may remain. Clubfoot is common, and approximately 10% have developmental dysplasia of the hip. The clubfoot is usually not rigid (261). Cervical spine fusions, usually involving C2 and C3, may be indicated by radiographs (260,262–266). These may resemble the picture seen in Klippel-Feil syndrome, but there are usually none of the other findings associated with that syndrome. Synostoses are also common in the upper extremity, with fusions involving the radial–ulnar articulation and the carpal bones, all without disability (262,265,267). Stippled epiphyses may be seen in the lower extremities, but rarely in the upper extremities (268).

The orthopaedic problems associated with fetal alcohol syndrome can be managed the same as these problems in children without this syndrome. The future for children with fetal alcohol is dim, despite placement out of the alcoholic home. Intellect remains retarded, with little catch up. Social services departments should be involved in these children's care.

NAIL-PATELLA SYNDROME

Children with nail-patella syndrome have a quartet of findings that include nail dysplasia, patellar hypoplasia, elbow dysplasia, and iliac horns (269). The most prominent feature is dystrophic nails (Fig. 9-30A). The nail may be com-

pletely absent, hypoplastic, or show grooves and distortions in its surface (270). The thumb is more involved than the small finger, and the ulnar border more involved than the radial. The hands are often very symmetric, and fingernails are more involved than toenails.

The second cardinal feature is hypoplastic patellae (271). They are quite small, and may be entirely absent (Fig. 9-30B). They are unstable, and may be found in a position of fixed dislocation. The patellar abnormality highlights the total knee dysplasia, with an abnormal femoral condyle and a curious septum running from the patella to the intercondylar groove (septum interarticularis), dividing the knee into two compartments. Abnormalities in varus and valgus alignment occur, with valgus more common because of the small, flat lateral femoral condyle (271).

A third feature is a dislocated radial head (271,272) (Fig. 9-30C). The elbow joint is dysplastic, with abnormalities in the lateral humeral condyle, mimicking in many ways the dysplasia of the knee. The trochlea is large and the capitellum hypoplastic, creating an asymmetric shape that may predispose the radial head to dislocation.

The fourth and pathognomonic feature is iliac horns: bony exostoses on the posterior surface of the ilium (273) (Fig. 9-30D). They are asymptomatic and require no treatment.

Nail-patella syndrome is caused by a mutation in the *LMX1B* gene. This gene is a homeodomain protein, which plays a role regulating transcription in limb-patterning during fetal development. Mutation in the gene will disrupt normal limb patterning and alter kidney formation, resulting in extremity deformities and an associated nephropathy (274).

Children have short stature, with the height falling be-

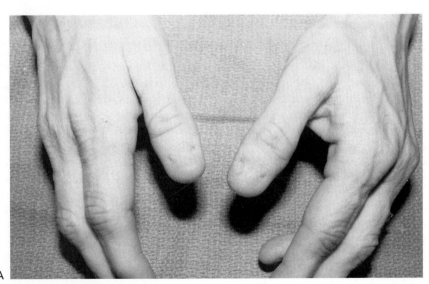

A

FIGURE 9-30. Nail-patella syndrome. The classic quartet of features consists of dystrophic nails shown in **A**. *(continued)*

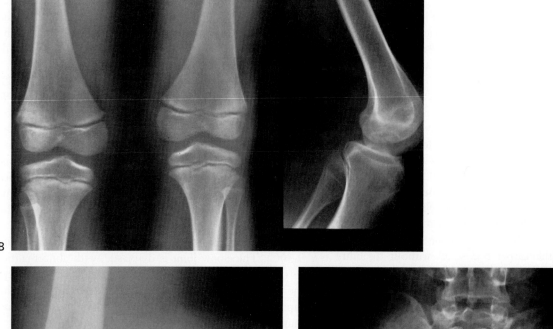

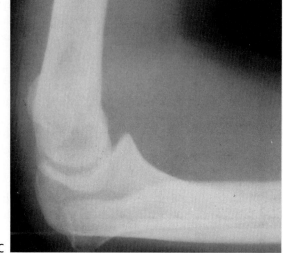

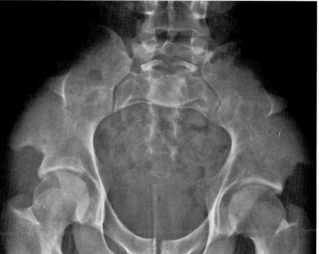

B

C

D

FIGURE 9-30. *(continued)* Absent patellae (notice the region of osteochondritis dissecans on the lateral film) are shown in **B**, posterior dislocation of the radial head in **C**, and iliac horns in **D**.

tween the third and tenth percentiles. There is shoulder girdle dysplasia that represents curious radiographic features, and not any significant functional disability (275). There is a foot deformity that is sometimes the chief presenting complaint of children with nail-patella syndrome (271,276). The foot deformities include variations of stiff calcaneal valgus, metatarsus adductus, and clubfeet.

There is a restricted range of motion and contractures affect several large joints, including knee-flexion deformities and external rotation contracture of the hip. When these contractures are severe and accompanied by stiff clubfeet, the diagnosis may be mistaken for arthrogryposis multiplex congenita. Madelung deformity, spondylolysis, and in some adults, inflammatory arthropathy may be present (269, 277, 278).

The knee disability is variable and related to the magnitude of quadriceps dysfunction and the dislocated patella.

Poor femoral condyles challenge achieving patella stability. As a rule, limited soft tissue or capsular releases are ineffective, but combined proximal and distal patella realignments have an overall favorable outcome [➡5.1, 5.2] (271). A contracted and fibrotic quadriceps may result in a knee extension contracture, and in such cases, quadricepsplasty is indicated along with the patella realignment. More commonly, an associated knee-flexion deformity may require hamstring release and posterior capsulotomy [➡4.23], although results have been inconsistent (271). Residual deformity, which is usually flexion or rotational, is managed by femoral osteotomy toward the end of the first decade. Osteochondritis dissecans of the femoral condyle is relatively common (Fig. 9-30B). An intraarticular septum makes arthroscopic management difficult, but the septum can be removed arthroscopically.

The radial head dislocation is asymptomatic in young

children, but may become symptomatic with time. In symptomatic individuals, excision of the radial head will improve symptoms arising from the prominent lateral bump, but the range of motion is rarely improved. Although traditional teaching advocates performing radial head excision after skeletal maturity, earlier excision in symptomatic children does not seem to be associated with significant problems (271). Clubfeet can be managed the same as idiopathic clubfeet [➥7.1].

The most important nonorthopaedic condition is kidney failure. The nephropathy of nail-patella syndrome causes significant morbidity, affecting the patient's longevity. There is great variability in the age at onset and severity of the nephropathy (279). All patients should be referred for a nephrology evaluation when this diagnosis is made. Patients can go on to chronic renal failure, requiring long-term nephrology management.

DE LANGE SYNDROME

The exceptionally characteristic face of a child with growth retardation makes the clinical diagnosis of de Lange syndrome reasonably reliable (280). The face has immediately recognizable down-turned corners of the mouth, single eyebrow (synophrys), elongated philtrum, and long eyelashes (281,282) (Fig. 9-31).

The syndrome itself is clinically defined, with the cause unknown. Duplication or deletion of the chromosome band 3q25-29 produces a phenotype similar to de Lange syndrome (283,284). In these instances, the mother is always the transmitting parent, suggesting genomic imprinting. The syndrome is relatively common, occurring 1 in 10,000 live births, and it is possible to make a prenatal diagnosis by ultrasound (285,286).

Most have mild orthopaedic deformities of the upper extremities (286–292) (Fig. 9-32). They form a curious constellation of a small hand, a proximally placed thumb, clinodactyly of the small finger, and decreased elbow motion, usually caused by a dislocated radial head. This combination rarely causes any disability. Some patients, however, have severe deformities of the upper extremity in the form of an absent ulna and a monodigital hand, a condition that can be unilateral or bilateral (Fig. 9-32).

The lower extremities are usually spared. Tight heel cords and other cerebral palsy-like contractures are seen occasionally. Syndactyly of the toes is fairly constant. Aplasia of the tibia has been reported rarely. There is possibly a higher incidence of Legg-Perthes disease, approaching about 10%.

The small size begins with intrauterine growth retardation. Children remain small, with a delayed skeletal age. The mortality rate in the first year of life is high because of defective swallowing mechanisms (293), gastroesophageal reflux (294), aspiration, and respiratory infections. If the children survive their first year, they usually do well, but the long-term outcome is not well known. Almost all walk, but their milestones are delayed. There is retarded mentation, but the added features of no speech and no interactions cause major disability (295). Self-mutilating behavior can be an obstacle to orthopaedic care (296,297).

Because of the mental retardation, the failure of developing speech and paucity of social interactions raise questions about the suitability of these patients for some types of orthopaedic treatment. Braces, physical therapy, and surgery for tight heel cords are justifiable. Upper-extremity surgery is not indicated unless improved performance capacity is ensured. Patients with de Lange syndrome do not use upper-extremity prostheses. Lower-extremity prostheses, however, should be prescribed for the rare case with tibial deficiency. Because the gastroesophageal reflux and swallowing disor-

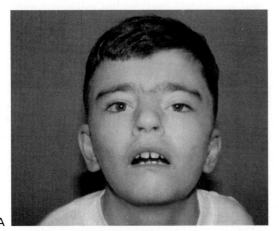 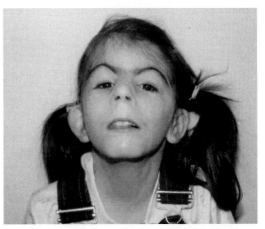

FIGURE 9-31. Cornelia de Lange syndrome. Notice the classic facial features of heavy eyebrows meeting in the midline, upturned nose, downturned corners of the mouth, and long eyelashes in a 13-year-old boy (**A**) and a 7-year-old girl (**B**). (From ref. 1, with permission.)

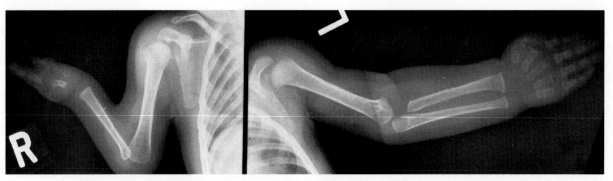

FIGURE 9-32. Cornelia de Lange syndrome in a child demonstrating a severely affected upper extremity on her right side (i.e., absent ulna and fingers) and a mildly affected arm on her left (i.e., short thumb and dysplasia of proximal radius). (From ref. 1, with permission.)

ders may persist well past the first year, there is a higher risk of anesthesia complications (298).

FAMILIAL DYSAUTONOMIA

Familial dysautonomia, also called Riley-Day syndrome, is an autosomal recessive disorder occurring primarily in Jews tracing their ancestry to Eastern Europe. Among such individuals, the incidence is estimated to be about 1 in 3,700. The clinical manifestations are caused by defective functioning of the autonomic nervous system and sensory system. The autonomic dysfunction causes labile blood pressure, dysphagia, abnormal temperature control, and abnormal gastrointestinal motility. Infants have difficulty swallowing, with misdirected fluids going to the lungs, resulting in pneumonia. There is a poor suck response and a curious absence of tears. During childhood, the autonomic dysfunction becomes more apparent, with wide swings in blood pressure and body temperature. There are cyclic vomiting episodes; these crises often last hours or days. Swallowing remains poor. The skin is blotchy. There is relative insensitivity to pain, and poor hot-cold distinction. Intelligence is normal, but the children exhibit emotional lability, and may have unusual personality development, especially in the teenage years. The diagnosis is made on clinical findings, and based on the presence of five signs: (i) lack of axon flare after intradermal injection of histamine, (ii) absence of fungiform papillae on the tongue, (iii) miosis of the pupil after conjunctival installation of methacholine chloride, (iv) absent deep tendon reflexes, and (v) diminished tear flow (299–301).

Linkage studies show the gene locus to be on chromosome 9 (9q31-33), but the actual gene has not yet been identified (302). The information about the locus, however, has been successfully utilized in prenatal diagnosis. Pathologic anatomy reveals a paucity of neurons in cervical sympathetic ganglia, dorsal sensory roots, and abdominal para-

sympathetic nerves (303). The number of small axons is depleted from the sensory nerves and the dorsal columns. Because of a primary failure to develop axons, the symptoms are present at birth, and there is a loss of nerve cells and progression of symptoms as the patient ages.

Musculoskeletal manifestations include scoliosis, fracture susceptibility, avascular necrosis, and a Charcot joint-like process. Although scoliosis affects a majority of patients, approximately one-fourth will need operative intervention (302,304–306) [➡2.9]. It has an early onset, and progression is often rapid. Kyphosis, accentuated by tight anterior pectoralis muscles, appears in approximately one-half of patients. Bracing does not work well, because of the underlying gastrointestinal and emotional problems. Anesthesia can be challenging in individuals with such autonomic lability, but with proper techniques, operative intervention is successful. Surgery seems to give better results if performed early in the course of the disease (307–309).

Fractures occur frequently, and often go unrecognized because of the insensitivity to pain (310). The physician should be suspicious of occult fractures in patients who have had trauma and swelling, but experience minimal tenderness. Fractures usually heal quite well, but early diagnosis and avoiding displacement is the goal.

Radiographic evidence of avascular necrosis is common, but the pathobiology is entirely unknown (302,306,311). There are Legg-Perthes changes in the hips. Osteochondritis dissecans of the knees is often extensive, involving both femoral condyles (Fig. 9-33). It may be difficult to differentiate the ossification changes in the knee due to osteochondritis dissecans from what may be an early Charcot joint (312,313). Hip dysplasia may be seen in patients with this syndrome.

The natural history of familial dysautonomia is characterized by a relatively high mortality rate in infancy, attributed to aspiration pneumonia (301). Sudden death in childhood and adolescence occurs because the child is unable to respond appropriately to stress or hypoxia. Early recognition

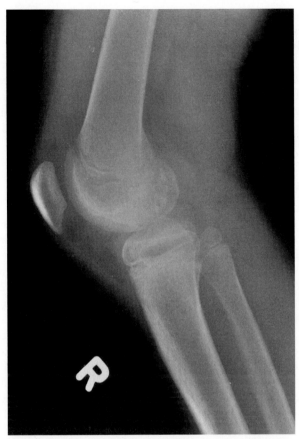

FIGURE 9-33. Familial dysautonomia. Irregular ossifications of the distal femoral epiphysis mimic osteochondritis dissecans.

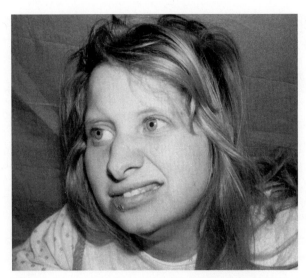

FIGURE 9-34. Rubinstein-Taybi syndrome. In a 10-year-girl, the characteristic Cyrano de Bergerac-like nose has a septum that extends below the nostrils.

of this syndrome and appropriate care, lead to a life expectancy of many decades. Management of the gastrointestinal problems, and the use of gastrostomy and fundoplications have been extremely successful in this regard. There have been successful pregnancies brought to term in affected mothers (314).

RUBINSTEIN-TAYBI SYNDROME

The Rubinstein-Taybi syndrome is characterized by mental retardation associated with characteristic digital changes, consisting mainly of broad thumbs and large toes (315). It is relatively common in the mentally retarded population, with an incidence of 1 in 500 in this population (316). Most cases are sporadic, although there is the possibility of autosomal dominant inheritance (317).

One of the most characteristic clinical features is the comical face with a Cyrano de Bergerac-like nose and the nasal septum extending below the nostrils (Fig. 9-34). The face may change with time, making this a less reliable finding (318). Broad terminal phalanges of the thumb are present in 87% of patients, and the great toe is affected in 100%.

One-half of the patients have radially angulated thumbs, a source of disability. Hallux varus is common, and the physician should consider Rubinstein-Taybi syndrome whenever congenital hallux varus is encountered. Patients have ligamentous laxity and pronated feet, and an increased incidence of fractures (316).

The radiographs are rather characteristic. The thumb shows a wide distal phalanx, with soft tissue hypertrophy and a triangular proximal phalanx (i.e., delta phalanx) that accounts for the radial deviation (Fig. 9-35A). The toe demonstrates duplicated or broad distal phalanx, but true polydactyly is not part of this syndrome (Fig. 9-35B). There is an assortment of insignificant other skeletal anomalies, many in the axial skeleton (319).

Patients with Rubinstein-Taybi syndrome have been shown to have breakpoints in, and microdeletions of, chromosome 16p13.3. This region contains the gene for CREB-binding protein, a nuclear protein participating as a co-activator in cyclic-AMP-regulated gene expression. This protein plays an important role in the development of the central nervous system, head, and neck, thus explaining the facial malformation and mental retardation. The propensity to develop tumors in these regions is probably caused by malregulation of cyclic-AMP-regulated gene expression (320).

Birth weight and size are normal, but growth retardation is noticed at the end of the first year, and there is no true pubertal growth spurt (321). The patients are mentally retarded, many with microcephaly. IQ can range from 35 to 80, with a delay in acquiring skills. However, these features vary. Associated medical problems include visual disturbances, congenital heart disease, and gastrointestinal abnormalities. Later in life, frequent upper respiratory infections

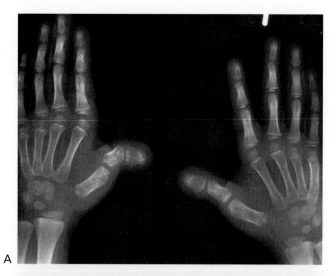

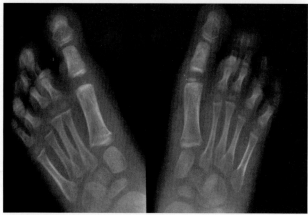

FIGURE 9-35. Rubinstein-Taybi syndrome in a 7-year-old patient. **A:** The thumbs are malformed, with a trapezoid proximal phalanx. The epiphysis extends around the radial side. **B:** The feet are more symmetric. Notice the broadening of the distal phalanx of the great toe. (From ref. 1, with permission.)

are related to abnormal craniofacial features, severe dental caries are common, and other infections lead to morbidity (322–324). Individuals with this syndrome are predisposed to certain types of central nervous system and head and neck tumors (325).

The thumb is treated if the radial deviation interferes with pinch, in which case osteotomy of the proximal phalanx should be performed. The deformity is progressive, and recurrence is common, as with any delta phalanx. The toe rarely requires treatment unless there is a significant congenital hallux varus. Patellar dislocation occurs in this syndrome. Although reports suggest that early surgical intervention might improve function, there are no data comparing early treatment with other managements to support this concept. If surgery is performed, the addition of an extensive quadriceps mobilization seems to decrease the revision rate (326,327) [➥5.1, 5.2]. We reserve surgical in-

tervention for the patella dislocation for symptomatic cases, or for cases in which the dislocation is clearly interfering with a patient's function.

Approximately one-third of patients have structural or conductive heart defects. Patients are sensitive to many anesthesia drugs, including neuromuscular blocking agents, which tend to induce arrhythmias and prolong awakening from anesthesia (328,329). Keloid formation is common (330).

PROGERIA

Progeria (i.e., Hutchinson-Gilford syndrome) is the best-known of many syndromes characterized by premature aging. It is exceedingly rare, with fewer than 30 affected children in North America. The cause is entirely unknown. Autosomal dominant (331) and autosomal recessive (332) inheritance patterns have been proposed, but a sporadic mutation is more likely (333).

These individuals have very abnormal levels of growth hormones, and hormone supplementation will increase growth velocity, but not result in improved survival (334). The cause is not known, but tissues from these patients have been used in a variety of reports to study the aging process. Fibroblasts from cultures derived from these indi-

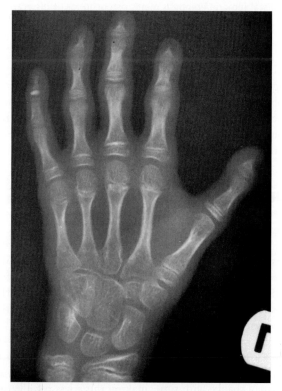

FIGURE 9-36. Progeria. The radiograph shows distal acrolysis, with resorption of the distal phalanges. (From ref. 1, with permission.)

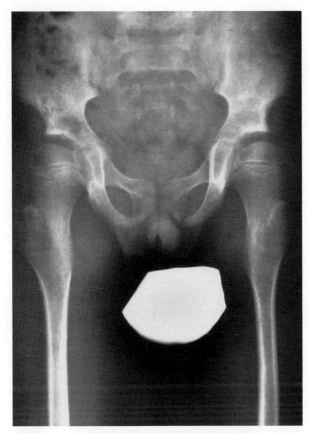

FIGURE 9-37. Progeria in an 11-year-old patient. The radiograph shows a marked degree of coxa valgus and some femoral head uncovering.

viduals have a variety of abnormalities, including a deficient ability to clear free radicals (335).

Children with progeria are diagnosed between 1 and 2 years of age, according to their clinical features alone. There is severe growth retardation and an inability to gain weight. If there is survival to adolescence, there is no pubertal growth spurt. Alopecia and a loss of subcutaneous fat is dramatic, and accounts for the distinctive appearance of a skinny old man or woman (336,337). These patients have joint stiffness that is not arthritis; it is a periarticular fibrosis. Osteolysis occurs in the fingertips, clavicle, and proximal humerus (331,338,339) (Fig. 9-36). The vertebrae may become osteopenic, creating fish-mouth vertebral bodies on radiographs (331,337,340). Fractures are common, often with delayed union. There is late developmental dysplasia of the hip, and the onset of a rather significant coxa valga (340,341) (Fig. 9-37). The children do not live long enough to develop arthritis secondary to the acetabular dysplasia. Not all systems age. There are no cataracts; there is no senility. Rather than aging, the normal tissues undergo an atrophic or degenerative change that mimics normal aging. The principal histopathologic atrophic changes occur in the skin, subcutaneous tissue, bone, and cardiovascular system. Ath-

erosclerosis with myocardial infarction by 10 years of age is the rule, and life expectancy rarely exceeds 20 years.

The children are vital until struck down by myocardial infarction. Despite a short life, it is imperative not to permit any suffering. Hip surgery is indicated only if there is a documented functional impairment. Surgery is not indicated to prevent future arthritis. There is no medical treatment for the basic disease process.

RUSSELL-SILVER DWARFISM

The patient with Russell-Silver syndrome is defined clinically as a short child with body asymmetry and a characteristic face (342–344) (Fig. 9-38). The cause is unclear. Some suggest autosomal dominant inheritance, and others an abnormal intrauterine environment (343,344). The associated genitourinary malformations and the variation in the pattern of sexual maturation chemically (increased gonadotropin secretion) or clinically (precocious sexual development) have suggested hypothalamic or other endocrine disturbance contributing to the pathogenesis. Affected children are small at birth and remain below the third percentile throughout growth, with a marked delay in skeletal maturation. Body asymmetry with hemihypertrophy affects 80%. It averages about 2 cm at maturity, but can be as much as 6 cm. Regardless of the magnitude of the discrepancy, it is clinically more apparent because the child is small. The face is characteristically triangular and seemingly too small for the cranial vault. There have been several reports of variations in sexual maturation pattern, chemically or clinically. Malformations of the genitourinary systems have been described (345,346).

Radiologic analysis discloses a remarkable array of orthopaedic findings, but it is not clear which are part of the

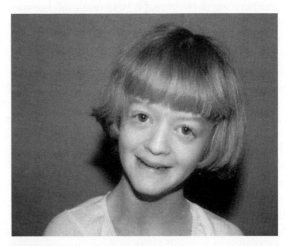

FIGURE 9-38. Russell-Silver syndrome. The triangular face is seemingly small for the size of the skull.

syndrome and which are coincidental (347–349). Scoliosis is usually idiopathic. Hand and foot abnormalities include clinodactyly, polydactyly, and hallux varus. Developmental hip dysplasia, avascular necrosis of the femoral head, and slipped capital femoral epiphysis may be present (332). Many radiographic changes, such as the minor hand abnormalities, suggest a disturbed morphogenesis.

Treatment consists of managing leg-length equality. This can be difficult because individual growth curves may vary, the skeletal age is very retarded, and puberty may be very abnormal. It is easy to miss the appropriate timing for epiphysiodesis. Growth hormone has been administered to improve stature. Although the use of growth hormone will increase growth velocity, it is not yet known if ultimate height is increased (350).

It is not known if screening for Wilms tumor, as is performed in other forms of hemihypertrophy, is necessary. However, there is a case report of Wilms tumor in an affected patient (351). Thus, it is safest to screen these patients as one would with any other hemihypertrophy (see Beckwith-Wiedemann syndrome below).

TURNER SYNDROME

This syndrome is present only in girls, and consists of short stature, sexual infantilism, a webbed neck, and cubitus valgus. It is a relatively common chromosome disorder affecting 1 of 2,500 live births, but the rate of intrauterine lethality is 95%. The syndrome is caused by a single X chromosome. In two-thirds of cases, all cells are XO, and parental origin of the single X chromosome is the mother in 70% of the cases (352). XO mosaicism occurs in about one-third of patients, and in 1% there is deletion of only a part of an X chromosome (352,353). Cytogenetic studies will confirm this diagnosis.

The affect of the single X chromosome may be different, depending on whether it is derived from the father or from the mother, which is probably the result of imprinting (354). Recent studies, based on individuals with partial loss of the X chromosome, suggest a critical region at Xp11.2–p22.1 responsible for the disease (355).

The identification of particular features at a particular age raises suspicion for this syndrome. At birth, the child has a webbed neck, widely spaced nipples, and edema of the hands and feet. The foot edema may persist for several months. During childhood, the low hairline, webbed neck, cubitus valgus, and short stature become more apparent. The adolescent has short stature and sexual infantilism. The most important features that call for chromosome analysis are edema of the hands and feet at birth, short stature in childhood, and sexual infantilism as an adolescent.

Growth retardation is a cardinal feature, with an ultimate height of about 140 cm (56 in.) (356). Bone maturation is normal until 8 to 9 years of age, then, because sex hormone stimulation is absent, there is neither skeletal maturation nor pubertal growth spurt. There is no puberty at all, and the girls remain without secondary sexual characteristics unless exogenous estrogen is administered. The web neck looks like a feature of Klippel-Feil syndrome, but the cervical spine radiographs are normal. It is a cutaneous web only, and the cause may be related to an intrauterine cystic hygroma (357). It is cosmetically unsightly, and plastic surgery is effective (358).

Idiopathic scoliosis is common, and the curve usually develops in juveniles. The delayed skeletal maturation allows a long period for curve progression. Growth hormone, which is almost always administered to girls with this syndrome, accelerates curve progression. Although the scoliosis can be managed the same way as idiopathic scoliosis, patients must be observed more frequently during growth hormone administration. Cubitus valgus is present in 80%, but there is a normal range of elbow motion and no disability (359). Genu valgum is also apparent, but the vast majority of cases are asymptomatic. Osteotomy is performed for the rare symptomatic case [➥4.17, 4.19]. There is a medial bony protuberance not unlike an osteochondroma, arising off the proximal tibia in some (360).

Osteoporosis is a significant problem because of the low estrogen and an altered renal vitamin D metabolism, which is correctable with the administration of growth hormone and sex steroid supplementation (361–364). Even in childhood, there may be the sequelae of osteoporosis, with a high incidence of wrist fractures reported (365).

Intelligence is normal, but there is a high frequency of learning disabilities (366,367). The life expectancy is normal, overall medical status is excellent, and social acceptance is good (368). There are some heart and kidney abnormalities reported at a somewhat higher incidence than for the normal population (369). Having only one X chromosome enables the patient to have X-linked recessive disorders, such as Duchenne muscular dystrophy.

Children with Turner syndrome are treated with growth hormone through adolescence, which results in a modest increase in growth velocity and final height from an average of 140 cm (55 in.) to just under 149 cm (58.5 in.) (370,371). Cyclic sex hormones are administered during adolescence and throughout adulthood. Estrogen is necessary for the development of secondary sexual characteristics, and the estrogen, and possibly the previously administered growth hormone, help to prevent osteoporosis. Many with Turner syndrome marry, and obstetric techniques of hormone supplementation and ovum transplantation can result in pregnancy.

NOONAN SYNDROME

The phenotype of Noonan syndrome is reminiscent of Turner syndrome, with short stature, webbed neck, cubitus valgus, and sexual immaturity (372,373). However, the chromosomes are normal. This syndrome affects boys and girls. The incidence is 1 in 1,000, and it is an autosomal dominant disorder (374). Many clinical features are shared with the Turner phenotype, but what distinguishes this syndrome are the normal gonads, a high incidence of mental retardation, and right-sided congenital heart defects, often with hypertrophic cardiomyopathy (375,376). Scoliosis is more common (40%) than in Turner patients, and more severe (377). Minor to major vertebral abnormalities may be seen on radiographs. Skeletal maturation is delayed despite normal puberty and menarche. Noonan syndrome is often misdiagnosed, and most frequently confused with King-Denborough syndrome, a myopathic arthrogryposis syndrome characterized by short stature, web neck, spinal deformity, and contractures. Recognizing the difference is important, because a malignant hyperthermia-like picture is part of the King-Denborough syndrome. Linkage analysis identified loci for Noonan syndrome at 12q22, and at 12q24 (378).

PRADER-WILLI SYNDROME

Prader-Willi is a syndrome of hypotonia, obesity, hypogonadism, short stature, small hands and feet, and mental deficiency (379–381). The incidence is 1 in 5,000 births, with a prevalence in the population of 1 in 16,000 to 25,000. As newborns, those with Prader-Willi syndrome are floppy babies, having hypotonia, poor feeding, and delayed milestones (382). They may mimic infants with spinal muscular atrophy. Approximately 10% have developmental dysplasia of the hip. The syndrome may be remembered with an "H" mnemonic: hypotonia, hypogonadism, hyperphagia, hypomentation, and small hands, all probably based on a hypothalamic disorder.

After 1 or 2 years of age, a different clinical picture appears (383). A characteristic face of upward-slanting, almond-shaped eyes becomes apparent (Fig. 9-39). Obesity begins, and a Prader-Willi diagnosis is usually suspected because of the onset of a voracious eating disorder. The patient has a preoccupation with food and an insatiable appetite (384,385). Obesity has a central distribution, sparing the distal limbs. Complex behavioral modification programs are occasionally effective, and a trial using fenfluramine has had limited success (386). The patient has short stature, below the 10th percentile, with an ultimate height of 150 cm (59 in.). There is no adolescent growth spurt. The genitalia are hypoplastic, and the patient has small hands and feet (387). Mental retardation is present, but it is extremely variable. Nevertheless, skills for independent living are almost nonexistent, and most reside in sheltered homes (384,388).

Prader-Willi syndrome is caused by a deletion of a

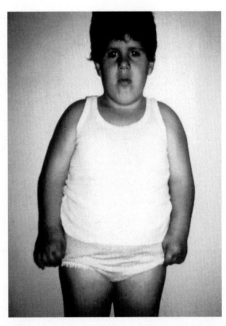

FIGURE 9-39. Prader-Willi syndrome in a 7-year-old patient. The features include truncal obesity and a round face with almond-shaped eyes. (From ref. 1, with permission.)

small part of chromosome 15 (15q11-13) of paternal origin (389,390). This is an example of genomic imprinting, because only missing DNA from the father causes the syndrome (391). Genomic imprinting is a process by which genes of maternal origin have different affects than genes of paternal origin. Angelman syndrome, or happy puppet syndrome, is phenotypically dissimilar to Prader-Willi syndrome. Angelman syndrome patients are small and mentally retarded, and they have athetosis and seizures. However, they have the exact chromosome deletion that occurs in Prader-Willi syndrome (15q11-13), except that the deleted DNA is of maternal origin (390).

The most significant orthopaedic problem is juvenile-onset scoliosis, which affects 50 to 90% (Fig. 9-40). It is difficult to control with an orthosis because of the truncal fat (392–395). Those who come to surgery have a significant anesthesia risk because of morbid obesity (396) [➡2.9]. The legs are malaligned, with genu valgum and pes planus, but the condition has limited or no effect on functional health and physical performance.

Although comparative studies are not available, case series suggest that growth hormone improves body composition, fat utilization, physical strength and agility, and growth in this syndrome (397,398). The lack of controlled trials, and ethical issues related to its use in this patient population, make the use of growth hormone in Prader-Willi syndrome of uncertain benefit.

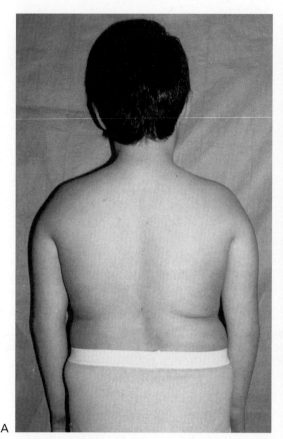
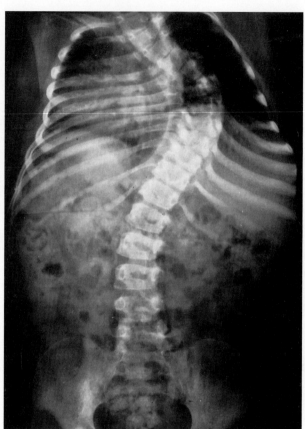

FIGURE 9-40. Prader-Willi syndrome in a 6-year-old patient. **A:** Scoliosis is difficult to detect because of the truncal obesity. **B:** The roentgenogram of this patient discloses a 50-degree thoracic curve. (**B** from ref. 1, with permission.)

BECKWITH-WIEDEMANN SYNDROME

Beckwith-Wiedemann syndrome is a triad of organomegaly, omphalocele, and a large tongue (399). The incidence is 1 in 14,000, and it is probably an autosomal dominant trait of variable expression. Patients are large, although this feature is not always noticed at birth (400). The child is in the 97th percentile by 1 year of age. The tongue is gigantic at birth, and although it tends to regress, hemiglossectomy is sometimes needed. Omphalocele is common, and 15% of the babies born with omphaloceles have Beckwith-Wiedemann syndrome. The abdominal viscera are enlarged, and a single-cell hypertrophy accounts for the large organs: in the adrenals, giant cortical cells; in the gonads, increased number of interstitial cells; and in the pancreas, islet cell hyperplasia. This underlies the 10% risk of developing benign or malignant tumors. Wilms tumor is the most common.

Beckwith-Wiedemann is linked to chromosome 11p15, which is near the Wilms tumor gene (11p13) and the insulin-like growth factor gene (11p15.5) (401). There may be some paternal genomic imprinting (see the section on Prader-Willi Syndrome, above) (402,403). The closeness of the Beckwith-Wiedemann gene locus and the embryonal tumor gene loci accounts for the higher incidence of tumors seen in this syndrome.

Pancreatic islet cell hyperplasia causes hypoglycemia. It is critical for the neonatologist to diagnose this syndrome early to prevent the consequences of hypoglycemia. If it is not managed properly, seizures occur at day 2 or 3. Central nervous system damage from the hypoglycemia leads to a cerebral palsy-like picture. The cerebral palsy-like findings confuse the diagnosis of this syndrome, and make the management of these patients more complex. The diagnosis can occasionally be made prenatally by ultrasound (404,405).

The clinical feature that make the orthopaedist suspect this diagnosis is the unusual combination of two otherwise common problems: spastic cerebral palsy and hemihypertrophy (Fig. 9-41). The spasticity is thought to be a result of the neonatal hypoglycemic episodes, especially if accompanied by neonatal seizures, but spastic hemiplegia is most commonly seen. In general, children with cerebral palsy tend to be small; Beckwith-Wiedemann syndrome should be suspected if a large child has spastic cerebral palsy. Asym-

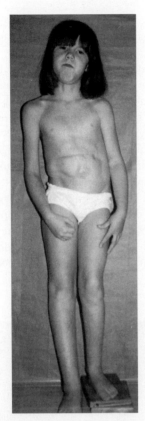

FIGURE 9-41. Beckwith-Wiedemann syndrome in an 8-year-old patient. Hemihypertrophy on right, a part of this syndrome, is combined with hemiatrophy on left, due to acquired encephalopathy secondary to hypoglycemic seizures as a newborn, yielding a significant leg-length discrepancy of 4.6 cm. Abdominal scars are a consequence of omphalocele repair. (From ref. 1, with permission.)

metric growth affects about 20%. It is usually true hemihypertrophy, but it can be significant if the spastic hemiplegia affects the smaller side.

Children with Beckwith-Wiedemann syndrome are predisposed to a variety of neoplasms, most notably Wilms tumor. Abdominal ultrasounds at regular intervals until the age of 6, to screen for Wilms tumor, are advocated. A series comparing a screened population (ultrasounds every 4 months) with a population that was not screened, showed that none of the children in the screened group presented with late-stage Wilms tumor, although one-half of the children who developed Wilms tumor in the nonscreened group presented with late-stage disease. This study suggests that screening every 4 months will identify early disease. However, a larger study is needed to determine if screening improves patient survival (406,407).

Scoliosis is common; it is usually idiopathic, but there may be insignificant morphogenic variations, such as 13 ribs. It is managed as any idiopathic curve. Other orthopaedic findings include cavus feet, dislocated radial heads, and occasional cases of polydactyly (408).

VACTERLS AND VATER ASSOCIATION

VATER, as the syndrome was previously known, has been expanded to VACTERLS (409). The letters of VACTERLS in this syndrome's name constitute an acronym for the systems and defects involved: vertebral, anus, cardiac, tracheal, esophageal, renal, limb, and single umbilical artery. The physician does not need to find examples of all seven categories of anomalies to diagnose the syndrome. The syndrome can be diagnosed prenatally by visualizing several of the malformations on ultrasound. The most obvious physical finding at birth is the radial ray defect. Between 5 and 10% of radial club hands are associated with VACTERLS.

The cause is unknown, but it is a nonrandom association, whose simultaneous occurrence by chance is unlikely (410). The current thought is that these structures are either all formed at the same time, or are all patterned by the same developmental signaling pathway. An event occurring during fetal development that disrupts either the common signaling pathway, or a variety of susceptible pathways operating at the same time, is probably responsible for the associated malformations.

The vertebral defects include disturbed spinal segmentation, with vertebral bars and blocks (411,412). Thoracic anomalies are worse in those with tracheoesophageal fistula, and lumbar anomalies are more common with those who have an imperforate anus. Occult intraspinal pathology is common (413,414), and a screening MR study of the spine is recommended, especially in patients who require operative management for their scoliosis. The curves can be managed like other types of congenital scoliosis [➥2.9, 2.11, 2.12].

Congenital heart defects are present in one-half of these patients. Ventricular septal defect is the most common problem. Duodenal atresia may be found in this syndrome. The VACTERLS patient often has a single kidney. Other collecting-system anomalies occur frequently among this group.

The limb anomalies range from a hypoplastic thumb to a radial club hand. The defect may be unilateral or bilateral; bilateral defects are always asymmetric (411). The legs are spared 80% of the time. When the lower extremities are involved, a duplicated hallux is the most common finding.

The normal umbilical cord has two arteries and one vein. The absence of an artery, detectable only at the time of delivery or in the immediate newborn period, reflects the broad range of morphologic defects dating back to placental formation.

Developmental delay may be observed, and is thought to be the consequence of skeletal anomalies of the arms, scoliosis, and surgery for gastrointestinal or genitourinary malformations. Nevertheless, several central nervous system malformations (e.g., encephalocele hydrocephalus) may be associated with VACTERLS, and must be excluded (413,414). If the patient survives the gastrointestinal anomalies and correction of the cardiac defects, the prognosis for a normal life is excellent. Each orthopaedic abnormality can be treated as an isolated problem. Sections on congenital scoliosis (see Chapter 18) and radial clubhand (see Chapter 22) contain detailed information. The key point is to recognize this association, and to identify other abnormalities that might interfere with treatment.

GOLDENHAR SYNDROME

The name "ocular-auricular-vertebral dysplasia" points to the areas in which anomalies are found: the eye, ear, and vertebrae (415). The defects vary in severity and frequently are associated with other malformations (416,417). It is not a rare syndrome, with an incidence of 1 in 3,000 to 5,000 births. The cause is unknown, but marked geographic variation and segregation analysis suggests a genetic disorder (418).

The typical eye defect is an epibulbar dermoid on the conjunctiva (Fig. 9-42A). Preauricular fleshy skin tags are found in front of the ear, and pits extend from the tragus to the corner of the mouth (Fig. 9-42B). In some patients, the ear may be hypoplastic or absent. The eye and ear anomalies are unilateral in 85% of these children, and facial asymmetry is the result of a hypoplastic mandibular ramus, invariably on the same side as the ear anomalies (Fig. 9-42C).

The vertebral anomalies may occur anywhere along the spine, although the lower cervical and upper thoracic predominate (Fig. 9-42C). Hemivertebrae are the most common defect, with an occasional block fusion found. Neural tube defect occurs more often than expected in the general

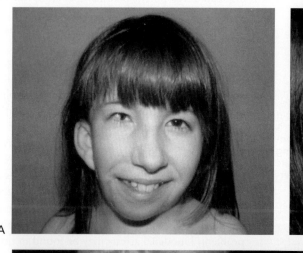

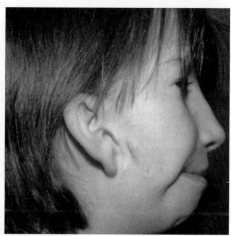

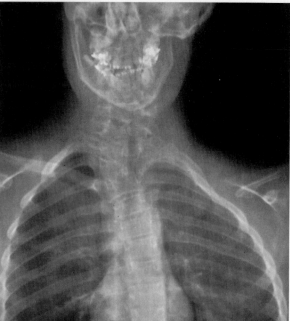

FIGURE 9-42. Goldenhar syndrome. **A:** Facial asymmetry and epibulbar dermoid of the right eye. **B:** Malformed ears with preauricular tags and sinuses. **C:** The x-ray film demonstrates the congenital anomalies of the lower cervical and upper thoracic spine. Hypoplasia of the ascending ramus of the mandible accounts for the facial asymmetry. The clavicle is absent on the same side as the deformed face. (From ref. 1, with permission.)

population, and it may involve lumbar spine, cervical spine, or the skull (i.e., encephalocele). Approximately one-half of patients have clinically detectable scoliosis (419). An idiopathic, compensatory curve below the congenital curve is often more troublesome than the congenital curve itself. Sprengel deformity and rib anomalies may be present in association with the congenital curves in the cervical-thoracic region. Orthotic management of scoliosis is difficult, and has no effect on the congenital portion of the curve. The location of the scoliosis is often too high for brace management. Early fusion should be performed for progression of the congenital curve. Preoperative CT and MRI are recommended to delineate the anatomy of the congenital curve and determine if there is any intraspinal pathology. There may be occult posterior element defects that will also be identified on CT.

Intubation for anesthesia may be difficult because of the small jaw, stiff neck, and upper airway dysmorphology (420). Other anomalies include congenital heart disease (e.g., ventricular septal defect) (416), cleft lip, and cleft palate (421). Mental retardation, affecting 10 to 25% of patients, is usually limited to cases involving microphthalmia or an encephalocele (422).

TRICHORHINOPHALANGEAL SYNDROME

The name of this syndrome causes confusion, because textbooks describe trichorhinophalangeal syndrome, trichorhinophalangeal syndrome with exostosis, and Langer-Giedion syndrome. It is best to think of two relatively distinct trichorhinophalangeal (TRP) syndromes: types I and II. Despite the clinical overlaps between the two, there are enough features to separate them into distinct syndromes.

Patients with TRP-I have a pear-shaped, bulbous nose, prominent ears, sparse hair, and cone epiphyses. They have mild growth retardation. The thumbs are broad, and the fingers are often angled at the distal interphalangeal and proximal interphalangeal joints. The hips mimic a Perthes-like disease in radiographs and symptoms (423). There may be lax ligaments.

The key feature distinguishing TRP-II from TRP-I is the presence of multiple exostoses, especially involving the lower extremities. Those with TRP-II have facial features and cone epiphyses similar to patients with TRP-I. There is a higher chance of mental retardation in TRP-II. Langer-Giedion syndrome and TRP-II are identical (424). Patients with TRP-II also have microcephaly, large and protruding ears, a bulbous nose, and sparse scalp hair. In infancy, the skin is redundant and loose, which may be severe enough to mimic Ehlers-Danlos syndrome. Marked ligamentous laxity may further support this error in diagnosis. There is a tendency toward fractures. Similar to TRP-I, the Perthes-like picture is expressed in TRP-II, as well as all the hand anomalies (425).

Both TRP-I and TRP-II are due to mutation or loss of

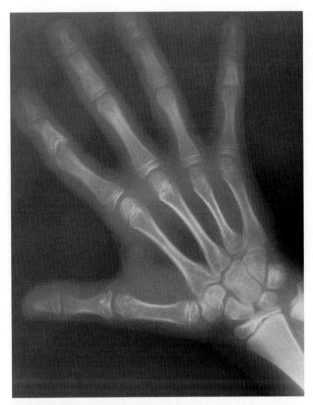

FIGURE 9-43. Trichorhinophalangeal syndrome. This 11-year-old patient has cone- or chevron-shaped epiphyses in the hand, and a broad thumb and distal phalanx.

the *TRSP1* gene (424). However, TRP-II is due to a larger loss of the chromosomal region, with loss of the adjacent gene, *EXT-1*, as well. The *EXT-1* gene is one of the genes responsible for hereditary exostoses, explaining the associated exostoses. The *TRSP1* gene is responsible for the fascial malformation and cone epiphyses present in both disorders. Individuals with loss of a large portion of a chromosome are more likely to have mental retardation, thus explaining the mental retardation in some patients with TRP-II, which has a larger region of chromosomal deletion. TRP-II is one of the few disorders actually known to be due to two contiguous genes (5).

Radiographically, the hand in a patient with TRP-I or TRP-II shows short fourth and fifth metacarpals, cone epiphyses, a short and broad thumb, and fingers with angled proximal and distal interphalangeal joints (426) (Fig. 9-43). The cone epiphyses, so characteristic of this syndrome, are not seen until after 3 or 4 years of age. The pelvis shows the unilateral or bilateral changes of Perthes in TRP-I and TRP-II, but rather than resolution, the Perthes-like picture persists, evolving into a pattern more like multiple epiphyseal dysplasia with precocious arthritis (Fig. 9-44). Despite the wealth of radiographic abnormalities, the hands rarely have functional disturbances. Osteotomy of the thumb is occasionally needed. If symptomatic, we recommend man-

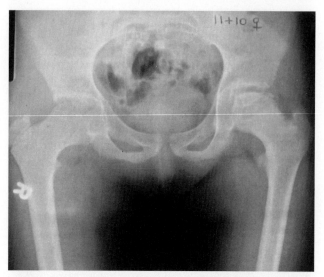

FIGURE 9-44. Trichorhinophalangeal syndrome, type I. The changes mimic Legg-Perthes disease, but by 12 years of age, they did not resolve. On the right is a small but spherical epiphysis. On the left, the changes are similar to those seen in Perthes disease and in multiple epiphyseal dysplasia.

aging the hips as in symptomatic Perthes, but there are insufficient data about outcome. Occasionally, an exostosis may be large or symptomatic enough to require excision.

MUCOPOLYSACCHARIDOSES

This group of genetic disorders is characterized by mucopolysaccharide excretion in the urine (427). There are at least 13 types (Table 9-2). The mild-to-severe mucopolysaccharidoses have similar radiographs and various clinical features, but each produces a particular sugar in the urine because of a specific enzyme defect (427,428). Changes in the naming and numbering of systems over the years have introduced considerable confusion in understanding the mucopolysaccharidoses. The incidence is 1 in 10,000.

The patients have somewhat thickened and coarse facial features and short stature, and many develop stiff joints (Fig. 9-45), especially in the hands. Stiffness is postulated to be the result of the deposition of mucopolysaccharide in the capsule and periarticular structures, and to reflect the loss of joint congruity. Radiographs reveal oval vertebral bodies that often are beaked anteriorly; a pelvis with wide, flat ilia; capacious acetabuli; unossified femoral head cartilage; and coxa valga. The radiographic and clinical features are usually not apparent at birth, but become more apparent as the child gets older. Thus, it may be difficult to diagnose a mucopolysaccharidosis during the first year of life.

All the mucopolysaccharides are autosomal recessive except for mucopolysaccharidosis type II (Hunter syndrome), which is X-linked. The most common mucopolysaccharidoses are type I (Hurler syndrome) and type IV (Morquio syndrome).

The mucopolysaccharidoses can be diagnosed by urine screening, using a toluidine blue-spot test. If the initial results are positive, specific blood testing is done for the associated sugar abnormality. Although spot tests are quick and inexpensive, they have high false-positive and high false-negative rates. They are the initial test that should be ordered.

The pathobiologic mechanisms are similar for the mucopolysaccharidoses. Each has a deficiency of a specific lysosomal enzyme that degrades the sulfated glycosamine glycans: heparan sulfate, dermatan sulfate, keratan sulfate, and chondroitin sulfate. The incomplete degradation product accumulates in the lysozymes themselves. The mucopolysac-

TABLE 9-2. MUCOPOLYSACCHARIDOSES

Designation	Name	Enzyme Defect	Stored Substance	Inheritance Pattern
MPS I	Hurler/Scheie	α-L-iduronidase	HS + DS	autosomal recessive
MPS II	Hunter	Iduronidase-2-sulfatase	HS + DS	X-linked recessive
MPS IIIA	Sanfilippo A	Heparin-sulfatase (sulfamidase)	HS	autosomal recessive
MPS IIIB	Sanfilippo B	α-N-acteylglucosamidase	HS	autosomal recessive
MPS IIIC	Sanfilippo C	Acetyl-CoA: α-glucosaminide-N-acetyltransferase	HS	autosomal recessive
MPS IIID	Sanfilippo D	Glucosamine-6-sulfatase	HS	autosomal recessive
MPS IVA	Morquio A	N-acetyl galactosamine-6-sulfate sulfatase	KS, CS	autosomal recessive
MPS IVB	Morquio B	β-D-galactosidase	KS	autosomal recessive
MPS IVC	Morquio C	Unknown	KS	autosomal recessive
MPS V	Formerly Scheie disease, no longer used.			
MPS VI	Moroteux-Lamy	Arylsulfatase B, N-acetylgalactosamine-4-sulfatase	DS, CS	autosomal recessive
MPS VII	Sly	β-D-glucuronidase	CS, HS, DS	autosomal recessive
MPS VIII		Glucoronate-2-sulpitase	CS, HS	autosomal recessive

CS, chondroitan sulfate; *DS,* dermatan sulfate; *HS,* heparin sulfate; *KS,* keratin sulfate; *MPS,* mucopolysaccharidosis.

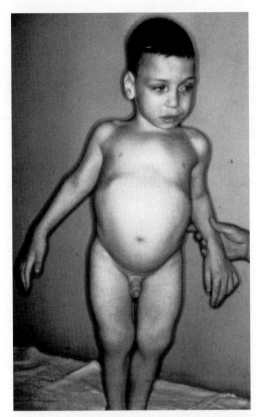

FIGURE 9-45. The classic appearance of a mucopolysaccharidosis in a 3-year-old patient includes facial features that are mildly coarsened, an abdominal protuberance from an enlarged spleen and liver, a short trunk, and stiff interphalangeal joints of the fingers.

charidoses are part of a larger group of disorders known as the lysosomal storage diseases. The incomplete product accumulates in the tissues, such as the brain, the viscera, and the joints. This unremitting process leads to the clinical progression of the disease. The child is normal at birth, but a problem may be chemically detectable by 6 to 12 months of age, and clinical progression is apparent by 2 years of age.

Mucopolysaccharidosis Type I

Mucopolysaccharidosis type I is the clinical prototype. It is characterized by a deficiency of L-iduronidase, the enzyme that degrades dermatan sulfate and heparan sulfate. The Hurler and Scheie forms represent the severe and mild ends of the clinical spectrum in mucopolysaccharidosis type I. Children with the Hurler form have progressive mental retardation; severe, multiple skeletal deformities; considerable organ and soft tissue deformities; and death before 10 years of age. The Scheie form is characterized by joint stiffness, corneal clouding, and no mental retardation; the diagnosis is usually made at about 15 years of age, and the patient has a normal life expectancy. Many patients with mucopolysaccharidosis I fall in the middle of this clinical spectrum. The clinical variation is determined by where and what kind of mutation occurs along the gene for L-iduronidase (429,430).

Marrow transplantation is used in more severe forms (Hurler syndrome), however, the results on the bones are variable (431). This may be due to the poor penetration of the enzyme derived from the transplanted leukocytes to the osseous cells (431). Initial studies suggested an improvement in most of the nonosseous manifestations of the disease with marrow transplant. More recent, longer-term studies cast doubt on the long-term effectiveness (432). Despite these disappointing longer-term results, marrow transplant may provide short-term improvement, especially in the nonosseous manifestations. The musculoskeletal deformities that persist after marrow transplant still require treatment.

Malalignment of the limbs can occur, and epiphyseal stapling, or osteotomies, may be necessary for genu valgum (433) [➡**4.17, 4.19, 6.1–6.4, 6.14**]. Approximately one-fourth have an abnormality of the upper cervical spine. Odontoid hypoplasia and a soft tissue mass in the canal can be managed like those in Morquio syndrome (below). The accumulation of degradation products in closed anatomic spaces, such as the carpal tunnel, causes triggering of the fingers and carpal tunnel syndrome. These can be managed operatively (434,435).

Mucopolysaccharidosis Type IV

Between 1929 and 1959, there was a miscellany of skeletal diseases described as "Morquio syndrome," including several types of spondyloepiphyseal dysplasia. Morquio syndrome is an autosomal recessive disorder with an incidence of 3 per 1,000,000 members of the population. Three types of Morquio syndrome are classified as subtypes of mucopolysaccharidosis type IV. All are caused by enzyme defects involved in degradation of keratan sulfate (427–429).

Patients with severe classic mucopolysaccharidosis type IVA are short-trunked dwarfs, although they appear normal at birth. They develop corneal opacities. The bone dysplasia is radiographically obvious, and the final height is less than 125 cm (50 in.). Patients have abnormal dentition. The deficient enzyme is *N*-acetylgalactosamine-6-sulfate sulfatase, and the chromosomal defect occurs at 16q24.3 (436). Patients with intermediate mucopolysaccharidosis type IVB have the same but milder phenotypes as those with type IVA. They are taller, with final heights greater than 125 cm (50 in.), and they have normal dentition. Here the enzyme defect is *β*-D-galactosidase. Patients with mild mucopolysaccharidosis type IVC have very mild clinical manifestations.

The three forms of Morquio mucopolysaccharidoses type IV can be separated by the severity of symptoms and the patient's age at detection. All patients are normal at birth. For patients with the severe type IVA, the diagnosis is made between 1 and 3 years of age; those with the mild type IV are diagnosed as teenagers; and those with the intermediate form are diagnosed somewhere in the middle of this age range. The three forms may also be separated by the severity of the radiographic changes.

Intelligence is normal in all of the mucopolysaccharidosis IV types, and only rarely are the facial features coarsened. Similarly, all are short-trunked dwarfs with ligamentous laxity; the laxity is rather profound in mucopolysaccharidosis type IVA. The degree of genu valgus is significant, aggravated by the lax ligaments (437–440).

Management of the knee proves difficult because of the osseous malalignment and the lax ligaments. Despite the observation that the fingers and joints are becoming stiff, the medial and lateral instability of the knee remains. Realignment osteotomies can restore plumb alignment [➡4.17, 6.1–6.5], but braces may be needed to control the instability during ambulation. The prophylactic use of braces, to prevent initial valgus or recurrent deformity after surgery, has not been effective (437–440). The hips and knees develop

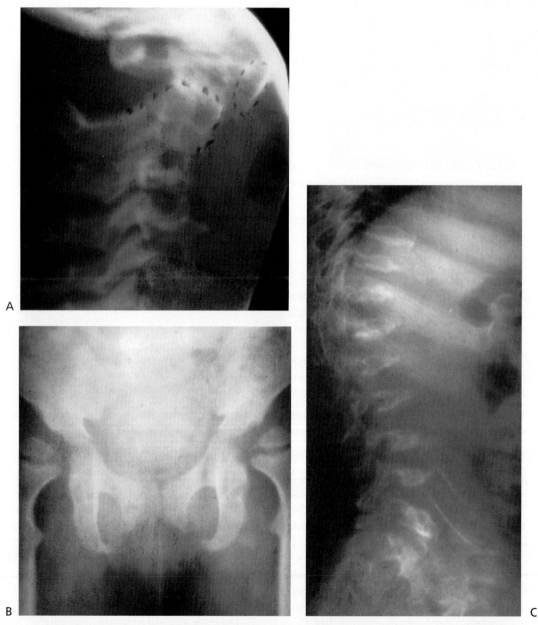

FIGURE 9-46. Morquio syndrome. The radiographic features include an absent odontoid (**A**), a pelvis with capacious acetabuli and coxa valga (**B**), and a marked platyspondyly at 12 years of age (**C**). It is difficult to imagine these vertebrae were normal at birth.

early arthritis. The hips show a progressive acetabular dysplasia. Early arthrograms may show substantial cartilage modeling within the capacious bony acetabulum, but in time, it disappears. The femoral capital epiphyses are initially advanced for the patient's age, but between 4 and 9 years of age, the femoral heads grow smaller, then disappear altogether (Fig. 9-46B, C). The pathophysiology of the progressive hip disease is not completely understood, and neither medication nor surgery have been shown to improve the prognosis (437–440).

Odontoid hypoplasia or aplasia is universal, with resultant C1–2 instability (439–442) (Fig. 9-46A). There is a soft tissue mass in the spinal canal, contributing to cord compression (442,443). This soft tissue mass can make the space available for the cord smaller than one would expect, based on radiographs alone. Neurologic function, especially of upper-extremity strength and tone, is probably more important than measuring distances on dynamic cervical spine films. The upper and lower extremity findings are often of flaccidity, rather than spasticity. The onset of the myelopathy can occur as early as the first decade of life, progressing as the soft tissue hypertrophies, with the C1–2 instabilities aggravating the situation. Sudden deaths of patients with Morquio disease have been reported, and they are typically attributed to the C1-2 subluxation. C1–2 fusion before the onset of symptoms is controversial, but promoted by some (442,443) [➡2.17]. Others think the best surgery is occipital cervical fusion because it reduces the anterior soft tissue mass (443,444) [➡2.18]. There are no comparative studies evaluating the outcomes of each of the different management approaches. Based on the available information, it is reasonable to obtain MRI studies on symptomatic individuals, or on those with radiographic evidence of instability. C1–2 fusions are recommended for asymptomatic in-

dividuals with MRI evidence of cord compression. Symptomatic individuals should be fused throughout the region of instability and cord compression.

Elsewhere in the spine, the vertebrae show a progressive platyspondylia with a thoracic kyphosis. No treatment is effective. Despite these problems, many patients with Morquio disease live for decades. Cardiorespiratory disease is common, but the problems at the upper cervical spine account for most disabilities.

HADJU-CHENEY SYNDROME

Hadju-Cheney syndrome, also called arthrodentosteodysplasia, consists of acroosteolysis, with osteoporosis and hypoplastic changes in the skull and mandible. The osteoporosis leads to multiple fractures of the skull, spine, and digits. The cranial sutures persist; wormian bones are seen on the skull radiographs. Basilar impression is a common finding, often requiring operative intervention. The terminal digits exhibit gradual loss of bone mass, sometimes called "pseudo-osteolysis." Patients tend to have a deep voice (445–449).

Orthopaedic manifestations include loose jointedness, patellar dislocations, scoliosis, frequent fractures, and basilar impression (449). The basilar invagination can cause hydrocephalus and an Arnold-Chiari malformation (450). This is usually managed by decompression and an occiput to upper cervical spine fusion (Fig. 9-47) [➡2.18]. Little data is available on the management of other musculoskeletal problems. Scoliosis can be managed as in idiopathic scoliosis, although the underlying osteopenia and associated spinal fractures may make nonoperative management more difficult.

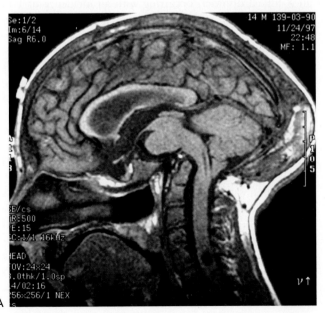

A

FIGURE 9-47. Hadju-Cheney syndrome. **A:** MRI of the head shows marked basilar invagination with an associated syrinx in the cervical cord. *(continued)*

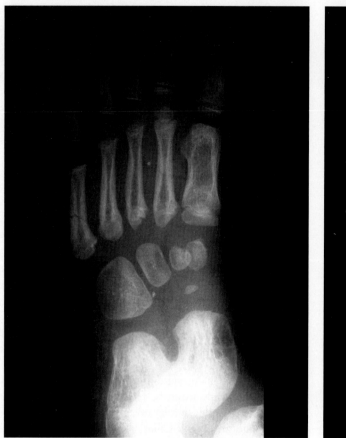

B

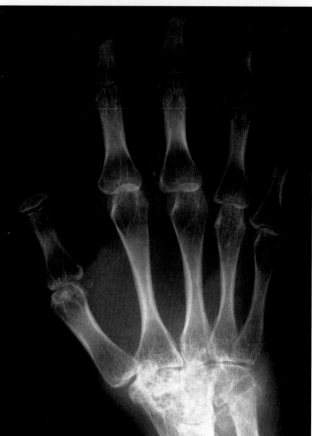

C

FIGURE 9-47. *(continued)* Radiographs show osteoporosis with pathologic fractures **(B)** and loss of bone mass in the terminal digits **(C)**, termed "pseudo-osteolysis."

Polycystic kidney disease and cardiac valvular disease are reported in some individuals, and cardiac and renal function should be evaluated before undergoing anesthesia (451,452). The disorder can be inherited in an autosomal dominant manner, but the causative gene is unknown.

RETT SYNDROME

Rett syndrome is an X-linked disorder, present almost exclusively in girls, that is characterized by normal development for the first 6 to 18 months, followed by rapid deterioration of higher brain functions. This is accompanied by dementia, autism, loss of purposeful use of the hands, and ataxia. After the initial rapid decline, the deterioration slows dramatically, so that effected individuals may have a relatively stable picture for several decades (453). There is variability in the severity of the decline, so that some girls are still walking as teenagers, whereas others stop ambulating in early childhood. A hand radiograph may help with the diagnosis, because 60% will have either negative ulnar variance or a short fourth metacarpal (454,455).

Children with this syndrome were initially thought to

have cerebral palsy with a movement disorder. Andreas Rett, a pediatrician practicing in Austria, noted that these girls all had normal development in the first month of life, and was thus able to separate them from cerebral palsy. This is an X-linked disorder, occurring with an incidence of 1 in 40,000. In some patients, it is caused by a mutation in the *MECP2* gene, which encodes X-linked methyl-CpG-binding protein 2. MeCP2 binds to a certain DNA sequence, and, through interaction with other factors, alters the way certain genes are transcribed. Mutations in this gene likely change the expression pattern of a wide variety of other genes (456), ultimately resulting in Rett syndrome. X-linked dominant diseases are more severe in boys, and Rett is probably fatal in the vast majority of male cases. Despite this, there are few cases of affected males reported (457).

Children with Rett syndrome present to the orthopaedist with a clinical picture similar to that of a total-body-involved cerebral palsy patient. Scoliosis occurs in over half the affected girls (457–461). Orthotic management probably does not alter the progression of the curve. There is a typical, usually long "c" pattern to the curves. These can be stabilized surgically, when they reach a magnitude that interferes with sitting or balance [➥**2.1, 2.5, 2.6, 2.9**]. However, as in cerebral palsy, there are no comparative studies showing improved function following spinal surgery. Spinal instrumentation and fusion should include the whole curve and any kyphotic segments. Although walking ability theoretically can worsen following extensive fusions, this has not occurred in the relatively small number of cases in which spinal surgery was undertaken in ambulatory girls with Rett syndrome (456,458). Coxa valga and lower-extremity contractures can occur, and these should be managed as in cerebral palsy, with emphasis placed on operative procedures that will improve function or decrease pain (459,461,462).

The life span in Rett syndrome is not known, but there are some affected individuals with a normal life span. There are a variety of nonorthopaedic problems, including cardiac conduction abnormalities, epilepsy, and vasomotor instability of the lower limbs. Some of these put the patients at increased risk when undergoing anesthesia (453).

References

1. Goldberg MJ. *The dysmorphic child: an orthopedic perspective.* New York: Raven, 1987.
2. Hecht JT, Scott CI Jr. Genetic study of an orthopedic referral center. *J Pediatr Orthop* 1984;4:208.
3. Jones KL. *Smith's recognizable patterns of human malformation.* 4th ed. Philadelphia: WB Saunders, 1992.
4. Jones KL, Robinson LK. An approach to the child with structural defects. *J Pediatr Orthop* 1983;3:238.
5. Online Mendelian Inheritance in Man, OMIM. Center for Medical Genetics, Johns Hopkins University and National Center for Biotechnology Information, National Library of Medicine (Bethesda, MD), 1999. Available at: http://www.ncbi.nlm.nih.gov/omim. Accessed February 24, 2000.
6. Van Regemorter N, Dodion J, Druart C, et al. Congenital malformations in 10,000 consecutive births in a university hospital: need for genetic counseling and prenatal diagnosis. *J Pediatr* 1984;104:386.

Neurofibromatosis

7. Riccardo VM, Eichner JE. *Neurofibromatosis: phenotype, national history, and prognosis.* Baltimore: Johns Hopkins University Press, 1986.
8. Riccardo WM. Neurofibromatosis: clinical heterogeneity. *Curr Probl Cancer* 1982;7:34.
9. Elster AD. Radiologic screening in the neurocutaneous syndromes: strategies and controversies. *Am J Neuroradiol* 1992;13:1078.
10. Kaufman A, Sherman FC, Black W, et al. Osseous destruction by neurofibroma diagnosed in infancy as "desmoplastic fibroma." *J Pediatr Orthop* 1984;4:239.
11. Kozlowski K, Lipson A. Bony tuberculosis misinterpreted—a cautionary tale. *Aust Radiol* 1993;37:119.
12. Locht RC, Huebert HT, McFarland DF. Subperiosteal hemorrhage and cyst formation in neurofibromatosis: a case report. *Clin Orthop* 1981;155:141.
13. Joseph KN, Bowen JR, MacEwen GD. Unusual orthopedic manifestations of neurofibromatosis. *Clin Orthop Rel Res* 1992; 278:17.
14. Mandell GA, Harcke T, Scott CI, et al. Protrusio acetabuli in neurofibromatosis: nondysplastic and dysplastic forms. *Neurosurgery* 1992;30:552.
15. Lubs MC, Bauer MS, Formes ME, Djokic B. Lisch nodules in neurofibromatosis type I. *N Engl J Med* 1991;324:1266.
16. Riccardo VM. Neurofibromatosis: past, present and future. *N Engl J Med* 1991;324:1285.
17. Huson SM, Compston DAS, Harper PS. A genetic study of von Recklinghausen neurofibromatosis in south east Wales. II. Guidelines for genetic counseling. *J Med Genet* 1989;26:712.
18. Riccardi VM. Type 1 neurofibromatosis and the pediatric patient. *Curr Probl Pediatr* 1992;66.
19. Samuelsson B, Riccardi VM. Neurofibromatosis in Gothenburg, Sweden. *Neurofibromatosis* 1989;2:78.
20. Graham PW, Oehlschlaeger FH. *Articulating the Elephant Man. Joseph Merrick and his interpreters.* Baltimore: Johns Hopkins University Press, 1992.
21. Xu G, O'Connell P, Viskochil D. The neurofibromatosis type 1 gene encodes a protein related to GAP. *Cell* 1990;62:608.
22. Li Y, Bollag G, Clark R. Somatic mutations in the neurofibromatosis 1 gene in human tumors. *Cell* 1992;69:281.
23. The I, Hannigan GE, Cowley GS. Rescue of a drosophila NF1 mutant phenotype by protein kinase A. *Science* 1997;276:794.
24. Gutmann DH, Collins FS. Recent progress toward understanding the molecular biology of von Recklinghausen neurofibromatosis. Brief review. *Ann Neurol* 1992;31:555.
25. Hruban RH, Shiu MH, Senie RT, et al. Malignant peripheral nerve sheath tumors of the buttock and lower extremity. A study of 43 cases. *Cancer* 1990;66:1253.
26. Viskochil D, White R, Cawthon R. The neurofibromatosis type 1 gene. *Ann Rev Neurosci* 1993;16:183.
27. Zlotogora J. Mutations in von Recklinghausen neurofibromatosis: an hypothesis. *Am J Med Genet* 1993;46:182.
28. Akbarnia BA, Gabriel KR, Beckman E, et al. Prevalence of scoliosis in neurofibromatosis. *Spine* 1992;17:S244.
29. Calvert PT, Edgar MA, Webb PJ. Scoliosis in neurofibromatosis. The natural history with and without operation. *J Bone Joint Surg Br* 1989;71:246.
30. Crawford AH Jr, Bagamery N. Osseous manifestations of neurofibromatosis in childhood. *J Pediatr Orthop* 1986;6:72.
31. Crawford AH. Pitfalls of spinal deformities associated with neurofibromatosis in children. *Clin Orthop Rel Res* 1989;245:29.
32. Funasaki H, Winter RB, Lonstein JB, et al. Pathophysiology of spinal deformities in neurofibromatosis. An analysis of 71 patients who had curves associated with dystrophic changes. *J Bone Joint Surg Am* 1994;76:692.
33. Sirois JL III, Drennan JC. Dystrophic spinal deformity in neurofibromatosis. *J Pediatr Orthop* 1990;10:522.
34. Winter RB, Moe JH, Bradford DS, et al. Spine deformity in neurofibromatosis. A review of one hundred and two patients. *J Bone Joint Surg Am* 1979;61:677.
35. Kim HW, Weinstein SL. Spine update. The management of scoliosis in neurofibromatosis. *Spine* 1997;22:2770.
36. Betz RR, Iorio R, Lombardi AV, et al. Scoliosis surgery in neurofibromatosis. *Clin Orthop Rel Res* 1989;245:53.
37. Hsu LCS, Lee PC, Leong JCY. Dystrophic spinal deformities in neurofibromatosis. Treatment by anterior and posterior fusion. *J Bone Joint Surg Br* 1984;66:495.
38. Shufflebarger HL. Cotrel-Dubousset instrumentation in neurofibromatosis spinal problems. *Clin Orthop Rel Res* 1989;245:24.
39. Craig JB, Govender S. Neurofibromatosis of the cervical spine. *J Bone Joint Surg Br* 1992;74:575.
40. Isu T, Miyasaka K, Abe H, et al. Atlantoaxial dislocation associated with neurofibromatosis. Report of three cases. *J Neurosurg* 1983;58:451.
41. Rockower S, McKay D, Nason S. Dislocation of the spine in neurofibromatosis. A report of two cases. *J Bone Joint Surg Am* 1982;64:1240.
42. Winter RB. Spontaneous dislocation of a vertebra in a patient

who had neurofibromatosis. Report of a case with dural ectasia. *J Bone Joint Surg Am* 1991;73:1402.

43. Wong-Chung J, Gillespie R. Lumbosacral spondyloptosis with neurofibromatosis. *Spine* 1991;16:986.

44. Bensaid AH, Dietemann JL, Kastler B, et al. Neurofibromatosis with dural ectasia and bilateral symmetrical pedicular clefts: report of two cases. *Neuroradiology* 1992;34:107.

45. Chee CP. Lateral thoracic meningocele associated with neurofibromatosis: total excision by posterolateral extradural approach. A case report. *Spine* 1989;14:129.

46. Dolynchuk KN, Teskey J, West M. Intrathoracic meningocele associated with neurofibromatosis: case report. *Neurosurgery* 1990;27:485.

47. Egelhoff JC, Bates DJ, Ross JS, et al. Spinal MR findings in neurofibromatosis types 1 and 2. *AJNR Am J Neuroradiol* 1992; 13:1071.

48. So CB, Li DKB. Anterolateral cervical meningocele in association with neurofibromatosis: MR and CT studies. *J Comput Assist Tomogr* 1989;13:692.

49. Winter R. Spontaneous dislocation of a vertebrae in a patient who had neurofibromatosis: report of a case with dural ectasia. *J Bone Joint Surg Am* 1991;73:1404.

50. Eichorn C, Wendt G, Staudte H-W, et al. Dural ectasia in von Recklinghausen's disease of the lumbar spine: a case report. *J Bone Joint Surg Br* 1995;77:835.

51. Morrissy RT, Riseborough EJ, Hall JE. Congenital pseudarthrosis of the tibia. *J Bone Joint Surg Br* 1981;63:367.

52. Morrissy RT. Congenital pseudarthrosis of the tibia. A long-term follow-up study. *Clin Orthop* 1982;166:14.

53. Alldred AJ. Congenital pseudarthrosis of the clavicle. *J Bone Joint Surg Br* 1963;45:312.

54. Bayne LG. Congenital pseudarthrosis of the forearm. *Hand Clin* 1985;1:457.

55. Gregg PJ, Price BA, Ellis HA, Stevens J. Pseudarthrosis of the radius associated with neurofibromatosis. A case report. *Clin Orthop* 1982;171:175.

56. Kaempffe FA, Gillespie R. Pseudarthrosis of the radius after fracture through normal bone in a child who had neurofibromatosis. A case report. *J Bone Joint Surg Am* 1989;71:1419.

57. Kameyama O, Ogawa R. Pseudarthrosis of the radius associated with neurofibromatosis: report of a case and review of the literature. *J Pediatr Orthop* 1990;10:128.

58. Maffulli N, Fixsen JA. Pseudoarthrosis of the ulna in neurofibromatosis. A report of four cases. *Arch Orthop Trauma Surg* 1991;110:204.

59. Ostrowski DM, Eilert RE, Waldsten G. Congenital pseudarthrosis of the ulna: a report of two cases and a review of the literature. *J Pediatr Orthop* 1985;5:463.

60. Craigen MA, Clarke NM. Familial congenital pseudarthrosis of the ulna. *J Hand Surg Br* 1995;20:331.

61. Ezekowitz RA, Mulliken JB, Folkman J. Interferon alpha-2a therapy for life threatening hemangiomas of infancy. *N Engl J Med* 1992;326:1456.

62. Folkman J. Successful treatment of an angiogenic disease. *N Engl J Med* 1989;320:1211.

63. Brill CB. Neurofibromatosis: clinical overview. *Clin Orthop Rel Res* 1989;245:10.

64. Mapstone TB. Neurofibromatosis and central nervous system tumors in childhood. *Neurosurg Clin North Am* 1992;3:771.

65. Sorensen SA, Mulvihill JJ, Nielsen A. Long-term follow-up of von Recklinghausen neurofibromatosis. Survival and malignant neoplasms. *N Engl J Med* 1986;314:1010.

66. Warrier RP, Kini KR, Ragu U, et al. Neurofibromatosis and malignancy. *Clin Pediatr* 1985;24:584.

67. Zoller M, Rembeck B, Akesson HO. Life expectancy, mortality and prognostic factors in neurofibromatosis type 1. A twelve-year follow-up of an epidemiological study in Goteborg, Sweden. *Acta Derm Venereol* 1995;75:140.

68. Listernick R, Charrow J, Greenwald M. Emergence of optic pathway gliomas in children with neurofibromatosis type 1 after normal neuroimaging results. *J Pediatr* 1992;121:584.

69. Coleman BG, Arger PH, Dalinka MK, et al. CT of sarcomatous degeneration in neurofibromatosis. *AJR Am J Roentgenol* 1983; 140:383.

70. Gutmann DH, Collins FS. The neurofibromatosis type 1 gene and its protein product, neurofibromin. Review. *Neuron* 1993; 10:335.

71. Meis JM, Enzinger FM, Martz KL, Neal JA. Malignant peripheral nerve sheath tumors (malignant schwannomas) in children. *Am J Surg Pathol* 1992;16:694.

72. Wanebo JE, Malik JM, VandenBerg SR, et al. Malignant peripheral nerve sheath tumors. A clinicopathologic study of 28 cases. *Cancer* 1993;71:1247.

73. Coleman BG, Arger PH, Dalinka MK. CT of sarcomatous degeneration in neurofibromatosis. *AJR Am J Roentgenol* 1983; 140:387.

74. Konishi K, Nakamura M, Yamakawa H, et al. Case report: hypophosphatemic osteomalacia in von Recklinghausen neurofibromatosis. *Am J Med Sci* 1991;301:322.

75. Weinstein RS, Harris RL. Hypercalcemic hyperparathyroidism and hypophosphatemic osteomalacia complicating neurofibromatosis. *Calcif Tissue Int* 1990;46:361.

76. Habiby R, Silverman B, Listernick R. Precocious puberty in children with neurofibromatosis type 1. *J Pediatr* 1995;126: 367.

77. Hofman KJ, Harris EL, Bryan RN. Neurofibromatosis type 1: the cognitive phenotype. *J Pediatr* 1994;124:S8.

78. Ferner RE, Hughes RA, Weinman J. Intellectual impairment in neurofibromatosis 1. *J Neurol Sci* 1996;138:133.

Proteus Syndrome

79. Barkmakian JT, Posner MA, Silver L, et al. Proteus syndrome. *J Hand Surg* 1992;17:32.

80. Kalen V, Burwell DS, Omer GE. Macrodactyly of the hands and feet. *J Pediatr Orthop* 1988;8:311.

81. Lacombe D, Taieb A, Vergnes P, et al. Proteus syndrome in 7 patients: clinical and genetic considerations. *Genet Couns* 1991; 2:93.

82. Biesecker LG, Happle R, Milliken JB, et al. Proteus syndrome: diagnostic criteria, differential diagnosis, and patient evaluation. *Am J Med Gene* 1999;84:389.

83. Aylsworth AS, Friedmann PA, Powers SK, et al. New observations with genetic implications in two syndromes: (1) father to son transmission of the Nager acrofacial dysostosis syndromeå (2) parental consanguinity in the Proteus syndrome. *Am J Hum Genet* 1987;41:A43.

84. Cremin BJ, Viljoen DL, Wynchank S, et al. The Proteus syndrome: the magnetic resonance and radiological features. *Pediatr Radiol* 1987;17:486.

85. Goodship J, Redfearn A, Milligan D, et al. Transmission of Proteus syndrome from father to son? *J Med Genet* 1991;28: 781.

86. Wiedemann HR, Burgio GR, Alenjoff P, et al. The Proteus syndrome: partial gigantism of the hands and/or feet, nevi, hemihypertrophy, subcutaneous tumors, macrocephaly or other skull anomalies and possible accelerated growth and visceral affections. *Eur J Pediatr* 1983;140:5.

87. Tibbles JA, Cohen MM. The Proteus syndrome: the Elephant Man diagnosed. *Br Med J* 1986;293:683.

88. Clark RD, Donnai D, Rogers J, et al. Proteus syndrome: an expanded phenotype. *Am J Med* 1987;25:99.

89. Hotamisligil GS. Proteus syndrome and hamartoses with overgrowth. *Dysmorphol Clin Genet* 1990;4:87.

90. Demetriades MD, Hager J, Nikolaides N, et al. Proteus syndrome: musculoskeletal manifestations and management: a report of two cases. *J Pediatr Orthop* 1992;12:106.

91. Stricker S. Musculoskeletal manifestations of Proteus syndrome: report of two cases with literature review. *J Pediatr Orthop* 1992; 12:667.

92. Azouz EM, Costa T, Fitch N. Radiologic findings in the Proteus syndrome. *Pediatr Radiol* 1987;17:481.

93. Turra S, Santini S, Cagnoni G. Gigantism of the foot: our experience in seven cases. *J Pediatr Orthop* 1998;18:337.

94. Ring D, Snyder B. Spinal canal compromise in Proteus syndrome: a case report and review of the literature. *Am J Orthop* 1997;26:275.

95. Choi ML, Wey PD, Borah GL. Pediatric neuropathy in Proteus syndrome. *Ann Plast Surg* 1998;40:528.

96. Malamitsi-Puchner A, Dimitriadis D, et al. Proteus syndrome: course of a severe case. *Am J Med Genet* 1990;35:283.

Arthrogryposis

97. Goldberg MJ. *The dysmorphic child: an orthopedic perspective.* New York: Raven, 1987:1.

98. Hall JG. Genetic aspects of arthrogryposis. *Clin Orthop* 1985; 194:44.

Contracture Syndromes Involving All Four Extremities

99. Hall JG, Reed SD, Driscoll EP. Part I. Amyoplasia: a common, sporadic condition with congenital contractures. *Am J Med Genet* 1983;15:571.

100. Sarwark JF, MacEwen GD, Scott CI. Current concepts review. Amyoplasia (a common form of arthrogryposis). *J Bone Joint Surg Am* 1990;72:465.

101. Otto AW. A human monster with inwardly curved extremities. *Clin Orthop* 1985;194:4.

102. Hall JG, Reed SD, McGillvray BC, et al. Part II. Amyoplasia: twinning in amyoplasia-a specific type of arthrogryposis with an apparent excess of discordantly affected identical twins. *Am J Med Genet* 1983;15:591.

103. Weston PJ, Ives EJ, Honore RL. Monochromonic diamniotic minimally conjoined twins. *Am J Med Genet* 1990;37:558.

104. Fahy MJ, Hall JG. A retrospective study of pregnancy complications among 828 cases of arthrogryposis. *Genet Couns* 1990;1: 3.

105. Hall JG, Reed SD. Teratogens associated with congenital contractures in humans and animals. *Teratology* 1982;25:173.

106. Robertson WL, Glinski LP, Kirkpatrick SJ, et al. Further evidence that arthrogryposis multiplex congenita in the human sometimes is caused by an intrauterine vascular accident. *Teratology* 1992;45:345.

107. Swinyard CA, Bleck EE. The etiology of arthrogryposis (multiplex congenita contracture). *Clin Orthop* 1985;194:15.

108. Jacobson L, Polizzi A, Morriss-Kay G. Plasma from human mothers of fetuses with severe arthrogryposis multiplex congenita causes deformities in mice. *J Clin Invest* 1999;103:1038.

109. Banker BQ. Neuropathologic aspects of arthrogryposis multiplex congenita. *Clin Orthop* 1985;194:30.

110. Clarren SK, Hall JG. Neuropathologic findings in the spinal cords of 10 infants with arthrogryposis. *J Neurol Sci* 1983;58: 89.

111. Quinn CM, Wigglesworth JS, Heckmatt J. Lethal arthrogryposis multiplex congenita: a pathological study of 21 cases. *Histopathology* 1991;19:155.

112. Brown LM, Robson MJ, Sharrard WJW. The pathology of arthrogryposis multiplex congenita neurologica. *J Bone Joint Surg Br* 1980;62:291.

113. Robinson RO. Arthrogryposis multiplex congenita: feeding, language and other health problems. *Neuropediatrics* 1990;21: 177.

114. Carlson WO, Speck GJ, Vicari V, et al. Arthrogryposis multiplex congenita. A long-term follow-up study. *Clin Orthop* 1985; 194:115.

115. Davidson J, Beighton P. Whence the arthrogrypotics? *J Bone Joint Surg Br* 1976;58:492.

116. Hoffer MM, Swank S, Eastman F, et al. Ambulation in severe arthrogryposis. *J Pediatr Orthop* 1983;3:293.

117. Hahn G. Arthrogryposis. Pediatric review and rehabilitative aspects. *Clin Orthop* 1985;194:105.

118. Thompson GH, Bilenker RM. Comprehensive management of arthrogryposis multiplex congenita. *Clin Orthop* 1985;194:6.

119. Diamond LS, Alegado R. Perinatal fractures in arthrogryposis multiplex congenita. *J Pediatr Orthop* 1981;1:189.

120. Palmer PM, MacEwen GD, Brown JR, et al. Passive motion therapy for infants with arthrogryposis. *Clin Orthop* 1985;194: 54.

121. Huurman WW, Jacobsen ST. The hip in arthrogryposis multiplex congenita. *Clin Orthop* 1985;194:81.

122. St. Clair HS, Zimbler S. A plan of management and treatment results in the arthrogrypotic hip. *Clin Orthop* 1985;194:74.

123. Staheli LT, Chow DE, Elliott JS, et al. Management of hip dislocations in children with arthrogryposis. *J Pediatr Orthop* 1987;7:681.

124. Williams P. The management of arthrogryposis. *Orthop Clin North Am* 1978;9:67.

125. Akazawa H, Oda K, Mitani S. Surgical management of hip dislocation in children with arthrogryposis multiplex congenita. *J Bone Joint Surg Br* 1998;80:636.

126. Szoke G, Staheli LT, Jaffer K, et al. Medial-approach open reduction of hip dislocation in amyoplasia-type arthrogryposis. *J Pediatr Orthop* 1996;16:127.

127. Guidera JK, Kortright L, Barber V, et al. Radiographic changes in arthrogrypotic knees. *Skeletal Radiol* 1991;20:193.

128. Sodergard J, Ryoppy S. The knee in arthrogryposis multiplex congenita. *J Pediatr Orthop* 1990;10:177.

129. Thomas B, Schopler S, Wood W, et al. The knee in arthrogryposis. *Clin Orthop* 1985;194:87.

130. Murray C, Fixsen JA. Management of knee deformity in classical arthrogryposis multiplex congenita (amyoplasia congenita). *J Pediatr Orthop B* 1997;6:191.

131. Brunner R, Hefti F, Tgetgel JD. Arthrogrypotic joint contracture at the knee and the foot: correction with a circular frame. *J Pediatr Orthop B* 1997;6:192.

132. Guidera KJ, Drennan JC. Foot and ankle deformities in arthrogryposis multiplex congenita. *Clin Orthop* 1985;194:93.

133. Zimbler S, Craig CL. The arthrogrypotic foot. Plan of management and results of treatment. *Foot Ankle* 1983;3:211.

134. Green ADL, Fixsen JA, Lloyd-Roberts GC. Talectomy for arthrogryposis multiplex congenita. *J Bone Joint Surg Br* 1984; 66:697.

135. Hsu LCS, Jaffray D, Leong JCY. Talectomy for club foot in arthrogryposis. *J Bone Joint Surg Br* 1984;66:694.

136. Niki H, Staheli LT, Mosca VS. Management of clubfoot deformity in amyoplasia. *J Pediatr Orthop* 1997;17:803.

137. Chang CH, Huang SC. Surgical treatment of clubfoot deformity in arthrogryposis multiplex congenita. *J Formos Med Assoc* 1997;96:30.

138. D'Souza H, Aroojis A, Chawara GS. Talectomy in arthrogryposis: analysis of results. *J Pediatr Orthop* 1998;18:760.

139. Bennet JB, Hansen PE, Granberry WM, et al. Surgical management of arthrogryposis in the upper extremity. *J Pediatr Orthop* 1985;5:281.

140. Williams PF. Management of upper limb problems in arthrogryposis. *Clin Orthop* 1985;194:60.

141. Doyle JR, James PM, Larsen W, et al. Restoration of elbow flexion in arthrogryposis multiplex congenita. *J Hand Surg* 1980;5:149.

142. Van Heest A, Waters PM, Simmons BP. Surgical treatment of arthrogryposis of the elbow. *J Hand Surg Am* 1998;23:1063.

143. Axt MW, Niethard FU, Doderlein L. Principles of treatment of the upper extremity in arthrogryposis multiplex congenita type I. *J Pediatr Orthop B* 1997;6:179.

144. Atkins RM, Bell MJ, Sharrard WJW. Pectoralis major transfer for paralysis of elbow flexion in children. *J Bone Joint Surg Br* 1985;67:640.

145. Bayne LG. Hand assessment and management of arthrogryposis multiplex congenita. *Clin Orthop* 1985;194:68.

146. Yonenobu K, Tada K, Swanson B. Arthrogryposis of the hand. *J Pediatr Orthop* 1984;4:599.

147. Daher YH, Lonstein JE, Winter RB, et al. Spinal deformities in patients with arthrogryposis. A review of 16 patients. *Spine* 1985;10:608.

148. Larsen LJ, Schottstaedt ER, Bost FC. Multiple congenital dislocations associated with characteristic facial abnormality. *J Pediatr* 1950;37:574.

149. Houston CS, Reed MH, Desautels JEL. Separating Larsen syndrome from the "arthrogryposis basket." *J Can Assoc Radiol* 1981;32:206.

150. Klenn PJ, Iozzo RV. Larsen's syndrome with novel congenital anomalies. *Hum Pathol* 1991;22:1055.

151. Laville JM, Lakermance P, Limouzy F. Larsen's syndrome: review of the literature and analysis of thirty-eight cases. *J Pediatr Orthop* 1994;14:63.

152. Oki T, Terashima Y, Murachi S, et al. Clinical features and treatment of joint dislocations in Larsen's syndrome. Report of three cases in one family. *Clin Orthop* 1976;119:206.

153. Steel HH, Koh EJ. Multiple dislocations associated with other skeletal anomalies (Larsen's syndrome) in three siblings. *J Bone Joint Surg Am* 1972;54:75.

154. Habermann ET, Sterling A, Dennis RI. Larsen's syndrome: a heritable disorder. *J Bone Joint Surg Am* 1976;58:558.

155. Marques MdeNT. Larsen's syndrome: clinical and genetic aspects. *J Genet Hum* 1980;28:83.

156. Stanley D, Seymour N. The Larsen syndrome occurring in four generations of one family. *Int Orthop* 1985;8:267.

157. Vujic M, Hallstensson K, Wahlstrom J. Localization of a gene for autosomal dominant Larsen syndrome to chromosome region 3p21.1–14.1 in the proximity of, but distinct from, the COL7A1 locus. *Am J Hum Genet* 1995;57:1113.

158. Munk S. Early operation of the dislocated knee in Larsen's syndrome. A report of two cases. *Acta Orthop Scand* 1988;59:582.

159. Bowen JR, Ortega K, Ray S, et al. Spinal deformities in Larsen's syndrome. *Clin Orthop* 1985;197:159.

160. Micheli LJ, Hall JE, Watts HG. Spinal instability in Larsen's syndrome. Report of three cases. *J Bone Joint Surg Am* 1976;58:562.

161. Johnston CE 2nd, Birch JG, Daniels JL. Cervical kyphosis in patients who have Larsen syndrome. *J Bone Joint Surg Am* 1996;78:545.

162. Stevenson GW, Hall SC, Palmieri J. Anesthetic considerations for patients with Larsen's syndrome. *Anaesthesia* 1991;75:142.

163. Kiel EA, Frias JL, Victorica BE. Cardiovascular manifestations in the Larsen syndrome. *Pediatrics* 1983;71:942.

Contracture Syndromes Involving Predominantly the Hands and Feet

164. Dhaliwal AS, Myers TL. Digitotalar dysmorphism. *Orthop Rev* 1985;14:90.

165. Kasai T, Oki T, Nogami H. Familial arthrogryposis with distal involvement of the limbs. *Clin Orthop* 1982;166:182.

166. Salis JG, Beighton P. Dominantly inherited digito-talar dysmorphism. *J Bone Joint Surg Br* 1972;54:509.

167. Hall JG, Reed SD, Greene G. The distal arthrogryposes: delineation of new entities—review and nosologic discussion. *Am J Med Genet* 1982;11:185.

168. Zancolli E, Zancolli E Jr. Congenital ulnar drift of the fingers. Pathogenesis, classification, and surgical management. *Hand Clin* 1985;1:443.

169. Hageman G, Jenekens FGI, Vette JK, et al. The heterogeneity of distal arthrogryposis. *Brain Dev* 1984;6:273.

170. McCormack MK, Coppola-McCormack P, Lee M. Autosomal-dominant inheritance of distal arthrogryposis. *Am J Med Genet* 1980;6:163.

171. Robinow M, Johnson GF. The Gordon syndrome: autosomal dominant cleft palate, camptodactyly, and club feet. *Am J Med Genet* 1981;9:139.

172. Rozin MM, Hertz M, Goodman RM. A new syndrome with camptodactyly, joint contractures, facial anomalies, and skeletal defects: a case report and review of syndromes with camptodactyly. *Clin Genet* 1984;26:342.

173. Bui TH, Lindholm H, Demir N, et al. Prenatal diagnosis of distal arthrogryposis type I by ultrasonography. *Prenat Diagn* 1992;12:1047.

174. Freeman EA, Sheldon JH. Cranio-carpo-tarsal dystrophy. An undescribed congenital malformation. *Arch Dis Child* 1938;13:277.

175. Walker BA. Whistling face-windmill vane syndrome (craniocarpotarsal dystrophy; Freeman-Sheldon syndrome). *Birth Defects* 1969;5:228.

176. Dallapiccola B, Giannotti A, Lembo A, Sagni L. Autosomal recessive form of whistling face syndrome in sibs. *Am J Med Genet* 1989;33:542.

177. Malkawi H, Tarawneh M. The whistling face syndrome, or craniocarpaltarsal dysplasia. Report of two cases in a father and son and review of the literature. *J Pediatr Orthop* 1983;3:364.

178. Wettstein A, Buchinger G, Braun A, Bazan UB. A family with whistling face syndrome. *Hum Genet* 1980;55:177.

179. Rinsky LA, Bleck EE. Freeman-Sheldon ("whistling face") syndrome. *J Bone Joint Surg Am* 1976;58:148.

180. Estrada R, Rosenfeld W, Salazar JD, et al. Freeman-Sheldon syndrome with unusual hand and foot anomalies. *J Natl Med Assoc* 1981;73:664.

181. O'Connell DJ, Hall CM. Cranio-carpo-tarsal dysplasia. A report of seven cases. *Radiology* 1977;123:719.

182. Wenner SM, Shalvoy RM. Two stage correction of thumb adductor contracture in Freeman-Sheldon syndrome. *J Hand Surg* 1989;14:937.

183. Marasovich WA, Mazaheri M, Stool SE. Otolaryngologic findings in whistling face syndrome. *Arch Otolaryngol Head Neck Surg* 1989;115:1373.

184. Duggar RG, DeMars PD, Bolton VE. Whistling face syndrome: general anesthesia and early postoperative caudal analgesia. *Anesthesiology* 1989;70:545.

185. Galaini CA, Matt BH. Laryngomalacia and intraneural striated muscle in an infant with Freeman-Sheldon syndrome. *Int J Pediatr Otolaryngol* 1993;25:243.

186. Jones R, Dolcourt JL. Muscle rigidity following halothane in two patients with Freeman-Sheldon. *Anesthesiology* 1992;77:599.

187. Sauk JJ, Delaney JR, Reaume C, et al. Electromyography of oral-facial musculature in craniocarpotarsal dysplasia (Freeman-Sheldon syndrome). *Clin Genet* 1974;6:132.

Contracture Syndromes with Skin Webs

188. Hall JG, Reed SD, Rosenbaum KN, et al. Limb pterygium syndromes: a review and report of 11 patients. *Am J Med Genet* 1982;12:377.
189. De Die-Smulders CE, Schrander-Stompel CT, Fryns JP. The lethal multiple pterygium syndrome: a nosological approach. *Genet Couns* 1990;1:13.
190. De Die-Smulders CE, Vonsee MJ, Zandvoort JA, Fryns JP. The lethal multiple pterygium syndrome: prenatal ultrasonographic and postmortem findings. *Eur J Obstet Gynecol Reprod Biol* 1990;35:283.
191. Hall JG. Genetic aspects of arthrogryposis. *Clin Orthop* 1985; 194:44.
192. Hartwig NG, Vermeij-Keers C, Bruijn JA, et al. Case of lethal multiple pterygium syndrome with special references to the origin of pterygia. *Am J Med Genet* 1989;33:537.
193. McCall RE, Buddon J. Treatment of multiple pterygium syndrome. *Orthopedics* 1992;15:1417.
194. Penchaszadeh VB, Salszberg B. Multiple pterygium syndrome. *J Med Genet* 1981;18:451.
195. Winter RB. Scoliosis and the multiple pterygium syndrome. *J Pediatr Orthop* 1983;3:125.
196. Escobar V, Weaver D. Popliteal pterygium syndrome. A phenotypic and genetic analysis. *J Med Genet* 1978;15:35.
197. Froster-Iskenns VG. Popliteal pterygium syndrome. *J Med Genet* 1990;27:320.
198. Herold HZ. Popliteal pterygium syndrome. *Clin Orthop* 1986; 299:194.
199. Hunter A. The popliteal pterygium syndrome: report of a new family and review of literature. *Am J Med Genet* 1990;36:196.
200. Oppenheim WL, Larson KR, McNabb MB, et al. Popliteal pterygium syndrome: an orthopaedic perspective. *J Pediatr Orthop* 1990;10:58.
201. Koch H, Grzonka M, Koch J. Popliteal pterygium syndrome with special consideration of the cleft malformation. Cleft palate. *Craniofac J* 1992;29:80.
202. Wynne JM, Fraser AG, Herman R. Massive oral membrane in the popliteal web syndrome. *J Pediatr Surg* 1982;17:59.
203. Cunningham LN, Keating MA, Snyder HM, et al. Urologic manifestations of the popliteal pterygium syndrome. *J Urol* 1989;141:910.
204. Addison A, Webb PJ. Flexion contractures of the knee associated with popliteal webbing. *J Pediatr Orthop* 1983;3:376.
205. Crawford A. Treatment of popliteal pterygium syndrome. *J Pediatr Orthop* 1982;2:443.
206. Hansson LI, Hansson V, Jonsson K. Popliteal pterygium syndrome in a 74-year-old woman. *Acta Orthop Scand* 1976;47:525.
207. Saleh M, Gibson MF, Sharrard WJ. Femoral shortening in correction of congenital knee flexion deformity with popliteal webbing. *J Pediatr Orthop* 1989;9:609.
208. Brunner R, Hefti F, Tgetgel JD. Arthrogrypotic joint contracture at the knee and the foot: correction with a circular frame. *J Pediatr Orthop B* 1997;6:192.

Down Syndrome

209. Gath A. Parental reactions to loss and disappointment: the diagnosis of Down's syndrome. *Dev Med Child Neurol* 1985;27:392.
210. Barden HS. Growth and development of selected hard tissues in Down syndrome: a review. *Hum Biol* 1983;55:539.
211. Caffey J, Ross S. Pelvic bones in infantile mongoloidism: roentgenographic features. *AJR Am J Roentgenol* 1958;80:458.
212. Cronk C, Crocker AC, Pueschel SM, et al. Growth charts for children with Down syndrome: 1 month to 18 years of age. *Pediatrics* 1988;81:102.
213. Wald NJ, Watt HC, Hackshaw AK. Integrated screening for Down's syndrome on the basis of tests performed during the first and second trimesters. *N Engl J Med* 1999;341:461.
214. Brock DJH. *Molecular genetics for the clinician.* Cambridge, UK: Cambridge University Press, 1993.
215. Kolata G. Down syndrome–Alzheimer's linked. *Science* 1985; 230:1152.
216. MacLachlan RA, Fidler KE, Yeh H, et al. Cervical spine abnormalities in institutionalized adults with Down's syndrome. *J Intellect Disabil Res* 1993;37:277.
217. Pueschel SM, Scola FH, Tupper TB, et al. Skeletal anomalies of the upper cervical spine in children with Down syndrome. *J Pediatr Orthop* 1990;10:607.
218. Pueschel SM, Moon AC, Scola FH. Computerized tomography in persons with Down syndrome and atlantoaxial instability. *Spine* 1992;17:735.
219. Selby KA, Newton RW, Gupta S, et al. Clinical predictors and radiological reliability in atlantoaxial subluxation in Down's syndrome. *Arch Dis Child* 1991;66:876.
220. Tredwell SJ, Newman DE, Lockitch G. Instability of the upper cervical spine in Down syndrome. *J Pediatr Orthop* 1990;10:602.
221. White KS, Ball WS, Prenger EC, et al. Evaluation of the craniocervical junction in Down syndrome: correlation of measurements obtained with radiography and MR imaging. *Radiology* 1993;186:377.
222. Gabriel KR, Mason DE, Carango P. Occipito-atlantal translation in Down's syndrome. *Spine* 1990;15:997.
223. Menezes AH, Ryken TC. Craniovertebral abnormalities in Down's syndrome. *Pediatr Neurosurg* 1992;18:24.
224. Stein SM, Kirchner SG, Horev G, et al. Atlanto-occipital subluxation in Down syndrome. *Pediatr Radiol* 1991;21:121.
225. Ohsawa T, Izawa T, Kuroki Y, et al. Follow-up study of atlantoaxial instability in Down's syndrome without separate odontoid process. *Spine* 1989;14:1149.
226. Martich V, Ben-Ami T, Yousefzadeh DK, et al. Hypoplastic posterior arch of C-1 in children with Down syndrome: a double jeopardy. *Radiology* 1992;183:125.
227. Fidone GS. Degenerative cervical arthritis and Down's syndrome. *N Engl J Med* 1986;314:320.
228. Tangerud A, Hestnes A, Sand T, et al. Degenerative changes in the cervical spine in Down's syndrome. *J Ment Defic Res* 1990;34:179.
229. Cremers MJ, Beijer HJ. No relation between general laxity and atlantoaxial instability in children with Down syndrome. *J Pediatr Orthop* 1993;13:318.
230. Pueschel SM, Herndon JH, Gelch MM, et al. Symptomatic atlanto-axial subluxation in persons with Down syndrome. *J Pediatr Orthop* 1984;4:682.
231. Pueschel SM, Scola FH, Pezzullo JC. A longitudinal study of atlanto-dens relationships in asymptomatic individuals with Down syndrome. *Pediatrics* 1992;89:1194.
232. Pueschel SM. Should children with Down syndrome be screened for atlantoaxial instability? *Arch Pediatr Adolesc Med* 1998;152:123.
233. Diamond LS, Lynne D, Sigman B. Orthopedic disorders in patients with Down's syndrome. *Orthop Clin North Am* 1981; 12:57.
234. Hresko MT, McCarthy JC, Goldberg MJ. Hip disease in adults with Down syndrome. *J Bone Joint Surg Br* 1993;75:604.
235. Roberts GM, Starey N, Harper P, et al. Radiology of the pelvis

and hips in adults with Down's syndrome. *Clin Radiol* 1980; 31:475.

236. Shaw ED, Beals RK. The hip joint in Down's syndrome. A study of its structure and associated disease. *Clin Orthop Rel Res* 1992;278:101.

237. Greene WB. Closed treatment of hip dislocation in Down syndrome. *J Pediatr Orthop* 1998;18:643.

238. Aprin H, Zink WP, Hall JE. Management of dislocation of the hip in Down syndrome. *J Pediatr Orthop* 1985;5:428.

239. Bennet GC, Rang M, Roye DP, et al. Dislocation of the hip in trisomy 21. *J Bone Joint Surg Br* 1982;64:289.

240. Gore DR. Recurrent dislocation of the hip in a child with Down's syndrome. *J Bone Joint Surg Am* 1981;63:823.

241. Nogi J. Hip disorders in children with Down's syndrome. *Dev Med Child Neurol* 1985;27:86.

242. Dugdale TW, Renshaw TS. Instability of the patellofemoral joint in Down syndrome. *J Bone Joint Surg Am* 1986;68:405.

243. Herring JA, Fielding JW. Cervical instability in Down's syndrome and juvenile rheumatoid arthritis. *J Pediatr Orthop* 1982; 2:205.

244. Miele JF, Piasio MA, Goldberg MJ. Orthopedic deformity occurring in Down syndrome patients with juvenile rheumatoid arthritis. *Orthop Trans* 1986;10:130.

245. Sherk HH, Pasquariello PS, Watters WC. Multiple dislocations of the cervical spine in a patient with juvenile rheumatoid arthritis and Down's syndrome. *Clin Orthop* 1982;162:37.

246. Levack B, Roper BA. Dislocation in Down's syndrome. *Dev Med Child Neurol* 1984;26:122.

Fetal Alcohol Syndrome

247. Day NL, Richardson GA. Prenatal alcohol exposure: a continuum of effects. *Semin Perinatol* 1991;4:271.

248. Ernhart CB. Clinical correlations between ethanol intake and fetal alcohol syndrome. *Recent Dev Alcohol* 1991;9:127.

249. Knupfer G. Abstaining for foetal health: the fiction that even light drinking is dangerous. *Br J Addiction* 1991;86:1057.

250. Rosett HL, Weiner L, Lee A, et al. Patterns of alcohol consumption and fetal development. *Obstet Gynecol* 1983;61:539.

251. Rosett HL, Weiner L. Prevention of fetal alcohol effects. *Pediatrics* 1982;69:813.

252. Abel EL, Sokol RJ. A revised conservative estimate of the incidence of FAS and its economic impact. *Alcoholism* 1991;15: 514.

253. Little RE, Wendt JK. The effects of maternal drinking in the reproductive period: an epidemiologic review. *J Subst Abuse* 1991;3:187.

254. Smith DF, Sandor GG, MacLeod PM, et al. Intrinsic defects in the fetal alcohol syndrome: studies on 76 cases from British Columbia and the Yukon Territory. *Neurobehav Toxicol Teratol* 1981;3:145.

255. Streissguth AP, Clarren SK, Jones KL. Natural history of the fetal alcohol syndrome: a 10-year follow-up of eleven patients. *Lancet* 1985;2:85.

256. Autti-Ramo I, Gaily E, Granstrom ML. Dysmorphic features in offspring of alcoholic mothers. *Arch Dis Child* 1992;67:712.

257. Rostand A, Kaminski M, Lelong N, et al. Alcohol use in pregnancy, craniofacial features, and fetal growth. *J Epidemiol Commun Health* 1990;44:302.

258. Crain LS, Fitzmaurice NE, Mondry C. Nail dysplasia and fetal alcohol syndrome. *Am J Dis Child* 1983;137:1069.

259. Van Rensburg LJ. Major skeletal defects in the fetal alcohol syndrome. *J Afr Med J* 1981;59:687.

260. West JR, Black AC Jr, Reimann PC, et al. Polydactyly and polysyndactyly induced by prenatal exposure to ethanol. *Teratology* 1981;24:13.

261. Halmesmaki E, Raivio K, Ylikorkala O. A possible association between maternal drinking and fetal clubfoot. *N Engl J Med* 1985;312:790.

262. Cremin BJ, Jaffer Z. Radiological aspects of the fetal alcohol syndrome. *Pediatr Radiol* 1981;11:151.

263. Lowry RB. The Klippel-Feil anomalad as part of the fetal alcohol syndrome. *Teratology* 1977;16:53.

264. Neidengard L, Carter TE, Smith DW. Klippel-Feil malformation complex in fetal alcohol syndrome. *Am J Dis Child* 1978; 132:929.

265. Spiegel PG, Pekman WM, Rich BH, et al. The orthopedic aspects of the fetal alcohol syndrome. *Clin Orthop* 1979;139: 58.

266. Tredwell SJ, Smith DF, MacLeod PJ, Wood BJ. Cervical spine anomalies in fetal alcohol syndrome. *Spine* 1982;7:331.

267. Jaffer Z, Nelson M, Beighton P. Bone fusion in the foetal alcohol syndrome. *J Bone Joint Surg Br* 1981;63:569.

268. Leicher-Duber A, Schumacher R, Spranger J. Stippled epiphyses in fetal alcohol syndrome. *Pediatr Radiol* 1990;20:369.

Nail-patella Syndrome

269. Beals RK, Eckhardt AL. Hereditary onycho-osteodysplasia (nail-patella syndrome). A report of nine kindreds. *J Bone Joint Surg Am* 1969;51;505.

270. Daniel CR III, Osment LS, Noojin RL. Triangular lunulae. A clue to nail-patella syndrome. *Arch Dermatol* 1980;116:448.

271. Guidera KJ, Satterwhite Y, Ogden JA, et al. Nail-patella syndrome: a review of 44 orthopaedic patients. *J Pediatr Orthop* 1991;11:737.

272. Yakish SD, Fu FH. Long-term follow-up of the treatment of a family with nail-patella syndrome. *J Pediatr Orthop* 1983;3:360.

273. Darlington D, Hawkins CF. Nail-patella syndrome with iliac horns and hereditary nephropathy. Necropsy report and anatomical dissection. *J Bone Joint Surg Br* 1967;49-B:164.

274. Dreyer SD, Zhou G, Baldini A, et al. Mutations in LMX1B cause abnormal skeletal patterning and renal dysplasia in nail-patella syndrome. *Nat Genet* 1998;19:47.

275. Loomer RL. Shoulder girdle dysplasia associated with nail-patella syndrome. A case report and literature review. *Clin Orthop Rel Res* 1989;238:112.

276. Hogh J, Macnical MF. Foot deformities associated with onycho-osteodysplasia. A familial study and a review of associated features. *Int Orthop* 1985;9:135.

277. Letts M. Hereditary onycho-osteodysplasia (nail-patella syndrome). A three generation familial study. *Orthop Rev* 1991; 20:267.

278. Papadakos VT, Swan A, Bhalla AK. Nail-patella syndrome associated with mixed crystal deposition arthropathy. *Clin Rheumatol* 1992;11:413.

279. Lommen EJ, Hamel BC, te Slaa RL. Nephropathy in hereditary osteo-onycho dysplasia (HOOD): variable expression or genetic heterogenity. *Prog Clin Biol Res* 1989;305:157.

de Lange Syndrome

280. Filippi G. The de Lange syndrome. Report of 15 cases. *Clin Genet* 1989;35:343.

281. De Die-Smulders C, Theunissen P, Schranger-Stumpel C, et al. On the variable expression of the Brachmann-de Lange syndrome. *Clin Genet* 1992;41:42.

282. Greenberg F, Robinson LK. Mild Brachmann-de Lange syndrome: changes of phenotype with age. *Am J Med Genet* 1989; 32:90.

283. Ireland M, English C, Cross I, et al. A de novo translocation t(3;17)(q26.a3;q3.1) in a child with Cornelia de Lange syndrome. *J Med Genet* 1991;28:639.

284. Lakshminarayana P, Nallasivam P. Cornelia de Lange syndrome with ring chromosomes 3. *J Med Genet* 1990;27:405.

285. Bruner JP, Hsia YE. Prenatal findings in Brachmann-de Lange syndrome. *Obstet Gynecol* 1990;76:966.

286. Drolshagen LF, Durmon G, Berumen M, et al. Prenatal ultrasonographic appearance of "Cornelia de Lange" syndrome. *J Clin Ultrasound* 199;220:470.

287. Condron CJ. Limb anomalies in Cornelia de Lange syndrome infant patient. *Birth Defects* 1969;5:226.

288. Curtis JA, O'Hara AE, Carpenter GG. Spurs of the mandible and supracondylar process of the humerus in Cornelia de Lange syndrome. *AJR Am J Roentgenol* 1977;129:156.

289. Filippi G, Renuart AW. Limb anomalies in the Cornelia de Lange syndrome: adult patient. *Birth Defects* 1969;5:228.

290. Halal F, Preus M. The hand profile in de Lange syndrome: diagnostic criteria. *Am J Med Genet* 1979;3:317.

291. Joubin J, Pettrone CF, Pettrone FA. Cornelia de Lange's syndrome. A review article (with emphasis on orthopedic significance). *Clin Orthop* 1982;171:180.

292. Pashayan HM, Fraser FC, Pruzansky S. Variable limb malformations in the Brachmann-Cornelia de Lange syndrome. *Birth Defects* 1975;11:147.

293. Rosenbach Y, Zahavi I, Dinari G. Gastroesophageal dysfunction in Brachmann-de Lange syndrome. *Am J Med Genet* 1992;42:379.

294. Cates M, Billmire DF, Bull MJ, Grosfeld JL. Gastroesophageal dysfunction in Cornelia de Lange syndrome. *J Pediatr Surg* 1989;24:248.

295. Fraser WI, Campbell BM. A study of six cases of de Lange Amsterdam dwarf syndrome, with special attention to voice, speech and language characteristics. *Dev Med Child Neurol* 1978;20:189.

296. Dossetor DR, Couryer S, Nicol AR. Massage for very severe self-injurious behaviour in a girl with Cornelia de Lange syndrome. *Dev Med Child Neurol* 1991;33:636.

297. Shear CS, Nyhan WL, Kirman BH, et al. Self-mutilative behavior as a feature of the de Lange syndrome. *J Pediatr* 1971;78:506.

298. Sargent WW. Anesthetic management of a patient with Cornelia de Lange syndrome. *Anesthesiology* 1991;74:1162.

Familial Dysautonomia

299. Axelrod FB, Porges RF, Stein ME. Neonatal recognition of familial dysautonomia. *J Pediatr* 1987;110:946.

300. Clayson D, Welton W, Axelrod FB. Personality development and familial dysautonomia. *Pediatrics* 1980;65:274.

301. Axelrod FB, Abularrage JJ. Familial dysautonomia: a prospective study of survival. *J Pediatr* 1982;101:234.

302. Blumenfeld A, Slaughenhaupt SA, Liebert CB, et al. Precise genetic mapping and haplotype analysis of the familial dysautonomia gene on human chromosome 9q31. *Am J Hum Genet* 1999;64:1110.

303. Pearson J, Pytel BA, Grover-Johnson N, et al. Quantitative studies of dorsal root ganglia and neuropathologic observations on spinal cords in familial dysautonomia. *J Neurol Sci* 1978;35:77.

304. Hensinger RN, MacEwen GD. Spinal deformity associated with heritable neurological conditions: spinal muscular atrophy, Friedreich's ataxia, familial dysautonomia, and Charcot-Marie-Tooth disease. *J Bone Joint Surg Am* 1976;58:13.

305. Robin GC. Scoliosis in familial dysautonomia. *Bull Hosp Joint Dis Orthop Inst* 1984;44:16.

306. Yoslow W, Becker MH, Bartels J, et al. Orthopaedic defects in familial dysautonomia. A review of sixty-five cases. *J Bone Joint Surg Am* 1971;53:1541.

307. Albanese SA, Babechko WP. Spine deformity in familial dysautonomia (Riley-Day syndrome). *J Pediatr Orthop* 1979;7:183.

308. Robin GC. Scoliosis in familial dysautonomia. *Bull Hosp Joint Dis Orthop Inst* 1984;44:26.

309. Rubery PT, Speilman JH, Hester P. Scoliosis in familial dysautonomia. *J Bone Joint Surg Am* 1995;77:1369.

310. Guidera KJ, Multhopp H, Ganey T, et al. Orthopaedic manifestations in congenitally insensate patients. *J Pediatr Orthop* 1990;10:514.

311. Mitnick JS, Axelrod FB, Genieser NB, et al. Aseptic necrosis in familial dysautonomia. *Radiology* 1982;142:89.

312. Brunt PW. Unusual cause of Charcot joints in early adolescence (Riley-Day syndrome). *Br Med J* 1967;4:277.

313. Chillag KJ, Stevens DB. Idiopathic neurogenic arthropathy. *J Pediatr Orthop* 1985;5:597.

314. Porges RF, Axelrod FB, Richards M. Pregnancy in familial dysautonomia. *Am J Obstet Gynecol* 1978;132:485.

Rubinstein-Taybi Syndrome

315. Rubinstein JH. Broad thumb-hallux (Rubinstein-Taybi) syndrome 1957–1988. *Am J Med Genet* 1990;6(suppl):3.

316. Hennekam RC, Van Den Boogaard MJ, Sibbles BJ, et al. Rubinstein-Taybi syndrome in The Netherlands. *Am J Med Genet* 1990;6(suppl):17.

317. Marion RW, Garcia DM, Karasik JB. Apparent dominant transmission of the Rubinstein-Taybi syndrome. *Am J Med Genet* 1993;46:284.

318. Allanson JE. Rubinstein-Taybi syndrome: the changing face. *Am J Med Genet* 1990;6(suppl):38.

319. Robson MJ, Brown LM, Sharrad WJW. Cervical spondylolis syndrome and other skeletal abnormalities in Rubinstein-Taybi syndrome. *J Bone Joint Surg Br* 1980;62:297.

320. Petrij F, Giles RH, Dauwerse HG. Rubinstein-Taybi syndrome caused by mutations in the transcriptional co-activator CBP. *Nature* 1995;376:351.

321. Stevens CA, Hennekam RC, Blackburn BL. Growth in the Rubinstein-Taybi syndrome. *Am J Med Genet* 1990;6(suppl):51.

322. Hennekam RC, Van Doorne JM. Oral aspects of Rubinstein-Taybi syndrome. *Am J Med Genet* 1990;6(suppl):42.

323. Partington MW. Rubinstein-Taybi syndrome: a follow-up study. *Am J Med Genet* 1990;6(suppl):65.

324. Stevens CA, Carey JC, Blackburn BL. Rubinstein-Taybi syndrome: a natural history study. *Am J Med Genet* 1990;6(suppl):30.

325. Miller RW, Rubinstein JH. Tumors in Rubinstein-Taybi syndrome. *Am J Med Genet* 1995;56:115.

326. Mehlman CT, Rubinstein JH, Roy DR. Instability of the patellofemoral joint in Rubinstein-Taybi syndrome. *J Pediatr Orthop* 1998;18:511.

327. Stevens CA. Patellar dislocation in Rubintein-Taybi syndrome. *Am J Med Genet* 1997;72:190.

328. Stirt JA. Anesthetic problems in Rubinstein-Taybi syndrome. *Anesth Analg* 1981;60:534.

329. Stirt JA. Succinylcholine in Rubinstein-Taybi syndrome. *Anesthesiology* 1982;57:429.

330. Selmanowitz VJ, Stiller MJ. Rubinstein-Taybi syndrome. Cutaneous manifestations and colossal keloids. *Arch Dermatol* 1981;117:504.

Progeria

331. Monu JU, Benka-Coker LB, Fatunde Y. Hutchinson-Gilford progeria syndrome in siblings. Report of three new cases. *Skeletal Radiol* 1990;19:585.

332. Khalifa MM. Hutchinson-Gilford progeria syndrome: report of

a Libyan family and evidence of autosomal recessive inheritance. *Clin Genet* 1989;35:125.

333. Brown WT. Progeria: a human-disease model of accelerated aging. *Am J Clin Nutr* 1992;55(suppl 6):1222S.

334. Abdenur JE, Brown WT, Friedman S, et al. Response to nutritional and growth hormone treatment in progeria. *Metabolism* 1997;46:851.

335. Yan T, Li S, Jiang X, et al. Altered levels of primary antioxidant enzymes in progeria skin fibroblasts. *Biochem Biophys Res Commun* 1999;257:163.

336. Badame AJ. Progeria. *Arch Dermatol* 1989;125:540.

337. Gillar PJ, Kaye CI, McCourt JW. Progressive early dermatologic changes in Hutchinson-Gilford progeria syndrome. *Pediatr Dermatol* 1991;8:199.

338. Moen C. Orthopaedic aspects of progeria. *J Bone Joint Surg Am* 1982;64:542.

339. Reichel W, Bailey JA II, Zigel S, et al. Radiological findings in progeria. *J Am Geriatr Soc* 1971;19:657.

340. Fernandez-Palazzi F, McLaren AT, Slowie DF. Report on a case of Hutchinson-Gilford progeria, with special reference to orthopedic problems. *Eur J Pediatr Surg* 1992;2:378.

341. Gamble JG. Hip disease in Hutchinson-Gilford progeria syndrome. *J Pediatr Orthop* 1984;4:585.

Russell-Silver Dwarfism

342. Angehrn V, Zachmann M, Prader A. Silver-Russell syndrome. Observations in 20 patients. *Helv Paediatr Acta* 1979;34:297.

343. Saal HM, Pagon RA, Pepin MG. Reevaluation of Russell-Silver syndrome. *J Pediatr* 1985;107:733.

344. Tanner JM, Lejarraga H, Cameron N. The natural history of the Silver-Russell syndrome: a longitudinal study of thirty-nine cases. *Pediatr Res* 1975;9:611.

345. Escobar V, Gleiser S, Weaver DD. Phenotypic and genetic analysis of the Silver-Russell syndrome. *Clin Genet* 1978;13:278.

346. Samn M, Lewis K, Blumberg B. Monozygotic twins discordant for the Russell-Silver syndrome. *Am J Med Genet* 1990;37:543.

347. Limbird TJ. Slipped capital femoral epiphysis associated with Russell-Silver syndrome. *South Med J* 1989;82:902.

348. Moss SH, Switzer HE. Congenital hypoplastic thumb in the Silver syndrome: a case report and review of upper extremity anomalies in the world literature. *J Hand Surg* 1983;8:480.

349. Spect EE, Hazelrig PE. Orthopaedic considerations of Silver's syndrome. *J Bone Joint Surg Am* 1973;55:1502.

350. Stanhope R, Ackland F, Hamill G, et al. Physiological growth hormone secretion and response to growth hormone treatment in children with short stature and intrauterine growth retardation. *Acta Paediatr Scand* 1989;349(suppl):47.

351. Bruckheimer E, Abrahamov A. Russell-Silver syndrome and Wilms tumor. *J Pediatr* 1993;122:165.

Turner Syndrome

352. Jacobs PA, Betts PR, Cockwell AE, et al. A cytogenetic and molecular reappraisal of a series of patients with Turner's syndrome. *Ann Hum Genet* 1990;54:209.

353. Gicquel C, Cabrol S, Schneid H, et al. Molecular diagnosis of Turner's syndrome. *J Med Genet* 1992;29:547.

354. Pagel M. Mother and father in surprise genetic agreement. *Nature* 1999;397:19.

355. Zinn AR, Tonk VS, Chen Z, et al Evidence for a Turner syndrome locus or loci at Xp11.2–p22.1. *Am J Human Genet* 1998; 63:1757.

356. Naeraa RW, Nielsen J. Standards for growth and final height in Turner's syndrome. *Acta Paediatr Scand* 1990;79:182.

357. Mostello DJ, Bofinger MK, Siddiqi TA. Spontaneous resolution of fetal cystic hygroma and hydrops in Turner syndrome. *Obstet Gynecol* 1989;73:862.

358. Thomson SJ, Tanne NS, Mercer DM. Web neck deformity: anatomical considerations and options in surgical management. *Br J Plast Surg* 1990;43:94.

359. Beals RK. Orthopedic aspects of the XO (Turner's) syndrome. *Clin Orthop* 1973;97:19.

360. Kosowicz J. The deformity of the medial tibial condyle in nineteen cases of gonadal dysgenesis. *J Bone Joint Surg Am* 1960; 42:600.

361. Mora S, Weber G, Guarneri MP, et al. Effect of estrogen replacement therapy on bone mineral content in girls with Turner syndrome. *Obstet Gynecol* 1992;79:747.

362. Naeraa RW, Nielsen J. Standards for growth and final height in Turner's syndrome. *Acta Paediatr Scand* 1990;79:182.

363. Neely EK, Marcus R, Rosenfeld RG, et al. Turner syndrome adolescents receiving growth hormone are not osteopenic. *J Clin Endocrinol Metab* 1993;76:861.

364. Saggese G, Federico G, Bertelloni S, et al. Mineral metabolism in Turner's syndrome: evidence for impaired renal vitamin D metabolism and normal osteoblast function. *J Clin Endocrinol Metab* 1992;75:998.

365. Ross JL, Long LM, Feuillan P, et al. Normal bone density of the wrist and spine and increased wrist fractures in girls with Turner's syndrome. *J Clin Endocrinol Metab* 1991;73:355.

366. Rovet JF. The psychoeducational characteristics of children with Turner syndrome. *J Learn Disabil* 1993;26:333.

367. Swillen A, Fryns JP, Kleczkowska A, et al. Intelligence, behaviour and psychosocial development in Turner syndrome. A cross-sectional study of 50 pre-adolescent and adolescent girls (4–20 years). *Genet Couns* 1993;4:7.

368. Sylven L, Hagenfeldt K, Brondum-Neilsen K, et al. Middle-aged women with Turner's syndrome. Medical status, hormonal treatment and social life. *Acta Endocrinol* 1991;125:359.

369. Subramaniam PN. Turner's syndrome and cardiovascular anomalies: a case report and review of the literature. *Am J Med Sci* 1989;297:260.

370. Rosenfeld RG. Growth hormone therapy in Turner's syndrome: an update on final height. *Acta Paediatr* 1992;383(suppl):3.

371. Rosenfeld RG, Frane J, Attie KM, et al. Six year results of a randomized, prospective trial of human growth hormone and oxandrolone in Turner syndrome. *J Pediatr* 1992;121:49.

Noonan Syndrome

372. Collins E, Turner G. The Noonan syndrome: a review of the clinical and genetic features of 27 cases. *J Pediatr* 1973;83:941.

373. Sharland M, Burch M, McKenna WM, et al. A clinical study of Noonan syndrome. *Arch Dis Child* 1992;67:178.

374. Sharland M, Morgan M, Smith G, et al. Genetic counselling in Noonan syndrome. *Am J Med Genet* 1993;45:437.

375. Burch M, Mann JM, Sharland M, et al. Myocardial disarray in Noonan syndrome. *Br Heart J* 1992;68:586.

376. Campbell AM, Bousfield JD. Anaesthesia in a patient with Noonan's syndrome and cardiomyopathy. *Anaesthesia* 1992;47:131.

377. Wedge JH, Khalifa MM, Shokeir MHK. Skeletal anomalies in 40 patients with Noonan's syndrome. *Orthop Trans* 1987;11: 40.

378. Legius E, Schollen E, Matthijs G, Fryns J-P. Fine mapping of Noonan/ cardio-facio cutaneous syndrome in a large family. *Eur J Hum Genet* 1998;6:32.

Prader-Willi Syndrome

379. Cassidy SB. Prader-Willi syndrome. *Curr Probl Pediatr* 1984; 14:1.

380. Gavranich J, Selikowitz M. A survey of 22 individuals with Prader-Willi syndrome in New South Wales. *Aust Paediatr J* 1989;25:43.

381. Holm VA, Cassidy SB, Butler MG, et al. Prader-Willi syndrome: consensus diagnostic criteria. *Pediatrics* 1993;91:398.

382. Aughton DJ, Cassidy SB. Physical features of Prader-Willi syndrome in neonates. *Am J Dis Child* 1990;144:1251.

383. Char F. A photographic study: the natural history of Prader-Willi syndrome. *J Clin Dysmorphol* 1984;2:2.

384. Borghgraef M, Fryns JP, Van den Berghe H. Psychological profile and behavioral characteristics in 12 patients with Prader-Willi syndrome. *Genet Couns* 1990;1:141.

385. Curfs LM, Verhulst FC, Fryns JP. Behavioral and emotional problems in youngsters with Prader-Willi syndrome. *Genet Couns* 1991;2:33.

386. Selikowitz M, Sunman J, Pendergast A, et al. Fenfluramine in Prader-Willi syndrome: a double blind, placebo controlled trial. *Arch Dis Child* 1990;65:112.

387. Hudgins L, Cassidy SB. Hand and foot length in Prader-Willi syndrome. *Am J Med Genet* 1991;41:5.

388. Waters J, Clarke DJ, Corbett JA. Educational and occupational outcome in Prader-Willi syndrome. *Child Care Health Dev* 1990;16:271.

389. Cassidy SB, ed. *Prader-Willi syndrome and other chromosome 15q deletion disorders. NATO ASI series H: cell biology.* vol 61. Heidelberg: Springer, 1992:265.

390. Knoll JH, Wagstaff J, Lalande M. Cytogenetic and molecular studies in the Prader-Willi and Angelman syndromes: an overview. *Am J Med Genet* 1993;46:2.

391. Nicholls RD. Genomic imprinting and uniparental disomy in Angelman and Prader-Willi syndromes: a review. *Am J Med Genet* 1993;46:16.

392. Gurd AR, Thompson TR. Scoliosis in Prader-Willi syndrome. *J Pediatr Orthop* 1981;1:317.

393. Holm VA, Laurnen EL. Prader-Willi syndrome and scoliosis. *Dev Med Child Neurol* 1981;23:192.

394. Rees D, Jones MW, Owen R, et al. Scoliosis surgery in the Prader-Willi syndrome. *J Bone Joint Surg Br* 1989;71:685.

395. Soriano RM, Weisz I, Houghton GR. Scoliosis in the Prader-Willi syndrome. *Spine* 1988;13:211.

396. Mayhew JF, Taylor B. Anaesthetic considerations in the Prader-Willi syndrome. *Can Anaesth Soc J* 1983;30:565.

397. Carrel AL, Myers SE, Whitman BY. Growth hormone improves body composition, fat utilization, physical strength and agility, and growth in Prader-Willi syndrome: A controlled study. *J Pediatr* 1999;134:221.

398. Davies PS, Evans S, Broomhead S. Effect of growth hormone on height, weight, and body composition in Prader-Willi syndrome. *Arch Dis Child* 1998;78:476.

Beckwith-Wiedemann Syndrome

399. Martinez y Martinez R, Martinez-Carboney R, Ocampo-Campos R, et al. Wiedemann-Beckwith syndrome: clinical, cytogenetical and radiological observations in 39 new cases. *Genet Couns* 1992;3:67.

400. Goldberg MJ. Beckwith-Wiedemann syndrome. In: Goldberg MJ, ed. *The dysmorphic child. An orthopedic perspective.* New York: Raven, 1987:175.

401. Ping AJ, Reeve AE, Law DJ, et al. Genetic linkage of Beckwith-Wiedemann syndrome to 11p15. *Am J Hum Genet* 1989;44:720.

402. Brown KW, Gardner A, Williams JC, et al. Paternal origin of 11p15 duplications in the Beckwith-Wiedemann syndrome. A new case and review of the literature. *Cancer Genet Cytogenet* 1992;58:66.

403. Viljoen D, Ramesar R. Evidence for paternal imprinting in familial Beckwith-Wiedemann syndrome. *J Med Genet* 1992; 29:221.

404. Lodeiro JG, Byers JW III, Chuipek S, et al. Prenatal diagnosis and perinatal management of the Beckwith-Wiedemann syndrome: a case and review. *Am J Perinatol* 1989;6:446.

405. Shah YG, Metlay L. Prenatal ultrasound diagnosis of Beckwith-Wiedemann syndrome. *J Clin Ultrasound* 1990;18:597.

406. Shah KJ. Beckwith-Wiedemann syndrome: role of ultrasound in its management. *Clin Radiol* 1983;34:313.

407. Choyke PL, Siegel MJ, Craft AW. Screening for Wilms tumor in children with Beckwith-Wiedemann syndrome or idiopathic hemihypertrophy. *Med Pediatr Oncol* 1999;32:200.

408. Lee FA. Radiology of the Beckwith-Wiedemann syndrome. *Radiol Clin North Am* 1972;10:261.

VACTERLS and VATER Association

409. Quan L, Smith DW. The VATER association: vertebral defects, anal atresia, T-E fistula with esophageal atresia, radial and renal dysplasia: a spectrum of associated defects. *J Pediatr* 1973;82:104.

410. Beals RK, Rolfe B. VATER association. A unifying concept of multiple anomalies. *J Bone Joint Surg Am* 1989;71:948.

411. Lawhorn SM, MacEwen GD, Bunnell WP. Orthopaedic aspects of the VATER association. *J Bone Joint Surg Am* 1986;68:424.

412. Wulfsberg EA, Phillips-Dawkins TL, Thomas RL. Vertebral hypersegmentation in a case of the VATER association. *Am J Med Genet* 1992;42:766.

413. Chestnut R, James HE, Jones KL. The VATER association and spinal dysraphia. *Pediatr Neurosurg* 1992;18:144.

414. Raffel C, Litofsky S, McComb JG. Central nervous system malformations and the VATER association. *Pediatr Neurosurg* 1990;16:170.

Goldenhar Syndrome

415. Sherk HH, Whitaker LA, Pasquariello PS. Facial malformations and spinal anomalies. A predictable relationship. *Spine* 1982;7:526.

416. Morrison PJ, Mulholland HC, Craig BG, et al. Cardiovascular abnormalities in the oculo-auriculo-vertebral spectrum (Goldenhar syndrome). *Am J Med Genet* 1992;44:425.

417. Van Bever Y, van den Ende JJ, Richieri-Costa A. Oculo-auriculo-vertebral complex and uncommon associated anomalies: report on 9 unrelated Brazilian patients. *Am J Med Genet* 1992; 44:683.

418. Kaye CI, Martin AO, Rollnick BR, et al. Oculoauriculovertebral anomaly: segregation analysis. *Am J Med Genet* 1992;43:913.

419. Darling DB, Feingold M, Berkman M. The roentgenological aspects of Goldenhar's syndrome (oculoauriculovertebral dysplasia). *Radiology* 1968;91:254.

420. Madan R, Trikha A, Venkataraman RK, et al. Goldenhar's syndrome: an analysis of anaesthetic management. A retrospective study of seventeen cases. *Anaesthesia* 1990;45:49.

421. Sherk HH, Whitaker LA, Pasquariello PS. Facial malformations and spinal anomalies. A predictable relationship. *Spine* 1982;7:526.

422. Schrander-Stumpel CT, de Die-Smulders CE, Hennekam RC, et al. Oculoauriculovertebral spectrum and cerebral anomalies. *J Med Genet* 1992;29:326.

Trichorhinophalangeal Syndrome

423. Minguella I, Ubierna M, Escola J, et al. Trichorhinophalangeal syndrome, type I, with avascular necrosis of the femoral head. *Acta Paediatr* 1993;82:329.

424. Ludecke HJ, Johnson C, Wagner MJ, et al. Molecular definition of the shortest region of deletion overlap in the Langer-Giedion syndrome. *Am J Hum Genet* 1991;49:1197.

425. Bauermeister S, Letts M. The orthopaedic manifestations of the Langer-Giedion syndrome. *Orthop Rev* 1992;21:31.

426. Burgess RC. Trichorhinophalangeal syndrome. *South Med J* 1991;84:1268.

Mucopolysaccharidoses

427. Hopwood JJ, Morris CP. The mucopolysaccharidoses. Diagnosis, molecular genetics and treatment. *Mol Biol Med* 1990;7:381.

428. Scriver CR, Beaudet AL, Sly WS, Valle D, eds. *The metabolic basis of inherited disease*, 6th ed. New York: McGraw-Hill, 1989.

429. Fukada S, Tomatsu S, Masue M, et al. Mucopolysaccharidosis type IVA. N-acetyl galactosamine-6-sulfate sulfatase exonic point mutations in classical Morquio and mild cases. *J Clin Invest* 1992;90:1049.

430. Jin WD, Jackson CE, Desnick RJ. Mucopolysaccharidosis type VI: identification of three mutations in the arylsulfatatase B gene of patients with severe and mild phenotypes provides molecular evidence for genetic heterogeneity. *Am J Hum Genet* 1992;50:795.

431. Field RE, Buchanan JA, Copplemans MG, et al. Bone marrow transplantation in Hurler's syndrome. Effect on skeletal development. *J Bone Joint Surg Br* 1994;76:957.

432. Guffon N, Souillet G, Maire I, et al. Follow-up of nine patients with Hurler syndrome after bone marrow transplantation. *J Pediatr* 1998;133:119.

433. Odunusi E, Peters C, Krivit W, et al. Genu valgum deformity in Hurler syndrome after hematopoietic stem cell transplantation: correction by surgical intervention. *J Pediatr Orthop* 1999;19:270.

434. Haddad FS, Hill RA, Jones DH. Triggering in the mucopolysaccharidoses. *J Pediatr Orthop B* 1998;7:138.

435. Haddad FS, Jones DH, Vellodi A, et al. Carpal tunnel syndrome in the mucopolysaccharidoses and mucopolipidoses. *J Bone Joint Surg Br* 1997;79:576.

436. Baker E, Guo XH, Orsborn AM, et al. The Morquio A syndrome (mucopolysaccharidosis IVA) gene maps to 16q24.3. *Am J Hum Genet* 1993;52:96.

437. Bassett GS. Orthopaedic aspects of skeletal dysplasias. *Instruct Course Lect, AAOS*. 1990;39:389.

438. Bassett GS. Lower-extremity abnormalities in dwarfing conditions. *Instruct Course Lect* 1990;39:389.

439. Goldberg MJ. Orthopaedic aspects of bone dysplasia. *Orthop Clin North Am* 1976;7:445.

440. Kopits SE. Orthopaedic complications of dwarfism. *Clin Orthop* 1976;114:153.

441. Bethem D, Winter RB, Luther L, et al. Spinal disorders of dwarfism: review of the literature and report of eighty cases. *J Bone Joint Surg Am* 1981;63:389.

442. Nelson J, Thomas PS. Clinical findings in 12 patients with MPS IVA (Morquio's disease): further evidence for heterogenity. Part III: odontoid dysplasia. *Clin Genet* 1988;33:126.

443. Stevens JM, Kendall BE, Crockard HA. The odontoid process in Morquio-Brailsford disease. The effects of occipitocervical fusion. *J Bone Joint Surg Br* 1991;73:851.

444. Stevens JM, Kendall BE, Crockard HA, et al. The odontoid process in Morquio-Brailsford's disease. The effects of occipitocervical fusion. *J Bone Joint Surg Br* 1991;73:851.

Hadju-Cheney Syndrome

445. Brown DM, Bradford DS, Gorlin RJ. The acro-osteolysis syndrome: morphologic and biochemical studies. *J Pediatr* 1976;88:580.

446. Elias AN, Pinals RS, Anderson HC. Hereditary osteodysplasia with acro-osteolysis (the Hadju-Cheney syndrome). *Am J Med* 1978;65:636.

447. Kawamura J, Miki Y, Yamazaki S. Hadju-Cheney syndrome: MR imaging. *Neuroradiology* 1991;33:442.

448. O'Reilly MAR, Shaw DG. Hadju-Cheney syndrome. *Ann Rheum Dis* 1994;53:279.

449. Weleber RG, Beals RK. Hadju-Cheney syndrome report of 2 cases and review of literature. *J Pediatr* 1976;88:249.

450. Ades LC, Morris LL, Haan EA. Hydrocephalus in Hadju-Cheney syndrome: brief report. *J Bone Joint Surg Br* 1988;70:674.

451. Kaler SG, Geggel RL, Sadehgi-Nejad A. Hadju-Cheney syndrome associated with severe cardiac valvular and conduction disease. *Am J Med Genet* 1995;56:30.

452. Kaplan P, Ramos F, Zackai EH. Cystic kidney disease in Hadju-Cheney syndrome. *Am J Med Genet* 1995;56:30.

Rett Syndrome

453. Hagberg B, Aicardi J, Dias K. A progressive syndrome of autism, dementia, ataxia, and loss of purposeful hand use in girls: Rett's syndrome: report of 35 cases. *Brain Dev* 1985;14:479.

454. Leonard H, Thomson M, Bower C. Skeletal abnormalities in Rett syndrome: increasing evidence for dysmorphogenetic defects. *Am J Med Genet* 1995;58:285.

455. Leonard H, Thomson M, Glasson E. Metacarpophalangeal pattern profile and bone age in Rett syndrome: further radiological clues to the diagnosis. *Am J Med Genet* 1999;83:95.

456. Amir RE, Van den Veyver IB, Wan M, et al. Rett syndrome is caused by mutations in X-linked MECP2, encoding methyl-CpG-binding protein 2. *Nat Genet* 1999;23:185.

457. Coleman M. Is classical Rett syndrome ever present in males? *Brain Dev* 1990;12:32.

458. Huang TJ, Lubicky JP, Hammerberg KW. Scoliosis in Rett syndrome. *Orthop Rev* 1994;23:937.

459. Guidera KJ, Borrelli J Jr, Raney E. Orthopaedic manifestations of Rett syndrome. *J Pediatr Orthop* 1991;11:208.

460. Harrison DJ, Webb PJ. Scoliosis in the Rett syndrome: natural history and treatment. *Brain Dev* 1990;12:156.

461. Loder RT, Lee CL, Richards BS. Orthopaedic aspects of Rett syndrome: a multicenter review. *J Pediatr Orthop* 1989;9:562.

462. Roberts AP, Conner AN. Orthopaedic aspects of Rett's syndrome: brief report. *J Bone Joint Surg Br* 1988;70:674.

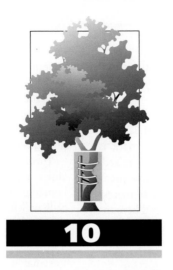

10

LOCALIZED DISORDERS OF BONE AND SOFT TISSUE

WILLIAM G. MACKENZIE
PETER G. GABOS

This chapter focuses on the congenital, developmental or acquired disorders that affect localized or regional areas of the pediatric musculoskeletal system. These entities often share a common clinical presentation and underlying pathologic process, yet are not confined to any one part of the skeleton nor are caused by a recognized systemic abnormality.

CONGENITAL AND DEVELOPMENTAL DISORDERS

Vascular Tumors and Malformations

Vascular anomalies are seen commonly in orthopaedic practice. Most are of no clinical importance, but, occasionally

W. G. Mackenzie: Orthopaedic Department, Thomas Jefferson Medical College, Philadelphia, Pennsylvania 19107; Department of Orthopaedics, Alfred I. duPont Hospital for Children, Wilmington, Delaware 19803.
P. G. Gabos: Department of Orthopaedic Surgery, Jefferson Medical College, Thomas Jefferson University Hospital, Philadelphia, Pennsylvania 19107; Department of Orthopaedic Surgery, Alfred I. duPont Hospital for Children, Wilmington, Delaware 19899.

these anomalies can be deforming or life threatening and require interdisciplinary management. These anomalies may be solitary or the organizing features of various syndromes (1).

The term "vascular anomalies" is used here to describe pediatric vascular disorders with primarily dermatologic or visceral manifestations, excluding abnormalities of the heart and great vessels. The term "hemangioma" has been traditionally used for every type of vascular anomaly, but Mulliken et al. have recently devised a classification system to better clarify these lesions based on their endothelial characteristics (2–4). Two main groups of disorders have been identified; the hemangiomas of infancy, vascular tumors with an early proliferative and later involuting stage; and vascular malformations, a heterogeneous group of vascular lessions comprised of dysplastic vessels, which can be capillary, venous, arterial, lymphatic, or a combination.

Vascular Tumors

Hemangiomas may be cutaneous, subcutaneous, intramuscular, or visceral. The location is most commonly in the head and neck (60%) followed in frequency by the trunk and extremities. The majority occur singly but 20% proliferate in multiple sites.

Cutaneous hemangiomas (formerly called "strawberry" or "capillary hemangiomas") are present in up to 12% of children at 1 year of age (5). A small cutaneous mark is present early in life, which grows rapidly to become a raised, bosselated, vivid red color that blanches poorly. Subsequent slow, spontaneous involution occurs with complete regression in 70% of children by 7 years (3). Lumbosacral hemangiomas and other lesions such as hypertrichosis and dimpling should alert the orthopaedist to an underlying occult spinal dysraphism.

Deep hemangiomas (formerly termed "cavernous hemangiomas") occur in the lower dermis or muscle. The overlying skin may be only slightly raised or bluish. On palpation, the mass is fibrofatty, similar to the superficial hemangioma. These deep hemangiomas can be confused with venous or lymphatic malformations which are usually soft and compressible unless thrombosed. Spontaneous involution usually occurs with deep hemangiomas. Sonography can differentiate between a hemangioma and vascular malformation but MRI is considered the gold standard (5,6).

Most hemangiomas resolve uneventfully with occasional scarring. Superficial ulceration and bleeding is uncommon. Up to 20% of hemangiomas can have significant complications including destruction of involved tissues or obstruction of a vital structure such as the eye or airway (5). High-output congestive heart failure can result from large hemangiomas and gastrointestinal bleeding from intestinal involvement. Kasabach-Merritt syndrome or thrombocytopenic coagulopathy was recently shown to be associated with a rare vascular tumor known as "kaposiform hemangioendothelioma," and not with the common hemangioma (7).

Intralesional or systemic corticosteroids and interferon-alpha are used for large, problematic or life-threatening hemangiomas (5). Factors that inhibit growth of endothelial cells will likely be used in the future (8).

Vascular Malformations

Vascular malformations are subcategorized by the type of vessel abnormality and its flow characteristics (5). The slow-flow anomalies include capillary malformations (CM) (port wine stains and telangiectasias), venous malformations (VM), and lymphatic malformations (LM) (previously known as "lymphangiomas" and "cystic hygromas"). Arterial (AM) and arteriovenous malformations (AVM) are fast-flow anomalies. Unlike the vascular tumors, vascular malformations do not regress spontaneously but can worsen depending on the type. Combined, complex malformations occur. An example of this is the Klippel-Trenaunay syndrome, a slow-flow, capillary–venous and often lymphatic malformation (CVLM), which results in limb overgrowth. Typical vascular malformations are outlined in Table 10-1.

Capillary malformations are usually referred to as "port wine stains." Most are cosmetic vascular birthmarks but

TABLE 10-1. ASSOCIATIONS OF VASCULAR MALFORMATIONS IN CHILDREN

Syndrome	Type and Location	Clinical Problems	Orthopaedic Concerns	Mode of Inheritance
Vascular malformations on limbs				
Klippel-Trenaunay	Capillary venous malformation anywhere, arteriovenous malformations in the extremities	Varicose veins, cardiac overload	Limb hypertrophy, macrodactyly	
Blue rubber bleb nevus	Multifocal cutaneous and visceral venous malformations	Gastrointestinal bleeding	Limb hypertrophy, hemarthrosis	Autosomal dominant
Maffucci	Venous malformations in subcutaneous tissue and intraosseous enchondromas	Malignant tumors	Enchondroma with skeletal deformity, overgrowth, and sarcoma	
Central hemangiomas with indirect effects on skeleton				
Rendu-Osler-Weber (hereditary hemorrhagic telangiectasia)	Capillary malformations on the lips, tongue, mucous membranes, and gastrointestinal and genitourinary systems	Bleeding from all sites, anemia, pulmonary arteriovenous malformations	Skeletal vascular malformations (hands, wrist, axial skeleton)	Autosomal dominant
Sturge-Weber	Capillary malformation on face, vascular malformation on brain	Seizures, mental retardation, glaucoma	Hemiplegia, hemiatrophy (neurogenic)	
Ataxia-telangiectasia	Capillary malformations on conjunctivae, face, neck, and arms	Progressive ataxia, sinus and pulmonary infections, lymphomas	Mimics Friedreich ataxia: foot and ankle contractures	Autosomal recessive

some indicate an underlying condition such as Sturge-Weber syndrome. This is a nonhereditary syndrome characterized by a capillary malformation in the trigeminal nerve distribution, and more importantly, an associated vascular anomaly of the ipsilateral choroid and leptomeninges (1,4,5). These children may develop seizures, hemiplegia, developmental delay and retinal damage. This disorder must be considered when assessing a child with apparent cerebral palsy. Magnetic resonance imaging (MRI) of the brain is usually diagnostic. Facial and limb capillary malformations can be associated with soft tissue and bone hypertrophy, which are usually seen at birth. These malformations may be part of a complex vascular anomaly such as Klippel-Trenaunay syndrome, which will be discussed later. Pulsed dye laser will improve the appearance of these lesions.

Cutis marmorata telangiectatica congenita is a rare disorder seen at birth, characterized by a deep purple, serpiginous, reticulated cutaneous pattern, usually involving the trunk and extremities (4,9). The cutaneous findings usually improve spontaneously but venous dilation becomes more prominent and atrophy of the involved limb with leg-length discrepancy can occur (9). There are no reports in the literature on the efficacy of epiphysiodesis in this disorder.

Hereditary hemorrhagic telangiectasia or Rendu-Osler-Weber syndrome is an autosomal dominant disorder characterized by spider-like, red maculopapules on the face and mucous membrane in the first decade (5). The resultant arteriovenous fistulas in the lungs and gastrointestinal tract can lead to hemorrhage and cardiac failure.

Ataxia-telangiectasia or Louis-Bar syndrome is an autosomal recessive condition that causes cerebellar ataxia followed by progressive neuromotor degeneration. Telangiectasias develop on the upper part of the body: the face, neck, arms, and conjunctiva. Contractures may develop at the foot and ankle.

Venous malformations are the most common of all vascular anomalies. They are typically cutaneous but can also be skeletal or visceral. Most are solitary but multiple lesions can occur which may indicate an autosomal dominant condition called "multiple glomangiomas" (5). Venous malformations manifest as easily compressible masses with blue coloration if superficial (Fig. 10-1A–C). The swelling is worse when the limb is dependent and improves with elevation. These lesions cause aching discomfort and usually enlarge gradually as the child matures. Subcutaneous lesions can cause local sensory nerve irritation (10). Activity-related pain mimicking a chronic compartment syndrome is often associated with intramuscular lesions and diagnosis can be difficult (10). Thrombosis is common and phleboliths can be present as early as 2 years of age (4,5). Periarticular lesions can cause recurrent hemarthroses.

The options for imaging include plain films, which show abnormalities in most cases of deep venous malformations including phleboliths and enlargement or distortion of soft tissue planes (1,11). Ultrasound and computed tomography

(CT) scans with intravenous contrast demonstrate similar findings but do not add significant new information to the plain films. They may be used to direct aspiration or needle biopsy if a limited specimen is useful. MRI and magnetic resonance angiography add significant anatomic detail and are the most informative diagnostic modalities (6). Hemangiomas produce a very high T2 signal, presumably because of the pooling of blood with low flow. The signal is nonuniform because of the fibrous and fatty septae within the hemangioma. MRI can determine the extent of deep hemangiomas and differentiate the vascular elements from surrounding tissues. However, MRI cannot differentiate feeding arteries from veins, and angiography is the only way to obtain this information. Venography may not demonstrate the lesion if the flow is slow (12,13). Angiography is helpful if an arteriovenous fistula is suspected, if sclerotherapy is planned or if surgical resection is being considered.

A low-grade, localized intravascular coagulopathy can occur in children with extensive venous malformations (2,5,14). The platelet count is normal in contrast to the Kasabach-Merritt phenomenon, and the prothrombin time and D-dimers are elevated. Heparin may be required for treatment (2).

Elastic support stockings control swelling and discomfort in the extremity. Sclerotherapy, the injection of an irritating solution, is an effective intervention, but the venous malformations can recur (5). Surgical resection, often done after sclerotherapy, is considered for large, painful lesions. Incomplete exsanguination under tourniquet control allows dissection in a relatively bloodless field and better visualization of the margins (10). Recurrence is common, and was noted in 48% of patients in one study (10). Pharmacologic treatment is indicated in vascular tumors with active angiogenesis but has not been successful in the management of vascular malformations (2).

Blue rubber bleb nevus syndrome, or Bean syndrome, is a multifocal, cutaneous, and visceral venous malformation (2,4,15,16). The lesions are usually present at birth and are raised soft, blue, compressible nodules that blanch. The nodules become more numerous as the child grows older. The main risk arises from gastrointestinal hemorrhage but there are significant orthopaedic problems. The cutaneous lesions in the hands and feet cause pain and interfere with function (15,17). Hemarthrosis and stiffness can result from articular involvement. Skeletal deformities may be secondary to pressure from adjacent lesions or hypertrophy may occur because of hypervascularity (15). Significant hypertrophy may require amputation.

Maffucci syndrome is characterized by venous malformations in the subcutaneous tissues, along with multiple intraosseous enchondromas. There is no consistent genetic basis (1). The hemangiomas are present at birth in only 25% of patients; in the remainder, the lesions become evident by 5 years of age. The clinical appearance is of a blue discoloration on the skin. X-ray films may show calcified thrombi in

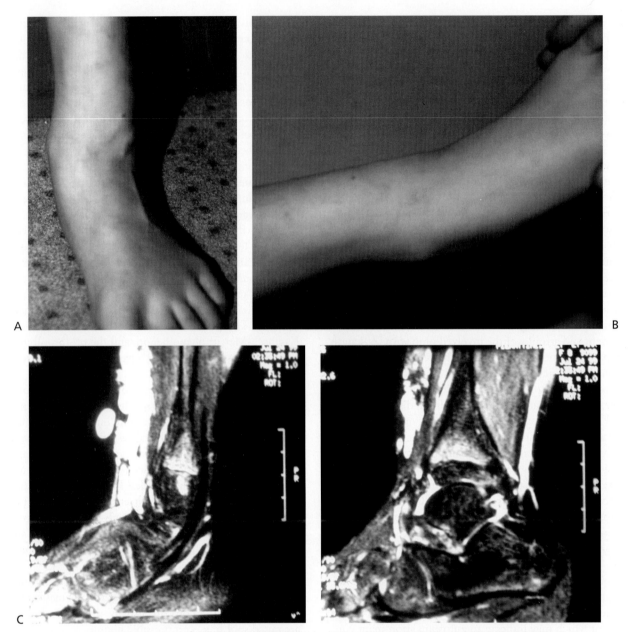

FIGURE 10-1. Eight-year-old girl with vascular malformation complaining of aching discomfort above the ankle. **A:** Standing clinical photograph demonstrating swelling and superficial irregularity over the anterolateral aspect of the ankle. This was nontender and easily compressible. **B:** With elevation of the limb, the lesion drained and was not palpable except for deep thick structures. **C:** MRI demonstrating high T2 signal typical of a vascular malformation.

addition to the enchondromas. The skeletal manifestations include short stature, limb-length inequality, angular deformities, and scoliosis. The patient's risk potential for malignant transformation is 30%; this may include the vascular lesions undergoing transformation to spindle cell hemangioendothelioma (2).

Lymphatic malformations may affect any area of the body, although they are most commonly seen in the cervicofacial region, axilla, mediastinum, and pelvis (18,19). Al-

though usually falling within the province of the general pediatric surgeon, a lymphatic malformation may first be noticed as a mass of unknown origin in a limb or as a cause of osteolysis or nerve compression. Most are present at birth or are detected in the first two years of life (5).

These malformations are slow-flow lesions that consist of anomalously formed lymphatic channels, described as microcystic, macrocystic, or a combination thereof (3–5). Superficial lymphatic malformations are recognized by clear, small vesicles. Intravesicular bleeding often occurs resulting in red nodules that are seen typically in combined lesions such as Klippel-Trenaunay syndrome. Large, deep malformations (also known as cystic hygromas or lymphangiomas) present as ballottable masses with an underlying blue hue. Although they are benign, they are locally aggressive and may compress adjacent structures. Airway compression by cervicofacial lesions can be life-threatening. Soft tissue and skeletal overgrowth is seen in association with these lesions. Chronic disseminated intravascular coagulation, as described previously in venous malformations, can also occur in large lymphatic malformations (2,5).

Diagnosis may be aided by transillumination, ultrasound, nuclear imaging, CT, or MRI. Lymphangiomas tend to have a characteristic MRI appearance, with a heterogeneous low signal on T1-weighted images, lower than that of muscle, but a very high T2-weighted signal, greater than that of fat (20). Enhancement with gadolinium did not occur in pure lymphatic malformations (6,21). Other congenital anomalies may affect these children.

A small percentage of lymphatic malformations may regress spontaneously. Staged surgical resection of the involved tissues should be done for symptomatic lesions. Sclerotherapy is useful in isolated lesions. Radical procedures, with removal of important adjacent structures, are not indicated to alter the course of the disease.

Lymphedema may occur at various ages. If present in childhood, it is called Milroy disease, a congenital lymphedema, which is autosomal dominant. Cases with onset slightly later in the first or in the second decade are called Meige disease and have the same inheritance pattern. Lymphedema is also seen as part of Turner syndrome and Noonan syndrome (i.e., Turner phenotype with normal-appearing chromosomes and mental retardation). Treatment in all of these cases is conservative: elevation when possible and compression with a Jobst stocking or intermittent pneumatic compression (13,22).

Osseous lymphatic malformations may include solitary intraosseous or more extensive forms. Solitary intraosseous lesions are extremely rare (23). They are lytic and well-demarcated but variably circumscribed. The appearance resembles a simple cyst, but involvement within bone is more extensive. Curettage and bone grafting has been reported with success (23).

Complex-combined Vascular Malformations

Several complex, combined vascular malformations exist, which have a mix of capillary, venous, lymphatic, or arterial malformations. They share a propensity for soft tissue and skeletal overgrowth.

Klippel-Trenaunay Syndrome

In 1900, Klippel and Trenaunay described their eponymous disorder, which has three essential features: a cutaneous capillary-venous malformation, varicose veins, and hypertrophy of soft tissue and bone in the involved limbs (Fig. 10-2A–C). The vascular malformation is usually seen early in life and typically does not cross the midline of the body (24–27). The entire limb is not uniformly affected. The severity of the varicose veins varies, but they tend to get larger with age and are always present by 12 years (28). Abnormalities in arteries and lymphatic vessels are also frequently seen. If clinically significant arteriovenous shunting is present in addition to the typical triad, the additional name "Parkes-Weber" has been applied (Klippel-Trenaunay-Parkes-Weber) (29). Some authors suggest that the Parkes-Weber syndrome should be considered distinct from Klippel-Trenaunay syndrome (5). Overgrowth usually occurs on the limb affected by the vascular malformations but may not. The mechanism leading to overgrowth involves increased bulk or girth and increased length and width of the bone. Most of the size discrepancy seen is in girth, secondary to soft tissue hypertrophy (sparing muscles) and lymphatic abnormalities (28).

Klippel-Trenaunay syndrome may be due to a somatic mutation for a factor critical to the endothelial activity necessary for vasculogenesis and angiogenesis in embryonic development (28,30,31). It is presumed that this vascular malformation induces the hypertrophy of other tissues, but there also may be primary mesodermal abnormalities in these cases (32). The absence of deep venous drainage and venous hypertension is not likely to be a causative factor, because deep veins are missing in only 14% of patients and venous flow is normal (24). Baskerville et al. suggest that increased flow through the abnormal capillary network and venous channels may promote overgrowth (24).

Clinical Features. Although most cases are evident from the time of birth or infancy, a few cases have been reported in which features appeared as late as 6 years of age. There is no recognized pattern of inheritance. The lower extremities are affected at least ten times more often than the upper extremities. The affected limb is longer than normal in 90% of patients (11,28,33). Usually, all bones and soft tissues are involved in the hypertrophy (Fig. 10-2).

The growth patterns of the involved limbs have not been rigorously studied over time, but there are enough reported cases of nonuniform overgrowth to caution the physician that prediction of an eventual discrepancy should be done only as a rough estimate. McCullough and Kenwright described two patients with a decreasing discrepancy with growth (34). Severe leg-length discrepancy is uncommon. In one study only 10% of the children had a discrepancy greater than 3 cm (28). In addition to the extremity hypertrophy, there is evidence of fundamental embryologic regulatory defects, especially distally, with 25% of patients having anomalies of fingers or toes, such as macrodactyly, syndactyly, polydactyly, and clinodactyly (33). Scoliosis affects at least 5% of patients, although it rarely requires sur-

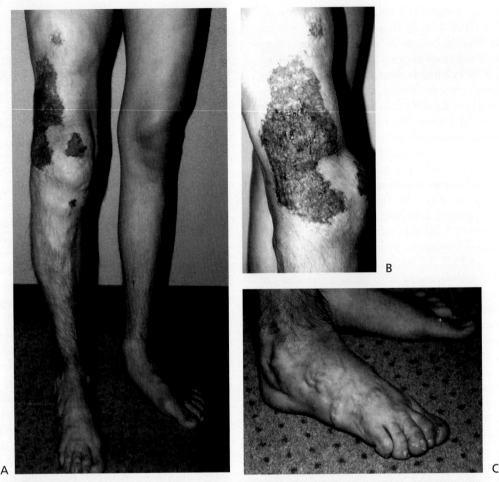

FIGURE 10-2. **A:** Fifteen-year-old boy with Klippel-Trenaunay syndrome of his right lower extremities with typical findings of hypertrophy, varicosities, and superficial complex combined vascular malformations. **B, C:** He had aching discomfort from the varicosities, intermittent pain from thrombophlebitis and drainage from the superficial vascular malformations.

gery. Systemic involvement may occur. In the central nervous system, arteriovenous malformations and cerebral and cerebellar hypertrophy have been described (35,36). The gastrointestinal and genitourinary system may be involved, resulting in bleeding in some cases. Surface bleeding from the hemangioma occurs in 25% of patients, and 15% have clinical pulmonary emboli, spontaneously or after operation (24). Congestive heart failure may occur in patients with large vascular malformations. Despite these complications, the life expectancy is not markedly decreased. The impact of this complex medical condition on the child's psychosocial development cannot be underestimated.

Pathology. Most notably, venous fibromuscular dysplasia, consisting of hypertrophied, irregular, or absent medial layers of the veins, allows dilatation. Valves are anomalous; they are absent or obstructed. Deep venous channels are usually present, and arteriovenous malformations are uncommon (31). Lymphatic hypoplasia is common. Other

tissues, such as nerve and subcutaneous tissue, may be hypertrophied.

Differential Diagnosis. Neurofibromatosis may produce massive hypertrophy without prominent nevi. Maffucci syndrome often includes limb-length inequality with vascular malformations, but it is differentiated by the presence of intraosseous enchondromas. Beckwith-Wiedemann syndrome involves localized overgrowth but also includes neonatal hypoglycemia, visceromegaly, macroglossia, and a predisposition for Wilms tumor. Proteus syndrome is a more severe disorder involving virtually all the features of Klippel-Trenaunay, but it also includes soft tissue tumors, pigmented skin lesions, and thickened palms and soles (25). Bannayan-Zonana syndrome is characterized by thoracic and abdominal lipomatosis, vascular malformations, and macrocephaly (37).

Imaging. Plain radiographs, limb-length evaluation, color duplex ultrasonography, MRI, MR angiography, MR lymphangiography, and lymphoscintigraphy can provide sufficient information for diagnosis and planning in most cases (21,28,37–39). Lymphatic imaging is particularly useful in the evaluation of children with massive hypertrophy (28). Arteriography may be helpful in planning for hemipelvectomy or hip disarticulation to map major vessels and anticipate significant bleeding (11). Contrast angiography is also useful for percutaneous treatment of a vascular malformation.

Treatment. The skeletal and vascular abnormalities of Klippel-Trenaunay syndrome are usually not dramatically progressive. Surgery has a limited role in this condition. It should be done only for disabling problems and when the benefit is fairly predictable (39). Instead, initial therapy of the aching, hypertrophic limb with varicosities should consist of compression. Intermittent pneumatic compression should be applied at night, using a custom-fitted garment and a home pump, inflated every 90 s to a pressure midway between diastolic and systolic (40). Just before arising, a Jobst compression garment is applied, then worn throughout the day. A marked decrease in limb girth, resolution of cardiac overload and dependent syncope, reduced discomfort, and marked improvement in function can be seen. A technique of manual lymphatic drainage can also be used, if there is a significant lymphatic component to the malformation (22). Thrombophlebitis and pulmonary embolism are common. Consultation with a vascular surgeon may be beneficial for most of these patients.

Surgery is beneficial in selected situations, including cardiac failure from shunting in children, not responding to compressive therapy; rapid enlargement in limb size; bleeding from abnormal vessels in the gut, kidney, or genitalia; coagulopathy; reconstruction of selected cases of syndactyly or polydactyly; and for severely disfiguring dysfunctional limbs, for which reconstruction is not an option and amputation may provide a more functional limb. The level of amputation is often dictated by the extent and severity of the vascular malformation. A knee disarticulation is preferred to a midthigh amputation because it is an end-bearing stump with rotational control, better suspension, the distal femoral physis is preserved and overgrowth is avoided. Midthigh amputation requires ischial weightbearing, which may be a problem in the presence of any scarring or gluteal vascular malformations (25,41,42). Risks of surgery include infection, particularly in children with abnormal lymphatic drainage and delayed wound healing, which is common after transverse amputations (43). Occasionally, a proximal limb disarticulation is needed in neonates as a lifesaving procedure. For patients in this age group, hypothermia and total circulatory arrest for up to 60 min has been successful as an adjunct to minimize blood loss (44). Pulsed-dye laser treatments can be used to treat the cutaneous vascular malformations over limited areas (28).

Certain procedures have low success rates. Surgery to debulk the extremities has usually resulted in recurrence or minimal improvement. Varicose vein ligation may provide relief of local symptoms, but the varicosities often recur, and ligation should be avoided if the deep venous system is not patent. Epiphysiodesis has a limited role because growth patterns are unpredictable, and the procedure does not decrease width of the involved extremities. Limb-shortening at skeletal maturity may be the most accurate technique. If surgery is planned, the involved skin should be protected, and the increased risk of deep thrombosis borne in mind.

Proteus Syndrome

Proteus syndrome is a sporadic vascular, skeletal, and soft tissue disorder characterized by vascular anomalies, macrodactyly, exostoses, asymmetric hypertrophy, subcutaneous tumors, scoliosis, and other anomalies (45–49). The name is derived from the Greek god, Proteus, who could change shape at will to avoid capture. This syndrome may result from somatic mosaicism (45). The cutaneous vascular malformations include capillary, lymphatic, capillary-venous, and capillary-lymphatic-venous types. Subcutaneous tumors, found most commonly on the trunk, are composed of adipose and fibrous tissue, Schwann cell structures, and vascular tissue. A symptomatic lipofibromatosis hamartoma of the median nerve in the carpal tunnel has been described in a child (50). MRI is helpful in delineating the nature and extent of the subcutaneous tumors as well as aiding in the diagnosis of the syndrome (45,51).

Macrodactyly is a common manifestation and can occur in the hands and feet (45). The enlarged digits may not be located on the same side of the hemihypertrophy. The macrodactyly progresses rapidly in the first few years of life, and slows in later childhood and adolescence. Severe cosmetic and functional problems can result. The histology is a hamartomatous proliferation of all mesenchymal tissues, especially the osseous and fibrofatty components (48). Treatment will be discussed in the section on macrodactyly later in this chapter. Another striking finding in the foot is plantar hypertrophy, resulting in cerebriform or gyriform creasing (Fig. 10-3).

Hemihypertrophy may be partial, complete, or crossed, and results in limb-length discrepancy, which varies greatly. Overgrowth and progressive atrophy have been described (46). Because skeletal age may be delayed and the rate of progression is not well understood, planning treatment can be difficult. Extensive overgrowth and joint contractures can result in amputation.

Angular upper- and lower-limb deformities are seen in Proteus syndrome. Genu valgum occurs commonly, recurs after bracing, and has required repeated osteotomies (46,48) (Fig. 10-4) [➡6.1–6.5]. Joint contractures and angular deformities may be caused by epiphyseal exostoses (46).

Scoliosis or kyphoscoliosis occurs in approximately 50% of children with Proteus syndrome and may require fusion (45–49). The effect of bracing is not known. Spondylomeg-

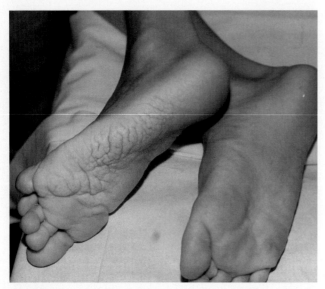

FIGURE 10-3. Adolescent male with Proteus syndrome with typical gyriform creasing of the sole of his foot.

aly, or localized spinal overgrowth, has been reported. This can result in progressive compressive neuropathy (48).

Gorham Disease

Gorham disease, or massive osteolysis, has also been called "disappearing bone disease" (52). This has been classified here as a complex, combined lymphatic venous malformation but the pathogenesis has not been fully elucidated. Osteolysis is initially localized to one bone and may subsequently involve adjacent bones. The joints and intervertebral discs do not act as barriers to extension. Progressive

bone resorption typically occurs and the bone is replaced by fibrous tissue. The resorption can stop spontaneously on rare occasions. Peak age of onset is in the second and third decades of life (53). Gorham disease is differentiated from other forms of idiopathic osteolysis based on its lack of association with neuropathy or a genetic mode of transmission (54). It may involve any area of the skeleton but is most common in the shoulder, pelvic girdles, and spine (53,55–57). It may present as dull, aching weakness in involved segments, with increasing deformity, or with pathologic fracture. Patients with lesions extending outside of bone have a high mortality rate, approaching 50% from chylothorax, chylopericardium, chyloperitoneum, and cachexia (18,55,58).

Radiographic Findings. On plain radiographs, single or multiple intramedullary and subcortical radiolucent foci are seen, which eventually coalesce (59). There is subsequent disappearance of contiguous bones and tapering of the bony remnants (Fig. 10-5A). No sclerosis or osteoblastic reaction is seen. If a pathologic fracture occurs, the bony lesion may be overlooked initially, if the lysis is minimal. Unlike normal fracture healing, the bone ends eventually become tapered, and there is no evidence of new callus forming. Computerized tomography is the best method to evaluate the extent of bone destruction. Arteriography, venography, and lymphangiography do not demonstrate the intraosseous lesion (56). Nuclear medicine scans are inconsistent in showing the lesion; MRI is very helpful, but the signal characteristics vary, depending on the stage of the disease process (54,55). The neovascular tissue is bright on T1 and T2 imaging early, but the predominant fibrous tissue present late in the process is dark on T1 and T2 imaging (Fig. 10-5B). The differential diagnosis includes other rare causes of idiopathic osteolysis, including hereditary multicentric

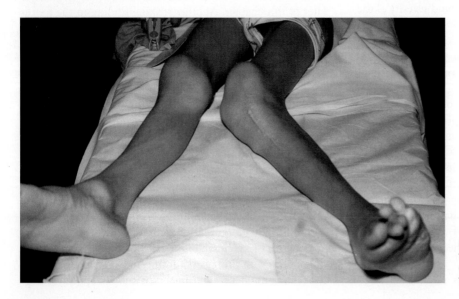

FIGURE 10-4. Adolescent male with Proteus syndrome with recurrent left genu valgum after a high tibial osteotomy just prior to repeat osteotomy.

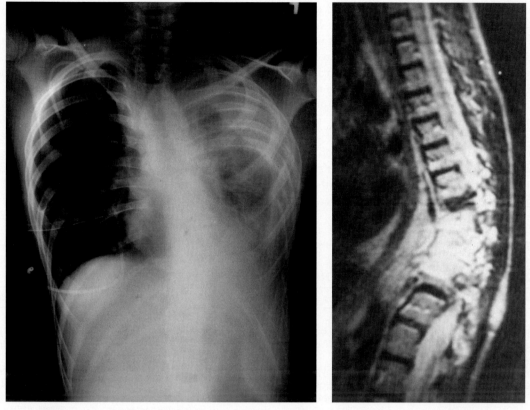

FIGURE 10-5. Twelve-year-old male with Gorham disease. **A:** Chest x-ray demonstrates loss of ribs 8, 9, and 10, and a chylothorax. **B:** The neovascular tissue is bright on T2 and on this MRI, there is extensive vertebral destruction and paravertebral involvement. This boy died from this process.

osteolysis (i.e., carpotarsal type), nonhereditary multicentric osteolysis with nephropathy, and others.

Histopathology. Histologic studies demonstrate numerous thin-walled vessels, lined by endothelial cells. The vessels may be empty or contain proteinaceous fluid and/or blood cellular elements (58). Fibrous connective tissue replaces the bone. There is no evidence of malignancy or inflammation. The histologic changes are similar to benign hemangioma or venous malformation of bone, but there is much more extensive bone destruction (53). The bone shows extensive osteoclastic activity. The cause is unclear, but perivascular cells of the lesion show the characteristics of osteoclast precursors (56).

Treatment. No treatment has been shown to be consistently successful, but surgery, with or without radiation therapy, has been the mainstay of treatment. Some cases, especially those without significant involvement of chest or abdominal cavities, stabilize spontaneously, although return of the "vanished" bone does not occur. This complicates the evaluation of published treatment protocols. Local resection and bone grafting, with or without internal fixation, has not been consistently successful (53). Most grafts are re-

sorbed, but there is one report of the successful use of a vascularized fibular graft in pelvic-femoral reconstruction (60). Wide resection and limb salvage, with or without prosthetic reconstruction, can be successful (53,54). Amputation has been required to achieve a satisfactory margin and improved function (53,60). Radiation therapy has proven effective in some cases, when doses of 30 Gy or more are used (53,61). Management of vertebral and rib involvement with chylothorax is frustrating. Resection with adequate margins is usually not possible. Pleural adhesion therapy with bleomycin and irradiation successfully managed the chylothorax in one patient (55).

Hemihypertrophy and Hemihypotrophy

Hemihypertrophy and hemihypotrophy are defined as asymmetries between the right and left sides of the body to a greater degree than can be attributed to normal variation. This may involve the length and girth of the limbs as well as the head, trunk, and internal organs.

The difficulty for the surgeon is deciding what is normal and what is not, that is, to determine whether the larger limbs are hypertrophic or the smaller limbs hypotrophic (62). Differentiation of overgrowth from undergrowth is based on comparison of the limb with its expected length, in proportion to the rest of the body. This may be visually obvious and straightforward for typical cases, or it may be difficult to discern in milder cases. The examiner may search for anomalies that herald the abnormal limb. Vascular malformations and associated digital malformations or macrodactyly usually signify overgrowth conditions; obvious muscle hypotrophy, focal neurologic abnormality, mental retardation, or joint abnormality may accompany undergrowth. If no such clues are found, a graph of normative sitting heights can be used to determine the patient's trunk height percentile, and a graph of normal lengths of the tibia and femur can be used to see which side falls on a percentile that most closely matches it (34).

To determine normal variation in limb size, Pappas and Nehme referred to an unpublished survey from the growth study at Children's Hospital, Boston (63). The maximum mean discrepancy seen at different ages for 95.5% of the population was approximately 1.4% (0.4 centimeter difference at 1 year, 0.8 centimeter at 10 years, and 1.1 centimeters at skeletal maturity) (63). Similar data have been reported in a group of young adult army recruits (64). Pappas and Nehme have defined abnormal asymmetry as a 5% or greater difference in length and/or circumference (63). MRI and other imaging techniques can assess the tissues in the extremities and aid in establishment of the diagnosis (37,62).

Hemihypertrophy and hypotrophy can be initially classi-

TABLE 10-2. DIFFERENTIAL DIAGNOSIS OF HEMIHYPERTROPHY AND HEMIHYPOTROPHY

Condition	Features	Growth Pattern	Treatment Implication
Hypertrophy of normal tissues			
Idiopathic hemihypertrophy	Increase in length and breadth of one extremity or one-half of body ± renal malformation	Proportionate, linear	Monitor for increased risk of Wilms or other neoplasm
Beckwith-Weidemann Syndrome	Large body size, hemihypertrophy of whole body, macroglossia, omphalocele, pancreatic hyperplasia	Irregular	Risk of Wilms or embryonal tumors
Hamartomatous disorders			
Klippel-Trenaunay syndrome	Limb-length discrepancies; combined, complex vascular malformation (may be on long or short side); varicosities	Often irregular, does not affect all segments equally	Prediction for epiphysiodesis inaccurate; operate for function; amputation sometimes needed; compression therapy
Neurofibromatosis	Café-au-lait spots (>5) plus family history of subcutaneous neurofibroma, dystrophic bone changes	Irregular	
Proteus syndrome	Vascular anomalies, asymmetric hypertrophy, macrodactyly, exostoses, subcutaneous masses	Irregular	Valgus often coexists; skeletal age delayed or disassociated
Hemi-3 syndrome	Hemihypertrophy, hemihyperesthesia, hemiareflexia	Hypertrophy of girth, not length	
Undergrowth of limb			
Idiopathic hemihypotrophy	Greater dysmorphism than hemihypertrophy, congenital scoliosis, genitourinary malformation	Proportionate	Discrepancy rarely exceeds 2 cm by maturity; treatment rarely indicated
Turner/mosaic (XO/XX)	Short stature, low hairline, peripheral edema, valgus of knees or elbows	Discrepancy accelerated near puberty	Keloids common
Russell-Silver syndrome	Very short stature (<3%), small, triangular face, one limb or whole side short, developmental dysplasia of the hip, scoliosis, genitourinary anomalies common	Eventual limb length discrepancy of 1–6 cm	Skeletal age is delayed
Neurogenic (e.g., hemiplegic, polio)	Undergrowth if proportional to weakness	Proportionate, affects weakest limb segments	Lengthening rarely indicated in weak limb
Skeletal dysplasia or dyostoses	Polyostotic fibrous dysplasia, multiple exostoses, multiple enchondromas		

fied as congenital or acquired. Acquired asymmetry can result from injury, infection, radiation, or inflammation (65,66). Congenital forms may be classified as total or limited, total having involvement of all organ systems, including the ipsilateral paired organs. Limited forms have only muscular, vascular, skeletal, or neurologic involvement and are also subdivided by the area of involvement: classic (ipsilateral upper and lower limbs), segmental (a single limb), facial or crossed (65–67). These disorders can also be classified as nonsyndromic (isolated) or syndromic (part of a clinical syndrome). Table 10-2 outlines the differential diagnosis of hemihypertrophy and hemihypotrophy.

Overgrowth may be seen in idiopathic or nonsyndromic hypertrophy, associated with Beckwith-Wiedemann syndrome, neurofibromatosis, Bannayan-Zonana syndrome, or vascular malformations such as Klippel-Trenaunay and Proteus syndromes and lymphatic malformations (see Table 10-2). Undergrowth may be secondary nonsyndromic hypotrophy, mosaicism for Turner syndrome, Russell-Silver syndrome, neurologic asymmetry (cerebral palsy, polio), osteochondromatosis, enchondromatosis, or polyostotic fibrous dysplasia (68).

Idiopathic or nonsyndromic hemihypertrophy is a condition of unknown cause affecting approximately 1 per 50,000 people (63,65,67,69). There is no clear inheritance pattern.

The hemihypertrophy is rarely apparent at birth but becomes evident during the early years of growth. The unilateral enlargement may include the ear, one-half of the tongue, the pupil, the nipple, the thorax, the abdomen, the internal organs, and the arm and leg (66,70) (Fig. 10-6A and B). Mental capacities are usually normal, unlike those of patients with idiopathic hemihypotrophy, and contrary to earlier reports (48,69). Cutaneous vascular lesions are not associated with nonsyndromic hemihypertrophy. Compensatory scoliosis secondary to the leg-length discrepancy is common but the incidence of structural scoliosis is also increased, even after leg-length equalization and may be the result of vertebral body asymmetry. Uncommon skeletal anomalies are syndactyly, lobster-claw hand, developmental dysplasia of the hip, and clubfoot (68). Genitourinary abnormalities are a common association, and can include inguinal hernias, cryptorchidism, and medullary sponge kidney (65,69).

These children are at increased risk for malignant tumors, such as Wilms, adrenal carcinoma, hepatoblastoma, and leiomyosarcoma (65). A recent study suggested an incidence of 5.9% (71). It is possible that the same abnormal cellular growth control mechanism that results in overgrowth also predisposes these children to tumor formation (65,71). Abdominal sonographic screening has been recommended for

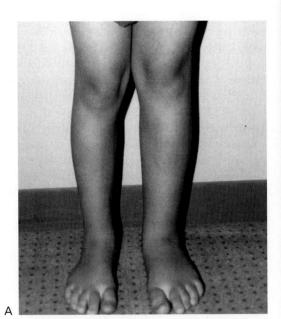

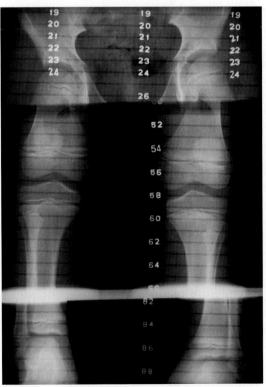

FIGURE 10-6. Eight-and-a-half-year-old boy with idiopathic hemihypertrophy. **A:** Note enlargement of the entire left lower extremity. The left upper extremity was enlarged as well. **B:** The lower extremity orthoroentgenogram demonstrates the leg-length discrepancy.

children with hemihypertrophy, to detect these tumors as early as possible (65,72). This is controversial, because there is little evidence that this results in a better clinical outcome for children with Wilms or other tumors, it will not diagnose extraabdominal tumors, and the hemihypertrophy is only recognized in 30% of children prior to the tumor diagnosis (65,73,74). Nevertheless, current recommendations are for regular screening: abdominal ultrasound every 3 months until age 7, then physical exam every 6 months, until skeletal maturity (72).

The leg-length discrepancy in nonsyndromic hemihypertrophy rarely exceeds 5 cm by skeletal maturity (34,63,70,75). The discrepancy usually increases continually with time, at the same proportionate rate (75). There are cases of resolution of inequality in early childhood and those with reduction of the rate of increase in adolescence, which can make an accurate prediction of discrepancy difficult (34,67). The tibia is overgrown as much as, or slightly more than, the femur (63). Limb girth is increased by an average of 10%, primarily due to muscle hypertrophy (63). Epiphysiodesis [➡4.19, 4.20, 6.12, 6.13] has resulted in satisfactory limb equalization at skeletal maturity in most children (63,70).

Beckwith-Wiedemann syndrome is a congenital overgrowth syndrome usually diagnosed at birth, and characterized by neonatal hypoglycemia, macroglossia, visceromegaly, omphalocele, hemihypertrophy, and a predisposition for embryonal tumors, most frequently Wilms tumor (76). The risk of Wilms tumor, hepatoblastoma, and neuroblastoma is higher than in nonsyndromic hemihypertrophy, and in one study, 13 of 183 children developed a tumor by age 4 years (77). Hemihypertrophy only occurs in about 13% of these children but puts them at greater risk of developing a cancer (77,78). These children must be carefully monitored for the development of embryonal tumors.

Other disorders with limb-length inequality include neurofibromatosis, Proteus syndrome, Klippel-Trenaunay syndrome, and lymphangiomas (51).

A rare disorder, known as the hemi-3 syndrome, may be associated with hemihypertrophy, mostly of limb width (79). Its other features include hemihyperesthesia, hemiareflexia, and scoliosis. It appears to be a neural crest disorder.

Hemihypotrophy is more likely to be associated with diffuse skeletal abnormalities than is hemihypertrophy (67). The term "hypotrophy" is preferred to atrophy, because there is decreased development, instead of a loss of previous normal tissue bulk.

Idiopathic hemihypotrophy appears to be about one-half as frequent as idiopathic hemihypertrophy (67). These patients, however, have a higher incidence of other dysmorphic features, including cleft palate and facial malformations, congenital scoliosis, and genitourinary malformations. Mental retardation is common, but Wilms tumor is not associated with the condition (80). Rarely does this syndrome require orthopaedic treatment, because, in most cases, the discrepancy is less than 2.5 cm.

Russell-Silver syndrome has some features in common with idiopathic hemihypotrophy, but it is characterized by overall short stature, with most patients never exceeding a height of 152 cm (5 feet). These patients have a characteristic small, triangular face, and renal and genital malformations (80). Scoliosis is common and may be congenital or idiopathic-like. The limb hypotrophy is usually minimal, but as much as 5 cm has been reported.

Patients who are mosaic for the Turner syndrome (XO/XX) may have hemihypotrophy, as may patients who have multiple enchondromas or osteochondromas, with mean discrepancies of 9 and 3.5 cm, respectively, for those patients with limb-length inequality. Neurogenic inequalities vary in proportion to the asymmetry of the neurologic involvement, rarely exceeding 2.5 cm in the lower extremities in cerebral palsy or 6 centimeters in polio patients (75). In assessing patients with localized overgrowth or undergrowth, it should not be assumed that the growth alteration is proportional. Shapiro described five patterns of limb-length discrepancy, and, even within a given diagnosis, multiple patterns may be seen (75). Periodic assessment should be done, if possible, during growth to determine the pattern being followed. Predictions are then more accurate. If significant joint contractures are present, plain radiographs or scans may not measure limb length accurately, and CT scans may be needed. For treatment of significant upper-extremity inequalities, normative growth data is also available (81).

Localized Gigantism and Macrodactyly

Macrodactyly is an uncommon anomaly characterized by an increase in the size of the constituent elements of a single or several adjacent digits of the hand or foot. Two types exist: the more common static type, which enlarges from birth; the increase in size being proportional with growth; and the progressive type, in which there is disproportionate growth of the involved digit (82). Localized gigantism is a term used inconsistently in the literature, which describes macrodactyly, as well as enlargement of tissues of the hands and feet proximal to the digits.

Macrodactyly, or localized gigantism, can occur as an isolated or idiopathic condition. Macrodystrophica-lipomatosa (fibrolipomatosis) is a nonhereditary overgrowth of all mesenchymal elements of the digit, particularly the fibroadipose tissue (37,83). Macrodactyly may also occur in association with neurofibromatosis and vascular malformations (capillary, venous, arterial, or lymphatic), such as Klippel-Trenaunay and Proteus syndrome (82–85). Children with multiple enchondromatosis, Maffucci syndrome, and tuberous sclerosis can have enlarged digits. It may be difficult to make a diagnosis in infancy because of the delayed manifestations in these syndromes such as the café-au-lait spots in neurofibromatosis. MRI evaluation of the tissues involved in the macrodactyly can be helpful in establishing a diagnosis in the absence of specific clinical features (37).

Clinical Features. Most cases of macrodactyly are evident soon after birth, although occasionally the dynamic type may not become apparent until later in infancy, when relentless enlargement occurs (Fig. 10-7A–D). The upper extremities are more commonly affected than lower extremities. Unilateral involvement occurs in 95% of cases, although, in two-thirds of patients, more than one digit on the involved side, usually adjacent, is affected (82). The second ray is the most commonly enlarged, followed in descending frequency by the third, first, fourth, and very rarely fifth rays. Syndactyly may coexist. Usually, the palmar or plantar surface is more hypertrophied than the dorsal,

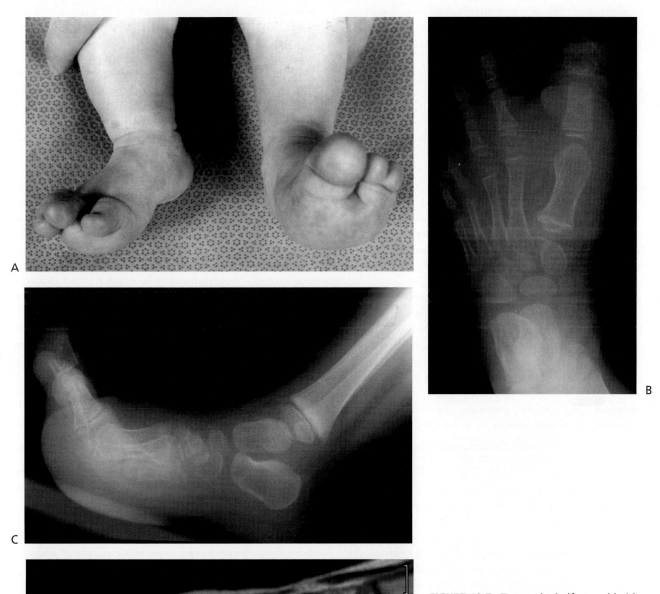

FIGURE 10-7. Two-and-a-half-year-old girl with progressive macrodactyly of both feet with macrodystrophica-lipomatosa. **A:** There is significant plantar hypertrophy, resulting in hyperextension of the digits, and there is marked asymmetry in the digital enlargement. **B, C:** The plain radiographs demonstrate the soft tissue enlargement, as well as the underlying bony enlargement. **D:** The MRI demonstrates overgrowth of essentially all elements in the digit, particularly the fibroadipose tissue typically seen in macrodystrophica-lipomatosa.

resulting in hyperextension of the metatarsal or metacarpophalangeal joints (86,87). If two adjacent digits are affected, they grow apart from each other. In static macrodactyly, the involved digits are about 1½ times the normal length and width. In the dynamic type, even more striking enlargement may occur. The bone age may be advanced in the involved phalanges (86,88). The metacarpals or metatarsals can be enlarged, widening the hand or foot (86). The width of the unilateral forearm, leg, thigh, or arm may also be subtly increased (88). Not long after skeletal maturity, interphalangeal joint stiffness and degenerative changes may supervene prematurely, even in untreated cases (82).

Pathology. The pathology varies, depending on the etiology of the macrodactyly. The most consistent feature is overgrowth of the fibro-fatty tissue but all tissues are enlarged in the involved digit (82,86,88). Fibrous bands and hypertrophied adipose tissue infiltrate muscle and nerve. A proliferation of fibroblastic tissue between the cortex and periosteum may account for the phalangeal overgrowth (86,88). The digital nerves are more prominent than usual, particularly in the hand, with proliferation of epineural and perineural tissue (82,83,86). Plexiform neurofibromas are typical in neurofibromatoses (83). Macrodactyly in children who have met strict criteria for the diagnosis of Proteus syndrome is not associated with enlarged digital nerves or fibroadipose tissue proliferation (85).

The pathogenesis of macrodactyly is unknown but neuroinduction is considered a possibility (83,86). Occult neurofibromatosis was once thought to be the cause, but long-term follow-up studies, including one of 26 years, have failed to reveal development of other features of neurofibromatosis besides the macrodactyly itself (89).

Treatment. The operative treatment varies, depending on the location, type, and severity of the macrodactyly. Management considerations are very different for the hand and foot. In the hand, function is paramount, and a significant increase in the width and length of a digit can be tolerated, whereas, in the foot, accommodating even a small excess of width in a shoe may be difficult. A good cosmetic result can be difficult to achieve. In the static type of macrodactyly, debulking and shortening procedures, such as phalangeal resection and epiphysiodesis, are successful. In contrast, the deformity seen in progressive forms will usually require ray resection. Extensive debulking can interfere with the blood supply to the skin and result in delayed wound healing.

Mild-to-moderate macrodactyly can be managed by a two stage (3 months apart) soft tissue debulking procedure, if length is not a problem (82). If length is a problem, then epiphysiodesis of the proximal phalanx, and the metacarpal or metatarsal, if involved, will be effective in the young child (less than 6–8 years) (82,86,90,91). In the older child, bone shortening by phalangeal resection can be combined with staged debulking (92,93). Ligament reconstruction or fu-

sion with Kirschner wire fixation will avoid the reported complications of floppy toes or secondary deformities (89). Isolated phalangeal amputation should be avoided because of subsequent angular deformities of the adjacent toes (84,89).

Digital shortening and debulking has not been effective, in the long term, for excessive forefoot widening. Ray resection is a more definitive solution to the multiple dimensions of enlargement often encountered (83,89,94,95). One or two rays may be taken, although the first ray of the foot should not be amputated in isolation because of its unique function in balance and weightbearing. To improve correction and avoid recurrence, it has been suggested to resect a wedge of adjacent tarsal bones, when doing a ray resection (83). Ray resection prevents crossover of the adjacent digits and eliminates "gap" formation and soft tissue enlargement. A three-ray foot is the minimum that is functionally serviceable. In the foot, more extensive involvement would necessitate midfoot or Syme disarticulation, depending on the extent of overgrowth.

As the patient matures, a subtle increase in width may be seen in all levels of the limb. Herring reported a case of macrodactyly with width increase, in the absence of any overall limb-length discrepancy (96). The family should be counseled from the first visit that this condition is complex and involves multiple tissues and levels. They need to know that multiple procedures may be necessary and that early, appropriate, aggressive resections, involving all affected dimensions, may decrease the total number of surgeries required. For example, as soon as it becomes apparent that length and width may be excessive, resection of one or several rays, with shortening or epiphysiodesis of an adjacent ray, may be appropriate. Often, several consultations with one or different surgeons may be necessary to help families achieve this realization.

Congenital Constriction Band Syndrome

Congenital constriction band syndrome, otherwise known as amniotic band syndrome, is a common cause of terminal congenital malformation of limbs, with a reported incidence of 1 in 5,000 to 10,000 children (97,98). The three main manifestations include acrosyndactyly, superficial or deep constriction bands involving a digit or extremity, and intrauterine amputation (97,99–101).

Clinical Features. The clinical presentation of congenital constriction band syndrome is quite variable. The bands may be superficial and incomplete or extend deeply to the underlying bone, and be circumferential. Two bands may be present in one extremity. Distal to the band, there may be significant neurovascular impairment (98–103). Impaired venous and lymphatic drainage causes swelling of the limb distal to the constriction. With growth, the constriction band occasionally gets more severe and becomes symptomatic (98). Upper-extremity involvement is more frequent than the lower extremity. Head, neck, or trunk constriction bands are very uncommon (104). The distal aspect of the limb, particularly the longest digits (index, long, and ring fingers, and great, second, and third toes) are most frequently affected (97–99,105).

Patterson developed a classification system based on the severity of the syndrome: simple constriction rings; constriction rings associated with deformity of the distal part, with or without lymphedema; and constriction rings associated with syndactyly and intrauterine amputation (106).

Amputations and syndactyly are seen in more than one-half of affected children. Transverse, terminal, digital amputations, with normal proximal skeletal development, are typical (97–99,105) (Fig. 10-8A). Simple syndactyly is common, whereas complex syndactyly with bony fusions is rare (99). Acrosyndactyly or fenestrated syndactyly, in which there is an open cleft between digits joined distally, can be seen. Hypoplastic or absent nails are consistently present.

The incidence of clubfoot in constriction band syndrome ranges from 12 to 56% (97–99,101,102,106) (Fig. 10-8B). These feet are often rigid and more difficult to treat than the idiopathic clubfoot. Approximately 30 to 50% of the clubfeet are classified as paralytic (100,101,103,107). These

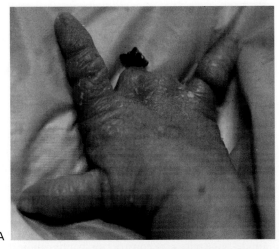

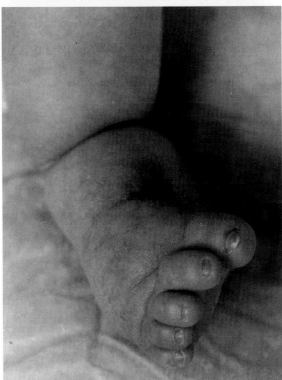

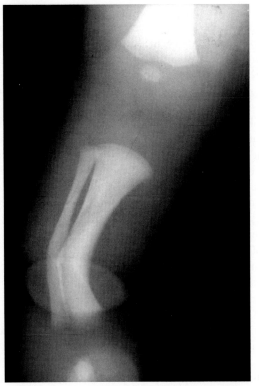

FIGURE 10-8. Child with congenital constriction band syndrome. **A:** Clinical photo demonstrating autoamputation of the long and ring digits through the proximal phalanges, and a circumferential constriction band in the proximal segment of the small finger. **B:** Clinical photograph demonstrating circumferential constriction band involving the distal lower leg, and an associated talipes equinovarus deformity. **C:** The radiograph of the same patient demonstrates an uncommon finding of angulation of the bone underlying the circumferential band.

feet have weakness of the peroneal muscles and are always associated with ipsilateral constriction bands. The deep constriction bands are thought to cause a compression neuropathy, direct muscle injury or perhaps a compartment syndrome. The nonparalytic clubfeet may or may not have ipsilateral constriction bands and are considered to be idiopathic clubfeet or resulting from oligohydramnios (99).

Angular deformity, bone dysplasia, and pseudarthrosis can occur deep to constriction bands in the upper and lower extremities (106,108,109). The anterolateral tibial bowing appears similar to that seen in congenital pseudarthrosis of the tibia associated with neurofibromatosis but in contrast remodeling can occur and realignment osteotomies, if required, will heal (108) (Fig. 10-8C). Rapid, spontaneous healing of osseous defects in the forearm and tibia of infants have been described (108,109). Zionts et al. prefer the term "discontinuity," rather than "pseudarthroses," in describing these defects, because of the spontaneous healing (109).

Leg-length discrepancy exceeding 2.5 cm, in 25% of children with constriction bands, has been reported (99). Surgical management will be required in some of these children, depending on the predicted discrepancy at skeletal maturity. Craniofacial abnormalities, including cleft lip and palate, are seen in 7% of children with constriction band syndrome (98,101).

Etiology. Despite many theories, the etiology and pathogenesis of constriction band syndrome remains unclear. Although the two main conflicting theories focus on whether the band formation is the result of factors intrinsic or extrinsic to the embryo or fetus, the disorder may be more heterogeneous than considered in the past.

The extrinsic theories have the widest acceptance. Torpin has proposed that entanglement of the limbs in defects or free strands of amnion result in constriction band syndrome (110,111). Supportive evidence includes the lack of hereditary factors, the ultrasonographic demonstration of prenatal amniotic bands, the involvement of the longer digits and the histologic demonstration of amnion in constriction bands. Amniocentesis in animals produces fetal malformations that resemble constriction band syndrome in humans. Kino demonstrated in rats that the malformations result from subcutaneous hemorrhages that are caused by excessive uterine contractions after amniocentesis (97). In a study reviewing children with clubfeet and constriction band syndrome, there was a history of attempted first-trimester abortion in 60% of the children (103).

The intrinsic theory by Streeter proposed that a defect of the subcutaneous germ plasm caused soft tissue necrosis and subsequent healing, with the formation of constriction bands (112). There is evidence that *in utero* vascular disruption from the death of a co-twin, or from placentally derived embolic infarcts, can cause constriction band syndrome (113). In these children, there was no ultrasound evidence of amniotic bands. It appears this syndrome may result from factors other than amniotic entanglement.

The differential diagnosis is limited, but there are some interesting conditions to consider. The "Michelin tire baby syndrome" consists of multiple benign circumferential skin creases. This is an autosomal dominant condition that has been traced through as many as four generations in one family. These creases are present from birth, disappear by 5 years of age, and predominantly involve the extremities (114). Hair-thread constriction may occur in infants, usually younger than 2 years of age, and cause circulatory compromise (115). Strands of hair or fabric strands may become wrapped around fingers and toes tightly enough to cause distal swelling and circumferential laceration of the skin. At that time, it may be difficult to visualize the hair causing the problem to differentiate it from congenital constriction bands. Ainhum is a disorder characterized by ulceration at the base of the fifth toe on the plantar surface, which progresses to a circumferential constriction ring with autoamputation. It is mainly seen in Africa (116).

Treatment. Superficial, asymptomatic constriction bands do not require treatment. Excision of the band, and closure with multiple Z-plasties, is indicated in bands that extend to the deep subcutaneous tissue or fascia, if there is edema distal to the band, in the presence of vascular insufficiency or neurologic deficit, and if the band is increasing in severity [➡1.3]. The surgical release has been traditionally staged, releasing one-half of the band at a time with a 6- to 12-week interval (99,106,117). There was concern that impaired venous or lymphatic flow and skin-flap necrosis would result, if the band was released in one stage, but single-stage release of constriction bands can be done safely (117) (Fig. 10-9A and B).

The constriction band and underlying fibrous tissue in the subcutaneous tissue, fascia, and muscle should be completely excised with an adjacent 1- to 2-mm cuff of normal tissue. The compressed neurovascular structures can be difficult to distinguish, and may be inadvertently damaged. To avoid injury, the nerves and vessels should be exposed proximally or distally and followed under the band. The wound should be closed with Z-plasties fashioned with large flaps at a 60-degree angle. In children with ischemia of the distal limb, a fasciotomy may be required.

Clubfeet in neonates with an ipsilateral constriction band can be treated by serial manipulation and casting, if there is no significant foot edema or evidence of neurovascular compromise. Resection of the constriction band should be done prior to surgical release of the clubfoot. Nonoperative management is rarely successful in these children (102,103,107). The severity of the clubfoot is more important than the presence or severity of the constriction band in predicting the outcome of surgical treatment (102,107). Rigid clubfoot with deep bands usually has a poor outcome. Muscle imbalance of the foot, resulting from peroneal weakness, should be managed by a split transfer of the tibialis anterior tendon (101,107).

Surgical intervention in children with acrosyndactyly is

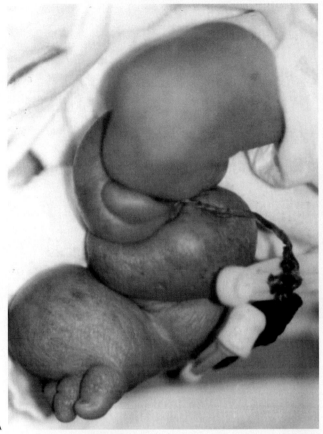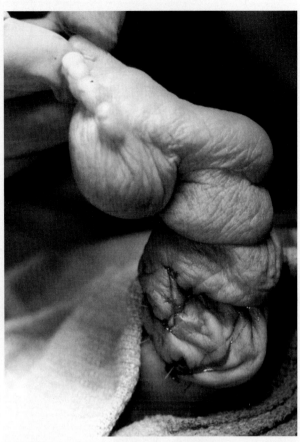

A

B

FIGURE 10-9. One-day-old female born at 28 weeks' gestation. An amniotic band around the umbilical cord led to fetal distress and precipitous delivery. **A:** Clinical photograph of the right lower extremity, with multiple deep circumferential bands. Marked distal swelling and vascular compromise with petechial formation is present. **B:** Clinical photograph immediately following emergent single-stage circumferential release of amniotic bands, with Z-plasty of the skin. Note decompression and reperfusion of all segments distal to the resected bands.

generally done between the ages of 6 months and 1 year because of the severity of the deformity and to allow for longitudinal growth and function (105).

Disorders Involving Joint and Bone

Progressive Diaphyseal Dysplasia

Progressive diaphyseal dysplasia, or Camurati-Engelmann syndrome, is a sclerosing bone dysplasia characterized by progressive diaphyseal thickening and sclerosis, bone pain and weakness (118,119).

Clinical Features. This autosomal dominant disorder is very rare (1 per 1 million) with boys being affected more often than girls (3:2 ratio) (120). The age at the onset of symptoms is highly variable, with the majority presenting in the first decade. In one study, the mean age of onset was 15 years and 4 months, with the age range from 1 to 70 years (120). The clinical and radiological manifestations are also variable. The most common symptoms are limb pain,

easy fatigability, headache, poor appetite, and difficulty running. Clinical signs include muscle weakness and atrophy, thickening of the long bones, genu valgum, waddling gait, and exophthalmus (120). These children can have mistaken diagnoses of neuromuscular disorders when radiographs are not done (121). Basilar skull sclerosis can lead to narrowing of cranial foramina with symptomatic auditory and optic nerve compression (122). Progression usually occurs in a slow, unpredictable fashion but occasionally will spontaneously stop. There is a normal life span.

Laboratory studies are not helpful for diagnosis. The alkaline phosphatase is elevated in 40% of patients (123). Biochemical markers of bone turnover may be useful for assessment of disease activity.

Radiographic Features. The plain radiographs demonstrate symmetric, periosteal and endosteal diaphyseal sclerosis and diaphyseal widening. The tibia is most frequently involved, but all the long bones in the upper and lower extremities, and the clavicle, can be affected early in the course of the disease. The cortex becomes wide and irregular

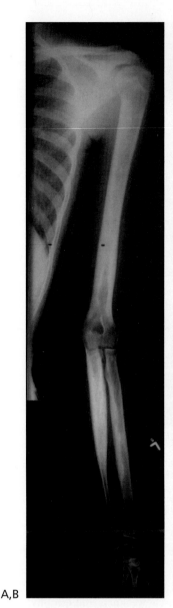
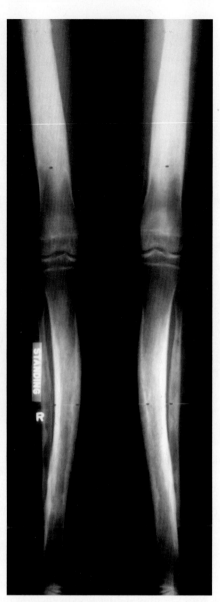

A,B

FIGURE 10-10. A, B: Seventeen-year-old female with diaphyseal dysplasia. Radiographs demonstrate wide and irregular cortices and marked narrowing of the medullary cavity of the long bones in the upper and lower extremities; typical finding of genu valgum is demonstrated.

with narrowing of the medullary cavity (Fig. 10-10A and B). Computerized tomography has shown that the thickening and sclerosis are not uniformly distributed in the long bones (124). Sclerosis at the base of the skull is common but is not an early finding. The radiological evolution is usually progressive, increasing sclerosis of the bone, with extension to the metaphysis and epiphysis and eventual involvement of the metacarpals and metatarsals, pelvis, and spine (120,123,125,126). In the spine, only the posterior elements and the posterior aspect of the vertebral body are affected with no stenosis (124,126). Technetium-99m bone scans demonstrate uptake in the middiaphysis of the involved long bones early in the disease, often before changes on the plain radiographs. MRI shows cortical involvement with sparing of the medullary cavities but is not helpful for diagnosis or management (126).

Pathology. Other than the thickened cortex, there is no histologic abnormality unique to progressive diaphyseal dysplasia. Early changes are typical of recent bone formation, with woven bone and lack of haversian system development, but later modeling occurs (122). Marrow fibrosis and narrowing of the medullary canal can occur, which may explain the occasional patient with anemia (125).

Etiology. The cause of this autosomal dominant disorder and the variability of its expression has not yet been explained. The more severe involvement in males who inherited the disease from the father has suggested the presence of a dynamic mutation with triplet repeat expansion (122). The candidate gene should have a function in endochondral and intramembranous bone formation.

Differential Diagnosis. Other sclerosing bone dysplasias with normal stature should be considered. Considerable overlap exists in the classification of sclerosing bone dysplasias (127). The diagnosis can be made by determining the inheritance pattern, clinical and radiological characteristics, and laboratory findings or lack thereof. Ribbing disease has a similar radiological appearance but affects only the lower extremities and is not always symmetrical. Extensive early cranial and facial involvement, an autosomal recessive inheritance pattern, and mental retardation differentiates craniodiaphysial dysplasia from progressive diaphyseal dysplasia. Osteopetrosis is differentiated by sclerosis throughout the skeleton. Hyperphosphatasia can have similar radiological findings but the alkaline phosphatase level is markedly increased. Hardcastle syndrome is an autosomal dominant disorder with diaphyseal medullary stenosis and sclerosis with pathologic fractures and malignant transformation (128). Juvenile Paget disease, infantile cortical hyperostosis, hypervitaminosis A, and fluorosis should also be considered in the differential diagnosis.

Treatment. There is no cure for this disorder but treatment can improve pain and function. Nonsteroidal antiinflammatories will alleviate limb pain and physical therapy may maximize function.

Corticosteroid administration results in reduced pain and fatigue and better function, such as the ability to run (129). It does not alter the natural history of the osseous changes.

Successful surgical realignment of the lower extremities has been described by Clawson and Loop (125). Knee flexion deformities, genu valgum, and external tibial torsion were corrected by distal femoral and proximal tibial and fibular osteotomies. The bone was described as being soft and vascular but healed uneventfully.

Melorheostosis

Melorheostosis, first described by Leri and Joanny in 1922, is a rare sclerosing skeletal dysplasia characterized by soft tissue contractures in childhood overlying slowly evolving linear hyperostosis (130). The name is derived from the Greek words *melos* meaning "limb" and *rhein* meaning "to flow," as in wax.

Clinical Features. This nonhereditary disorder affects both sexes equally. The typical presentation is with painless, asymmetric joint contractures prior to 6 years of age (131,132). The lower extremities are much more frequently involved than the upper extremities. The underlying hyperostosis develops slowly and progresses with age, usually more rapidly in childhood. The overlying soft tissues may be thickened with lymphedema, or have sclerodermatous skin changes or vascular malformations (133–136). There is also associated muscle atrophy and periarticular fibrosis

with contractures. Flexion contractures at the knee, hip, finger, ankle equinus and patellar dislocation are the most common joint deformities (132). Paraarticular ossification and synovitis can further impair joint motion (137,138). Limb-length discrepancy, and varus and valgus deformity about the knee and ankle, are caused by fibrosis and physeal abnormalities. A mean of 4 centimeters of shortening was noted in one study of 11 children but one patient had overgrowth of the affected limb (132). Melorheostosis does not shorten life span but the morbidity may be considerable.

Etiology. The etiology of this disorder is not known. It has been observed that distribution of the lesions correspond to sclerotomes (138). A hypothesis is that an infection, analogous to herpes zoster, occurs and lesions spread along the distribution of affected nerve roots with resultant scarring and osseous changes.

Radiographic Features. The classic radiographic appearance of melorheostosis is asymmetrical bands of sclerosis in an irregular, linear pattern often described as molten wax flowing down the side of a candle (Fig. 10-11A–C). In children the hyperostosis is endosteal, unlike adults, in whom it is in an extracortical, subperiosteal location (136,137). The hyperostosis can be located throughout the skeleton, typically on one side of the diaphysis of long bones, the pelvis and in the hands and feet. The ribs, skull, and spine are affected least often. Patches of hyperostosis, rather than a linear pattern, are present in the carpal and tarsal bones and the epiphyses. This is similar to that seen in osteopoikilosis. Increased uptake is noted in involved areas on bone scan.

The hyperostosis consists of woven or nonlamellar dense bone with thickened, sclerotic and irregular laminae (137).

Differential Diagnosis. The differential diagnosis includes osteomyelitis, osteopetrosis, osteopoikilosis, and osteopathia striata, all of which can have similar radiographic findings. Mixed sclerosing bone dysplasia is comprised of melorheostosis, osteopoikilosis and/or osteopathia striata in the same individual (127). These three rare bone dysplasias are postulated to have a close association. The transient periosteal reaction in infantile cortical hyperostosis is less dense and is found in different locations. Focal scleroderma may cause soft tissue fibrosis and contractures but the bones are radiologically normal (139).

Treatment. The soft tissue contractures are resistant to manipulation, bracing and serial casting (140). Nonsteroidal antiinflammatory medications can improve the discomfort. Surgical treatment including soft tissue releases, capsulotomies, and osteotomies are difficult and incomplete correction or rapid recurrence of the deformity is common, sometimes necessitating an amputation (132,137). Distal limb ischemia can occur when the chronically contracted and

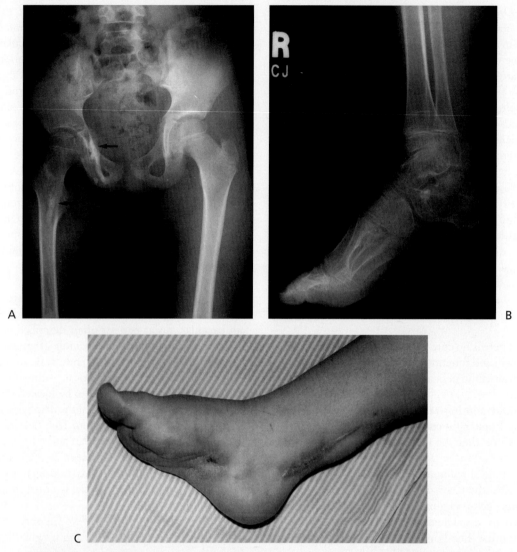

FIGURE 10-11. Eight-year-old girl with melorheostosis who presented with an equinovarus foot deformity. **A:** The classical findings of irregular linear hyperostosis are seen at the arrows. **B:** Patches of hyperostosis are seen in the talus and calcaneus and this is typical of melorheostotic involvement of the tarsals. **C:** There was pain and swelling about the equinovarus foot. Previous surgical releases resulted in rapid recurrence of the deformity.

flexed joint is extended. Osteotomies that permit shortening may avoid this complication.

The Ilizarov technique has been used in a small number of children for lengthening [➡4.16, 6.9], realignment of angular deformities and correction of joint contractures (140–143). Realignment and lengthening have been done successfully but complications include pseudarthrosis, and, in one child, ischemia with pain and loss of function and eventual amputation (141,143).

Osteopoikilosis

Osteopoikilosis, or osteopathia condensans disseminata, is an uncommon, autosomal dominant, sclerosing bone dys-

plasia characterized by numerous small foci of increased radiodensity in the periarticular regions.

Clinical Features. This disorder develops during childhood and persists through life. The children have normal stature and most are asymptomatic, but up to 20% will have mild articular discomfort with a joint effusion (144). The diagnosis is often made as an incidental radiological finding. Fractures heal uneventfully and pathological fractures have not been reported. The risk of malignancy is probably not higher than the normal population. Osteopoikilosis is frequently seen in association with a hereditary dermatologic condition, dermatofibrosis lenticularis disseminata, or Buschke-Ollendorf syndrome, which is marked

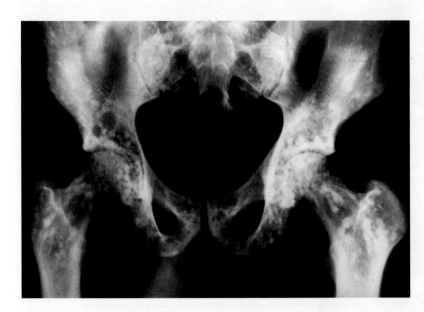

FIGURE 10-12. Osteopoikilosis. Extensive involvement of the pelvis in this asymptomatic patient.

by the presence of papular fibromas (145,146). This syndrome is usually asymptomatic but soft tissue fibrosis and joint contractures can occur in these children that appear clinically similar to that seen in melorheostosis.

Radiographic Features. The osteosclerotic nodules are well-defined, homogeneous, bilateral, circular- to ovoid-shaped from 1 to 15 mm, and are located in the metaphyses and epiphyses of long bones, the carpus, the tarsus, the pelvis, and the scapulae (Fig. 10-12). The ribs, clavicle, and skull are not involved (144,147). The lesions may increase or decrease in size or number (147).

The bone scan usually does not demonstrate increased uptake in the lesions (148). This is useful, to differentiate this condition from metastatic breast or prostate carcinoma. Mastocytosis should also be considered in the differential diagnosis.

The etiology and pathogenesis of osteopoikilosis is not clear. The sclerotomal distribution and association with abnormalities of mesodermal tissues suggests a relationship between this condition and other osteosclerotic disorders (145,147,149).

Pathologic Features. The sclerotic areas consist of focal condensations of compact lamellar bone within the spongiosa (144,149).

Treatment. There is no treatment for this benign disorder. In the rare cases of associated fibrosis and joint contracture, the management is the same as for melorheostosis.

Osteopathia Striata

Osteopathia striata, or Voorhoeve disease, is another of the sclerosing bone dysplasias and is characterized by dense linear striations in bone (150,151).

Clinical Features. This is a rare, autosomal dominant disorder that exhibits no physical or laboratory abnormalities. The diagnosis is usually made on an incidental radiograph.

Radiographic Features. The radiographic hallmark is dense linear striations in the tubular and flat bones with the exception of the skull and clavicles. These lesions do not change with time. In the long bones, the striations are parallel to the long axis and affect principally the metaphyses but may extend into the epiphyses (Fig. 10-13A and B). A fan-shaped pattern of linear striations can be seen in the iliac wings, likely reflecting the growth pattern of the pelvis (151). There is no increased uptake on the bone scan.

Osteopathia striata occasionally is an osseous constituent in more complex sclerosing bone dysplasias, such as osteopathia striata with cranial sclerosis and mixed sclerosing bone dysplasia; nonsclerosing bone dysplasias, such as spondastrime dysplasia; and congenital malformation syndromes, such as focal dermal hypoplasia (149,151,152).

Treatment. Treatment is not required for asymptomatic isolated osteopathic striata.

Congenital Pseudarthrosis of the Clavicle

Congenital pseudarthrosis of the clavicle is a rare disorder of formation of the clavicle that is recognizable at birth. The right clavicle is most commonly affected, although bilateral involvement has been reported in approximately 10% of cases, and rare examples of isolated left-sided involvement have been documented. The absence of birth trauma and subsequent lack of exuberant early callus formation distinguish it from acute neonatal fracture. The roentgenographic appearance of the clavicular defect and lack of other charac-

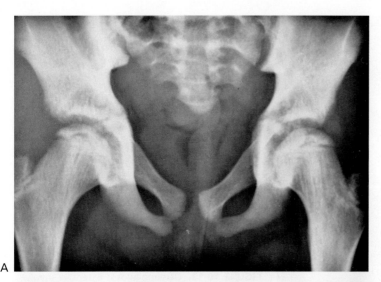

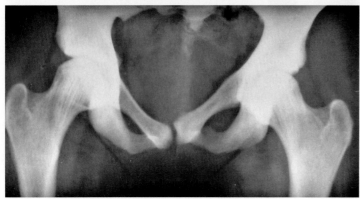

FIGURE 10-13. Osteopathia striata. The streaking of the proximal femurs did not change much in this patient between the ages of 12 years (**A**) and 25 years (**B**). Note the flattened femoral epiphysis.

teristic bony malformations of the skull and pelvis distinguish it from cleidocranial dysplasia.

Etiology. A genetic basis for congenital pseudarthrosis of the clavicle is unclear. Most cases are felt to arise sporadically, although familial cases demonstrating autosomal dominant inheritance have been reported (153,154). Congenital pseudarthrosis of the clavicle is thought to occur either by a primary intrinsic failure of clavicular development or as a result of external compressive forces. The development of the clavicle from two separate centers of intramembranous ossification was first recognized by Mall (154), and has been confirmed by others (155,156). It has been postulated that an intrinsic failure of coalescence of these two centers is responsible for the development of the pseudarthrosis (157). Lloyd-Roberts and colleagues postulated that extrinsic compression by the subclavian artery, alone or in combination with a cervical rib, was responsible for the defect. This interesting concept is supported by the overwhelming frequency of right-sided involvement, and the normally higher location of the right subclavian artery compared to the left, and the location of the artery directly

below the area of the defect. Rare cases of left-sided involvement have been associated with dextrocardia, and bilateral cases have been associated with cervical ribs (158).

Clinical Features. Congenital pseudarthrosis of the clavicle typically presents in infancy or in early childhood, with a painless prominence and hypermobile segment over the middle-third of the clavicle. Radiographs may be necessary to distinguish the lesion from birth fracture or cleidocranial dysplasia. The majority of lesions involve only the right clavicle, although bilateral cases and rarer left-sided cases have been described. The cosmetic deformity tends to be slowly progressive, with an increase in noticeable prominence over the pseudarthrosis and foreshortening and dropping of the shoulder girdle over time. The pseudarthrosis can become painful with certain overhead activities, or with direct compression or palpation. Shoulder motion is typically regarded as normal, and significant functional disability is unusual. Several cases of later development of thoracic outlet compression syndrome have been reported in association with congenital pseudarthrosis of the clavicle (153,159–164).

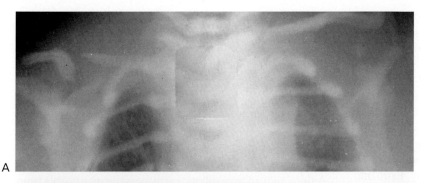

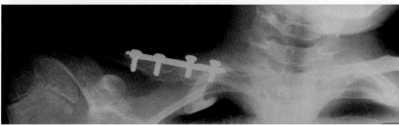

A

B

FIGURE 10-14. Pseudarthrosis of the right clavicle. **A:** Congenital pseudarthrosis of the right clavicle. There are no signs of healing. **B:** Radiographic appearance after solid union achieved by open reduction, internal fixation, and autogenous bone grafting in a different 8-year-old boy.

Radiographic Features. The radiographic findings in congenital pseudarthrosis are characteristic. The clavicle typically displays a definite separation in its midportion, with the medial aspect lying superior to the lateral aspect, owing to muscle forces and the weight of the upper extremity. The bone ends appear bulbous, with sclerotic closure of the marrow cavity and no evidence of callus formation or reactive bones (Fig. 10-14A). The disorder is easily distinguishable from cleidocranial dysplasia, due to the lack of other characteristic radiographic abnormalities of the skull and pelvis, including wide cranial sutures, coxa vara, failure of pubic ossification, and hypoplastic ilia. If necessary, subsequent radiographs of the clavicle will fail to demonstrate callus formation, thereby distinguishing early cases from acute neonatal fracture.

Histopathology. Histopathologic specimens from resected lesions have demonstrated hyaline cartilaginous caps at both ends of the pseudarthrosis, often joined by dense fibrous and fibrocartilaginous tissue (165). Hirata and colleagues demonstrated columnar distribution of chondrocytes in different stages of maturation at the ends of the pseudarthrosis, similar to that seen in a developing cartilaginous physis. Endochondral ossification at these terminal ends was confirmed by tetracycline labeling (166).

Treatment. Most cases of congenital pseudarthrosis of the clavicle that are described in the literature have undergone some form of operative treatment [➥1.2], and therefore the true natural history of untreated cases is unknown. Indications for operative management have included progressive pain and unacceptable cosmetic deformity at the site of the pseudarthrosis, functional limitations and later onset

of thoracic outlet compression syndrome (153,157, 159–168). Most authors advocate delaying surgery until the patient is approximately 3 to 6 years of age, using a technique of resection of the pseudarthrosis, bone grafting, and internal fixation, most commonly with use of a plate and screws (153,156,162,168) (Fig. 10-14B). Solid union of the pseudarthrosis and acceptable cosmesis using these methods has been uniformly achieved. However, the patient should be counseled preoperatively that they would effectively be trading a "bump" for a "scar." Grogan and colleagues reported on early operative treatment of this condition, with 6 of 8 patients below the age of 30 months (167). They demonstrated union in all 8 patients using a technique of careful preservation of the periosteal sleeve, resection of the pseudarthrosis, and approximation of the bone ends without bone grafting or internal fixation. Toledo and MacEwen pointed out the hazards of using an intramedullary pin for fixation after operative treatment of this condition (169).

Dysplasia Epiphysealis Hemimelica

Dysplasia epiphysealis hemimelica is a rare disorder of localized osteochondral overgrowth, involving single or multiple epiphyses or ossification centers. First reported by Mouchet and Belot as "tarsomegalie," the disorder was later clarified by Trevor, who termed the disorder "tarso-epiphysial aclasis" (170,171). Fairbank later suggested the term "dysplasia epiphysialis hemimelica," to deemphasize tarsal involvement, and to describe the predilection for unilateral involvement of the medial or lateral aspect of one or more epiphyses (172). Although the lesion most commonly affects the medial aspect of the epiphysis, lateral involvement, as well as involvement of entire epiphyses, has been reported. Unilateral distribution when multiple sites are involved is common, and the lesion can present on both sides of an affected joint.

Etiology. The etiology of dysplasia epiphysealis hemimelica is unknown. Trevor considered dysplasia epiphysealis hemimelica to be a congenital error of skeletal development, in which an altered process of cell division at the superficial zone of articular cartilage allows for persistent proliferation and production of a large cartilaginous mass (171). Fairbank hypothesized that the disorder was due to a localized disturbance of the pre- or postaxial part of the apical cap of the limb bud in early fetal development (172). To date, no clear genetic transmission of the disorder has been described.

Clinical Features. The incidence of the disorder has been estimated at 1 per 1 million, with the majority of cases affecting males. Presentation is usually in childhood or early adolescence, although presentations in older adulthood have been described (173). In cases of multiple sites of involvement, the lesions are characteristically unilateral, although bilateral cases are reported. Azouz et al. classified dysplasia epiphysealis hemimelica into three types: localized (involving only one epiphysis), classic (involving more than one bone in a single limb), and generalized (involving an entire lower extremity from the pelvis to foot), with the classic form being most common (174). Clinical features vary, depending on the location of the lesion, but patients typically complain of painless swelling or a mass on one side of a joint, limitation of motion, and occasionally locking, angular deformity, limp, regional muscle wasting, or limb-length discrepancy. The lower extremities are affected most commonly, predominantly at the knee and ankle (171,172, 175,176). Other reported sites have included the capital femoral epiphysis and acetabulum, sacroiliac joint, metacarpophalangeal joint, wrist, shoulder, and subtalar joint (177–183).

Radiographic Features. The radiographic features of dysplasia epiphysealis hemimelica can vary depending on the age of the patient and maturation of the lesion. The radiologic diagnosis is fairly straightforward when the lesion is fully calcified or ossified, appearing as an irregular, often multicentric, lobulated mass protruding directly from one side of the affected epiphysis or tarsal bone (Fig. 10-15A–C). The affected ossification center will often appear prematurely, and may be larger than the contralateral side. Modeling abnormalities of the adjacent metaphysis have also been reported. However, early lesions may present only with joint space enlargement or small foci of irregular calcification, and may resemble paraarticular tumors or other disorders with ectopic ossification or calcification. With maturation, the lesion enlarges and ossifies, and becomes

confluent with the underlying epiphyseal bone (184). MRI has proven useful in demonstrating the extent of the lesion, and in identifying a potential cleavage plane between the lesion and the underlying epiphysis (175,184–186).

Histopathology. On gross and microscopic examination, the lesion will resemble an osteochondroma, although no discrete stalk is present. Microscopically, one may find a boundary of cartilage separating the lesion from the underlying bony epiphysis, if the lesion has not yet fully ossified. A thick zone of hyperplastic cartilage is distinguishable from the rest of the cartilaginous epiphysis only by some irregularity in the size and distribution of the chondrocytes (172). Malignant degeneration of the lesion has not been reported.

Treatment. Treatment of dysplasia epiphysealis hemimelica should be directed at addressing the patient's complaints, while preserving the integrity of the affected joint as much as possible. Most of the reported cases of dysplasia epiphysealis hemimelica have been treated surgically, and therefore the long-term prognosis for untreated lesions involving the weightbearing surface of the joint (i.e., articular lesions) is mostly unknown. Fairbank predicted that involved joints would go on to early degenerative joint disease, and this has been demonstrated in some patients after surgical intervention (175,176,181,187). If the cartilaginous overgrowth is not on the weightbearing surface of the joint (i.e., juxtaarticular lesions), simple excision is warranted to relieve pain and improve function. However, recurrence of the lesion prior to skeletal maturity has been reported (176,177). Fairbank described spontaneous correction of associated angular deformities after excision, but this has not been a consistent finding (154). The treatment of articular lesions remains somewhat controversial. Kuo and colleagues did not recommend excision of articular lesions due to unsatisfactory results in 3 of 9 patients with lesions involving the distal tibia and talus (176). Keret and colleagues performed corrective osteotomies without excision for angular deformity associated with articular lesions if an arthrogram demonstrated a smooth joint surface (175). The authors noted recurrence of valgus deformity at the knee after varus osteotomy in 1 of 3 patients, requiring repeat osteotomy.

Fibrodysplasia Ossificans Progressiva

Fibrodysplasia ossificans progressiva is a genetic disorder characterized by congenital malformations of the great toes and by later development of a predictable pattern of heterotopic endochondral osteogenesis of tendons, ligaments, fasciae and striated muscles. Although most patients present as new mutations, autosomal dominant transmission and variable expressivity has been confirmed by several authors (188–191). The incidence of this condition is extremely rare, affecting less than 1 in 1 million persons (192).

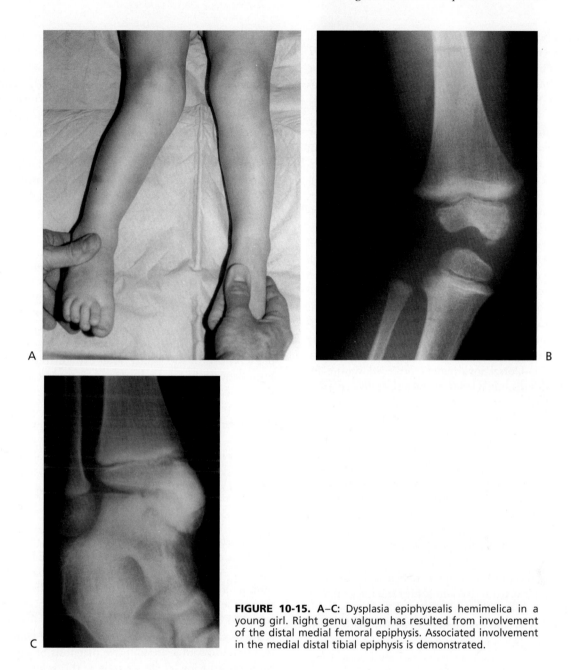

FIGURE 10-15. A–C: Dysplasia epiphysealis hemimelica in a young girl. Right genu valgum has resulted from involvement of the distal medial femoral epiphysis. Associated involvement in the medial distal tibial epiphysis is demonstrated.

Etiology. The genetic defect and pathophysiology responsible for fibrodysplasia ossificans progressiva are unknown at this time. The combination of the congenital malformation of the great toe and the postnatal development of heterotopic bone, in characteristic patterns of developmental gradients, suggests a possible role of the bone morphogenetic proteins in the etiology of fibrodysplasia ossificans progressiva. Bone morphogenetic proteins have been implicated in several embryonic epithelial and mesenchymal interactions, such as limb formation, and have the potential to transdifferentiate myoblasts in culture into osteoblast-like cells. Shafritz and colleagues demonstrated overexpres-

sion of bone morphogenetic protein 4 (BMP 4) and its messenger ribonucleic acid (mRNA) in cells derived from an early fibroproliferative lesion in a patient with fibrodysplasia ossificans progressiva (193). Expression of this mRNA was noted in lymphoblastoid cell lines from 26 of 32 patients with the disorder, compared to only 1 of 12 normal subjects. Lanchoney and colleagues have identified elevated steady-state levels of BMP 4 mRNA and BMP 4 receptor mRNA in lesional and nonlesional muscle cell lines from patients with fibrodysplasia ossificans progressiva, suggesting that molecular deregulation of BMP 4 signaling pathways could lead to the disease phenotype (194). Although the gene for

BMP 4 has been mapped to chromosome 14q22-q23, Xu and Shore were unable to identify a mutation in the *BMP 4* gene or its upstream flanking region, in a family showing autosomal-dominant inheritance of fibrodysplasia ossificans progressiva (195).

Clinical Features. The earliest recognizable manifestation of fibrodysplasia ossificans progressiva involves aberrant morphology of the great toe, which demonstrates shortening of the first ray, delta-shaped proximal phalanx, interphalangeal joint fusion, and varying degrees of hallux valgus, either alone or in combination (196). Progressive heterotopic ossification becomes evident at a mean age of 5 years, but may be seen shortly after birth, or as late as the second decade of life. Most lesions arise spontaneously, although blunt trauma can trigger the onset. Individual nodules can regress, although most progress to form mature bone. In their review of 44 patients with fibrodysplasia ossificans progressiva, Cohen and colleagues noted a predictable pattern of involvement of heterotopic ossification, proceeding from axial to appendicular, cranial to caudad, and proximal to distal (197). Dorsal involvement preceded ventral involvement, with the initial lesion characteristically occurring as a painful, erythematous, subfascial nodule in the posterior aspect of the neck, spine, or shoulder girdle. Kaplan and colleagues described the early, intermediate, and late progression of a typical lesion in fibrodysplasia ossificans progressiva (191). The early lesion is heralded by pain, erythema, swelling, warmth, and tenderness, and may resemble an infectious process. After several weeks, the swelling and pain begin to subside, but an increase in induration occurs (the intermediate lesion). The late lesion is present by 12 weeks, and consists of a hard, painless mass that is evident roentgenographically (Fig. 10-16A–G).

Severe disability ensues secondary to extraarticular ankylosis of the major diarthrodial joints. Hip and knee involvement can impair walking and sitting ability. Progressive spinal deformity is common, and can be particularly severe when unilateral pelvis-to–chest-wall synostosis is present (198). Humeral-to–chest-wall synostosis can lead to superior subluxation of the glenohumeral joint (199). Involvement of the temporomandibular joint may lead to inanition with resultant poor nutrition. Decubiti often develop due to a combination of underlying bony prominences, poor nutrition, and lack of mobility. Other associations have included shortened thumbs, fifth-finger clinodactyly, conductive hearing loss, diffuse thinning of the hair on the scalp, premature cessation of menses in female patients, and, uncommonly, mental retardation. Exacerbating factors may include trauma to the muscles, biopsy of lesions, surgical attempts at bone removal, intramuscular injections, careless venipuncture, and dental therapy (196). New lesions can occur throughout the patient's lifetime, and most patients become completely immobilized and confined to a wheelchair by their third decade. The diaphragm, extraocular

muscles, cardiac muscle, and smooth muscle are characteristically spared in the disorder.

Cardiopulmonary dysfunction can play a role in the shortened survival of some patients with fibrodysplasia ossificans progressiva. Heterotopic ossification involving the chest wall and spine can lead to impaired chest wall dynamics and reliance on diaphragmatic breathing (192,197). Kussmaul and coworkers found a high incidence of right ventricular abnormalities on electrocardiographic evaluation of their patients with fibrodysplasia ossificans progressiva who had severely restrictive chest wall disease (200). The investigators raise the possibility that cor pulmonale could eventually develop in such patients.

Radiographic Features. The areas of heterotopic ossification in fibrodysplasia ossificans progressiva are initially similar in radiographic appearance to myositis ossificans, with diffuse calcification developing progressive zonal osseous maturation. Sheets of mature skeletal bone eventually form along striated muscles, fasciae, tendons, and ligaments, causing ankylosis of the joints. Solid extraosseous bridges can form between bones, leading to characteristic synostoses of the cervical spine to occiput, scapula and chest wall to humerus, spine to pelvis, and pelvis to femur. In addition to the characteristic great toe deformities, abnormal cervical vertebrae with small bodies, large posterior elements and fused lateral masses, shortened first metacarpals, fifth-finger clinodactyly, short and broad femoral necks, and exostoses of the proximal tibiae have been reported (Fig. 10-16C–F) (196).

Histopathology. Erroneous biopsies of the lesions in fibrodysplasia ossificans progressiva have provided insight into the pathogenesis of the ossification. Histopathologic and immunohistochemical studies of specimens from early pre-osseous lesions reveal an abundance of primitive vascular cells and angiogenesis, with a conspicuous absence of an acute or chronic inflammatory process. The clinician may be misled toward a presumptive diagnosis of aggressive fibromatosis or low-grade sarcoma at this stage, if fibrodysplasia ossificans progressiva is not considered. Intermediate lesions exhibit scattered cartilaginous foci and evidence of endochondral ossification, proceeding in a sequence that appears entirely normal. Late lesions demonstrate histologically normal lamellar bone, with fatty marrow encased in fibrous connective tissue (201).

Treatment. There is presently no effective treatment for fibrodysplasia ossificans progressiva. Treatment is largely supportive, with attempts at limiting the exacerbating factors of ectopic bone formation, such as trauma, intramuscular injections, careless venipuncture and dental extractions. Padding of bony prominences and nutritional support may be useful in preventing decubiti. Biopsy of lesions or surgery

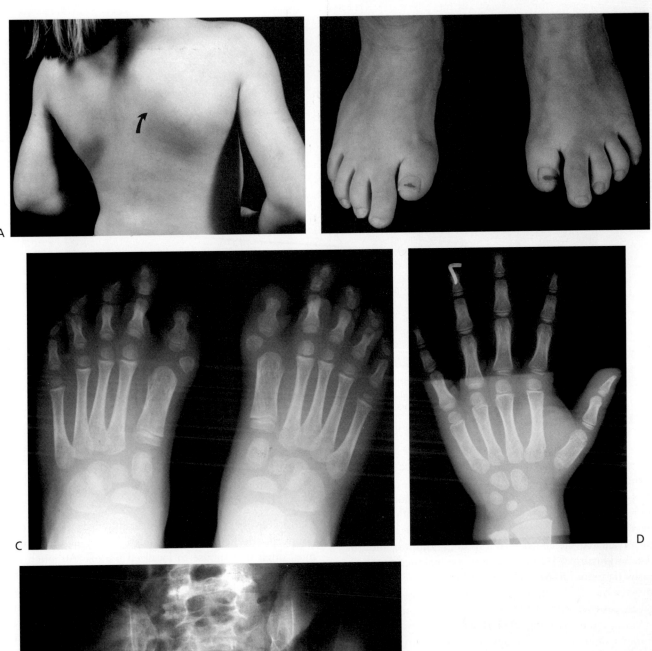

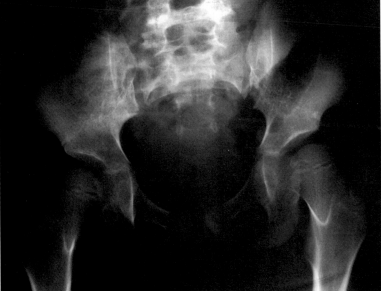

FIGURE 10-16. Fibrodysplasia ossificans progressiva. Four-year-old female at the time of presentation. She complained of right periscapular swelling, warmth, and tenderness. **A:** Clinical photograph demonstrating the area of right periscapular involvement (*arrow*). **B:** Characteristic great toe morphology, demonstrating shortening of the great toes bilaterally. **C:** Bilateral radiographs of the feet demonstrating shortened great toes, with bilateral delta phalanges and shortened first metatarsals. **D:** Anteroposterior radiograph of the hand, demonstrating characteristic shortening of the thumb metacarpal. **E:** Anteroposterior radiograph of the pelvis, demonstrating short, broad femoral necks, and exostoses. *(continued)*

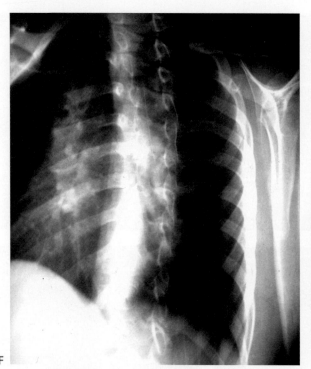

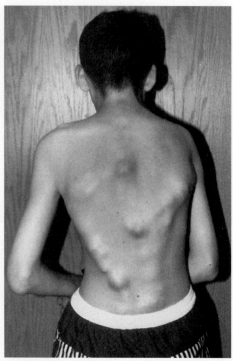

FIGURE 10-16. *(continued)* **F:** Early spontaneous fusion along the posterior elements and lateral masses is demonstrated. **G:** Clinical appearance of an older individual with advanced subcutaneous ossification and characteristic dorsal-to-ventral pattern.

to excise ectopic bone must be avoided, because they uniformly precipitate new bone formation (196).

The administration of high doses of oral diphosphonates and corticosteroids has not been shown to influence the development of the ectopic ossifications. Brantus and Meunier evaluated the effects of intravenous administration of ethane-1-hydroxy-1-diphosphonate and oral prednisone on early flare-ups in patients with fibrodysplasia ossificans progressiva (202). During a mean follow-up of 6 years in seven patients with the disorder, the symptoms of local swelling and pain during 29 of 31 acute flare-ups were ameliorated, and, in 21 flare-ups, no ossification appeared. However, the percentage of acute flare-ups that normally result in ossification is unknown, and so the effect of intravenous diphosphonates during early flare-ups on subsequent progression to ossification cannot be confirmed. As well, during the period of study, 10 new ossifications were observed that resulted in severe deterioration of joint mobility, and there was no change in the radiographic appearance of preexisting ossifications.

Future direction of medical therapies in fibrodysplasia ossificans progressiva will likely center around inhibitors of endochondral osteogenesis. Proposed treatments have included the use of *BMP 4* inhibitors, isotretinoin (an inhibitor of mesenchymal tissue differentiation into cartilage and bone), and antiangiogenic factors (202–205). To date, such treatments should be regarded as investigational.

ACQUIRED DISORDERS

Myositis Ossificans

Myositis ossificans refers to the acquired development of nonneoplastic heterotopic ossification within soft tissues, most often in response to localized trauma. Although the process most commonly develops within skeletal muscle, the term itself is a misnomer, because nonmuscular tissue may be involved, and inflammation is rare. Adolescents and young adults, predominantly male, are affected most frequently, although myositis ossificans has been reported in infancy (206).

Etiology

Precipitating factors in myositis ossificans include single or repetitive trauma in up to 70% of cases (207). The development of heterotopic ossification has also been reported after severe thermal injury, in neurologic diseases, and posttraumatic paraplegia and brain injury, and after some orthopaedic operations, such as total hip arthroplasty (208–216). Rarer genetic and developmental forms of heterotopic ossification exist, including fibrodysplasia ossificans progressiva, progressive osseous heteroplasia, pseudomalignant heterotopic ossification, Albright hereditary osteodystrophy, and parosteal fasciitis (196,203,217–220).

The origin of the bone-forming cells in myositis ossificans remains unknown. Recent investigations into the role of extraskeletal osteogenic precursor cells, and the local factors that induce them, may provide insight into the origins of ectopic bone formation in myositis ossificans, and in other disorders characterized by the formation of heterotopic ossification (221,222).

Clinical Features

Signs and symptoms of myositis ossificans typically include localized pain and a palpable mass which begin to occur approximately 1 to 3 weeks after injury. Increased warmth, swelling, and limitation of motion of the affected area may be noted. A low-grade fever and a mildly elevated erythrocyte sedimentation rate may be present. Limb involvement predominates, most commonly in the quadriceps or brachialis muscles, although virtually any region of the body can been affected. A decrease in pain and increased firmness to the lesion occur over an 8- to 12-week period, with the development of varying degrees of contracture of the affected part.

Radiographic Features

Early plain radiographs in myositis ossificans may demonstrate a noncalcified mass in the soft tissues, typically over the diaphyseal region of the extremity. Within 2 to 4 weeks from injury, floccular calcifications begin to appear within the mass, and a periosteal reaction of the underlying bone may be seen if the cambium layer of the periosteum was involved in the initial injury. Over a 6- to 8-week period, serial radiographs obtained at 1- to 2-week intervals characteristically demonstrate peripheral osseous maturation of the lesion, with a central lucent zone and a lucent line separating it from the underlying cortex, and should be helpful in distinguishing the lesion from an extraosseous sarcoma (Fig. 10-17A and B). By 5 to 6 months, mature bone is evident, and the lesion may show a decrease in overall size. Computed tomography may be particularly helpful in delineating the zonal maturation and cortical separation in myositis ossificans, when the diagnosis is unclear (Fig. 10-18A and B) (207). Other imaging modalities that have been utilized in the diagnosis of myositis ossificans include bone scintigraphy, ultrasound, MRI, leukocyte scanning, and angiography, particularly in early lesions or in difficult cases (207,220). In cases with the typical history of trauma and localized findings, and with roentgenographic evidence of progressive peripheral osseous maturation, the use of these other imaging modalities is infrequently required.

Histopathology

The hallmark of myositis ossificans on histopathologic examination is the presence of zonal phenomenon, as de-

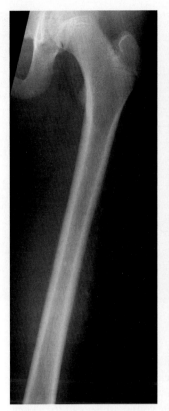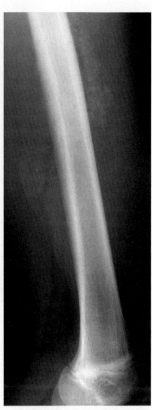

A,B

FIGURE 10-17. Adolescent male complaining of quadriceps tightness, swelling, and discomfort, 6 weeks after sustaining an impact to his thigh during a football game. **A, B:** Anteroposterior and lateral radiographs of the femur demonstrate floccular calcifications within the soft tissue of the thigh, with underlying periosteal reaction in the femoral diaphysis.

scribed by Ackerman (223). The typical lesion consists of a central (inner) zone of undifferentiated cells and atypical mytotic figures, which may be impossible to distinguish from a sarcoma; an adjacent (middle) zone of well-oriented osteoid formation in a nonneoplastic stroma; and a peripheral (outer) zone of well-oriented lamellar bone, clearly demarcated from the surrounding tissue. Although rarely required, when biopsy is performed in cases of myositis ossificans, a specimen of sufficient size and orientation is important in establishing the architectural pattern of the lesion.

Treatment

Prevention of heterotopic ossification at the site of initial injury would ideally be preferable. Nonsteroidal antiinflammatory agents can be utilized to help diminish symptomatology in the early stages of myositis ossificans. Hughston and colleagues suggested that strict rest of the affected part, through the use of splinting, would allow for more complete resorption of the hematoma, and discourage formation of heterotopic bone (224). Thorndike advocated a combina-

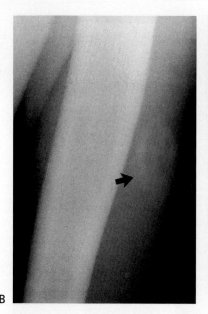
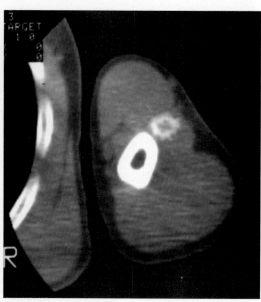

A,B

FIGURE 10-18. Myositis ossificans. **A:** Anteroposterior radiograph demonstrating myositis ossificans in the left upper arm (*arrow*). **B:** CT scan of the same patient, delineating peripheral maturation and clear separation of the lesion from the underlying cortex of the humerus.

tion of rest, icing, compression bandaging, and avoidance of massage therapy (225). Jackson and Feagin developed a treatment strategy for the prevention of myositis ossificans after quadriceps contusions in young athletes (226). They recommended a three-phase program of 24 to 48 h of strict rest of the extremity, elevation and icing (phase I), followed by restoration of motion (phase II), and progressive resistance strengthening (phase III). However, there is presently no clear evidence that such measures alter the development of myositis ossificans, or modify its severity.

The extent of the ossification in myositis ossificans can be deceiving until maturation of the lesion occurs. Similarly, areas of mature ossification can regress partially or totally over time. Many of these lesions will become asymptomatic, and not interfere with function of the affected part. It is therefore advisable, when considering excision of heterotopic bone, to wait until full maturation of the lesion is demonstrated roentgenographically, or on bone scintigraphy (typically 12 to 18 months after injury), and to remove lesions only when they interfere with function or cause persistent local symptomatology.

The Osteochondroses

Osteochondrosis is characterized by a disturbance in endochondral ossification, including both chondrogenesis and osteogenesis, in a previously normal endochondral growth region. The condition is considered idiopathic, and has been described in nearly every growth center of the body, including epiphyses, apophyses, and physes. The various osteochondroses often have associated eponyms, and their clinical features are related to their area of occurrence. As a group, the osteochondroses have relatively well-defined natural his-

tories, and generally predictable outcomes (227). The more clinically significant osteochondroses are described throughout this text according to anatomic region, but are highlighted here for their features as localized disorders of bone and cartilage (Table 10-3).

Etiology

The initial event, or combination of events, leading to the process of disordered endochondral ossification and subsequent necrosis remains unknown. Traumatic and vascular etiologies have been proposed. It has been suggested that the normal process of chondrification of cartilage canals in

TABLE 10-3. EXAMPLES OF OSTEOCHONDROSES BY REGION

Upper Extremity
    Capitellum (Panner)
    Carpal navicular (Kienboch)
    Phalangeal epiphysis (Theemann)
    Distal radial epiphysis (Madelung)

Vertebral end plates
    Schuermann

Lower extremity
    Capital femoral epiphysis (Legg-Perthes)
    Proximal tibial physis (Blount)
    Tibial tubercle (Osgood-Schlatter)
    Calcaneal apophysis (Sever)
    Tarsal navicular (Köhler)
    Metatarsal heads, 2, 3, or 4 (Freiberg)

General
    Osteochondritis dissecans, especially knee, ankle, elbow

the growth center fails, leading to necrosis of cartilage canal vessels in the subchondral bone and adjacent epiphyseal cartilage, or to failed enlargement of the bony centrum and disordered proliferation of cartilage cells within the epiphysis (227,228). In the case of lesions involving segmental epiphyseal necrosis of the subchondral bone and overlying cartilage, so-called "osteochondritis dissecans," it is not clear whether the vascular necrosis precedes or is subsequent to necrosis of the cartilage. The osteochondroses affecting non-articular cartilage, so-called "traction apophysitis," may be related to mechanical disruption of the endochondral mechanism from longitudinally directed shear forces along tendonous or ligamentous attachments.

Clinical Features

The clinical presentation of the various osteochondroses are dependent on the site and degree of involvement, but may include local or referred pain, inflammation, effusion, limitation of motion, gait disturbance, or, in the case of physeal involvement such as Blount disease, visible disturbance in growth.

Radiographic Features

Although the exact imaging features of an osteochondrosis are characteristic for the anatomic area involved, they do share some common radiographic features. Early involvement may appear as a decrease in size, increase in density, or irregular architecture of the involved centrum. Resorption of necrotic bone may lead to apparent worsening of the radiographic appearance, with return of radiographically evident bone, as revascularization and reossification occurs (Fig. 10-19A–C). The resultant area may come to appear radiographically normal, or demonstrate permanently altered anatomy. Delay in complete revascularization of a fragmented necrotic centrum may result in separation of an ununited segment, as in osteochondritis dissecans.

Histopathology

In general, all stages of the process have been described, including necrosis of bone and cartilage, revascularization, granulation tissue invasion, osteoclastic resorption of necrotic segments, osteoid replacement along necrotic trabeculae, and, eventually, formation of mature lamellar bone (227). Biopsy of an area of involvement is rarely indicated, however, due to the characteristic clinical and radiographic findings. Of interest is that in osteochondritis dissecans, in which it is largely accepted that necrosis of the underlying subchondral bone leads to the separation of an osteocartilaginous fragment from the surrounding viable bone, the specimen may be purely cartilaginous, and if bone is present, it is not always necrotic (229).

Treatment

In children, the majority of osteochondroses are self-limiting, and will respond to symptomatic, nonoperative treatment with complete resolution (229–232). A combination of rest, icing, and rehabilitation of the affected part can help decrease the duration of symptoms, but may not influence the final outcome (230). Surgical intervention is typically reserved for more clinically severe forms, often to reduce causative stress, such as bony realignment in some cases of Blount disease, or to stimulate healing or remove intraarticular fragments, as in some cases of osteochondritis dissecans.

Infantile Quadriceps Fibrosis

Infantile quadriceps fibrosis refers to a condition of congenital or acquired contracture of all or part of the extensor mechanism of the knee. This entity has been called "congenital fibrosis" by some authors; however, we prefer the term "infantile quadriceps fibrosis" to distinguish this entity from congenital dislocation of the knee, which may have quadriceps fibrosis as a feature (233–235).

Clinical Features

The clinical features include varying degrees of limitation of knee flexion, thigh atrophy, genu valgum or recurvatum, high-riding patella, and habitual patellar dislocation, which are felt to be directly related to the extent of the quadriceps fibrosis (233,234,236). In some patients, increases in knee flexion are possible only after obligate lateral dislocation of the patella (236). There may be a history of repeated intramuscular injections of the thigh and gluteal muscles in early infancy, often in relation to severe or prolonged illness (236–238). In some children, the etiology cannot be established, but may be due to some other form of direct or indirect injury to the quadriceps mechanism. The physician should consider mild forms of arthrogryposis, congenital dislocation of the knee or patella, or spinal dysraphism, in the differential diagnosis.

Etiology

Early descriptions of infantile quadriceps fibrosis implied that the disorder was due to a muscular dysplasia of congenital origin, superficially resembling an incomplete syndrome of arthrogryposis (233,234,239). Gunn established the role of intramuscular injections in infancy as the major cause of the fibrosis, and this has since been confirmed by others (236–238,240,241).

Pathology

On gross and histologic examination, diffuse fibrosis and fatty replacement of muscle are present, most commonly

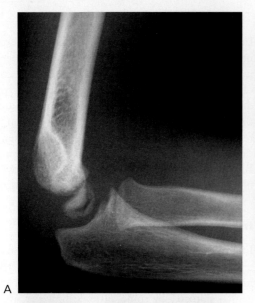

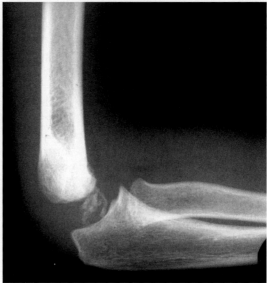

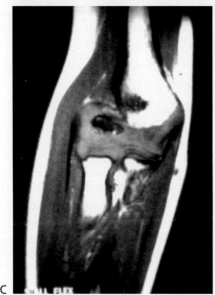

FIGURE 10-19. Seven-year-old male complaining of right elbow pain. **A:** Lateral radiograph of the elbow when the child was initially seen, demonstrating intraarticular effusion, subchondral lucency, and sclerosis of the capitellar ossification center. **B:** Lateral radiograph obtained approximately 4 months later, demonstrating fragmentation of the capitellar ossification center. **C:** MRI demonstrating avascular changes within the capitellar ossification center.

involving the vastus lateralis, vastus intermedius, and iliotibial tract (233,236). An "abnormal" attachment of the iliotibial tract to the superolateral patella was noted by Jeffreys, which more likely represented a mechanically hypertrophied epicondylopatellar ligament (242,243).

Treatment

Nonoperative treatment, in the form of manipulation, splinting, and stretching, has not been successful in addressing the condition (233). Surgical intervention has included various forms of distal muscle and fascia release, lengthening of the quadriceps tendon, and rebalancing of the extensor mechanism, depending on the extent of involvement and clinical features (233,234,236,244). In selected cases, early

release of the muscles, through a limited subtrochanteric exposure, has been described, with good results reported (237).

Reflex Sympathetic Dystrophy

Reflex sympathetic dystrophy is a syndrome characterized by pain in an extremity and associated dysfunction of the autonomic nervous system. This syndrome usually follows a minor trauma, but has been associated with many medical and surgical conditions, and with certain drugs. Although thought to be rare in children, it is being recognized with increasing frequency (245,246). The syndrome has been given a variety of names, including posttraumatic pain syndrome, algoneurodystrophy, shoulder–hand syndrome, Sudeck atrophy, and causalgia. The term "causalgia" has been primarily used to describe the burning pain following a peripheral nerve injury, while "reflex sympathetic dystrophy" has been reserved for cases that resemble causalgia, but do not have a vascular or neural lesion (247). To clarify the picture, the term "complex regional pain syndrome" has been proposed to correspond with "reflex sympathetic dystrophy (type I)" and "causalgia (type II)" (248).

Clinical Features

Girls are much more likely to be affected with reflex sympathetic dystrophy than boys, and the lower extremities are much more frequently involved than the upper extremities (245,246,249,250).

The cardinal symptoms and signs include pain, vasomotor abnormalities, trophic changes, and motor manifestations (251). The pain is disproportionate in duration, severity, and distribution to that which would be expected in response to the initiating noxious event. It may be spontaneous and aggravated by dependency or touch, or evoked by mechanical or thermal stimuli. Hyperpathia, or pain that persists after the stimulus has been removed, and allodynia, or pain that is produced by a nonnoxious stimulus, such as light touch, are common complaints. Edema is a common early finding. The temperature of the affected extremity may be colder or warmer than the uninvolved side, and have a different skin color. Although chronic trophic changes are reported as being rare in children (249), one study reported a 15% incidence of trophic changes (245). Skin, hair, and nail growth changes, subcutaneous tissue and muscle atrophy, and leg-length discrepancy can be seen. Motor changes include weakness, tremor, dystonia, and reduced movement.

Although it has been commonly held that children who develop this syndrome have predisposing psychogenic factors (252), several recent studies have concluded there are no predisposing traits (245,253). Psychological stressors can modify the severity of the symptoms and the continuous pain, and accompanying disability may result in anxiety disorders and depression.

Reflex sympathetic dystrophy has been classically described as evolving through characteristic stages: the acute stage, followed by the dystrophic period, and, finally, by atrophy (254). The staging system has been shown recently to not consistently describe the evolution of the disorder (255).

The diagnosis of reflex sympathetic dystrophy is primarily clinical. The current diagnostic criteria (256) require:

1. The presence of an initiating noxious event or a cause of immobilization.
2. Continuing pain, allodynia, or hyperalgesia in which the pain is disproportionate to the inciting event.
3. Evidence at some time of edema, changes in skin blood flow, or abnormal sudomotor activity in the painful region.

4. The diagnosis is excluded by the existence of conditions that would otherwise account for the degree of pain and dysfunction.

There are no specific diagnostic studies available. Plain radiographs, bone scan, and thermography are rarely required for diagnosis in children.

The diagnosis is typically delayed, occasionally for a year or more (245,246,250,257). Reflex sympathetic dystrophy can be localized to the knee, and may be misdiagnosed as anterior knee pain syndrome.

The differential diagnosis includes trauma, stress fracture, infection, tumor (such as osteoid osteoma), and psychological disorders with somatic manifestations.

Radiographic Features

Plain radiographs may be normal or demonstrate osteopenia in children (250). The patchy osteopenia typical in adults is not often present in children. Bone scan has been advocated as a diagnostic tool in adults, however, in children, the results are highly variable, demonstrating increased, decreased, or normal uptake in the involved extremities (250,258). The sensitivity and specificity of the bone scan are not sufficient for its routine use in the diagnosis of reflex sympathetic dystrophy (246,250). The bone scan is useful though, to rule out occult skeletal disorders such as stress fracture or neoplasm (245).

Etiology

The etiology and pathogenesis of reflex sympathetic dystrophy is unknown. Many theories suggest dysfunction of the sympathetic nervous system but this is controversial (247). Ochoa has demonstrated, in human studies that the pain and accompanying features that resemble sympathetically mediated disturbances may be due instead to sensitization of peripheral nociceptors and mechanoreceptors, and to the effects of vasoactive substances released at the endings of small sensory afferent fibers (259).

Treatment

The goal of treatment is to restore function. This is ideally achieved through a coordinated, staged, progressive approach that uses treatment modalities required to achieve both remission and rehabilitation (245,251,260).

A 1998 consensus report, by Stanton-Hicks and others, outlines a treatment algorithm for reflex sympathetic dystrophy in adults and children (251). It focuses on the principles of patient motivation, mobilization, and desensitization facilitated by the relief of pain. Physical therapy is the cornerstone of treatment, with pharmacologic management (nonsteroidal antiinflammatories, opioids, tricyclic antidepressants, steroids, and drugs such as carbamazepine), regional anesthesia (for analgesia and sympathetic blockade), neuromodulation, and psychotherapy used as adjuncts to facilitate management. Casts and splints should not be used in the treatment because immobilization may exacerbate the problem (249). An interdisciplinary team approach is most likely to succeed. The initial treatment for children should be physical therapy. It is necessary to educate the patient and the family about the nonprotective nature of the neuropathic pain to help them work through the discomfort (251). More than 50% of the children will respond to physical therapy alone (249,250), or in combination with transcutaneous electrical nerve stimulation (TENS), psychotherapy, and the use of oral medication (245). Treatment early in the course of the disease gives the best results. Sympathetic nerve blocks may be useful if the abovementioned treatment is not successful. A continuous block with a catheter technique may be preferable to intermittent blocks (251,261). Physical rehabilitation and behavioral therapy are continued under the sympathetic nerve block.

The typical outcome is one of improvement, but children can have long-term persistent pain and dysfunction (245).

References

Congenital and Developmental Disorders

Vascular Tumors and Malformations

1. Goldberg M. Hemangioma syndromes. In: Goldberg M, ed. *The dysmorphic child*. New York: Raven, 1987.
2. Enjolras O. Vascular tumors and vascular malformations: are we at the dawn of a better knowledge? *Pediatr Derm* 1999;16: 238.
3. Mulliken JB, Glowacki J. Hemangiomas and vascular malformations in infants and children: a classification based on endothelial characteristics. *Plast Reconstr Surg* 1982;69:412.
4. Mulliken JB, Young AE, et al. *Vascular birthmarks: hemangiomas and malformations*. Philadelphia: WB Saunders, 1988.
5. Fishman SJ, Mulliken JB. Vascular anomalies, a primer for pediatricians. *Pediatr Clin North Am* 1998;45:455.
6. Meyer JJ, Hoffer FA, Barnes PD, et al. Biologic classification of soft tissue vascular anomalies: MR correlation. *Am J Radiol* 1991;157:559.
7. Enjolras O, Wassef M, Majoyer E, et al. Infants with Kasabach-Merritt syndrome do not have "true" hemangiomas. *J Pediatr* 1997;130:631
8. Folkman J. Angiogenesis in cancer, vascular, rheumatoid and other diseases. *Nature Med* 1995;1:27

Vascular Malformations

9. Dutkowsky JP, Kasser JR, Kaplan LC. Leg length discrepancy associated with vivid cutis marmorata. *J Pediatr Orthop* 1993; 13:456.
10. Rogalski R, Hensinger R, Loder R. Vascular abnormalities of the extremities: clinical findings and management. *J Pediatr Orthop* 1993;13:9.
11. Yousem DM, Scott WW Jr, Fishman EK. Case report 440: Klippel-Trenaunay syndrome of right lower extremity. *Skeletal Radiol* 1987;16:652.
12. Levine C. Imaging of body asymmetry and hemihypertrophy. *Crit Rev Diagn Imaging* 1990;31:1.

13. Stringel G. Hemangiomas and lymphangiomas. In: Ashcroft KW, Haldor TM, eds. *Pediatric surgery*. Philadelphia: WB Saunders, 1993.
14. Enjolras O, Ciabrini D, Mazoyer E, Laurian C. Pure venous malformations in the limbs (27 cases). *J Am Acad Dermatol* 1997;36:219.
15. McCarthy JE, Goldberg MJ, Zimbler S. Orthopaedic dysfunction in the blue rubber-bleb nevus syndrome. *J Bone Joint Surg Am* 1982;64:280.
16. Moodley M, Ramdial P. Blue rubber bleb nevus syndrome: case report and review of the literature. *Pediatrics* 1993;92:160.
17. Pasaboc LG, Gibbs PM, Kwan W. Blue rubber bleb nevus syndrome in the foot. *J Foot Ankle Surg* 1994;33:271.
18. Gupta AK, et al. Mediastinal and skeletal lymphangiomas in a child. *Pediatr Radiol* 1991;21:129.
19. Hoeffel JG, Marchal AC, Pierre E, et al. Cystic lymphangioma of the pelvis in childhood. *Br Radiol* 1990;63:813.
20. Siegel MJ, Glazer HS, St. Amour TF, et al. Lymphangiomas in children: MRI imaging. *Radiology* 1989;170:467.
21. Mandell GA, Alexander MA, Harcke HT. A multiscintigraphic approach to imaging of lymphedema and other causes of the congenitally enlarged extremity. *Semin Nucl Med* 1993;23:334.
22. Boris M, Weindorf S, Lasinski B, et al. Lymphedema reduction by non-invasive complex lymphedema therapy. *Oncology* 1994; 8:95.
23. Jumbelic M, Feuerstein M, Dorfman HD. Solitary intraosseous lymphangioma. *J Bone Joint Surg Am* 1984;66:1479.

Complex-combined Vascular Malformations

24. Baskerville PA, Ackroyd JS, Lea Thomas M, et al. The Klippel-Trenaunay syndrome. Clinical, radiological and hemodynamic features and management. *Br J Surg* 1985;72:232.
25. Guidera KJ, Brinker MR, Koussoff BG, et al. Overgrowth management in Klippel-Trenaunay and Proteus syndromes. *J Pediatr Orthop* 1993;13:459.
26. Klippel M, Trenaunay P. Du naevus variquex ostephypertrophique. *Arch Gen Med (Paris)* 1900;185:641.
27. Lindenauer SM. The Klippel-Trenaunay syndrome. *Ann Surg* 1965;162:303.
28. Berry SA, Peterson C, Mize W, et al. Klippel-Trenaunay syndrome. *Am J Med Gen* 1998;79:312.
29. Parkes-Weber F. Hemangiectatic hypertrophy of limbs: congenital phlebarteriectasis and so-called congenital varicose veins. *Br J Child Dis* 1918;15:13.
30. Baskerville PA, Ackroyd JS, Browse NL. The etiology of the Klippel-Trenaunay syndrome. *Ann Surg* 1985;292:624.
31. Lie JT. Pathology of angiodysplasia in Klippel-Trenaunay syndrome. *Pathol Res Pract* 1988;183:747.
32. Pelleren D, Martelli H, Lutoiche X, et al. Congenital soft tissue dysplasia: a new malformation entity and concept. *Prog Pediatr Surg* 1989;22:1.
33. Moor JJ, Warren FH, Arensman RM. Klippel-Trenaunay syndrome: rarely a surgical disease. *South Med J* 1988;81:83.
34. McCullough CJ, Kenwright J. The prognosis in congenital lower limb hypertrophy. *Acta Orthop Scand* 1979;50:307.
35. Anlar B, Yalaz R, Erzen C. Klippel-Trenaunay-Weber syndrome: a case with cerebral and cerebellar hemihypertrophy. *Neuro Radiology* 1988;30:360.
36. Oyesiku NM, Gahm NJ, Goldman RL. Cerebral arteriovenous fistula in Klippel-Trenaunay-Weber syndrome. *Dev Med Child Neurol* 1988;30:245.
37. D'Costa H, Hunter JD, O'Sullivan G, et al. Magnetic resonance imaging in macromelia and macrodactyly. *Br J Radiol* 1996;69: 502.
38. Laor T, Hoffer FA, Burrows PE, Kozakewick HP. MR lymph-

angiography in infants, children and young adults. *AJR Am J Roentgenol* 1998;171:1111.

39. McCarthy RE, Lytle JD, VanDevanter S. The use of total circulatory arrest in the surgery of giant hemangioma and Klippel-Trenaunay syndromes in neonates. *Clin Orthop* 1983;289:237.

40. Stringel G, D'Astous J. Klippel-Trenaunay syndrome and other cases of lower limb hypertrophy: pediatric surgical implications. *J Pediatr Surg* 1987;22:645.

41. Letts RM. Orthopaedic treatment of hemangiomatous hypertrophy of the lower extremity. *J Bone Joint Surg* 1997;59:777.

42. Sooriakumaran S, Landham TL. The Klippel-Trenaunay syndrome. *J Bone Joint Surg* 1991;73B:169.

43. Gates PE, Drvaric DM, Kruger L. Wound healing in orthopaedic procedures for Klippel-Trenaunay syndrome. *J Pediatr Orthop* 1996;16:723.

44. McGrory BJ, Amadio PC, Dobyns JH, et al. Anomalies of the fingers and toes associated with Klippel-Trenaunay syndrome. *J Bone Joint Surg Am* 1991;73:1537.

45. Biesecker LG, Happle R, Mulliken JB, et al. Proteus syndrome: diagnostic criteria, differential diagnosis, and patient evaluation. *Am J Med Genet* 1999;84:389.

46. Demetriades D, Hager J, Nikolaudes N, et al. Proteus syndrome: musculoskeletal manifestations and management: a report of two cases. *J Pediatr Orthop* 1992;12:106.

47. Samlaska CP, Levin SW, James WD, et al. Proteus syndrome. *Arch Dermatol* 1989;125:1109.

48. Stricker S. Musculoskeletal manifestations of Proteus syndrome: report of two cases with literature review. *J Pediatr Orthop* 1992; 12:667.

49. Wiedemann HR, Burgio GR, Aldenhoff P. The Proteus syndrome. *Eur J Pediatr* 1983;140:5.

50. Choi ML, Wey PD, Borah GL. Pediatric peripheral neuropathy in proteus syndrome. *Ann Plast Surg* 1998;40:528.

51. Cremin BJ, Viljoen DL, Wynchank S, et al. The Proteus syndrome: MR and radiological features. *Pediatr Radiol* 1987;17: 486.

52. Gorham LW, Stout AP. Massive osteolysis. *J Bone Joint Surg Am* 1955;37:985.

53. Shives TC, Beabout JW, Unni KK. Massive osteolysis. *Clin Orthop Rel Res* 1993;294:267.

54. Remia LF, Richolt J, Buckley KM, et al. Pain and weakness of the shoulder in a 16-year-old boy. *Clin Orthop Rel Res* 1998; 347:268.

55. Aoki M, Kato F, Saito H, et al. Successful treatment of chylothorax by bleomycin for Gorham's disease. *Clin Orthop Rel Res* 1996;330:193.

56. Heyden G, Knidblom LG, Nielson M. Disappearing bone disease. *J Bone Joint Surg Am* 1977;59:57.

57. Mendez AA, Keret D, Robertson W, et al. Massive osteolysis of the femur. *J Pediatr Orthop* 1989;9:604.

58. Joseph J, Bartal EG. Disappearing bone disease. *J Pediatr Orthop* 1987;7:584.

59. Johnson PM, McClure JG. Observations on massive osteolysis. *Radiology* 1958;71:28.

60. Picault C, Comtet JJ, Imbert JC, et al. Surgical repair of extensive idiopathic osteolysis of the pelvic girdle. *J Bone Joint Surg Br* 1984;66:148.

61. Dunbar SF, Rosenberg A, Mankin H, et al. Gorham's massive osteolysis. The role of radiation therapy and a review of the literature. *Int Radiol Oncol Biol Phys* 1993;26:491.

62. Levine CL. The imaging of body asymmetry and hemihypertrophy. *Crit Rev Diagn Imaging* 1990;31:1.

63. Pappas AM, Nehme AM. Leg length discrepancy associated with hypertrophy. *Clin Orthop* 1979;144:198.

64. Rush WA, Steiner HA. A study of lower extremity length inequality. *AJR Am J Roentgenol* 1946;56:616.

65. Ballock RT, Wiesner GL, Myers MT, et al. Hemihypertrophy. Concepts and controversies. *J Bone Joint Surg Am* 1997;79: 1731.

66. Ward J, Lerner HH. A review of the subject of congenital hemihypertrophy and a complete case report. *J Pediatr* 1947;31:403.

67. Beals RK. Hemihypertrophy and hemihypotrophy. *Clin Orthop* 1992;166:200.

68. Phelan EM, Carty HM, Kalos S. Generalized enchondromatosis associated with hemangiomas, soft tissue calcifications and hemihypertrophy. *Br J Radiol* 1986;59:69.

69. Viljoen D, Pearn J, Beighton P. Manifestations and natural history of idiopathic hemihypertrophy. *Clin Genet* 1984;26:81.

70. MacEwen GD, Case JL. Congenital hemihypertrophy. *Clin Orthop* 1967;50:147.

71. Hoyme HE, Seaver LH, Jones KL, et al. Isolated hemihyperplasia (hemihypertrophy): report of a prospective multicenter study of the incidence of neoplasia and review. *Am J Med Genet* 1998;79:274.

72. Clericuzio CL, Johnson C. Screening for Wilms tumor in high risk individuals. *Hematol Oncol Clin North Am* 1995;9:1253.

73. Green DM, Breslow NE, Beckwith JB, et al. Screening of children with hemihypertrophy, aniridia and Beckwith-Wiedemann syndrome in patients with Wilms tumor: a report from the national Wilms tumor study. *Med Pediatr Oncol* 1993;21: 188.

74. Janik JS, Steeler RA. Delayed onset of hemihypertrophy in Wilms' tumor. *J Pediatr Surg* 1976;11:581.

75. Shapiro F. Developmental patterns in lower extremity length discrepancies. *J Bone Joint Surg Am* 1992;64:639.

76. Elliot M, Bayley R, Cole T, et al. Clinical features and natural history of Beckwith-Wiedemann syndrome: presentation of 74 new cases. *Clin Genet* 1994;46:168.

77. Debaun MR, Zucker MA. Risk of cancer during the first four years of life in children from the Beckwith-Wiedemann syndrome registry. *J Pediatr* 1998;132:398.

78. Wiedemann HR. Tumors and hemihypertrophy associated with Wiedemann-Beckwith syndrome. *Eur J Pediatr* 1983;141:129.

79. Nudleman K, Andermann E. Hemi-3 syndrome. *Brain* 1984; 107:533.

80. Goldberg MJ. Syndromes of overgrowth. In: Goldberg M, ed. *The dysmorphic child.* New York: Raven, 1987.

81. Bortel DT, Pritchett JW. Straight-line graphs for prediction of growth of the upper extremity. *J Bone Joint Surg Am* 1993;75: 885.

82. Barsky AJ. Macrodactyly. *J Bone Joint Surg Am* 1967;49:1255.

83. Turra S, Santini S, Cagnoni G, et al. Gigantism of the foot: our experience in seven cases. *J Pediatr Orthop* 1998;18:337.

84. Ackland MK, Uthoff HK. Idiopathic localized gigantism: a 26-year follow-up. *J Pediatr Orthop* 1988;8:618.

85. Miura H, Uchida Y, Iharak, et al. Macrodactyly in Proteus syndrome. *J Hand Surg Br* 1993;18:308.

86. Dennyson WG, Bear JN, Bhoola KD. Macrodactyly in the foot. *J Bone Joint Surg Br* 1977;59:355.

87. Stevens PM. Toe deformities. In: Drennan JC, ed. *The child's foot and ankle.* New York: Raven, 1984.

88. Ben-Bassat M, Casper J, Laron Z. Congenital macrodactyly. *J Bone Joint Surg Br* 1966;48:359.

89. Grogan DP, Bernstein RM, Habal MB, et al. Congenital lipofibromatosis associated with macrodactyly of the foot. *Foot Ankle Int* 1991;12:40.

90. Jones KG. Megalodactylism. *J Bone Joint Surg Am* 1963;45: 1704.

91. Topoleski TA, Ganel G, Grogan DP. Effect of proximal phalangeal epiphysiodesis in the treatment of macrodactyly. *Foot Ankle Int* 1997;18:500.

92. Kotwal PP, Farooque M, Macrodactyly. *J Bone Joint Surg Br* 1998;18:337.

93. Tsuge K. Treatment of macrodactyly. *Plast Reconstr Surg* 1967; 39:590.

94. Dedrick DP, Kling TF Jr. Ray resection in the treatment of macrodactyly of the foot in children. *Orthop Trans* 1985;9:145.

95. Kalen V, Burwell DS, Omer GE. Macrodactyly of the hands and feet. *J Pediatr Orthop* 1988;8:311.

96. Herring JA, Tolo VT. Instructional case: macrodactyly. *J Pediatr Orthop* 1984;4:503.

97. Kino Y. Clinical and experimental studies of the congenital constriction band syndrome with an emphasis on its etiology. *J Bone Joint Surg Am* 1975;57:636

98. Moses JM, Flatt AE, Cooper RR. Annular constricting bands. *J Bone Joint Surg Am* 1979;61:562.

99. Askins G, Ger E. Congenital constriction band syndrome. *J Pediatr Orthop* 1988;8:461.

100. Cowell HR, Hensinger RN. The relationship of clubfoot to congenital annular bands. In: Bateman JE, ed. *Foot science*. Philadelphia: WB Saunders, 1976.

101. Tada K, Yonenobu K, Swanson AB. Congenital constriction band syndrome. *J Pediatr Orthop* 1984;4:726.

102. Allington NJ, Jay Kumar S, Guille JT. Clubfeet associated with congenital constriction bands of the ipsilateral lower extremity. *J Pediatr Orthop* 1995;15:599.

103. Gomez VR. Clubfeet in congenital annular constricting bands. *Clin Orthop* 1996;323:155.

104. Bahadoran Ph, Lacour J Ph, Terrisse A, et al. Congenital constriction band of the trunk. *Pediatr Dermatol* 1997;6:470.

105. Wiedrich TA. Congenital constriction band syndrome. *Hand Clin* 1998;14:29.

106. Patterson TJS. Congenital ring constrictions. *Br J Plast Surg* 1961;14:1.

107. Chang C, Huang S. Clubfoot deformity in congenital constriction band syndrome: manifestations and treatment. *J Formos Med Assoc* 1998;97:328.

108. Bourne MH, Klassen RA. Congenital annular constricting bands. *J Bone Joint Surg* 1987;7:218.

109. Zionts LE, Osterkamp JA, Crawford TO, Harvey JP. Congenital annular bands in identical twins. *J Bone Joint Surg Am* 1984; 56:450.

110. Torpin R. Amniochorionic mesoblastic fibrous strings and amniotic bands: associated constricting fetal malformations or fetal death. *Am J Obstet Gynecol* 1965;91:65.

111. Torpin R. *Fetal malformations caused by amnion rupture during gestation*. Springfield, IL: Charles C Thomas, 1968.

112. Streeter GL. Focal deficiencies in fetal tissues and their relationship to intrauterine amputation. *Contrib Embryol* 1930;22:1.

113. VanAllen MI, Siegel-Bartelt J, Dixon J, et al. Constriction bands and limb reduction defects in two newborns. *Am J Med Genet* 1992;44:598.

114. Bass HN, Caldwell S, Brooks BS. Michelin tire baby syndrome. *Am J Med Genet* 1993;45:370.

115. Abel M, McFarland R. Hair and thread constriction in infants. *J Bone Joint Surg Am* 1993;75:915.

116. Keane BH, Tucker HA. Etiologic concepts and pathologic aspects of ainhum. *Arch Pathol* 1986;41:639.

117. Greene WB. One-stage release of congenital circumferential constriction bands. *J Bone Joint Surg Am* 1993;75:650.

Disorders Involving Joint and Bone

118. Camurati M. Dilulraro caso di osteite simmetrica ereditaria degli arti inferiori. *Chir Organi Mov* 1922;6:662.

119. Engelmann G. Ein von osteopathia hyperostica (sclerotisans) multiples infantiles. *Fortschr Rontgenstr* 1929;39:1101.

120. Naveh Y, Kaftori JK, Alon U, et al. Progressive diaphyseal dysplasia: genetics and clinical and radiologic manifestations. *Pediatrics* 1984;74:399.

121. Stenzler S, Grogan DP, Frenchman SM, et al. Progressive diaphyseal dysplasia presenting as neuromuscular disease. *J Pediatr Orthop* 1989;9:463.

122. Saraiva JM. Progressive diaphyseal dysplasia: a three-generation family with markedly variable expressivity. *Am J Med Gen* 1997; 71:348.

123. Hundley JD, Wilson FC. Progressive diaphyseal dysplasia: review of the literature and report of seven cases in one family. *J Bone Joint Surg Am* 1973;55:461.

124. Kaftori JK, Kleinhaus A, Naveh Y. Progressive diaphyseal dysplasia: radiographic follow-up and CT findings. *Radiology* 1987; 164:772.

125. Clawson DK, Loop JW. Progressive diaphyseal dysplasia (Engelmann's disease). *J Bone Joint Surg Am* 1964;46:143.

126. Grey AC, Wallace R, Crone M. Engelmann's disease. A 45 year follow-up. *J Bone Joint Surg Br* 1996;78:488.

127. Nevin NC, Thomas PS, Davis RI, et al. Melorheostosis in a family with autosomal dominant osteopoikilosis. *Am J Med Genet* 1999;82:409.

128. Norton KI, Wagreich JM, Granowetter L, Martignetti JA. Diaphyseal medullary stenosis (sclerosis) with bone malignancy (malignant fibrous histrocytoma): Hardcastle syndrome. *Pediatr Radiol* 1996;26:675.

129. Naveh Y, Alon U, Kafton JK, Berant M. Progressive diaphyseal dysplasia: evaluation of corticosteroid therapy. *Pediatrics* 1985; 75:321.

130. Leri A, Joanny J. Un affection non decrite des os: Hyperostose "en coulee: sur toute la longeur d'un membre ou melorheostose." *Bul Mem Soc Hop Paris* 1922;46:1141.

131. Rozencwaig R, Wilson NR, McFarland GB Jr. Melorheostosis. *Am J Orthop* 1997;26:83.

132. Younge D, Drummond D, Herring J, et al. Melorheostosis in children. Clinical features and natural history. *J Bone Joint Surg Br* 1979;61:415.

133. Alvarez MJ, Lazaro MA, Espada G, et al. Linear scleroderma and melorheostosis: case presentation and literature review. *Clin Rheumatol* 1996;15:389.

134. Fryns JP, Pedersen JC, Vanfleteren L, et al. Melorheostosis in a 3-year-old girl. *Acta Pediatr Belg* 1980;33:185.

135. Ippolito V, Mirra JM, Motta C, et al. Case report 771: melorheostosis in association with desmoid tumor. *Skeletal Radiol* 1993;22:284.

136. Moris JM, Samilson RL, Corley CL. Melorheostosis: review of the literature and report of an interesting case with a nineteen year follow-up. *J Bone Joint Surg Am* 1963;45:1191.

137. Campbell CJ, Papademetriou T, Bonfiglio M. Melorheostosis: a report of clinical, roentgenographic and pathological findings in fourteen cases. *J Bone Joint Surg Am* 1968;50:1281.

138. Murray RO, McCreadie J. Melorheostosis and sclerotomes: a radiological correlation. *Skeletal Radiol* 1979;4:57.

139. Buckley SL, Skinner S, James P, Ashley RK. Focal scleroderma in children. *J Pediatr Orthop* 1993;13:784.

140. Atar D, Lehmann WB, Grant AD, et al. The Ilizarov apparatus for treatment of melorheostosis. *Clin Orthop* 1992;281:163.

141. Griffet J, El Hayek T, Giborn P. Melorheostosis: complications of a tibial lengthening with the Ilizarov apparatus. *Eur J Pediatr Surg* 1998;8:186.

142. Marshall JH, Bradish CF. Callotasis in melorheostosis: a case report. *J Bone Joint Surg Br* 1993;75:155.

143. Naudie D, Hamdy RC, Fassier F, et al. Complications of limb lengthening in children who have an underlying bone disorder. *J Bone Joint Surg Am* 1998;80:18.

144. Benli IT, Akalin S, Boysan E, et al. Epidemiological, clinical

and radiological aspects of osteopoikilosis. *J Bone Joint Surg Br* 1992;74:504.

145. Al Attia HM, Sherif AM. Buschke-Ollendorf syndrome in a grade multipara: a case report and short review of the literature. *Clin Rheumatol* 1998;17:172.

146. Walpole IR, Manners PJ. Clinical considerations in Buschke-Ollendorf syndrome. *Clin Genet* 1990;37:59.

147. Chigira M, Kati K, Mishio K, et al. Symmetry of bone lesions in osteopoikilosis. *Acta Orthop Scand* 1991;62:495.

148. Whyte MP, Murphy WA, Siegel BA: 99m Tc–pyrophosphate bone imaging in osteopoikiliosis, osteopathia striata and melorheostosis. *Radiology* 1988;127:439.

149. Walker GF. Mixed sclerosing bone dystrophies. *J Bone Joint Surg Br* 1964;46:546.

150. Fairbanks HAT. Osteopathia striata. *J Bone Joint Surg Br* 1950;32:117.

151. Greenspan A. Sclerosing bone dysplasias. A target-site approach. *Skeletal Radiol* 1991;20:561.

152. Nishimura G, Okada T, Tachibana K, et al. Osteopathia striata short stature, and characteristic facies: a previously unknown skeletal dysplasia. *Eur J Pediatr* 1997;156:631.

153. Gibson DA, Carroll N. Congenital pseudarthrosis of the clavicle. *J Bone Joint Surg Br* 1970;52:629.

154. Mall FP. On ossification centers in human embryos less than one hundred days old. *Am J Anat* 1906;5:433.

155. Gardner E. The embryology of the clavicle. *Clin Orthop Rel Res* 1968;58:9.

156. Lombard JJP. Pseudarthrosis of the clavicle. *South Afr Med J* 1984;66:151.

157. Alldred AJ. Congenital pseudarthrosis of the clavicle. *J Bone Joint Surg Br* 1963;45:312.

158. Lloyd-Roberts GC, Apley AG, Pyrford OR. Reflections on the etiology of congenital pseudarthrosis of the clavicle. *J Bone Joint Surg Br* 1975;57:24.

159. Bargar WL, Marcus RE, Ittleman FP. Late thoracic outlet syndrome secondary to pseudarthrosis of the clavicle. *J Trauma* 1984;24:857.

160. de Gauzy JS, Baunin C, Puget C, et al. Congenital pseudarthrosis of the clavicle and thoracic outlet syndrome in adolescence. *J Pediatr Orthop* 1999;8:299.

161. Hahn K, Shah R, Shalev Y, et al. Congenital clavicular pseudarthrosis associated with vascular thoracic outlet syndrome: case presentation and review of the literature. *Cathet Cardiovasc Diagn* 1995;35:321.

162. Schoenecker PL, Johnson GE, Howard B, et al. Congenital pseudarthrosis. *Orthop Rev* 1992;21:855.

163. Valette H. Pseudarthrose congenitale de la clavicule et syndrome de la traversee thoraco-brachiale. Revue de la litterature a propos d'un cas. *J Mal Vasculaires* 1995;20:51.

164. Young MC, Richards RR, Hudson AR. Thoracic outlet syndrome with congenital pseudarthrosis of the clavicle: treatment by brachial plexus decompression, plate fixation and bone grafting. *Can J Surg* 1988;31:131.

165. Behringer BR, Wilson FC. Congenital pseudarthrosis of the clavicle. *Am J Dis Child* 1972;123:511.

166. Hirata S, Miya H, Mizuno K. Congenital pseudarthrosis of the clavicle. Histologic examination for the etiology of the disease. *Clin Orthop Rel Res* 1995;315:242.

167. Grogan DP, Love SM, Guidera KJ, et al. Operative treatment of congenital pseudarthrosis of the clavicle. *J Pediatr Orthop* 1991;11:176.

168. Schnall SB, King JD, Marrero G. Congenital pseudarthrosis of the clavicle: a review of the literature and surgical results of six cases. *J Pediatr Orthop* 1988;8:316.

169. Toledo LC, MacEwen GD. Severe complications of surgical treatment of congenital pseudarthrosis of the clavicle. *Clin Orthop Rel Res* 1979;139:64.

170. Mouchet A, Belot J. La tarsomegalie. *J Radiol Electrologie* 1926;10:289.

171. Trevor D. Tarso-epipysial aclasis. A congenital error of epiphysealis development. *J Bone Joint Surg Br* 1950;32:204.

172. Fairbank TJ. Dysplasia epiphysialis hemimelica. *J Bone Joint Surg Br* 1956;32:237–257.

173. DeVine JH, Rooney RC, Carpenter C, et al. Dysplasia epiphysealis hemimelica in an elderly patient. *Am J Orthop* 1997;26:223.

174. Azouz RM, Slomic AM, Marton D, et al. The variable manifestations of dysplasia epiphysealis hemimelica. *Pediatr Radiol* 1985;15:44.

175. Keret D, Spatz DK, Caro PA, et al. Dysplasia epiphysealis hemimelica: diagnosis and treatment. *J Pediatr Orthop* 1992;12:365.

176. Kuo RS, Bellemore MC, Monsell FP, et al. Dysplasia epiphysealis hemimelica: clinical features and management. *J Pediatr Orthop* 1998;18:543.

177. Graves SC, Kuester DJ, Richardson EG. Dysplasia epiphysealis hemimelica (Trevor disease) presenting as peroneal spastic flatfoot deformity: a case report. *Foot Ankle* 1991;12:55.

178. Heiple KG. Carpal osteochondroma. *J Bone Joint Surg Am* 1961;43:861.

179. Levi N, Ostgaard SE, Lund B. Dysplasia epiphysealis hemimelica (Trevor's disease) of the distal radius. *Acta Orthop Belgica* 1998;64:104.

180. Maylack FH, Manske PR, Strecker WB. Dysplasia epiphysealis hemimelica at the metacarpophalangeal joint. *J Hand Surg Am* 1988;13:916.

181. Mendez AA, Keret D, MacEwen GD. Isolated dysplasia epiphysealis hemimelica of the hip joint. *J Bone Joint Surg Am* 1988;70:921.

182. Saxton HM, Wilkinson JA. Hemimelica skeletal dysplasia. *J Bone Joint Surg Br* 1964;46:608.

183. Segal LS, Vrahas MS, Schwentker EP. Dysplasia epiphysealis hemimelica of the sacroiliac joint. *Clin Orthop Rel Res* 1996;333:202.

184. Iwasawa T, Aida N, Kobayashi N, et al. MRI findings of dysplasia epiphysealis hemimelica. *Pediatr Radiol* 1996;26:65.

185. Lang IM, Azouz EM. MRI appearances of dysplasia epiphysealis hemimelica of the knee. *Skeletal Radiol* 1997;26:226.

186. Peduto AJ, Frawley KJ, Bellemore MC, et al. MR imaging of dysplasia epiphysealis hemimelica: bony and soft-tissue abnormalities. *Am J Radiol* 1999;172:819.

187. Connor JM, Horan FT, Beighton P. Dysplasia epiphysealis hemimelica: clinical and genetic study. *J Bone Joint Surg Br* 1983;65:350.

188. Burton-Fanning FW, Vaughan AL. A case of myositis ossificans. *Lancet* 1901;2:849.

189. Gastor A. A case of myositis ossificans. *West London Med J* 1905;10:37.

190. Harris NH. Myositis ossificans progressiva. *Proc R Soc Med* 1961;54:70.

191. Kaplan FS, McCluskey W, Hahn G, et al. Genetic transmission of fibrodysplasia ossificans progressiva. *J Bone Joint Surg Am* 1993;75:1214.

192. Connor JM, Evans CC, Evans DAP. Cardiopulmonary function in fibrodysplasia ossificans progressiva. *Thorax* 1981;36:419.

193. Shafritz AB, Shore EM, Gannon FH, et al. Overexpression of an osteogenetic morphogen in fibrodysplasia ossificans progressiva. *N Engl J Med* 1996;335:555.

194. Lanchoney TF, Olmstead EA, Shore EM, et al. Characterization of bone morphogenetic protein 4 receptor in fibrodysplasia ossificans progressiva. *Clin Orthop Rel Res* 1998;346:38.

195. Xu M, Shore EM. Mutational screening of the bone morpho-

genetic protein 4 gene in a family with fibrodysplasia ossificans progressiva. *Clin Orthop Rel Res* 1998;346:53.

196. Connor JM, Evans DAP. Fibrodysplasia ossificans progressiva: the clinical features and natural history of 34 patients. *J Bone Joint Surg Br* 1982;64:76.

197. Cohen RB, Hahn GV, Tabas JA, et al. The natural history of heterotopic ossification in patients who have fibrodysplasia ossificans progressiva. A study of forty-four patients. *J Bone Joint Surg Am* 1993;75:215.

198. Shah PB, Zasloff MA, Drummond D, et al. Spinal deformity in patients who have fibrodysplasia ossificans progressiva. *J Bone Joint Surg Am* 1994;76:1442.

199. Sawyer JR, Klimkiewicz JJ, Iannotti JP, et al. Mechanism for superior subluxation of the glenohumeral joint in fibrodysplasia ossificans progressiva. *Clin Orthop Rel Res* 1998;346:130.

200. Kussmaul WG, Esmail AN, Sagar Y, et al. Pulmonary and cardiac function in advanced fibrodysplasia ossificans progressiva. *Clin Orthop Rel Res* 1998;346:104.

201. Kaplan FS, Tabas JA, Gannon FH, et al. The histopathology of fibrodysplasia ossificans progressiva. An endochondral process. *J Bone Joint Surg Am* 1993;75:220.

202. Brantus J, Meunier PJ. Effects of intravenous etidronate and oral corticosteroids in fibrodysplasia ossificans progressiva. *Clin Orthop Rel Res* 1998;346:117.

203. Kaplan FS, Sawyer J, Connors S, et al. Urinary basic fibroblast growth factor. A biochemical marker for preosseous fibroproliferative lesions in patients with fibrodysplasia ossificans progressiva. *Clin Orthop Rel Res* 1998;346:59.

204. Olmstead EA, Gannon FH, Wang Z, et al. Embryonic overexpression of c-fos protooncogene. A murine stem cell chimera applicable to the study of fibrodysplasia ossificans progressiva in humans. *Clin Orthop Rel Res* 1998;346:81.

205. Zasloff MA, Rocke DM, Crofford LJ, et al. Treatment of patients who have fibrodysplasia ossificans progressiva with isotretinoin. *Clin Orthop Rel Res* 1998:346:121.

Acquired Disorders

206. Heifetz SA, Galliana CA, DeRosa GP. Myositis (fasciitis) ossificans in an infant. *Pediatr Pathol* 1992;12:223.

207. Cushner FD, Morwessel RM. Myositis ossificans traumatica. *Orthop Rev* 1992;21:1319.

208. Boyd BM Jr, Roberts WM, Miller GR. Periarticular ossification following burns. *South Med J* 1959;52:1048.

209. Costello FV, Brown A. Myositis ossificans complicating anterior poliomyelitis. *J Bone Joint Surg Br* 1951;33:594.

210. Damanski M. Heterotopic ossification in paraplegia. A clinical study. *J Bone Joint Surg Br* 1961;43:286.

211. Evans EB. Orthopaedic measures in the treatment of severe burns. *J Bone Joint Surg Am* 1966;48:661.

212. Garland DE, Blum CE, Waters RL. Periarticular heterotopic ossification in head-injured adults. *J Bone Joint Surg Am* 1980; 62:1143.

213. Hardy AG, Dickson JW. Pathological ossification in traumatic paraplegia. *J Bone Joint Surg Br* 1963;45:76.

214. Ritter MA, Vaughn RB. Ectopic ossification after total hip arthroplasty. Predisposing factors, frequency, and effect on results. *J Bone Joint Surg Am* 1977;59:345.

215. Warren SB. Heterotopic ossification after total hip replacement. *Orthop Rev* 1990;19:603.

216. Wharton GW, Morgan TH. Ankylosis in the paralyzed patient. *J Bone Joint Surg Am* 1070;52:105.

217. Brook CG, Valman HB. Osteoma cutis and Albright's hereditary osteodystrophy. *Br J Dermatol* 1971;85:471.

218. Kaplan FS, Craver R, MacEwen GD, et al. Progressive osseous heteroplasia: a distinct developmental disorder of heterotopic ossification. *J Bone Joint Surg Am* 1994;76:425.

219. Letts M, Pang E, Carpenter B, et al. Parosteal fasciitis in children. *Am J Orthop* 1995;24:119.

220. Ogilvie-Harris DJ, Fornasier VL. Pseudomalignant myositis ossificans. Heterotopic new bone formation without a history of trauma. *J Bone Joint Surg Am* 1980;62:1274.

221. Illes T, Dubousset J, Szendroi M, et al. Characterization of bone-forming cells in post-traumatic myositis ossificans by lectins. *Pathol Res Pract* 1992;188:172.

222. Reilly TM, Seldes R, Luchetti W, et al. Similarities in the phenotype expression of pericytes and bone cells. *Clin Orthop Rel Res* 1998;346:95.

223. Ackerman LV. Extra-osseous localized non-neoplastic bone and cartilage formation. *J Bone Joint Surg Am* 1958;40:279.

224. Hughston J, Whatley G, Stone M. Myositis ossificans traumatica. *South Med J* 1962;55:1167.

225. Thorndike A. Myositis ossificans traumatica. *J Bone Joint Surg* 1940;22:315.

226. Jackson P, Feagin JA. Quadriceps contusion in young athletes: relationship of severity of injury to treatment and prognosis. *J Bone Joint Surg Am* 1973;55:95.

227. Siffert RS. Classification of the osteochondroses. *Clin Orthop Rel Res* 1981;158:10.

228. Carlson CS, Meuten DJ, Richardson DC. Ischemic necrosis of cartilage in spontaneous and experimental lesions of osteochondrosis. *J Orthop Res* 1991;9:317.

229. Chiroff RT, Cooke CP. Osteochondritis dissecans: a histologic and microradiographic analysis of surgically excised lesions. *J Trauma* 1975;15:689.

230. Borges JLP, Guille JT, Bowen JR. Kohler's bone disease of the tarsal navicular. *J Pediatr Orthop* 1995;15:596.

231. Green WT, Banke HH. Osteochondritis dissecans in children. *J Bone Joint Surg Am* 1953;35:26.

232. Van Demark RE. Osteochondritis dissecans with spontaneous healing. *J Bone Joint Surg Am* 1952;34:143.

233. Hnevkovsky O. Progressive fibrosis of the vastus intermedius muscle in children. *J Bone Joint Surg Br* 1961;43:318.

234. Karlen A. Congenital fibrosis of the vastus intermedius muscle. *J Bone Joint Surg Br* 1984;46:488.

235. Uhthoff HK, Ogata S. Early intrauterine presence of congenital dislocation of the knee. *J Pediatr Orthop* 1994;14:254.

236. Gunn DR. Contracture of the quadriceps muscle. A discussion on the etiology and relationship to recurrent dislocation of the patella. *J Bone Joint Surg Br* 1964;46:492.

237. Sengupta S. Pathogenesis of infantile quadriceps fibrosis and its correction by proximal release. *J Pediatr Orthop* 1985;5:187.

238. Shanmugasundaram TK. Post-injection fibrosis of skeletal muscle: a clinical problem. A personal series of 169 cases. *Int Orthop* 1980;4:31.

239. Fairbank TJ, Barrett AM. Vastus intermedius contracture in early childhood. *J Bone Joint Surg Br* 1961;43:326.

240. Hollaert P, Adijns P, Destoop N, et al. Review of the literature on quadriceps fibrosis and study of 11 cases. *Acta Orthop Belg* 1975;41:255.

241. Makhani JS. Quadriceps fibrosis. A complication of intramuscular injections in the thigh. *Indian J Pediatr* 1971;38:54.

242. Fulkerson JP, Gossling HR. Anatomy of the knee joint lateral retinaculum. *Clin Orthop Rel Res* 1980;153:183.

243. Jeffreys TE. Recurrent dislocation of the patella due to abnormal attachment of the iliotibial tract. *J Bone Joint Surg Br* 1963;45:740.

244. Williams PF. Quadriceps contractures. *J Bone Joint Surg Br* 1968;50:278.

245. Wilder RT, Berde CB, Wolohan M, et al. Reflex sympathetic dystrophy in children. *J Bone Joint Surg Am* 1992;74:910.

246. Cimaz R, Matucci-Cerinic M, Zulian F, et al. Reflex sympathetic dystrophy in children. *J Child Neurol* 1999;14:363.

247. Schott GD. An unsympathetic view of pain. *Lancet* 1995;345:634.

248. Stanton-Hicks M, Janig W, Hassenbusch S, et al. Reflex sympathetic dystrophy: changing concepts and taxonomy. *Pain* 1995;63:127.

249. Bernstein BH, Singsen BH, Kent TJ, et al. Reflex sympathetic dystrophy in children. *J Pediatr* 1978;43:211.

250. Dietz FR, Matthews KD, Montgomery WJ. Reflex sympathetic dystrophy in children. *Clin Orthop* 1990;258:225.

251. Stanton-Hicks M, Barn R, Boas R, et al. Complex regional pain syndromes: guidelines for therapy. *Clin J Pain* 1998;14:155.

252. Sherry DD, Weisman R. Psychological aspects of childhood reflex neurovascular dystrophy. *Pediatrics* 1988;81:572.

253. Lynch ME. Psychological aspects of reflex sympathetic dystrophy: a review of the adult and paediatric literature. *Pain* 1992;49:337.

254. Schwartzman RJ, McLellan TL. Reflex sympathetic dystrophy: a review. *Arch Neurol* 1987;44:555.

255. Veldman PHJM, Reynen HM, Arntz IE, et al. Signs and symptoms of reflex sympathetic dystrophy: prospective study of 829 patients. *Lancet* 1993;342:1012.

256. Merskey H, Bagduk N, eds. *Classification of chronic pain,* 2nd ed. Seattle, WA: IASP, 1994.

257. Pillemer FG, Micheli LJ. Psychological considerations in youth sports. *Clin Sports Med* 1988;7:679.

258. Laxer RM, Allen RC, Malleson PN. Technetium 99m–methylene diphosphonate bone scans in children with reflex neurovascular dystrophy. *J Pediatr* 1985;106:437.

259. Ochoa JL. Pain mechanisms in neuropathy. *Curr Opin Neurol* 1994;7:407.

260. Silber JJ, Magid M. Reflex sympathetic dystrophy in children and adolescents. *Am J Dev Child* 1988;142:1325.

261. Berde CB, Sethna NF, Micheli LJ. A technique for continuous lumbar sympathetic blockade for severe reflex sympathetic dystrophy in children and adolescents. *Anesth Analg* 1988;67(suppl):514.

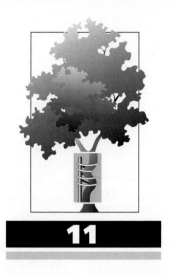

11

DISEASES RELATED TO THE HEMATOPOIETIC SYSTEM

WALTER B. GREENE

The hematopoietic system includes the circulating blood, the bone marrow, the spleen, the lymph nodes, and reticuloendothelial cells scattered throughout the body. The multiple cells that compose the hematopoietic system lead to a large number and variety of disorders. This chapter focuses on pediatric disorders of the hematopoietic system that affect the musculoskeletal system

W. B. Greene: Department of Orthopaedic Surgery, University of Missouri Health Science Center, Columbia, Missouri 65212.

BONE MARROW FAILURE SYNDROMES

Erythrocytes, granulocytes, and platelets develop in the bone marrow, and bone marrow failure syndromes are characterized by failure of the bone marrow to produce these cells (1). Some of these disorders cause a pancytopenia, and some syndromes affect only one or two of the bone marrow cell lines. Fanconi anemia, Diamond-Blackfan anemia, Schwachman-Diamond syndrome, cartilage-hair hypoplasia, and thrombocytopenia with absent radius syndrome are the five inherited bone marrow failure syndromes that have a significant association with congenital skeletal abnormalities (2). It is important for the orthopaedic surgeon to understand these syndromes, because the hematologic abnormalities associated with these disorders typically present after the skeletal problems have been diagnosed.

Fanconi Anemia

Fanconi anemia is an autosomal recessive disorder that ultimately causes pancytopenia (1,3). Onset of the pancytopenia is typically delayed, and in 995 patients, the average age at diagnosis of aplastic anemia was 7.8 years in boys and 8.8 years in girls (1). A few patients have onset of hematologic abnormalities in either infancy or the adult years, with 4% having these disorders diagnosed in the first year of life and 10% after 15 years of age.

The classic anomalies associated with Fanconi anemia include short stature, hypoplastic or absent thumbs, café-au-lait or hypopigmented spots, and a characteristic facial appearance with a broad nose, epicanthal folds, and micrognathia. Children who develop the pancytopenia at an early age are more likely to have associated abnormalities. For example, upper-limb anomalies occur in 48% of all patients, but are noted in 68% of patients who are diagnosed before 1 year of age (1). The most common skeletal anomaly is hypoplasia, or absence of the thumb. Radial hemimelia may also occur. In a review of 68 patients with Fanconi anemia, hypoplasia was seen in 25 patients, and radial hemimelia associated with absence or deficiency of the thumb was observed in 9 patients (3). Other skeletal abnormalities are less frequent, and include Klippel-Feil syndrome, Sprengel deformity, hip dislocation, and syndactyly of the second and third toes.

Thrombocytopenia is usually the first hematologic manifestation. Granulocytopenia and anemia follow, in that order. The cause of the anemia is not well understood, but the diagnosis of Fanconi anemia can be confirmed by detecting chromosome breaks after culturing the lymphocytes with DNA cross-linking agents.

If treatment of the pancytopenia is limited to blood transfusions, 80% of patients die within 2 years. Androgens, combined with corticosteroids, are the first line of therapy, and may result in remission; however, almost all responders must remain on androgen therapy. Bone marrow transplantation offers a cure for the aplastic anemia and leukemia. The International Bone Marrow Transplant Registry reported a 66% 2-year probability of survival in 151 patients transplanted from a human leukocyte antigen (HLA)–identical sibling, and 29% survival in 48 patients transplanted from an alternative donor (4).

Fanconi anemia is a premalignant condition; at least 15% of patients develop leukemia, myelodysplastic syndrome, liver tumors, or other cancers (1). To decrease the risk of DNA damage to other tissues, pretransplantation preparation of patients with Fanconi anemia should include a lower dose of cyclophosphamide, and no irradiation. However, a

secondary malignancy after transplantation is still relatively common in Fanconi anemia (5).

Diamond-Blackfan Anemia

Diamond-Blackfan anemia is a rare, single cytopenic type of bone marrow failure. The anemia develops by 1 year of age in 90% of patients (6). In a review of 527 cases, associated malformations were observed in 24% of patients (1). Dysmorphic facial features, upper limb anomalies, and short stature are most common. Anomalies of the thumb are the most common skeletal abnormality, with triphalangeal thumbs present in 19 of the 527 patients (1). Other anomalies of the radial aspect of the hand include subluxed or hypoplastic thumbs, and flattening of the thenar eminence. Incomplete radial hemimelia has been reported, but forearm deficits are uncommon in Diamond-Blackfan anemia (7). Klippel-Feil syndrome occurs in approximately 1% of patients.

Infants with Diamond-Blackfan syndrome typically are healthy at birth, but develop the insidious onset of listlessness, irritability, and pallor by the age of 2 to 3 months, or later in the first year of life. The anemia, however, may be present at birth, or may develop after 1 year of age. Laboratory studies demonstrate a striking normocytic anemia, with hemoglobin levels of 3 to 4 g/dL. Platelet and white blood cell counts are usually normal. Bone marrow aspirates typically show erythroid hypoplasia, but no depression of granulocyte or platelet precursors. Some cases are familial, and some of the inherited cases have been linked to chromosome 19q (6). The pathogenesis of Diamond-Blackfan anemia is uncertain, but the variable presentations and the variable responses to hematopoietic growth factors suggest multiple causes (1,8).

The first line of therapy is corticosteroids, and the overall response rate is approximately 70%. The most common pattern of the responders is a long-term dependence on steroid medications, but at a reduced dosage. Supportive transfusions and chelation therapy are necessary for patients who do not respond to steroids. Experience with bone marrow transplantation is limited, but six of eight children who underwent transplantation from HLA-identical siblings were reported to be alive 5 to 87 months after surgery, with no evidence of anemia (9). Leukemia (nine cases) and osteogenic sarcoma (one case) have been described in patients who did not respond to steroids (10).

Schwachman-Diamond Syndrome

Schwachman-Diamond syndrome is an autosomal recessive disorder characterized by exocrine pancreatic insufficiency and neutropenia. Except for cystic fibrosis, Schwachman-Diamond syndrome is the most common cause of pancreatic insufficiency in children (1). These children present during the first year of life with failure to thrive, malabsorption, steatorrhea, and frequent respiratory and cutaneous infections (1,11,12).

Musculoskeletal problems are common in Schwachman-Diamond syndrome (1,11–13). In a review of 21 patients that included routine skeletal surveys, all patients were noted to have skeletal abnormalities, ranging from metaphyseal chondrodysplasia to delayed bone maturation (11). Proportionate short stature and delayed bone age were always present, and were initially noted between the first and second year of life. Metaphyseal chondrodysplasia, mainly affecting the hips, was observed in 13 of the 21 patients; however, this may be an underestimation, because the radiographic features of metaphyseal chondrodysplasia may not be obvious in older adolescents or adults. Marked coxa vara was noted in 4 of the 13 patients with metaphyseal chondrodysplasia. Clinodactyly (48%), long-bone tubulation associated with genu varum (33%), and abnormally short ribs with flared anterior ends (47%) also were observed (11). A type II bifid thumb also has been reported (14).

In addition to the pancreatic insufficiency, neutropenia associated with skin and respiratory infections is typically found during infancy or early childhood. Laboratory studies show normal sweat chloride tests, but excessive fecal fat and deficient pancreatic trypsin, lipase, and amylase in the stool and duodenal secretions. Pancreatic biopsies demonstrate preservation of the islets of Langerhans, but fatty tissue replacement of the remainder of the organ.

Intermittent neutropenia, with the neutrophil count periodically being less than 1500/mm^3, is seen in approximately two-thirds of patients, and is constant in the remainder. Impaired chemotaxis is present in all patients (12). Intermittent thrombocytopenia and mild anemia also may develop. Pancytopenia was noted in 44 of 200 patients, at an average age of 9 years (1). Bone marrow aspirates may appear normal, but they usually show decreased cellularity or myeloid maturation arrest.

Treatment for patients with Schwachman-Diamond syndrome includes high doses of oral pancreatic enzymes (1). This significantly improves the malabsorption, but does not affect either limb growth or neutropenia. Respiratory and sinus tract infections are frequent, but these respond to prompt treatment with antibiotics. Although the malabsorption seems to improve with age, infections continue to be a problem.

Leukemia develops in 5 to 10% of patients (1), but this may be an underestimation, because in one study, myelodysplastic syndrome was found in 7 of 21 patients (12).

Cartilage-hair Hypoplasia

Cartilage-hair hypoplasia is an autosomal recessive, short-limbed, metaphyseal chondrodysplasia associated with defective cell-mediated immunity. McKusick and colleagues (15) originally described the clinical and genetic characteristics of this disorder in 77 patients belonging to the Old Amish sect. Cartilage-hair hypoplasia has subsequently been described in the non-Amish population, and a review of 63 such patients found similar clinical and laboratory manifestations to those of the Amish population (16). Of note, more than 100 Finnish patients have also been described (17).

Hair that is fine, sparse, and unpigmented, as well as short stature (lower than the third percentile), are consistent findings (15,16). The limbs are disproportionately short. These patients superficially resemble people with achondroplasia; however, the sparse, unpigmented hair and normal-sized skull permit ready differentiation. Furthermore, narrowing of the interpedicular distance is absent.

Immunodeficiency in cartilage-hair hypoplasia was first suspected because of an atypical response to varicella infection. McKusick and colleagues (15) observed that two patients died of this disease, and three others had such virulent attacks that smallpox was seriously considered. The immunologic defects are quite variable, ranging from mild lymphopenia to severe combined immunodeficiency syndrome. Chronic neutropenia and anemia may also occur (16–18). Recurrent viral respiratory tract infections are common during childhood, but in many patients the impaired cellular immunity is mild enough that adults with cartilage-hair hypoplasia have no health problems. Some children, however, have severe problems with recurrent respiratory tract infections and failure to thrive. Bone marrow transplantation may be required (19,20). Although bone marrow transplantation may correct the immune deficiency, it does not change the deficient growth and chondrodysplasia (19). Because vaccine-related illness may occur, vaccination should be performed only with attenuated virus.

The gene for cartilage-hair hypoplasia has been localized to 9p21-p13 (21). Selective defective expression of early-activation genes may be the underlying defect in cartilage-hair hypoplasia (20). This could explain the multisystem nature of the disease.

Thrombocytopenia with Absent Radius Syndrome

Thrombocytopenia with absent radius (TAR) syndrome is a unique autosomal recessive condition characterized by bilateral absence of the radius, with the thumbs being present. Retention of the thumbs distinguishes TAR from Fanconi anemia and trisomy 18. In the latter two diseases, the thumbs are absent if the radius is absent (1). The diagnosis of TAR also is aided by early manifestations of thrombocytopenia (22,23). Sixty percent of these patients have hemorrhagic problems within the first week of life, and 95% by 4 months (1).

The anomalies in 100 patients with TAR have been reviewed and summarized (24) (Table 11-1). In addition to the intercalary radial hemimelia, other anomalies of the upper extremity may occur, including hypoplasia of the

TABLE 11-1. SKELETAL DEFICIENCY IN THROMBOCYTOPENIA WITH ABSENT RADIUS SYNDROME

Deficiency	Presence/Number of Patients with Adequate Documentation
Upper extremity	
Bilateral absent radius	99/100
Unilateral absent radius	1/100
Thumbs present	100/100
Thumbs hypoplastic	48/92
Ulnar involvement	50/68
Short and bowed	35
Unilaterally absent	3
Bilaterally absent	12
Humerus involvement	36/87
Hypoplastic	22
Absent	14
Shoulder girdle involvement (hypoplastic or absent scapula and clavicle)	10/49
Middle phalanx of the little finger (hypoplastic and absent)	35/41
Lower extremity	
Hip dislocation	6/79
Lower extremity phocomelia	5/100
Stiff knee	9/100
Genu varum	29/92
Patella abnormalities	13/92
Clubfoot	4/100
Face	
Mandibular hypoplasia	11/79

(Adapted from ref. 24, with permission.)

thumb, clinodactyly of the little finger associated with hypoplasia of the middle phalanx, ulnar shortening and bowing, and short or absent humeri that are typically bilateral. Klippel-Feil syndrome and/or scapular hypoplasia also is observed.

Lower-extremity abnormalities occur in 40% of patients (1). Most lower-extremity abnormalities in TAR syndrome are concentrated at the knee, but dislocation of the hip and clubfoot may occur. Genu varum, associated with flexion contracture and internal tibial torsion, was the most common abnormality recorded by Schoenecker and colleagues (25) in their detailed description of 21 patients. Absence or hypoplasia of the patella, sometimes accompanied by either lateral or medial dislocation, also was observed.

Hypoplasia of the medial femoral condyle is a primary factor in the genu varum and joint malalignment. Recurrent varus is a frequent finding after osteotomies and patella realignment procedures (25). Gounder and colleagues (26) reported on soft tissue release of the knee, followed by postoperative bracing, but did not provide adequate information concerning long-term follow-up to determine whether soft tissue release performed at an early age is better than osteotomy for the knee deformities in TAR.

Micrognathia secondary to mandibular hypoplasia also may be present (Table 11-1). Cardiac anomalies have been reported in 10% of patients, with tetralogy of Fallot, atrial septal defect, and ventricular septal defect being the most common lesions (1).

Thrombocytopenia may necessitate a delay in centralization of the hand and wrist (Fig. 11-1). Early and prolonged splinting, combined with frequent stretching exercises, will prevent progressive contractures (27). With shortening of the humerus and the ulna, centralization may be contraindicated.

Thrombocytopenia in patients with TAR syndrome tends to be episodic and is precipitated by nonspecific stresses, such as upper respiratory tract infections and gastrointestinal disturbances (1,23). During infancy, the platelet count is typically in the range of 15,000 to 30,000/mm³ but may be more depressed. Periodic leukemoid reactions may be observed, and may temporally correlate with the thrombocytopenic episodes. Because platelet function is normal, bleeding tendencies correlate with platelet counts. Supportive therapy with platelet transfusions has significantly altered the mortality risk during infancy. Steroids or splenectomy is not necessary.

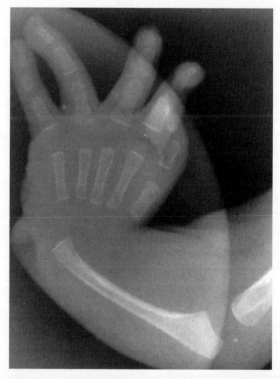

FIGURE 11-1. Anteroposterior radiograph of the left hand of a 1-month-old infant with bilateral radial hemimelia and essentially normal thumbs. Patient was started on a program of progressive casting and splinting, with anticipation of centralization at 6 months of age. At age 2 months, laboratory studies, obtained for evaluation of gastroenteritis, revealed thrombocytopenia with a platelet count of 17,000/mm³. Low platelet count continued, and centralization of the wrist was delayed.

The prognosis for patients with TAR syndrome is good. Only one case of leukemia has been reported (28). The thrombocytopenia typically resolves by early childhood, and platelet counts of more than 100,000 cells/μL are typical after the first year. Reconstructive operations can be performed at that time.

DISORDERS OF ERYTHROCYTES

The erythrocyte, with its unique hemoglobin molecule, delivers oxygen from the lungs to the tissue, and transports carbon dioxide in the opposite direction. The intravascular journey of an erythrocyte is approximately 175 miles in its normal life span of 120 days. Anemia is the result of a reduced number of erythrocytes, or of a reduced life span of the erythrocyte, or both. Any process that disrupts production, alters the structure of the erythrocyte, or impairs the function of the hemoglobin molecule can cause anemia.

Iron-deficiency Anemia

Iron-deficiency anemia (IDA) is the most common nutritional deficiency in the western world, and the most common cause of anemia (29). The peak incidence is between 4 months and 3 years of age, and during adolescence. Iron-deficiency anemia causes lethargy, easy fatigability, blue sclerae, koilonychia, and, during infancy, growth retardation and impaired cognitive development. The mechanism by which IDA impairs cognitive development is unclear. Marrow hyperplasia accompanies severe IDA, and radiographs of the skull may show widening of the diploic space with striations (30). Although skeletal abnormalities and low body weight resolve with treatment, developmental deficiencies, secondary to chronic IDA in young children, are not fully reversible (31,32).

Prevention is critically important, and includes iron supplementation during pregnancy, and selective screening (29,33,34). Risk factors during early childhood include the following: premature and low-birth-weight infants; infants fed a diet of non–iron-fortified infant formula for more than 2 months; infants introduced to cow's milk before age 12 months; breast-fed infants who, after age 6 months, do not receive supplemental iron-fortified food or formula; children who consume more than 24 oz of cow's milk daily; and children who have special health care needs (29,33). Adolescent girls also develop IDA. Risk factors for this group include poor nutrition, increased duration or frequency of menstrual flow, chronic use of certain analgesic medications, and prolonged training for long-distance running (35,36).

The orthopaedic surgeon most likely will encounter iron-deficiency anemia during the preoperative evaluation; however, determination of hemoglobin levels for all preoperative patients is not necessary (37). The author performs this test on adolescent girls who have started menstruating, or who have other risk factors, on infants at risk, who did not receive adequate supplementation, and on any patient whose history or physical examination suggests anemia. Hemoglobin levels of less than 11 g/dL in infants, and less than 12 g/dL in adolescents, should be evaluated and treated. Patients who have mild anemia can be given a 4-week therapeutic trial of iron. An increase in hemoglobin of 1 g/dL is considered diagnostic of iron-deficiency anemia (29). Severe anemia, or anemia occurring during the middle period of growth, requires more extensive laboratory studies to exclude other diagnostic possibilities.

Sickle Cell Disease

Approximately 1 of every 300 African-American people has sickle cell disease (38). The three common genotypes for sickle cell disease are:

- SS disease, which is homozygous for hemoglobin S
- SC disease, which is heterozygous for hemoglobin S and hemoglobin C
- Sβ disease, which is heterozygous for hemoglobin S and hemoglobin β-thalassemia

People with the sickle cell trait are heterozygous for hemoglobin S and a normal β-globulin chain. They have no clinical problems under physiologic conditions, and may participate in athletic events without restriction.

Hemoglobin S results from an abnormality of the β-globulin gene on chromosome 11, which causes substitution of valine for glutamic acid at the sixth codon from the amino terminus (39). Hemoglobin C occurs when lysine is substituted for the same glutamic acid affected in hemoglobin S (40). Patients with SC disease have similar, but less frequent, complications than patients with SS disease. The *β-thalassemia* gene causes reduced synthesis of the β-globulin polypeptide. Patients with Sβ disease have clinical manifestations that depend on the output of the *β-thalassemia* gene. If no hemoglobin A is produced, the patients are listed as having Sβ^0 disease, and have a clinical course comparable to that of patients with SS disease. If there is some production of hemoglobin A from the *β-thalassemia* gene, the patients are classified as having Sβ^+ disease, and have a milder clinical course, similar to that seen with SC disease.

Vasoocclusion and hemolysis are the basic pathologic events in sickle cell disease. When hemoglobin S is deoxygenated, it polymerizes and changes to a gel of intertwined fibers (39). As a result, the erythrocyte becomes distorted, fragile, and is rapidly destroyed. The paradox is that sickle cells are not only more fragile, but are relatively rigid and more viscous. Therefore, in addition to increased hemolysis, these erythrocytes clog small blood vessels and infarct tissues. Other factors, such as cellular dehydration from enhanced potassium chloride cotransport, and adhesion of SS erythrocytes to the endothelium, play a role in the vasoocclusion.

The rate and extent of polymer formation depends on the degree of deoxygenation of the cell, the intracellular concentration of hemoglobin, and the amount of hemoglobin F. Because the transit time in the microcirculation is typically short, polymers do not form in most SS cells as they complete the circulatory route. However, anything that retards the transit time can affect the degree of polymerization. In addition, the relatively slow circulation in bone makes it a target organ for vasoocclusion.

Considerable heterogeneity is observed in patients with sickle cell disease. The basis of this clinical variability is not fully understood, but probably involves a variety of genetic and environmental factors. Patients who have hereditary persistence of fetal hemoglobin have mild disease. The concomitant presence of *α-thalassemia* genes in patients with hemoglobin SS causes the erythrocytes to be smaller and lighter. These patients have higher hemoglobin levels and fewer reticulocytes, but are at greater risk for vasoocclusive disorders (41). Environmental factors, such as nutrition, public health measures, rates of immunization, and access to medical care, affect the rate and degree of complications. In the United States, 50% of patients with sickle cell disease survive beyond the fifth decade, but less than 2% survive to the age of 5 years in parts of Africa (42,43).

The clinical manifestations of sickle cell disease in children are listed in Table 11-2. Good pediatric preventive care minimizes the risk of some of these complications (44).

Vaccinations for pneumococcus, hepatitis B, and *Haemophilus influenzae* should be given in a timely fashion. Prophylactic penicillin, started at the time of diagnosis and continued until 5 years of age, diminishes the risk of bacteremia. Early evaluation and treatment of febrile illnesses reduces the risk of sepsis.

Although their birth weight is normal, subsequent growth and development are delayed in children with sickle cell disease. The salient findings of the Cooperative Study of Sickle Cell Disease, sponsored by the National Institutes of Health, include the following: weight is affected more than height; patients with SS and $S\beta^0$ disease demonstrate more delay in growth than patients with SC and $S\beta^+$ disease; and, in general, by the end of adolescence patients have caught up with controls in height, but not weight (45). Increased hemolysis and greater metabolic requirements for erythropoiesis, as well as a greater number of infectious episodes, probably explain the delay in growth. Sexual development is also delayed in sickle cell disease, and the delay in attaining different Tanner stages also is affected by the type of sickle cell disease (45).

Sickle cell disease is the most common cause of stroke in children (46), and, in 4,082 patients, the incidence of cerebrovascular events was highest during the childhood years (47). Exchange transfusion at the time of the acute infarction minimizes the risk of permanent impairment (40). The risk of recurrent stroke is approximately 50 to 70%, if children with sickle cell disease are untreated. A prophylactic transfusion program, which keeps hemoglobin

TABLE 11-2. CLINICAL FEATURES OF SICKLE CELL DISEASE IN CHILDREN

Vasoocclusive complications	
Crises	Frequent in some, uncommon in others
Dactylitis	In children younger than 6 years old
Osteonecrosis	Prognosis and manifestations less severe, compared with adults
Priapism	Onset after age 10 years; in children, episodes tend to be muliple short episodes
Splenic sequestration	More common in children younger than 2 years of age, often preceded by infection
Stroke	Four to 8% of children with SS disease; peak incidence is at 3 to 8 years of age; silent central nervous system damage and cognitive impairment more frequent
Acute chest syndrome	More common in children, but more severe in adults; may occur in postoperative period; most common cause of death after 10 years of age
Complications of hemolysis	
Anemia	Hematocrit = 15 to 30 in SS disease, higher in SC disease
Cholelithiasis	May occur in children, present in most adults
Acute aplastic episodes	Associated with parvovirus
Infection complications	
Sepsis	Most common cause of death in young children; *Streptococcus pneumoniae* most common
Osteomyelitis	*Salmonella* and *Staphylococcus aureus*
Septic arthritis	Relatively uncommon
Reactive arthritis	May be triggered by *Salmonella enteritidis*

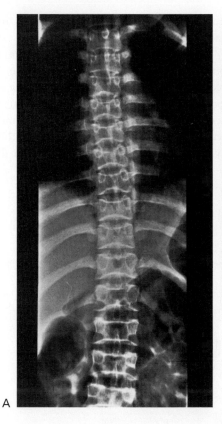

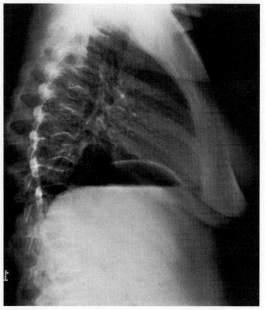

FIGURE 11-2. Sixteen-year-old girl with sickle cell anemia. Anteroposterior (**A**) and lateral (**B**) radiographs of the spine show the typical biconcavity of multiple vertebrae.

S levels at less than 30%, reduces the rate of recurrent infarction to approximately 10 to 15% (40,48). More controversial is whether children at risk for stroke, as identified by Doppler ultrasonography, should undergo the potentially harmful long-term prophylactic transfusion therapy (49,50).

Bone and joint problems in sickle cell disease include the sickle cell crises, dactylitis, osteonecrosis, osteomyelitis, septic arthritis, reactive arthritis, and leg ulcers. In addition, hemolytic anemia in these patients causes erythroid hyperplasia of the bone marrow, with resultant increased size of the medullary spaces, and osteopenia. The spine is more likely to demonstrate the effect of marrow hyperplasia. Thinning of the cortices and trabeculae lead to collapse, with development of a biconcave "fish" vertebra and mild structural changes (Fig. 11-2). Two studies have shown decreased bone mineral density in children with sickle cell disease (51,52), but, fortunately, the osteopenia in most patients has limited clinical significance.

A sickle cell crisis is the most common cause of extremity and spinal pain in patients with sickle cell disease. In a study of 3,578 patients, the average rate of crisis requiring medical treatment was 0.8 per year in SS disease, 1.0 per year in Sβ^0 disease, and 0.4 per year in SC and Sβ^+ disease (53). An elevated fetal hemoglobin level was associated with a lower rate of crises. Considerable variation, however, occurs within groups, and 39% of the SS disease patients recorded no painful episodes requiring treatment.

A sickle cell crisis results from a localized area of infarction. Back or extremity pain is secondary to bone marrow infarction, whereas abdominal pain is most likely secondary to infarction in the intestines (54,55). The excruciating pain associated with a crises is secondary to the resultant inflammatory response. Levels of substance P, a known stimulator of tumor necrosis factor and interleukin-8, are elevated in patients with sickle cell disease, and increase further during a crisis (56).

The humerus, tibia, and femur are the most common sites of long-bone infarction in children (54). Swelling and limitation of motion are typically mild. Temperature elevation is usually low grade, but 21% of the episodes reported by Keeley and Buchanan (54) involved a temperature greater than 39°C. A sickle cell crisis typically lasts 3 to 5 days. Supportive measures are the mainstay of therapy. With severe pain, parenteral opiates should be given at frequent, fixed intervals until the pain has diminished (43).

Dactylitis, or hand–foot syndrome, is secondary to infarction of a bone in the hand or foot, and frequently is the first clinical manifestation seen after hemoglobin F has been replaced by hemoglobin S. The typical patient is a child younger than 2 years of age, who presents with an acutely swollen hand or foot (57–59). In a prospective study, Stevens and colleagues (59) reported a 45% incidence of dactylitis, with 41% of the affected patients demonstrating recurrent episodes until 4 years of age. Radiographic findings are similar in dactylitis and osteomyelitis, with initial radiographs demonstrating soft tissue swelling, and subsequent examinations characterized by periosteal elevation, subperiosteal bone reaction, bone lysis, and ultimately, bone reformation (58). The problem of dactylitis ceases with the disappearance of hematopoietic marrow in the hands and feet,

and no series has reported this condition in patients older than 6 years of age.

The risk of osteomyelitis and other infections is more common in patients with sickle cell disease. This is attributable to a combination of factors, including splenic dysfunction, defective mechanisms of opsonization and complement function, and episodes of bacteremia secondary to localized bowel infarction. Fortunately, the rate of osteomyelitis is relatively low, compared with the incidence of

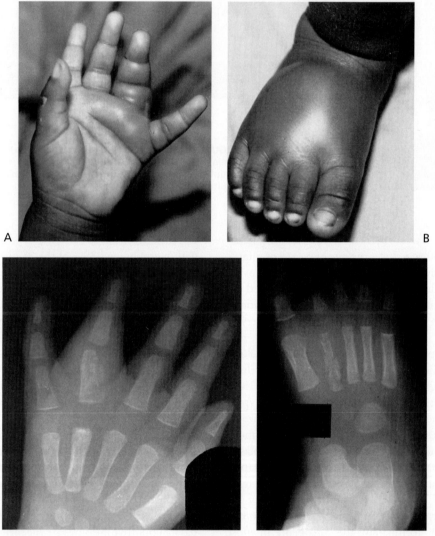

FIGURE 11-3. Osteomyelitis in a 7-month-old boy with sickle cell anemia. Patient presented with swelling of the hand and foot. Initial diagnosis was dactylitis. Because of persistent swelling and elevated temperature, aspiration was performed 48 h after admission. Purulent material was obtained, and cultures demonstrated *Salmonella* organisms. Antibiotic therapy, and surgical drainage of the hand and foot, successfully resolved the infection. **A:** Forty-eight h after admission, the hand shows marked swelling in the region of the ring finger. **B:** Forty-eight h after admission, there is swelling on the dorsum of the foot. **C:** Anteroposterior radiograph of the hand on the 15th hospital day. **D:** Anteroposterior radiograph of the foot on the 15th hospital day. Osteolysis and periosteal elevation are noted in the proximal phalanx of the ring finger and the second metatarsal. Although this patient had osteomyelitis, the radiographic appearance also is consistent with a healing dactylitis. (From ref. 62, with permission.)

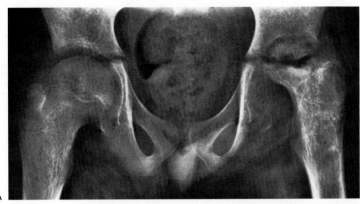
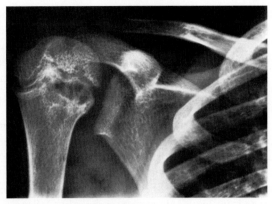

A

B

FIGURE 11-4. Eight-year-old boy with sickle cell anemia, who presented with high fever and bilateral shoulder and left hip pain. Cultures from the left hip and right shoulder demonstrated *Salmonella* organisms. **A:** Pelvic radiograph 4 months after diagnosis demonstrates progressive destruction of the left femoral head, as a result of osteonecrosis from the concomitant septic arthritis and osteomyelitis. **B:** Anteroposterior radiograph of the right shoulder demonstrates osteolytic changes in the humeral head and the metaphysis. Similar changes were observed on the contralateral side.

sickle cell crises. Dalton and colleagues (60) observed a 1.6% incidence of osteomyelitis per admission for musculoskeletal complaints in children with sickle cell disease.

The unique features of osteomyelitis in sickle cell anemia include a high incidence of *Salmonella* and multifocal infections, and delay in diagnosis. In reviewing the nine studies of osteomyelitis in sickle cell anemia, published from 1981 to 1996, Burnett et al. (61) observed that *Salmonella* was the most common infecting organism, and that the overall ratio of *Salmonella* to *Staphylococcus aureus* was 1.4 to 1. Interestingly, the incidence of *Salmonella* was relatively high in studies from centers in the United States, the ratio of *Salmonella* to *S. aureus* being 5.1 to 1 in this population. Other Gram-negative enteric bacilli are almost as common as *S. aureus* as a cause of osteomyelitis in sickle cell disorders. Capillary occlusion and infarction of gut mucosa account for the high incidence of both *Salmonella* and the other Gram-negative enteric organisms.

The key to minimizing complications, such as chronic osteomyelitis and multifocal sites, is early recognition (Figs. 11-3 and 11-4). However, differentiating a sickle cell crisis or dactylitis from osteomyelitis may be difficult. The degrees of fever and leukocytosis overlap, and the initial radiographs do not show abnormalities in either disorder. In addition, because of the shape of the erythrocyte, the erythrocyte sedimentation rate is unreliable in sickle cell disorders. Furthermore, the usual radionuclide and magnetic resonance imaging studies are inconclusive (63). As a result, appropriate treatment of osteomyelitis may be delayed (62,64,65). Although various combinations, such as sequential gallium scans, have been reported to be useful, the reliability and radiation exposure of these techniques have led experienced observers to comment that these tests, as well as magnetic resonance imaging, do not reliably differentiate infarction from infection (63,66,67).

Osteomyelitis should be considered when a child presenting with an apparent crisis or dactylitis, has a temperature greater than 39°C, an unusual degree of pain, and a "left shift" in the peripheral leukocyte count (62,66). Blood cultures, as well as aspiration or open biopsy of the affected bone, may be necessary to differentiate these two clinical problems, and should be performed whenever the diagnosis is uncertain. Ultrasonography also should be considered in the evaluation process. In a recent study, Sadat-Ali et al. (68) observed that ultrasonography routinely demonstrated periosteal elevation in sickle cell patients who had osteomyelitis, but did not show abnormalities in patients with infarction.

If osteomyelitis is a possibility, antibiotic therapy is instituted with chloramphenicol or ampicillin to cover *Salmonella*, and with oxacillin to provide protection against *S. aureus*. The emergence of resistant *Salmonella* species has caused some authors to suggest that a newer β-lactam or quinolone should be used as the initial antibiotic (69,70). With a delay in diagnosis, surgical drainage and prolonged parenteral antibiotic therapy is needed. The wound should be left open when a large subperiosteal abscess is present (65).

Pathologic fractures complicating long-bone osteomyelitis are more common in patients with sickle cell anemia (65,71), and occurred in 10% of patients in one large series (69). In that study, fractures were more common in the first decade of life, in acute, compared with chronic, osteomyelitis, and in patients whose treatment was delayed. Delayed union, malunion, or joint stiffness complicated approximately 10 to 15% of the fractures.

Compared with osteomyelitis, septic arthritis is relatively

uncommon in sickle cell disease (58,72). Unless the joint infection is secondary to direct penetration from an adjacent osteomyelitis, most cases of septic arthritis are caused by organisms other than *Salmonella* (72). Because of delay in diagnosis, septic arthritis of the hip in patients with sickle cell disease is more likely to be complicated by avascular necrosis or dislocation (71).

Reactive arthritis, causing a sterile joint effusion, also may occur in children with sickle cell anemia (73,74). The knees and elbows are most frequently involved, but symptoms may occur in other joints. Acute onset of pain occurs in one or more joints. Fever is commonly present, and may range from low-grade to greater than 39°C. Synovial fluid analysis typically reveals a leukocyte count of less than 20,000/mm³. Joint effusions usually last 1 to 2 weeks, and the duration of arthralgia ranges from a few days to 2 months. The cause of reactive arthritis is unknown, but may be associated with minor episodes of *Salmonella* enteritis or microvascular thrombosis in the synovial tissue. Treatment for reactive arthritis is splinting and analgesic medication.

Osteonecrosis of the femoral and humeral heads is common in sickle cell disease. In radiographic studies of more than 2,500 patients older than 5 years of age, the prevalence was dependent on the patient's age and the type of sickle cell disease (75,76). The prevalence was higher in the proximal femur, averaging 9.7% at this location, compared with 5.6% in the humerus (Tables 11-3 and 11-4). Patients with the SC or $S\beta^+$ genotype had a lower incidence of osteonecrosis, and tended to develop this problem at a later age. Within the SS group, patients homozygous for the α-thalassemia gene were more likely to develop osteonecrosis. This provides further evidence that the association of the α-thalassemia gene increases the risk of vasoocclusion. Bilateral osteonecrosis of the humeral head was more common, occurring in 67% of patients, compared with a 54% incidence of bilateral involvement of the femoral head. Concomitant humeral and femoral head osteonecrosis was common, occurring in 76% of SS patients and 75% of SC patients.

Osteonecrosis of the femoral head may not cause symptoms for several years. In a large radiographic study, almost one-half of the patients were asymptomatic at the time of diagnosis, but 21% of this group became symptomatic in the follow-up period, which averaged 5.6 years (75). Children have a better prognosis. In the study by Hernigou and colleagues (77), when the osteonecrosis developed before 10 years of age, only 5 of 14 hips had a Harris hip score lower than 80 points, at an average follow-up of 19 years. In comparison, 51 of 81 hips had a low hip rating when the osteonecrosis developed between 10 and 14 years of age. Therefore, young children with sickle cell disease have a reasonable potential for healing avascular necrosis of the femoral head, but the prognosis is guarded when osteonecrosis develops during adolescence.

Although not particularly useful in the very early detection of osteonecrosis, magnetic resonance imaging (MRI) is helpful in defining the extent of the infarct (78) (Fig. 11-5). Furthermore, MRI frequently shows that segments of the femoral head are involved to varying degrees, suggesting that different segments of the femoral head are infarcted at different times (80).

Several series have documented poor results after total joint arthroplasty in patients with sickle cell disease (81–83). Both acute and late complications are increased, with the incidence of infection and early revision being alarmingly high. This factor, and the poor long-term results for children older than 10 years of age, necessitate consideration of realignment osteotomy for this group. Radiography and MRI should define the extent of the avascular necrosis. With extensive involvement of the femoral head, or deficiency of the lateral pillar, a femoral or pelvic osteotomy should be considered. Abduction bracing is a better alternative for younger children (Fig. 11-5), but loss of motion and total head involvement require consideration of other therapeutic alternatives.

Compared with osteonecrosis of the femoral head, disability and pain are less frequent with osteonecrosis of the humeral head. In a large radiographic survey, more than 79% of the patients were asymptomatic at diagnosis (76).

TABLE 11-3. PREVALENCE OF FEMORAL HEAD OSTEONECROSIS IN SICKLE CELL DISEASE

Age (years)	Percent with Femoral Head Osteonecrosis	Type of Sickle Cell Disorder	
		Genotype	Percent[a]
5–9	1.3	$S\beta^0$	13.1
10–14	4.6	SS	10.2
15–24	8.2	SC	8.8
25–34	18.8	$S\beta^+$	5.8
35–44	21.9		
≥45	32.5		

[a] Age-adjusted rate.
(Adapted from ref. 75, with permission.)

TABLE 11-4. PREVALENCE OF HUMERAL HEAD OSTEONECROSIS IN SICKLE CELL DISEASE

Age (years)	Percent with Humeral Head Osteonecrosis	Type of Sickle Cell Disease	
		Genotype	Percent[a]
5–9	1.2	SS	6.0
10–14	2.6	$S\beta^0$	5.7
15–24	3.8	SC	4.6
25–34	9.7	$S\beta^+$	3.6
35–44	18.7		
≥45	22.0		

[a] Age-adjusted rate.
(Adapted from ref. 76, with permission.)

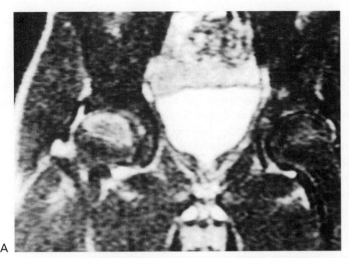
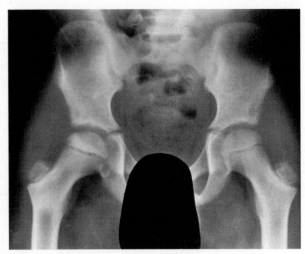

A

B

FIGURE 11-5. A: Magnetic resonance image of a 7-year, 4-month-old boy with sickle cell anemia. Patient complained of pain in the right hip. The T2-weighted image is consistent with avascular necrosis of the right femoral head. On other views, abnormal signals also were present in the left femoral head, although not to the degree seen in the right femur. **B:** Anteroposterior radiograph of the pelvis 5 months later demonstrates sclerosis of the lateral and inferior margins of the epiphysis, consistent with the creeping substitution healing of osteonecrosis. Patient had been maintained in an abduction brace. (Adapted from ref. 79, with permission.)

The disease process, however, may progress. The crescent sign and collapse of the humeral head typically begin in the superior medial quadrant. Further fragmentation and joint incongruity will cause symptoms and restricted motion, but the need for prosthetic replacement is uncommon.

Hydroxyurea stimulates hemoglobin F synthesis in many patients with sickle disease, and in a study of 299 adult patients, the frequency of crisis, acute chest syndrome, and hospitalization and the need for blood transfusion were significantly reduced by hydroxyurea (84). Similar findings have been observed in children, although these studies involved an earlier phase (85–87). The major short-term toxicity of hydroxyurea is reversible neutropenia, but whether this drug will prove to be carcinogenic over the long term is unknown. For that reason, hydroxyurea is not used in patients with minimal symptoms. It is hoped that hydroxyurea and other medications will prevent the organ damage and mortality associated with sickle cell disorders.

The use of bone marrow transplantation in patients with sickle cell disease is controversial (88). Complications are less frequent if the patient is young without major chronic organ damage, and is being transplanted from a healthy HLA-identical relative. In a series of 22 children with sickle cell disease who received marrow transplants from HLA-matched siblings, Walters et al. (89) observed that 15 were cured, 4 had recurrent disease with unknown effect of the conditioning chemotherapy on their sickle cell disease, 1 had mixed results, and 2 died after transplantation. Successful transplantation will cure the patient of the sickle cell disease and its associated pain. Furthermore, Hernigou et al. (90) reported significant healing of humeral head os-

teonecrosis after bone marrow transplantation in a 13-year-old boy. On the other hand, even if transplantation is successful, these patients are likely to be infertile, and to have an uncertain future risk of chemotherapy inducing malignancy.

Intraoperative considerations for patients with sickle cell disease include adequate hydration, avoidance of hypothermia and deoxygenation, and maintenance of blood volume. The use of a tourniquet does not cause increased sickling (91), but special efforts should be made to exsanguinate the limb before inflating the pneumatic tourniquet. In a study of 1,079 surgical procedures performed on 717 sickle cell patients, the only association between preoperative hemoglobin A level and complication rate was the reduction in painful crises (92). Of note, complications after operation were more common in patients receiving regional, rather than general, anesthesia.

Thalassemia

The thalassemias are an extremely heterogeneous group of inherited anemias caused by mutations in the synthesis of hemoglobin (93). Normal hemoglobin is a tetramer consisting of two α-like and two β-like globin polypeptides. Hemoglobin A, a highly soluble and stable polypeptide formed by two α-globulin and two β-globulin chains, is the predominant hemoglobin found in normal red blood cells after the age of 6 months. Two minor hemoglobins, hemoglobin A2 ($\alpha2\delta2$) and hemoglobin F ($\alpha2\gamma2$), normally constitute a small fraction of the hemoglobin found in red blood cells, with the proportion of hemoglobin A2 being about 2.5%

and that of hemoglobin F being less than 1% after the age of 6 months.

Thalassemia is characterized by absent or deficient synthesis of one or more globin chains. The consequences range from severe anemia to laboratory abnormalities of no clinical significance.

The gene for α-globulin is duplicated on chromosome 16. Therefore, each human cell contains four copies of the *α-globulin* gene. The four α-thalassemia syndromes are based on whether one, two, three, or four of the α-globulin genes are defective (93). If all four α-globulin genes are affected, the result is hydrops fetalis and death *in utero*. Otherwise, patients with α-thalassemia have significantly fewer problems than patients with β-thalassemia. This is because unpaired β-globulin chains can form a relatively stable tetramer (hemoglobin H). A person with one affected gene has the silent carrier syndrome, which is characterized by no anemia and normal red blood cells. In the thalassemia trait syndrome, two genes are affected; these patients have mild anemia with hypochromic and microcytic red blood cells. In practical terms, thalassemia trait at the time of diagnosis requires differentiation from iron-deficiency anemia (94). Patients with three affected *α-globulin* genes have hemoglobin H disease, a syndrome characterized by moderate anemia, chronic hemolysis, and a relatively benign course. As a result of different mutations, clinical heterogeneity is seen within each α-thalassemia syndrome. Individuals who are heterozygous for β-thalassemia are sometimes classified as having thalassemia minor.

Cooley anemia or severe β-thalassemia is secondary to homozygous mutations of the *β-globulin* gene, with a resultant absent or severely deficient synthesis of the β-polypeptide chain. Therefore, in β-thalassemia, many of the hemoglobin molecules are composed of unpaired α-globulin chains. This molecule is extremely insoluble and causes intracellular precipitates. The circulating erythrocytes are distorted, extremely small, and have a markedly reduced amount of hemoglobin. In addition, increased hemolysis occurs because these damaged erythrocytes are removed at an accelerated rate. The clinical consequences are severe anemia, growth retardation, hepatosplenomegaly, and bone marrow expansion, with its associated complications.

Current use of the term "thalassemia major" implies a homozygous β-thalassemia that requires regular blood transfusion (93). "Thalassemia intermedia" is applied to a group of homozygous β-globin patients who maintain hemoglobin levels of 6 to 10 g/dL, except during periods of infection or surgery. Severity of disease is related to the relative imbalance between α-globin and total non-α-globin synthesis. This is determined by the specific mutation(s) in the β- and *α-globin* genes, as well as by the ability of the individual to synthesize hemoglobin F.

Untreated patients with thalassemia major present with severe anemia during the first months of life, and most will die during the first 5 years of life. Transfusion programs to maintain hemoglobin levels between 9.5 and 11.5 mg/dL, and chelation therapy to minimize the effect of iron overload, have markedly altered life expectancy and other problems seen in thalassemia; however, even when serial transfusions are begun at an early age, patients still may develop growth retardation and endocrine abnormalities, and may die of cardiac dysfunction in middle age (95).

Skeletal abnormalities seen in sporadically treated thalassemia result from extreme erythroid hyperplasia, which causes widening of the marrow space, thinning of the cortex, and striking osteoporosis (96). The earliest changes are noted in the hands and feet. The metacarpals, metatarsals, and phalanges are expanded to a rectangular, then a convex shape. The changes observed in these peripheral areas diminish in older children as the distal red marrow is replaced by fatty marrow; however, the skull, the spine, and the pelvis in these patients may show progressive radiologic changes (Figs. 11-6 and 11-7).

Earlier studies noted that fractures after minimal trauma occurred in 40 to 50% of patients with thalassemia at an average age of 10 to 16 years (97–99). Transfusion therapy has decreased the incidence and nature of this complication. For example, Michelson and Cohen (100) recorded a fracture incidence of 21%, at an average age of 25 years, when a transfusion program was started during early childhood. Furthermore, fractures in these patients occurred after a more appropriate level of trauma, and healed within an expected time and without the deformity commonly seen in earlier studies.

Premature fusion of the physis also was observed in earlier studies of thalassemia patients (97,101). This problem was noted in 15 to 20% of the patients, and was particularly common in the proximal humeral physis. The cause of the premature physeal fusion was unclear, but the problem was observed more frequently in the patients who had a delay in beginning transfusion therapy (101).

Iron overload in thalassemia results from transfusion therapy and excessive absorption of iron in the gut (102). Excessive catabolic iron overwhelms the iron-binding capacity of transferrin. Free iron is toxic to cells, promoting hydroxyl radical formation. Hemosiderin deposits accumulate in the reticuloendothelial cells, leading to hepatomegaly. Iron deposition also occurs in the central and peripheral bone marrow (103). Most importantly, free iron in the heart impairs the function of the mitochondrial respiratory chain. As a result, fatal cardiomyopathy occurs during the adolescent years unless treatment is instituted. Chelation therapy with deferoxamine markedly delays or prevents cardiac disease. The prognosis for survival without cardiac disease is particularly good for patients whose serum ferritin concentrations remain less than 2,500 ng/mL (104). Chelation therapy is best started at a young age, but even then it may not always prevent growth failure and/or delayed or absent puberty (105).

Spinal cord compression, secondary to extramedullary

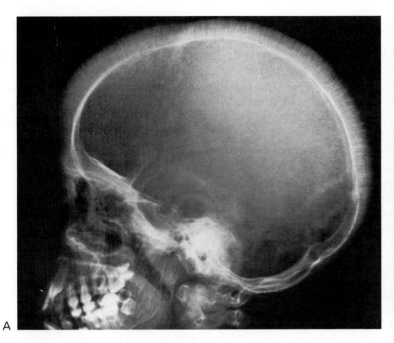

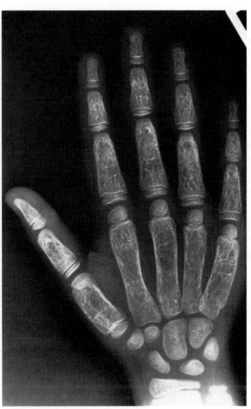

B

FIGURE 11-6. A: Lateral radiograph of the skull, showing the radial striations of the calvarium in an 11-year-old boy with thalassemia major. **B:** Note the widened marrow cavities of the metacarpals and phalanges, and the marked osteoporosis.

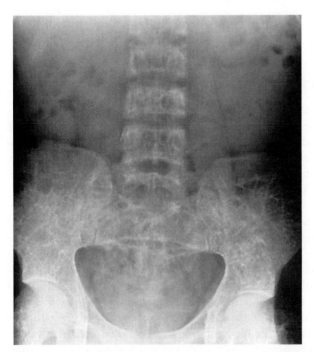

FIGURE 11-7. Anteroposterior radiograph of the lumbar spine and pelvis in a 26-year-old man with homozygous β-thalassemia. Radiographs show marked osteoporosis and lacy trabeculae secondary to marrow hypoplasia. (From ref. 79, with permission.)

hematopoiesis, is an uncommon complication typically seen in adult patients with thalassemia intermedia (106–108). Treatment is controversial. MRI should be performed. Surgical decompression, radiotherapy, and transfusion therapy are treatment alternatives.

Owing to the long-term problems of chronic transfusion therapy and the risk of blood-borne diseases, bone marrow transplantation increasingly is being used for patients with thalassemia major (93,109). The best results are seen in patients younger than 16 years who have not developed hepatomegaly or portal fibrosis, who have received regular chelation treatment before transplantation, and who receive a bone marrow transplant from an HLA-identical donor after undergoing a preoperative conditioning regimen. In this group, 12-year Kaplan-Meier analysis in 111 patients showed a 96% survival rate, a 90% disease-free survival rate, a 7% rejection mortality, and a 4% nonrejection mortality. After successful bone marrow transplantation, chelation treatment may improve liver and cardiac function (110).

Anemia of Chronic Inflammation

Anemia of chronic inflammation (ACI) is a well-recognized, but imperfectly understood, disorder associated with disorders of chronic infection, serious trauma, malignancy, and inflammation, such as juvenile rheumatoid arthritis (94,111,112). Although, in the past this disorder was frequently called anemia of chronic disease, the change in nomenclature reflects a shift in understanding that inflammation is the key component. Chronic diseases without an inflammatory component are not ACI (111). Furthermore, within a particular disease, the patients who develop anemia are the patients who have a more serious course of their underlying disease (113).

In patients with ACI, the anemia is typically mild (hemoglobin greater than 9 g/dL) and nonprogressive. The erythrocytes are normocytic or mildly microcytic. However, the most characteristic laboratory findings in ACI are an elevated plasma ferritin level and normal-to-low transferrin saturation. These parameters allow differentiation from iron-deficiency anemia, in which both ferritin and transferrin levels are low, and distinguish ACI from iron-overload disorders, in which both levels are high.

ACI is a multifactorial process reflecting impaired release of iron from storage sites, and inhibition of erythroid progenitors. In ACI, large deposits of iron remain stored as hemosiderin in the reticuloendothelial cells (111,112). Inflammatory mediators, such as interluekin-1 and tumor necrosis factor, stimulate ferritin synthesis, and excessive ferritin shells are probably the cause of iron remaining in storage (114). As a result, there is impaired transport of iron from storage sites to developing erythrocytes. Patients with ACI also have low levels of erythropoietin, which is consistent with cell culture studies demonstrating suppression of erythropoietin production by inflammatory cytokines (115).

Treatment of ACI is most effective when the source of inflammation can be eliminated. Iron therapy is of no value, and observation is often chosen when the anemia is mild. Blood transfusion or erythropoietin may be necessary when the anemia is compromising postoperative management or other aspects of treatment (94,111).

DISORDERS OF NEUTROPHILS

Phagocytic white blood cells include two groups: granulocytes (neutrophils, eosinophils, and basophils) and mononuclear cells (monocytes and tissue macrophages). Neutrophils are the first line of defense against bacterial and fungal infections, and as such, their specialized machinery is focused to seek out, ingest, and kill microorganisms (116,117). While circulating in the bloodstream, neutrophils detect and respond to chemotactic substances released from a site of infection. As a result, a chain of complex and overlapping reactions ensue (117):

- Loose adhesions are made and broken between the neutrophil and the postcapillary venule endothelium. As a result, neutrophil movement is slowed (leukocyte rolling), and the cells gain a more intense exposure to the activating factors.
- Blood flow is reduced by tighter adhesions formed be-

tween neutrophils and platelets, between neutrophils and endothelium, and by neutrophils adhering to each other.
- Adhesions are then loosened, and the neutrophils migrate between endothelial cells to sites of infection, in a complex process of receptor engagement, signal transduction, and cytoskeleton remodeling. Secretion of gelatinase, heparinase, and other enzymes facilitates this migratory process.
- On reaching the site of infection, neutrophils adhere to microorganisms by several different types of receptors.
- Neutrophils engulf most bacteria (phagocytosis), with the microorganism sequestered in a closed vacuole called a "phagosome." Organisms that are too large, such as fungi, are covered by a firmly adherent layer of neutrophils, which then proceed with phagocytosis in a similar, collective manner at the neutrophil–hyphae interface.
- Neutrophils have different types of granules, which contain a variety of antimicrobial proteins. Optimal killing requires concurrent degranulation and activation of nicotinamide adenine dinucleotide phosphate (NADPH) oxidase, with injection of their products into the phagosome.
- Activation of NADPH oxidase at the phagosome membrane sets off the respiratory burst reaction. NADPH reacts with oxygen to generate superoxide, which combines with water to produce hydrogen peroxide (H_2O_2). Myeloperoxidase, an azurophil granule component, catalyzes H_2O_2 to combine with chloride anions to form hypochlorous acid (HOCl). The oxidants H_2O_2 and HOCl not only kill bacteria, but also activate neutrophil granule proteases and, more importantly, denature bacterial proteins, making them susceptible to proteolysis. Finally, these oxidants inactivate chemotactic factors, thereby serving to terminate the neutrophil invasion.

Chronic Granulomatous Disease

Inherited defects of neutrophils may affect various components of neutrophil function and structure (117). Chronic granulomatous disease (CGD) is the most common congenital disorder of neutrophils, occurring in 1 per 200,000 to 250,000 live births. Osteomyelitis is relatively common in CGD and has some unique features in this disorder.

CGD is actually a group of four related diseases characterized by deficiency in NADPH oxidase. Defects in four *phox* proteins (phagocyte oxidase proteins that participate in the activation of NADPH) have been identified as causes of CGD (117–120). Inactive NADPH includes three cytosolic components (p47 *phox*, p67 *phox*, and p21 *rac*) and cytochrome *b*, which is plasma-membrane–bound, and is composed of the larger gp91 *phox* and the smaller p22 *phox* subunits. During activation of NADPH oxidase, the cytosolic components migrate and attach to the membrane components.

CGD is most commonly transmitted by sex-linked recessive inheritance as a result of a mutation in the X chromosome gene for gp91 *phox* (117). Other types of CGD are autosomal recessive disorders. Approximately 60 to 65% of CGD is secondary to a defect in gp91 *phox*, and 30% is secondary to a defect in the gene encoding p47 *phox* (chromosome 7). Defects in p67 *phox* (chromosome 1) or p22 *phox* (chromosome 16) account for the remaining cases of CGD.

Phagocytosis is normal in CGD, but the neutrophils have decreased ability to kill microbes that are catalase-positive. Therefore, infections with *Staphylococcus aureus, Aspergillus* species, *Escherichia coli, Klebsiella* species, *Salmonella* species, *Berkholdaria cepacia, Pseudomonas aeruginosa, Serratia marcescens, Enterobacter* species, *Proteus* species, and *Nocardia* species are common in CGD. With an infection by a catalase-negative microbe, the H_2O_2 produced by the bacterium may be used by the CGD neutrophils as a bypass to complete the killing process.

A typical patient with CGD is a boy who develops symptoms of recurrent skin and pulmonary infections associated with persistent lymphadenopathy in the first or second year of life. Girls may be affected if the CGD is secondary to the less common autosomal recessive disorders. Nitroblue tetrazolium dye is a useful screening test for CGD, but it is being supplanted by the more accurate flow cytometry test using dihydrorhodamine 123 fluorescence, which detects oxidant production (117).

Recurrent infections include superficial infections, such as skin abscess, lymphadenitis, and perirectal abscess, or deep infections, such as pneumonia, otitis media, osteomyelitis, and liver abscess (116,121) (Fig. 11-8). The severity of CGD is not uniform. An adverse prognostic indicator is development of symptoms before 1 year of age (122), a factor that probably reflects the site of mutation, and whether any residual NADPH oxidase activity is present.

Osteomyelitis can be particularly problematic in CGD, and has been noted in 20 to 30% of these patients (116). Earlier reports of osteomyelitis in CGD indicated that the bones of the hands and feet were most commonly involved (123), but in a later review of 13 children who developed 20 episodes of osteomyelitis (124), the spine and the ribs were the most common sites of infection. Direct spread from a contiguous lung or hepatic abscess is the usual cause of spine or rib involvement, whereas hematogenous spread causes long-bone infections. *Aspergillus* is a common cause of vertebral osteomyelitis in CGD (116,124), and, as one might expect, the diagnosis of vertebral osteomyelitis is often delayed in these children. Sponseller and colleagues (124) found that these patients did not respond to antibiotics alone, and noted that their best results were obtained with preoperative imaging to define the extent of the bony infection, temporary withholding of antibiotics to obtain reliable intraoperative cultures, thorough debridement of the infected tissue, and leaving the wound open to allow healing by secondary intention. However, other authors have reported successful medical cure of extensive *Aspergillus*

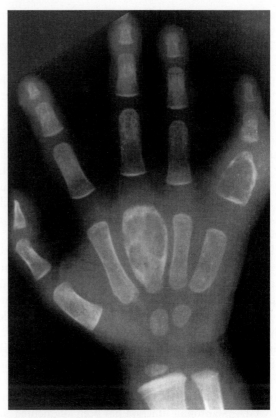

FIGURE 11-8. Fifteen-month-old boy with a 2-month history of progressive swelling of the right hand. Anteroposterior radiograph of the hand demonstrates fusiform swelling and osteolysis of the third metacarpal and proximal phalanx of the little finger. The patient had a past history of tuberculosis meningitis. Because the chest radiograph demonstrated infiltrates, the preoperative diagnosis was tuberculosis dactylitis. A drainage procedure was performed. Cultures demonstrated *Serratia marcescens*; subsequent tests confirmed the diagnosis of chronic granulomatous disease.

osteomyelitis of the spine, using recombinant γ-interferon and antifungal agents (125–127).

A 50% survival rate at 10 years of age was noted in one retrospective study published in 1989 (128), but most CGD patients now survive into adulthood (117). Principles of the comprehensive management of a child with CGD include the following (117):

■ Prevention of infections by timely immunizations, compulsive hygiene (hand washing, dental cleaning, careful anal washing, prompt cleansing of any skin damage), and avoidance of possible sources of pathogens (passive smoke, bedside humidifiers, decaying plants)

■ Prophylaxis with trimethoprim-sulfamethoxazole or dicloxacillin; studies have shown an approximately 50% reduction in infections in children with CGD on prophylactic antibiotics

■ Use of recombinant human γ-interferon; a multicenter, double-blind, randomized study demonstrated a 70% reduced infection risk when interferon was administered prophylactically (129)

- Early administration of parenteral antibiotics that cover *S. aureus,* as well as Gram-negative bacteria
- Prompt drainage of abscesses and selected surgical biopsy for culture and definitive diagnosis; the latter is particularly true with suspected fungal infections.

Formation of granulomas, probably secondary to chronic inflammation from inadequate immunologic debridement, may complicate CGD. As a result, gastric outlet obstruction, ileocolitis, chronic cystitis, hepatosplenomegaly, and other chronic inflammatory problems may develop. Cyclosporine has been reported as an effective treatment for retractable colitis in one child with CGD (130).

Heterozygous carriers of X-linked CGD may sustain some infectious problems if they have a relatively large number of abnormal cells (116). Female carriers may also develop the autoimmune disorder discoid lupus erythematosus. This and other autoimmune disorders, although less likely, also have been noted in patients with CGD (131).

Bone marrow transplantation is controversial in CGD, but it has been performed successfully with an HLA-compatible sibling and preconditioning therapy (132,133). Clinical trials of gene therapy are under way in patients with CGD. Neutrophil function has been augmented in a small percentage of cells for a few months (134), but high-level, permanent gene transfer to hematopoietic cells has not been achieved.

DISORDERS OF LYMPHOCYTES AND THE IMMUNE SYSTEM

Lymphocytes can be divided into two main categories. Bone marrow-derived lymphocytes, the B cells, are precursors for humoral immunity cells (i.e., plasma cells that secrete antibodies). Thymus-derived lymphocytes, or T cells, control cell-mediated immunity, and have both effector and regulatory functions. Effector functions include delayed hypersensitivity and graft-versus-host reactivity. Regulatory functions include enhancement and suppression of both cell-mediated and humoral immunity.

X-linked Agammaglobulinemia

X-linked agammaglobulinemia is a sex-linked recessive disorder manifested by recurrent bacterial infections that typically begin after 6 months of age, when maternal immunoglobulins have essentially disappeared (135). Physical findings are sparse. Tonsils and palpable lymph nodes are virtually absent. The history of recurrent dermatitis, otitis media, pneumonia, and meningitis initiates appropriate laboratory studies. The disease is confirmed by profound hypo-

gammaglobulinemia, absence of B lymphocytes, and a normal number of T cells and lymphocytes (136). Defective production of cytoplasmic tyrosine kinase, a signaling protein that is necessary for the maturation at the pre-B-cell stage, is the cause of X-linked agammaglobulinemia (137).

Without circulating B lymphocytes, children are susceptible to infection by pyogenic encapsulated bacteria (135,137). Response to fungal and viral infections is normal, except for enterovirus and vaccine-associated poliomyelitis. Delayed hypersensitivity and allograft rejection are also normal. Untreated, patients with agammaglobulinemia usually develop bronchiectasis and die of pulmonary complications. The prognosis is significantly improved with immunoglobulin therapy and prompt institution of antibiotics for infections.

The unique musculoskeletal problem seen in agammaglobulinemia, and in other disorders causing hypogammaglobulinemia, is an arthropathy that resembles juvenile rheumatoid arthritis. In a review of 69 patients with X-linked agammaglobulinemia, 11 had aseptic arthritis and 4 had septic arthritis at presentation, and 3 patients subsequently developed aseptic arthritis (138). The arthritis is usually nonerosive, and either oligoarticular or polyarticular, and it most commonly affects the knees, the wrists, the ankles, and the fingers (139). The cause of the arthritis is unclear, but the presence of excessive suppressor T cells in the synovial tissue clearly makes the arthritis in these patients different from classic rheumatoid arthritis (140).

Although the arthritis in most patients responds to immunoglobulin therapy, chronic synovitis persists in a few patients (139). Atypical infections undoubtedly account for some of these cases. In a survey of 358 patients with primary antibody deficiency, Franz and colleagues (141) found that mycoplasmal infection was the most common cause of severe chronic erosive arthritis.

Acquired Immunodeficiency Syndrome

Through 1997, it is estimated that 12 million people worldwide have died of acquired immunodeficiency syndrome (AIDS), and 3 million of these deaths were in children (142). Children younger than 13 years of age account for 1% of the AIDS cases in the United States, but even in this country, AIDS is one of the top ten causes of death between the ages of 1 and 13 years (143). The rate in children is much higher in sub-Saharan Africa, where two-thirds of the 30 million people with human immunodeficiency virus (HIV) infections reside.

Perinatal transmission is the cause of most HIV infections in children younger than 13 years of age. Congenital HIV infection can be acquired in the intrauterine environment, during delivery, or after delivery (through breast feeding) (144). Studies suggest that the most common route of vertical transmission is intrapartum, and the least common is by breast feeding.

When the patient is infected, viremia occurs. HIV binds to cells expressing CD4 molecules on their surface, primarily CD4 lymphocytes, but also cells of the monocyte-macrophage lineage (144). Cells of the central nervous system, such as microglia, astrocytes, and oligodendroglia, also may be affected. CD4 lymphocytes accumulate in the lymph nodes, where they proliferate, resulting in a generalized lymphadenopathy. During this period of clinical latency, there is a reduction in the measurable level of HIV in the blood but also a gradual deterioration of the immune system, which is characterized by depletion of CD4 cells trapped in the lymph nodes. In the later phase of the disease, the dendritic meshwork of the lymph nodes deteriorates, and HIV levels in the bloodstream again increase.

Untreated, the duration between infection and AIDS-related illnesses is shorter in children than in adults (144,145). However, great strides have been made in the prevention of vertical HIV transmission, as well as in the treatment of infected infants (146–148). In one study, antiretroviral treatment of the mother, during pregnancy, and of the infant decreased the transmission rate from 25.5% in the placebo group to 8.3% in the group receiving zidovudine (147). The use of prophylactic antibiotics, a consistent immunization program, and aggressive therapy for *Pneumocystis carinii* pneumonia and other infections, also extend the life expectancy of these infants. Approximately 70% survive until their fifth birthday, and these figures are continuing to change (149). As a result, the diagnosis of congenital HIV infection by itself should not be a contraindication to elective surgery.

Encephalopathy is common in congenital HIV infection (144,145). The most common manifestation is a progressive disorder, but some children have a static encephalopathy that is similar to spastic diplegic or quadriplegic cerebral palsy. If gross motor development is stymied by muscle imbalance and contractures, and if the immunologic status is satisfactory, then surgical procedures will improve motor function. The CD4 count and viral load should be assessed preoperatively. Absolute CD4 counts are higher in infants, and severe depression of CD4 lymphocytes is considered to be present when there are counts of less than $750/mm^3$ in children younger than 12 months of age, less than $500/mm^3$ in children 1 to 5 years old, and less than $200/mm^3$ in children 6 years of age or older.

Although the incidence of vertical transmission of HIV infection is decreasing in the United States, the incidence in adolescents is increasing (150). In addition, compared with adults, the infection rate is higher in adolescent girls, indicating a larger proportion of heterosexual transmission in this group. The elimination of contaminated clotting factors has virtually eradicated HIV infection in children with hemophilia.

DISORDERS OF THE MONOCYTE-MACROPHAGE SYSTEM

The mononuclear phagocytic system includes monocytes and macrophages, cells that are critical components of the immune system. Macrophages ingest and kill invading organisms, and also are important in tissue breakdown and remodeling. The mononuclear phagocytic system also functions in antigen presentation, cellular cytotoxicity, and modulation of lymphocytes.

Cells of the monocyte-macrophage system arise from a common stem cell in the bone marrow. After differentiation into monocytes, these cells circulate in the peripheral blood, and migrate to different tissues where they reside, and may change and develop highly specialized functions. Although widely distributed, macrophages are particularly abundant in the spleen, liver (Kupffer cells), lymph nodes, lungs, and bone. Osteoclasts are also derived from monocytes, and, as such, are an example of a highly specialized resident macrophage. Osteopetrosis (Chapter 7) is secondary to a deficiency in osteoclast function, and, therefore, could be classified as a disorder of the monocyte-macrophage system.

Dendritic cells are clearly derived from bone marrow cells. Furthermore, there is supporting but not conclusive evidence that monocytes and dendritic cells develop from a common precursor. Dendritic cells are antigen-presenting but are nonphagocytic. Types of dendritic cells include: (a) follicular dendritic cells found in germinal centers, and thought to function as presenting antigens to B cells; (b) interdigitating reticulum cells, also found in lymph nodes, and thought to function as presenting antigens to T cells; and (c) Langerhans cells of the skin (151).

Storage diseases of the reticuloendothelial system, also called "lysosomal storage diseases," have profound effects on the mononuclear phagocytic system, including the organs housing the reticuloendothelial system. Storage diseases may affect other organ systems, particularly the central nervous system. The common pathogenesis in the storage diseases is a deficiency of a catabolic enzyme normally found in lysosomal particles of the cell cytoplasm (151,152). As a result, products of cellular metabolism accumulate, which would normally be degraded and excreted. The lysosomes are overloaded, and the cell eventually disrupts. Abnormal accumulation of macrophages and organ dysfunction subsequently occur.

The different types of lysosomal storage diseases seen in children and their associated skeletal abnormalities are listed in Table 11-5. Type 1 Gaucher disease, as well as various types of mucopolysaccharidosis and mucolipidosis, are commonly evaluated and treated by orthopaedic surgeons. Gaucher disease will be discussed in this chapter.

Gaucher Disease

Gaucher disease, initially described in 1882 by Philippe Charles-Ernest Gaucher, is the most common lysosomal

TABLE 11-5. STORAGE DISEASES IN CHILDREN, AND ASSOCIATED MUSCULOKELETAL ABNORMALITIES

Disease	Age at Onset	Stored Material	Enzyme Deficiency	Presenting Symptoms	Additional Skeletal Manifestations
Sphingolipidoses					
Gaucher disease, type 1	Childhood	Glucocerebroside	Glucocerebrosidase	Splenomegaly, anemia, thrombocytopenia	Gaucher crises, widened metaphysis, osteopenia, pathologic fracture, osteonecrosis
Gaucher disease, type 2	Infancy	Glucocerebroside	Glucocerebrosidase	Central nervous system signs, failure to thrive, hepatomegaly	Not significant, death by age 2 years
Gaucher disease, type 3	Adolescence	Glucocerebroside	Glucocerebrosidase	Hepatosplenomegaly, neurologic manifestations	Most have only neurologic manifestations
Niemann-Pick disease, type A (acute neuronopathic form)	Infancy	Sphingomyelin	Sphingomyelinase (severe)	Developmental delay, hepatosplenomegaly	Wasting of the extremities
Niemann-Pick disease, type B (chronic without central nervous system involvement)	Second year	Sphingomyelin	Sphingomyelinase (severe)	Hepatosplenomegaly	Osteopenia, modeling defects with metaphyseal flaring, sea-blue histiocytes in bone marrow, long vertebral pedicles secondary to sphingomyelin in spinal cord
Niemann-Pick disease, types C and D (chronic neuropathic)	Childhood	Sphingomyelin; unesterified cholesterol accumulates in lysosomes	Sphingomyelinase	Considerable variability; infantile group has psychomotor delay; juvenile has ataxic gait; late onset has apparent psychiatric disturbance	No apparent problems from bone marrow infiltration
Farber disease	Infancy	Ceramide	Ceramidase	Painful swelling in the hands and feet, hoarseness, vomiting	Periarticular nodules associated with joint contractures
G_{M1}-gangliosidosis, type 1	Infancy	G_{M1}-ganglioside, glycoprotein	G_{M1}-ganglioside-β-galactosidase	Slow development, spastic quadriplegia, hepatosplenomegaly	Stubby hands, broad wrists, widening of the midshaft of the humerus, anterior breaking of the lumbar vertebrae, spatulate ribs
G_{M1}-gangliosidosis, type 2	1–3 years of age	G_{M1}-ganglioside, glycoprotein	G_{M1}-ganglioside-β-galactosidase	Cessation and regression of motor development	Not significant
G_{M1}-gangliosidosis, type 3	3–30 years of age	G_{M1}-ganglioside, glycoprotein	G_{M1}-ganglioside-β-galactosidase	Progressive pyramidal and extrapyramidal disease	Not significant
G_{M2}-gangliosidosis	Infancy	G_{M2}-ganglioside, globoside	Hexosaminidase A (Tay-Sach disease), hexosaminidase A and B (Sandhoff disease)	Slow development, progressive motor dysfunction, cherry-red macula	Sandhoff disease has foam cells in bone marrow

TABLE 11-5. *(continued)*

Disease	Age at Onset	Stored Material	Enzyme Deficiency	Presenting Symptoms	Additional Skeletal Manifestations
Mucopolysaccharidoses					
Type I, Hurler syndrome	Infancy	Dermatan sulfate, heparan sulfate	α-Iduronidase	Coarse facial features, corneal opacities, hearing loss, enlarged tongue, frontal bossing, hepatosplenomegaly, joint stiffness	Dysostosis multiplex with rounding and anterior beaking of vertebrae, lumbar kyphosis secondary to hypoplasia of the lumbar vertebrae, shortening of metacarpals and phalanges
Type 1, Scheie syndrome	After 5 years of age	Dermatan sulfate, heparan sulfate	α-Iduronidase	Joint stiffness, claw hands and feet	Carpal tunnel syndrome
Type I, Hurler-Scheie syndrome	3–8 years of age	Dermatan sulfate, heparan sulfate	α-Iduronidase	Progressive corneal clouding, deafness, hepatosplenomegaly, joint stiffness, valvular heart disease	Skeletal changes similar, but less severe than Hurler syndrome, progressive mental retardation
Type II, Hunter syndrome	2–4 years of age	Dermatan sulfate, heparan sulfate	Iduronate sulfatase	Coarse facial features, progressive deafness, stiff joints, hepatosplenomegaly	Dysostosis multiplex as in type I, short stature, degenerative arthritis of the hips
Type III, Sanfilippo syndrome types A, B, C, and D	2–6 years of age	Heparan sulfate	A, heparan-*N*-sulfatase; B, *N*-acetyl-α-glucosaminidase; C, acetyl coenzyme A; α-glucosaminide acetyltransferase; D, *N*-acetyl-α-glucosamine-6-sulfatase	Delayed development, marked hyperactivity, sleep disorders, hirsutism, joint stiffness	Mild dysostosis multiplex with thickening of the calvaria and biconvex configuration of thoracolumbar vertebrae, stature within normal limits
Type IV, Morquio syndrome (type A)	1–2 years of age (severe form)	Keratan sulfate	Galactosamine-6-sulfatase	Short stature, dwarfism, loose joints	Short neck, aplasia odontoid process with C1–C2 subluxation, kyphosis, waddling gait, bowed knee
Type IV, Morquio syndrome (type B)	Variable, usually later than type A	Keratan sulfate	β-galactosidase	Similar but usually less severe than type A Morquio syndrome	Similar but usually less severe than type A Morquio syndrome
Type VI, Maroteaux syndrome	1–2 years of age (severe form)	Dermatan sulfate	Galactosamine-4-sulfatase	Coarse facies, joint stiffness, corneal clouding, deafness	Short stature, C1–C2 subluxation, crouched stance with hip and knee contractures
Type VII, Sly syndrome	Variable	Dermatan sulfate, keratan sulfate	β-Glucuronidase	Coarse facies, cloudy corneas, short stature	Dysostosis multiplex
Mucosulfatidosis (multiple sulfatase deficiency)	Neonatal, late infantile, and juvenile forms	Sulfatides, mucopolysaccharides	Arylsulfatase A, B, and C, other sulfatases	Prominent forehead, flattened nose, short neck, delayed development, hepatomegaly	Dysostosis multiplex

(continued)

TABLE 11-5. *(continued)*

Disease	Age at Onset	Stored Material	Enzyme Deficiency	Presenting Symptoms	Additional Skeletal Manifestations
Mucolipidoses					
Sialidosis type I	Late childhood	Sialyloligosaccharides, glycoproteins	Neuraminidase specific for glycoproteins and oligosaccharides, with a terminal sialic acid	Falls, decreased visual acuity, myoclonus	Often absent, scoliosis may develop
Sialidosis type II	Congenital, infantile, and juvenile types	Sialyoligosaccharides, glycoproteins	Same as above	Dysmorphic facies, short stature, developmental delay	Dysostosis multiplex, stippled epiphyses, ovoid vertebral bodies
Type II mucolipidosis (I-cell disease)	Infancy	Sialyloligosaccharides, glycoproteins, glycolipids	High serum, but deficient fibroblast levels of variety of acid hydrolases	Wizened face at birth, gingival hyperplasia, stiff joints	Delayed conversion of cartilage to bone, osteopenia, V-shaped deformity of the wrist, acetabular dysplasia, short rounded vertebral bodies, anteroinferior beaking T12 or L1
Type III mucolipidosis (pseudo-Hurler polydystrophy)	2–4 years of age	Glycoproteins, glycolipids	Same as above	Stiffness in hands and shoulders	Short stature, scoliosis, progressive joint stiffness, destruction of hip joints, carpal tunnel syndrome, claw hands
Type IV mucolipidosis (short stature)	Infancy	Glycolipids, glycoproteins	Unknown	Slow development, corneal clouding	
Other Diseases					
Fucosidosis	Type I, 6–18 months; type 2, 2–3 years; type 3, later childhood	Fucoglycolipids, fucosylotigosaccharides	α-Fucosidase	Slow development, developmental deterioration	Dysostosis multiplex
α-Mannosidosis	Type 1, infantile; type 2, juvenile-adult	Mannosyloligosaccharides	α-Mannosidase	Slow development, coarse facies, hepatosplenomegaly	Dysostosis multiplex, severe in type 1 and mild in type 2
Aspartylglucosaminosis	Second year	Aspartylglucosamine	Aspartylglucosaminase	Recurrent infection, diarrhea, hernias, hypotonia, progressive mental retardation	Mild dysostosis multiplex with wedge-shape vertebrae
Wolman disease	Infancy	Cholesterol esters, triglycerides	Acid lipase	Vomiting, diarrhea, hepatosplenomegaly, calcified adrenals	Not significant
Neuronal ceroid lipofuscinoses (five types)	Variable, related to type	Ceroid lipofuscin pigments	CLN-1-palmitoyl-protein thioesterase; others unknown	Progressive neurologic dysfunction	Not significant

storage disease, with an overall incidence of approximately 1 per 40,000 (152). A sentinel study by Brady and colleagues (153) proved that Gaucher disease was caused by a deficiency of glucocerebrosidase, the lysosomal enzyme that hydrolyzes glucocerebroside, an important component of cell wall membranes. In patients with Gaucher disease, the normal necrosis of cells, especially leukocytes, causes a gradual accumulation of glucocerebroside in macrophages. The resultant Gaucher cell is a large, lipid-laden cell found mostly in the red pulp of the spleen, the liver sinusoids, and the bone marrow. Clinical manifestations of Gaucher

disease are either attributable to accumulation of these abnormal macrophages or a secondary consequence of the resultant organ dysfunction. For example, thrombocytopenia and clotting deficiency resulting from hepatosplenomegaly may precipitate severe leg or back pain, the so-called "bone or Gaucher crisis."

Three forms of Gaucher disease are recognized. All are characterized by autosomal recessive inheritance. Type I is by far the most common, and is characterized by splenomegaly with resultant pancytopenia, hepatomegaly, and infiltration of the bone marrow, with multiple skeletal manifestations. Type II disease, also known as the acute neuropathic or infantile type, is rare, involves the central nervous system, and causes death before age 2 years. Type III disease, also called the chronic neuronopathic type, is typified by the development of hepatosplenomegaly during the first decade, and by neurologic problems during adolescence. All types of Gaucher disease are panethnic, but type I is particularly prevalent among Ashkenazi Jews. The incidence of Gaucher disease in this population has been calculated to be 1 per 450 live births, with a carrier frequency of 9% (154). The prevalence of type III is particularly high in Norrbotten, a northern district of Sweden.

The gene for glucocerebrosidase has been mapped, and more than 109 mutations have been described in patients with Gaucher disease (155). Most are missense mutations causing substitution of one amino acid for another, but insertions, deletions, and crossover recombinations also occur (152). The most common mutations in Jewish patients are 1226G and 84G, whereas 1448C and 1226G are most common in non-Jewish patients (156). The 1226G mutation is an alanine-to-glycine transition at base 1226 that results in an asparagine-to-serine substitution at amino acid 370. This substitution is associated with residual enzyme activity, and patients homozygous for 1226G either remain asymptomatic or have onset of symptoms in the adult years. In contrast, patients homozygous for the 1448T allele have severe loss of enzyme activity, and develop either type II or type III disease. Individuals carrying a 1226G/1448T combination have type I disease, with earlier and more severe involvement. Of note, the presence of the 1226G mutation precludes the development of neurologic problems (157).

Obviously, the type of mutation and its effect on enzyme activity correlate best with clinical severity and age at presentation. However, considerable heterogeneity also is noted among patients with the same genotype (157,158). Possible explanations for this variability include the effect of unknown modifying genes that link with the cerebroside enzyme, and the effect of nongenetic events, such as the influence of viral infections on splenomegaly, and traumatic injuries on the skeletal manifestations of the disease.

Age at onset of symptoms ranges from early childhood to the older adult years. In the study by Zimran and colleagues (158), the age at diagnosis averaged 25 years (range, 8 months to 70 years). The most common symptom at presentation was an abnormality of coagulation, such as epistaxis, easy bruising, or prolonged bleeding after superficial wounds. An incidental finding of splenomegaly or thrombocytopenia prompted diagnosis in some patients before symptoms occurred. Bone pain or fracture may herald the disease, but this was uncommon, noted in only 13% of patients.

Splenomegaly is a cardinal feature of Gaucher disease (158,159). The spleen may be enormous, occupying one-half of the abdomen, with resultant protuberant abdomen,

aching pain, and altered posture. Pancytopenia may occur, although thrombocytopenia and mild anemia are more common. Drug therapy has virtually eliminated the development of hypersplenism and the need for splenectomy in Gaucher disease.

Hepatomegaly also occurs, because glucocerebroside accumulates in Kupffer cells, the specialized macrophage cells that line the walls of the sinusoids of the liver. Compared with the spleen, the degree of liver dysfunction is not as severe (152). Abnormal liver function tests are common, but these abnormalities are of limited consequence. An exception is the effect of liver dysfunction on clotting factors. The resultant coagulopathy may complicate treatment of fractures or operations for arthritic conditions. Drug therapy can reverse these abnormalities.

The skeletal changes seen in Gaucher disease include abnormal widening of the metaphysis, osteopenia, Gaucher crisis or pseudoosteomyelitis, osteomyelitis, pathologic fractures, hemorrhagic cysts, avascular necrosis, and subsequent arthritis.

Infiltration of the bone marrow by the Gaucher cells is the primary cause of the skeletal problems. Triglyceride-rich adipocytes in the bone marrow are progressively replaced by Gaucher cells, and MRI studies show decreased intensity of involved marrow signals on both the T1 and T2 images (160,161). Quantitative MRI studies also correlate with disease severity, as measured by splenic enlargement and other complications (161–163).

Abnormal flaring of the metaphysis, the so-called Erlenmeyer-flask deformity, develops in approximately 70% of patients (158) (Fig. 11-9). This bony deformity most likely

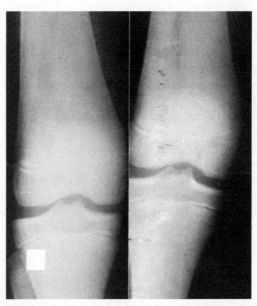

FIGURE 11-9. Flaring of the distal femoral metaphysis, known as Erlenmeyer-flask deformity, in a child with Gaucher disease. (Courtesy of Henry J. Mankin, M.D.)

results from expansion of a relatively weak metaphyseal cortex by the abundant Gaucher cells. The distal femur is most often involved, but the proximal tibia and the proximal humerus also may exhibit a widened metaphysis (164).

Osteopenia is most obvious in the axial and proximal portions of the appendicular skeleton. The osteopenia, however, is diffuse. Bone density measurements in 61 adult patients showed significant decrease at the lumbar spine, femoral neck, and distal radius, and the severity of the osteoporosis correlated with other disease indicators (165). Patients with osteopenia may complain of aching in the bones or loss of height secondary to vertebral wedging; however, the primary consequence of osteopenia is its predisposition to pathologic fractures.

A Gaucher crisis is characterized by acute, intense pain that is relatively well localized (159,166,167). Common sites include the distal femur, the proximal tibia, and the proximal femur. Mild swelling, localized tenderness, and fever are often present. The leukocyte count is elevated, ranging from 13,100 to 19,800 units in one series (166). Likewise, the erythrocyte sedimentation rate is elevated, typically in the range of 40 to 120 mm/h. These symptoms mimic osteomyelitis; hence, the alternative term for a Gaucher crisis is "pseudoosteomyelitis." Although uncommon, a crisis may be the first clinical manifestation of Gaucher disease. The finding of concomitant splenomegaly will suggest the correct diagnosis.

The cause of a crisis is hemorrhage in the intramedullary canal and, on occasion, the subperiosteal space (161,168). Thrombocytopenia and deficient clotting factors, in the environment of bone marrow crowded with Gaucher cells, lead to intramedullary bleeding. Blood under pressure and the inflammatory reaction explain the intense pain, and why the acute symptoms mimic osteomyelitis. Intramedullary hemorrhage also may cause localized ischemia and subsequent osteonecrosis.

At the onset of a crisis, radiographs are normal, but technetium bone scans demonstrate decreased uptake, and MRI scans show edema, as well as intramedullary and subperiosteal hemorrhage (166–168). Consistent with the subsequent inflammatory and remodeling responses, radiographs a few weeks after onset demonstrate periosteal elevation and lytic areas within the medullary canal (164) (Fig. 11-10). Bone scans at this time show increased uptake surrounding a central photopenic area (166). Several months later, the bone scans return to normal, but radiographs may show areas of sclerosis in the intramedullary canal, or areas of osteonecrosis in the femoral head, the tibial plateau, the femoral condyles, or the humeral head (Fig. 11-11).

Treatment for a crisis is supportive. The pain is typically severe for 1 to 3 days, and, during this time, intravenous narcotics are required. High-dose prednisolone has been reported to be effective at providing pain relief within a few hours (169). This therapy theoretically reduces bone and subperiosteal edema. With conventional treatment, the pain

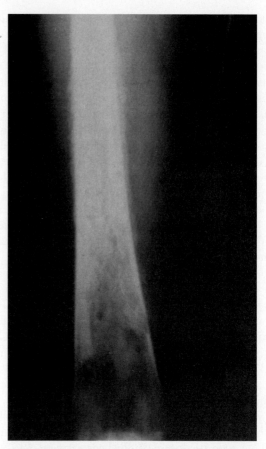

FIGURE 11-10. Bone destruction, sclerosis, and periosteal new bone formation in the femoral shaft after a Gaucher crisis. (Courtesy of Henry J. Mankin, M.D.)

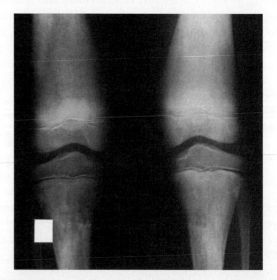

FIGURE 11-11. Radiolucency and osteosclerosis in the proximal tibial metaphysis are a result of Gaucher crisis. Note the Erlenmeyer-flask appearance of the distal femur. (Courtesy of Henry J. Mankin, M.D.)

gradually subsides over 2 to 4 weeks. Continued observation is needed to determine whether a complication, such as osteonecrosis of the femoral head, develops.

Osteomyelitis in Gaucher disease is uncommon, but it is characterized by a delay in diagnosis because it often follows a crisis. Furthermore, there is an increased prevalence of anaerobic organisms that is most likely related to the ischemic bone marrow. Laboratory and imaging studies may not differentiate a crisis from osteomyelitis. A bone biopsy may be required, but should be performed with caution, and using strict aseptic technique, because these patients are susceptible to developing infections after aspiration or surgical drainage (170).

Pathologic fractures may occur in children with Gaucher disease. Katz and colleagues (171) analyzed 23 fractures occurring in nine children with an average age of 12 years (range, 6 to 18 years). Common locations included the distal femur, the proximal tibia, and the base of the femoral neck. Fifteen fractures (65%) occurred at a site that had been affected by a crisis 2 to 12 months previously. Fractures of the femoral neck occur more often in children younger than 10 years of age, and may be complicated by coxa vara, pseudarthrosis, and avascular necrosis (164). Delayed union and nonunion are common in patients with Gaucher disease who are not on drug therapy.

Back pain in patients with Gaucher disease may be severe and secondary to either a crisis or a pathologic fracture (Fig. 11-12), or the pain may be mild and presumably secondary to osteopenia. In a series of 19 children and adolescents with spinal involvement, 9 episodes of nonspecific mild pain, which lasted for 2 to 5 days, occurred in the thoracic spine, and 3 patients had severe pain that was typical of a Gaucher crisis (172). One of the latter patients developed increased kyphosis. Pathologic fractures presented with an insidious onset of pain 1 to 2 months before diagnosis. The most common fracture pattern was rectangular compression and a "bone-within-a-bone" appearance of two to three adjacent vertebrae. In these patients, the vertebra healed with a central depression, and kyphosis or scoliosis was an infrequent complication. Anterior wedge compression fracture of one or more vertebrae also may occur, and these patients may develop severe kyphosis and spinal cord compression (172).

Osteonecrosis may develop in the femoral head, the femoral condyles, the tibial plateau, and the humeral head (159,164,167). In 53 patients evaluated at an average age of 33 years (range, 1 to 72 years), Zimran and colleagues (158) observed avascular necrosis of the femoral head in 11 patients. Two patients had total hip arthroplasty, and two patients had total knee replacement. Children who develop avascular necrosis of the femoral head have a guarded prognosis (Fig. 11-13). By their young adult years, they are mostly asymptomatic with daily activities, but have poor radiographic ratings (173). Osteonecrosis of the humeral head in patients with Gaucher disease is similar to sickle cell anemia, in that joint incongruity may cause limitation of motion, but the disability usually is not severe enough to limit routine activities or require total joint arthroplasty.

In the past, operative intervention in patients with Gaucher disease was complicated by excessive bleeding and

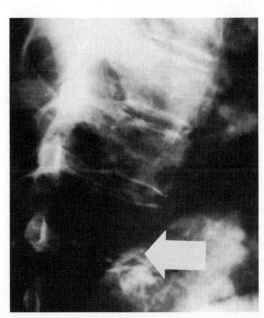

FIGURE 11-12. Compression fracture of a vertebra in Gaucher disease. (Courtesy of Henry J. Mankin, M.D.)

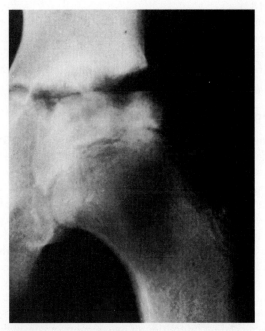

FIGURE 11-13. Late phases of osteonecrosis of the femoral head demonstrate flattening and incongruity. (Courtesy of Henry J. Mankin, M.D.)

osteopenic bone-limiting fixation (164,167). New drug therapy markedly decreases these problems.

Developments in medical therapy are exciting but expensive. In 1991, Barton and colleagues (174) reported that glucocerebrosidase could be altered, and the resultant enzyme, alglucerase, could be transported across the cell membrane. In addition to the placenta-derived enzyme, a recombinant form of the enzyme is now available. Studies of patients treated with alglucerase have consistently found normalization of hematologic parameters, decreased splenomegaly and hepatomegaly volume, and increased hemoglobin concentrations (175,176). Changes in the skeleton were not obvious in early studies, but with therapy for more than 3.5 years, Rosenthal and colleagues (177) noted marked improvement in both marrow composition and bone mass.

The cost of enzyme replacement therapy for Gaucher disease is very expensive, particularly when administered using a regimen of 60 U/kg every 2 weeks, which is the amount initially described. For a 70-kg patient, the wholesale cost of the medication alone is $382,000 (U.S.) per year. Several studies have reported that a low-dose/high-frequency protocol (2.3 U/kg three times per week; 30 U/kg/month) provides equivalent normalization of blood counts and decrease in the size of the liver and spleen (178–181). Indeed, some patients are satisfactorily managed using 15 U/kg/month. Home transfusion is a necessary component of this treatment. Skeletal symptoms are also reduced on the low-dose/high-frequency protocols, but whether the reduced dosage will be as effective in altering the skeletal changes is still unanswered. In addition, normalization of growth retardation was only noted in children receiving higher doses (60 to 120 U/kg/month) of alglucerase (182).

Bone marrow transplantation can be successful in type I Gaucher disease, but with the success of enzyme therapy, this treatment modality is used infrequently (183). Gene transfer trials have been initiated, and preliminary results are encouraging (184).

Langerhans Cell Histiocytosis

Eosinophilic granuloma of bone was first described in 1940 by Lichenstein and Jaffe (185) and Otani and Ehrlich (186). Green and Faber (187), in 1942, observed that the histopathology of eosinophilic granuloma was similar to that seen in Hand-Schüller-Christian disease and the more severe Letterer-Siwe disease. Because proliferating histiocytes are common to all three disorders, Lichenstein (188) designated this group of diseases "histiocytosis X." Because the Langerhans cell histiocyte is unique to these disorders, the Histiocyte Society, in 1985, recommended the term "Langerhans cell histiocytosis" (189), and that term is preferred.

Langerhans cell histiocytosis (LCH) is a disease complex characterized by infiltration of one or more organs by large mononuclear cells with benign-appearing nuclei that often have a central groove (151). Compared with other histiocytes, the unique structural aspect of the Langerhans cell is tubular or racket-shaped granules seen on electron microscopy. These granules, or organelles, apparently result from internalization of antigen complexes formed at the cell membrane (190). Enzymatic and monoclonal antibody studies have confirmed that these Langerhans cells have features of dendritic cells (191,192).

Not all of the histiocytes in LCH lesions are Langerhans cells; the typical granules are found in 2 to 79% of the histiocytes (193). Other cell types found in LCH lesions include lymphocytes, eosinophils, neutrophils, and, on occasion, multinucleated giant cells. Eosinophils are the predominant other cells, although they may be sparse or virtually absent.

Histopathologic features vary depending on the stage of the disease, the tissue involved, and unknown factors (151,194). Early in the disease process, the bony lesions typically are dominated by histiocytes. More mature lesions may be difficult to differentiate from a subacute or chronic osteomyelitis, but foci of necrosis, granulomatous changes with variable amounts of fibrosis, multinucleated giant cells, and the presence of the Langerhans cell usually distinguish the lesion as LCH.

The pathogenesis of LCH is still speculative. The disease is not a neoplasm, at least not in the classic sense; there is no evidence of aneuploidy and, although Langerhans cells within a lesion are clonal, this is not enough to define LCH as a neoplasm (195). A reactive immunologic process, causing bone and soft tissue destruction, is the probable cause. Some stimulus, perhaps a virus, triggers proliferation of the Langerhans cells; however, sensitive *in situ* hybridization and polymerase chain reaction techniques failed to find evidence of viruses in 56 cases of LCH (196). Cytokines are abundant in LCH tissue (197), and these enzymes probably play a major role in the inflammatory and osteolysis response. A loss of a "down-regulatory" signal could result in a proliferation of abnormal Langerhans cells.

LCH is more common in children, and, in this group, the median age of onset is 2 to 3 years (151). The clinical manifestations of LCH are protean, and every patient at presentation needs a thorough evaluation to determine the extent of the disease. Furthermore, ongoing evaluation is needed because the extent of the disease and its classification may change. The extent of the disease is classified as solitary bone involvement, multiple bone involvement without soft tissue involvement, bone and soft tissue involvement, or soft tissue involvement alone. Common sites of soft tissue involvement include the skin, lymph nodes, lungs, liver, ears, and pituitary stalk. The extent of soft tissue involvement, and the presence of organ dysfunction, usually are classified by the criteria described by Lahey (198) (Table 11-6). Skin involvement may vary from a few discrete pinhead lesions to a generalized pustular eczematous eruption. Generalized skin disease is a typical presenting feature in children younger than 2 years of age, and is a poor prognostic

TABLE 11-6. CRITERIA OF ORGAN DYSFUNCTION IN LANGERHANS CELL HISTIOCYTOSIS

Liver
    Albumin < 2.5 g/dL
    Bilirubin > 1.5 mg/dL
    Edema
    Ascites

Pulmonary system[a]
    Cough
    Cyanosis
    Dyspnea
    Pleural effusion
    Pneumothorax

Hematopoietic system
    Anemia < 10 mg/dL[b]
    Leukopenia < 4,000/dL
    Neutropenia < 1,500/dL
    Thrombocytopenia < 100,000/dL

[a] Not secondary to pulmonary infection.
[b] Not attributable to iron-deficiency anemia.
(Adapted from ref. 198, with permission.)

factor (199). Fatal dissemination occurs more often in children younger that 2 years of age at onset, but it also may occur when the disease is diagnosed in later childhood, or even in the adult years (200). Failure of organs, such as the lungs, liver, spleen, and bone marrow, is the usual cause of death (198,199,201–203). Generalized involvement of the brain often occurs in adults and in children with disseminated disease.

Diabetes insipidus occurs in 12 to 50% of children with multiple system involvement (201,204). It may be the only abnormality at the onset of the disease (205), but more often it occurs after LCH has been diagnosed. Diabetes insipidus is the most frequent abnormality that subsequently develops in patients who have only bone involvement at the onset of disease (206).

Skeletal lesions are common, occurring in 80 to 97% of patients with LCH (199,203,204,207,208). The skull, spine, pelvis, ribs, and femur are the common sites of bony lesions (209). Other long bones may be involved, but lesions in the hands and feet are rare. Skull lesions have a well-defined, punched-out appearance (Fig. 11-14). Vertebra plana, first described by Compere and colleagues (210), is the typical spinal lesion. The vertebral body is markedly collapsed, but in contrast to an infectious process, the adjacent disc space is preserved. Posterior elements usually are spared. In the series by Ruppert and colleagues (211), a thoracic vertebra was most often affected (54%), and a cervical vertebra was least often involved (11%).

Long-bone lesions are typically lytic, and located in the diaphysis or metaphysis (Fig. 11-14). Other radiographic features include endosteal scalloping, cortical thinning, and widening of the medullary cavity (211). Lamellated eleva-

tion of the periosteum (onion skinning), simulating Ewing sarcoma or osteomyelitis, accounts for approximately 5% of the solitary eosinophilic granulomas (Fig. 11-15). In a series of 25 children presenting with diaphyseal periosteal elevation, ten cases were secondary to Ewing sarcoma and seven were diagnosed as eosinophilic granuloma (212). Patients with Ewing sarcoma are more likely to show definite Codman triangles, as well as intramedullary and cortical destruction. Epiphyseal or transphyseal involvement is uncommon, but has been reported (211,213,214). In a series of 15 solitary lucent epiphyseal lesions, only one case was secondary to eosinophilic granuloma (213).

Skeletal surveys should be combined with bone scans, because both modalities can give false-negative results (207,215). In a study that compared bone scans with skeletal surveys in 42 patients, 36 (19%) of the 191 lesions were missed on bone scans, and 55 (29%) were missed on routine skeletal surveys (215). Bone scans were more sensitive in detecting LCH lesions in the ribs, spine, and pelvis, but less sensitive in detecting lesions in the skull. Both modalities have similar sensitivity in the extremities. MRI changes are nonspecific, because the low signal intensity on T1-weighted images, and the high signal intensity on T2-weighted images, do not differentiate eosinophilic granuloma from osteomyelitis or Ewing sarcoma (216). On the other hand, bone scans, computed tomography, and MRI may be useful in localizing a site of unexplained pain, or in finding spinal cord compression.

A bony lesion without soft tissue involvement is the most common presentation of LCH, accounting for 50 to 77% of the pediatric cases (203,204,207,208). Patients with solitary bone involvement at disease onset have the best prognosis, and, in this group, no deaths have been reported (201,203,204,207,217). In comparison, patients with organ dysfunction at disease onset have a mortality rate of 30 to 70% (201–204). Evolution to multiple bone lesions or soft tissue involvement is also uncommon. Bollini and colleagues (207) reviewed 216 patients from eight series who had solitary bone involvement. Evolution to multiple bone lesions occurred in 7% of patients, mostly during the first year after diagnosis, and only 1% of patients developed soft tissue involvement. Dimentberg and Brown (208) found a 30% incidence of new bony lesions in patients with initial solitary involvement. Their protocol, however, included periodic skeletal surveys, and 55% of their new lesions were asymptomatic.

Multiple bone involvement without soft tissue involvement has a good prognosis. However, the incidence of additional bone lesions and subsequent soft tissue involvement is higher in this group (208). Development of diabetes insipidus is the most common soft tissue problem. The mortality rate of this group is low, being only 1 of 22 patients in the series reported by Raney and D'Angio (203).

The presenting complaints of patients with a solitary

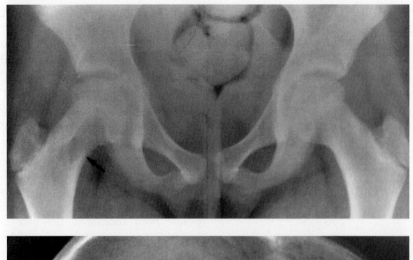

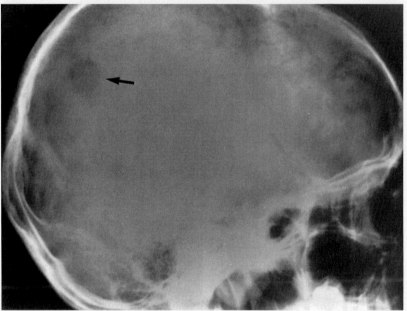

FIGURE 11-14. Eosinophilic granuloma, with multiple bone involvement, in a 9-year-old girl who had progressive symptoms of pain and limp involving the right hip. **A:** Anteroposterior radiograph of the pelvis demonstrates a lytic lesion in the right femoral neck. Biopsy defined the diagnosis. Follow-up radiographs, taken 5 months later, show complete resolution of the lesion. **B:** Lateral radiograph of the skull 5 months after biopsy of the femur. At that time, the patient had a sore spot on the back of the head. Radiographs show the typical "punched-out" appearance of eosinophilic granuloma. Three months later, the patient developed a third bony lesion in the left proximal femur. Subsequent follow-up showed a full resolution of symptoms without therapy.

bone lesion are localized swelling, pain, or limp (Fig. 11-16). The child also may be asymptomatic, with the diagnosis being made from radiographs obtained for unrelated reasons. In any circumstance, these patients should be evaluated for possible additional bone lesions. Inquire concerning symptoms of lethargy, polyuria or polydipsia, chronic cough, dyspnea, and feeding difficulties. Examine for the possibility of skin rash, otitis, exophthalmos, tachypnea, sinusitis, hepatomegaly, jaundice, splenomegaly, growth retardation, and swelling or tenderness over the skull, facial bones, spine, and extremities. A lateral skull radiograph is

a good screening study for a child with a solitary bone lesion of unknown cause. Additional laboratory studies that should be considered for a child with known LCH include a complete blood count and smear, liver function tests, serum and urine osmolarity, and radiographic survey of the chest and skeleton (208). Unless clinically indicated, hand and foot radiographs are not necessary because these regions are rarely involved. For patients with significant risk of organ dysfunction, such as those with obvious soft tissue involvement or those younger than 3 years of age who have multiple bone lesions, Dimentberg and Brown (208) recommend

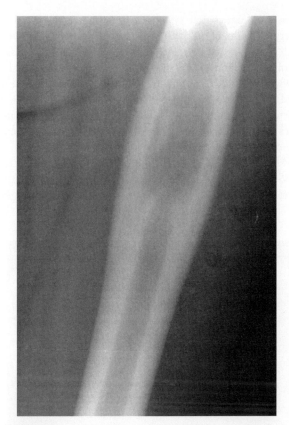

FIGURE 11-15. Eosinophilic granuloma in a 12-year-old girl who had pain in the thigh for 3 to 4 months. Radiograph of the femur shows an expansile lesion with periosteal reaction.

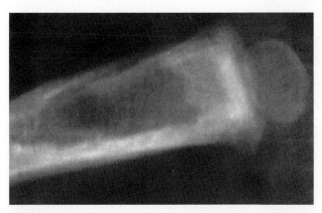

FIGURE 11-16. Eosinophilic granuloma in a 9-month-old boy who had a 2-week history of a mass in the thigh. Before transfer, the patient had received several days of antibiotic therapy. Lateral radiograph of the distal femur shows a large lytic lesion with periosteal elevation. After biopsy and curettage, the femur was protected with a spica cast. No other lesions developed, and follow-up 10 years later demonstrated no abnormalities.

additional studies, including arterial blood gas, bone marrow aspirate, computed tomography of the chest, abdominal ultrasonography, audiology assessment, dental assessment, and immunologic profile.

A biopsy is necessary to confirm the suspected diagnosis. The exception is the patient with classic multifocal radiographic findings. When the skin is involved, it is the preferred site of biopsy. A typical lytic lesion of bone can be biopsied by transcutaneous needle aspiration (207). Open biopsy is preferred when curettage is indicated, or for mid-diaphyseal lesions characterized by periosteal elevation.

Treatment of bone lesions in patients without soft tissue involvement should be limited to observation, medical management, steroid injection, or curettage. The rate of healing was not significantly different in a study evaluating treatment versus observation of bony lesions (218). Observation is indicated when the patient is asymptomatic or has only mild symptoms, and when the lesion does not have a high risk of fracture. Curettage is an adjunct to open biopsy. In addition, this mode of therapy, with or without supplemental bone grafting, may be selected for lesions associated with intense pain or significant risk of fracture. Intralesional steroid injections have been reported to provide good results (219). Owing to the variable rate of healing and the self-limited nature of LCH, it is difficult to know whether this treatment influences the natural history. Steroid injections, however, may be preferred for lesions with persistent pain and slow healing after curettage. Based on the abundant production of cytokines and prostaglandin E_2 in bone lesions of LCH, Munn and colleagues (220) treated ten symptomatic children with indomethacin (1 to 2.5 mg/kg/day in divided doses). Eight patients had complete response to treatment. Whether indomethacin has a specific role in slowing disease progression or merely acts as an analgesic has not yet been established. Of note, low-dose radiotherapy should not be used because there are two reports documenting secondary malignancy after this therapy was used for solitary bone involvement (208,221).

Solitary spinal lesions typically cause pain, and may be associated with postural adaptations, such as torticollis or scoliosis. However, LCH in the spine may also be asymptomatic. Indeed, multiple sites of asymptomatic spinal involvement may be present in patients with disseminated soft tissue involvement. Vertebra plana without posterior arch involvement is the most common pattern, but cases have been reported of lesions limited to the posterior arch, of lesions involving the vertebral body that did not cause collapse, and of lesions in the spinal cord without bony involvement (211,222,223). Most patients do not have neurologic deficits, and can be treated symptomatically by short-term immobilization in plaster casts, and orthoses after the diagnosis has been confirmed (224). Reconstitution of vertebral height to a variable but effective amount is the natural history, and long-term follow-up studies have not observed back or neck dysfunction (223).

Although uncommon, eosinophilic granuloma of the spine may cause neurologic deficit (223,225). In these patients, clinical and MRI examinations should be able to differentiate nerve root involvement from spinal cord compression. With nerve root impingement, treatment should include bed rest, immobilization, and perhaps steroid injection. For patients with spinal cord compression, surgical decompression and stabilization should be considered, unless there is disseminated disease and an unfavorable prognosis. Radiotherapy may be indicated with this degree of involvement.

Chemotherapy has a limited role in LCH, and most au-

thors now agree that systemic chemotherapy generally is reserved for patients who have constitutional symptoms, such as fever and weight loss, and those who have severe skin involvement and organ dysfunction, as defined by Lahey (198,202,226,227). Even in this group, a short course of prednisolone may be the best initial treatment (202). Bone marrow transplantation also has been reported in isolated cases of patients who did not respond to multiple-regimen chemotherapy (228,229).

The earliest radiographic finding denoting healing of appendicular skeletal lesions is development of a trabecular pattern (Fig. 11-17). In a study by Alexander and colleagues

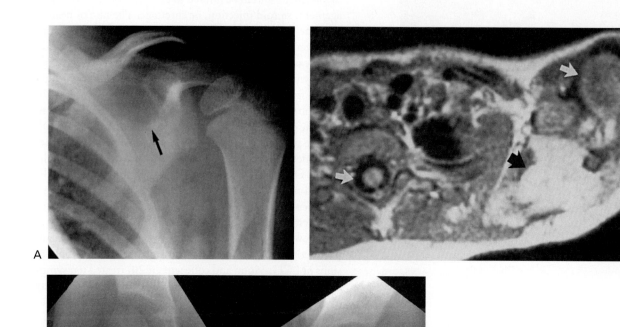

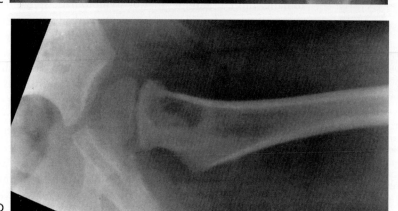

FIGURE 11-17. A 2-year, 6-month-old girl who presented with swelling in the posterior region of the scapula. **A:** Anteroposterior view of the scapula demonstrates a lytic lesion (*arrow*). Biopsy showed Langerhans cell histiocytosis. **B:** Four months later, the patient developed recurrent swelling and drainage from the left scapular biopsy site. Magnetic resonance image before the second biopsy of the scapula shows increased signal intensity with spread into soft tissues anterior and posterior to the scapula. *White arrow* points to the humeral head and spinal cord. *Black arrow* points to the mass invading the scapula. Repeat biopsy also demonstrated Langerhans cell histiocytosis. The scapular lesion subsequently resolved without problems. **C:** Anteroposterior radiograph of the pelvis at age 3 years, 4 months. At that time, the patient had developed a limp and pain in the left leg. Radiographs show a lytic lesion in the proximal femur. Spica cast immobilization was used for 7 weeks. **D:** Frog-leg lateral radiograph of the left hip at age 3 years, 4 months. *(continued)*

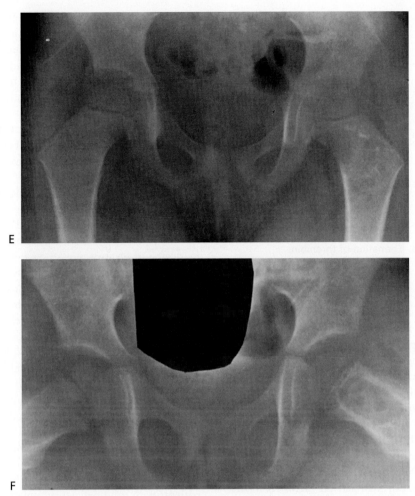

FIGURE 11-17. *(continued)* **E:** Anteroposterior radiograph of the pelvis at age 3 years, 6 months. **F:** Frog-leg lateral radiograph of the pelvis at age 3 years, 6 months. Trabecular pattern indicates progressive healing of the Langerhans cell histiocytosis. (Courtesy of Gary D. Bos, M.D.)

(230), the trabecular pattern was observed 6 to 10 weeks after diagnosis in patients who had uneventful healing. Complete healing then occurred within the next 36 to 40 weeks. Therefore, it is reasonable to repeat radiographs of the involved lesion approximately 2 months after diagnosis. If a trabecular pattern has developed, the next radiologic examination can be scheduled at the 6-month interval. However, if no evidence of trabeculation has occurred, repeat radiographs are warranted in another 2 months. If there is no evidence of healing at 4 months after diagnosis, additional therapy may be indicated. Routine skeletal surveys, as well as a complete physical examination, should be performed every 6 months for at least 2 years (208). These surveys will diagnose new bony and soft tissue lesions in a timely fashion.

In summary, Langerhans cell histiocytosis is a fascinating disorder that is probably secondary to an aberrant reactive immunologic process. Solitary bony involvement is most common. In these patients, treatment probably does not

influence healing, and making a diagnosis and classifying the extent of involvement is more important. Periodic reexamination is needed, because the disease classification may change. Patients with organ dysfunction have a guarded prognosis, and systemic chemotherapy is indicated.

DISORDERS OF HEMOSTASIS

Hemostasis protects us from the many bumps of everyday activity and permits safe surgery. Injury to a blood vessel initiates a highly integrated set of reactions to restore hemostasis. Although the reactions overlap, it is helpful to divide the clotting process into vascular, platelet, and plasma components.

The vascular component includes the grossly evident vasoconstriction, as well as exposure of tissue elements that activate platelets, and the coagulation cascade. The platelet component includes adhesion of platelets to vascular tissues

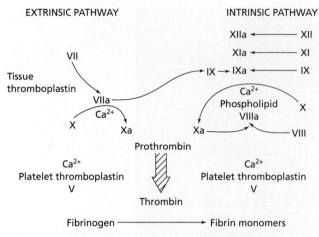

FIGURE 11-18. Formation of thrombin.

(assisted by factor VIII–related von Willebrand factor), aggregation of platelets to each other to form a platelet plug, and stabilization of the platelet plug by deposition of fibrin within it.

The plasma component of restoration of hemostasis has an extrinsic or membrane surface pathway and an intrinsic pathway. Because it is now evident that activated factor VII can activate both factor X and factor IX, the relative value of the intrinsic versus the extrinsic pathway is considered less important. In the extrinsic pathway, tissue factor binds activated factor VII on membrane surfaces. The tissue factor–factor VIIa complex can then activate factor IX in the intrinsic pathway and factor X in the standard extrinsic pathway (Fig. 11-18). Factor IXa combines with activated factor VIII to form a complex that also activates factor X. In the intrinsic pathway, exposure to collagen activates factor XII, which then activates factor XI; this is followed by activation of factor IX. Factor VIII is important, because once it is activated, this factor accelerates the activation of factor X by activated factor IX. Activated factor Xa forms a complex with activated factor V, to convert prothrombin to thrombin, which then converts fibrinogen to fibrin.

Hemophilia

Any of the 14 coagulation factors may be deficient, but musculoskeletal problems are primarily found in patients with deficits of either factor VIII, also known as hemophilia A, or factor IX, also known as hemophilia B. Both factor VIII and factor IX deficiencies are transmitted by a sex-linked recessive gene; therefore, both disorders are largely restricted to the male population. The other inherited coagulation disorders are very uncommon, and, more importantly, are characterized by mucosal hemorrhages, such as epistaxis and menorrhagia, and rarely demonstrate hemorrhage into a joint, except after major trauma. A surveillance

study of people with hemophilia A or B in six U.S. states found that 2,156 (79%) had factor VIII deficiency (231). The age-adjusted prevalence of hemophilia A and B was 13.4 cases per 100,000 males, and the average incidence was estimated to be 1 in 5,032 live male births. Hemophilia occurs in all ethnic groups, and shows no significant racial predilection.

The diagnosis of hemophilia is suggested in infants who have atypical bleeding at the time of circumcision or atypical bruising with neonatal immunizations, and in toddlers who develop lip lacerations and unusual bruising while learning to walk. A history of affected males on the maternal side of the family is another clue. The partial thromboplastin time is abnormal in both factor VIII and IX deficiency, and specific factor assays are used to establish the diagnosis and its degree of severity.

Coagulation factors are quantitated in units: 1 U is equal to the activity of the clotting factor in 1 mL of pooled, normal plasma. The concentration of factors VIII and IX is commonly designated as a percentage of activity, representing units per deciliter. Therefore, factor VIII and IX activity in a normal person should be 100%, but a range from 50 to 200% is within normal limits. Deficiencies of coagulation factors are graded as severe (less than 1% activity), moderate (1 to 5% activity), and mild (more than 5% activity) (232). In a surveillance study, 43% of patients had severe, 26% had moderate, and 31% had mild hemophilia (231). In patients with severe hemophilia, a hemarthrosis may occur with minimal trauma, or spontaneously during normal daily activities, but joint bleeds rarely develop in patients with mild deficiency, unless significant trauma occurs. Patients with moderate deficiency have intermediate symptoms but typically develop significantly less arthropathy than patients with severe disorders.

Neither acute bleeding episodes nor surgery can be managed effectively in hemophiliacs without appropriate replacement of the missing clotting factor. When only whole blood or plasma was available, the volume requirements for even a single transfusion were so great that transfusions were administered only in limb-threatening and life-threatening situations. The discovery of cryoprecipitate, in 1965 (233), and the subsequent development of concentrates (234,235), radically expanded treatment options for hemophiliacs. With concentrates, it was possible to deliver a total blood volume of clotting factor in a 50-mL solution. As a result, transfusion therapy at home and elective operations were widely instituted in the 1970s.

Both factor VIII and factor IX concentrates were initially prepared from plasma that was pooled from many donors, a process that allowed transmission of blood-borne diseases. In the 1970s, hepatitis was a recognized complication of transfusion therapy, and most hemophiliacs at that time had hepatitis-associated antibodies. In the early 1980s, AIDS clearly was identified in hemophiliacs. Heat treatment of the concentrates, however, virtually eliminated HIV, so that hemophiliacs who received their initial transfusion after 1984 were not infected by HIV (232). Both factor VIII and factor IX can now be manufactured using recombinant DNA techniques that produce a purified product. Therefore, virtually all pediatric patients with hemophilia are now seronegative for both HIV and hepatitis viruses.

Inhibitors are antibodies that develop to the infused product. They develop in about 15% of patients with severe factor VIII deficiencies, but their frequency is much lower in patients with factor IX deficiency (236,237). Patients with an inhibitor do not bleed more frequently, but have limited options for transfusion. The potency of a patient's inhibitor status is defined in Bethesda units per milliliter of plasma. High responders have inhibitor titers of greater than 10 Bethesda units, and develop an anamnestic response with subsequent exposure. Low responders maintain an inhibitor titer of less than 10 Bethesda units, even when exposed to repeated doses of factor VIII. Of note, the likelihood of developing a high-titer inhibitor is remote if a patient has received 100 transfusions, and elective surgery may proceed in these patients without apprehension that this complication will develop in the postoperative period (232).

Low responders can undergo elective surgery, using higher doses of factor VIII transfusion. In high responders, elective surgery is not feasible unless the patient has undergone multiple, sequential transfusions to induce immune tolerance. The overall success rate for immune tolerance in hemophilia A is 63 to 83% (238). Daily factor transfusions increase the likelihood of success, and the duration of transfusions is typically several months. The other option under investigation is activated factor VII. Factor VIIa is thought to interact with tissue factor at the site of bleeding, then to activate factor X, thereby bypassing factor VIII. Intraoperative hemostasis was achieved with recombinant factor VIIa

in 28 of 29 inhibitor patients undergoing elective surgery (239).

Hemophilic arthropathy begins with a hemarthrosis, particularly when two or three bleeding episodes occur in a joint within a short period. As the blood inside the joint is catabolized, the breakdown products must be absorbed by the synovium. Iron is the most damaging element (232,240–242). Synovial cells can absorb a limited amount of iron, but when that quantity is exceeded, the cell disintegrates and releases lysosomes that not only destroy articular cartilage, but inflame the synovial tissue. The result is a hypertrophic and hypervascular synovium that, in a person with a clotting deficiency, is friable, and tends to bleed easily (Fig. 11-19). Thus begins a vicious cycle of recurrent hemarthrosis followed by more synovitis and joint destruction.

Blood-breakdown products also affect the chondrocytes. Even in the early stage of joint disease, the chondrocytes contain siderosomes (secondary lysosomes containing iron ferritin granules), and show intracellular evidence of cell disruption (232,243). With disintegration of the chondrocyte, not only are lysosomes released to destroy the matrix of the cartilage, but the factory (the chondrocyte) also is destroyed (Fig. 11-20).

As hemophilic arthropathy progresses, the synovium loses its marked villous formation, and is mostly replaced by fibrous tissue. This, in combination with erosion of the articular surfaces, causes loss of joint motion. The end result may be a disabling arthritis at an early age (Fig. 11-21).

Radiographic changes in the early stages of hemophilic arthropathy are similar to those observed in rheumatoid arthritis. Soft tissue swelling, osteopenia, and overgrowth of the epiphysis are observed with the initiation of synovitis. As the disease progresses, marginal erosions, subchondral cysts, subchondral irregularity, widening of the intercondylar notch of the femur, squaring of the patella, enlargement

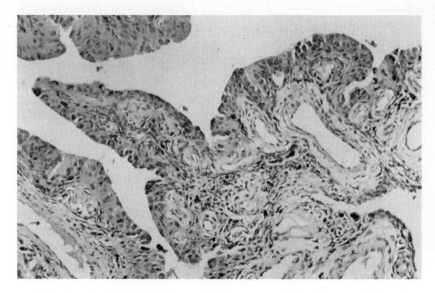

FIGURE 11-19. Synovium from an 8-year-old boy with hemophilia who had an 18-month history of hypertrophic synovitis and recurrent hemarthrosis in the knee. Note villous formation, markedly increased vascularity, and chronic inflammatory cell infiltrates. (From ref. 232, with permission.)

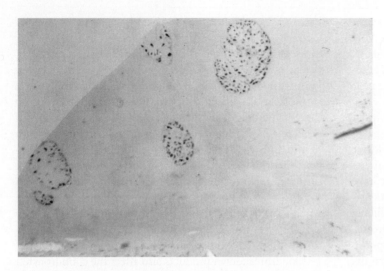

FIGURE 11-20. Cartilage shaving from patellar erosions in an 11-year-old boy with factor IX hemophilia. The patient had only a 9-month history of difficulty with this knee. Chondrocytes demonstrate disintegration, with iron deposition around the periphery (Perls stain). (From ref. 232, with permission.)

of the radial head, and widening of the trochlear notch of the olecranon are characteristic changes (Fig 11-22). With end-stage arthropathy, narrowing of the articular cartilage is obvious, but the subchondral bone is more sclerotic in hemophiliacs than in patients with rheumatoid arthritis. Hemophilic arthropathy may be staged by radiographs, and a four-part, seven-point classification has shown good correlation with joint function, as measured by range of motion and muscle torque (244) (Table 11-7).

The knee, ankle, and elbow are the joints most commonly affected in hemophiliacs (245–247). In small children, the ankle is frequently the target. In one series (245), the elbow was the most common site of bleeding during

adolescence, but other studies (246,247) have noted that the knee is more frequently affected at that age. The shoulder, hip, and wrist rarely are affected by a hemarthrosis, and, in this era of home therapy, these joints rarely progress to significant arthropathy.

The physical signs of hemarthrosis include increased warmth, swelling, and some limitation of motion. A prodrome of pain or discomfort frequently is perceived before the joint swelling is obvious. Transfusion as soon as possible is most critical in the management of any bleeding episode, and with concentrates home therapy is feasible. For routine treatment of muscle or joint hemorrhage, the patient or the patient's parents transfuse 20 to 25 U of factor per kilogram of body weight. This amount of transfusion typically keeps the clotting factor greater than 1% for at least 48 hours (Fig. 11-23).

Home transfusion therapy, with treatment on demand, has certainly reduced the severity and incidence of hemophilic arthropathy, but has not eliminated this problem. Prophylactic transfusions, a concept initiated in some northern European centers, are being used increasingly in the United States. Transfusions (25 U/kg) are typically given three times per week. This keeps factor levels greater than 1%, an amount that should prevent joint bleeds that occur with trivial trauma. Theoretically, if the joints are normal at the end of childhood, then the mature, adult person with hemophilia could function quite well within the confines of his or her coagulopathy.

To maintain essentially normal radiologic outcomes, prophylactic transfusions must be started in most patients by the age of 2 to 3 years (248,249). Even a small number of joint bleeds (one to four), before the initiation of continuous prophylaxis, will adversely influence the subsequent progression of arthropathy. Venous access, therefore, is a problem when transfusions are administered three times per week in a small child. Implantable devices are required.

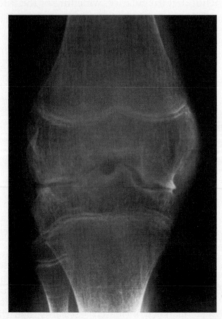

FIGURE 11-21. Radiograph of the knee of a 14-year-old boy with advanced hemophilic arthropathy.

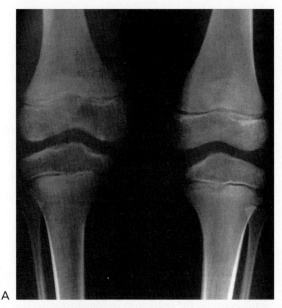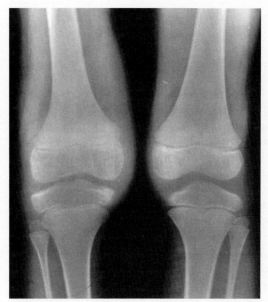

FIGURE 11-22. A: Anteroposterior standing radiograph of the knee in a 7-year, 2-month-old boy with factor VIII deficiency. Early changes of hypertrophic synovitis and hemophilic arthropathy are present in the right knee. Note the widening of the intercondylar notch. **B:** Anteroposterior standing radiograph of both knees 8 months later. The arthropathy has progressed despite good compliance with home transfusion therapy and 6 months of prophylactic transfusions. Significant joint narrowing and cartilage erosions are observed in the right knee. (From ref. 79, with permission.)

These devices are effective, but have a risk of bacteremia with long-term use, the rate, over approximately 3 years, ranging from 12 to 56% (250–252). The treatment is also expensive, primarily because of the cost of recombinant factors VIII and IX. The cost of the factor itself, if administered three times per week between the ages of 2 and 18 years in

TABLE 11-7. RADIOGRAPHIC GRADING OF HEMOPHILIC ARTHROPATHY

Classification	Score
Subchondral irregularity	
Absent	0
Mild (≤50% of joint surface)	1
Pronounced	2
Joint space narrowing	
Absent	0
≤50%	1
>50%	2
Joint margin erosion	
Absent	0
Present	1
Joint surface incongruity	
Absent	0
Mild	1
Pronounced	2

(Adapted from ref. 244, with permission.)

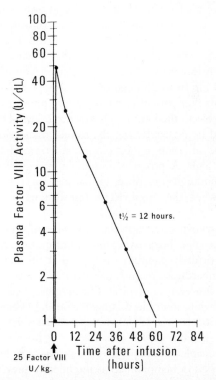

FIGURE 11-23. Typical falloff curve after infusion of 25 U/kg body weight of factor VIII in a patient with severe hemophilia. $t^{1/2}$, half-life. (From ref. 79, with permission.)

an average-size child, is approximately $3 million (U.S.). Therefore, studies that include issues such as costs of hospitalization, surgery, and days lost from school or work still find that prophylactic transfusion is significantly more expensive than episodic care (253,254).

Another approach to preventing disabling hemophilic arthropathy is to use different treatment protocols for minor versus major joint bleeds. A minor hemarthrosis can be treated at home by transfusing the appropriate concentrate as soon as possible. Ice packs, mild analgesics, crutches, and splints are useful adjuncts in controlling pain and swelling.

A major hemarthrosis is different. This type of bleed usually occurs after significant trauma, or as a recurrent hemarthrosis in a joint that already is affected by synovitis. A major hemarthrosis is painful. Furthermore, with a large amount of blood in the joint, hypertrophic synovitis and recurrent hemarthrosis are likely sequelae. In addition to transfusion, a major hemarthrosis should be treated with aspiration, short-term splinting, a defined rehabilitation program, and, most importantly, repeated transfusions, to minimize the risk of developing hypertrophic synovitis.

Aspiration is critical in treating a major hemarthrosis (232). Removing the bulk of blood within the joint greatly reduces the amount of iron that must be absorbed, the risk of developing hypertrophic synovitis, and recurrent hemorrhage. Aspiration also dramatically reduces the severe pain associated with a major hemarthrosis. After routine factor transfusion (25 U/kg), the joint is aspirated using local anesthetic agents and other analgesic measures.

Prophylactic transfusions are needed to protect the joint while it is recovering from a major hemarthrosis. Transfusions are repeated every 48 hours. This schedule keeps factor levels greater than 1%, an amount that usually prevents recurrent hemorrhage. The prophylactic transfusions are continued for 10 to 28 days, or even longer if synovitis is still present. For patient comfort, and to minimize risk of an early rebleed, the joint is splinted for 2 days. The splint is removed immediately after the second transfusion. This enables the initiation of joint motion at a time when factor levels are high. A program of muscle strengthening and range of motion is prescribed, so that the joint is fully rehabilitated when the prophylactic transfusions are discontinued.

When synovitis develops, the affected joint is swollen by the hypertrophic, boggy synovium. Joint motion, however, is not particularly painful or restricted at this early stage, unless a hemarthrosis recently has occurred. Recurrent hemarthroses, however, are typical. Furthermore, between episodes of obvious joint bleeds, ongoing oozing of blood from the hypervascular friable synovium perpetuates the synovitis and joint effusion.

The principle of nonoperative management of hypertrophic synovitis in hemophiliacs is intended to prevent joint bleeds so that the synovitis may resolve. In a study of prophylactic transfusions for hypertrophic synovitis and recurrent hemarthrosis, the rate of hemarthrosis in the affected joint was reduced, but only 36% (12 of 33 joints) achieved a good result (defined as 0 to 0.5 bleeding episodes per month and decreased synovial hypertrophy) (255). It is uncommon for prophylactic transfusions to resolve subacute synovitis completely, particularly if the synovial hypertrophy is moderate or severe.

Synovectomy in hemophiliacs initially was reported by Storti and colleagues (256) in 1969. Since then, many centers have reported the results of this operation in hemophiliacs. Reduction in the rate of hemarthrosis is a consistent result, and is the only noncontroversial aspect of this procedure. This is important, however, because reducing the incidence of joint bleeds has both functional and economic benefits. An acute hemarthrosis is painful, and will limit ambulation and function for 1 to 10 days, even when transfusions are administered promptly (245). Therefore, when hemarthroses are occurring three to six times per month, the child is severely disabled. In addition, by 1 year after synovectomy, the reduction in transfusion requirements actually offsets the cost of transfusion required to perform the operation (257).

Whether synovectomy stops the progression of hemophilic arthropathy is more difficult to answer. Although the data are not conclusive, the reports of knee synovectomy, with long-term follow-up (258–265), and my personal observations, support the concept that the procedure delays but does not eliminate the progression of arthropathy. Joints with less-advanced changes at the time of synovectomy have demonstrated less progression (258,260,262,265). Although recurrent synovitis is uncommon, it is not surprising that the arthropathy continues to progress because articular cartilage erosions already are present in many hemophiliacs at the time of synovectomy.

Most synovectomies have been performed on the knee. The initial technique was an open procedure managed with conventional postoperative therapy. In these cases, loss of motion was common and significant, even with prolonged inpatient therapy. For example, in a series of 13 patients, Montane and colleagues (260) observed that 11 patients lost an average of 43 degrees of motion. Continuous passive motion, and the use of arthroscopic technique to perform the operation, have improved the results of knee synovectomy in hemophiliac patients (258,265–269). Most authors who advocate arthroscopic knee synovectomy also recommend postoperative continuous passive motion (258,266, 268,269). By using these techniques, the range of knee motion can be maintained. Arthroscopic synovectomy of the knee in a hemophiliac is a demanding and time-consuming procedure. The hypertrophic, fibrotic synovium can be difficult to remove, and thorough removal is necessary to prevent recurrent hemarthroses. In addition, arteriovenous fistula has been reported after this procedure in hemophiliac patients (270).

Open synovectomy of the knee has some advantages. It permits more effective and less traumatic removal of the synovium, particularly where the synovium inserts at the margin of the articular cartilage. Joint motion is maintained by preserving the joint capsule in the suprapatellar region and instituting continuous passive motion immediately after the operation. Preserving the suprapatellar capsule provides an interface for movement of the quadriceps tendon over the distal femur. This tissue, however, has become attenuated by the hypertrophic synovium, and must be dissected carefully from the underlying synovium. Because articular erosions and fibrillations typically are present in these patients at the time of synovectomy, it is mandatory that an arc of motion be established immediately. Otherwise, adhesions develop and it is difficult to rehabilitate the joint.

Elbow synovectomy usually is accompanied by radial head excision in the older adolescent or adult. The enlarged and incongruent radial head is probably secondary to the hypervascular synovium stimulating aberrant growth. After the radial head has been removed, it is easy to excise the remainder of the synovium. For a younger child, excision of the radial head is contraindicated. In this situation, it is difficult to perform an open synovectomy without taking down the collateral ligaments. Arthroscopic synovectomy would seem to be a better approach in younger children, and Busch and Kurczynski (271) have reported good results in three patients treated with arthroscopic synovectomy of the elbow.

The limited experience with ankle synovectomy in children suggests that the results are good and that rehabilitation is relatively easy, using either open or arthroscopic technique. Greene (272) described a three-incision technique that allowed a complete synovectomy. Continuous passive motion was not required, and rehabilitation was easy and effective, even though three of the five children were younger than 5 years of age. The rate of hemarthrosis in the involved ankle averaged 3.4 per month before synovectomy, compared with 0.1 per month after the operation. In addition, the range of ankle motion increased by an average of 10 degrees. Busch and Kurczynski (271) have presented similar results after arthroscopic synovectomy of the ankle. Of note, 1 of their 17 ankle synovectomy patients developed a pseudoaneurysm of the anterior tibial artery.

Radiosynovectomy is an alternative and may be the only option for a patient with an inhibitor. Radioactive isotopes cause fibrosis of synovial tissue; however, articular cartilage is relatively resistant to the effects of radiation, and joint function is maintained. The cost of a radiosynovectomy is significantly lower. The procedure can be performed on an outpatient basis, and, more importantly, transfusion of the expensive clotting factor is only necessary for 1 to 3 days. Therefore, even a patient with a high-responding inhibitor can undergo radiosynovectomy. The disadvantages are the higher rate of recurrent hemarthrosis and the theoretical concerns of causing chromosomal damage and subsequent malignancy.

Gold (^{198}Au), yttrium (^{90}Y), rhenium (^{186}Re), chromic phosphate (^{32}P), and dysprosium (^{165}Dy) are the radioisotopes that have been used in hemophiliac patients. ^{165}Dy has a short half-life (2.3 h) and therefore can be used only in centers that are adjacent to nuclear reactors. For that reason, it has been reported in only a few patients with hemophilia (273). ^{198}Au and ^{186}Re have relatively short half-lives (2.7 and 3.7 days, respectively) and have been used successfully in patients with hemophilia (274–276). These agents, however, have the disadvantage of a relatively shallow depth of penetration; therefore, they may not be optimal for large joints. Furthermore, leakage outside the joint may be higher with these agents.

Good results in patients with hemophilia have been reported with ^{90}Y (277–279), an agent that has a relatively short half-life of 2.7 days, but a greater depth of penetration (mean of 3.6 versus 1.2 mm for ^{198}Au and ^{186}Re). Heim and colleagues (279) used ^{90}Y in 50 joints of 43 hemophilia patients, 4 of whom had inhibitors. The rate of hemarthrosis of the affected joint decreased from one bleed per week to one bleed per month. Eight joints required a second injection. Erken (278) reported on 58 joints in 35 hemophiliacs, ranging in age from 5 to 20 years. Factor levels were increased to 80% at the time of injection and were maintained at more than 50% for 3 days. An estimated dose of 5 mCi of ^{90}Y was injected into the knee joint, and less into smaller joints. The joints were immobilized for 48 to 60 h to minimize leakage of radioisotope from the joint. The frequency of hemorrhage decreased from 4 per month, before the injection, to 0.2 per month at a mean follow-up of 7 years. Eight patients required repeat injection. After the second injection, the rate of hemarthrosis was decreased in four patients and unchanged in four patients.

Some authors favor ^{32}P, a radioactive agent that has a half-life of 14 days. The theoretical advantage of a prolonged half-life is that an acute inflammatory reaction and subsequent hemorrhage would not occur. Therefore, ^{32}P could be safer for patients with an inhibitor. The long half-life also means that only a single transfusion is necessary before the injection. The theoretical disadvantage is the greater risk of this agent accumulating in tissues outside the joint. Two centers have reported good results with ^{32}P in patients with hemophilia (280,281).

The role of radioactive synovectomy in hemophilia is evolving. The percentage of patients with recurrent hemarthrosis is higher than that observed after surgical synovectomy, but the results are acceptable. The expense of transfusion therapy for surgical synovectomy, and the low morbidity of the procedure, are obvious advantages that are particularly germane in developing countries. In centers performing these procedures, careful monitoring is needed to document the possible side effects of radiotherapy on children.

Muscle hemorrhages are common in patients with severe factor VIII or IX deficiency, and may occur after minimal trauma. Characteristic sites include the volar compartment of the forearm, the iliopsoas, the quadriceps, and the anterior and posterior calf muscles. Clinical symptoms progress from stiffness, to pain on movement, to pain at rest. In a study of lower-extremity muscle bleeds in children, the quadriceps muscle was involved in 44%, the posterior calf muscles in 35%, the adductors in 7%, and the anterior calf muscles in 7% (282). Most patients with bleeding episodes in this study were transfused within 3 h, and the time for complete restoration of joint motion averaged 3.5 days.

Home transfusion therapy is effective for minor muscle bleeds. A single infusion usually is adequate if it is administered soon after the onset of the hemorrhage. For lower-extremity bleeds, crutches are used until normal range of motion has been regained. Patients or parents are instructed to call their physicians if they have symptoms of severe pain or neurologic dysfunction. With symptoms suggestive of a compartment syndrome in a hemophiliac who does not have an inhibitor, the factor levels are increased to 100%, then evaluation and management should be routine. This means that compartment pressures are measured, and fasciotomy is performed when indicated.

Patients with a high-titer inhibitor are at increased risk for complications from muscle hemorrhage (Fig. 11-24). These patients should seek medical attention early, so that alternative transfusions can be started. To minimize the risk of a compartment syndrome and contractures, nonoperative modalities, such as protective dressings, elevation, and splinting, should be aggressively pursued.

An iliopsoas bleed, sometimes called a "retroperitoneal hemorrhage," may be associated with femoral nerve paralysis and, as such, demands more intensive therapy. Hemorrhage into the iliacus compartment causes femoral nerve paralysis. Because the iliacus muscle is confined between the pelvic wall and the overlying fascia, a relatively small hemorrhage in this muscle also will cause marked pain. The patient holds the hip in a flexed position, and the pain is markedly increased by attempts at hip extension. Hemarthrosis into the hip joint can be differentiated by flexing the hip. In this position, rotation of the hip will be relatively normal with an iliopsoas hemorrhage, but rotation will remain limited with a bleed into the joint. If the location of the hemorrhage is unclear, ultrasonography or computed tomography may be used to define the site of bleeding. In the 1970s, femoral nerve palsies were found in approximately 60% of iliacus bleeds (247). The increased use of home therapy has reduced the incidence of this complication.

The standard treatment for femoral nerve palsy associated with an iliopsoas bleed is bed rest and continuous transfusion, to maintain factor levels at 50% or higher, for 7 to 14 days. With this therapy, the femoral nerve paralysis resolves, but several months may elapse before the quadriceps muscle regains sufficient strength to extend the knee against gravity. Growe and Meek (283) reported a case that was treated by open decompression of the iliopsoas muscle. This patient had symptoms for 5 days, a severe flexion contracture, paralysis of the femoral nerve, and a compartment pressure measurement of 166 mm Hg with the hip in extension, and 60 mm Hg with the hip flexed. At operation, a large organized clot was evacuated from the interval between the psoas and iliacus muscles. The patient's hip flexion contracture resolved within 1 week, and the quadriceps muscle function was normal within 1 month.

An equinus contracture may develop after hemorrhage into the gastrocnemius soleus muscle, particularly when there is a delay in transfusion for more than 6 to 12 hours (Fig. 11-25). Aggressive use of sequential splints and casts prevents this problem, even in patients with inhibitors. After a single transfusion, the leg should be immobilized in a compressive dressing and posterior splint. If an equinus contracture is present after 48 hours, a short-leg walking cast is applied with the ankle held in maximum dorsiflexion. The cast aids ambulation, but more importantly, minimizes the establishment of an equinus contracture, as the hematoma organizes. The cast is changed every few days, until the ankle can be positioned in neutral dorsiflexion with the knee extended. Stretching exercises then are used to gain further dorsiflexion.

Fixed knee-flexion contractures rarely develop in patients on home transfusion therapy. The exception is the patient with an inhibitor. In these patients, the alternatives to transfusion are not always effective, and an acute hemarthrosis may evolve into a fixed knee-flexion contracture. Traction, if instituted in an early and timely fashion, will allow the patient to regain full knee extension in 3 to 7 days.

Severe knee-flexion contractures that are chronic may be complicated by posterior subluxation of the tibia (232,285). If the patient also has an inhibitor that precludes elective

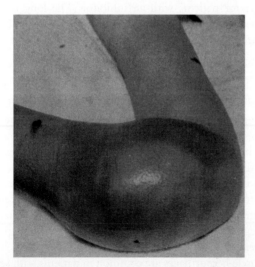

FIGURE 11-24. Massive soft tissue hemorrhage in the forearm of a 5-year-old patient with hemophilia can lead to Volkmann contractures.

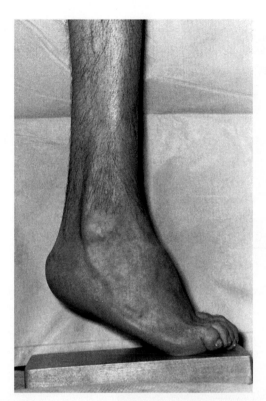

FIGURE 11-25. A 29-year-old man, with hemophilia and high-titer inhibitor, sustained multiple calf hemorrhages during childhood, which resulted in a fixed equinus contracture. Consistent and persistent treatment with serial casts could have greatly minimized the deformity and enhanced the patient's lower extremity function. (From ref. 284, with permission.)

surgery, the flexion contracture and subluxation of the tibia may be corrected with a Quengel cast (232) (Fig. 11-26). Offset subluxation hinges pull the proximal tibia forward, and the toggle stick allows windlass correction of the flexion deformity. The Quengel cast usually can correct the contracture to approximately 15 degrees. Further extension is attained with standard cast-wedging techniques.

Whether using traction or casting, the goal is to correct the knee-flexion contracture to 5 to 10 degrees. If less correction is attained, recurrent contractures are more likely. Furthermore, a typical patient will subsequently lose a few degrees of correction, but if the knee-flexion contracture remains less than 15 degrees, knee function is maximized, and stress across the joint is minimized. Therefore, after the contracture is corrected, a period of bracing is necessary. Over several months, the patient gradually is weaned from the brace, while a program of strengthening and range of motion is instituted.

The necessity of Quengel casting and bracing for a chronic contracture does not mean that the knee will be ankylosed. In my experience, approximately half of the patients ultimately regained more than 100 degrees of knee

motion, despite having a flexion contracture of more than 40 degrees at the start of treatment (285). Factors associated with good results included no significant joint erosions at the initiation of therapy, no breakthrough bleeding during treatment, and good compliance during the period of bracing.

A pseudotumor, or hemophiliac cyst, starts as a hemorrhage that is intramuscular, subperiosteal, or intraosseous. A fibrous capsule eventually surrounds and sequesters the large mass of blood, which ultimately is transformed to necrotic erythrocytes and reactive tissues. Pseudotumors continue to enlarge. The capsule of the pseudotumor has a relatively sparse vasculature, but the coagulation defects in these patients allow ongoing small and asymptomatic hemorrhages, probably secondary to altered pressure gradients that develop when the extravasated blood is catabolized. As the pseudotumor expands, the surrounding soft tissue is displaced and erosion of adjacent bones occurs (Fig. 11-27). Eventually, a clinically apparent mass or pathologic fracture causes the patient to seek evaluation. The radiographs of a pseudotumor typically demonstrate a soft tissue mass, areas of soft tissue calcification, varying degrees of osseous destruction, and reactive new bone formation. The differential diagnosis includes aneurysmal bone cysts, osteomyelitis, and some types of sarcoma.

Pseudotumors were more common before the development of effective concentrates. At that time, pseudotumors in young children were more likely in the bones of the hands and feet. In a series of 19 pseudotumors, Martinson (287) observed that 9 occurred in the carpometacarpal or tarsometatarsal bones. In my experience, which is during the era of concentrates and home transfusion therapy, most pseudotumors have been located in the pelvis, and probably originated from a bleed in the iliacus muscle. Other sites may be involved, however, and I have treated hemophiliacs with pseudotumors of the proximal humerus, the olecranon, and the proximal femur.

The pseudotumor should be excised, if at all possible. Delay in operation will only allow further expansion of the pseudotumor and destruction of surrounding structures. Computed tomography is adequate to demonstrate the extent of the mass (288). In most situations, a lesional excision is indicated, but in large pseudotumors of the pelvis, some of the inner wall of the pseudotumor capsule may be left to minimize the risk of massive hemorrhage from adherent internal iliac vessels.

Fracture patterns are different in hemophiliacs who have significant arthropathy of the lower extremities. Limited mobility of their lower extremities, coupled with disuse osteoporosis, make supracondylar fracture of the femur and fractures of the femoral neck more likely. Fracture in these patients, even if nondisplaced, will cause more bleeding, swelling, and risk of compartment syndrome. Transfusion therapy should be instituted immediately, and most of these

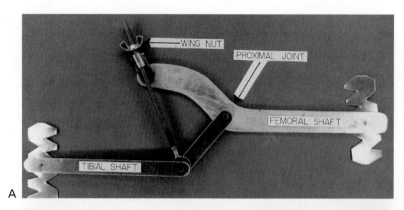

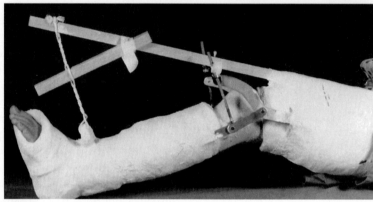

FIGURE 11-26. **A:** Quengel cast antisubluxation hinge. **B:** Completed Quengel cast applied to a patient. (From ref. 286, with permission.)

patients will need to be admitted to the hospital at least overnight for observation. For fractures that can be treated by nonoperative means, the amount and duration of transfusion are individualized, depending on the location of the fracture, the amount of apparent hemorrhage, and the social situation. Patients who require open reduction should be transfused using standard protocols for surgical procedures.

ACUTE LEUKEMIA

Acute leukemia is the most common neoplasm in children, accounting for approximately one-third of pediatric cancer cases (289). "Acute leukemia" is used for diseases that have a predominance of immature hematopoietic or lymphoid precursors, whereas "chronic leukemia" describes conditions characterized by proliferation of mature marrow elements. Acute lymphoblastic leukemia (ALL) accounts for approximately 80% of the leukemias seen in children. The peak incidence of ALL is between the ages of 1 and 5 years, and the frequency declines progressively in the older childhood age groups. With intensive combination chemotherapy and central nervous system prophylaxis, the survival rate of ALL has improved significantly, and the current rate of cure is approximately 80% (290). Adverse risk factors include a white blood cell count greater than 50,000/mm^3 at

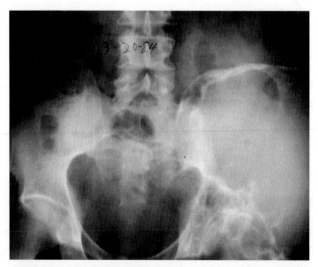

FIGURE 11-27. Pseudotumor of the ilium in a 39-year-old man with severe factor VIII deficiency and low-titer inhibitor. There is marked destruction of the left ilium.

TABLE 11-8. SIGNS AND SYMPTOMS OF DIAGNOSIS OF ACUTE LYMPHOBLASTIC LEUKEMIA IN 137 CHILDREN

Signs and Symptoms	Patients[a] (%)
Lethargy or malaise	36
Fever or infection	31
Extremity or joint pain	23
Bleeding manifestation	18
Anorexia	12
Abdominal pain	7
Central nervous system manifestation	2

[a] Some patients presented with more than one sign or symptom.
(Adapted from ref. 291, with permission.)

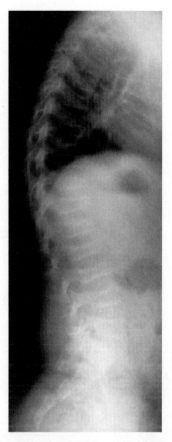

FIGURE 11-28. A 6-year-old girl presented with acute pain and an inability to walk. Radiographic examination revealed diffuse osteopenia and multiple compression fractures. Diagnostic evaluation revealed acute leukemia. (From ref. 297, with permission.)

diagnosis, patients with mature B-cell ALL, specific genetic abnormalities, age younger than 1 year at diagnosis, and a poor early response to induction therapy.

Although ALL is primarily a disease of the bone marrow, any organ may be infiltrated by the malignant cells. For that reason, the signs and symptoms at diagnosis can vary (Table 11-8). Pain in the extremities, or a limp, may be the initial manifestation of ALL, and the first physician evaluating these children may be an orthopaedic surgeon. In a representative study of 296 patients, a limp or extremity pain was the chief complaint at diagnosis in 52 patients (18%), and was an associated symptom in 65 patients (22%) (292). In another study of 40 ALL patients, 5 presented with refusal to walk and 13 had gait abnormalities (293). Pain is most common in the lower extremities, but it also may be present in the upper extremities. A history of night pain is significant, but is not always present or obtainable in these young children. Back pain also may be noted, and pathologic fracture of the vertebral body is found at diagnosis in 2 to 7% of children with ALL (294–296) (Fig. 11-28).

Arthritis or painful swelling of a joint may herald the onset of leukemia (298,299), and in one series, they were observed in 11% of ALL patients (299). Multiple joints may be involved, and migratory joint pain may occur. Asymmetric involvement of the large joints is characteristic. The cause of the arthritis is uncertain, but may be related to infiltration of the synovium by leukemic cells or by the hyperuricemia often observed at diagnosis.

Infiltration of the bone marrow by the leukemic cells explains the limb and back pain. Radiographic changes at diagnosis are even more frequent than musculoskeletal symptoms (294,295,300,301). Characteristic findings include localized and generalized osteoporosis, radiolucent metaphyseal bands, osteolytic defects, cortical defects, osteosclerosis, and periosteal reactions (Figs. 11-29 and 11-30). Osteopenia and metaphyseal lucent bands are the most common findings. Fractures also may be present. Typical patterns include: impaction fracture in the femur or tibia and vertebral compression fractures. Radiologic skeletal

changes do not portend a worse prognosis (300), and some studies have observed that, on average, ALL children with skeletal changes have more normal hematologic indexes and enhanced survival (294). However, the presence of five or more skeletal lesions at diagnosis is associated with a delay in diagnosis, and decreased survival (294,300).

Mineral homeostasis may be abnormal at diagnosis. In a prospective study of 40 children with ALL, low levels of 1,25-dihydroxyvitamin D and osteocalcin with hypercalciuria, were observed in approximately two-thirds of the patients (302). Bone density Z scores correlated with plasma 1,25-dihydroxyvitamin D concentrations. The cause of the defective mineralization at diagnosis is unclear, because renal tubular studies and 25-vitamin D levels were normal.

Children with ALL who present with bone pain often incur a delay in diagnosis, and may be misdiagnosed as having osteomyelitis, septic arthritis, or juvenile rheumatoid arthritis (292,295,298). This possibility may be minimized by inquiring about symptoms such as lethargy, fever, headache, vomiting, night pain, and easy bruising, and by including examination of the lymph nodes and abdominal organs in a child who presents with unexplained limb or

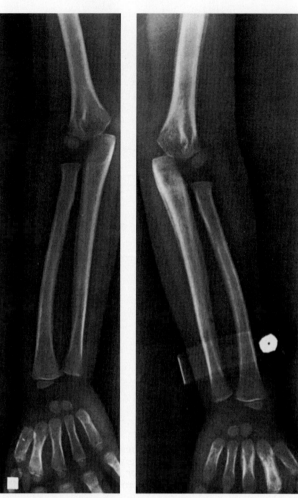

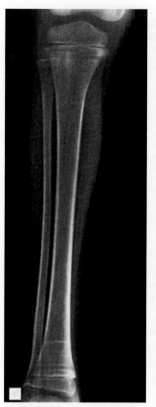

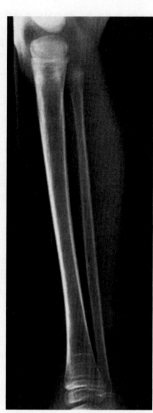

FIGURE 11-30. A 6-year-old girl with acute myelogenous leukemia shows multiple growth rest lines, generalized osteopenia, and a metaphyseal band.

FIGURE 11-29. A 3-year-old boy with acute lymphocytic leukemia shows periosteal new bone formation, involving large segments of the radius, the ulna, and the humerus. A metaphyseal band is present at the distal radius.

back pain. A complete blood count may be helpful, particularly if the white blood cell count is markedly elevated or significantly depressed, or if blast forms are noted. However, children with ALL also may have a nondiagnostic leukocyte count that is normal or only slightly elevated, as well as an elevated erythrocyte sedimentation rate. In this situation, radiographs showing a greater degree of osteopenia than one would expect will suggest the correct diagnosis. Radiographs also should be carefully examined for the presence of more characteristic lesions, such as metaphyseal lucent bands. Bone scans in children with leukemia are inconsistent, and may show increased uptake in an asymptomatic region, or normal or decreased uptake in areas that have obvious lysis on plane radiographs (289). With any suspicion, diagnostic bone marrow aspiration should be considered.

Distinguishing systemic juvenile rheumatoid arthritis from ALL in children who present with fever and multiple joint pain may be challenging. Lymphadenopathy, spleno-

megaly, and hepatomegaly are equivalent in both groups (298). Musculoskeletal night pain, however, is observed frequently in ALL, whereas morning stiffness is common in juvenile rheumatoid arthritis. Nonarticular bone pain, in addition to the joint symptoms, is found in ALL, but is absent in juvenile rheumatoid arthritis. Radiographic findings are limited to joint effusions in juvenile rheumatoid arthritis patients, whereas other abnormalities are frequently observed in children with leukemia.

The basic approach to therapy for leukemia involves a relatively brief induction phase, followed by intensification (consolidation) treatment, then prolonged continuation therapy (289,290). The goal of induction therapy is to reduce the leukemic cell load, so that there are normal blood cell counts and a normocellular bone marrow with less than 5% blasts. A typical regimen includes a glucocorticoid (dexamethasone), vincristine, and asparaginase. Intrathecal chemotherapy is included. Intensification therapy also incorporates combination chemotherapy. To prevent relapse, therapy at lower dosage levels is continued for 2.5 to 3 years, even in children showing a good response.

Leukemic bone and joint pain typically resolves with the institution of chemotherapy; however, during chemotherapy, osteoporosis may increase and pathologic fractures may occur. In a prospective study of 40 ALL children during 24 months of chemotherapy, Atkinson and colleagues (302) observed that 64% had a significant reduction in bone mineral content, as measured by Z scores. Bone density was most severely affected in children older than 11 years of age. During the 2-year treatment period, fractures occurred in 15 patients, and a reduction in bone mineral content during the first 6 months of treatment had a 64% positive predictive value for this complication. Although rare, severe osteoporosis and multiple vertebral body collapse during treatment of ALL also have been reported (303). After therapy is completed, the bone mineral content improves, but long-term survivors of ALL remain relatively osteopenic compared with controls (304,305). Whether this will have any long-term consequences is unclear at this time.

Symptomatic osteonecrosis is more likely to develop in adults with leukemia, but has also been reported in the pediatric population. Murphy and Greenberg (306) found multifocal, symptomatic osteonecrosis in 5 of 228 children with ALL. Sites of involvement included the femoral condyle, femoral head, humeral condyle, talus, and capitellum. These patients were older at diagnosis, ranging from 9.5 to 16.7 years of age. Dexamethasone was thought to be the causative agent. Recent MRI studies indicate that osteonecrosis is more common than previously realized. In a prospective MRI study of 24 ALL patients, 9 patients (38%) developed osteonecrosis during treatment, and 6 of them were asymptomatic (307).

Allogenic bone marrow transplantation, with its greater risk of osteonecrosis, may be necessary for ALL patients who relapse, or who are in high-risk categories. Multiple osteochondromas were observed in nine ALL patients (23%) at a mean 6 years after total body irradiation (308). At a mean follow-up of 2.5 years after diagnosis of the osteochondromata, no lesion had demonstrated malignant change. Short stature also occurs as a consequence of treating ALL. This complication has been greatly reduced by treatment protocols that lessen the need for or the degree of cranial irradiation (309).

References

Bone Marrow Failure Syndromes

1. Alter BP, Young NS. The bone marrow failure syndromes. In: Nathan DG, Oski SH, eds. *Hematology of infancy and childhood*, 5th ed. Philadelphia: WB Saunders, 1998:237.
2. Alter BP. Arms and the man or hands and the child: congenital anomalies and hematologic syndromes. *J Pediatr Hematol Oncol* 1997;19:287.
3. Minagi H, Steinbach HL. Roentgen appearance of anomalies associated with hypoplastic anemias of childhood: Fanconi's anemia and congenital hypoplastic anemia (erythrogenesis imperfecta). *Am J Roentgenol* 1966;97:100.
4. Gluckman E, Auerbach AD, Horowitz MM, et al. Bone marrow transplantation for Fanconi anemia. *Blood* 1995;86:2856.
5. Deeg HJ, Socie G, Schock G, et al. Malignancies after marrow transplantation for aplastic anemia and Fanconi anemia: a joint Seattle and Paris analysis of results in 700 patients. *Blood* 1996;87:386.
6. Willig TN, Ball SE, Tchernia G. Current concepts and issues in Diamond-Blackfan anemia. *Curr Opin Hematol* 1998;5:109.
7. Hurst JA, Baraitser M, Wonke B. Autosomal dominant transmission of congenital erythroid hypoplastic anemia with radial abnormalities. *Am J Med Genet* 1991;40:482.
8. McGuckin CP, Ball SE, Gordon-Smith EC. Diamond-Blackfan anemia: three patterns of in vitro responses to haemopoietic growth factors. *Br J Hematol* 1995;89:457.
9. Mugishima H, Gale RP, Rowlings PA, et al. Bone marrow transplantation for Diamond-Blackfan anemia. *Bone Marrow Transplant* 1995;15:55.
10. Aquino VM, Buchanan GR. Osteogenic sarcoma in a child with transfusion-dependent Diamond-Blackfan anemia. *J Pediatr Hematol Oncol* 1996;18:230.
11. Aggett PJ, Cavanagh NPC, Matthew DJ, et al. Schwachman's syndrome. *Arch Dis Child* 1980;55:331.
12. Smith OP, Hann IM, Chessells JM, et al. Haematological abnormalities in Schwachman-Diamond syndrome. *Br J Haematol* 1996;94:279.
13. Dhar S, Anderton JM. Orthopaedic features of Schwachman syndrome. *J Bone Joint Surg Am* 1994;76:278.
14. Dror Y, Durie P, Marcon P, et al. Duplication of distal thumb phalanx in Schwachman-Diamond syndrome. *Am J Med Genet* 1998;78:67.
15. McKusick VA, Eldridge R, Hostetler JA, et al. Dwarfism in the Amish. *Bull Johns Hopkins* 1965;116:285.
16. van der Burgt I, Haraldsson A, Oosterwijk JC, et al. Cartilage hair hypoplasia, metaphyseal chondrodysplasia type McKusick: description of seven patients and review of the literature. *Am J Med Genet* 1991;41:371.
17. Makitie O, Kaitila I. Cartilage-hair hypoplasia: clinical manifestations in 108 Finnish patients. *Eur J Pediatr* 1993;152:211.
18. Beals RK. Cartilage-hair hypoplasia: a case report. *J Bone Joint Surg Am* 1968;50:1245.
19. Berthet F, Siegrist CA, Ozsahin H, et al. Bone marrow transplantation in cartilage-hair hypoplasia: correction of the immuno-deficiency but not of the chondrodysplasia. *Eur J Pediatr* 1996;155:286.
20. Castigli E, Irani AM, Geha RS, et al. Defective expression of early activation genes in cartilage-hair hypoplasia (CHH) with severe combined immunodeficiency (SCID). *Clin Exp Immunol* 1995;102:6.
21. Sulisalo T, Francomano CA. High-resolution genetic mapping of the cartilage-hair hypoplasia (CHH) gene in Amish and Finnish families. *Genomics* 1994;20:347.
22. Hall JG, Levin J, Kuhn JP, et al. Thrombocytopenia with absent radius (TAR). *Medicine* 1969;48:411.
23. Hall JG. Thrombocytopenia and absent radius (TAR). *J Med Genet* 1987;24:79.
24. Hedberg VA, Lipton JM. Thrombocytopenia with absent radii. *Am J Pediatr Hematol Oncol* 1988;10:51.
25. Schoenecker PL, Cohn AK, Sedgwick WG, et al. Dysplasia of the knee associated with the syndrome of thrombocytopenia and absent radius. *J Bone Joint Surg Am* 1984;66:421.
26. Gounder DS, Ockelford PA, Pullon HW, et al. Clinical manifestations of the thrombocytopenia and absent radii (TAR) syndrome. *Aust NZ J Med* 1989;19:479.
27. Dell PC, Sheppard JE. Thrombocytopenia, absent radius syndrome: report of two siblings and a review of the hematologic and genetic features. *Clin Orthop* 1982;162:129.
28. Camitta BM, Rock A. Acute lymphoidic leukemia in a patient

with thrombocytopenia/absent radii (Tar) syndrome. *Am J Pediatr Hematol Oncol* 1993;15:335.

Disorders of Erythrocytes

29. Oski FA. Iron deficiency in infancy and childhood. *N Engl J Med* 1993;329:190.

30. Lanzkowsky P. Radiological features of iron-deficiency anemia. *Am J Dis Child* 1968;116:16.

31. Filer LJ. Iron needs during rapid growth and mental development. *J Pediatr* 1990;117:S143.

32. Hurtado EK, Claussen AH, Scott KG. Early childhood anemia and mild or moderate mental retardation. *Am J Clin Nutr* 1999; 69:115.

33. Morey SS. CDC guidelines for prevention, detection, and treatment of iron deficiency. *Am Fam Physician* 1998;58:1475.

34. Preziosi P, Prual A, Galan P, et al. Effect of iron supplementation on the iron status of pregnant women: consequences for newborns. *Am J Clin Nutr* 1997;66:1178.

35. Ballin A, Berar M, Rubinstein U, et al. Iron state in female adolescents. *Am J Dis Child* 1991;146:803.

36. Raunikar RA, Sabio H. Anemia in the adolescent athlete. *Am J Dis Child* 1992;146:1201.

37. Roy WL, Lerman J, McIntyre BG. Is preoperative haemoglobin testing justified in children undergoing minor elective surgery? *Can J Anaesth* 1991;38:700.

38. Schneider RG, Hightower B, Hosty TS, et al. Abnormal hemoglobins in a quarter million people. *J Am Soc Hematol* 1976; 48:629.

39. Bunn HF. Pathogenesis and treatment of sickle call disease. *N Engl J Med* 1997;337:762.

40. Dover GJ, Platt OS. Sickle cell disease. In: Nathan DG, Oski SH, eds. *Hematology of infancy and childhood*, 5th ed. Philadelphia: WB Saunders, 1998:762.

41. Serjeant GR. Natural history and determinants of clinical severity of sickle cell disease. *Curr Opin Hematol* 1995;2:103.

42. Steinberg MH. Management of sickle cell disease. *N Engl J Med* 1998;340:1021.

43. Platt OS, Brambilla DJ, Rosse WF, et al. Mortality in sickle cell disease: life expectancy and risk factors for early death. *N Engl J Med* 1994;330:1639.

44. McKie VC. Sickle cell anemia in children: practical issues for the pediatrician. *Pediatr Ann* 1998;27:521.

45. Platt OS, Rosenstock W, Espeland MA. Influence of sickle cell hemoglobinopathies on growth and development. *N Engl J Med* 1984;311:7.

46. Earley CJ, Kittner SJ, Feeser BR, et al. Stroke in children and sickle-cell disease: Baltimore-Washington cooperative young stroke study. *Neurology* 1998;51:169.

47. Ohene-Frempong K, Weiner SJ, Sleeper LA, et al. Cerebrovascular accidents in sickle cell disease: rats and risk factors. *Blood* 1998;91:288.

48. Pegelow CH, Adams RJ, McKie V, et al. Risk of recurrent stroke in patients with sickle cell disease treated with erythrocyte transfusions. *J Pediatr* 1995;126:896.

49. Adams RJ, McKie VC, Hsu L. Prevention of a first stroke by transfusions in children with sickle cell anemia and abnormal results on transcranial Doppler ultrasonography. *N Engl J Med* 1998;339:5.

50. Cohen AR. Sickle cell disease: new treatments, new questions. *N Engl J Med* 1998;339:42.

51. Brinker MR, Thomas KA, Meyers SJ, et al. Bone mineral density of the lumbar spine and proximal femur is decreased in children with sickle cell anemia. *Am J Orthop* 1998;27:43.

52. Soliman AT, Berehi H, Darwish A, et al. Decreased bone mineral density in prepubertal children with sickle cell disease: corre-

lation with growth parameters, degree of siderosis and secretion of growth factors. *J Trop Pediatr* 1998;44:194.

53. Platt OS, Thorington BD, Brambilla DJ, et al. Pain in sickle cell disease: rates and risk factors. *N Engl J Med* 1991;325:11.

54. Keeley K, Buchanan GR. Acute infarction of long bones in children with sickle cell anemia. *J Pediatr* 1982;101:170.

55. Mankad VN, Williams JP, Harpen MD, et al. Magnetic resonance imaging of bone marrow in sickle cell disease: clinical, hematologic, and pathologic correlations. *Blood* 1990;75:274.

56. Michaels LA, Ohene-Frempong K, Zhao H, et al. Serum levels of substance P are elevated in patients with sickle cell disease and increase further during vaso-occlusive crisis. *Blood* 1998; 92:3148.

57. Babhulkar SS, Pande K, Babhulkar S. The hand-foot syndrome in sickle-cell haemoglobinopathy. *J Bone Joint Surg Br* 1995; 77:310.

58. Diggs LW. Bone and joint lesions in sickle-cell disease. *Clin Orthop* 1967;52:119.

59. Stevens MCG, Padwick M, Serjeant GR. Observations on the natural history of dactylitis in homozygous sickle cell disease. *Clin Pediatr* 1981;20:311.

60. Dalton GP, Drummond DS, Davidson RS, et al. Bone infarction versus infection in sickle cell disease in children. *J Pediatr Orthop* 1996;16:540.

61. Burnett NW, Bass JW, Cook BA. Etiology of osteomyelitis complicating sickle cell disease. *Pediatrics* 1998;101:296.

62. Greene WB, McMillan CW. *Salmonella* osteomyelitis and hand-foot syndrome in a child with sickle cell anemia. *J Pediatr Orthop* 1987;7:716.

63. Bonnerot V, Sebag G, de Montalembert M, et al. Gadolinium-DOTA enhanced MRI of painful osseous crises in children with sickle cell anemia. *Pediatr Radiol* 1994;24:92.

64. Bennett OM, Namnyak SS. Bone and joint manifestations of sickle cell anaemia. *J Bone Joint Surg Br* 1990;72:494.

65. Epps CH Jr, Bryant DOD III, Coles MJM, et al. Osteomyelitis in patients who have sickle-cell disease. *J Bone Joint Surg Am* 1991;73:1281.

66. Buchanan GR. Differentiation of bone infarct from infection in a child with sickle cell disease. *Pediatr Infect Dis J* 1996;15: 725.

67. Kahn CE Jr, Ryan JW, Hatfield MK, et al. Combined bone marrow and gallium imaging: differentiation of osteomyelitis and infarction in sickle hemoglobinopathy. *Clin Nucl Med* 1998;13:443.

68. Sadat-Ali M, al-Umran K, al-Habdan I, et al. Ultrasonography: can it differentiate between vasoocclusive crisis and acute osteomyelitis in sickle cell disease? *J Pediatr Orthop* 1998;18:552.

69. Anand AJ, Glatt AE. *Salmonella* osteomyelitis and arthritis in sickle cell disease. *Semin Arthritis Rheum* 1994;24:211.

70. Bryan JP, Rocha H, Scheld WM. Problems in salmonellosis: rationale for clinical trials with lower β-lactam agents and quinolones. *Rev Infect Dis* 1986;8:189.

71. Ebong WW. Pathological fracture complicating long bone osteomyelitis in patients with sickle cell disease. *J Pediatr Orthop* 1986;6:177.

72. Syrogiannopoulos GA, McCracken GH, Nelson JD. Osteoarticular infections in children with sickle cell disease. *Pediatrics* 1986;78:1090.

73. Hanissian AS, Silverman A. Arthritis of sickle cell anemia. *South Med J* 1974;67:28.

74. Schumacher HR, Andrews R, McLaughlin G. Arthropathy in sickle-cell disease. *Ann Intern Med* 1973;78:203.

75. Milner PF, Kraus AP, Sebes JI, et al. Sickle cell disease as a cause of osteonecrosis of the femoral head. *N Engl J Med* 1991; 325:1476.

76. Milner PF, Kraus AP, Sebes JI, et al. Osteonecrosis of the humeral head in sickle cell disease. *Clin Orthop* 1993;289:136.

77. Hernigou P, Galacteros F, Bachir D, et al. Deformities of the hip in adults who have sickle-cell disease and had avascular necrosis in childhood. *J Bone Joint Surg Am* 1991;73:81.

78. Ware HE, Brooks AP, Toye R, et al. Sickle cell disease and silent avascular necrosis of the hip. *J Bone Joint Surg Br* 1991; 73:947.

79. Greene WB. Disease of the hematopoietic system and chronic inflammatory arthritides: musculoskeletal complications in children. In: Bowen JR, Epps CE, eds. *Complications in pediatric orthopaedic surgery.* Philadelphia: JB Lippincott, 1995:715.

80. Rao VM, Mitchell DG, Steiner RM, et al. Femoral head avascular necrosis in sickle cell anemia: MR characteristics. *Magn Reson Imaging* 1988;6:661.

81. Acurio MT, Friedman RJ. Hip arthroplasty in patients with sickle-cell haemoglobinopathy. *J Bone Joint Surg Br* 1992;74: 367.

82. Bishop AR, Roberson JR, Eckman JR, et al. Total hip arthroplasty in patients who have sickle-cell hemoglobinopathy. *J Bone Joint Surg Am* 1988;70:853.

83. Clarke HJ, Jinnah RH, Brooker AF, et al. Total replacement of the hip for avascular necrosis in sickle cell disease. *J Bone Joint Surg Br* 1989;71:465.

84. Charache S, Terrin ML, Moore RD, et al. Effect of hydroxyurea on the frequency of painful crises in sickle cell anemia. Investigators of the Multicenter Study of Hydroxyurea in Sickle Cell Anemia. *N Engl J Med* 1995;332:1317.

85. Ohene-Frempong K, Smith-Whitley K. Use of hydroxyurea in children with sickle cell disease: what comes next? *Semin Hematol* 1997;34(Suppl 3):30.

86. Olivieri NF, Vichinsky EP. Hydroxyurea in children with sickle cell disease: impact on splenic function and compliance with therapy. *J Pediatr Hematol Oncol* 1998;20:26.

87. Rogers ZR. Hydroxyurea therapy for diverse pediatric populations with sickle cell disease. *Semin Hematol* 1997;34(Suppl 3): 42.

88. Platt OS, Guinan EC. Bone marrow transplantation in sickle cell anemia: the dilemma of choice. *N Engl J Med* 1996;335: 426.

89. Walters MC, Patience M, Leisenring W, et al. Bone marrow transplantation for sickle cell disease. *N Engl J Med* 1996;335: 369.

90. Hernigou P, Bernaudin F, Reinert P, et al. Bone-marrow transplantation in sickle cell disease: effect on osteonecrosis. A case report with a four-year follow-up. *J Bone Joint Surg Am* 1997; 79:1726.

91. Stein RE, Urbaniak J. Use of the tourniquet during surgery in patients with sickle cell hemoglobinopathies. *Clin Orthop* 1980; 151:231.

92. Koshy M, Weiner SJ, Miller ST, et al. Surgery and anesthesia in sickle cell disease. Cooperative Study of Sickle Cell Diseases. *Blood* 1995;86:3676.

93. Orkin SH, Nathan DG. The thalassemias. In: Nathan DG, Oski SH, eds. *Hematology of infancy and childhood*, 5th ed. Philadelphia: WB Saunders, 1998:811.

94. Abramson SD, Abramson N. 'Common' uncommon anemias. *Am Fam Physician* 1999;59:851.

95. Kattamis C, Liakopoulou T, Kattamis A. Growth and development in children with thalassaemia major. *Acta Pediatr Scand Suppl* 1990;366:111.

96. Caffey J. Cooley's anemia: a review of the roentgenographic findings in the skeleton. *Am J Roentgenol* 1957;78:381.

97. Dines DM, Canale VC, Arnold WD. Fractures in thalassemia. *J Bone Joint Surg Am* 1976;58:662.

98. Exarchou E, Politou G, Vretou E, et al. Fractures and epiphyseal deformities in beta-thalassemia. *Clin Orthop* 1984;189:229.

99. Finsterbush A, Farber I, Mogle P, et al. Fracture patterns in thalassemia. *Clin Orthop* 1985;192:132.

100. Michelson J, Cohen A. Incidence and treatment of fractures in thalassemia. *J Orthop Trauma* 1988;2:29.

101. Colavita N, Orazi C, Danza SM, et al. Premature epiphyseal fusion and extramedullary hematopoiesis in thalassemia. *Skeletal Radiol* 1987;16:533.

102. Hershko C, Link G, Cabantchik I. Pathophysiology of iron overload. *Ann NY Acad Sci* 1998;850:191.

103. Levin TL, Sheth SS, Ruzal-Shapiro C, et al. MRI marrow observations in thalassemia: the effects of the primary disease, transfusional therapy, and chelation. *Pediatr Radiol* 1995;25:607.

104. Olivieri NF, Nathan DG, MacMillan JH, et al. Survival in medically treated patients with homozygous beta-thalassemia. *N Engl J Med* 1994;331:574.

105. Giardina PJ, Grady RW. Chelation therapy in beta-thalassemia: the benefits and limitations of desferrioxamine. *Semin Hematol* 1995;34:304.

106. Aydingoz U, Oto A, Cila A. Spinal cord compression due to epidural extramedullary haematopoiesis in thalassemia: MRI. *Neuroradiology* 1997;39:870.

107. Coskun E, Keskin A, Suzer T, et al. Spinal cord compression secondary to extramedullary hematopoiesis in thalassemia. *Eur Spine J* 1998;7:501.

108. Lau SK, Chan CK, Chow YYN. Cord compression due to extramedullary hemopoiesis in a patient with thalassemia. *Spine* 1994;19:2467.

109. Lucarelli G, Giardini C, Baronciani D. Bone marrow transplantation in thalassemia. *Semin Hematol* 1995;32:297.

110. Mariotti E, Angelucci E, Agostini A, et al. Evaluation of cardiac status in iron-loaded thalassemia patients following bone marrow transplantation: improvement in cardiac function during reduction in body iron burden. *Br J Haematol* 1998;103:916.

111. Andrews NC, Bridges KR. Disorders of iron metabolism and sideroblastic anemia. In: Nathan DG, Oski SH, eds. *Hematology of infancy and childhood*, 5th ed. Philadelphia: WB Saunders, 1998:423.

112. Konijn M. Iron metabolism in inflammation. *Baillieres Clin Haematol* 1994;7:829.

113. Peeters HR, Jongen-Lavrencic M, Raja AN, et al. Course and characteristics of anaemia in patients with rheumatoid arthritis of recent onset. *Ann Rheum Dis* 1996;55:162.

114. Means RT Jr. Pathogenesis of the anemia of chronic disease: a cytokine-mediated anemia. *Stem Cells* 1995;13:32.

115. Means RT Jr. Erythropoietin in the treatment of anemia in chronic infectious, inflammatory, and malignant diseases. *Curr Opin Hematol* 1995;2:210.

Disorders of Neutrophils

116. Dinauer MC. The phagocyte system and disorders of granulopoiesis and granulocyte function. In: Nathan DG, Oski SH, eds. *Hematology of infancy and childhood*, 5th ed. Philadelphia: WB Saunders, 1998:889.

117. Malech HL, Nauseef WM. Primary inherited defects in neutrophil function: etiology and treatment. *Semin Hematol* 1997;34: 279.

118. Forehand JR, Johnston RB Jr. Chronic granulomatous disease: newly defined molecular abnormalities explain disease variability and normal phagocyte physiology. *Curr Opin Pediatr* 1994; 6:668.

119. Meischl C, Ross D. The molecular basis of chronic granulomatous disease. *Springer Semin Immunopathol* 1998;19:417.

120. Verhoeven AJ. The NADPH oxidase: lessons from chronic

granulomatous disease neutrophils. *Ann NY Acad Sci* 1997;832: 85

121. Eckert JW, Abramson SL, Starke J, et al. The surgical implications of chronic granulomatous disease. *Am J Surg* 1995;169: 320.

122. Finn A, Hadzic N, Morgan G, et al. Prognosis of chronic granulomatous disease. *Arch Dis Child* 1990;65:942.

123. Wolfson JJ, Kane WJ, Laxdal SD, et al. Bone findings in chronic granulomatous disease of childhood: a genetic abnormality of leukocyte function. *J Bone Joint Surg Am* 1969;51:1573.

124. Sponseller PD, Malech HL, McCarthy EF, et al. Skeletal involvement in children who have chronic granulomatous disease. *J Bone Joint Surg Am* 1991;73:37.

125. Heinrich SD, Finney T, Craver R, et al. *Aspergillus* osteomyelitis in patients who have chronic granulomatous disease. *J Bone Joint Surg Am* 1991;73:456.

126. Kline MW, Bocobo FC, Paul ME, et al. Successful medical therapy of *Aspergillus* osteomyelitis of the spine in an 11-year-old boy with chronic granulomatous disease. *Pediatrics* 1994; 93:830.

127. Pasic S, Abinun M, Pistignjat B, et al. *Aspergillus* osteomyelitis in chronic granulomatous disease: treatment with recombinant gamma-interferon and itraconazole. *Pediatr Infect Dis J* 1996; 15:833.

128. Mouy R, Fischer A, Vilmer E, et al. Incidence, severity, and prevention of infections in chronic granulomatous disease. *J Pediatr* 1989;114:555.

129. The International Chronic Granulomatous Disease Cooperative Study Group. Controlled trial of interferon gamma to prevent infection in chronic granulomatous disease. *N Engl J Med* 1991; 324:504.

130. Rosh JR, Tang HB, Mayer L, et al. Treatment of intractable gastrointestinal manifestations of chronic granulomatous disease with cyclosporine. *J Pediatr* 1995;126:143.

131. Lee BW, Yap HK. Polyarthritis resembling juvenile rheumatoid arthritis in a girl with chronic granulomatous disease. *Arthritis Rheum* 1994;37:773.

132. Calvino MC, Maldonado MS, Otheo E, et al. Bone marrow transplantation in chronic granulomatous disease. *Eur J Pediatr* 1996;155:877.

133. Ho CM, Vowels MR, Lockwood L, et al. Successful bone marrow transplantation in a child with X-linked chronic granulomatous disease. *Bone Marrow Transplant* 1996;18:213.

134. Malech HL, Bauer TR Jr, Hickstein DD. Prospects for gene therapy of neutrophil defects. *Semin Hematol* 1997;34:355.

Disorders of Lymphocytes and the Immune System

135. Bonilla FA, Rosen FS, Geha RS. Primary immunodeficiency diseases. In: Nathan DG, Oski SD, eds. *Hematology of infancy and childhood*, 5th ed. Philadelphia: WB Saunders, 1998:1023.

136. Conley ME. X-linked immunodeficiencies. *Curr Opin Genet Dev* 1994;4:401.

137. Manis J, Schwartz RS. Agammaglobulinemia and insights into B-cell differentiation. *N Engl J Med* 1996;335:1523.

138. Hansel TT, Haeney MR, Thompson RA. Primary hypogammaglobulinaemia and arthritis. *Br Med J* 1987;295:174.

139. Lee AH, Levinson AI, Schumacher HR Jr. Hypogammaglobulinemia and rheumatic disease. *Semin Arthritis Rheum* 1993;22: 252.

140. Chattopadhyay C, Natvig JB, Chattopadhyay H. Excessive suppressor T-cell activity of the rheumatoid synovial tissue in X-linked hypogammaglobulinaemia. *Scand J Immunol* 1980;11: 455.

141. Franz A, Webster AD, Furr PM, et al. Mycoplasmal arthritis in patients with primary immunoglobulin deficiency: clinical features and outcome in 18 patients. *Br J Rheumatol* 1997;36: 661.

142. Horowitz HW, Telzak EE, Sepkowitz KA, et al. Human immunodeficiency virus infection. Part I. *Dis Mon* 1998;44:545.

143. Centers for Disease Control. AIDS among children: United States, 1996. *MMWR* 1996;45:1005.

144. Chadwick EG, Yogev R. Pediatric AIDS. *Pediatr Clin North Am* 1995;42:969.

145. Miller CR. Pediatric aspects of AIDS. *Radiol Clin North Am* 1997;35:1191.

146. Andiman WA. Medical management of the pregnant woman infected with human immuno-deficiency virus type 1 and her child. *Semin Perinatol* 1998;22:72.

147. Connor EM, Sperling RS, Gelber R, et al. Reduction of maternal-infant transmission of human immunodeficiency virus type 1 with zidovudine treatment. Pediatric AIDS Clinical Trials Group Protocol 076 Study Group. *N Engl J Med* 1994;331: 1173.

148. Wu LR, Capparelli EV, Connor JD. Therapy of pediatric AIDS. *Curr Opin Pediatr* 1995;7:214.

149. Cooper A. Human immunodeficiency virus and acquired immunodeficiency syndrome: recent developments and their implications for pediatric surgeons. *Semin Pediatr Surg* 1995;4: 252.

150. Lindegren ML, Hanson C, Miller K, et al. Epidemiology of human immunodeficiency virus infection in adolescents, United States. *Pediatr Infect Dis J* 1994;13:525.

Disorders of the Monocyte-macrophage System

151. Sullivan JL, Woda BA. Lymphohistiocytic disorders. In: Nathan DG, Orkin SH, eds. *Hematology of infancy and childhood*, 5th ed. Philadelphia: WB Saunders, 1998:1359.

152. Kolodny EH, Lebron D. Storage diseases of the reticuloendothelial system. In: Nathan DG, Oski SH, eds. *Hematology of infancy and childhood*, 5th ed. Philadelphia: WB Saunders, 1998:1461.

153. Brady RO, Kanfer JN, Shapiro D. Metabolism of glucocerebrosides. II. Evidence of an enzymatic deficiency in Gaucher's disease. *Biochem Biophys Res Commun* 1965;18:221.

154. Beutler E, Nguyen NJ, Henneberger MW, et al. Gaucher disease: gene frequencies in the Ashkenazi Jewish population. *Am J Hum Genet* 1993;51:85.

155. Beutler E, Gelbart T. Hematologically important mutations: Gaucher disease. *Blood Cells Mol Dis* 1998;24:2.

156. Beutler E, Gelbart T. Gaucher disease mutations in non-Jewish patients. *Br J Haematol* 1993;85:401.

157. Beutler E. Gaucher disease. *Curr Opin Hematol* 1997;4:19.

158. Zimran A, Kay A, Gelbart T, et al. Gaucher disease: clinical, laboratory, radiologic, and genetic features of 53 patients. *Medicine* 1992;71:337.

159. Stowens DW, Teitelbaum SL, Kahn AJ, et al. Skeletal complications of Gaucher disease. *Medicine* 1985;64:310.

160. Miller SP, Zirzow GC, Doppelt SH, et al. Analysis of the lipids of normal and Gaucher bone marrow. *J Lab Clin Med* 1996; 127:353.

161. Herman G, Shapiro RS, Abdelwahab IF, et al. MR imaging in adults with Gaucher disease type I: evaluation of marrow involvement and disease activity. *Skeletal Radiol* 1993;22:247.

162. Johnson LA, Hoppel BE, Gerard EL, et al. Quantitative chemical shift imaging of vertebral bone marrow in patients with Gaucher disease. *Radiology* 1992;182:451.

163. Rosenthal DI, Barton NW, McKusick KA, et al. Quantitative imaging of Gaucher disease. *Radiology* 1992;185:841.

164. Amstutz HC, Carey EJ. Skeletal manifestations and treatment of Gaucher's disease. *J Bone Joint Surg Am* 1966;48:670

165. Pastores GM, Wallenstein S, Desnick RJ, et al. Bone density in type 1 Gaucher disease. *J Bone Miner Res* 1996;11:1801.

166. Katz K, Mechlis-Frish S, Cohen IJ, et al. Bone scans in the diagnosis of bone crisis in patients who have Gaucher disease. *J Bone Joint Surg Am* 1991;73:513.

167. Mankin HJ, Doppelt SH, Rosenberg AE, et al. Metabolic bone disease in patients with Gaucher's disease. In: Avioli LA, Krane SM, eds. *Metabolic bone disease and clinically related disorders*, 2nd ed. Philadelphia: WB Saunders, 1990:730.

168. Horev G, Kornreich L, Hadar H, et al. Hemorrhage associated with "bone crisis" in Gaucher's disease identified by magnetic resonance imaging. *Skeletal Radiol* 1991;20:479.

169. Cohen IJ, Kornreich L, Mekhmandarov S, et al. Effective treatments of painful bone crises in type I Gaucher's disease with high dose prednisone. *Arch Dis Child* 1996;75:218.

170. Bell RS, Mankin HJ, Doppelt SH. Osteomyelitis in Gaucher disease. *J Bone Joint Surg Am* 1986;68:1380.

171. Katz K, Cohen IJ, Ziv N, et al. Fractures in children who have Gaucher disease. *J Bone Joint Surg Am* 1987;69:1361.

172. Katz K, Sabato S, Horev G, et al. Spinal involvement in children and adolescents with Gaucher disease. *Spine* 1993;18:332.

173. Katz K, Horev G, Grunebaum M, et al. The natural history of osteonecrosis of the femoral head in children and adolescents with Gaucher disease. *J Bone Joint Surg Am* 1996;78:14.

174. Barton NW, Brady RO, Dambrosia JM, et al. Replacement therapy for inherited enzyme deficiency: macrophage-targeted glucocerebrosidase for Gaucher's disease. *N Engl J Med* 1991; 324:1464.

175. Barton NW, Brady RO, Dambrosia JM, et al. Dose-dependent responses to macrophage-targeted glucocerebrosidase in a child with Gaucher disease. *J Pediatr* 1992;120:277.

176. Pastores GM, Sibille AR, Grabowski GA. Enzyme therapy in Gaucher disease type 1: dosage efficacy and adverse effects in 33 patients treated for 6 to 24 months. *Blood* 1993;82:408.

177. Rosenthal DI, Doppelt SH, Mankin JH, et al. Enzyme replacement therapy for Gaucher disease: skeletal responses to macrophage-targeted glucocerebrosidase. *Pediatrics* 1995;96:629.

178. Beutler E, Demina A, Laubscher K, et al. The clinical course of treated and untreated Gaucher disease: a study of 45 patients. *Blood Cells Mol Dis* 1995;21:86.

179. Beutler E. Enzyme replacement therapy for Gaucher's disease. *Baillieres Clin Haematol* 1997;10:751.

180. Elstein D, Hadas-Halpern I, Itzchaki M, et al. Effect of low-dose enzyme replacement therapy on bones in Gaucher disease patients with severe skeletal involvement. *Blood Cells Mol Dis* 1996;22:104.

181. Zimran A, Hadas-Helpern I, Zevin S, et al. Low-dose high-frequency enzyme replacement therapy for very young children with severe Gaucher disease. *Br J Haematol* 1993;85:783.

182. Kaplan P, Mazur A, Manor O, et al. Accelerating of retarded growth in children with Gaucher disease after treatment with alglucerase. *J Pediatr* 1996;129:149.

183. Kaye EM. Therapeutic approaches to lysosomal storage diseases. *Curr Opin Pediatr* 1995;7:650.

184. Barranger JA, Rice EO, Dunigan J, et al. Gaucher's disease: studies of gene transfer to haematopoietic cells. *Baillieres Clin Haematol* 1997;10:765.

185. Lichenstein L, Jaffe H. Eosinophilic granuloma of bone with report of a case. *Am J Pathol* 1940;16:595

186. Otani S, Ehrlich J. Solitary granuloma of bone simulating primary neoplasm. *Am J Pathol* 1940;16:479

187. Green WT, Faber S. Eosinophilic or solitary granuloma of bone. *J Bone Joint Surg Am* 1942;24:499

188. Lichenstein L. Histiocytosis X (eosinophilic granuloma of bone, Letterer-Siwe disease, and Schüller-Christian disease). *J Bone Joint Surg Am* 1964;46:76.

189. D'Angio GJ, Favara BE, Ladisch W. Workshop on the childhood histiocytosis: concepts and controversies. *Med Pediatr Oncol* 1986;14:104.

190. Favara BE. Langerhans' cell histiocytosis pathobiology and pathogenesis. *Semin Oncol* 1991;18:3.

191. Beckstead JH, Wood GS, Turner RR. Histiocytosis X cells and Langerhans cells: enzyme histochemical and immunologic similarities. *Hum Pathol* 1984;15:826.

192. Cambazard F, Dezutter-Dambuyant C, Staquet MJ, et al. Eosinophilic granuloma of bone and biochemical demonstration of 49-kDa Cdla molecule expression by Langerhans cell histiocytosis. *Clin Exp Dermatol* 1991;16:377.

193. Mierau GW, Favara BE, Brenman JM. Electron microscopy in histiocytosis X. *Ultrastruct Pathol* 1982;3:137.

194. Makley JT, Carter JR. Eosinophilic granuloma of bone. *Clin Orthop* 1986;204:37.

195. Dehner LP. Morphologic findings in the histiocytic syndromes. *Semin Oncol* 1991;18:8.

196. McClain K, Jin H, Gresik V, et al. Langerhans cell histiocytosis: lack of a viral etiology. *Am J Hematol* 1994;47:16.

197. de Graaf JH, Tamminge RY, Dam-Meiring A, et al. The presence of cytokines in Langerhans' cell histiocytosis. *J Pathol* 1996; 180:400.

198. Lahey ME. Histiocytosis X: an analysis of prognostic factors. *J Pediatr* 1975;87:184.

199. Broadbent V. Favourable prognostic features in histiocytosis X: bone involvement and absence of skin disease. *Arch Dis Child* 1986;61:1219.

200. Novice FM, Collison DW, Kleinsmith DM, et al. Letterer-Siwe disease in adults. *Cancer* 1989;63:166.

201. Berry DH, Gresik MV, Humphrey GB, et al. Natural history of histiocytosis X: a pediatric oncology study. *Med Pediatr Oncol* 1986;14:1.

202. McLelland J, Broadbent V, Yeomans E, et al. Langerhans cell histiocytosis: the case for conservative treatment. *Arch Dis Child* 1990;65:301.

203. Raney RB, D'Angio GJ. Langerhans' cell histiocytosis (histiocytosis X): experience at the Children's Hospital of Philadelphia, 1970–1984. *Med Pediatr Oncol* 1989;17:20.

204. Leavey P, Varughese M, Breatnach F, et al. Langerhans cell histiocytosis: a 31-year review. *Ir J Med Sci* 1991;160:271.

205. Schmitts S, Martin E, Zachmann M, et al. Pituitary stalk thickening with diabetes insipidus preceding typical manifestations of Langerhans cell histiocytosis in children. *Eur J Pediatr* 1993; 152:399.

206. Grois N, Barkovich AJ, Rosenau W, et al. Central nervous system disease associated with Langerhans' cell histiocytosis. *Am J Pediatr Hematol Oncol* 1993;15:245.

207. Bollini G, Jouve JL, Gentet JC, et al. Bone lesions in histiocytosis X. *J Pediatr Orthop* 1991;11:469.

208. Dimentberg RA, Brown KLB. Diagnostic evaluation of patients with histiocytosis X. *J Pediatr Orthop* 1990;10:733.

209. Greis PE, Hankin FM. Eosinophilic granuloma: the management of solitary lesions of bone. *Clin Orthop* 1990;257:204.

210. Compere EL, Johnson WE, Coventry MB. Vertebra plana (Calve's disease) due to eosinophilic granuloma. *J Bone Joint Surg Am* 1954;36:969.

211. Ruppert D, Oria RA, Kumar R, et al. Radiologic features of eosinophilic granuloma of bone. *Am J Roentgenol* 1989;153: 1021.

212. Kozlowski K, Diard F, Padovani J, et al. Unilateral mid-femoral periosteal new bone of varying aetiology in children. *Pediatr Radiol* 1986;16:475.

213. Gardner DJ, Azouz EM. Solitary lucent epiphyseal lesions in children. *Skeletal Radiol* 1988;17:497.

214. Leeson MC, Smith A, Carter JR, et al. Eosinophilic granuloma of bone in the growing epiphysis. *J Pediatr Orthop* 1985;5:147.

215. Dogan AS, Conway JJ, Miller JH, et al. Detection of bone lesions in Langerhans cell histiocytosis: complementary roles of scintigraphy and conventional radiography. *J Pediatr Hematol Oncol* 1996;18:51.

216. Beltran J, Aparisi F, Bonmati LM, et al. Eosinophilic granuloma: MRI manifestations. *Skeletal Radiol* 1993;22:157.

217. Fiorillo A, Sadile F, De Chiara C, et al. Bone lesions in Langerhans cell histiocytosis. *Clin Pediatr* 1993;32:118.

218. Womer RB, Raney RB, D'Angio GJ. Healing rates of treated and untreated bone lesions in histiocytosis X. *Pediatrics* 1985; 76:286.

219. Egeler RM, Thompson RC Jr, Voute PA, et al. Intralesional infiltration of corticosteroids in localized Langerhans' cell histiocytosis. *J Pediatr Orthop* 1992;12:811.

220. Munn SE, Olliver L, Broadbent V, et al. Use of indomethacin in Langerhans cell histiocytosis. *Med Pediatr Oncol* 1999;32: 247.

221. Greenberger JS, Crocker AC, Vawter G, et al. Results of treatment of 127 patients with systemic histiocytosis (Letterer-Siwe disease, Schüller-Christian syndrome and multifocal eosinophilic granuloma). *Medicine* 1981;60:311.

222. Baber WW, Numaguchi Y, Nadell JM, et al. Eosinophilic granuloma of the cervical spine without vertebrae plana. *J Comput Tomogr* 1987;11:346.

223. Robert H, Dubousset J, Miladi L. Histiocytosis X in the juvenile spine. *Spine* 1987;12:167.

224. Mammano S, Candiotto S, Balsano M. Cast and brace treatment of eosinophilic granuloma of the spine: long-term follow-up. *J Pediatr Orthop* 1997;17:821.

225. Alley RM, Sussman MD. Rapidly progressive eosinophilic granuloma. *Spine* 1992;17:1517.

226. Raney RB. Chemotherapy for children with aggressive fibromatosis and Langerhans' cell histiocytosis. *Clin Orthop* 1991; 262:58.

227. Starling KA. Chemotherapy of histiocytosis-X. *Hematol Oncol Clin North Am* 1987;1:119.

228. Greinix HT, Storb R, Sanders JE, et al. Marrow transplantation for treatment of multisystem progressive Langerhans cell histiocytosis. *Bone Marrow Transplant* 1992;10:39.

229. Ringdén O, Åhström L, Lönnqvist B, et al. Allogenic bone marrow transplantation in a patient with chemotherapy-resistant progressive histiocytosis X. *N Engl J Med* 1987;316:733.

230. Alexander JE, Seibert JJ, Berry DH, et al. Prognostic factors for healing of bone lesions in histiocytosis X. *Pediatr Radiol* 1988; 18:326.

Disorders of Hemostasis

231. Soucie JM, Evatt B, Jackson D. Occurrence of hemophilia in the United States. The Hemophilia Surveillance System Project Investigators. *Am J Hematol* 1998;59:288.

232. Greene WB, McMillan CW. Nonsurgical management of hemophilic arthropathy. *Instructional Course Lect* 1989;38:367.

233. Pool JG, Shannon AE. Production of high-potency concentrates in antihemophilic globulin in a closed-bag system: assay in vitro and in vivo. *N Engl J Med* 1965;273:1443.

234. Brinkhouse KM, Shanbrom E, Roberts HR, et al. A new high-potency glycine-precipitated antihemophilic factor (AHF) concentrate. *JAMA* 1968;205:613.

235. Wagner RH, McLester WD, Smith M, et al. Purification of antihemophilic factor (factor VIII) by amino acid precipitation. *Thromb Diath Haemorrh* 1964;11:64.

236. McMillan CW, Green WB, Blatt PM, et al. The management of musculoskeletal problems in hemophilia. *Instructional Course Lect* 1983;33:210.

237. Shapiro SS. Antibodies to blood coagulation factors. *Clin Haematol* 1979;8:207.

238. DiMichele DM. Immune tolerance: a synopsis of the international experience. *Haemophilia* 1998;4:568.

239. Shapiro AD, Gilchrist GS, Hoots WK, et al. Prospective, randomized trial of two doses of rFVIIa (NovoSeven) in haemophilia patients with inhibitors undergoing surgery. *Thromb Haemost* 1998;80:773.

240. Mainardi CL, Levine PH, Werb Z, et al. Proliferative synovitis in hemophilia: biochemical and morphologic observations. *Arthritis Rheum* 1978;21:137.

241. Roosendaal G, Vianen ME, Wenting MJ, et al. Iron deposits and catabolic properties of synovial tissue from patients with haemophilia. *J Bone Joint Surg Br* 1998;80:540.

242. Stein H, Duthie RB. The pathogenesis of chronic haemophilic arthropathy. *J Bone Joint Surg Br* 1981;63:601.

243. Roy S. Ultrastructure of articular cartilage in experimental haemarthrosis. *Arch Pathol* 1968;86:69.

244. Greene WB, Yankaskas BC, Guilford WB. Comparison of radiologic classification of hemophilic arthropathy with clinical parameters. *J Bone Joint Surg Am* 1989;71:237.

245. Aronstam A, Browne RS, Wassef M, et al. Clinical features of early haemarthroses in severely affected adolescent haemophiliacs. *Clin Lab Haematol* 1984;6:9.

246. Gamble JG, Bellah J, Rinsky LA, et al. Arthropathy of the ankle in hemophilia. *J Bone Joint Surg Am* 1991;73:1008.

247. Houghton GR, Duthie RB. Orthopaedic problems in hemophilia. *Clin Orthop* 1979;138:197.

248. Funk M, Schmidt H, Escuriola-Ettingshausen C, et al. Radiological and orthopedic score in pediatric hemophilic patients with early and late prophylaxis. *Ann Hematol* 1998;77:171.

249. Kreuz W, Escuriola-Ettingshausen C, Funk M, et al. When should prophylactic treatment in patients with haemophilia A and B start? The German experience. *Haemophilia* 1998;4:413.

250. Ljung R, van den Berg M, Petrini P, et al. Port-A-Cath usage in children with haemophilia: experience of 53 cases. *Acta Paediatr* 1998;87:1051.

251. Miller K, Buchanan GR, Zappa S, et al. Implantable venous access devices in children with hemophilia: a report of low infection rates. *J Pediatr* 1998;132:934.

252. Perkins JL, Johnson VA, Osip JM, et al. The use of implantable venous access devices (IVAD's) in children with hemophilia. *J Pediatr Hematol Oncol* 1997;19:339.

253. Bohn RL, Avorn J, Glynn RJ, et al. Prophylactic use of factor VIII: an economic evaluation. *Thromb Haemost* 1998;75:932.

254. Smith PS, Teutsch SM, Shaffer PA, et al. Episodic versus prophylactic infusions for hemophilia A: a cost-effective analysis. *J Pediatr* 1996;129:424.

255. Greene WB, McMillan CW, Warren MW. Prophylactic transfusion for hypertrophic synovitis in children with hemophilia. *Clin Orthop* 1997;343:19.

256. Storti E, Traldi A, Tosatti E, et al. Synovectomy, a new approach to haemophilic arthropathy. *Acta Haematol* 1969;41:193.

257. Wilson FC, Mayhew DE, McMillan CW. Surgical management of musculoskeletal problems in hemophilia. *Instructional Course Lect* 1983;32:233.

258. Klein KS, Aland CM, Him HC, et al. Long-term follow-up of arthroscopic synovectomy for chronic hemophilic synovitis. *Arthroscopy* 1987;3:231.

259. Matsuda Y, Duthie DB. Surgical synovectomy for haemophilic arthropathy of the knee joint: long-term follow-up. *Scand J Haematol* 1984;33(Suppl 40):237.

260. Montane I, McCollough NC, Lian EC. Synovectomy of the

knee for hemophilic arthropathy. *J Bone Joint Surg Am* 1986; 68:210.

261. O'Connell FD. Open surgical synovectomy of the knee in hemophilia: long-term follow-up. In: Gilbert MS, Greene WB, eds. *Musculoskeletal problems in hemophilia.* New York: The National Hemophilia Foundation, 1989:91.

262. Post M, Watts G, Telfer M. Synovectomy in hemophilic arthropathy: a retrospective review of 17 cases. *Clin Orthop* 1986; 202:139.

263. Scarponi R, Silvello L, Landonio G, et al. Long-term evaluation of knee-joint function after synovectomy in haemophilia. *Br J Haematol* 1982;52:337.

264. Storti E, Ascari E, Gamba G. Postoperative complications of joint function after knee synovectomy in haemophiliacs. *Br J Haematol* 1982;50:544.

265. Triantafyllou SJ, Hanks GA, Handal JA, et al. Open and arthroscopic synovectomy in hemophilic arthropathy of the knee. *Clin Orthop* 1992;283:196.

266. Casscells CD. Commentary: the argument for early arthroscopic synovectomy in patients with severe hemophilia. *Arthroscopy* 1987;3:78.

267. Greene WB. Use of continuous passive slow motion in the postoperative rehabilitation of difficult pediatric knee and elbow problems. *J Pediatr Orthop* 1983;3:419.

268. Limbird TJ, Dennis SC. Synovectomy and continuous passive motion (cpm) in hemophilic patients. *Arthroscopy* 1987;3:74.

269. Wiedel JD. Arthroscopic synovectomy of the knee in hemophilia. *Clin Orthop* 1996;328:46.

270. Cohen B, Griffiths L, Dandy DJ. Arteriovenous fistula after arthroscopic synovectomy in a patient with haemophilia. *Arthroscopy* 1992;8:373.

271. Busch M, Kurczynski E. The role of arthroscopic synovectomy in the treatment of children with hemophilia. Presented at the Pediatric Orthopaedic Society of North America meeting, May 4, 1993, White Sulphur Springs, WV.

272. Greene WB. Synovectomy of the ankle for hemophilic arthropathy. *J Bone Joint Surg Am* 1994;76:812.

273. Zuckerman JD, Solomon GE, Shortkroff S, et al. Principles of radiation synovectomy. In: Gilbert MS, Greene WB, eds. *Musculoskeletal problems in hemophilia.* New York: The National Hemophilia Foundation, 1990:93.

274. Fernandez-Palazzi F, de Boscl NB, de Vargas AF. Radioactive synovectomy in haemophilic haemarthrosis: follow-up of fifty cases. *Scand J Haematol* 1984;33(Suppl 40):291.

275. Löfqvist T, Petersson C, Nilsson IM. Radioactive synoviorthesis in patients with hemophilia with factor inhibitor. *Clin Orthop* 1997;343:37.

276. Merchan EC, Magallon M, Martin-Villar J, et al. Long-term follow-up of haemophilic arthropathy treated by AU-198 radiation synovectomy. *Int Orthop* 1993;17:120.

277. Dawson TM, Ryan PF, Street AM, et al. Yttrium synovectomy in haemophilic arthropathy. *Br J Rheumatol* 1994;33:351.

278. Erken EHW. Radiocolloids in the management of hemophilic arthropathy in children and adolescents. *Clin Orthop* 1991;264: 129.

279. Heim M, Horoszowski H, Lieberman L, et al. Methods and results of radionucleotide synovectomies. In: Gilbert MS, Greene WB, eds. *Musculoskeletal problems in hemophilia.* New York: The National Hemophilia Foundation, 1990:98.

280. Rivard GE, Girard M, Belanger R, et al. Synoviorthesis with colloidal ^{32}P chromic phosphate for the treatment of hemophilic arthropathy. *J Bone Joint Surg Am* 1994;76:482.

281. Siegel ME, Siegel HJ, Luck JV Jr. Radiosynovectomy's clinical applications and cost effectiveness: a review. *Semin Nucl Med* 1997;27:364.

282. Aronstam A, Rainsford SG, Painter MJ. Patterns of bleeding in adolescents with severe haemophilia A. *Br Med J* 1979;1: 469.

283. Growe GH, Meek R. Decompression of the iliopsoas muscle. In: Gilbert MS, Greene WB, eds. *Musculoskeletal problems in hemophilia.* New York: The National Hemophilia Foundation, 1990:45.

284. Greene WB. Chronic inflammatory arthritides and diseases related to the hematopoietic system. In: Drennan JC, ed. *The child's foot and ankle.* New York: Raven, 1992:461.

285. Greene WB, Howes CL, Mathewson AB. Treatment of knee flexion contractures in hemophiliacs with inhibitors and pre-existent arthropathy. In: Gilbert MS, Greene WB, eds. *Musculoskeletal problems in hemophilia.* New York: The National Hemophilia Foundation, 1990:74.

286. Greene WB, Wilson FC. Nonoperative management of hemophilic arthropathy and muscle hemorrhage. *Instructional Course Lect* 1983;32:223.

287. Martinson A. Hemophilic pseudotumors. In: Boone DC, ed. *Comprehensive management of hemophilia.* Philadelphia: FA Davis, 1976:94.

288. Hermann G, Yeh HC, Gilbert MS. Computed tomography and ultrasonography of the hemophilic pseudotumor and their use in surgical planning. *Skeletal Radiol* 1986;15:123.

Acute Leukemia

289. Niemeyer CM, Sallan SE. Acute lymphoblastic leukemia. In: Nathan DG, Orkin SH, eds. *Hematology of infancy and childhood,* 5th ed. Philadelphia: WB Saunders, 1998:1245.

290. Pui CH, Evans WE. Acute lymphoblastic leukemia. *New Engl J Med* 1998;339:605.

291. Sallan SE, Weinstein HJ. Childhood acute leukemia. In: Nathan DG, Oski FA, eds. *Hematology of infancy and childhood,* 3rd ed. Philadelphia: WB Saunders, 1987:1028.

292. Jonsson OG, Sartain P, Ducore JM, et al. Bone pain as an initial symptom of childhood acute lymphoblastic leukemia: association with nearly normal hematologic indexes. *J Pediatr* 1990;117:233.

293. Halton JM, Atkinson SA, Fraher L, et al. Mineral homeostasis and bone mass at diagnosis in children with acute lymphoblastic leukemia. *J Pediatr* 1995;126:557.

294. Heinrich SD, Gallagher D, Warrior R, et al. The prognostic significance of the skeletal manifestations of acute lymphoblastic leukemia of childhood. *J Pediatr Orthop* 1994;14:105.

295. Rogalsky RJ, Black GB, Reed MH. Orthopaedic manifestations of leukemia in children. *J Bone Joint Surg Am* 1986;68:494.

296. Santangelo JR, Thomson JD. Childhood leukemia presenting with back pain and vertebral compression fractures. *Am J Orthop* 1999;28:257.

297. Greene WB. Idiopathic juvenile osteoporosis. In: Weinstein SL, ed. *The pediatric spine.* New York: Raven, 1994:933.

298. Ostrov BE, Goldsmith DP, Athreya BH. Differentiation of systemic juvenile rheumatoid arthritis from acute leukemia near the onset of disease. *J Pediatr* 1993;122:595.

299. Saulsbury FT, Sabio H. Acute leukemia presenting as arthritis in children. *Clin Pediatr* 1985;24:625.

300. Appell RG, Buhler T, Willich E, et al. Absence of prognostic significance of skeletal involvement in acute lymphocytic leukemia and non-Hodgkin lymphoma in children. *Pediatr Radiol* 1985;15:245.

301. Masera G, Carnelli V, Ferrari M, et al. Prognostic significance of radiological bone involvement in childhood acute lymphoblastic leukemia. *Arch Dis Child* 1977;52:530.

302. Atkinson SA, Halton JM, Bradley C, et al. Bone and mineral abnormalities in childhood acute lymphoblastic leukemia: influence of disease, drugs and nutrition. *Int J Cancer* 1998;11:35.

303. D'Angelo P, Conter V, Di Chiara G, et al. Severe osteoporosis and multiple vertebral collapses in a child during treatment for B-ALL. *Acta Haematol* 1993;38:38.

304. Arikoski P, Komulainen J, Voutilainen R, et al. Reduced bone mineral density in long-term survivors of childhood acute lymphoblastic leukemia. *J Pediatr Hematol Oncol* 1998;20:234.

305. Warner JT, Evans WD, Webb DK, et al. Relative osteopenia after treatment for acute lymphoblastic leukemia. *Pediatr Res* 1999;45:544.

306. Murphy RG, Greenberg ML. Osteonecrosis in pediatric patients with acute lymphoblastic leukemia. *Cancer* 1990;65:1717.

307. Ojala AE, Paakko E, Lanning FP, et al. Osteonecrosis during the treatment of childhood acute lymphoblastic leukemia: a prospective MRI study. *Med Pediatr Oncol* 1999;32:11.

308. Harper GD, Dicks-Mireaux C, Leiper AD. Total body irradiation-induced osteochondromata. *J Pediatr Orthop* 1998;18:356.

309. Mohnike K, Dorffel W, Timme J, et al. Final height and puberty in 40 patients after antileukaemic treatment during childhood. *Eur J Pediatr* 1997;156:272.

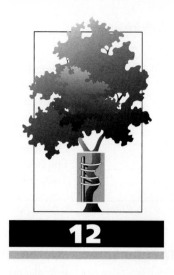

12

JUVENILE IDIOPATHIC ARTHRITIS

DOWAIN A. WRIGHT

D. A. Wright: Department of Pediatrics, University of California–San Francisco School of Medicine at Fresno, San Francisco, California 93638; Department of Rheumatology and Immunology, Valley Children's Hospital, Madera, California 93638.

OVERVIEW OF PEDIATRIC RHEUMATIC DISEASE ENCOUNTERED BY THE PEDIATRIC ORTHOPAEDIC SURGEON

Pain is a common complaint in childhood. Each year, as many as 1% of all children will have pains severe enough to be evaluated (1). Approximately 15% of healthy children reported episodes of musculoskeletal pain on a health questionnaire (2). Healthy children in daycare centers have approximately one painful episode every 3 h, related to play, discipline, or interaction with peers (3). The orthopaedic surgeon is often the first specialist to encounter the child with joint, limb, or back pain. They must be able to identify the most likely cause of the pain and initiate treatment or referral to an appropriate medical specialist.

Juvenile arthritis is the most common rheumatic disease of childhood. It is one of the most common chronic illnesses occurring in children. The annual incidence ranges from 10 to 14 per 100,000, with an overall prevalence of 1 to 2 per 1,000 (4,5). Although only 1 in 100 children evaluated by a physician for joint pain will ultimately be diagnosed with arthritis, the frequency of arthritis presenting to the orthopaedic specialist is surely higher.

The purpose of this chapter is to provide the orthopaedic surgeon with an in-depth understanding of the presentation, differential diagnosis, and management of children with arthritis. With this framework, the orthopaedic specialist should be able to identify children with juvenile arthritis, and to differentiate arthritis from benign pains of childhood, psychogenic pain syndromes, infection, malignancy, or other systemic autoimmune diseases (lupus, dermatomyositis, and vasculitis). Infection and malignancies, as well as congenital, mechanical, or traumatic causes of limb or joint pain, are presented only as a contrast to juvenile arthritis, because detailed presentations on these subjects are found elsewhere in this text.

CLASSIFICATION AND DIAGNOSIS OF JUVENILE IDIOPATHIC ARTHRITIS

The cause(s) of juvenile arthritis is not known. With the great heterogeneity of presentation and course, there will likely be multiple initiating factors in the setting of a suscep-tible host. There is no laboratory test that will make a definitive diagnosis of arthritis. A diagnosis of juvenile arthritis is made by taking a thorough history, performing a skilled and comprehensive physical examination, utilizing directed laboratory tests and imaging procedures, and following the child over time.

There have been two major sets of criteria for the diagnosis and classification for juvenile arthritis. The diagnostic criteria for juvenile chronic arthritis (JCA) were defined by the European League Against Rheumatism (EULAR) (6) (Table 12-1). In the EULAR criteria, JCA is differentiated into onset types of pauciarticular, polyarticular, juvenile rheumatoid (positive rheumatoid factor [RF]), systemic, juvenile ankylosing spondylitis, and juvenile psoriatic arthritis. In North America, the most frequently used criteria have been those by the American College of Rheumatology (ACR) for juvenile rheumatoid arthritis (JRA) (7) (Table 12-1). These criteria define the subtypes of JRA to be oligoarticular (pauciarticular), polyarticular, and systemic. They exclude other causes of juvenile arthritis, including spondyloarthropathies (juvenile ankylosing spondylitis, inflammatory bowel disease–associated arthritis, and related diseases), juvenile psoriatic arthritis, arthritis associated with other systemic inflammatory diseases (systemic lupus erythematosus, dermatomyositis, sarcoidosis, etc.) and infectious or neoplastic disorders.

These criteria, although similar, do not identify identical populations or spectra of disease, but have often been used interchangeably. This has led to confusion in interpretation of studies of the epidemiology, treatment, and outcome of juvenile arthritis. Recently, the International League of Associations of Rheumatologists (ILAR) has proposed (8) and revised (9) criteria for the diagnosis and classification of juvenile arthritis, or "Durban Criteria" (Table 12-2). The term "juvenile idiopathic arthritis" (JIA) has been proposed to replace both JRA and JCA, and will encompass all juvenile arthritides lasting greater than 6 weeks that are of unknown cause. This international compromise will allow uniform interpretation of clinical and therapeutic data. Although these criteria are not definitive, and some children will fit into either no category or two or more categories, they should be thought of as a work in progress. As techniques become available to better define the genetic risk factors and specific triggers of juvenile arthritis, uniform modifica-

TABLE 12-1. COMPARISON OF ACR AND EULAR CLASSIFICATION OF JUVENILE IDIOPATHIC ARTHRITIS

	ACR	EULAR
Age at onset:	<16 years	<16 years
Arthritis:	One or more joints	One or more joints
Duration of disease:	6 weeks or longer	3 months or longer
Onset type:	In first 6 months	
	Polyarthritis: 5 or more joints	Pauciarticular <5 joints
	Oligoarthritis: <5 joints	Polyarticular >4 joints, RF negative
	Systemic: arthritis with characteristic fever at onset	Juvenile rheumatoid arthritis >4 joints, RF positive
		Juvenile ankylosing spondylitis
		Juvenile psoriatic arthritis
Exclusions:	Other forms of juvenile arthritis	

ACR, American College of Rheumatology; *EULAR*, European League Against Rheumatism; *RF*, rheumatoid factor.

tions to the criteria can be made. At least now we are all starting with the same basic set of assumptions. In the remaining sections of this chapter, the term "juvenile arthritis" is used to denote any type of arthritis in childhood, "JIA" will be used as defined above, and the terms "JRA" and "JCA" will be used only when referring to specific epidemiologic, therapeutic, or outcome data.

Oligoarthritis

Oligoarticular onset of JIA is defined as arthritis affecting one to four joints during the first 6 months of disease. There are two subcategories: persistent oligoarthritis affects no more than four joints throughout the entire course of arthritis. Extended oligoarthritis affects a cumulative total of five

TABLE 12-2. CRITERIA FOR CLASSIFICATION OF JUVENILE IDIOPATHIC ARTHRITIS: DURBAN, 1997

Age at onset: before 16th birthday
Arthritis in one or more joints
Duration of disease: at least 6 weeks
Onset type:

Systemic Arthritis
Arthritis with or preceded by daily fever of at least 2 weeks' duration, accompanied by one or more of the following:
1. Evanescent, nonfixed erythematous rash
2. Generalized lymph node enlargement
3. Hepatomegaly or splenomegaly
4. Serositis

Polyarthritis (RF-negative)
Arthritis affecting five or more joints during the first 6 months of disease; tests for RF are negative

Psoriatic Arthritis
1. Arthritis and psoriasis, or
2. Arthritis and at least two of:
   a. dactylitis
   b. nail abnormalities (pitting or onycholysis)
   c. family history of psoriasis confirmed by a dermatologist in at least one first-degree relative

Other Arthritis
Children with arthritis of unknown cause that persists for at least 6 weeks, but that either:
1. does not fulfill criteria for any of the other categories, or
2. fulfills criteria for more than one of the other categories

Oligoarthritis
1. Persistent oligoarthritis: no more than four joints involved
2. Extended oligoarthritis: affects a cumulative total of five or more joints after the first 6 months of disease

Polyarthritis (RF-positive)
Arthritis affecting five or more joints during the first 6 months of disease, associated with positive RF tests on two occasions at least 3 months apart

Enthesitis-related Arthritis
Arthritis and enthesitis, or arthritis or enthesitis with at least two of:
1. Sacroiliac joint tenderness and/or inflammatory spinal pain
2. Presence of HLA-B27
3. Family history of HLA-B27–associated disease in at least one first- or second-degree relative
4. Anterior uveitis that is usually associated with pain, redness, or photophobia
5. Onset of arthritis in a boy after the age of 8 years

RF, rheumatoid factor; *CRP*, C-reactive protein.

joints or more after the first 6 months of disease. A child will be excluded from this diagnostic category if any of the following five conditions are met: a family history of psoriasis, confirmed by a dermatologist, in at least one first- or second-degree relative; family history of medically confirmed HLA-B27–associated disease in at least one first- or second-degree relative; HLA-B27–positive male with onset of arthritis after 8 years of age; a positive RF test; or systemic arthritis. Characteristics include the age at onset of arthritis. Also, the patterns of arthritis should be noted, including: large joints only, small joints only, limb predominance (upper, lower, both), specific joint involvement, and symmetry of arthritis. Finally, the occurrence of anterior uveitis, presence of antinuclear antibody (ANA), and any human leukocyte antigens (HLA) class I and II showing predisposing or protective alleles should be considered. This diagnostic subgroup will certainly contain some children with psoriatic arthritis who have not yet developed a psoriatic dermatitis. It will also exclude the few children with oligoarticular disease and a positive RF. However, these children are likely to have an early onset of RF-positive polyarticular arthritis, or at least would be predicted to have a more prolonged and severe course, and as such, should be excluded from the oligoarticular group.

Polyarthritis (RF −)

Polyarticular onset (RF-negative) JIA is defined as arthritis affecting five or more joints during the first 6 months of disease with a negative RF, and the absence of systemic arthritis. Descriptors for RF-negative polyarticular JIA include age at onset, symmetry of arthritis, presence of ANA, and occurrence of uveitis.

Polyarthritis (RF +)

RF-positive polyarticular JIA is defined as arthritis affecting five or more joints during the first 6 months of disease, associated with a positive RF test on two occasions at least 3 months apart, and the absence of systemic arthritis. Descriptors include age at onset of arthritis, symmetry, presence of ANA, and immunogenetic characteristics. This disease is likely to be the equivalent of early-onset adult rheumatoid arthritis.

Systemic Arthritis

Systemic JIA is characterized by arthritis with or preceded by daily fever of at least 2 weeks' duration, which is documented to be quotidian for at least 3 days, and accompanied by one or more of the following: evanescent, nonfixed, erythematous rash; generalized lymphadenopathy; hepato- or splenomegaly; or serositis. This type of arthritis can be described in terms of age at onset of arthritis and the pattern of arthritis during and after the first 6 months: oligoarthritis, polyarthritis, or arthritis present only after the first 6 months of systemic illness. Other descriptors include the features of systemic disease after the first 6 months of disease, the presence of RF, and the level of C-reactive protein (CRP).

Psoriatic Arthritis

Psoriatic arthritis is defined as arthritis and psoriasis, or arthritis and at least two other criteria, including: dactylitis, nail abnormalities (pitting or onycholysis), or a family history of psoriasis documented by a dermatologist in at least one first-degree relative. Exclusions include the presence of RF and systemic arthritis. Descriptors include the age at onset of arthritis or psoriasis, pattern of joint involvement, oligoarticular or polyarticular course, presence of ANA, or uveitis.

Enthesitis-related Arthritis

Enthesitis-related arthritis (ERA) is defined as arthritis and enthesitis (pain at insertion sites of tendons and ligaments), or arthritis or enthesitis with at least two of the following characteristics: sacroiliac joint tenderness and/or inflammatory spinal pain, presence of HLA-B27, family history in at least one first- or second-degree relative of a medically confirmed HLA-B27–associated disease (e.g., ankylosing spondylitis, sacroiliitis with inflammatory bowel disease, or acute [symptomatic] anterior uveitis associated with pain, redness, or photophobia), or onset of arthritis in a boy after the age of 8 years. Enthesitis is defined as tenderness at the insertion of tendon, ligament joint capsule, or fascia to bone. Descriptors for enthesitis-related arthritis include age at onset of arthritis or enthesitis, patterns of arthritis, symmetry of arthritis, oligoarticular or polyarticular disease course, and the presence of inflammatory bowel disease.

Other Juvenile Idiopathic Arthritides

Despite our best attempts to categorize children with idiopathic arthritis, there will inevitably be children who do not fit into any known category. This group of children with JIA will be considered to have undifferentiated or overlap arthritis. This category of other arthritis is defined as children with arthritis of unknown cause that persists for at least 6 weeks, but that either does not fulfill criteria for any other category, or fulfills criteria for more than one of the other categories.

APPROACH TO THE EVALUATION OF CHILDREN WITH LIMB PAIN, LIMP, OR JOINT PAIN WITH OR WITHOUT SWELLING

The evaluation of children with limb or back pain, a new limp, or joint pain with or without swelling, requires a comprehensive history and physical examination. The first

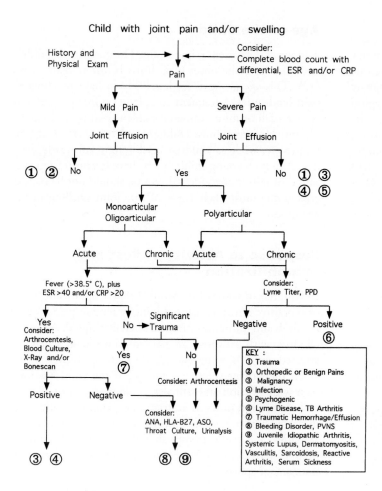

FIGURE 12-1. Algorithm for evaluation of a child with joint pain and/or swelling. Chronic is considered <6 weeks. *ANA*, antinuclear antibody; *ASO*, antistreptolysin-O; *PPD*, tuberculin skin test; *PVNS*, pigmented villonodular synovitis; *ESR*, erythrocyte sedimentation rate; *CRP*, C-reactive protein.

priority is to rule out an infection (osteomyelitis, septic arthritis, discitis), malignancy, or orthopaedic abnormality requiring prompt intervention. The causes of arthritis in children are extensive and many are rare. There are no pathognomonic presentations, and there is extensive overlap of all types of juvenile arthritis. Laboratory tests and radiologic studies are often uninformative, and should not be used to make or dismiss the diagnosis of juvenile arthritis. The purpose of this section is to provide the orthopaedist with an overview of the ways children present with arthritis, and to generate a framework for the logical identification of the appropriate diagnosis with a minimum of diagnostic procedures. The algorithm in Figure 12-1 provides a guide for the evaluation of children presenting with limb or joint pain. The first step in any evaluation of a child with possible arthritis is to obtain a thorough history and review of systems.

Timing of Pain or Disability

The timing of the pain is important. Children with arthritis will frequently have mild-to-moderate pain and stiffness (gelling) in the mornings, after a nap, sitting in class, after a long automobile ride, or other periods of inactivity. These complaints will generally improve within minutes or hours of renewed activity. Although there may be some residual limp or mild complaints of pain or stiffness, many children with JIA will be entirely asymptomatic on presentation to the physician's office. The major exception to this is the child with enthesitis-related arthritis, who may have morning pain and stiffness, but who will worsen throughout the day or with activities, because of repeated stress on inflamed tendons and entheses. A minority of children with JIA will have significant pain throughout the day, and the physical exam is likely to reveal severe arthritis in those with increased pain. It would be very unusual for the pain associated with JIA to keep a child from falling asleep or to wake the child from sleep. When a child has only afternoon, evening, and/or nighttime pains that resolve in the morning, this is typical for benign pains of childhood (growing pains). When pain is present both day and night, and interferes with sleep, it is unlikely to be due to JIA, but, depending on the duration and location, may be associated with malignancy, infection, or psychogenic pain syndromes.

Duration of Pain

The duration of pain is also important. Severe pain of new onset, which prompts immediate evaluation, may be due to infection, malignancy, or trauma. Pain that is slowly worsening or unchanged over weeks or months is typical of JIA. When pain has been present for many years, the cause is often psychogenic or mechanical. It is not unusual for a parent to note that a child has had pain, clumsiness, or difficulty walking from the time the child's first steps were taken. When neurologic abnormalities, including cerebral palsy, are excluded, the majority of these children have benign mechanical problems, or parental anxiety can be considered.

Location of Pain

The location of the pain is an important part of the history. Children with JIA will rarely have muscular pains. True weakness should suggest either an inflammatory or congenital myopathy. Long-bone or periarticular pain is often seen with trauma or malignancies. When pain is random, intermittent, or migratory, especially if it comes and goes during the clinic visit, it is often psychogenic in origin. Pain with JIA can be additive, and can have spontaneous improvement, but it is usually present consistently over weeks or months.

Intensity of Pain

The quality or intensity of the pain can be difficult to determine in children, especially for the preverbal child. Pain-rating scales for children have been developed to be sensitive to the cognitive-developmental conceptualizations of children (10). Children are asked to rate their pain on a visual analog scale (VAS), in terms of present pain and worst pain intensity for the previous week. Each VAS is a 10-cm horizontal line with no numbers or descriptors. The child VAS is anchored with the developmentally appropriate pain descriptors: happy and sad faces, corresponding to no pain and severe pain, respectively.

In general, the intensity of pain reported by children with JIA ranges from moderate to absent (11). Rarely, the child will report severe pain. Most children with JIA will maintain near-normal function. Acute arthritis, such as postinfectious reactive arthritis, including acute rheumatic fever, is typically much more painful than JIA. Intense pain that is nonmigratory and present night and day is more likely to represent infection or malignancy. However, severe pain that is intermittent or migratory, interferes with school, and causes sleep disturbance in a child with normal laboratories and growth, is usually psychogenic in origin. Children with psychogenic pain syndromes are often unable to perform normal daily activities, due to the high level of perceived pain.

Age of the Child

The age of the patient is important. The majority of children with JIA have the onset of arthritis before 6 years of age (12). This age group is far less likely to have psychogenic pain syndromes. A frequent complaint on first presentation is that a fall or injury caused a sudden swelling and pain in a joint. However, most children under 6 years of age fall frequently, whereas children aged 1 to 4 fall nearly every day. Although young children may have fractures from even innocent falls, nonaccidental trauma should not be considered as the most likely cause of true joint swelling in this age group.

Response to Activity or Rest and Immobilization

In children in whom it is possible that a significant injury or repetitive stress has caused joint or tendon pain, resting the limb and immobilization are often attempted. Although children with arthritis can have minimal pain when the affected joint is immobilized, they are uniformly worse when the cast or splint is removed. If the child has joint pain with effusion and stiffness, prolonged immobilization will often result in severe restriction in range of motion and increased pain. Children with arthritis usually improve with activities, and every attempt should be made to keep them mobile. We do not limit athletic activities but do encourage noncontact sports.

Associated Symptoms

Other associated symptoms can often be useful in guiding your evaluation of joint pain. Fevers, whether continuous or periodic, can be associated with infection and malignancies or systemic inflammatory disease. Weight loss, with laboratory evidence of inflammation, suggests the presence of a systemic illness, such as infection, malignancy, inflammatory bowel disease, or systemic onset JIA. Persistent fatigue, sleep disturbance, and depression are often signs of a psychogenic pain syndrome. Fatigue should not be confused with true weakness, which could represent the onset of an inflammatory myositis.

Family History

The family history is important in evaluation for suspected JIA. The presence of HLA-B27–associated diseases, chronic back pains, or psoriasis could suggest the onset of an associated disease. Other systemic autoimmune disorders, including adult rheumatoid arthritis, often group in families, but have no direct pattern of inheritance. Children with psychogenic pain syndromes are often found to have a relative, usually the mother, who has chronic pain and acts as a role model for the pain behavior.

Physical Exam

A comprehensive physical exam, when combined with a complete history and screening laboratory tests, will often be sufficient to diagnose the child with arthritis. The musculoskeletal exam will often allow differentiation between mechanical or psychogenic causes of pain and inflammatory etiologies. Children with functional pain syndromes will often have complaints of pain that are out of proportion to the exam and often are migratory or transient, even during the exam.

Arthritis

Arthritis is defined as swelling within a joint, or limitation in range of joint movement with joint pain or tenderness, that is observed by a physician, and which is not due to a primary mechanical disorder. Young children will often be difficult to examine, and should be observed closely for limp or joint swelling prior to approaching the child. It is often instructive to observe the child playing in the waiting area and walking to or from the exam room. All children with joint pain or swelling should have a comprehensive joint exam. Often, children with joint pain will be quite apprehensive about the exam. When a child presents with the complaint of a single swollen or tender joint, it is important to evaluate all joints for signs of arthritis. It is not infrequent that joints other that the presenting joint will be involved with arthritis. As such, it is wise to begin the exam at sites distant from the point of pain, and gain the trust of the child prior to approaching the painful site. Examination of a painful site will often end your ability to further examine the child.

Labs and Tests

There are no multitest panels appropriate for the evaluation of children with joint pain and swelling. Specific laboratory evaluations should be guided by the history and physical examination. For most children, a complete blood count with differential, CRP, and erythrocyte sedimentation rate (ESR) are indicated. This will help to identify hematologic abnormalities suggesting malignancy, and to document the presence or absence of systemic inflammation. The CRP is an acute-phase protein synthesized in the liver in response to proinflammatory cytokines. The ESR is an indirect measure of systemic inflammation and the acute-phase response. In most children, the ESR is below 15 mm/h. The ESR rises in response to the relative decline in concentration of serum albumin and increase in acute-phase proteins, including fibrinogen and others. The ESR may be elevated due to marked anemia, or by a low serum concentration of albumin due to decreased production or loss, as in nephrotic syndrome. Most children with arthritis will have an ESR less than 100 mm/h, whereas systemic arthritis, malignan-

cies, and infections are more likely with an ESR greater than 100 mm/h. However, many children with oligoarticular and some with polyarticular arthritis will have a normal ESR and CRP. The addition of a CRP can be helpful in situations in which infection is highly suspected, because the short half-life of this acute-phase protein results in a rapid decline in concentration with effective antibiotic treatment, whereas the ESR may even continue to rise.

The antinuclear antibody (ANA) titer is a measure of serum antibodies that can bind to one of many potential antigens present in the nucleus of normal human cells. ANA titers are usually considered to be elevated when they can be identified at a dilution of 1:40, or with an absolute value of 7.5 IU/mL. The presence of an elevated ANA should never be used to diagnose arthritis. However, the ANA does have some utility as a screening test for JIA (13,14). The frequency of ANA positivity is greatest in younger girls with oligoarticular disease, and represents an increased risk for anterior uveitis (15). When arthritis is suspected by history and physical exam, the presence of a positive ANA should prompt immediate referral to an ophthalmologist for a slit-lamp exam to evaluate for the presence of uveitis. Even in the absence of an ANA, children with confirmed arthritis should have a routine ophthalmologic exam with slit lamp. However, it is known that elevated ANA titers may be present in up to 20% of normal children (typically, at titers of 1:40 to 1:80), and may be induced by recent illness, or be present in first- or second-degree relatives of patients with systemic lupus erythematosus (SLE) (16,17). Children who have an ANA elevated to any level, with no evidence of systemic inflammation, and no arthritis on examination by a pediatric rheumatologist, are extremely unlikely to subsequently develop a significant autoimmune disease (16,18).

The rheumatoid factor (RF) is an autoreactive antibody, usually IgM, recognizing IgG that has bound to antigen. RF positivity is infrequent in children with arthritis, and rarely occurs in children younger than 7 years of age. When present in children with arthritis, the RF signifies a chronic inflammatory state, and has been associated with a higher frequency of erosive synovitis and poor prognosis (19,20). Studies in children and adults demonstrated that a positive RF is as likely to be present in children with diseases other than JIA as it is in those with JIA (21,22). Thus, there is no role for RF testing in the orthopaedic or pediatric office evaluation of children with possible arthritis.

The presence of HLA-B27 is highly associated with transient reactive arthritis, inflammatory bowel disease, and enthesitis-related arthritis. The high familial occurrence of ankylosing spondylitis is directly related to the presence of HLA-B27 (23). Although HLA-B27 is found in nearly 8% of the white population, it can be useful in the diagnosis of enthesitis-related arthritis. It is especially important in boys after the age of 8, when there is a family history of HLA-B27–associated illness, or sacroiliac joint or spinal inflammatory pain.

On rare occasions and in specific circumstances, children may develop gout (24). However, there is no utility in obtaining uric acid levels as a screening test for arthritis. The diagnosis of gout is made by documentation of the presence of urate crystals in synovial fluid, irrespective of serum uric acid levels.

Synovial Fluid Analysis

Arthrocentesis with synovial fluid analysis and culture should be performed in all children with an acute febrile monoarthritis. Infection should also be considered when a child with polyarticular arthritis has an acutely swollen and tender joint, usually accompanied by fever, because this may represent a secondary septic arthritis. The diagnosis and treatment of septic arthritis are discussed in detail in Chapter 13.

Synovial fluid analysis in children with JRA usually shows an inflammatory fluid. However, the total white blood cell count can range from 150 to greater than 100,000 cells/mm^3 (25–27), with average counts of between 10,000 and 12,000 cells/mm^3. There is often a neutrophil predominance, with a range of 18 to 88% and average of 56% (25). Synovial biopsy is obtained if the tuberculin test is positive, or if the diagnosis of sarcoidosis is being considered.

Radiographic Studies

Initial evaluation of children with joint pain and/or swelling by plain radiographs is useful, predominantly to identify periarticular osteopenia, fractures, or other bony lesions. In early JIA, there are no pathognomonic radiographic findings. The diagnosis of JIA is typically made long before bony changes are apparent. Ultrasound is often a rapid and noninvasive way to identify an intraarticular effusion. Radionucleotide imaging with ^{99m}Tc to evaluate for osteomyelitis will occasionally identify other joints with subclinical inflammation, suggesting a diagnosis of JIA. Although rarely required for diagnosis, magnetic resonance imaging

is the most sensitive technique for detecting early articular changes in JIA (28–30).

DIFFERENTIAL DIAGNOSIS OF JOINT PAIN AND SWELLING IN CHILDREN

A comprehensive differential diagnosis of arthritis in childhood is beyond the scope of this chapter. There are over 100 disorders in which arthritis may be a significant manifestation (31). The most common classes of disorders that must be considered in the differential diagnosis of JIA include mechanical or orthopaedic conditions, infection, trauma, psychogenic, and inflammatory. Often, the differential diagnostic considerations will be determined by whether the presentation is acute, subacute, or chronic, whether the child has monoarticular or polyarticular arthritis, and by the presence of systemic signs such as fever (Table 12-3).

Arthritis and Limb Pain Associated with Other Conditions

Children with an acute inflammatory oligo- or polyarthritis will often present with a sudden swollen and/or painful joint. This is in contrast to most children with JIA who, with the exception of systemic onset, often have a subacute or insidious onset. Children with injuries can often describe the exact time and place where the injury occurred, whereas children with benign pains will frequently have a history of pain from the time they could walk. Conversely, children with psychogenic pain frequently can also describe an event, minor or major injury, or illness as the initiator of their pain. However, many children fail to fit the expected profiles, and atypical presentations often occur. It is important to evaluate children with limb and joint pain with a broad differential diagnosis, which can be better defined with a thorough history and comprehensive physical exam. The presence or absence of fever, the age and sex of the child, and associated signs and symptoms will aid the con-

TABLE 12-3. CLASSES OF DISORDERS IN THE DIFFERENTIAL DIAGNOSIS OF JIA

Monoarticular	Polyarticular	Febrile Syndromes
Oligoarthritis	Polyarthritis	Systemic arthritis
Psoriatic arthritis	Psoriatic arthritis	Malignancy
Enthesitis-related arthritis	Enthesitis-related arthritis	Lymphoid
Sarcoidosis	Sarcoidosis	Neuroblastoma
Transient synovitis of the hip	Systemic lupus erythematosus	Systemic lupus erythematosus
Trauma	Juvenile dermatomyositis	Juvenile dermatomyositis
Hemophilia	Systemic vasculitis	Systemic vasculitis
Pigmented villonodular synovitis	Scleroderma	Infection: viral or bacterial
Septic arthritis	Gonococcal septic arthritis	Inflammatory bowel disease
Reactive arthritis	Reactive arthritis	Reactive arthritis

sultant in determining the optimal strategy for the selection of diagnostic testing.

Infectious Arthritis

Septic arthritis generally affects a single joint and is associated with fever, elevated neutrophil count, ESR, and CRP. This is in contrast to monoarticular JIA, which seldom has significant systemic inflammatory signs. Gonococcal arthritis in sexually active children, however, can present with an oligoarticular, polyarticular, or migratory pattern, with significant tenosynovitis. There are instances in which organisms such as *Staphylococcus aureus* can present with a subacute arthritis. However, this presentation is most common for mycobacterial infections or Lyme disease. In most cases, septic joints are extremely painful, but in JIA, swelling is often out of proportion to reported pain.

Lyme Disease

In early Lyme disease, the signs and symptoms of infection include fever and migratory arthralgia, with little or no joint swelling. Early localized disease is typically manifest by the presence of erythema migrans, the classic expanding rash that occurs most often at the site of the tick bite and develops within 7 days to 1 month after infection (32). Lyme arthritis occurs months to years after the initial infection. Many patients with untreated Lyme disease will complain of migratory arthralgias or arthritis (33). In a recent retrospective study of 90 children with Lyme arthritis, Gerber et al. (34) noted that the majority (63%) had monoarticular disease, but no children had greater than four joints involved. The knee was affected most often (90%), followed by hip (14%), ankle (10%), wrist (9%), and elbow (7%), whereas small joints were rarely involved. The majority of children with Lyme arthritis do not recall a tick bite or erythema migrans (34,35). This is in contrast to prospective studies in which 90% of children diagnosed with Lyme disease had a history of erythema migrans. The most likely reason for this discrepancy is that the majority of children with erythema migrans are identified and treated with antibiotics, and do not develop late complications of Lyme disease. Lyme arthritis is typically a low-grade inflammatory synovitis with a large and relatively painless joint effusion. The ESR can be normal or elevated, and 25% can have values greater than 60 mm/h (34). In both children and adults, a chronic form of Lyme arthritis can persist after treatment, and is associated with *HLA-DR4* and *HLA-DR2* alleles (36). The majority of children with Lyme arthritis can be effectively treated with a single, 4-week course of orally administered amoxicillin or doxycycline (34).

Postinfectious Arthritis

Postinfectious or reactive arthritis results in a sterile synovitis that occurs as the result of the immune response to a nonarticular infection. Most children have reactive arthritis following upper respiratory or gastrointestinal infections, rather than genitourinary disease, which is more common in adults (37–39). The classic presentation of reactive arthritis is the triad of conjunctivitis, urethritis, and arthritis found in Reiter's syndrome (RS). The complete triad of RS is very uncommon in childhood. Children account for less than 1% of all patients with complete RS, and the ratio of boys to girls is 4:1 (39,40). A history of sexual activity could suggest infection with *Chlamydia* (41). In patients with classic RS and other postinfectious reactive arthritis, a large majority carry the *HLA-B27* allele (39,42).

Transient Synovitis of the Hip

Transient synovitis of the hip (TSH) is a self-limited, postinfectious, inflammatory arthritis. TSH has a peak incidence, predominantly in boys (70%), between 3 and 10 years of age. It is an idiopathic disorder often preceded by a nonspecific upper respiratory tract infection (43). Trauma has frequently been associated with TSH, and may be a predisposing factor (44). The onset of pain is often gradual, may be focused to the hip, thigh, or knee, and lasts for an average of 6 days. Occasionally, TSH can be bilateral (4%). The child often presents with inability to walk or with a severe limp. There is a loss of internal rotation of the hip, and it is usually held in flexion, abducted, and externally rotated. There is often low-grade fever. The ESR and white blood cell count are normal to mildly elevated (45). Plain radiographs are often normal, or may show mild widening of the joint space. Ultrasound is a sensitive and reliable method to confirm the presence of an effusion (45). With rest and nonsteroidal antiinflammatory drugs (NSAIDs), the majority of children will have complete resolution of symptoms within 2 weeks. The majority of children with TSH will have a single event, with 4 to 17% having a recurrence usually within the first 6 months after the initial onset (44).

Acute Rheumatic Fever

Acute rheumatic fever (ARF) occurs as a postinfectious reaction to infection of the oropharynx with group A beta-hemolytic streptococcus. The incidence of ARF has remained relatively constant at around 1 per 100,000 children between the ages of 5 and 17 years (46). It is very unusual for ARF to occur before the age of 4 years. Although ARF is rare in developed countries, it remains the most common cause of acquired heart disease in the developing world. In South Africa, the prevalence of ARF has been estimated to be 690 per 100,000 (47).

Clinical Features of ARF

Arthritis. The classic arthritis of ARF is a migratory polyarthritis, usually affecting the legs first, and later the arms.

Joint involvement is the most common (75%) and often the first manifestation of the disease (48). The affected joints are often red and swollen, with pain out of proportion to the physical examination. The arthritis of ARF is exquisitely responsive to aspirin, and dramatic relief is often obtained within several hours after the first dose. Residual synovitis does not commonly develop.

Carditis. Rheumatic carditis occurs in nearly 65% of children with ARF (48), and is the only cause of significant morbidity and mortality. The use of Doppler echocardiography has increased the sensitivity of detection of valvar involvement in ARF, and abnormalities have been found in as many as 90% of patients with ARF (46). Arthralgia cannot be used as a minor criteria if arthritis is present. A prolonged PR interval is often seen in ARF, but is not associated with increased risk for carditis.

Subcutaneous Nodules. The subcutaneous nodules of ARF are typically small (<1 cm in diameter) and painless. They typically are present for 1 to 2 weeks. The overlying skin is not inflamed nor attached to the nodule. The most typical locations are over bony prominences. Nodules occur in less than 10% of patients, but are often associated with carditis.

Erythema Marginatum. Erythema marginatum is an irregular, nonpruritic skin rash, pink-to-red in color, usually affecting the trunk and occasionally the proximal limbs, but never the face. The rash occurs early in the disease, and when present may persist after all other manifestations of disease have resolved. It occurs in less than 10% of children with ARF, but is also associated with carditis.

Chorea. Sydenham's chorea is a neurologic disorder with choreiform movements and emotional lability. The movement disorder can often be unilateral. It cannot be suppressed voluntarily, but is not present during sleep. Chorea occurs in nearly 15% of children with ARF. The interval between the streptococcal pharyngitis and the onset of chorea can be as long as 3 months. When chorea is the only major manifestation there may be no markers of inflammation, and streptococcal pharyngitis can be difficult to identify.

The diagnosis of ARF is based on the application of the modified Jones criteria (49) (Table 12-4). The diagnosis requires the presence of two major criteria, or one major criterion and two minor criteria, and requires supportive evidence of a preceding streptococcal infection (increased ASO/anti-DNase B, positive rapid streptococcal antigen test or throat culture). It is clear that not all children who meet the Jones criteria will have ARF, and conversely, a small number of children with ARF will not meet these criteria.

Treatment. Treatment of ARF is usually with aspirin, 80 to 100 mg/kg/d in children (8 gm/day maximum), and

TABLE 12-4. THE MODIFIED JONES CRITERIA FOR DIAGNOSIS OF ACUTE RHEUMATIC FEVER

Major Manifestations	Minor Manifestations
Carditis	Fever
Polyarthritis	Arthralgia
Subcutaneous nodules	Prolonged PR interval
Erythema marginatum	Increased ESR or CRP
Chorea	

Diagnosis requires the presence of two major criteria, or one major and two minor criteria, with supporting evidence of a preceding streptococcal infection (rising streptococcal antibody titers, positive throat culture or rapid streptococcal test).

ESR, erythrocyte sedimentation rate; *CRP*, C-reactive protein.

serum salicylate concentrations of 20 to 30 mg/dL. In the presence of carditis, congestive heart failure, or heart block, corticosteroid therapy is added. The typical treatment doses are 2 mg/kg/day of prednisone for 2 to 3 weeks, then tapered over an additional 3 weeks. The aspirin is typically discontinued 3 weeks after stopping the corticosteroids. Eradication of streptococci by treatment with penicillin is indicated in all patients with ARF, even in the absence of a positive throat culture. Children with a history of ARF should receive prophylactic antibiotics: intramuscular benzathine penicillin every 3 to 4 weeks, oral penicillin V twice daily, or sulfadiazine once per day. Patients with documented rheumatic heart disease should continue prophylaxis indefinitely.

Poststreptococcal Arthritis

Recently, the entity of poststreptococcal-reactive arthritis (PSRA) has been characterized, and many investigators feel that it is a variant of ARF (50–52). PSRA typically presents as a nonmigratory oligo- or polyarthritis. It is differentiated from ARF by the frequent presence of tenosynovitis and the poor response to aspirin or other nonsteroidal drugs. In addition to arthritis, other clinical manifestations include erythema nodosum, livedo reticularis, cutaneous vasculitis, and systemic polyarteritis nodosa (53,54). Limited studies have suggested that there is increased risk for ARF and rheumatic carditis with further episodes of streptococcal pharyngitis, and that streptococcal prophylaxis is indicated (50,52). Children with PSRA were found to have a statistically significant increased frequency of HLA-DRB1*01, while those with ARF had an increased frequency of HLA-DRB1*16, and the frequency of HLA-B27 was not different than controls (55). The association of PSRA with HLA-DRB1*01, but not with HLA-B27, suggests that its pathogenesis may be more similar to that of ARF than to reactive arthritis. This would again support the recommendation for prophylaxis.

Serum Sickness

Serum sickness is a clinical syndrome resulting from an adverse immunologic response to foreign antigens mediated by the deposition of immune complexes. Although serum sickness was first described after injection of heterologous serum, today the most common causes are antibiotics (penicillins and sulfonamides) and viral infections (56–58). Serum sickness is characterized by fever, arthralgia or arthritis, lymphadenopathy, cutaneous eruptions (urticarial or morbilliform), and angioedema. Both serum sickness and allergic angioedema can be confused with acute-onset juvenile arthritis. However, the majority of children with serum sickness will spontaneously improve within a few days to weeks. For mild disease, removal of the offending antigen, and treatment with antihistamines and nonsteroidal antiinflammatory medications, is sufficient. In severe cases, a several-week course of corticosteroids may be required.

Other Inflammatory Arthropathies

Gout

Gouty arthritis is characterized by hyperuricemia and deposition of monosodium urate crystals into the joint. The major clinical manifestations include acute mono- or oligoarthritis, frequently involving the first metatarsophalangeal joint, resulting in podagra. Gout may result from either increased production or decreased excretion of uric acid. Gout is extremely rare in children (24). The diagnosis of gout can only be confirmed by demonstration of negatively birefringent, monosodium urate crystals in the synovial fluid when viewed under a polarized light microscope. Acute gout is treated with nonsteroidal antiinflammatory medications, colchicine, and occasionally prednisone. After the acute event has subsided, allopurinol is utilized to prevent recurrences by decreasing serum levels of uric acid. The use of allopurinol in acute gout is not recommended due to a paradoxical worsening of gout with a sudden decrease in uric acid levels.

Cystic Fibrosis-associated Arthritis

Children and young adults with cystic fibrosis (CF) have an increased incidence of musculoskeletal disorders. CF-associated arthritis is a transient reactive arthritis often associated with pulmonary exacerbations (59–63). Teenagers and older patients with CF have a higher-than-expected occurrence of RF-positive polyarticular JIA or adult rheumatoid arthritis (64). Finally, some children with CF develop secondary hypertrophic osteoarthropathy, demonstrable on radiographs (65,66).

Systemic Autoimmune Diseases

Many of the systemic autoimmune diseases can cause an acute or chronic arthritis. There are often signs, symptoms, or laboratory abnormalities that will aid in the diagnosis of these conditions. For a thorough discussion of these diseases in children, several excellent texts and reviews are available (31,67,68).

Systemic lupus erythematosus (SLE) is an episodic, autoimmune inflammatory disease characterized by multiorgan system inflammation. Arthralgia and arthritis affect 75% of the children with SLE. It is usually polyarticular, and the joint pain is often out of proportion to physical findings. The arthritis typically responds readily to corticosteroids, is rarely erosive (69), and does not typically result in deformity.

Sarcoidosis is uncommon in childhood (70). However, arthritis is frequent in childhood-onset sarcoidosis, and typically presents as an oligoarthritis affecting the knees, ankles, and/or elbows. It is characterized by very large effusions and boggy synovitis with minimal pain or loss of motion. A synovial biopsy will often be diagnostic, showing the presence of noncaseating sarcoid granulomas.

Vasculitis in childhood can be associated with arthritis. However, the disease most likely to be seen by the orthopaedic surgeon is Henoch-Schonlein purpura (HSP). HSP is the most common vasculitic syndrome in childhood, occurring in slightly more than 1 in 10,000 children per year (71). The classic manifestations of HSP are nonthrombocytopenic palpable purpura, arthritis, abdominal pain, gastrointestinal hemorrhage, and glomerulonephritis. In the complete syndrome the diagnosis is often clear. However, the arthritis can precede the appearance of the rash, and the rash may be unrecognized if a comprehensive skin examination is not done. The rash of HSP often begins on the lower extremities as an urticarial eruption, followed by petechiae and purpura, which are most often concentrated on the buttocks and lower extremities, especially the ankles. The purpura will frequently recur in crops over several weeks, resulting in multiple lesions in different stages of evolution. The arthritis of HSP presents as a periarticular swelling and tenderness, most commonly of large joints, with severe pain and limitation of motion. The younger child will often refuse to use the affected joint. The arthritis is usually transient, and resolves without sequelae in a few days to weeks. In most children, HSP will resolve completely within 4 weeks from onset.

Foreign Body Synovitis

Plant thorns and wood splinters may be introduced onto the joint space and cause a chronic synovitis or tendonitis (72). Typically, the injury has been long forgotten, because many months may pass between entry of the thorn into the skin and egress into the joint. Often, a careful history will uncover the past trauma. Surgical removal of the splinter and synovectomy are the only effective treatments.

Coagulopathies and Hemoglobinopathies

Children with congenital coagulopathies (hemophilia) and hemoglobinopathies (sickle cell disease) will present with acute joint pain and swelling, resulting from hemarthrosis and localized ischemia, respectively. A comprehensive discussion of these conditions is found in Chapter 11.

Malignancies

Leukemia in childhood frequently presents with musculoskeletal pain and arthritis (73,74). Although a joint effusion can occur, the pain is usually localized to the metaphyses of the long bones. The pain in children with malignancies is typically more severe than in JIA and will frequently be continuous. Another feature of children with malignancies is the extreme elevation of the ESR (often >100), whereas in JIA, the ESR is usually only moderately elevated, and may be normal. Plain radiographs may show subperiosteal elevation, osteolytic reaction, or metaphyseal rarefaction. In a recent study of 29 children with malignancy who were referred to pediatric rheumatologists, features suggestive of malignancy included nonarticular "bone" pain (68%), back pain as a major presenting feature (32%), bone tenderness (29%), severe constitutional symptoms (32%), and atypical clinical features (48%) (75). Atypical features included night sweats (14%), ecchymoses and bruising (14%), abnormal neurologic signs (13%), and abnormal masses (7%). Children with malignancy were more likely to have the combination of an elevated ESR with a low platelet count (28%).

Benign Tumors

Pigmented villonodular synovitis (PVNS) is a benign tumor of the synovium. Although PVNS is rare in childhood, it does frequently result in recurrent joint swelling (76,77). This usually results in recurrent effusions that are minimally painful, with progressive cartilage destruction and erosion of bone. A frequent finding is chocolate brown synovial fluid on joint aspiration. The diagnosis is often confirmed by synovial biopsy showing nodular hypertrophy, with proliferating fibroblasts and synovial cells and hemosiderin-laden macrophages. Surgical excision can be curative. However, many patients have recurrences, and occasionally multifocal disease can occur.

Benign Pains of Childhood

Growing Pains

Growing pains, or benign pains of childhood are common, and may affect up to 20% of all children at some time (78). The diagnosis of growing pains should be reserved for those children, typically from 2 to 12 years of age, who have benign pain, precipitated by exercise and routine physical activities. These pains usually occur in the afternoon, evening, or middle of the night, but are never present in the morning. They often respond well to massage or analgesics. The physical examination shows no sign of synovitis, and laboratory studies are always normal. Therapy for growing pains includes gentle massage and stretching. Children with recurring or daily pains often have significant benefit from a single bedtime dose of acetaminophen, ibuprofen, or naproxen. Frequently, acetaminophen 1 h before and after exercise can be beneficial.

Exaggerated Benign Pains of Childhood

There are children who have exaggerated but benign pains that are similar to growing pains. These pains are often more frequent, more intense, can be present at any time of the day, and are typically increased by physical activity. These children often have distinct physical exam findings that aid in diagnosis of this syndrome: hypermobile joints, pes planus, and/or leg-length discrepancy.

Hypermobility, either generalized or localized, is a common finding in children with pain (79). The diagnosis of hypermobility requires three of the following: opposition of the thumb to the flexor aspect of the forearm, hyperextension of the fingers parallel to the extensor aspect of the forearm, hyperextension of the elbows or knees by more than 10 degrees, or excessive dorsiflexion of the ankle and eversion of the foot (80). Children with hypermobility will often benefit from weight training, with strengthening about the hypermobile joints.

Ligamentous laxity in the feet can result in pes planus, with pronation and pain in the medial side of the arch. There are often associated mechanical strains resulting in pain in the ankles, knees, hips, and lower back. These children may benefit from the use of orthotic shoe inserts.

A congenital leg-length discrepancy is also frequently associated with benign pains of childhood. These children will often have a leg-length difference of less than 2.5 cm. However, this difference is more significant in proportion in small children. These children are often reported as clumsy from the time they began to walk. They will frequently benefit from the temporary use of sole inserts for the shoe of the shorter leg.

Pain Amplification Syndromes

Pain is an unpleasant sensory and emotional experience associated with real or potential injury, or is perceived in terms of such injury. The sensation of pain is a complex process dependent on multiple factors, including degree of injury, personal experience or knowledge of others' experience, and current emotional, as well as physical health. Psychogenic pain can develop without obvious cause, as a consequence of an acute or chronic illness, or following a severe or even mild injury, but persists or worsens long after any inciting factor has been relieved. This type of pain can be localized or diffuse. It is frequently described as more intense than other types of pain, and is often associated with changes in mood, sleep patterns, and vocational and avocational function. A comprehensive discussion of the psychogenic pain syndromes in childhood is beyond the scope of this chapter, so I refer the reader to a number of excellent reviews (81–86).

Chronic pain syndromes in children are a frequent diagnostic dilemma for pediatricians and pediatric subspecialists. Nearly all of these children present with the belief of the parents, and occasionally the child, that the pain must be due to arthritis. Much of the difficulty in categorization of children with chronic musculoskeletal pain results from the variable nomenclature used by different clinicians and researchers. Malleson et al. (87) have suggested the use of diffuse idiopathic pain syndrome, which includes primary fibromyalgia syndrome, and localized idiopathic pain syndrome, which includes reflex sympathetic dystrophy (RSD).

An alternative proposal (81) is to use the term "pain amplification syndrome" for all chronic idiopathic pain syndromes of childhood, and to subclassify them as: (a) with autonomic dysfunction (complex regional pain syndrome type 1 or 2, reflex neurovascular dystrophy, reflex sympathetic dystrophy, algodystrophy, sympathetically mediated pain syndrome, Sudeck atrophy, localized idiopathic pain syndrome); (b) without autonomic dysfunction—constant (psychogenic, psychosomatic, pseudodystrophy, localized idiopathic pain syndrome, diffuse idiopathic pain syndrome); (c) without autonomic dysfunction—intermittent (psychogenic, psychosomatic, growing pains); (d) with multiple painful points (fibromyalgia, diffuse idiopathic pain syndrome); and (e) hypervigilant (psychogenic, psychosomatic, growing pains). This system has some advantages in allowing classification of chronic pain that does not meet the well-defined criteria for fibromyalgia or RSD (88–90).

Despite the difficulty with nomenclature, the common symptomatology that pervades all these pain syndromes is the presence of noninflammatory pain that is disproportional to physical exam findings, and that most children display *la belle indifference*, an appearance of unconcern regarding the severe pain and disability they are experiencing. The majority of patients are female (80%), with onset typically after 6 years of age, but may be present in children as young as 3 years (83,86,91). Another very important aspect of these pain syndromes is the ability to move from one symptom complex to another, or to have characteristics of multiple psychogenic syndromes simultaneously. A child may present with localized limb pain without autonomic signs, then develop classic RSD, which resolves, only to be followed by diffuse pain with multiple painful points or fibromyalgia.

Reflex Sympathetic Dystrophy

RSD is likely underrecognized in children (84,86,91,92). The onset of RSD is often after minor trauma, or after a fracture that has healed and the cast has been removed. There is an initial pain that causes the child to stop using the affected limb. The disuse perpetuates the pain and the involved extremity becomes painful to even light touch (allodynia), swollen, cold, and discolored. Plain radiographs of the affected limb can show soft tissue swelling, and, after 6 to 8 weeks, a generalized osteoporosis. Technetium 99m bone scans can show either a diffuse increase or decrease in uptake of isotope (Fig. 12-2). Outcome for children with RSD is thought to be generally good when intensive physical and psychologic therapy is instituted within the first year (83,84,91). However, others have shown that more than 50% of children with RSD who presented after 1 year had elapsed between onset of symptoms and diagnosis continued to have pain and prolonged dysfunction (91). The most effective treatment for RSD is vigorous physical therapy and careful attention to the underlying psychosocial stressors (83,84,86). The affected limb should never be immobilized, because this will uniformly cause a worsening of the pain during or after the period of immobilization.

Childhood-onset Fibromyalgia

Fibromyalgia syndrome (FMS) is a common noninflammatory disorder characterized by chronic diffuse pain, and localized tender points with a decreased pain threshold. FMS accounted for 2.1% of new patient diagnoses by pediatric rheumatologists in a U.S. pediatric rheumatology disease registry (93). Childhood-onset FMS is similar to the adult disorder, which is characterized by diffuse pain, tender/trigger points, irritable bowel syndrome, headaches, fatigue, and nonrestorative sleep (89). Yunus and Masi (88) defined criteria for pediatric FMS, including diffuse pain and five or more tender points. They found prominent symptoms were nonrestorative sleep (100%), fatigue (91%), stiffness (79%), subjective swelling (61%), headaches (54%), paresthesias (36%), and irritable bowel syndrome (27%). It is the morning stiffness and generalized pains that may prompt the referral of a child with FMS to an orthopaedic surgeon. Therapy for FMS consists of physical therapy with stretching and aerobic exercise (including aqua therapy), stress reduction, and psychologic counseling.

JUVENILE IDIOPATHIC ARTHRITIS

Juvenile arthritis is one of the most frequent chronic illnesses of children. The majority of children with JIA have syndromes that are unique to childhood. Even in those types of JIA that have an adult equivalent, such as ankylosing spondylitis and psoriatic arthritis, children often have a dif-

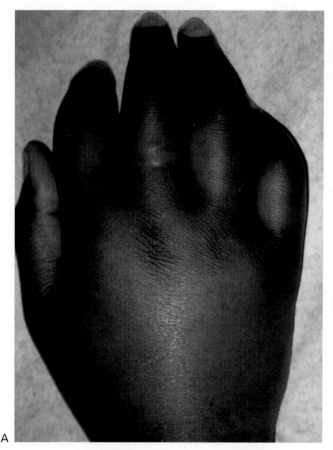

A

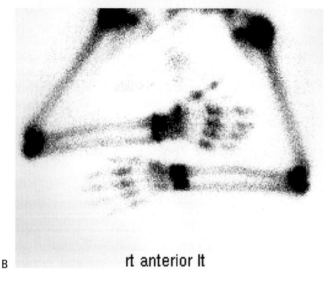

B   rt anterior lt

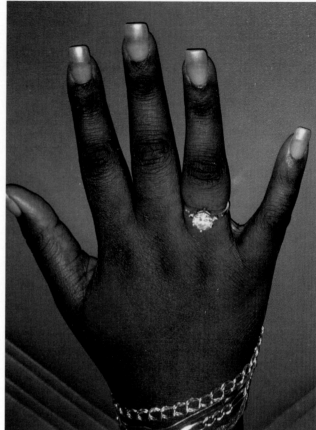

C

FIGURE 12-2. Reflex sympathetic dystrophy in a child with a 1-month history of hand-swelling and pain. **A:** Right hand after 1 month of illness. **B:** Technetium 99m bone scan showing diffuse increase in uptake of isotope in the affected hand. In some patients, isotope uptake is diffusely decreased. **C:** Right hand after three weeks of physical therapy and psychotherapy.

ferent pattern of onset and course than adults. Children with arthritis are also uniquely affected by articular inflammation which, due to their skeletal immaturity, can result in growth disturbances. As a result of localized inflammation, there can be acceleration of ossification centers, accelerated growth, or premature closure of epiphyses, resulting in diminished length.

Epidemiology

Juvenile arthritis is the most common rheumatic disease of childhood. The worldwide incidence ranges from 7 to 20 cases per 100,000 children at risk per year (1,5,94,95). Recent studies have suggested that the incidence of JRA may be decreasing (5). Alternatively, the improved recognition of Lyme disease, and the exclusion of psoriatic arthritis and juvenile spondyloarthropathies, may be a contributing factor.

The overall prevalence of JRA in the United States has been estimated to be between 57 and 113 per 100,000 children younger than 16 years old (96). The prevalence of childhood-onset psoriatic arthritis and enthesitis-related arthritis (spondyloarthropathies) is less well characterized. The prevalence of juvenile ankylosing spondylitis is reported to be 2 to 10 per 100,000, whereas juvenile psoriatic arthritis has a prevalence of 2 to 12 per 100,000 (97). The incidence of juvenile spondyloarthropathies in whites of Northern European ancestry is slightly greater than 1 per 100,000 (94,98). However, spondyloarthropathy is the most common form of juvenile arthritis in some Mexican and North American Indian children (99,100).

Etiology

The etiology of JIA is unknown. Chronic arthritis is a complex disorder requiring inappropriate immunologic activation, with failure of self-tolerance, in the setting of multiple host genetic and environmental factors. JIA is a heterogeneous disorder with multiple ages and patterns of onset, and with a highly variable course. It is likely that multiple initiating factors are involved, including infection, trauma, and autoimmunity, all in conjunction with genetic predilection for arthritis.

Genetics

There are many reported associations between HLA types and juvenile arthritis. Other than HLA-B27, the majority of the associations of JIA have been with the HLA class II antigens, which are restricted to cells of lymphoid origin (102). In oligoarticular arthritis, there is an increased association with HLA-DR8, HLA-DR6, and HLA-DR5, with relative risks of 2 to 27. This means that a child who carries one or more of these genes has a 2- to 27-fold increased risk of developing the disease, compared to the population as a whole. The presence of uveitis is correlated with HLA-DR5, whereas protection from uveitis is correlated with HLA-DR1 (102). Chronic uveitis has also been associated with HLA-DRB1 and HLA-DQA1 (103). Polyarticular onset with positive rheumatoid factor is associated with HLA-DR4, which parallels the association with adult rheumatoid arthritis, whereas HLA-DR7 seems protective. Rheumatoid factor negative polyarticular disease is associated with HLA-DR8, HLA-DPw3, and HLA-DQw4, with relative risk factors of 3 to 10. Systemic-onset disease has overlapping risk factors, showing an association with HLA-DR4, HLA-DR5, and HLA-DR8, with relative risks ranging from around 2 to 7 (101).

Juvenile ankylosing spondylitis (JAS) and related diseases show a striking familial occurrence. The only immunogenic factor in common in this class of diseases has been shown to be HLA-B27. Data from multiple immunogenetic studies have shown that 90% of patients with JAS express the HLA-B27 antigen (104,105). These data are supported by an animal model in which spontaneous inflammatory disease of the gastrointestinal tract, peripheral and vertebral joints, male genital tract, skin, nails, and heart were seen in transgenic rats expressing a functional human HLA-B27 allele (106).

Imbalances in levels of proinflammatory and antiinflammatory cytokines may be associated with chronic inflammation. A polymorphism in the *IL-1α* gene was found to be associated with uveitis and pauciarticular arthritis in Norwegians (107). Children who have an *IL-6* genotype, which has a relatively higher transcription rate when stimulated, may be at greater risk for systemic arthritis (108).

Infection as Trigger

Infection has been implicated in both the onset and exacerbation of chronic arthritis in children (109). Of all types of JIA, systemic onset has clinical features most consistent with an infectious process: acute onset, high fever, rash, lymphadenopathy, and arthritis. However, there has to date been no convincing laboratory evidence of infection in this relatively homogeneous disease. Multiple viral and bacterial agents have been associated with JIA (110). However, no single or even large group of agents has been convincingly implicated in any form of JIA. It is more probable that multiple conserved viral and bacterial antigens, with epitopes that crossreact with human antigens, may promote an inappropriate autoimmune response. This association is strongest for the HLA-B27–associated diseases (111) in which arthritogenic peptides from enteric pathogens have generated specific B27-restricted CD8$^+$ T lymphocytes that were isolated from arthritic joints (112).

CLINICAL SYNDROMES OF JIA

Clinical Onset Types

The relative prevalence of each of the subtypes of juvenile arthritis vary widely, depending on whether the EULAR or ACR are utilized. The onset diagnosis of children with JRA, over many years, has been relatively consistent, with approximately 50% of children having oligoarticular disease, 30 to 40% with polyarticular disease, and 10 to 20% systemic onset. Only recently has psoriatic arthritis been separated from the spondyloarthropathies and differentiated from JRA. The subtypes of JCA show similar figures for oligoarticular (50%) and systemic onset (11%). However, the prevalence of polyarticular disease is only 20% and the remaining is divided among undifferentiated spondyloarthropathy, JAS, juvenile psoriatic arthritis, and inflammatory bowel disease-associated arthritis (94) (Table 12-5). The most current summary of the prevalence of individual subtypes uti-

TABLE 12-5. FREQUENCY OF JUVENILE ARTHRITIS SUBTYPES

Subtypes	Symmons et al. (94) (%)	Subtypes	Bowyer and Roettcher (93) (%)
Systemic JCA	11	Systemic JRA	11
Polyarticular JCA		Polyarticular JRA	
RF-positive	3	RF-positive	1
RF-negative	17	RF-negative	24
Oligoarticular JCA	50	Oligoarticular JRA	38
Spondyloarthropathy[a]	11	Spondyloarthropathy[a]	24
Psoriatic arthritis	7	Psoriatic arthritis	3

[a] All spondyloarthropathies, including juvenile ankylosing spondylitis and inflammatory bowel disease-associated arthritis.

lizing the ACR criteria is from the Pediatric Rheumatology Data Base (93) (Table 12-5). Of 2,828 children with arthritis, 11% had systemic onset, 24% polyarticular (RF–), 1% polyarticular (RF+), 38% pauciarticular, 24% spondyloarthritis (11% JAS), and 3% psoriatic arthritis. Each subtype of juvenile arthritis has individual characteristics, and each type can have widely different courses and outcomes, which further emphasizes the heterogeneity of JIA.

Systemic Arthritis

Systemic onset juvenile arthritis (113) was first completely described by Still in 1897, and systemic arthritis has often been called "Still's disease." His classic article was reprinted in 1978 (114). Systemic arthritis is characterized by the presence of daily or twice-daily spiking fevers, usually to 39°C or higher (115). Children with systemic arthritis are frequently quite ill-appearing while febrile. The fever often responds poorly to NSAIDs, but will typically respond well to corticosteroids. In most children, the fever is accompanied by a characteristic rash (116) (Fig. 12-3). The rash consists of discrete, erythematous macules, which are blanching, transient, and frequently nonpruritic. The rash is often more pronounced on the trunk, but is often present on the extremities, and may occur on the face. Many children with systemic arthritis will have extraarticular manifestations, including hepatosplenomegaly, pericarditis, pleuritis, lymphadenopathy, and abdominal pain. The extraarticular features may be present for weeks, months, and occasionally, years prior to the onset of arthritis. Usually, the extraarticular manifestations of systemic arthritis are self-limited, and will resolve spontaneously or with corticosteroid therapy. Occasionally, the pericarditis can result in tamponade. Systemic arthritis can occur at any age, but is slightly more common before 6 years of age (94), and can occur rarely in adulthood, when it is referred to as "adult-onset Still's disease." There is an equal ratio of males to females, which may support the premise that there is an infectious trigger for systemic arthritis (117).

The laboratory features of systemic arthritis are notable for elevated acute-phase reactants. The ESR and CRP are greatly elevated. The disease is often accompanied by anemia of chronic disease (118–120), a leukocytosis, and a marked thrombocytosis, which may exceed 1 million/mm³. Clinical experience has shown that, when the platelet count remains greater than 500,000/mm³ after 5 years, remission is unlikely. Elevation of serum ferritin has been correlated with active inflammation in some children with systemic arthritis (121). Patients with systemic arthritis can have coagulation abnormalities with generation of fibrin split products, which have also been correlated with active disease (122). Children with systemic arthritis are rarely ANA- or RF-positive.

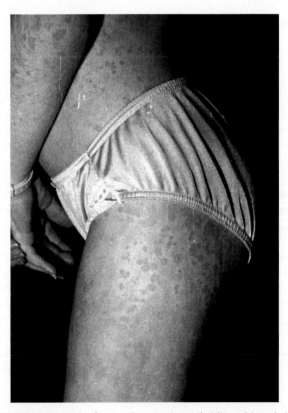

FIGURE 12-3. Rash of systemic-onset juvenile idiopathic arthritis.

The differential diagnosis of systemic arthritis is essentially the same as for fever of unknown origin. Systemic arthritis often presents the greatest challenge to the clinician during the phase prior to the onset of arthritis. The diagnostic possibilities that must be considered include infections, malignancy, inflammatory bowel disease, systemic lupus erythematosus, and vasculitides (polyarteritis nodosa, Kawasaki disease).

Clinical Course

One striking feature of systemic arthritis is arrest of linear growth during periods of active disease (123,124) (Fig. 12-4). The use of glucocorticoids also may result in growth retardation, as well as Cushing syndrome, in this same group of patients. When children with systemic arthritis have active inflammatory disease the use of human growth hormone fails to significantly increase linear growth (125,126). The prognosis of systemic arthritis is determined predominantly by the course of arthritis. Nearly 50% of children with systemic arthritis will have an oligoarticular course that is typically mild, and in the majority of these children, the arthritis will ultimately remit. The remaining half of the children with systemic onset will develop a polyarticular arthritis that can remit, but progresses in approximately 50% of cases (25% of all systemic-onset JIA) to a severe, unrelenting, and destructive course despite all current therapeutic interventions (127). Chronic anterior uveitis is extremely rare in systemic arthritis. Systemic amyloidosis, usually presenting with the onset of proteinuria and hypertension, can occur as a result of any chronic inflammatory disease. Nearly 8% of children with systemic arthritis, and to a lesser degree, the other subtypes of JIA, have been shown to develop this life-threatening complication (128). The incidence of amyloidosis in North America is significantly lower than that seen in Europe. The reason for this discrepancy remains unclear.

Macrophage activation syndrome (MAS) is a severe, potentially life-threatening complication seen nearly exclusively in systemic arthritis. It is characterized by macrophage activation with hemophagocytosis, and is associated with hepatic dysfunction, disseminated intravascular coagulation with a precipitous fall in the ESR secondary to hypofibrinogenemia, and encephalopathy (129). It has been suggested

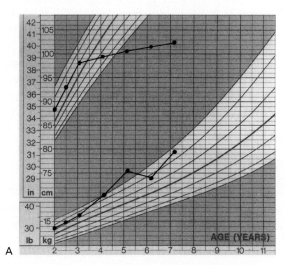

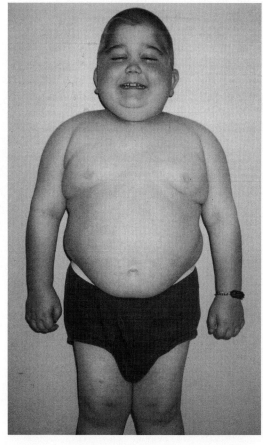

FIGURE 12-4. Child with systemic-onset juvenile idiopathic arthritis. **A:** Growth arrest due to systemic inflammation and chronic steroid use. **B:** The same child at age 7 with chronic polyarthritis, growth arrest, and Cushing syndrome.

that antiinflammatory medications and viral infections can induce this syndrome. High-dose corticosteroids and cyclosporine A have been shown to improve the outcome of MAS (130,131).

Oligoarthritis

Oligoarthritis is the most common subtype of JIA, and is characterized by arthritis in four or fewer joints during the first 6 months of disease. These children rarely have complaints of pain, do not have associated fever, and are not systemically ill. The knee is the most common joint affected, followed by ankles and elbows. The hips are only rarely affected. Small joints of the hands and feet are seldom affected in oligoarthritis. Asymmetric oligoarticular involvement of small joints, with or without large-joint arthritis, is most characteristic of psoriatic arthritis. The majority of children with oligoarthritis present before 6 years of age, and girls predominate (4 to 1). Although oligoarthritis can present in older children, the late-onset type, in which there is a male predominance and high incidence of HLA-B27, now should be classified as enthesitis-related arthritis.

Most children with oligoarthritis will have a mild elevation of the ESR (rarely above 80 mm/h), but it can be normal. The CRP is usually normal or mildly elevated. Antinuclear antibodies are found in 40 to 80% of children with oligoarthritis, and are associated with increased risk for anterior uveitis. An RF is generally absent in oligoarthritis. However, when an RF is present in children with chronic oligoarthritis, it has been associated with an aggressive and erosive disease (132).

The differential diagnosis of a child with a monoarticular arthritis depends on the duration of the joint involvement. In children with acute onset of joint pain and swelling, infections (septic arthritis or osteomyelitis), trauma, hematologic causes of hemarthrosis, and malignancy must be considered. These patients should have a thorough evaluation, including an arthrocentesis. If the arthritis is longstanding, these causes are less likely. However, both Lyme disease and mycobacterial infections can produce a prolonged monoarthritis indistinguishable from JIA.

Clinical Course

The majority of children with oligoarthritis have a mild and remitting course. However, in untreated children with longstanding unilateral knee arthritis, there can be overgrowth of the affected limb, resulting in a marked leg-length discrepancy (133,134). There is a subgroup of children with oligoarthritis that is indistinguishable within the first 6 months of disease, but progresses to polyarthritis (extended oligoarticular), which is usually most consistent with RF-negative polyarticular JIA.

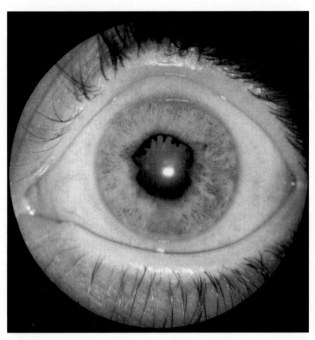

FIGURE 12-5. Iritis in oligoarticular juvenile idiopathic arthritis. Posterior synechiae are finger-like adhesions between the iris and lens, and result in an irregular pupil.

Chronic uveitis (Fig. 12-5) is the most serious complication seen in oligoarthritis, and occurs in 13 to 34% of all patients with juvenile arthritis. Nearly 80% of all cases of anterior uveitis in childhood are associated with JIA (135). Initially, the eyes of most patients with JIA-associated uveitis appear normal, and are asymptomatic. Of those children who will ultimately develop uveitis, it is already present in 6% of patients at onset of arthritis, but develops in a majority of children within 4 to 7 years after diagnosis. Although the overall incidence and severity of uveitis seems to be decreasing (136,137), even a low-grade chronic uveitis can result in a poor visual outcome (138). Current guidelines for ophthalmologic examination in children with juvenile arthritis recommend routine screening examinations, including slit-lamp evaluation, based on age and type of onset (139) (Table 12-6).

Polyarthritis

Polyarticular-onset JIA is characterized by the insidious, but occasionally acute, onset of a generally symmetric arthritis in five or more joints. It can involve both large and small joints, and frequently affects the cervical spine and temporomandibular joints. Typically, girls outnumber boys 3 to 1. Mild systemic features can be present in children with polyarthritis. They may have low-grade fevers, lymphadenopathy, and hepatosplenomegaly. The fevers are not typically the high quotidian temperature spikes that are diagnostic of systemic arthritis, and rash is rarely seen (7). There

TABLE 12-6. GUIDELINES FOR INITIAL FREQUENCY OF SCREENING EYE EXAMS IN JIA

Juvenile Arthritis Onset Type	Minimum Screening Frequency	
	Age at Onset	
	<7 years	≥7 years
Oligoarthritis		
ANA-positive	3 to 4 months	6 months
ANA-negative	6 months	6 months
Polyarthritis		
ANA-positive	3 to 4 months	6 months
ANA-negative	6 months	6 months
Systemic arthritis	1 year	1 year
Psoriatic arthritis		
ANA-positive	3 to 4 months	6 months
ANA-negative	6 months	6 months
Enthesitis-related arthritis	1 year	1 year

All patients with an irregular iris, or an acute red, painful, or photophobic eye, should be examined immediately.

ANA, antinuclear antibodies.

are at least two distinct subgroups of polyarthritis: those with and without the presence of RF.

RF-negative polyarthritis can occur at any age, with the median age of onset at 6.5 years (94). This subgroup can be ANA-positive (40 to 50%), and this is associated with an increased incidence of uveitis (5%) (135).

The second subgroup of polyarthritis includes those with a positive RF. This subtype occurs predominantly in older girls (>8 years) who are HLA-DR4–positive, and is indistinguishable from adult rheumatoid arthritis. These children are more likely to have a symmetric small-joint arthritis, rheumatoid nodules, and early erosive synovitis with a chronic course. However, these children rarely develop chronic uveitis.

Most patients with active polyarthritis will have an elevated ESR, typically 20 to 80 mm/h. The ESR is often a useful measure of disease activity in children with polyarthritis (14,140). Children with significant joint disease will often develop anemia of chronic disease, with hemoglobin in the range of 7 to 10 g/dL, although this is more marked in systemic arthritis (118,119).

The differential diagnosis of polyarthritis is quite different from that of monoarticular disease. Polyarticular septic arthritis is unusual, although an asymmetric polyarthritis and tenosynovitis can be caused by *Neisseria gonorrheae*. Systemic lupus should be considered, especially in adolescent and preadolescent girls. Reactive arthritis, inflammatory bowel-related arthritis, juvenile psoriatic arthritis, and enthesitis-related arthritis, including juvenile ankylosing spondylitis, should be considered. Although juvenile dermatomyositis and scleroderma may present with polyarthritis, the associated signs and symptoms of these disorders usually lead to a correct diagnosis.

Clinical Course

Children with polyarthritis that is rheumatoid-factor–positive are at risk for a prolonged and destructive course. These children are typically older girls with multiple joints involved (20 or greater), including the small joints of the hands and feet, early erosions, and rheumatoid nodules. The presence of hip arthritis has been shown to be a poor prognostic sign, and may lead to destruction of the femoral heads (141). If polyarthritis persists longer than 7 years remission is unlikely. The onset of puberty seems to have no relation to disease activity or remission (67). Severe polyarticular (polyarticular and systemic JIA) disease, with involvement of the temporomandibular joints prior to 5 years of age, can result in micrognathia (142).

Psoriatic Arthritis

The diagnosis of juvenile psoriatic arthritis was considered to be rare in children. Prior to 1982, there were fewer than 80 cases described in the English literature, when Shore and Ansell (143) published the first large collection of 60 children with psoriatic arthritis. The rarity of juvenile psoriatic arthritis was unusual, due to the relatively large number of children with psoriasis, and the fact that 7% of adults with psoriasis have arthritis (144). Juvenile psoriatic arthritis has historically been considered a juvenile spondyloarthropathy. However, recent studies have shown the juvenile psoriatic arthritis is a distinct entity that has been underdiagnosed, often due to the long period from onset of arthritis to onset of psoriasis (144,145).

Psoriatic arthritis may account for up to 7% of JIA. There is a mild female predominance (1.6 to 2.3 girls to 1 boy) and it often affects young children, with a median onset age of 5.9 to 10.1 years. The arthritis is often an asymmetric oligo- or polyarthritis affecting both large and small joints. At onset, the majority have nail pitting (67%) (Fig. 12-6), a family history of psoriasis (69%), or dactylitis (39%), and less than one-half of the children have the rash of psoriasis (13 to 43%) (94,144,145). Current criteria do not require the development of psoriasis to confirm a diagnosis of psoriatic arthritis (9) (Table 12-2).

Children with psoriatic arthritis usually do not develop an RF, but a positive ANA can be seen in 50%, and is a risk factor for uveitis. HLA-DR1 and HLA-DR6 were statistically significant risk factors for development of juvenile psoriatic arthritis (145). There is a mild, but not statistically significant, increase in the presence of HLA-B27 in children with psoriatic arthritis, and these children are more likely to have axial arthritis (143–145). The presentation of children under 5 years of age is often heralded by the involvement of a small number of fingers or toes that are relatively asymptomatic, but result in marked overgrowth of the digit(s).

The differential diagnosis of psoriatic arthritis is essentially the same as for polyarthritis. However, the diagnosis

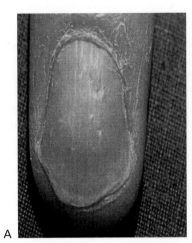
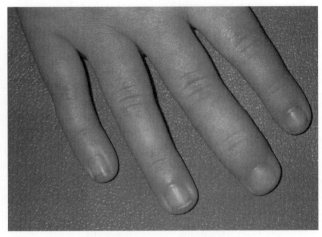

FIGURE 12-6. Juvenile psoriatic arthritis. **A:** Nail pitting associated with psoriasis. **B:** Swelling of a single distal interphalangeal joint in a child with juvenile psoriatic arthritis.

of psoriatic arthritis should be suspected in a child with dactylitis, nail pitting, asymmetric involvement of large and small joints, arthritis of the distal interphalangeal (DIP) joints (Fig. 12-6), or a first- or second-degree relative with psoriasis. There is rarely fever or systemic illness as may be seen in septic arthritis caused by *Neisseria gonorrheae.*

Clinical Course

Children with psoriatic arthritis can have a chronic lifelong arthritis that may follow a relapsing and remitting course. Arthritis mutilans and predominant DIP joint disease are unusual. However, many of the children will have prolonged polyarthritis that may result in irreversible joint damage (143). Amyloidosis has been noted in the European literature, and has resulted in the death of at least 3 children (143,146). Chronic anterior uveitis has been observed in up to 17% of children (144,145), is associated with a positive ANA titer, and is clinically indistinguishable from the uveitis in oligo- and polyarthritis. The uveitis associated with psoriatic arthritis may be more resistant to treatment than the other forms of chronic uveitis associated with childhood arthritis (67).

Enthesitis-related Arthritis

The criteria for classification of enthesitis-related arthritis (ERA) describes a group of arthritides that includes undifferentiated spondyloarthritis, ankylosing spondylitis, and inflammatory bowel disease-associated arthritis. At the onset, juvenile spondyloarthropathies are often undifferentiated, preventing the application of adult-onset criteria for diagnosis. The addition of criteria for the presence of HLA-B27, a family history of HLA-B27–associated disease, and

the onset of arthritis in a boy after 8 years of age, will increase the number of children included in this category (9). However, in an effort to better define the group of children who have psoriatic arthritis, the Durban criteria now excludes children from the diagnosis of ERA, even those with ankylosing spondylitis, if they have a first- or second-degree relative with psoriasis. This will likely contribute a significant number of children to the "Other Arthritis" category, in that they either fulfill no criteria or fulfill criteria for more than one category. It is probable that families with a genetic propensity for psoriasis, who also carry the *HLA-B27* gene, may have two distinct mechanisms contributing to the development of arthritis. These disorders will be better defined as the underling mechanisms are elucidated by molecular and genetic research. The current criteria will include many of those children previously diagnosed with a syndrome of seronegativity, enthesopathy, and arthropathy (SEA syndrome), who were shown to be at increased risk for development of classic spondyloarthritis or juvenile ankylosing spondylitis (147,148).

ERA is often associated with enthesitis and arthralgias or arthritis long before any axial skeletal involvement is identified (148). Enthesitis is identified when marked tenderness is noted at the 6, 10, and 2 o'clock positions on the patella, at the tibial tuberosity, iliac crest, or the attachments of the Achilles tendon or plantar fascia (67). In some children the only manifestation of ERA may be severe enthesopathy of the heel(s) (149) (Fig. 12-7).

Laboratory evaluation of children with ERA is relatively unremarkable. There is often systemic inflammation with thrombocytosis and an elevated ESR. A highly elevated ESR (>100) is more likely to be associated with inflammatory bowel disease in a child who meets the criteria for ERA. The RF is uniformly negative, but ANAs can be present in

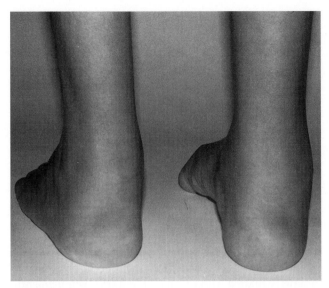

FIGURE 12-7. Achilles tendonitis and enthesitis in a child with enthesitis-related arthritis. (Courtesy of Dr. Ruben Burgos-Vargas.)

the same proportion as the childhood population (16,17,67).

The primary extraarticular manifestation of ERA is acute anterior uveitis (AAU), which can occur in up to 27% of children with ankylosing spondylitis (150). AAU is highly associated with the presence of HLA-B27 (50%) (151). It typically presents with an acute, painful, red, photophobic eye. Although AAU may resolve with no ocular residua, some children will have a persistent uveitis that is relatively resistant to therapy, and can result in blindness (152,153).

Juvenile Ankylosing Spondylitis

Children with juvenile ankylosing spondylitis (JAS) have often been diagnosed based on adult criteria that require radiographic evidence of sacroiliitis. JAS most often presents in late childhood or adolescence. Children with JAS and sacroiliac (SI) involvement are often HLA-B27-positive (82 to 95%), and the male-to-female ratio is 6:1 (97). Most children ultimately diagnosed with JAS will initially have an episodic arthritis of large joints of the lower extremities and the tarsal bones. Regardless of axial disease, the most reliable predictors to differentiate JAS from oligo- or polyarticular JIA are the presence of enthesitis and tarsal disease in children who have arthritis of the lower, but not of the upper extremities (154).

The presentation of JAS is most remarkable for the absence of axial involvement. Only 12.8 to 24% of children with JAS have pain, stiffness, or limitation of motion of the sacroiliac or lumbosacral spine at onset. A peripheral arthropathy or enthesopathy, affecting predominantly the lower limb joints and entheses, is seen in 79 to 89.4%.

These children tend to have fewer than five joints involved, and rarely more than ten. At presentation, the joint involvement is usually asymmetric, or even unilateral (155). Small joints of the toes are commonly involved in JAS, but are seldom affected in other forms of JIA, with the exception of psoriatic arthritis.

The diagnosis of JAS is often difficult at onset. However, the combination of peripheral joint arthritis, with a lower-extremity predominance, enthesitis, and SI, or lumbosacral disease, would strongly suggest the diagnosis of ERA and possible JAS. Septic SI joint disease and osteomyelitis can present with SI pain and limitation of motion.

Examination of the axial skeleton is important in the diagnosis of JAS. Pain may be elicited over the SI joints by direct pressure, lateral compression of the pelvis, or distraction of the SI joints (Patrick test). Quantitation of the normal lumbar spine flexion, by Macrae and Wright's modification of the Schober test (156), can identify children with limitation of lumbar spine flexion. With the child standing upright, an anchoring mark is made at the lumbosacral junction (dimples of Venus). A mark is then made 5 cm below and 10 cm above the lumbosacral junction. Then, with the child in maximal forward flexion, the distance between the upper and lower points is measured. In general, a modified Schober measurement of greater than 21 cm (i.e., an increase of 6 cm) is within normal limits (67). The measurement of fingertip to floor distance on forward flexion is not reproducible, reflects both hip and back flexion, and does not correlate with the Schober index. Chest expansion is also not a reliable test for spine involvement in JAS (155).

Clinical Course

The initial course of JAS is characterized by remitting and relapsing symptoms, which are frequently mild. This can not be differentiated from the child who seems to have recurrent bouts of reactive arthritis. However, the pattern of joint disease (which often progresses to become polyarticular) and axial disease is usually evident after the third year of illness (155). Children with long-standing JAS have been shown to develop tarsal bone coalition that has been termed "ankylosing tarsitis" (157) (Fig. 12-8).

Outcome data for JAS are incomplete and at times contradictory. The prognosis of JAS has been reported as both worse and better than adult-onset ankylosing spondylitis (158,159). Peripheral joint arthritis tends to be more common than that seen in adults (67). Hip disease had been associated with a poor functional outcome (158,160), and may require total hip arthroplasty.

Inflammatory Bowel Disease-associated Arthritis

The prevalence of arthritis in children with inflammatory bowel disease (IBD) has been reported to be 7 to 21%,

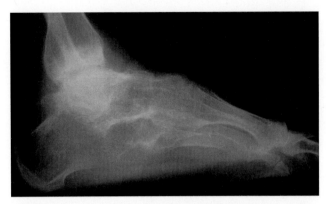

FIGURE 12-8. Ankylosing tarsitis, a complex disorder resulting in ankylosis of the foot in a child with juvenile ankylosing spondylitis. (Courtesy of Dr. Ruben Burgos-Vargas.)

and usually occurs after the diagnosis of the bowel disease (161–163). There are two different patterns of arthritis seen (67). The most common type is an oligo- or polyarticular arthritis of the lower limbs. This group is less likely to meet the criteria for ERA. This arthritis is often episodic, with exacerbation lasting 4 to 6 weeks, and rarely, for months. The activity of the peripheral arthritis often reflects the underlying activity of the IBD. The less-common type of IBD-associated arthritis is a HLA-B27–associated oligoarticular arthritis of the lower limbs, with sacroiliitis and enthesitis,

and no relationship to bowel inflammation (67). This form is more likely to persist and progress, despite control of the bowel disease, and seems identical to other ERAs.

RADIOLOGIC FINDINGS IN JIA

Early in the course of JIA, there are often no specific radiologic findings. As the disease progresses, there is often periarticular osteopenia, localized soft tissue swelling, and occasionally, joint space widening due to effusion or synovial hypertrophy. Late changes seen in JIA include joint space narrowing from cartilage loss, erosions, subluxation, and ultimately ankylosis (Figs. 12-9 and 12-10). Erosive changes do not typically occur before 2 years of active disease, and significant changes in radiographs rarely occur in less than 6 months. Children with chronic polyarthritis will frequently develop bony ankylosis of the carpal and tarsal joints, and in the cervical spine.

Radiologic abnormalities of cervical spine (Fig. 12-11) can result from apophyseal joint inflammation and bony fusion, often initially at the C2–C3 level. Atlantoaxial instability can be seen with chronic arthritis of the cervical spine. Symptoms can range from minimal to severe neck pain and limitation of movement of the cervical spine, to neurologic damage due to impingement of the spinal cord. Special precautions for children with JIA and cervical spine arthritis must be made prior to anesthesia, due to the rigid cervical spine and atlantoaxial instability, to avoid serious injury.

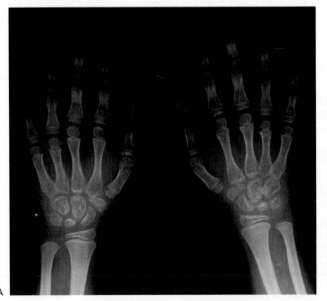

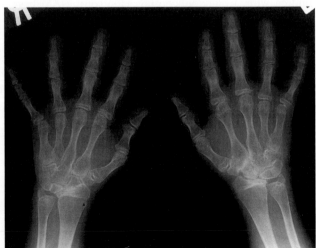

A   B

FIGURE 12-9. Polyarticular juvenile idiopathic arthritis with wrist and finger involvement. **A:** At 6 years of age, there is periarticular osteopenia and diffuse swelling of the wrist and fingers. **B:** At 20 years of age, there is significant carpal and carpometacarpal fusion.

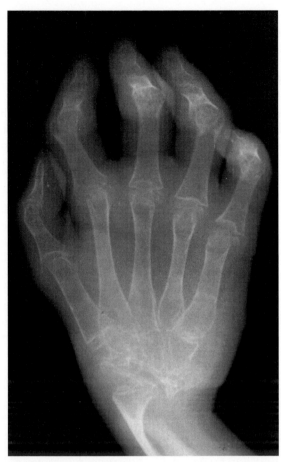

FIGURE 12-10. Systemic-onset polyarticular juvenile idiopathic arthritis with prolonged arthritis, resulting in severe osteopenia and destructive changes in the hand and wrist, with severe ulnar deviation.

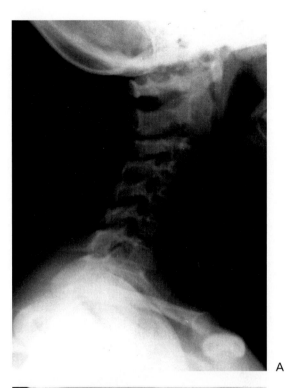

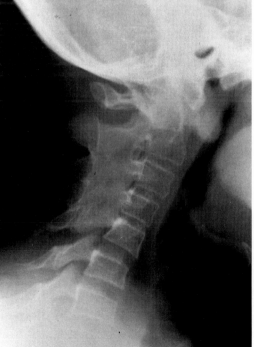

FIGURE 12-11. The cervical spine in a child with polyarticular JIA. **A:** At 6 years of age, there are no radiographic abnormalities. **B:** At 21 years of age, there is ankylosis of C2–C5.

Likewise, serious traumatic injuries have occurred after spontaneous cervical spinal fusion as a consequence of JIA, highlighting the vulnerable nature of these children (164).

Radiographs in psoriatic arthritis can show both asymmetric erosive disease, with or without regional osteoporosis, and periosteal new bone formation. The periostitis can lead to overgrowth of the affected bone. Although erosive changes of the DIP joints can be seen, this is a rare occurrence (67) (Fig. 12-12).

Children with ankylosing spondylitis will develop radiographic changes in the SI joints, but this may not occur for 1 to 15 (average 6.5) years after diagnosis (150). These findings can include pseudowidening due to erosions, sclerosis, and fusion (Fig. 12-13). Radiologic changes in the lumbosacral spine occur later in the course of JAS, and are less frequent (165). Chronic enthesitis, particularly at the

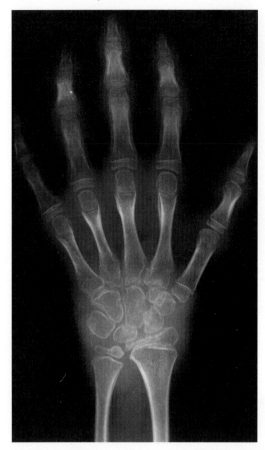

FIGURE 12-12. Juvenile psoriatic arthritis affecting the hand, with metacarpophalangeal, proximal, and distal interphalangeal joint involvement, with marked fusiform swelling, and periostitis.

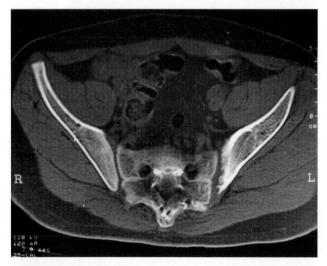

FIGURE 12-13. CT scan of the SI joints in a child with juvenile ankylosing spondylitis, showing erosions and sclerosis of the SI joints. (Courtesy of Dr. Ruben Burgos-Vargas.)

calcaneus, can result in erosion at the insertion of the Achilles tendon or plantar fascia.

TREATMENT OF JIA

The treatment of juvenile arthritis is best achieved with a multidisciplinary team approach. First and foremost, the child and family must participate in informed decision-making. The team of health care professionals can provide comprehensive care of all facets of this chronic disease. The team should include the primary care physician, to coordinate medical care, and the rheumatologist, for diagnosis and treatment plans. Other valuable members of the treatment team may include the rheumatology nurse, for education and family support; social worker, for monetary and school advocacy; dietitian, to minimize the effects of corticosteroid therapy; physical and occupational therapists, to maintain and improve strength and range of joint motion; ophthalmologist, for uveitis screening and treatment; and occasionally the pediatric orthopaedic surgeon, when surgical interventions are indicated.

Medications

There are many drugs available to treat arthritis. Often, two or more drug classes must be used simultaneously to achieve disease control. Many recent advances in understanding the mechanisms of inflammation in arthritis have led to novel therapeutic strategies. The fundamental purpose of pharmacologic therapy is to achieve pain control, decrease inflammation, promote, then maintain remission. The medications used are individualized for each patient, depending on their subtype of arthritis, degree of inflammation, and previous response to medications.

Nonsteroidal Antiinflammatory Drugs

The mechanism of action of NSAIDs is by inhibition of the biosynthesis of prostaglandins, by direct action on the enzyme cyclooxygenase (COX) (166). The recent discovery of a second COX enzyme (COX-2), which is induced in the proinflammatory cascade, and the differential inhibition of the two COX isoforms (COX-1 and COX-2) by individual NSAIDs, has provided the basis for the development of safer NSAIDs (167). At this time, no COX-2–specific NSAID is approved for use in children. However, this exciting scientific advance will likely change NSAID use in children in the near future.

NSAIDs are the initial therapeutic intervention in most children with JIA. NSAIDs provide both analgesia and an antiinflammatory effect. The average time-course for response to NSAIDs is 4 to 12 weeks (168). Thus, an NSAID is usually given for 4 to 8 weeks before substituting another, if there has not been sufficient improvement. NSAIDs are

TABLE 12-7. NSAIDS FOR THE TREATMENT OF JIA

Drug (brand)	Dosage (usual number of daily doses)
Choline magnesium trisalicylate[a–c] (Trilisate)	50 mg/kg/day (2)
Salicylsalicylic acid[a,b] (Disalcid)	50–100 mg/kg/day (2)
Ibuprofen[a,c] (Motrin, Advil, etc.)	40 mg/kg/day (4)
Naproxen[a,c] (Naprosyn)	10–20 mg/kg/day (2)
Tolmetin[a] (Tolectin)	15–30 mg/kg/day (3)
Indomethacin[a,c] (Indocin)	1–3 mg/kg/day (3)
Diclofenac (Voltaren)	2–3 mg/kg/day (2)
Nabumetone (Relafen)	20–25 mg/kg/day (1–2)

[a] FDA-labeled for use in children.
[b] No inhibition of platelet aggregation.
[c] Liquid preparation available.

generally safe and well tolerated in most children. Abdominal pain, nausea, and vomiting are common side effects, but gastrointestinal hemorrhage is rare (169). However, gastroduodenal injury is more frequent in children receiving high doses, or more than one NSAID (170). The use of aspirin for JIA is no longer recommended due to the risk of Reye syndrome, increased hepatotoxicity, bleeding, and four-times-per-day dosing.

The doses of NSAIDs in children are based on body weight, and are proportionally greater than in adult rheumatic diseases (Table 12-7). Preparations that come in a liquid form and have once to twice-daily dosing are preferred. In the United States, the most commonly used NSAID for JIA is naproxen (10 to 20 mg/kg/day, b.i.d.). In children with fevers and serositis associated with systemic arthritis and with JAS, indomethacin is often the most effective NSAID (67). Children on chronic NSAID therapy should have a complete blood count, renal and liver function tests, and urine analysis every 6 months.

Nearly two-thirds of children with juvenile arthritis are inadequately treated with NSAIDs alone (171). These children require additional pharmacologic interventions.

Corticosteroids

Intraarticular corticosteroid injections had been shown to be safe and effective in controlling the synovitis in JIA (172,173). Triamcinolone hexacetonide (1 mg/kg for large joints and 0.5 mg/kg for medium joints) is the most commonly used agent, and often provides long-term control of inflammation. The most frequent adverse consequence of intraarticular corticosteroids is development of subcutaneous atrophy at the site of injection. Systemic corticosteroids can be used for rapid control of severe arthritis. However, long-term use should be restricted to those children with severe arthritis or systemic features that do not respond to other interventions.

Methotrexate

Methotrexate is the most commonly used second-line agent for treatment of juvenile arthritis. It is typically given at 0.5 to 1 mg/kg (with a maximum of 20 to 30 mg) once weekly by mouth or subcutaneous injection. It has been shown to be superior to placebo in polyarticular and extended oligoarticular, but not systemic arthritis (174,175), and can produce radiologic improvement of erosions (176). Methotrexate has been shown to decrease the severity of uveitis in children with JIA who were dependent on topical corticosteroids (177).

The major side effects with methotrexate use are nausea, diarrhea, and oral ulcers. Supplementation with folic acid (1 mg/day) can usually prevent gastrointestinal complications. One of the most significant long-term side effects of methotrexate use is the development of liver fibrosis and cirrhosis (178–180). Serial abnormalities of hepatic enzymes were significantly associated with liver fibrosis in children taking methotrexate for juvenile arthritis (181), suggesting that the current guidelines for patients with rheumatoid arthritis are applicable to patients with JIA (182).

Sulfasalazine

Sulfasalazine has been used extensively in Europe, and increasingly in North America, for treatment of both spondyloarthropathies and JRA/JCA (183,184). It is typically given in the enteric-coated form, at a dose of 50 mg/kg/day in two divided doses. Recently, a randomized, double-blind, placebo-controlled trial showed that sulfasalazine is both safe and effective for the treatment of oligo- and polyarticular JCA (185). Serious side effects have been noted in children with systemic arthritis, and the routine use of sulfasalazine is not recommended for this subgroup (186,187).

Physical and Occupational Therapy

All children with prolonged arthritis should be evaluated by a physical and/or occupational therapist to provide an appropriate teaching and treatment program. Most treatment programs for JIA will include active and passive range of motion exercises, strengthening, and other modalities, such as a hot paraffin bath for relief of hand stiffness. Swimming has the advantage of providing muscle-strengthening and active range of motion without significant weight-bearing. Splinting may be used to maintain alignment, provide rest, and reduce flexion contractures. For children with severe flexion contractures, a dynamic tension splint or serial casting can be used to correct the contracture. Physical therapy for range of motion in JAS is primarily to prevent loss of mobility and poor functional positioning.

Surgical Interventions for Complications of JIA

For the majority of children with JIA, orthopaedic surgery has a limited role in the management plan. With early detection and aggressive medical management, including intra-articular corticosteroid injections, the majority of children with juvenile arthritis have a satisfactory outcome without significant disability. However, for those children with persistent arthritis, treated or untreated, continued presence of pain, joint contractures, and mechanical instability, there is often significant benefit from individualized orthopaedic surgical intervention. Many of the reports of surgery for juvenile arthritis actually refer to adults who have had arthritis since childhood. Surgical intervention in JIA presents several problems to the management team. The small size and growth potential of children must be considered. Also, in the postsurgical period, prolonged immobilization can lead to decreased strength and range of motion, with or without active arthritis. Often after a surgical procedure there will be intensive physical therapy required to mobilize the child's joints. There is no universal agreement about which procedures are indicated for the treatment of complications of chronic arthritis in childhood. However, the overall goal is to provide symptomatic relief and increased function.

Synovectomy

Synovectomy may be indicated in a minority of children with JIA for relief of pain, swelling, and impaired joint motion related to synovial hypertrophy. There may be short-term benefit in joint-swelling and pain, but range of motion may not improve, or may even worsen (188–192). The greatest benefit has been seen in large joints (193,194). But recurrences are common, and the ultimate outcome of children with JIA is not altered by prophylactic synovectomy (195,196).

Soft Tissue Release

Soft tissue release may rarely be useful in a child with a severe contracture of the knee or hip that has been resistant to splinting or serial casting. Initial observations regarding soft tissue release were encouraging (197). However, more recent reports have been less striking, with only a modest benefit and a tendency to deteriorate (198,199). In most cases, vigorous physical therapy will avoid the need for this frequently unsuccessful operation.

Arthrodesis

Arthrodesis is indicated for treatment of severe joint destruction of the ankle after prolonged synovitis in oligo- or poly-articular JIA. After puberty, a fixed and painful deformity of the ankle is best corrected by performing a triple arthrodesis. Occasionally, in children with isolated damage of the subtalar or talonavicular joint, a single joint fusion may be appropriate (200) [➥7.10, 7.11]. If required, these procedures may be later converted to a triple arthrodesis [➥7.9].

Although many children with JIA have cervical spine arthritis and atlantoaxial instability, there is no consensus on the indications for prophylactic fusion. In many cases a simple cervical orthosis may stabilize the neck and prevent further subluxation. However, fusion of the cervical spine (C1–C2) is indicated in children who have progressive neurologic involvement (201,202) [➥2.17].

Osteotomy

Osteotomy has only occasional utility in children with arthritis. In a younger child with a fixed deformity of the knee but good remaining joint surface and minimal active synovitis, a knee osteotomy may result in correction of the deformity (203). Unfortunately, the osteotomy makes a subsequent total knee arthroplasty more difficult due to the distorted anatomy.

Infrequently, a shortening osteotomy of the radius or lengthening of the ulna may be utilized to correct length discrepancies of the forearm bones. Recently, distraction lengthening of the ulna in six children (eight wrists), with severe destructive changes in the wrist due to JCA, was reported (204). This procedure was found to adequately correct the deformity with improved function, and in the majority no further splinting was required with an average follow-up of 70 months (range 12 to 152).

Epiphysiodesis

An appropriately timed epiphysiodesis has been successfully used to correct leg-length discrepancies in oligoarticular arthritis (205,206). The discrepancy can be predicted using the method of Moseley (207). Simon et al. (206) reported that 15 patients followed to skeletal maturity had satisfactory results.

Total Joint Arthroplasty

Total joint arthroplasty is indicated for children with JIA who have severe destructive joint changes with functional impairment or disabling pain. The most common joints replaced are the hip and knee, but there may be indications for shoulder and elbow arthroplasty.

Total hip replacement is typically performed due to severe destruction or ankylosis, resulting in functional impairment. Initial series using predominantly cemented hip replacements showed reduction in pain and improved functional ability, but with a significant rate of loosening and subsequent revision (208,209). Recent results have suggested an improved outcome with cementless arthroplasty of the hip, but poor bone stock remains an indication for cementing (210,211).

The knee is frequently involved in JIA, and when there is significant pain, deformity, and functional incapacity, a total knee replacement is indicated. Initial results of total knee arthroplasty in JIA have been encouraging, with few revisions required (212–214). Recent long-term follow-up of total knee arthroplasty in young adults and children with arthritis has been equally encouraging (215). Cementless total knee arthroplasty has been used in selected cases (216).

Total elbow replacement may be indicated in children with severe destruction of the elbow joint. In a recent review, Connor and Morrey (217) evaluated the long-term outcome of 19 children (23 elbows), who had been managed with total elbow arthroplasty and followed for at least 2 years. Only three (13%) had a poor result due to late complications: aseptic loosening, instability, and worn bushings.

Shoulder replacement in juvenile arthritis is indicated when there is prolonged pain, limitation of function, and significant joint destruction. There are not sufficient data to evaluate the efficacy of total shoulder arthroplasty in children. However, in studies of adults with rheumatoid arthritis, and in some including children, the results have been promising (218,219).

References

Overview of Pediatric Rheumatic Disease Encountered by the Pediatric Orthopaedic Surgeon

1. Kunnamo I, Kallio P, Pelkonen P. Incidence of arthritis in urban Finnish children: a prospective study. *Arthritis Rheum* 1986;29:2132.
2. Goodman JE, McGraft PJ. The epidemiology of pain in children and adolescents: a review. *Pain* 1991;46:247.
3. McGrath PJ, McAlpine L. Psychologic perspectives on pediatric pain. *J Pediatr* 1993;122:S2.
4. Kaipiainen-Seppanen O, Savolainen A. Incidence of chronic juvenile rheumatic diseases in Finland during 1980–1990. *Clin Exp Rheumatol* 1996;14:441.
5. Peterson LS, Mason T, Nelson AMO, et al. Juvenile rheumatoid arthritis in Rochester, Minnesota 1960–1993. Is the epidemiology changing? *Arthritis Rheum* 1996;39:1385.

Classification and Diagnosis of Juvenile Idiopathic Arthritis

6. European League Against Rheumatism (EULAR). Bulletin 4. Nomenclature and classification of arthritis in children. Basel: National Zeitung AG, 1977.
7. Cassidy JT, Levinson JE, Bass JC, et al. A study of classification criteria for a diagnosis of juvenile rheumatoid arthritis. *Arthritis Rheum* 1986;29:274.
8. Fink CW. Proposal for the development of classification criteria for idiopathic arthritides of childhood (published erratum appears in *J Rheumatol* 1995;22:2195). *J Rheumatol* 1995;22:1566.
9. Petty RE, Southwood TR, Baum J, et al. Revision of the proposed classification criteria for juvenile idiopathic arthritis: Durban, 1997. *J Rheumatol* 1998;25:1991.

Approach to the Evaluation of Children with Limb Pain, Limp, or Joint Pain with or without Swelling

10. Varni JW, Thompson KL, Hanson V. The Varni/Thompson Pediatric Pain Questionnaire. I. Chronic musculoskeletal pain in juvenile rheumatoid arthritis. *Pain* 1987;28:27.

11. Sherry DD, Bohnsack J, Salmonson K, et al. Painless juvenile rheumatoid arthritis. *J Pediatr* 1989;116:921.
12. Sullivan DB, Cassidy JT, Petty RE. Pathogenic implications of age of onset in juvenile rheumatoid arthritis. *Arthritis Rheum* 1975;18:251.
13. Haynes DC, Gershwin ME, Robbins DL. Autoantibody profiles in juvenile arthritis. *J Rheumatol* 1986;13: 58.
14. Petty RE, Cassidy JT, Sullivan DB. Serologic studies in juvenile rheumatoid arthritis. A review. *Arthritis Rheum* 1977;20(suppl):260.
15. Rosenberg AM. Uveitis associated with juvenile rheumatoid arthritis. *Semin Arthritis Rheum* 1987;16:158.
16. Cabral DA, Petty RE, Fung M, et al. Persistent antinuclear antibodies in children without identifiable inflammatory, rheumatic or autoimmune disease. *Pediatrics* 1992;89:441.
17. Allen RC, Dewez P, Stuart L. Antinuclear antibodies using HEp-2 cells in normal children and in children with common infections. *J Paediatr Child Health* 1991;27:39.
18. Deane PMG, Liard G, Siegel DM, et al. The outcome of children referred to a pediatric rheumatology clinic with a positive antinuclear antibody test but without an autoimmune disease. *Pediatrics* 1995;95:892.
19. Stillman JS, Barry PE. Juvenile rheumatoid arthritis: series 2. *Arthritis Rheum* 1977;20(suppl):171.
20. Schaller JG. Juvenile rheumatoid arthritis: series 1. *Arthritis Rheum* 1977;20(suppl):165.
21. Eichenfield AH, Athreya BH, Boughty RA. Utility of rheumatoid factor in the diagnosis of juvenile rheumatoid arthritis. *Pediatrics* 1986;78:480.
22. Shmerling RH, Delbanco TL. How useful is the rheumatoid factor? *Arch Intern Med* 1992;152:2417.
23. Petty R. HLA-B27 and rheumatic diseases of childhood. *J Rheumatol* 1990;17:7.
24. Howell RR. Juvenile gouty arthritis. *Am J Dis Child* 1985;139:547.
25. Cassidy JT, Brody GL, Martel W. Monarticular juvenile rheumatoid arthritis. *J Pediatr* 1967;70:867.
26. Baldassare AR, Chang F, Zuckner J. Markedly raised synovial fluid leukocyte counts not associated with infectious arthritis in children. *Ann Rheum Dis* 1978;37:404.
27. Zuckner J, Baldassare A, Chang F, et al. High synovial fluid leukocyte counts of noninfectious etiology. *Arthritis Rheum* 1977;20(suppl):270.
28. Senac MO, Deutsch D, Bernstein BH. MR imaging in juvenile rheumatoid arthritis. *AJR Am J Roentgenol* 1988;150:873.
29. Verbruggen LA, Shahabpour M, Van Roy P, et al. Magnetic resonance imaging of articular destruction in juvenile rheumatoid arthritis. *Arthritis Rheum* 1990;33:1426.
30. Yulish BD, Lieberman JM, Newman AJ. Juvenile rheumatoid arthritis: assessment with MR imaging. *Radiology* 1987;165:149.

Differential Diagnosis of Joint Pain and Swelling in Children

31. Klippel JH, Weyand CM, Wortmann RL. *Primer on the rheumatic diseases.* 11th ed. Atlanta: Arthritis Foundation, 1997:1.
32. Steere AC, Bartenhagen NH, Craft JE. The early clinical manifestations of Lyme disease. *Ann Intern Med* 1983;99:76.
33. Steere AC, Schoen RT, Taylor E. The clinical evolution of Lyme arthritis. *Ann Intern Med* 1987;107:725.
34. Gerber MA, Zemel LS, Shapiro ED. Lyme arthritis in children: clinical epidemiology and long-term outcomes. *Pediatrics* 1998;102:905.
35. Huppertz HI, Karch H, Suschke HJ, et al. Lyme arthritis in

European children and adolescents. *Arthritis Rheum* 1995;38: 361.

36. Steere AC, Dwyer E, Winchester R. Association of chronic Lyme arthritis with HLA-DR4 and HLA-DR2 alleles. *N Engl J Med* 1990;323:219.

37. Cuttica JJ, Schenines EJ, Garay SM, et al. Juvenile onset Reiter's syndrome: a retrospective study of 26 patients. *Clin Exp Rheumatol* 1992;10:285.

38. Smith RJ. Evidence for *Chlamydia trachomatis* and *Ureaplasma urealyticum* in a patient with Reiter's disease. *J Adolesc Health Care* 1989;10:155.

39. Rosenberg AM, Petty RE. Reiter's disease in children. *Am J Dis Child* 1979;133:394.

40. Wright V. Reiter's disease. In: Scott JT, ed. *Copeman's textbook of the rheumatic diseases.* London: Longmans Green, 1978:549.

41. Keat A, Maini RN, Nkwazi GC. Role of *Chlamydia trachomatis* and HLA B27 in sexually acquired reactive arthritis. *Br Med J* 1978;1:605.

42. Keat AC, Maini RN, Pegrum GD, et al. The clinical features and HLA associations of reactive arthritis associated with non-gonococcal urethritis. *Q J Med* 1979;190:323.

43. Harrersen D, Weiner D, Weiner S. The characterization of "transient synovitis of the hip" in children. *J Pediatr Orthop* 1986;6:11.

44. Koop S, Quanbeck D, Three common causes of childhood hip pain. *Pediatr Clin North Am* 1996;43:1053.

45. Wingstrand H. Transient synovitis of the hip in the child. *Acta Orthop Scand* 1986;57(suppl):219.

46. Veasy LG, Wiedmeier SE, Orsmond GS. Resurgence of acute rheumatic fever in the intermountain area of the United States. *N Engl J Med* 1987;316:280.

47. McLaren MJ, Hawkins DM, Koorhop HJ. Epidemiology of rheumatic heart disease in black school children of Soweto, Johannesburg. *Br Med J* 1975;3:474.

48. Veasy LG, Tani LY, Hill HR. Persistence of acute rheumatic fever in the intermountain area of the United States. *J E Pediatr* 1994;124:9.

49. Dajani AS, Ayoub E, Bierman FZ. Guidelines for the diagnosis of rheumatic fever. Jones criteria, 1992 update. *JAMA* 1992; 268:2069.

50. Schaffer FM, Agarwal R, Helm J, et al. Post-streptococcal-reactive arthritis and silent carditis: a case report and review of the literature. *Pediatrics* 1994;93:837.

51. Arnold MH, Tyndall A. Post-streptococcal-reactive arthritis. *Ann Rheum Dis* 1989;48:681.

52. De Cunto CL, et al. Prognosis of children with poststreptococcal reactive arthritis. *Pediatr Infect Dis J* 1988;7:683.

53. Bont L, Brus F, Dijkman-Neerincx RHM, et al. The clinical spectrum of post-streptococcal syndromes with arthritis in children. *Clin Exp Rheumatol* 1998;16:750.

54. Fink CW. The role of the *Streptococcus* in post-streptococcal reactive arthritis and childhood polyarteritis nodosa. *J Rheumatol* 1991;18(suppl.29):14.

55. Ahmed S, et al. Poststreptococcal reactive arthritis: clinical characteristics and association with HLA-DR alleles. *Arthritis Rheumatol* 1998;41:1096.

56. Beilory L, et al. Human serum sickness: a prospective analysis of 35 patients treated with equine anti-thymocyte globulin for bone marrow failure. *Medicine* 1988;67:40.

57. Weston WL, Brice SL, Jester JD, et al. Herpes simplex virus in childhood erythema multiforme. *Pediatrics* 1992;89:32.

58. Erffmeyer JE. Serum sickness. *Ann Allergy* 1986;56:105.

59. Schidlow DV, Goldsmith DP, Palmer J, et al. Arthritis in cystic fibrosis. *Arch Dis Child* 1984;59:377.

60. Summers GD, Webley M. Episodic arthritis in cystic fibrosis: a case report. *Br J Rheumatol* 1986;31:535.

61. Pertuiset E, Menkes CJ, Lenoi G. Cystic fibrosis arthritis. A report of five cases. *Br J Rheumatol* 1992;28:341.

62. Newman AJ, Ansell BM. Episodic arthritis in children with cystic fibrosis. *J Pediatr* 1979;94: 594.

63. Dixey J, Redington AN, Butler RC. The arthropathy of cystic fibrosis. *Ann Rheum Dis* 1988;47:218.

64. Sagransky DM, Greenwald RA. Seropositive rheumatoid arthritis in a patient with cystic fibrosis. *Am J Dis Child* 1980;129: 634.

65. Nathanson I, Riddlesberger MMJ. Pulmonary hypertrophic osteoarthropathy in cystic fibrosis. *Radiology* 1980;135:649.

66. Athreya BH, Borns P, Roselund ML. Cystic fibrosis and hypertrophic osteoarthropathy in children. *Am J Dis Child* 1973;129: 634.

67. Cassidy JT, Petty RE. *Textbook of pediatric rheumatology.* 3rd ed. Philadelphia: WB Saunders, 1995.

68. Isenberg DA, Miller JJ, eds. *Adolescent rheumatology.* London: Martin Dunitz, 1999.

69. Ragsdale CG, Petty RE, Cassidy JT. The clinical progression of apparent juvenile rheumatoid arthritis to systemic lupus erythematosus. *J Rheumatol* 1980;17:777.

70. Pattishall EN, Strope GL, Spinola AM. Childhood sarcoidosis. *J Pediatr* 1986;108:169.

71. Steward M, Savage JM, Bell B. Long term renal prognosis of Henoch-Schonlein purpura in an unselected childhood population. *Eur J Pediatr* 1988;147:113.

72. Barton LL, Saied KR. Thorn-induced arthritis. *J Pediatr* 1978; 93:322.

73. Costello PB, Brecker ML, Starr JL. A prospective analysis of the frequency, course, and possible prognostic significance of the joint manifestations of childhood leukemia. *J Rheumatol* 1983;10:753.

74. Saulsbury FT, Sabio G. Acute leukemia presenting as arthritis in children. *Clin Pediatr* 1985;24:625.

75. Cabral DA, Tucker LB. Malignancies in children who initially present with rheumatic complaints. *J Pediatr* 1999;134:53.

76. Flandry F, Hughston JC. Pigmented villonodular synovitis. *J Bone Joint Surg Am* 1987;69:942.

77. Walls JP, Nogi J. Multifocal pigmented villonodular synovitis in a child. *J Pediatr Orthop* 1985;5:229.

78. Peterson H. Growing pains. *Pediatr Clin North Am* 1986;33: 1356.

79. Gedalia A, Person DA, Brewer EJ. Hypermobility of the joints in juvenile episodic arthritis/arthralgia. *J Pediatr* 1985;107:873.

80. Carter C, Wilkinson J. Persistent joint laxity and congenital dislocation of the hip. *J Bone Joint Surg Br* 1964;46:40.

81. Sherry DD. Pain syndromes. In: Isenberg DA, Miller JJ, eds. *Adolescent rheumatology.* London: Martin Dunitz, 1999:197.

82. Yunus MB, Masi AT. Juvenile primary fibromyalgia syndrome. A clinical study of thirty-three patients and matched normal controls. *Arthritis Rheumatol* 1985;28:138.

83. Sherry DD, Weisman R. Psychologic aspects of childhood reflex neurovascular dystrophy. *Pediatrics* 1988;81:572.

84. Sherry DD, McGuire T, Mellins E, et al. Psychosomatic musculoskeletal pain in childhood: clinical and psychological analyses of 100 children. *Pediatrics* 1991;88:1093.

85. Sherry DD. Musculoskeletal pain in children. *Curr Op Rheumatol* 1997;9:465.

86. Bernstein BH, Singsen BH, Kent JT, et al. Reflex neurovascular dystrophy in childhood. *J Pediatr* 1978;93:211.

87. Malleson PN, Al-Matar M, Petty RE. Idiopathic musculoskeletal pain syndromes in children. *J Rheumatol* 1992;19:1786.

88. Yunus MB, Masi AT. Juvenile primary fibromyalgia syndrome. A clinical study of thirty-three patients and matched normal controls. *Arthritis Rheum* 1985;28:138.

89. Wolfe F, Smythe HA, Yunus MB, et al. The American College

of Rheumatology 1990 Criteria for the Classification of Fibromyalgia. Report of the Multicenter Criteria Committee. *Arthritis Rheum* 1990;33:160.

90. Bernstein BH, Singsen BH, Kent JT, et al. Reflex neurovascular dystrophy in childhood. *J Pediatr* 1978;93:211.

91. Wilder RT, Berde CB, Wolohan M, et al. Reflex sympathetic dystrophy in children. Clinical characteristics and follow-up of seventy patients. *J Bone Joint Surg Am* 1992;74:910.

92. Silber TJ, Majd M. Reflex sympathetic dystrophy syndrome in children and adolescents. Report of 18 cases and review of the literature. *Am J Dis Child* 1988;142:1325.

93. Bowyer S, Roettcher P. Pediatric rheumatology clinic populations in the United States: results of a 3 year survey. Pediatric Rheumatology Database Research Group. *J Rheumatol* 1996;23:1968.

Juvenile Idiopathic Arthritis

94. Symmons DP, Jones M, Osborne J, et al. Pediatric rheumatology in the United Kingdom: data from the British Pediatric Rheumatology Group National Diagnostic Register. *J Rheumatol* 1996;23:1975.

95. Towner SR, Michet CJJ, O'Fallen WM, et al. The epidemiology of juvenile arthritis in Rochester, Minnesota. *Arthritis Rheum* 1983;26:1208.

96. Singsen BH. Rheumatic diseases of childhood. *Rheum Dis Clin North Am* 1990;16:581.

97. Cabral DA, Malleson PN, Petty RE. Spondyloarthropathies of childhood. *Pediatr Clin North Am* 1995;42:1051.

98. Malleson PN, Fung MY, Rosenberg AM, et al. The incidence of paediatric rheumatic diseases: results from the Canadian Paediatric Rheumatology Association Disease Registry. *J Rheumatol* 1996;23:1981.

99. Burgos-Vargas R, Lardizabal-Sanabria J, Katona G. Ankylosing spondylitis and related diseases in the Mexican Mestizo. *Spine* 1990;4:665.

100. Goften JP, Chalmers A, Price GE, et al. HLA-B27 and ankylosing spondylitis in BC Indians. *J Rheumatol* 1975;2:328.

101. De Inocencio J, Giannini EH, Glass DN. Can genetic markers contribute to the classification of juvenile arthritis? *J Rheumatol* 1993;40(suppl):12.

102. Malagon C, Van Kerckhove C, Giannini EH. The iridocyclitis of early onset pauciarticular juvenile rheumatoid arthritis: outcome in immunogenetically characterized patients. *J Rheumatol* 1992;19:160.

103. Ploski R, Vinje O, Ronningen KS, et al. HLA class II alleles and heterogeneity of juvenile rheumatoid arthritis. *Arthritis Rheum* 199336:465.

104. Rubin LA, Amos CI, Wade JA, et al. Investigating the genetic basis for ankylosing spondylitis. Linkage studies with the major histocompatibility complex region. *Arthritis Rheum.* 1994;37:1212.

105. Burgos-Vargas R, Pacheco-Tena C, Vazquez-Mellado J. Juvenile-onset spondyloarthropathies. *Rheum Dis Clin North Am* 1997;23:569.

106. Hammer RE, Maika SD, Richardson JA, et al. Spontaneous inflammatory disease in transgenic rats expressing HLA-B27 and human β_2m: an animal model of HLA-B27–associated human disorders. *Cell* 1990;63:1099.

107. McDowell TL, Symons JA, Ploski R, et al. A genetic association between juvenile rheumatoid arthritis and a novel interleukin-1 alpha polymorphism. *Arthritis Rheum* 1995;38:221.

108. Martin K, Woo P. Juvenile idiopathic arthritides. In: Isenberg DA, Miller JJ, eds. *Adolescent rheumatology.* London: Martin Dunitz, 1999:78.

109. Kunnamo I. Infections and related risk factors of arthritis in children. *Scand J Rheumatol* 1987;16:93.

110. Pugh MT, Southwood TR, Gaston JS. The role of infection in juvenile chronic arthritis. *Br J Rheumatol* 1993;32:838.

111. Sieper J, Braun J. Pathogenesis of spondylarthropathies. *Arthritis Rheum* 1995;38:1547.

112. Hermann E, Yu DTY, Meyer KH, et al. HLA-B27-restricted CD8 T cells derived from synovial fluids of patients with reactive arthritis and ankylosing spondylitis. *Lancet* 1993;342:646.

Clinical Syndromes of JIA

113. Schneider R, Laxer RM. Systemic onset juvenile rheumatoid arthritis. *Baillieres Clin Rheum* 1998;12:245.

114. Still GF. On a form of chronic joint disease in children. *Am J Dis Child* 1978;132:195.

115. Calabro JJ, Marchesano JM. Fever associated with juvenile rheumatoid arthritis. *N Engl J Med* 1967;276:11.

116. Calabro JJ, Marchesano JM. Rash associated with juvenile rheumatoid arthritis. *J Pediatr* 1968;72:611.

117. Lang B, Shore A. A review of current concepts on the pathogenesis of juvenile rheumatoid arthritis. *J Rheumatol* 1990;17(suppl 21):1.

118. Vreugdenhil, G, Baltus CAM, Van Eijk HG, et al. Anaemia of chronic disease: diagnostic significance of erythrocyte and serological parameters in iron deficient rheumatoid arthritis. *Hum Nutr Clin Nutr* 1990;40C:57.

119. Prouse PJ, Harvey AR, Bonner B. Anaemia in juvenile chronic arthritis: serum inhibition of normal erythropoiesis in vitro. *Ann Rheum Dis* 1986;36:127.

120. Koerper MA, Stempel DA, Dallman PR. Anemia in patients with juvenile rheumatoid arthritis. *J Pediatr* 1980;92:930.

121. Pelkonen P, Swanljung K, Siimes MA. Ferritinemia as an indicator of systemic disease activity in children with systemic juvenile rheumatoid arthritis. *Acta Paediatr Scand* 1986;75:64.

122. Bloom BJ, Tucker LB, Miller LC, et al. Fibrin D-dimer as a marker of disease activity in systemic onset juvenile rheumatoid arthritis. *J Rheumatol* 1998;25:1620.

123. Bernstein BH, Stobie D, Singsen BH, et al. Growth retardation in juvenile rheumatoid arthritis (JRA). *Arthritis Rheum* 1977;20(suppl):212.

124. Woo PM. Growth retardation and osteoporosis in juvenile chronic arthritis. *Clin Exp Rheum* 1994;12(suppl 10):S87.

125. Davies UM, Rooney M, Preece MA, et al. Treatment of growth retardation in juvenile chronic arthritis with recombinant human growth hormone. *J Rheumatol* 1994;21:153.

126. Davies UM, Jones J, Reeve J, et al. Juvenile rheumatoid arthritis. Effects of disease activity and recombinant human growth hormone on insulin-like growth factor 1, insulin-like growth factor binding proteins 1 and 3, and osteocalcin. *Arthritis Rheum* 1997;40:332.

127. Schneider R, Lang BA, Reilly BJ. Prognostic indicators of joint destruction in systemic-onset juvenile rheumatoid arthritis. *J Pediatr* 1992;120:200.

128. David J, Vouyiouka O, Ansell BM, et al. Amyloidosis in juvenile chronic arthritis: a morbidity and mortality study. *Clin Exp Rheum* 1993;11:85.

129. Prieur AM, Stephan JL. Macrophage activation syndrome in children with joint diseases. *Rev Rheum Engl Ed* 1994;61:385.

130. Ravelli A, De Benedetti F, Viola S, et al. Macrophage activation syndrome in systemic juvenile rheumatoid arthritis successfully treated with cyclosporine. *J Pediatr* 1996;128:275.

131. Mouy R, Stephan JL, Pillet P, et al. Efficacy of cyclosporine A in the treatment of macrophage activation syndrome in juvenile arthritis: report of five cases. *J Pediatr* 1996;129:750.

132. Sailer M, Cabral D, Petty RE, et al. Rheumatoid factor positive,

oligoarticular onset juvenile rheumatoid arthritis. *J Rheumatol* 1997;24:586.

133. Bunger C, Bulow J, Tondebold E. Microcirculation of the juvenile knee in chronic arthritis. *Clin Orthop* 1986;204:294.

134. Vostrejs M, Hollister JR. Muscle atrophy and leg length discrepancies in pauciarticular juvenile rheumatoid arthritis. *Am J Dis Child* 1988;142:343.

135. Kanski JJ. Uveitis in juvenile chronic arthritis. *Eye* 1988;2:641.

136. Sherry DD, Mellins ED, Wedgewood RJ. Decreasing severity of chronic uveitis in children with pauciarticular arthritis. *Am J Dis Child* 1991;145:1026.

137. Chalom EC, Goldsmith DP, Koehler MA, et al. Prevalence and outcome of uveitis in a regional cohort of patients with juvenile rheumatoid arthritis. *J Rheumatol* 1997;24:2031.

138. Nguyen QD, Foster S. Saving the vision of children with juvenile rheumatoid arthritis-associated uveitis. *JAMA* 1998;280:1133.

139. American Academy of Pediatrics Section on Rheumatology and Section on Ophthalmology. Guidelines for ophthalmologic examinations in children with juvenile rheumatoid arthritis. *Pediatrics* 1993;92:295.

140. Olshaker JS, Jerrard DA. The erythrocyte sedimentation rate. *J Emerg Med* 1997;15:869.

141. Blane CE, Ragsdale CG, Hensinger RN. Late effects of JRA on the hip. *J Pediatr Orthop* 1987;7:677.

142. Olson L, Echerdal O, Hallonsten AL. Craniomandibular function in juvenile chronic arthritis. A clinical and radiographic study. *Swed Dent J* 1991;15:71.

143. Shore A, Ansell BM. Juvenile psoriatic arthritis—an analysis of 60 cases. *J Pediatr* 1982;100:529.

144. Southwood TR, Petty RE, Malleson PN, et al. Psoriatic arthritis in children. *Arthritis Rheum* 1989;32:1007

145. Roberton DM, Cabral DA, Malleson PN, et al. Juvenile psoriatic arthritis: followup and evaluation of diagnostic criteria. *J Rheumatol* 1996;23:166.

146. Wesolowska H. Clinical course of psoriatic arthropathy in children. *Mater Med Pol* 1985;55:185.

147. Rosenberg AM, Petty RE. A syndrome of seronegative enthesopathy and arthropathy in children. *Arthritis Rheum* 1982;25:1041.

148. Cabral DA, Oen KG, Petty RE. SEA syndrome revisited: a longterm followup of children with a syndrome of seronegative enthesopathy and arthropathy. *J Rheumatol* 1992;19:1282.

149. Gerster JC, Piccinin P. Enthesopathy of the heels in juvenile onset seronegative B-27 positive spondyloarthropathy. *J Rheumatol* 1984;12:310.

150. Ansell BM. Ankylosing spondylitis. In: Moll JMH, ed. *Juvenile spondylitis and related disorders*. Edinburgh: Churchill Livingstone, 1980:120.

151. Derhaag PJFM, Feltkamp TEW. Acute anterior uveitis and HLA-B27. *Inter Opth* 1990;14:19.

152. Rosenbaum JT. Acute anterior uveitis and spondyloarthropathies. *Rheum Dis Clin North Am* 1992;18:143.

153. Power WJ, Rodriguez A, Pedroza-Seres M, et al. Outcomes in anterior uveitis associated with the HLA-B27 haplotype. *Ophthalmology* 1998;105:1646.

154. Burgos-Vargas R, Vazquez-Mellado J. The early clinical recognition of juvenile-onset ankylosing spondylitis and its differentiation from juvenile rheumatoid arthritis. *Arthritis Rheum* 1995;38:835.

155. Burgos-Vargas R, Petty RE. Juvenile ankylosing spondylitis. *Rheum Dis Clin North Am* 1992;18:123.

156. Macrae IF, Wright V. Measurement of back movement. *Ann Rheum Dis* 1969;28:584.

157. Burgos-Vargas R. Spondyloarthropathies and psoriatic arthritis in children. *Curr Opin Rheum* 1993;5:634.

158. Garcia-Morteo O, Maldonado-Cocco JA, Suarez-Almazor ME, et al. Ankylosing spondylitis of juvenile onset: comparison with adult onset disease. *Scand J Rheumatol* 1983;12:246.

159. Calin A, Elswood J. The natural history of juvenile-onset ankylosing spondylitis: a 24-year retrospective case-control study. *Br J Rheumatol* 1988;27:91.

160. Marks SH, Barnett M, Calin A. A case-control study of juvenile- and adult-onset ankylosing spondylitis. *J Rheumatol* 1982;9:739.

161. Farmer RG, Michener WM. Prognosis of Crohn's disease with onset in childhood and adolescence. *Dig Dis Sci* 1979;24:752.

162. Lindsley C, Schaller J. Arthritis associated with inflammatory bowel disease in children. *J Pediatr* 1974;84:16.

163. Hamilton JR, Bruce MD, Abdourhamam M. Inflammatory bowel disease in children and adolescents. *Adv Pediatr* 1979;26:311.

Radiologic Findings in JIA

164. Vogel LC, Lubicky JP, Cervical spine fusion: not protective of cervical spine injury and tetraplegia. *Am J Orthop* 1997;26:636.

165. Ladd JR, Cassidy JT, Martel W. Juvenile ankylosing spondylitis. *Arthritis Rheum* 1971;14:579.

Treatment of JIA

166. Vane JR. Inhibition of prostaglandin synthesis as a mechanism of action for aspirin-like drugs. *Nat New Biol* 1971;231:232.

167. Vane J. Towards a better aspirin. *Nature* 1994;367:215.

168. Lovell D, Giannini E, Brewer E. Time course of response to nonsteroidal anti-inflammatory drugs in patients with juvenile rheumatoid arthritis. *Arthritis Rheum* 1984;27:1433.

169. Lindsley C. Uses of nonsteroidal anti-inflammatory drugs in pediatrics. *Am J Dis Child* 1993;147:229.

170. Mulberg AE, Linz C, Bern E, et al. Identification of nonsteroidal antiinflammatory drug-induced gastroduodenal injury in children with juvenile rheumatoid arthritis. *J Pediatr* 1993;122:647.

171. Giannini EH, Cawkwell GD. Drug treatment in children with juvenile rheumatoid arthritis. Past, present, and future. *Pediatr Clin North Am* 1995;42:1099.

172. Huppertz HI, Tschammler A, Horwitz AE, et al. Intraarticular corticosteroids for chronic arthritis in children: efficacy and effects on cartilage and growth. *J Pediatr* 1995;127:317.

173. Padeh S, Passwell JH. Intraarticular corticosteroid injection in the management of children with chronic arthritis. *Arthritis Rheum* 1998;41:1210.

174. Giannini EH, Brewer EJ, Kuzmina N, et al. Methotrexate in resistant juvenile rheumatoid arthritis. Results of the U.S.A.-U.S.S.R. double-blind, placebo-controlled trial. *N Engl J Med* 1992;326:1043.

175. Woo P, Wilkes H, Southwood T, et al. Low dose methotrexate is effective in extended oligoarticular arthritis but not in systemic arthritis of children. *Arthritis Rheum* 1997:40:S47.

176. Ravelli A, Viola S, Ramenghi B, et al. Radiologic progression in patients with juvenile chronic arthritis treated with methotrexate. *J Pediatr* 1998;133:262.

177. Weiss AH, Wallace CA, Sherry DD. Methotrexate for resistant chronic uveitis in children with juvenile rheumatoid arthritis. *J Pediatr* 1998;133:266.

178. Wallace CA, Sherry DD. A practical approach to avoidance of methotrexate toxicity. *J Rheumatol* 1995;22:1009.

179. Hashkes PJ, Balistreri WF, Bove KE, et al. The long-term effect of methotrexate therapy on the liver in patients with juvenile rheumatoid arthritis. *Arthritis Rheum* 1997;40:2226.

180. Kugathasan S, Newman AJ, Dahms BB, et al. Liver biopsy

findings in patients with juvenile rheumatoid arthritis receiving long-term, weekly methotrexate therapy. *J Pediatr* 1996;128:149.

181. Hashkes PJ, Balistreri WF, Bove KE, et al. The relationship of hepatotoxic risk factors and liver histology in methotrexate therapy for juvenile rheumatoid arthritis. *J Pediatr* 1999;131:47.

182. Kremer JM, Alarcon GS, Lightfoot RW, et al. Methotrexate for rheumatoid arthritis. Suggested guidelines for monitoring liver toxicity. *Arthritis Rheum* 1994;37:316.

183. Huang JL, Chen LC. Sulphasalazine in the treatment of children with chronic arthritis. *Clin Rheumatol* 1998;17:359.

184. Imundo LF, Jacobs JC. Sulfasalazine therapy for juvenile rheumatoid arthritis. *J Rheum* 1996;23:360.

185. van Rossum MA, et al. Sulfasalazine in the treatment of juvenile chronic arthritis: a randomized, double-blind, placebo-controlled, multicenter study. Dutch Juvenile Chronic Arthritis Study Group. *Arthritis Rheum* 1998;41:808.

186. Ansell BM, Hall MA, Loftus JK, et al. A multicenter pilot study of sulphasalazine in juvenile chronic arthritis. *Clin Exp Rheumatol* 1991;9:201.

187. Hertzberger-ten Cate R, Cats A. Toxicity of sulfasalazine in systemic juvenile chronic arthritis. *Clin Exp Rheumatol* 1991;9:85.

188. Eyring EJ, Longert A, Bass J. Synovectomy in juvenile rheumatoid arthritis. *J Bone Joint Surg Am* 1971;53:638.

189. Granberry WM, Brewer EJJ. Results of synovectomy in children with rheumatoid arthritis. *Clin Orthop* 1974;101:120.

190. Larsen EH, Reiman I, Revig O. Synovectomy in infantile arthritis. Proceedings of the British Orthopaedic Association. *J Bone Joint Surg Br* 1968;50:221.

191. McMaster M. Synovectomy of the knee in juvenile rheumatoid arthritis. *J Bone Joint Surg Br* 1972;54:263.

192. Mogensen B, Brattstrom H, Ekelund L, et al. Synovectomy of the hip in juvenile chronic arthritis. *J Bone Joint Surg Br* 1982;64:295.

193. Rydholm U, Elborgh R, Ranstam J, et al. Synovectomy of the knee in juvenile chronic arthritis. A retrospective consecutive follow-up study. *J Bone Joint Surg Br* 1986;68:223.

194. Kampner S, Ferguson AB. Efficacy of synovectomy in juvenile rheumatoid arthritis. *Clin Orthop* 1972;88:94.

195. Jacobsen ST, Levinson JE, Crawford AH. Late results of synovectomy in juvenile rheumatoid arthritis. *J Bone Joint Surg Am* 1985;67:8.

196. Kvien TK, Pahle JA, Hoyeraal HM. Comparison of synovectomy and no synovectomy in patients with juvenile rheumatoid arthritis. A 24-month controlled study. *Scand J Rheumatol* 1987;16:81.

197. Ansell BM. The management of chronic arthritis of children. *J Bone Joint Surg Br* 1983;65:536.

198. Rydholm U, Brattstrom H, Lidgren L. Soft tissue release for knee flexion contracture in juvenile chronic arthritis. *J Pediatr Orthop* 1986;6:448.

199. Swann M, Ansell BM. Soft-tissue release of the hips in children with juvenile chronic arthritis. *J Bone Joint Surg Br* 1986;68:404.

200. Sammarco GJ, Tablante EB. Subtalar arthrodesis. *Clin Orthop Rel Res* 1998;349:73.

201. Hensinger RN, Devito PD, Ragsdale CG. Changes in the cervical spine in juvenile rheumatoid arthritis. *J Bone Joint Surg Am* 1986;68:189.

202. Fried JA, Athreya B, Gregg JR. The cervical spine in juvenile rheumatoid arthritis. *Clin Orthop* 1983;179:102.

203. Swann M. Juvenile chronic arthritis. *Clin Orthop* 1987;219:38.

204. Mink van der Molen AB, Hall MA, Evans DM. Ulnar lengthening in juvenile chronic arthritis. *J Hand Surg Br* 1998;23:438.

205. Rydholm U, Brattstrom H, Bylander B, et al. Stapling of the knee in juvenile chronic arthritis. *J Pediatr Orthop* 1987;7:63.

206. Simon S, Whiffen J, Shapiro F. Leg-length discrepancies in monoarticular and pauciarticular juvenile rheumatoid arthritis. *J Bone Joint Surg Am* 1981;63:209.

207. Moseley CF. A straight line graph for leg length discrepancies. *J Bone Joint Surg Am* 1977;59:174.

208. Chmell MJ, Scott RD, Thomas WH, et al. Total hip arthroplasty with cement for juvenile rheumatoid arthritis. Results at a minimum of ten years in patients less than thirty years old. *J Bone Joint Surg Am* 1997;79:44.

209. Witt JD, Swann M, Ansell BM. Total hip replacement for juvenile chronic arthritis. *J Bone Joint Surg Br* 1991;73:770.

210. Kumar MN, Swann M. Uncemented total hip arthroplasty in young patients with juvenile chronic arthritis. *Ann Royal Col Surg Eng* 1998;80:203.

211. Haber D, Goodman SB. Total hip arthroplasty in juvenile chronic arthritis: a consecutive series. *J Arthroplasty* 1998;13:259.

212. Carmichael E, Chaplin DM. Total knee arthroplasty in juvenile rheumatoid arthritis. A seven-year follow-up study. *Clin Orthop* 1986;210:192.

213. Sarokhan AJ, Scott RD, Thomas WH, et al. Total knee arthroplasty in juvenile rheumatoid arthritis. *J Bone Joint Surg Am* 1983;65:1071.

214. Stuart MJ, Rand JA. Total knee arthroplasty in young adults who have rheumatoid arthritis. *J Bone Joint Surg Am* 1988;70:84.

215. Dalury DF, Ewald FC, Christie MJ, et al. Total knee arthroplasty in a group of patients less than 45 years of age. *J Arthroplasty* 1995;10:598.

216. Boublik M, Tsahakis PJ, Scott RD. Cementless total knee arthroplasty in juvenile onset rheumatoid arthritis. *Clin Orthop* 1993;286:88.

217. Connor PM, Morrey BF. Total elbow arthroplasty in patients who have juvenile rheumatoid arthritis. *J Bone Joint Surg Am* 1998;80:678.

218. Stewart MPM, Kelly IG. Total shoulder replacement in rheumatoid disease. *J Bone Joint Surg Br* 1997;79:68.

219. Thomas BJ, Amstuz HC, Cracchiolo A. Shoulder arthroplasty for rheumatoid arthritis. *Clin Orthop* 1990;265:125.

Lovell & Winter's Pediatric Orthopaedics, fifth edition, edited by Raymond T. Morrissy and Stuart L. Weinstein.
Lippincott Williams & Wilkins, Philadelphia © 2000

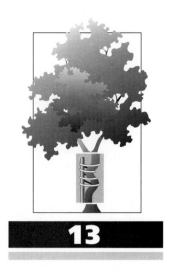

BONE AND JOINT SEPSIS

RAYMOND T. MORRISSY

BONE AND JOINT INFECTION

Bone and joint sepsis is a relatively common disorder in the pediatric population. This makes it likely that all orthopaedic surgeons will be faced with the problems inherent in the diagnosis and treatment of these disorders. If diagnosis was always easy this would be of little concern, but bone and joint sepsis in childhood is characterized by protean manifestations. The infant may only appear to be septic. The cause of the limp may not be obvious. The bone changes may resemble a tumor. The joint swelling may be due to an acute onset of juvenile rheumatoid arthritis (JRA).

After diagnosis, other problems remain. What antibiotic is correct for use before culture results are known? What should be done if the cultures are negative? What is the best way to administer the antibiotic, and for how long? When is surgery indicated? The diversity of organisms, the variety

R. T. Morrissy: Chief, Department of Orthopaedics, Children's Healthcare of Atlanta at Scottish Rite; Emory University, Atlanta, Georgia 30342.

of locations where infection is possible, and the numerous conditions associated with bone and joint sepsis increase the difficulty.

Definition

Osteomyelitis is an inflammation of the bone, and arthritis is an inflammation of the joint. Although it is assumed that osteomyelitis and septic arthritis are caused by bacteria, in certain cases the bacteria cannot be isolated, making it necessary to develop criteria that establish the diagnosis in the absence of a bacteria. A useful definition of osteomyelitis is proposed by Peltola and Vahvanen (1). They consider the diagnosis to be firm when two of the following four criteria are present: pus aspirated from bone; positive bone or blood culture; classic symptoms of localized pain, swelling, warmth, and limited range of motion (ROM) of the adjacent joint; and radiographic changes typical of osteomyelitis. Another useful classification is that proposed by Morey and Peterson (2) in which the diagnosis is considered to be definite, when an organism is isolated from the bone or adjacent soft tissue, or there is histologic evidence of osteomyelitis; probable, when there is a positive blood culture, in addition to clinical and roentgenographic features of osteomyelitis; or likely, when there are typical clinical findings in addition to definite roentgenographic evidence of osteomyelitis and a response to antibiotics.

Because so many patients with septic arthritis have negative cultures, it is important to use criteria that include those patients. Morey et al. included those patients with negative cultures when five of the following six criteria are present: temperature greater than 38.3°C, pain in the suspected joint that is made worse with motion, swelling of the suspected joint, systemic symptoms, absence of other pathologic processes, and a satisfactory response to antibiotics (3).

Epidemiology

Knowledge of the epidemiology of osteomyelitis and septic arthritis is derived from institutional studies and governmental morbidity data (4–6).

Osteomyelitis shows a clearly increased incidence in childhood, with a slight increase after 50 years of age. In contrast, the incidence of septic arthritis, although greatest in childhood, is markedly increased in the older age groups (7). In childhood, septic arthritis occurs about twice as often as osteomyelitis and tends to have its peak incidence in the early years of the first decade, whereas osteomyelitis has a peak incidence in the later years of the first decade. The disease is more common in males, and actually tends to increase with age through adolescence, according to hospital morbidity data (8).

There is an impression among clinicians, and in some institutional reports, of a seasonal variation in the incidence of acute hematogenous osteomyelitis (AHO). Gillespie (7) confirmed this, showing an increase in the early autumn and late summer, in both the Northern and Southern hemispheres.

Gillespie (7) has shown that incidence of AHO varies among races, with a higher incidence in New Zealand Maoris and Australian aboriginals than in children of European descent in these countries. At the same time, groups of similar ethnic background show differences in the incidence of AHO for which social or environmental factors may be responsible.

The idea that osteomyelitis is a changing disease is not new, and perhaps indicates that it is a disease that is capable of continuous change, depending on various circumstances. In the city of Glasgow, Scotland, the incidence of AHO in children younger than 13 years of age has dropped by more than 50%, due mainly to a decrease in long-bone infections. At the same time, the incidence of subacute infections increased from 12 to 42% during the period of study (4). Jones and colleagues (9) also suggest that the incidence of subacute osteomyelitis is increasing, while the incidence of acute AHO is decreasing. In a review of 60 patients having AHO between 1980 and 1985, 35% had subacute infection.

A study from Denmark, which reviewed 30 years' experience with bone and joint infection due to *Staphylococcus aureus*, found that although *S. aureus* bacteremia had increased over the last decade of the study (coinciding with an increase in hospital admissions), the prevalence of AHO in patients 1 to 20 years of age decreased. There was a significant increase in joint infections among patients between 1 and 20 years of age during a 4-year period in this decade. The investigators thought this likely to be due to a change in the type of *S. aureus* that was predominant during this period, illustrating the complex bacterial–host interaction (5).

In the 1970s, a change in the causative organism in septic arthritis was noted, with *Haemophilus influenzae* type B becoming the most common cause in children 1 and 4 years of age (5). The reason for this is not clear. Currently, *H. influenzae* has virtually disappeared as a cause of joint sepsis where the vaccine against *H. influenzae* has been administered (10). It has been replaced by *Kingella kingae* in the same age group. This is discussed later.

Etiology

Koch's postulates are the basis of the germ theory of infections:

- The organism must be identified at the site of the disease
- The organism must not be found in other diseases
- The organism must be able to produce the disease in other animals
- The organism must be identified in the disease that is produced (11).

Pasteur (12) failed to satisfy Koch postulates when he injected staphylococci intravenously into guinea pigs, as did many others after him. In attempting to produce hematogenous osteomyelitis, Rodet (13) was reportedly successful, but details in his report are sketchy. Others have reported variable success in producing hematogenous osteomyelitis (14).

The reproducible creation of a bone or joint infection requires some other intervention, usually something that has the potential to change the local environment. The standard model for the study of antibiotics for treatment of osteomyelitis involves the injection of sodium morrhuate directly into the bone to produce necrosis, followed by the injection of bacteria directly into the area (15).

Some of the earliest attempts to produce osteomyelitis in animals involved trauma to the bone, and many of these were reportedly successful. Trauma to the growth plate, followed by the intravenous injection of *S. aureus*, has produced an AHO that resembles the human form of the disease (16,17). These studies allow observations on the pathology of AHO.

How bacteria lodge in a bone or joint, then establish a clinical infection, cannot be completely explained. There are numerous bacteria in and on the body, and bacteremia is a daily event in childhood, giving ample opportunity for bacteria to gain access to the bones and joints (18). The answer lies in a better understanding of the factors that influence host resistance, of bacteria pathogenicity, and of factors that relate both—an exploration of which is beyond the scope of this chapter.

Among the factors that have been observed to be associated with infection, none is so common as trauma. The idea of trauma as a predisposing factor to infection is not new. As mentioned, it was one of the earliest methods in experimental efforts to produce AHO. The entire subject was summarized by Burrows (19) in 1932, when he popularized the term *locus minoris resistentiae,* to describe the effect injury had on decreasing resistance to infection. Clinically, trauma to the affected part is noted in 30 to 50% of those who have clinical AHO (20–24). Although there are no similar clinical data for septic arthritis, experimental models demonstrate the role of trauma in the production of the disease (25,26). The conclusion that may be drawn from the clinical and laboratory data is that trauma is not always essential for an infection to be established, but that it makes it easier in some circumstances.

Just as trauma is a factor, so is the function of the immune system. This is easily illustrated by the increased susceptibility to infections of all types in those patients with diseases characterized by deficient or altered immune function, and in the neonate with immature immune function.

More mysterious are those factors that may cause temporary and transient depression of immune function (e.g., intercurrent viral illness, anesthesia, surgery, trauma, and malnutrition); all are known to impair certain aspects of immune function, and have been related to an increased incidence of clinical infection.

Despite partial understanding of the interrelated factors

between host and bacteria, many aspects of AHO and septic arthritis in children remain unexplained; for example, the predilection for males, increased incidence of infection in the lower extremities, and peak age incidence.

Pathophysiology of Osteomyelitis

Bone is unique as a tissue and as an organ, not only for its rigid and variable structure, but also for its ability to heal and replace itself with entirely normal tissue without scar.

There are two types of cortical bone that are especially evident in childhood. That which is found in the metaphyseal region is little more than a compact version of cancellous bone. Its maze-like structure allows easy communication between the subperiosteal space and the medullary space. The cortical bone of the diaphysis is dense lamellar bone, which is relatively acellular. Consequently, it is impenetrable and renews itself more slowly. This structure is more obvious in the larger bones (Fig. 13-1A).

The cancellous bone that makes up the central part is also differentiated both by structure and function. The central cellular part, known as the medullary cavity, has little bone, but contains a rich reticuloendothelial system. The metaphyseal region has more bone structure, but is relatively acellular, containing few cells of the reticuloendothelial system. These differences are more pronounced in the long bones, particularly at the rapidly growing ends (Fig. 13-1A and B).

The periosteum of a child's bone is thick. Although it is easily separated from the bone, it is not easily penetrated by infection. Because its blood supply is from the outside, elevation from the bone does not impair function, and it continues to produce osteoid and bone. In children, this response of an elevated periosteum is often dramatic, producing a layer of bone around the original bone that is called the involucrum.

In a classic article, Hobo (27) described his experiments on the localization of both India ink particles and bacteria in bone after intravenous injection. He noted that, although most bacteria lodged in the medullary cavity, they were rapidly phagocytized, and no infection resulted. In the area beneath the epiphyseal plate, few bacteria lodged. These bacteria were not phagocytized, however, due to the absence of phagocytic cells in this region of the bone, and infection subsequently developed. Hobo thought that the vessels beneath the physeal plate were small arterial loops that emptied into venous sinusoids, and that the resulting turbulence was the cause of localization. However, electron microscopic studies have shown these to be small terminal branches (28). In addition, it has been demonstrated that the endothelial wall of new metaphyseal capillaries have gaps that allow the passage of blood cells and presumably, bacteria (29).

How and why bacteria lodge in the area beneath the epiphyseal plate and establish an infection in this region, is poorly understood. In closed experiments with trauma as a model, infection did not develop in fractures of the

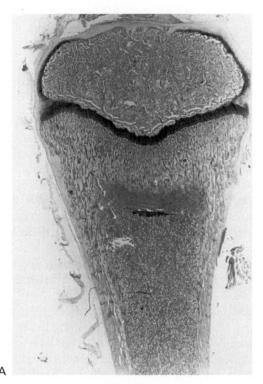
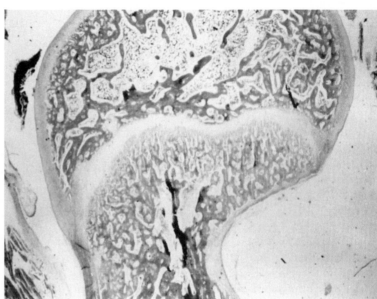

FIGURE 13-1. Proximal tibia (**A**) and proximal radius (**B**) of a 6-week-old rabbit, demonstrating the difference in the cortical bone between the metaphysis and the diaphysis. The diaphyseal cortex is composed of thick, relatively acellular bone, whereas the metaphyseal cortex is a condensation of the spongy metaphyseal bone. Also note the difference in the cellularity between the metaphyseal and the diaphyseal areas. The size of this metaphyseal area, separating the cellular marrow from the area beneath the epiphyseal plate, is different in the rapidly growing bones, such as the proximal tibia, than in the slow-growing bones, such as the proximal radius.

diaphysis of the fibula, or in the uninjured metaphysis of the tibia, but developed in the injured metaphysis (16,17). Thus, bacterial seeding of a hematoma cannot be the explanation. It is possible that specific bacteria–substrate interactions play a role (e.g., those that occur for the localization of certain bacteria in the nasopharynx or on damaged heart valves). This is illustrated in experiments with mice which suggest that substrate production by certain strains of *S. aureus* was related to their ability to lodge in the bone following intravenous administration (30). Possibly, the injury to the unique physeal plate cartilage produces a new substrate that is attractive to certain bacteria—specifically, those that cause AHO. There are numerous other as yet unexplored possibilities.

Trueta (31) was the first to note the importance of the changing anatomy of the interosseous blood supply with age. In the infant, before the ossific nucleus is formed, the vessels from the metaphysis penetrate directly into the cartilaginous anlage of the epiphysis (Fig. 13-2A). As the ossific nucleus develops, a separate blood supply to this epiphysis develops, and the metaphyseal vessels crossing the developing physeal plate disappear (Fig. 13-2B). The change is signaled by the development of the ossification of the epi-

physis, and is generally complete with the distinct formation of a physeal plate (Fig. 13-2C).

Because of this blood supply pattern in the infant, the initial bacterial localization is in the cartilaginous precursor of the epiphysis. Infection results in its early destruction, with the consequent alteration of future growth. When the physeal plate is formed, it provides a temporary barrier to the spread of infection into the epiphysis because the vessels end beneath the plate.

A unique characteristic of hematogenous osteomyelitis is its predilection for the most rapidly growing end of the large long bones, especially those of the lower extremity. This may be explained by the observation that in rapidly growing bones the phagocytic cells are further from where the bacteria localize, because of the structure of these bones (Fig. 13-1A,B). Thus, the inflammatory response takes longer to reach the bacteria, allowing a clinical infection to become established.

Bone formation and resorption are integrally linked. Diseases that result in net bone loss may be viewed as being processes that alter this linkage. The earliest change observed in osteomyelitis is the death of the osteoblasts, followed by resorption of the bony trabeculae by numerous osteoclasts

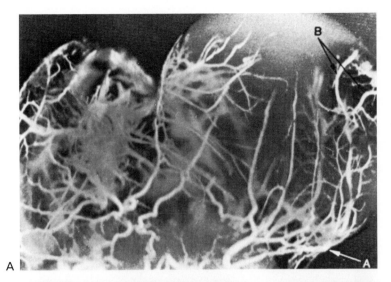

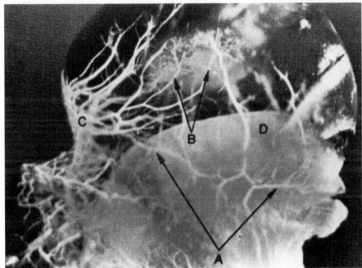

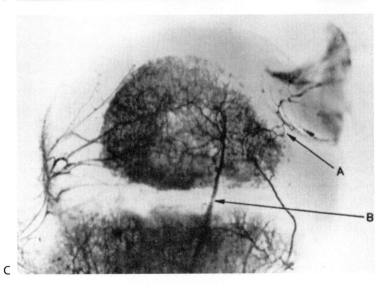

FIGURE 13-2. Human specimens of the proximal femur, which are injected with barium sulfate, demonstrate the changing blood supply to the developing femoral head with growth. **A:** In the 3-day-old infant, the vessels proceed directly from the metaphysis into the cartilaginous precursor of the femoral head. *B* represents two arteries penetrating from the ligamentum teres. **B:** By 9 months of age, separate vessels have developed to supply the ossifying nucleus of the femoral head. *A* represents a subsynovial ring that is intracapsular. *B* illustrates the separate vessels, which have developed to supply the ossific nucleus. These arteries in turn come from the ascending cervical arteries, which cross the periphery of the epiphysis (*C*). **C:** At 3 years, 4 months of age, the vessels crossing from the metaphysis have disappeared. Only peripheral vessels remain to supply the epiphysis. The supply from the ligamentum teres (*A*) is decreasing. The vessel *B* is actually a branch of the anterior cervical artery, which enters at the periphery, as seen on other views of the same specimen. (From ref. 182, with permission.)

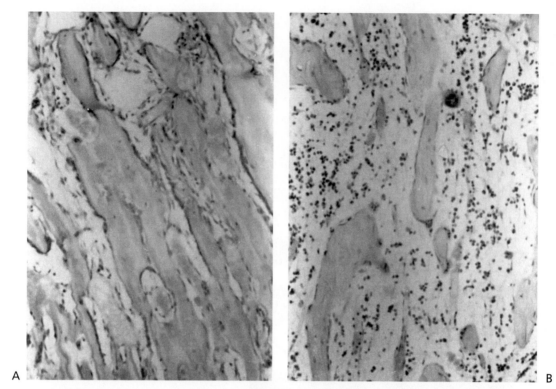

FIGURE 13-3. A: A photomicrograph of the proximal tibial metaphysis of a 6-week-old rabbit demonstrates trabecular bone lined with osteoblasts. **B:** Twenty-four hours after induction of experimental hematogenous osteomyelitis by injury to the physis and intravenous injection of *Staphylococcus aureus*, the osteoblasts have disappeared, and the trabeculae are being resorbed by osteoclasts.

(Fig. 13-3A and B). This occurs over a wide area of the metaphysis surrounding the infection, beginning within 12 to 18 h. In experimental situations, it has also been shown that lymphocytes may release an osteoclastic activating factor, whereas macrophages, monocytes, and vascular endothelial cells may all directly resorb both the crystalline and matrix components of bone.

Although the complete mechanism of this finding is yet to be elucidated, it is known that, in response to toxins and bacterial antigens, interleukin-1 is produced by macrophages and polymorphonuclear leukocytes (32). Interleukin-1 is known to cause most of the events known as inflammation, and to stimulate the production of prostaglandin E_2, which stimulates osteoclast bone resorption (33). In response to these stimuli, inflammatory cells accumulate and migrate to the area of bacterial localization beneath the physis. As these inflammatory cells migrate to the accumulating bacteria, the bone in the path of the migration is resorbed (Fig. 13-4A and B).

In response to products liberated by the increasing number of bacteria, as well as host factors, inflammatory cells begin to accumulate (34). Because there are few such cells in the area of bacterial localization beneath the physeal plate, this response begins in a region closer to the medullary

cavity. Over the next few days, this inflammatory response migrates to the area of the bacteria, and the bone in its path is resorbed (Fig. 13-5A). As the accumulation of pus continues, it finds egress through the maze-like cortex of the metaphysis (Fig. 13-5A). If the infection continues, a subperiosteal abscess forms, the periosteum is elevated, and new osteoid is formed under the elevated periosteum (Fig. 13-5B).

If the metaphysis lies within the joint, septic arthritis results early in the process, because the periosteum within the joint is thin, and the pus quickly ruptures through it. This occurs in four locations in the older child: proximal femur, proximal humerus, distal lateral tibia, and proximal radius. As the periosteum is elevated, the cortical bone is deprived of its blood supply, and may become necrotic, forming a sequestrum. Because the blood supply to the periosteum comes from the muscle side, it remains healthy, and begins to lay down new bone, known as the involucrum.

It is important to note that the pus does not usually spread down the medullary cavity, because it is successfully walled off by the inflammatory response (Fig. 13-5B). Contrary to how it may first appear, in the presence of a healthy inflammatory response the path of least resistance is through the metaphyseal cortex. The spread of pus into the medul-

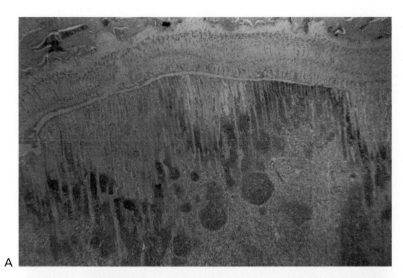

A

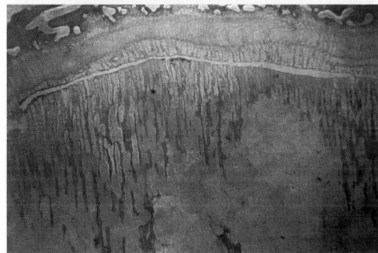

B

FIGURE 13-4. A: In a hematoxylin and eosin-stained specimen of a 3-day-old hematogenous infection in the proximal tibia of a rabbit, the accumulation of inflammatory cells and microabscesses can be seen. **B:** In an adjacent Gram-stained section, the remaining bony and cartilaginous columns and microabscesses can be seen. In addition, small clumps of organisms can be seen beneath the physis.

lary cavity is seen either in a neglected case or in a patient whose immunity is impaired.

Pathophysiology of Septic Arthritis

As in bone, the unique anatomic features of a joint should be considered in relation to infection. The synovial lining of the joint is a unique and vascular tissue that does not have a basement membrane. It secretes a fluid that is essentially a transudate of serum. The remainder of the joint surface is avascular cartilage. The interior of the joint provides a unique environment for bacterial proliferation, similar to a culture tube.

It is probable that the transient bacteremia experienced by children results in bacteria entering the joint. It has been demonstrated that the joint has the ability to clear bacteria from itself, thus avoiding clinical infection (35). There are two important limitations to this ability: The mechanism is not so effective with pathogenic bacteria (e.g., *S. aureus*),

and there is a limit to the amount of bacteria that can be cleared.

Localization of bacteria in a joint is not so well understood as it is in bone. Although trauma has been implicated as being a factor (26), it may not completely explain the propensity for large joints and those of the lower extremity to be involved. What is apparent, however, is that bacteria are present not only in the synovium, but they also gain access to the joint cavity early in the process. Within a matter of hours, this is associated with a synovitis and fibrinous exudate, followed shortly by areas of synovial necrosis.

The mechanisms of cartilage destruction have been extensively studied in both bacterial and nonbacterial arthritis. Although the specific mechanisms of cartilage destruction may differ depending on the infecting organism, it is important that the clinician understand the biology of the process that she/he is attempting to alter.

A large variety of enzymes (e.g., proteases, peptidases, collagenases) are released from the leukocytes, the synovial

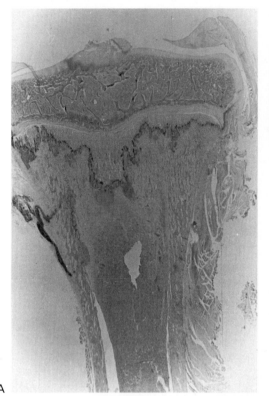
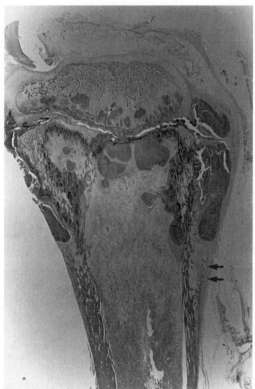

FIGURE 13-5. A: Rabbit's tibia with 3-day-old hematogenous osteomyelitis. A small amount of pus has found its way through the metaphyseal cortex into the subperiosteal space. **B:** Rabbit's tibia with 7-day-old infection. Note the well-developed intraosseous abscesses, in addition to the large subperiosteal abscess. New bone formation is occurring beneath the elevated periosteum (*arrows*). (From ref. 16, with permission.)

cells, and the cartilage. These enzymes are capable of degrading the matrix and the collagen of articular cartilage. In addition, organisms (e.g., *S. aureus*, several Gram-negative bacteria) liberate extracellular proteolytic enzymes (36–41).

These enzymes initiate the first measurable change in the articular cartilage, the loss of glycosaminoglycan. This can occur as early as 8 h in experimental models, and is not detectable by visual inspection (42). It renders the cartilage less stiff and perhaps subject to increased wear. Collagen destruction occurs later in the process, and is responsible for the visual changes that may be seen (43–45). It is important to understand that these destructive mechanisms do not require the continued presence of live organisms to be sustained.

DIAGNOSIS

History

Among the expected symptoms in any case of bone or joint sepsis, pain leads the list (46,47). This common symptom is not always verbalized by children. Thus, it is important

for the physician to realize that it may be expressed in many different ways: refusal to walk, refusal to bear weight, limping, or simple disuse of a part.

A careful history should do more than lead to a suspicion of infection. It should lead to the consideration of the possible organism and to any circumstances that may predispose to that organism, the duration of the infectious process, and the likely location of the process.

Although it is difficult to relate the stage of infection seen in experimental animals to the onset of clinical symptoms of a child, there seems to be a relatively close correlation, which suggests that symptoms begin shortly after the establishment of the inflammatory reaction in the bone or joint. The ease of access to expert medical care in some parts of the United States demonstrates this. It is no longer unusual to see children within 12 h of the onset of limp, who have only normal or mildly elevated laboratory values and a positive bacterial aspirate from the bone or joint.

A good clinical correlation is that pus is seldom found on aspiration of bone with fewer than 3 days of symptoms. The same is not true for joints, wherein elevated leukocyte counts are found in the joint fluid within 24 h of symptoms. This response is frequently blunted by the unintentional or ill-advised use of antibiotics before establishing the diagnosis of bone or joint infection. Thus, when recent antibiotic administration is a part of the history, care must be taken in interpreting each clinical symptom, sign, and laboratory value.

In the history, a careful search should be made for concomitant infections, recent infection, or reasons for lowered resistance to infection. A history of recent upper respiratory infection or other seemingly unrelated illness is frequent, and may explain an organism's access to the circulation. Recent rashes or swollen nodes are important for their association with diseases such as rheumatoid arthritis, Lyme arthritis, or leukemia.

Chickenpox is probably the most common childhood illness that produces a temporary suppression of immunity, leading to an increased incidence of skin infections, usually due to *S. aureus* and group A *Streptococcus*. This in turn leads to an increased opportunity for bone or joint infections with these organisms (48).

Trauma has been mentioned as a possible etiologic factor in both osteomyelitis and septic arthritis. Its importance in the history is twofold. First, it should be recognized that symptoms after trauma may not be due to trauma, particularly when they are more severe day-by-day or fail to improve as expected. Second, the history of trauma may successfully direct the search for the location in children too young to communicate.

Examination

The entire purpose of the examination is to search for signs of infection and to localize the process. The typical child who is seen in the first 3 to 4 days of osteomyelitis or septic arthritis may appear unhappy and out of sorts, but rarely appears to be ill or moribund, as has often been described. Fever is not a consistent accompaniment of what would seem to be such a serious infection (46,47). Children with subacute osteomyelitis may remain relatively active, favoring only the affected part, and showing no systemic symptoms of infection.

Because most cases of AHO and septic arthritis involve the lower extremities, a common finding is limp. This usually is an antalgic limp, defined by a shortened stance phase on the affected leg. Failure to use an upper extremity in the usual manner, or discomfort noted by the parent in dressing the child, are common symptoms in the upper extremity.

Swelling and erythema, cardinal signs of infection, are of value early in the process only in bones that are not covered by muscles and in joints that are easily palpated. Loss of normal concavities and loss of normal skin wrinkles may be the only subtle clues. Visual comparison of the normal and affected limb, symmetrically positioned, should always be done.

After the affected part is identified by limp or disuse, palpation of the bones and joints is used to identify the specific location of the inflammation. In the case of small children who cry at the mere presence of a stranger and panic at being touched, it is often beneficial to instruct the parent how to elicit the tender area. After showing the parent how to palpate the area, the physician should leave the room and allow the parent to first examine the unaffected, then the affected part, and report the results.

Joints are more effectively examined by ROM than tenderness, although palpation of those joints that are not covered by muscle may reveal both the presence of an effusion, and tenderness. Involvement of large joints covered by large amounts of tissue is detected by a decreased ROM. In the axial skeleton, such as the spine and the sacroiliac (SI) region, percussion and compression, respectively, are more effective in eliciting symptoms than is palpation.

An infected joint usually has neither full flexion nor extension, and may be painful through anything but a small ROM. In the case of the hip, internal rotation, abduction, and extension, all of which tighten the hip capsule, are painful and limited.

Laboratory

The leukocyte count is not a reliable indication of inflammation in its early stages, and when normal, often leads the physician away from the correct diagnosis of sepsis. In a series from the Mayo clinic, only 25% of infants and children with osteomyelitis had a leukocyte count above normal for their age, and only in 65% was the differential count abnormal (2). The results were similar for a series of patients from the same institution with septic arthritis (3). This has been confirmed in other series (20,46,47).

The most useful laboratory tests used in the diagnosis of bone or joint sepsis are those that measure the acute phase response. These responses are discussed in recent review articles (49,50). This acute phase response is actually the increase or decrease in a variety of plasma proteins, in response to cytokine production secondary to acute or chronic inflammation. In addition to being responsible for many of the systemic symptoms seen in infection, e.g., fever, anorexia, lethargy, and anemia, an increase of many of these proteins can be measured in the blood. The two most common tests to measure the acute phase response today are the C-reactive protein (CRP) and the erythrocyte sedimentation rate (ESR). There is evidence that this acute phase response may differ in different inflammatory conditions. For example, CRP will be elevated in trauma whereas the ESR will not.

The ESR is one of the nonspecific acute-phase reactants found in the serum in response to inflammation. The test measures the rate at which the erythrocytes fall through plasma, and is dependent mostly on the concentration of fibrinogen. However, the result can be greatly affected by the size, shape, and number of erythrocytes present, as well as other proteins in the plasma. The ESR is unreliable in the neonate, in the presence of significant anemia, in patients with sickle cell disease, or when the patient is taking steroids.

The ESR is almost always elevated within 48 to 72 h of the onset of infection, and returns to normal over a period of 2 to 4 weeks after elimination of the infection. The ESR is less reliable in the first 48 h of the infection than after 48 h. In the Mayo clinic series, the ESR was below 20 mm/hr in only 5 of 76 patients with septic arthritis (3). It appears that an elevated ESR can be anticipated in about 90% of cases that subsequently prove to be AHO (46,47). Although noted to be elevated just as often in patients with osteomyelitis, the ESR was significantly higher in those with septic arthritis (3). Those authors did not find the value of the ESR diminished by previous antibiotic therapy.

An additional problem in the clinical usefulness of the ESR is that it continues to rise for 3 to 5 days after institution of successful therapy. Although a continuing rise beyond the fourth to fifth day of treatment is an indication of failure to eradicate the infection, it is because of this delayed response that the ESR is not a good means of assessing the resolution of sepsis during the first week of treatment (51).

The CRP is a substance found in the serum in response to inflammation and trauma. The CRP may begin to rise within 6 h of the triggering stimulus, then increases several hundred-fold, reaching a peak within 36–50 h. Because of the short half-life of the protein (47 h), it will also fall quickly to normal with successful treatment, in contrast to the ESR. This makes the CRP of greater value than the ESR, not only for earlier diagnosis of infection, but also for determining resolution of the inflammation (52).

One report comparing serial determinations of ESR and CRP in 44 children with proved bacteriologic osteomyelitis demonstrated the ESR to be elevated initially in 92% of the patients, and the CRP to be elevated in 98% (53). The peak ESR was measured on days 3 through 5, whereas the peak CRP was measured on day 2. Thereafter, it took the ESR about 3 weeks to return to normal, whereas the CRP returned to normal within 1 week. Thus, the CRP is more likely to be helpful in diagnosing the early case of infection, and is more useful after its resolution.

The question is often raised as to whether or not the CRP is useful in separating a musculoskeletal infection from an otitis media, which is commonly seen in children. Elevated CRP values are reported in 22% of those with a bacteria otitis media, and 65% of those with a viral otitis media (54). Thus, it would seem that an elevated CRP may be due to otitis media.

Blood cultures are indispensable, because they frequently demonstrate the organism. In most series, the yield from blood culture ranges between 30 and 50% in both septic arthritis and osteomyelitis (47). The yield from both blood culture and aspirated material decreases with previous antibiotic therapy (3). Even with previous antibiotic treatment,

however, the chances of obtaining positive cultures, when all sources (blood, bone, and joint fluid) are cultured, remain high (47).

The importance of needle aspiration of the bone or direct biopsy at the time of surgery, before antibiotic administration, is emphasized by the frequency with which positive cultures are obtained. In 91 aspirations of bone for osteomyelitis, pus was obtained in 58%, and positive cultures were obtained in 70% of these aspirates, yielding 40 positive cultures from all aspirates (47). In other series, the yield of positive cultures from bone has been even higher, ranging from 51 to 73% (46,51).

Aspiration of joint fluid provides the opportunity to gather more information than does bone aspiration. The question, however, is which tests, in addition to the culture and Gram stain, are worthwhile. The answer appears to be that only the leukocyte count and the percentage of polymorphonuclear cells are of value (55,56). Because fluid from an infected joint frequently clots, it may be helpful to rinse the syringe with heparin before aspirating the joint. Because only a small amount of fluid may be obtained, care must be taken not to leave any significant volume of heparin in the syringe, which may alter the cell count.

Although it is generally assumed that septic joints have a leukocyte count from 80,000/mL to more than 100,000/mL, and other inflammatory disorders in the differential diagnosis have counts of 50,000/mL and less, there is considerable overlap (Table 13-1). In a series of 126 bacteriologically proved cases of septic arthritis, Fink and Nelson (55) found leukocyte counts of 50,000 mL or less in 55%, with 34% having counts less than 25,000/mL. Only 44% of the patients had counts of 100,000/mL. At the same time, inflammatory diseases (e.g., rheumatoid arthritis) may have counts in excess of 80,000/mL (58).

As in osteomyelitis, the frequency of positive cultures seems to be slightly higher with open biopsy than with needle biopsy, but the difference is not great. In addition,

TABLE 13-1. SYNOVIAL FLUID ANALYSIS

Disease	Leukocytes*	Polymorphs* (%)
Normal	<200	<25
Traumatic	<5,000 with many erythrocytes	<25
Toxic synovitis	5,000–15,000	<25
Acute rheumatic fever	10,000–15,000	50
Juvenile rheumatoid arthritis	15,000–80,000	75
Septic arthritis	>80,000	>75

* The leukocyte count and percentage of polymorphs can vary in most diseases, depending on the severity and duration of the process. Overlap greater than shown in these averages is possible. (From ref. 57, with permission.)

the positive yields are generally not as high as in osteomyelitis, ranging in various reports from 36 to 80% (46,51,59).

The importance of obtaining material from blood and bone or joint aspiration is emphasized in a report by Vaughan and colleagues (60), in which many children with osteomyelitis had only positive blood cultures, whereas others had only positive bone cultures.

Gram staining is the only opportunity for presumptive identification of the organism within a few hours of initial patient contact, and is thus a valuable test that should not be ignored. It appears from reports of both septic arthritis and osteomyelitis that the Gram stain demonstrates an organism in about one-third of the bone or joint aspirates (46,47,55).

Certain bacteria growing in the body release their type-specific polysaccharide capsule into the circulation. Detection of this antigen, by either counterimmunoelectrophoresis or cold agglutination tests, can provide presumptive evidence for the organism (61,62). The release of this antigen does not depend on the presence of live organisms. Therefore, this test has the potential of rapid identification of the organism, and may be especially useful in patients who have received previous antibiotics. However, the yield from this test has been low, and it is not used in the diagnosis of bone or joint sepsis.

Offering promise for the future are molecular diagnostic tests to identify the presence of bacteria, along with the species and its sensitivities. These tests rely on the identification of specific DNA and RNA in the samples. The tests can be performed in an hour (rather than a day or more) for positive cultures. They also have the theoretical advantage of identifying the organism even if treatment with antibiotics has begun, since they do not depend on live bacteria for culture. However, to date these tests have not proven specific or sensitive enough for reliable clinical use (63).

Imaging

The imaging of musculoskeletal sepsis is discussed in more detail in Chapter 3.

Plain Radiographs

Deep soft tissue swelling is the earliest radiographic evidence of osteomyelitis (64). The role of radiography in the diagnosis of early bone and joint sepsis is often undervalued. This is because it is often considered only to seek changes in the bone, which in osteomyelitis may not occur for at least 5 to 7 days after the onset of symptoms. Radiographs are a two-dimensional representation of density difference, and as such, can detect changes in the soft tissues as well as in the bone. Because the inflammation in the bone or joint produces edema in the soft tissues adjacent to the area of inflammation, there is swelling in this region, with enlargement of this muscle layer detectable on the radiograph. In addition, the edema obliterates the normal fat planes that can be seen between the muscle layers. All of this can be detected with routine radiographs if they are properly obtained.

Detection of deep soft tissue swelling and loss of normal fat planes depends on comparison of one limb with the other. Therefore, radiographs of symmetrically positioned views of both limbs should be ordered, using a technique to demonstrate the soft tissues (Fig. 13-6).

Radiographs to detect deep soft tissue swelling are of most value in suspected sepsis of the long bones. The technique becomes less useful in the axial skeleton, because of the large overlapping muscles. An additional problem in interpretation occurs around the hip. In this location, the normal external rotation and abduction position assumed by the irritable hip (regardless of the cause) causes the appearance of capsular bulging (65). Another sign that is often

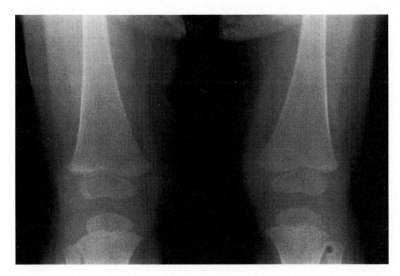

FIGURE 13-6. Plain radiograph of a 16-month-old toddler with a 36-h history of increasing difficulty bearing weight and pain in the region of the left knee. Note the deep soft tissue swelling about the medial side of the distal left femur. Deep soft tissue swelling is the earliest finding in osteomyelitis.

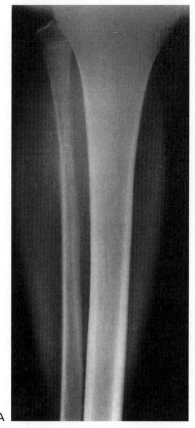

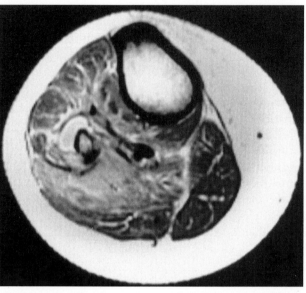

FIGURE 13-7. A: Radiograph of the leg of a 14-year-old boy who presented with swelling and pain for the past 6 weeks. He related the onset to twisting his leg when he fell into a hole. Is this osteomyelitis or tumor? Note the deep soft tissue swelling, the bone destruction, and the periosteal new bone around the fibula. **B:** The magnetic resonance imaging scan demonstrated bone destruction, fluid in one area around the fibula, and extensive edema in the surrounding muscles, all of which suggest that osteomyelitis is more likely. The fibula was biopsied as though the lesion were malignant. Pus and Gram-positive staphylococci were identified.

sought in suspected sepsis of the hip joint is joint space widening. Although this may be seen frequently in the neonate, it is often lacking in older children. It is a late sign, and its absence is not to be interpreted as lack of sepsis (66).

The more classic radiographic signs of osteomyelitis—resorption of bone and periosteal new bone formation—are easily recognized. The forms that the bone destruction can take are myriad, however, and particularly in children, can be confused with bone neoplasms (67–69). This is another point that illustrates the importance of a definitive tissue or bacteriologic diagnosis before treatment can be confidently pursued (Fig. 13-7).

Bone Scan

Radionuclide scanning of the skeleton is done with three different radiopharmaceuticals: technetium 99m (99mTc) diphosphonate, gallium 67 citrate, and indium 111. Because of 99mTc diphosphonate's high diagnostic accuracy, easy availability, relatively low cost compared with other

methods, and rapidity, it is the clear choice for detecting physiologic alterations in the skeletal tissues of children. Bone scintigraphy is discussed in more detail in Chapter 3.

There are several facts about bone scintigraphy that the orthopaedist needs to understand and evaluate. First is the mechanism of isotope uptake. Isotope uptake depends on both vascularity and calcium phosphate deposition (70). Isotope uptake is greater, the newer the calcium phosphate deposition. Second, the bone scan consists of three phases: an angiogram, performed immediately after injection; immediately followed by the second or "blood pool" phase; and 2 to 3 h later, the mineral phase, which reflects uptake in the bone. All three phases are helpful, especially in distinguishing cellulitis from osteomyelitis. Third, the quality of the bone scan should be evaluated. The bladder should be empty, so that accumulated isotope does not obstruct the sacrum. It is important that symmetrically positioned views of both sides be obtained. In children, it is important that pinhole or converging-collimator images be obtained of suspected areas of infection. Because most AHO occurs in the metaphysis adjacent to the physeal plate, such views are necessary to separate early metaphyseal changes from the large amount of uptake found in the physeal plate (Fig. 13-8A and B). Because these images are time-consuming to obtain and may require that the child be sedated, it is important that the physician communicate the desired areas of interest to the radiologist.

The value of radionuclide scans differs in children with suspected bone or joint sepsis, depending on the diagnosis. In a large series of 280 patients referred with a clinical diagnosis of osteomyelitis, the scan correctly identified osteomyelitis at 55 of 62 sites of proved osteomyelitis in the appendicular skeleton (71). This report demonstrated a sensitivity of 89% and a specificity of 94%, with an overall accuracy of 92% for this method. Considering differences in populations and methodologies, these results are not too different from other reports in the literature.

The accepted criterion for diagnosis of septic arthritis on radionuclide scan is equally increased uptake on both sides of the joint. The interpretation is not so simple in practice. Compared with osteomyelitis, the diagnosis of septic arthritis presents a different problem: Although the scan may correctly identify the site of joint sepsis in about 90% of infected joints, it does not accurately separate bone from joint sepsis, nor differentiate infectious from noninfectious arthritis (71,72). This is a particular problem in the hip, in which the differential diagnoses may include transient synovitis, septic arthritis, or osteomyelitis of the femoral neck.

Not all positive scans indicate infection, and because skeletal scintigraphy is interpreted, it suggests that many factors need to be included if the scan is to be helpful (73,74). Foremost among these factors is that the scan should be interpreted in the context of the clinical facts. This was illustrated by McCoy and colleagues, who demonstrated improved specificity and sensitivity when the scan was interpreted with knowledge of the clinical findings and initial laboratory studies, compared to when the interpretation was a blind reading of the scan (75). The importance of this has been emphasized by others (71,72).

The interpretation of the scan is important. There is a tendency on the part of many orthopaedic surgeons to call a bone scan "positive" or "negative," depending on areas of increased, normal, or decreased uptake. Linking knowledge of the pathophysiology of the disease process to the scan, which actually reflects localized physiologic changes in the bone, is more useful and more accurate.

Although localized increased isotope uptake may be due

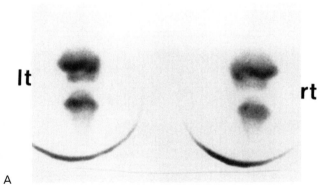

A

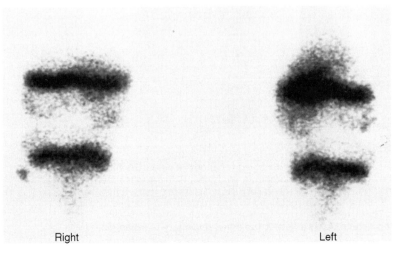

B   Right   Left

FIGURE 13-8. **A:** Bone scan of lower extremities of the same patient in Fig. 13-6. Note the activity around the physis. Differences in isotope uptake between the two sides are equivocal. **B:** Pinhole views of the distal femurs clearly demonstrate a difference between the left and right. In addition, the pattern of "peaking" in the metaphysis is typical of early osteomyelitis and corresponds to the expected pathologic process.

to osteomyelitis, it may also be due to any other process that increases the vascularity or deposition of calcium phosphate. Among the most common disorders seen in children are tumors and bone resorption due to disuse. Therefore, the bone scan can localize the area of the skeleton where there is altered physiology, but it cannot determine the cause (Fig. 13-9A and B).

The importance of a cold scan, in which there is an area of decreased isotope uptake, has been recognized as a serious problem, indicating acute devascularization of the bone caused by subperiosteal abscess (71,72,76,77).

The diagnosis and treatment of an acute bone or joint infection should not be delayed by the bone scan. In many institutions today, it may be easier to obtain an MRI during the evening or weekend hours. This, and the value of the MRI in detecting marrow changes early, may change the role of bone scintigraphy. Regardless of these changes, bone scintigraphy is still the method of choice when multiple sites are in question, or the site is unknown.

In requesting or waiting for a bone scan, the question often arises whether aspiration of the bone or joint alters the results of the scan. McCoy and colleagues (75) demonstrated in the clinical situation that the aspiration did not alter the scan, whereas Canale and colleagues (78) showed the same results in an experimental situation. This suggests that when the site of pathology is known and aspiration is indicated it need not, and in many cases probably should not, be delayed while waiting for a bone scan.

Computed Tomography

CT is valuable in the detection of focal areas of bone destruction, as well as detection and delineation of soft tissue abscess associated with bone and joint infection. Positive bone scans of the spine and pelvis often fail to provide the surgeon with the exact location of the lesion, which would permit either aspiration or planning of a surgical approach. In such circumstances, CT examination of the area localized by the bone scan can prove useful (79). Compared to MRI, its advantages are its greater availability and lower cost, both of which come at the disadvantage of being unable to detect early changes within the marrow in early cases.

Magnetic Resonance Imaging

MRI is a useful technique in the evaluation of both acute and chronic osteomyelitis because of its ability to provide good anatomic detail in many planes, and to detect pathologic changes within the marrow and soft tissues. Its actual use, however, is mitigated by its cost and the frequent necessity for sedation or general anesthesia in small children. It is simply not necessary for the diagnosis and treatment of the usual case of osteomyelitis or septic arthritis, but can

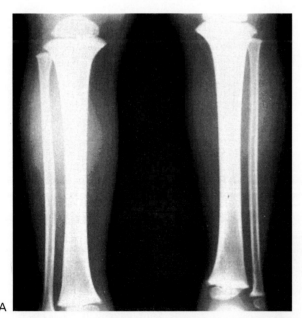
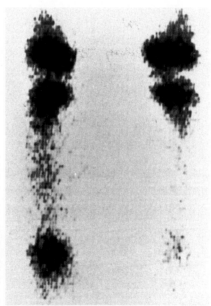

A

B

FIGURE 13-9. A: A seven-year-old girl complained of pain in her leg for about 24 hours. Examination revealed diffused swelling in the leg and a rapidly spreading erythema. Radiographs show superficial soft tissue swelling on the right leg, but the deep soft tissue layers are not swollen. This appearance indicates cellulitis. **B:** Bone scan was obtained on this patient and mistakenly interpreted as showing osteomyelitis. The diffused pattern of uptake is not typical of osteomyelitis, but represents the effects of increased circulation throughout the bone, secondary to inflammation and acute disuse.

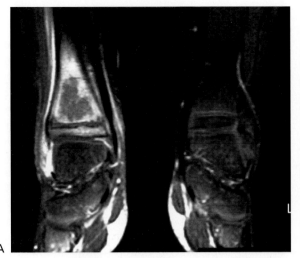 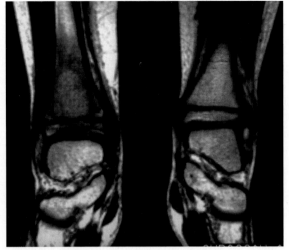

FIGURE 13-10. A: T1 MRI of the distal tibia in an 11-year-old female with right ankle pain and limp. She was started on oral antibiotic, but failed to resolve. The MRI demonstrates the edema in the distal right tibia, compared to the normal marrow signal from the left tibia. **B:** The spin echo postcontrast T1 images show enhancement due to the contrast material, and the absence of the bright fat signal. Note the center of the lesion, which suggests abscess formation.

prove very helpful in those cases in which uncertainty exists but the location of the disease process is known.

MRI for the evaluation of sepsis should include both T1- and T2-weighted sequences, because the difference between the two is important (Fig. 13-10). In acute osteomyelitis the low-intensity signal seen on the T1-weighted image becomes a high-intensity signal on the T2-weighted image. These changes reflect the increased water in the marrow produced by the edema, hyperemia, and purulent exudate that characterize the pathologic process (80) (see Chapter 3).

In a group of 43 children admitted to the hospital with the diagnosis of musculoskeletal infection, Mazur and colleagues showed the MRI had a sensitivity of 97% and a specificity of 92% (81). The indications for MRI in the diagnosis of acute bone or joint sepsis remain those cases in which the diagnosis cannot be made by the usual means. These will be cases in which there is confusion with neoplasia, cases previously treated, suspected sepsis in the axial skeleton, or when there is conflicting information (Fig. 13-7).

Ultrasound

Following its use in evaluation of developmental dislocation of the hip, ultrasound examination has been suggested as a tool for diagnosis of septic arthritis of the hip. Several reports leave no doubt that ultrasound can detect the presence of fluid within the hip, as well as the presence of a bulging capsule (82–84).

Ultrasound examination can be useful when the physician is unable to elicit the clinical signs of an irritable hip (limited and painful internal rotation) that accompany a joint effusion. Despite reports to the contrary, it does not seem possible to separate pus in septic arthritis from synovial fluid due to toxic synovitis, thus limiting the value of the test once irritability of the hip is established by clinical examination (85,86). It would seem to find it greatest use in the irritable hip that may be secondary to extracapsular irritation, e.g., early pelvic osteomyelitis with irritation of the surrounding muscles.

Ultrasound also has been applied to the diagnosis of osteomyelitis, based on the ultrasound detection of the soft tissue changes in the periosteum and surrounding soft tissues, including subperiosteal abscess (87). This may prove of value in guiding aspiration in some cases, but is of limited value due to its inability to detect changes within the bone.

Aspiration

The history, physical examination, and all of the radiographic procedures have been used to locate the area of abnormality. None of these examinations has the ability to confirm whether this abnormal area is caused by infection or some other process, such as neoplasia. In addition, none of these modalities allow identification of the organism—an essential step in confirming the diagnosis, selecting the correct antibiotic, and determining the need for surgical debridement.

Aspiration is the step most often omitted in the workup of a suspected osteomyelitis and, to a lesser extent, septic arthritis. The reasons are many: The physician is reluctant to introduce a needle into the bone or joint for fear of causing an infection; the physician is afraid of hurting the patient; the physician does not believe that it is necessary. None of these are valid reasons. There is little risk of introducing new organisms when sterile technique is used. With intravenous sedation and local anesthetic the aspiration of bone or joint can be performed with little discomfort. Aspiration of the bone or joint often yields organisms that are not found by culture of blood and other materials (46,47,51).

Aspiration of joints is a relatively simple matter, causing no more discomfort than placing an intravenous needle. Aspiration of the bone may be more difficult. Depending on the age and cooperation of the patient, various amounts of sedation may be necessary. Oral or intravenous midazolam (Versed) has proven to be quick and effective. After the area is prepared with a skin disinfectant, sterile towels are used to drape the area. A large-bore, cannulated, shallow tapered needle is used. The needle is first inserted into the most likely area until it contacts bone. Aspiration at this point may withdraw pus, indicating a subperiosteal abscess. If no pus is obtained, the needle is twisted like a drill until it is felt to penetrate the bone. Aspiration is again performed. The needle easily penetrates the thin metaphyseal bone.

Any material obtained should be sent for both culture and Gram staining, even if it does not appear to be purulent, because it may contain organisms. It is an unfortunate mistake to think that it is only blood and to discard it. The next most common error is to be too far from the metaphysis. Fear of being in the physis or epiphysis, coupled with difficulty in discerning the landmarks in a small, fat, and swollen extremity, leads to this error. The physician knows this is the case when it is difficult to penetrate the bone with the needle because the metaphyseal bone is easy to penetrate, whereas the cortical bone of the diaphysis is impenetrable with the usual needle (Fig. 13-1A).

DIFFERENTIAL DIAGNOSIS

Osteomyelitis

Although most cases of osteomyelitis in infants and children are relatively easy to diagnose, there are always cases having an atypical presentation and appearance, and osteomyelitis can be a great imitator. It is therefore helpful for the physician to always keep in mind those conditions that may present with the characteristics of bone infection, and thus be mistaken for infection.

Trauma is perhaps the most common. It is easily confused with osteomyelitis, because the latter often presents with a history of injury to the part, and is characterized by the same features: pain, swelling, tenderness, and soft tissue swelling on radiographs. In trauma, the symptoms are of sudden onset, whereas in infection, the symptoms usually begin more gradually. Trauma may be associated with an elevation of the CRP, but not of the ESR, whereas both are usually elevated in osteomyelitis. The pain of trauma

usually improves within 36 to 48 h, whereas that of osteomyelitis worsens.

Most troublesome are those cases that are difficult to distinguish from neoplasia (68,69). The most common malignancy in childhood is leukemia, and approximately 30% of these children present with bone pain (88). To complicate matters even more, 39% of these children present with constitutional symptoms such as lethargy, 18% with fever, and 60% have an elevated leukocyte count and elevated ESR (89). Although lucent metaphyseal bands are said to be characteristic of leukemia, other bone changes are also seen. One study found lytic lesions in 19%, sclerotic lesions in 4%, and periosteal new bone in 2% (89).

The treating physician should be suspicious when other signs associated with leukemia are noted (e.g., bleeding, easy bruising, bone pain in multiple sites). A low leukocyte count, seen in 35% of patients presenting with leukemia, should also raise suspicion, although this finding may also indicate serious systemic sepsis. An anemia that is not explained by acute symptoms of osteomyelitis or abnormally low platelets should also arouse suspicion. An additional clue is when the bone scan does not demonstrate the findings that would be expected in the presence of osteomyelitis. The typical finding in leukemia is a lytic lesion without increased uptake, because the lesion is purely lytic, without new bone formation or reaction (90).

Other less common neoplasms may mimic osteomyelitis (67–69). Whenever the characteristic appearance of one of these neoplasms is recognized, the physician should immediately run through the differential diagnosis in his or her mind, remembering that the differential diagnosis is the possibilities arranged in order of probability. In the younger child, an irregular lytic lesion and/or the presence of periosteal new bone, with or without a lytic lesion, should always suggest osteomyelitis, metastatic neuroblastoma, and eosinophilic granuloma, along with leukemia. In the older child and adolescent, the various forms of subacute osteomyelitis, discussed below, most often mimic tumors. The most difficult to differentiate from osteomyelitis, when periosteal new bone characterizes the lesion, is Ewing sarcoma (91). In all such cases, the diagnosis must be established before treatment is begun. The lesion should be approached as a malignancy, with complete radiographic staging and a biopsy approach that would not jeopardize limb salvage surgery, if the lesion is malignant. In cases in which trauma or infection is as likely as tumor, and the situation is not acute, it may be advisable to follow the course for 1 or 2 weeks. In this situation, occult trauma will show rapid resolution of symptoms and maturation of new bone, while the signs of infection will become more obvious.

Bone infarction can mimic AHO. (The differential diagnosis of bone infarct and osteomyelitis in sickle cell disease is discussed later.) Gaucher disease is another less-common disorder in which acute bone infarction occurs. Similar to those with sickle cell disease, these patients can also have

AHO, although it is less common than bone infarction. In one series of 49 patients with Gaucher disease, 11 were admitted to the hospital with acute lower-extremity pain, constitutional symptoms, fever, an elevated leukocyte count, and an elevated ESR (92). Of these, 5 were diagnosed as AHO, whereas the others had a bone infarction. There was no difference between the clinical signs and laboratory data for the two groups. Because bone destruction was rapid in those with osteomyelitis, the authors recommended early biopsy for culture. Because these patients seem to be unusually susceptible to infection after bone surgery, it is best to perform this biopsy by aspiration and in the sterile environment of the operating room.

Septic Arthritis

The differential diagnoses of septic arthritis, which is that of an acutely swollen and painful joint, include many more possibilities than that for osteomyelitis. The culture results are even more important, because many disorders mimicking septic arthritis are not diagnosed by biopsy but by many complex laboratory tests, and often by the passage of time. In considering the differential diagnoses of septic arthritis, the urgency of making the correct diagnosis is important. The physician should always consider what must be diagnosed today, what can be diagnosed tomorrow, and what can be diagnosed next week. For example, septic arthritis, particularly of the hip, should be diagnosed as soon as possible, whereas there is little harm to the patient if JRA is diagnosed next week.

One of the most difficult and yet important differentials is between septic arthritis of the hip and toxic synovitis, a condition thought to be caused by a postinfectious arthritis (see Chapter 12). The importance of this diagnosis is the need for immediate drainage of the hip in the presence of bacterial sepsis, whereas the treatment of toxic synovitis is observation. Both may present with a history of a few to several days of hip pain, with limp progressing to the inability to walk. The physical signs are similar in both, with limited and painful internal rotation, abduction, and extension. A longer history of symptoms, with cyclic improvement and worsening, suggests toxic synovitis. The pain is usually worse and the motion more restricted in septic arthritis.

One study comparing 94 patients with toxic synovitis and 38 with septic arthritis found that there was significant overlap of the temperature, leukocyte count, and ESR between the two groups (93). That the ESR is often elevated in toxic synovitis is not always appreciated. A more recent study by Kocher et al. found four independent multivariate clinical predictors to help distinguish septic arthritis from toxic synovitis: history of fever, nonweightbearing, ESR greater than 40 mm/h, and WBC greater than 12,000/mm^3 (94). An algorithm for the probability of a patient having septic arthritis is shown in Table 13-2.

JRA is frequently a consideration, especially when it presents as a single acutely swollen joint (see Chapter 12). Clinically different from septic arthritis, the history is often a more gradual onset, particularly regarding pain. The patient usually remains ambulatory. The examination is characterized by motion that is good with surprisingly little pain, compared with the large amount of swelling that is usually present. The joint is only mildly tender and the synovium may be thickened. Initial laboratory tests are not helpful in

TABLE 13-2. ALGORITHM FOR PROBABILITY OF SEPTIC ARTHRITIS

	Multivariate Predictor			
History of Fever	Nonweight-bearing	Erythrocyte Sedimentation Rate ≥40 mm per hr	Serum White Blood Cell Count >12,000 cells per mm³ (12.0 × 10⁹ cells per L)	Predicted Probability of Septic Arthritis (%)
Yes	Yes	Yes	Yes	99.8
Yes	Yes	Yes	No	97.3
Yes	Yes	No	Yes	95.2
Yes	Yes	No	No	57.8
Yes	No	Yes	Yes	95.5
Yes	No	Yes	No	62.2
Yes	No	No	Yes	44.8
Yes	No	No	No	5.3
No	Yes	Yes	Yes	93.0
No	Yes	Yes	No	48.0
No	Yes	No	Yes	33.8
No	Yes	No	No	3.4
No	No	Yes	Yes	35.3
No	No	Yes	No	3.7
No	No	No	Yes	2.1
No	No	No	No	0.1

(From ref. 107, with permission.)

the differential diagnosis. The synovial fluid leukocyte count usually contains fewer than 100,000 leukocytes/mL, whereas in sepsis, the count is typically more than 100,000 leukocytes/mL. This is not always true, however, and the leukocyte count can be more than 100,000 leukocytes/mL in JRA (58). In many cases, the aspirate from the joint has the appearance of pus from a septic joint; in such cases, the physician has little choice but to begin treatment for septic arthritis, while searching for other clues.

Rheumatic fever, a sequela of group A streptococcal infection, is another childhood illness that often is associated with swollen and painful joints. For reasons that are not clear, there was a resurgence of rheumatic fever beginning in the late 1980s, after years of decline (95). The problem for the orthopaedic surgeon is to think of this disorder in the initial evaluation, because those additional findings that lead to the diagnosis must be sought. The joint pain is typically in the large joints (knees, ankles, elbows, and wrists), and is evanescent and migratory. Also characteristic is that the pain, which is severe, is out of proportion to the amount of swelling, which is usually mild. The history should seek evidence of an untreated pharyngitis or febrile illness, a rash, or some other infection due to group A *Streptococcus* approximately 2 weeks before the onset of joint swelling. Inquiry should also be made about any joint symptoms preceding the presenting complaint, especially the involvement of multiple joints.

The diagnosis of rheumatic fever is based on the Jones criteria. The major criteria are carditis, arthritis, chorea, subcutaneous nodules, and erythema marginatum. The minor criteria are fever; arthralgia; elevated ESR or CRP; heart block, as evidenced on an electrocardiogram; and a previous history of rheumatic fever. The diagnosis is made when there are two major or one major and two minor criteria. A heart murmur usually is not present this early in the course of the disease. Rheumatic fever is one diagnosis that must be considered in the differential diagnosis of any patient with septic arthritis.

Another disorder that causes either arthralgia or arthritis is Henoch-Schönlein purpura. This disorder is a vasculitis of unknown origin (possibly allergic), which affects mainly children between the ages of 2 and 11 years of age. In the full-blown case having all of the clinical manifestations (nonthrombocytopenic purpuric rash, abdominal pain, arthritis, and nephritis), the diagnosis is not difficult. The joint manifestations, which occur in up to 75% of the patients, precede the other symptoms in about 25% of those affected. For this reason, the orthopaedist should be familiar with the features of the joint findings. The joints most commonly involved are the knees and ankles. The swelling and tenderness are more periarticular than that in septic arthritis, and if an effusion is present, it is usually mild. Joint fluid will not contain blood. The earliest signs of purpura must be sought, which may be fine pinpoint hemorrhagic lesions, usually seen below the waist. The joint symptoms do not require treatment, and usually disappear within days. These

patients require medical management for the other, sometimes more serious, manifestations of the disease.

There are many other causes of joint swelling that merit consideration. Enteroarthritis secondary to *Salmonella* or *Yersinia* infection may be suspected when abdominal symptoms coincide. The arthritis may precede the abdominal symptoms, however. These patients can be confused with those having septic arthritis, because as with septic arthritis, the ESR and CRP are often elevated to high levels. Kawasaki disease, a vasculitis of unknown etiology, may present with joint symptoms in its early stage. It is characterized by a rash with red eyes and lips, erythema of the palms and soles with edema, and lethargy. The child does not like to be moved, and may seem to be more ill than the visible signs suggest. Serum sickness, which is often manifest by joint swelling and an urticarial rash, usually affects more than one joint, and most commonly follows treatment with penicillin or a cephalosporin antibiotic, especially Ceclor. Other considerations are discussed later in this chapter.

TREATMENT

There are four principles that the physician must always keep in mind when treating an infection:

1. Identify the organism.
2. Select the correct antibiotic.
3. Deliver the antibiotic to the organisms.
4. Stop the tissue destruction.

Organism Identification

The first principle, to identify the organism, is the ultimate purpose of diagnosis. The diagnosis of musculoskeletal sepsis, and septic arthritis in particular, is difficult to establish with certainty unless an organism is identified. Likewise, it is even more difficult to treat the infection with certainty until the specific organism is identified.

Select Correct Antibiotic

The value of knowing the relative incidence of causative organisms in a particular case is to aid in selecting a likely effective antibiotic before the organism is positively identified by culture, and to understand the unique characteristics of the organism, including antibiotic resistance, so that initial treatment may be modified accordingly. The antibiotics commonly used in the treatment of musculoskeletal sepsis are listed in Table 13-3.

When hematogenous osteomyelitis and septic arthritis are considered apart from any unique circumstances, age is the most important factor in the incidence of a particular organism. In reviewing different series, there are often wide variations in the percentage of cases caused by a particular

TABLE 13-3. ANTIBIOTICS COMMONLY USED IN THE TREATMENT OF BONE AND JOINT SEPSIS

Drug[1]	Route	Dosage[2,3]	Comments
Amoxicillin	Oral	80 mg/kg/d q8h	
Ampicillin	IV	100–150 mg/kg/d q6h	
Dicloxacillin	Oral	100 mg/kg/d q6h	
Methicillin	IV	150 mg/kg/d q6h	
Nafcillin	IV	150 mg/kg/d q6h	
Penicillin G	IV	150,000 U/kg/d q4–6h	
Penicillin V	Oral	100 mg/kg/d q6h	
Oxacillin	IV	150 mg/kg/d q6h	
Cefazolin (Ancef, Kefzol)	IV	100 mg/kg/d q8h	Max dose 6 gm/d
Cephalexin (Keflex)	Oral	100 mg/kg/d q6h	
Cefotaxime (Claforan)	IV	150 mg/kg/d q6–8h	
Cefprozil (Cefzil)	Oral	60 mg/kg/d q12h	
Ceftazidime (Fortaz)		100–150 mg/kg/d q8h	Max dose 8 gm/d
Ceftriaxone (Rocephin)	IV/IM	50–75 mg/kg/d q24h	Max dose 2 gm/d
Cefuroxime (Zinacef)	IV	100–150 mg/kg/d q8h	
Cefuroxime axetil (Ceftin)	Oral	60 mg/kg/d q12h	
Ciprofloxacin (Cipro)	IV/Oral	30 mg/kg/d q12h	Max 800 mg/d
		30 mg/kg/d q12h	Max 1500 mg/d
Clindamycin	IV/Oral	25–40 mg/kg/d q6h	
Gentamicin	IV	7.5 mg/kg/d q8h	Monitor peak and trough start at third dose
Vancomycin	IV	40 mg/kg/d q6h	Administer over 1 h monitor peak and trough start at fourth dose
Bactrim	IV/Oral	10 mg/kg/d (of trimethroprim component) bid	

[1] CBC should be monitored weekly for neutropenia or anemia, in any patient on high-dose IV penicillin or cephalosporin therapy. It should be monitored monthly on high-dose oral therapy.

[2] Doses recommended are for normal children with normal renal function for the treatment of bone and joint infections. Recommended doses for the treatment of other conditions may be lower or higher.

[3] For doses in the neonatal period, see: Nelson, JD. *Pocket book of pediatric antimicrobial therapy*, 10th ed. Baltimore: Williams & Wilkins, 1998–1999.

organism. This may be because of the years over which the data were gathered, the population being evaluated, on the diligence in identifying the organisms. Despite these variations, some generalizations can be made based on age that are very useful in the initial selection of an antibiotic.

The most useful age divisions are: premature neonates, term neonates, children under 3 to 4 years of age, and children older than 4 years of age. The reasons for this have to do with the organisms that predominate in these age groups. The premature infant is discussed later as a special problem.

The term "neonate" may be considered as any child from birth to 6 weeks of age. Although the neonatal period is considered the first 28 days it is more helpful, when thinking of infection, to think of the neonate being any infant up to 6 weeks of age. The particular organisms that affect this population are group A and group B streptococcus, *Streptococcus pneumoniae*, and *Escherichia coli,* in addition to *Staphylococcus aureus*. In this age group, cefotaxime (Claforan) is the first drug of choice. Ceftriaxone (Rocephin) is also a good choice in a child without jaundice.

Prior to the use of the vaccine against *H. influenzae* type b (HIB), it was the most common organism causing septic arthritis in patients younger than 5 years of age, whereas *S.*

aureus was, and remains, the most common organism in children older than 5 years of age (55,96,97). This made it important to select an initial antibiotic that was effective against HIB in this age group. Today, HIB is a rare cause of bone or joint sepsis because of the immunization. HIB may still be suspected in the newborn or in the unusual child who today has not received immunization. It is important to recognize that as many as 30% of children with HIB septic arthritis may also have meningitis (97,98). This is especially likely to occur in children younger than 2 years of age. Several other organisms (e.g., group B streptococci and *Escherichia coli*) found in septic arthritis also show a predilection for the younger age groups, and may also cause meningitis.

An organism that is increasingly identified in osteoarticular infections, particularly in the younger child under the age of 3 or 4 years, is *Kingella kingae* (99). This organism was initially identified and characterized in the late 1960s. It has been isolated in slightly more than 1% of pharyngeal cultures, but may be more prevalent. In one series of infections due to *K. kingae*, 56% of the patients had a respiratory infection (100). This predilection for the respiratory tract, and the increased incidence of musculoskeletal infection with this organism during the winter months, is noted in other reports (59,99). The organism is described as an opportunistic pathogen, and is thought to colonize the nasopharynx then invade the bloodstream. Favored sites are bone, joints, disc spaces, and heart.

The increased incidence of *K. kingae* infection may be due to better methods of isolation. It has been demonstrated that inoculation of the material into a BACTEC culture bottle (Johnston Laboratories, Towson, MD) can dramatically increase the rate of recovery of *K. kingae* (100).

Like *H. influenzae*, *K. kingae* infections most often occur in children younger than 4 years of age. Most children are healthy before the onset of the infection. The organism affects joints most frequently. The clinical course and laboratory findings do not differ significantly from septic arthritis caused by other organisms. The bone infections are often insidious and frequently occur in the epiphysis.

K. kingae is sensitive to penicillin and many of the semisynthetic penicillins and cephalosporins that are used to treat bone and joint infections (101,102). It is possible that in the past many of the culture-negative cases of musculoskeletal sepsis resolved with these commonly used antibiotics, without *K. kingae* being identified. A second organism seen in septic arthritis in this age group is *Streptococcus pneumoniae*. Currently 30 to 50% of these organisms are relatively resistant to the semisynthetic penicillins and cephalosporins (103).

Today, ceftriaxone (Rocephin) is an excellent drug for initial treatment of bone and joint sepsis in children under the age of 4 years of age. The fact that it is effective against most of the common organisms seen in this age group; the fact that it can be administered once a day, significantly reducing costs; and the very high minimal inhibitory concentrations that are reached in the blood, all favor this antibiotic.

It is important to remember that despite the variety of organisms responsible for bone and joint sepsis in the younger child, *S. aureus* is still the most common causative organism in AHO after infancy, and particularly over the age of 5 years. The reported incidence ranges between 25 and 64%, depending largely on the age mix of the patients in the study (20,46,47,51). However, streptococcal organisms, including group A *Streptococcus* and *S. pneumoniae*, are also found in the child older than 5 years of age, with the reported incidence ranging from 4 to 21%. Infections with streptococcal organisms tend to occur in the younger age range (20,49,51,165), whereas *Staphylococcus aureus* becomes more common with increasing age. In this older age range in which *Staphylococcus* predominates, a semisynthetic penicillin, e.g., oxacillin or a cephalosporin, e.g., cefazolin (Ancef, Kefzol) or cefuroxime (Zinacef), are good initial choices.

Preferably, children between birth and 2 to 3 years of age are managed along with a pediatrician or pediatric specialist. One of the important reasons, other than the management of the antibiotics, is that these children more frequently have other sites of involvement, e.g., meningitis. They require a good clinical examination for meningitis and other problems which may not be commensurate with the best skills of the orthopaedist.

It needs to be understood that these are initial choices which are made before culture results are available. Once the organism is identified, the antibiotic choice is changed to one that is effective but narrower in its range of activity. The antibiotics most commonly used to treat bone and joint infections in children are listed in Table 13-3.

The selection of an oral antibiotic should be based on Gram stain and culture results. For the child younger than the age of 5 years, cefuroxime axetil (Ceftin) and cefprozil (Cefzil) are good choices. For the older child, cephalexin suspension or dicloxacillin capsules are a good choice (see Table 13-3).

Antibiotic Delivery

Giving an antibiotic to a patient who has an infection is not sufficient. The physician must ensure that the antibiotic both reaches all of the organisms and effectively kills them. This involves several issues. Does it matter whether the antibiotic is given intravenously or orally? How long should the antibiotic be given, and why? Where can the antibiotic be expected to penetrate? Can it kill the organism when it gets there? In this era of cost containment, and with the worthwhile goal of keeping children out of the hospital, the real questions are, how long does the patient have to remain in the hospital, and when can intravenous administration of antibiotic be switched to oral administration?

Route of Administration

Initial antibiotic therapy for bone or joint infections should always begin with intravenous administration. The question of how soon the intravenous route can be switched to the oral, in any particular case, is a question for which no data are available. Intravenous administration is more expensive than oral administration, however, and certainly less convenient for the patient (104). An advantage to intravenous administration is that high concentrations of antibiotic can be achieved quickly with certainty. These levels exceed those usually necessary, whereas the levels achieved with oral administration are usually adequate. The difficulty with oral administration is in ensuring that absorption from the gut is adequate, and that the patient is compliant. Despite these potential pitfalls, the efficacy of oral antibiotics in the treatment of bone and joint sepsis has been well documented (104–107), and represents an acceptable method of treatment following an initial course of intravenous antibiotics.

An additional troublesome problem with prolonged intravenous administration in small children, is maintaining vascular access. This usually requires that these children have a peripheral indwelling catheter (PIC line) placed. While lessening the problems, these lines are not without problems, e.g., clotting and becoming infected, as well as requiring a certain level of skill on the part of the home health agency that is managing the line. Thus, they are not a reason to give intravenous antibiotic longer than necessary.

The successful administration of oral therapy requires the same conditions as for intravenous therapy, i.e., that the antibiotic reach the organisms in sufficient concentration and be in the bone for a sufficient length of time to kill the organisms. Patients may generally be switched to oral antibiotics therapy when the course of the disease is resolving, abscess formation is not present or has been debrided, or the antibiotic is well-tolerated orally by the patient, and the parents are reliable.

In one series about 10% of the patients failed to achieve adequate serum concentrations of the antibiotic after oral administration (107). Reports such as this led to the recommendation that the peak serum level be measured to verify that adequate antibiotic was present. There is some evidence that it may actually be the trough level that is more significant (109,110). In practices in which measurement of bactericidal concentration of antibiotic has been measured as a routine in the past, it is now used more often only for more difficult situations. This has evolved because, with adequate oral doses, it is very unusual to find insufficient levels of antibiotic or treatment failures that can be attributed to insufficient levels of antibiotic. Experience has taught that, to achieve adequate serum levels of antibiotic, larger oral doses (usually two times larger) are needed than those commonly recommended (Table 13-3).

Although it is decreasing as a routine practice, at times it will be necessary or advisable to measure the concentration of the antibiotic. Because the direct measurement in the blood of the level of commonly used antibiotics (e.g., semisynthetic penicillins, cephalosporins) is not feasible, it is measured indirectly by the serum bactericidal test. This test uses serial dilutions of patient serum to test against the bacteria, which is isolated to determine the minimal dilution that is bactericidal for the organism (111,112).

Blood is drawn after the administration of the oral antibiotic to determine the peak level. For antibiotic given in suspension, the blood is drawn 1 h after administration; for antibiotic administered in capsule or tablet, blood is drawn approximately 1.5 to 2 h after administration. If the trough level is to be measured, blood is drawn just before the next dose. Dilutions of the serum are prepared and tested against the isolated organism. If an organism is not isolated, a representative laboratory strain of the presumed organism is used. Although it is controversial regarding how much the peak serum level should exceed the bactericidal concentration, a 1:8 dilution is generally accepted as being effective. When adequate levels are not present, the dose may be increased: probenecid (Benemid) to inhibit renal excretion may be added, or intravenous therapy may be reinstituted.

The serum level of other antibiotics (e.g., gentamicin, vancomycin) can and should be monitored in all cases. These antibiotics can be measured directly in the blood.

Not only does the blood level of these intravenous antibiotics vary significantly between individuals, but their toxic side effects are significant. Both the peak and trough levels need to be measured and monitored. For gentamicin, blood is drawn approximately 30 min after administration, and just before the next dose. The peak level should be between 5 and 10 μg/mL, and the trough should be 1.9 μg/mL or less. For vancomycin, blood is drawn 1 h after administration, and just before the next dose. The peak level should be between 20 and 40 μg/mL and the trough between 5 and 10 μg/mL.

Generally, blood levels of gentamicin or vancomycin should be measured every 3 to 4 days, in addition to those of blood urea nitrogen (BUN) and creatinine. For prolonged (longer than 3 weeks) or recurrent therapy with these drugs, it is wise to monitor the patient for ototoxicity also. Vancomycin should be infused over no less than 1 h to avoid the release of histamine by the drug (red man syndrome) or serious hypotension. If a rash occurs, it usually can be circumvented by administering the drug over 90 to 120 min, or by the use of intravenous diphenhydramine (Benadryl) 1 mg/kg (total dose not to exceed 50 mg) just before the infusion.

Penetration

After an adequate serum level of the antibiotic is achieved, it must reach all of the areas harboring bacteria. In evaluating data on antibiotic penetration, it is necessary to consider the antibiotic in addition to the methods used to measure its concentration (113). Methicillin, dicloxacillin, cephaloridine, and cefazolin all penetrate into pus and bone in children with osteomyelitis in concentrations several times greater than the mean inhibitory and mean bactericidal concentrations for *S. aureus* (114). The same is true for orally administered ampicillin, cephalexin, cloxacillin, dicloxacillin, and penicillin G in the synovial fluid of children with septic arthritis (115). There is no evidence that antibiotics penetrate into dead bone.

Efficacy of Antibiotic

The treatment of musculoskeletal sepsis presents a paradox. If the antibiotics kill the bacteria, and there is a sufficient serum concentration in the absence of dead bone, why is not antibiotic administration more rapidly and universally successful? The answer lies in understanding that there are several factors that may interfere with the antibiotic action. One factor that is poorly studied is the effect the local environment has on the ability of the antibiotic to kill bacteria. It is known that the interaction of purulent material from some Gram-negative organisms can interfere with the action of certain antibiotics (116,117).

With a large inoculum and the production of large amounts of β-lactamase, β-lactam antibiotics, such as semisynthetic penicillins and cephalosporins, are susceptible to breakdown, rendering them ineffective (118–120). In addition, the low pH at the site of infection is known to interfere with the action of some antibiotics. These factors suggest that the local environment is important to the effective action of the antibiotic, and that the site of infection may not be the ideal environment.

Duration of Administration

There are no good data that indicate how long antibiotics should be administered in any particular case. The old recommendation of 6 weeks of intravenous administration is often based on difficult and complicated referral cases from large tertiary medical centers, which do not represent the "usual" case (121). Conversely, there is no evidence, other than clinical experience, that a shorter duration can be effective. More important than rigid rules is an understanding of the pathophysiology of each case, so that the treatment can be based on the particulars of that case. The correct answer is that the antibiotic should be continued until all of the organisms have been killed.

To illustrate, consider two different cases. A 5-year-old boy presents with a history of increasing pain in the distal thigh for 3 days, and inability to walk on the day of presentation. His radiographs are normal, except for deep soft tissue swelling. Aspiration demonstrates pus, and he undergoes surgical debridement the same day. He is started on the correct antibiotic. Over the next 5 days, the pain, swelling, and fever subside, the CRP is falling, and he begins to walk. He can be safely treated with 5 days (perhaps less) of intravenous antibiotics, followed by oral antibiotics for an additional 3 or 4 weeks.

Another 5-year-old boy is seen 2 weeks after the onset of pain in the distal thigh. His physician had placed him on oral antibiotics after 3 days, but the pain and limp continued to worsen. His radiographs show extensive involvement of the distal femoral metaphysis, with radiolucent areas and periosteal new bone. He undergoes surgical debridement, but it is not deemed possible to debride all of the bone that is involved. At the end of 7 days, his fever is decreasing, the CRP has not fallen, and although his signs and symptoms are improving, he still has some swelling and tenderness. This patient should remain on intravenous antibiotics.

These two cases illustrate the factors to consider when deciding the duration of antibiotic therapy. How long has the infection been present, and how much bone is involved? Is there abscess formation? Has the patient had adequate surgical debridement to remove the pus and other materials that interfere with effective antibiotic action? Has all of the dead bone been removed to expose organisms to antibiotic? Is the patient getting better? These clinical observations can be aided to a limited extent by radiographic and laboratory studies, remembering that radiographic changes lag behind the actual bone changes, and that the ESR and, to a lesser degree, the CRP also lag behind resolving infection during the first week (51).

Current practice is a sequential course of intravenous antibiotic, followed by an oral course. Clinical parameters determine when oral antibiotics begin. In the typical case which resolves quickly with treatment, oral therapy starts after 5 days of intravenous antibiotic administration; in the case of osteomyelitis, it continues for 4 to 6 weeks and, in septic arthritis, for an additional 2 to 3 weeks.

Surgery

Destruction of tissue is the final result of infection. Although bone has the ability to repair itself, articular and epiphyseal cartilage do not. Therefore, one of the main goals of treatment is to stop tissue destruction. Killing the bacteria is the first part of the treatment, but not the only part. Tissue destruction is mainly the result of the complex process known as the "inflammatory reaction." Although this reaction is initiated by bacteria, the presence of live bacteria is not necessary for its continuation. It is well recognized that the products liberated by bacteria, cell wall fragments of dead bacteria, products liberated from leukocytes, and products of tissue destruction are all capable of causing an inflammatory reaction, which results in tissue destruction (37,40,122–124).

With an understanding of the mechanisms of tissue destruction and the delivery of antibiotic to the bacteria in an environment where it can be effective, the basis for surgery becomes more meaningful. Surgery is for debridement. It removes the inflammatory products more rapidly than the host defense mechanisms. In so doing, it provides a more effective environment in which antibiotics can work. It reduces the size of the inoculum, ensuring more effective antibiotic action of many commonly used antibiotics. Lastly, it removes all of the dead and avascular bone or the thick fibrinous exudate from joints, thus exposing all of the organisms to antibiotic. This provides a more rapid end to tissue destruction, and requires a shorter course of antibiotic therapy.

The indications for surgical debridement of AHO remain controversial and in flux. Difficulty in evaluating published reports and recommending various points of view arise because of failure to identify the important characteristics of those who were treated with surgery and those who were not. Among those factors that are important to evaluate are the duration and severity of infection, the type of organism, appropriateness of antibiotic use, the duration of intravenous antibiotic versus oral, and length of hospitalization.

The author has used the aspiration of pus, or failure of signs and symptoms to resolve within 36 to 48 h, as an indication for surgical debridement. This practice is based on the same principles used to treat infection in other parts of the body. Especially important is the age-old wisdom of draining an abscess, regardless of location. With these criteria, many cases avoid surgery, few require prolonged intravenous therapy, and recurrence is distinctly unusual. This is a mainstream opinion that is evolving in clinical practice, and that is supported by others (125,126).

Surgical debridement of a focus of hematogenous osteomyelitis requires an incision only large enough to expose the area of bone involved. Incision of the periosteum in the involved area is performed first, to drain the subperiosteal abscess. Stripping of the periosteum to expose additional periosteal abscess should be done sparingly, to avoid devascularization of the bone. Next, using a drill an entry hole is made into the bone. This can be enlarged with a rongeur to allow access with a curet, but this hole should not be any larger than necessary to curet the involved bone. The diseased area is easily distinguished from more normal bone by "feel" with the curet and the appearance of the material removed.

Specimens should be sent for both culture and routine histology. The importance of routine histologic examination of material from the bone is twofold. Some tumors have a tendency to become necrotic and, when surgically explored, may look similar to pus; the most common is metastatic neuroblastoma, followed by Ewing sarcoma. In addition, if positive identification of the organism is not obtained, it is reassuring to have a histologic diagnosis of osteomyelitis.

The indications for arthrotomy in the treatment of septic arthritis are perhaps even more controversial (except for the hip), although more sharply divided between the orthopaedic and pediatric literature. Experimental evidence supports lavage of the joint, but individual experiences constitute the evidence that drives clinical decisions.

In experimental staphylococcal septic arthritis in rabbits that were treated with antibiotic, the beneficial effect of surgical lavage was demonstrated (45). During the first arthrotomy at 4 days, all of the material in the knee could be washed out; at 7 days, it had to be removed manually. All cultures were negative at 7 days. Both the surgically treated and nonsurgically treated animals showed loss of glycosaminoglycan. There was no collagen degradation in those treated by surgical lavage, however. A similar study has shown that arthrotomy and irrigation may be more effective than repeated aspirations, as the above data suggest (127).

In the author's experience, there is no question that some joint infections can be cured with antibiotics alone. This seems to be especially true in the smaller joints, such as the wrist, and in younger children. Attempts to treat joints such as the knee without drainage have never been as prompt to resolve as those treated with a small arthrotomy and irrigation, followed by a brief period of splinting.

Effective drainage of most joints can be performed through a small incision. The incision should be large enough to permit a small retractor to be inserted into the joint. On the knee of a small child, this can be accomplished with an incision of no more than 2.5 cm. After suctioning the purulent material from the joint, a swab of the synovium is obtained for culture. A small biopsy of the synovium may also be sent for culture. Irrigation is then performed with saline through a small rubber catheter directed into all of the recesses of the joint. A drain (or irrigation system, if preferred) is inserted into the joint, and the wound is closed (128,129).

Repeated aspiration has been recommended, but suffers from two drawbacks: it is ineffective in draining the joint (Fig. 13-11), and it becomes a difficult trial for both the patient and the physician because it must be repeated at least daily for several days. Arthroscopy has also been recommended (130,131). Morbidity following arthroscopy does

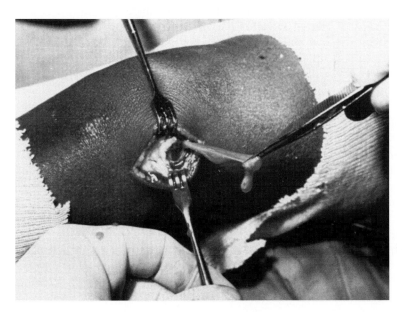

FIGURE 13-11. This patient with 3 days of symptoms was diagnosed as having septic arthritis after aspiration of the joint. Within 2 h of aspiration, the knee joint was opened through a small arthrotomy, with the patient under general anesthesia. Before and after irrigation, large amounts of thick fibrinous pus were removed with a forceps, illustrating the inadequacy of aspiration as a method to debride the joint.

not seem to be any different than for open arthrotomy in septic joints, whereas the operative time and resources are more costly for arthroscopy.

RESULTS

Most children who are seen for AHO or septic arthritis can expect to recover without sequelae. These disorders are curable. Untoward consequences are usually due to advanced disease at the time of presentation, or problems in the initial management. Other than these two factors, the literature sheds little light on other reasons for failure, because the reports cover decades during which organisms, antibiotics, and principles of management changed (20,60,120,126,132–134).

Most complications from musculoskeletal sepsis occur in the hip for reasons documented elsewhere in this chapter. Other than the hip, joint destruction is expected only in the late-presenting and neglected case. Chronic osteomyelitis remains distinctly unusual, probably because of the rapid bone turnover in children. Epiphyseal destruction with growth arrest is occasionally seen, but usually in cases in which appropriate treatment is delayed.

SPECIAL CONDITIONS

Spine

For decades, physicians have recognized hematogenous infections of both the disc space and the vertebral body. Descriptions of the disorder as "a benign form of osteomyelitis of the spine" provide a clue to its natural history (135), whereas the various descriptions in the literature of vertebral osteomyelitis and discitis, over the past several decades, reflect the uncertainty that these are indeed two separate conditions (136,137). Modern imaging modalities, such as scintigraphy, CT scanning, and MRI have resolved the confusion by demonstrating evidence of bone involvement in children with the clinical presentation of discitis (138,139). It thus appears that both vertebral osteomyelitis and discitis are the result of a hematogenous infection beginning in the bone adjacent to the cartilaginous vertebral end plate.

The vascular anatomy of the vertebral body and disc has been well studied (140–143). These studies demonstrate that the blood supply to the disc comes from the contiguous bone of the vertebral bodies. In the young child, vessels can be identified traversing the cartilaginous vertebral end plate and entering the annulus. By the age of 8 years, these vessels have largely disappeared, but a rich anastomotic network of vessels remains along the periphery of the disc that can persist until 30 years of age.

The etiology of the syndrome of discitis is most likely infectious. Occasionally, the question of traumatic injury to

the vertebral end plate, similar to a Salter-Harris I fracture, is raised; however, substantial proof is lacking. The different presentations, the characteristic age range (average age, 7 years), and the isolation of bacteria from many cases also militates against this being a traumatic disorder. It is recognized, however, that this is an infection that behaves differently than most musculoskeletal infections.

The presentation of patients with discitis is variable and insidious, with fewer than one-half presenting with the characteristic symptoms of refusal to walk or back pain (144). In addition, signs of infection, such as fever, are usually minimal or absent. Despite this, three different patterns of clinical presentation have been described (145,146). The first presentation is in the younger child, usually younger than 3 years of age, who has difficulty walking. In the very young child this may begin with a reluctance, then refusal to walk, and may be confused with more common causes, such as a septic hip. In the child who is attempting to walk, there is often a characteristic gait, with the child bending forward and hands on the thighs for support.

The second presentation, usually occurring in children 7 to 15 years of age, is abdominal pain. This can be vague and associated with a poor appetite and listlessness. Sometimes the pain radiates anteriorly and can be confused with an intraabdominal condition, although localized physical signs in the abdomen are lacking.

The final presentation is back pain. In the classic presentation, the patient complains of back pain, has loss of the normal lumbar lordosis, and is painful to percussion. In some children, this onset may be gradual, whereas in others who often have radiographic evidence of vertebral osteomyelitis, the onset may be rapid and may suggest infection. In most cases, fever is absent or low. It is also important to remember that these presentations may overlap greatly in age, symptoms, and findings.

The laboratory evaluation, as with most cases of skeletal sepsis, is not helpful unless the underlying disease is suspected and all of the correct tests are obtained. The leukocyte count may or may not be elevated or show a leftward shift. The ESR and CRP are usually elevated, and blood cultures may be positive, but not so reliably as in the usual infection involving a major bone or joint.

Radiographs at the initial presentation are often normal, and usually show no changes in the first 1 to 3 weeks of symptoms. One of the earliest findings, often seen only in retrospect, is an irregularity of the vertebral end plate. This is followed by narrowing of the disc space, then erosion of the vertebral end plate, as evidence of involvement of more than just the disc space (Fig. 13-12).

Bone scintigraphy is useful in suspected cases, demonstrating increased isotope uptake at the affected disc space. This usually occurs sooner than the radiographic changes, but the author has seen negative bone scans after 2 weeks of symptoms in patients with proved discitis. CT scanning is a useful technique to delineate the anatomic changes in

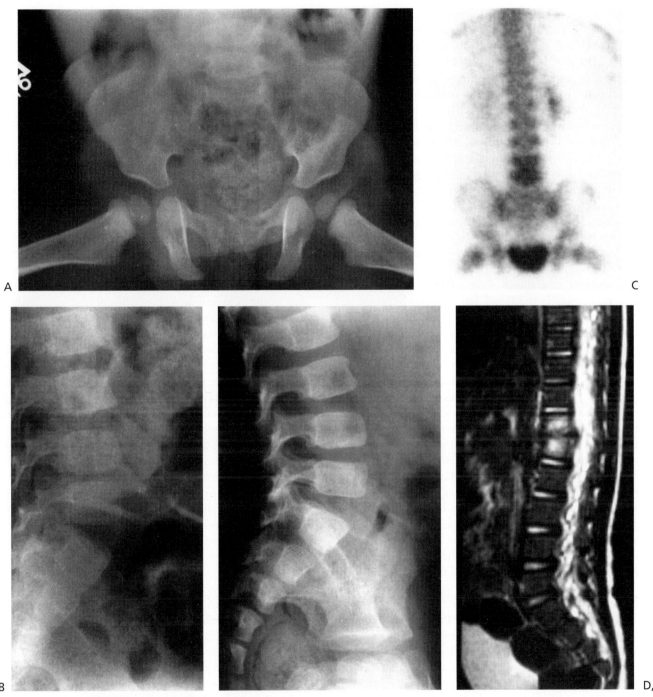

FIGURE 13-12. A: AP view of the pelvis of a 14-month-old child who stopped walking after several days of limping, falling, and irritability. This radiograph was ordered by the initial treating physician because of the suspicion of hip infection. Note the narrowing of the L4–L5 disc space. **B:** The lateral view was taken subsequently, when examination by the orthopaedic surgeon demonstrated pain on percussion of the lower spine. Again, note the narrowing of the L4–L5 disc space. **C:** Increased isotope uptake in the vertebral bodies of L4 and L5, which is typical of discitis, is demonstrated. **D:** At 10-month follow-up, the disc space has almost recovered its normal height. **E:** A fast spin-echo T2 MRI of a 22-month-old child with a similar story. Note the more significant changes in the disc than expected on the radiographs. The enhancement of the vertebral bodies demonstrates that the process is not confined to the disc as described in the past.

the vertebral bodies. When performed on patients having classic disc space narrowing, it usually shows unsuspected areas of vertebral involvement. Although it is not often necessary, MRI is a useful tool in the case that is difficult to diagnose. In addition, it gives so much clear information that it is hard to resist using this as the first imaging test following the plain radiograph. MRI clearly demonstrates the involvement of the adjacent vertebrae (138,139).

Differential diagnosis between tumor and infection is usually not difficult on the plain radiographs. Collapse of the vertebral body, with preservation of the disc space, is seen in eosinophilic granuloma (vertebra plana) and, to a lesser extent, in leukemia. Neither of these conditions demonstrates increased isotope uptake on bone scan early in their course. Destruction of bone, with subsequent involvement of one or two disc spaces, suggests infection. A large amount of bone destruction, especially in adjacent vertebrae, suggests tuberculosis. Primary bone tumors of the spine are unusual in childhood, but must also be considered when bone destruction is present. MRI offers more detail about the extent of both bone and surrounding soft tissue involvement, and for that reason is a very useful test when a question arises as to the possibility of tumor (147).

In almost all other cases of musculoskeletal infection, aspiration or biopsy for culture is considered to be mandatory. With infections of the vertebrae and disc, however, difficulty, potential complications, morbidity, and cost are factors that usually lead to treatment without biopsy. This course is supported by the usually benign natural history of this condition, and by the excellent results that are achieved with empiric treatment in the absence of positive cultures. In those series in which biopsy has been performed, the yield of positive cultures is slightly less than 50%. Open biopsy is more likely to yield positive cultures than needle biopsy, and there is a trend toward better identification of organisms in more recent series. The results of the positive biopsies show a preponderance of *S. aureus* as the causative organism (144–146,148).

The treatment of disc space infections reflects both past observations and contemporary knowledge. Past observations of this disease demonstrated that it was largely self-limited, with occasional morbidity, and was successfully treated with rest, despite recognition of a likely infectious etiology (136,149). Current treatment consists of antistaphylococcic antibiotics (e.g., a semisynthetic penicillin or first-generation cephalosporin, as used in the initial treatment of AHO) (146). This has resulted in less morbidity (138). Antibiotic therapy is usually started intravenously, with hospitalization and bed rest. Careful observation for the onset of neurologic signs that would indicate epidural abscess formation is advisable until the patient shows resolution of symptoms. Immobilization may also be used, but the trend is to avoid it. If the patient's symptoms resolve, intravenous antibiotics are switched to oral antibiotics after 5 to 7 days. Oral antibiotics are continued for 3 to 5 weeks.

Resolution of symptoms usually occurs within the first 72 h. If this is not the case, the physician should begin to question the diagnosis or the specific bacterial etiology. Further imaging studies, such as CT scan or MRI, may be justified in such circumstances to search for tumor or abscess formation. Biopsy is indicated in a patient who fails to respond to antibiotics and bed rest, or has findings on imaging studies that suggest a diagnosis other than typical discitis.

Pelvis and Sacroiliac Joint

Infections of the pelvis and SI joint share two features with each other and with discitis: They present with a wide variety of symptoms, and are thus difficult to diagnose, and they can usually be treated successfully without surgery. However, unlike discitis, pelvic infections can occur in many locations within the pelvis, making diagnosis and localization more difficult. The debate over whether the process in the SI joint is an osteomyelitis or true septic arthritis is largely irrelevant to the clinician. Both are possible and probably occur, and both are treated in the same way.

The presentation is not always acute, as in most forms of septic arthritis and osteomyelitis. In one series, only one-third of the cases were acute, and the average time from onset to diagnosis was 3.9 weeks (150). Morgan and Yates (151) described four different presentations of osteomyelitis of the pelvis, depending on the initial area of pain: hip joint, abdominal, buttocks, and sciatic. In addition, they described a systemic presentation with malaise and fever. Beaupre and Carrol (152) described three presentations of SI joint osteomyelitis, which they termed gluteal, abdominal, and lumbar disc. The lumbar disc syndrome presents with pain in the lower back, hip, and thigh; the gluteal syndrome presents with pain, and possibly a mass in the buttocks; and the abdominal syndrome can mimic acute appendicitis.

The most important step in the diagnosis of pelvic osteomyelitis is to consider it as a possibility. Failure to perform an adequate examination for symptoms in the SI joint by compression and careful palpation of the other pelvic bones is a common cause of delay in diagnosis and confusion with other sites of infection. At the same time, it is important to remember that the pelvis and the SI joint are the site for many different pathologic processes, of which infection is only one (153).

Perhaps the most common diagnosis that is confused with SI joint sepsis is septic hip. SI joint infection is generally seen in older children, with the mean age being 10 years, whereas septic hip is more common in the younger child (150). Despite the complaint of pain around the hip, children with SI joint infection often remain ambulatory, and have relatively free internal rotation of the hip, in contrast to those with a septic hip. Conversely, patients with SI joint infection frequently experience greater pain on external rotation of the hip than internal rotation. If the

FABER test (flexion, abduction, external rotation) is performed, it usually elicits pain in the presence of SI joint sepsis, as does compression of the pelvis (Gaenslen test). Tenderness almost always is found over the SI joint, if sought. Other areas (e.g., the ischium, pubis, ilium) should always be palpated for tenderness in children with gait disturbance or hip pain.

It is important to remember that osteomyelitis can occur in any location in any pelvic bone, and failure to elicit symptoms in the SI joint does not rule out pelvic osteomyelitis (154,155). Bony tenderness is usually present at the site of involvement, emphasizing the importance of suspicion, followed by a careful examination (155).

Osteomyelitis of the ischiopubic synchondrosis presents a confusing picture, despite tenderness being present. This synchondrosis, which fuses between 5 and 12 years of age, and occasionally later, shows a radiographic picture of expansion, and uneven mineralization before fusion. In addition, it is often asymmetric to the opposite side, which may have fused earlier, and radioisotope uptake is increased in many cases (156). Kloiber and colleagues report that, if the radioisotope activity at the ischiopubic synchondrosis is equal to or greater than that adjacent to the triradiate cartilage, or if the activity extends into the adjacent pubic ramus or ischium, it is indicative of a pathologic process (157).

Oblique radiographic views demonstrating the SI joint may be obtained, but their value today in making an early diagnosis with better imaging techniques is doubtful. In most cases of pelvic osteomyelitis, the initial radiographs are normal. This is especially true when symptoms have been present for fewer than 1 or 2 weeks. The earliest sign of infection on the radiograph is disappearance of the subchondral margins and erosion; however, this should be considered to be a late finding. If radiographic changes are present with less than 1 week of symptoms, careful consideration should be given to other disorders, such as tumor or chronic inflammatory SI disease. Until recently, the ^{99m}Tc bone-scanning was the most effective test in localizing a focus of pathology within the pelvic bones, but this may be changing, with further experience with MRI (158–161). Single photon emission computed tomography (SPECT) scanning should be utilized in the pelvis, as in the spine.

CT scans likewise can be helpful in several respects, but are not necessary in all cases (159,161,162). CT scans can better delineate the extent of bone involvement than can the radionuclide scan.

More recently, the value of MRI has become apparent in not only localizing the location and extent of bone involvement, but also in better delineating soft tissue changes, e.g., abscess formation (163) (Fig. 13-13).

Schaad and colleagues reported that the bacterial etiology was established in 57% of the cases they studied from their own patients, and from a literature review (150). In most cases, *S. aureus* is the organism that is cultured from blood, direct aspiration, or biopsy (150,152,159,161,164). *Staph-*ylococcus epidermidis* and *Streptococcus* species are also reported, but, in many cases, may be contaminants (159). An occasional *Salmonella* species may be isolated in patients who are not otherwise predisposed (150,161,165).

Laboratory findings in SI joint sepsis and pelvic osteomyelitis parallel other bone and joint infections, with the leukocytes often being normal and the ESR and CRP levels usually elevated. Blood cultures are positive in about 50% of cases; therefore, considering the difficulty in obtaining cultures from the SI joint and pelvis, they should always be obtained. *Salmonella* is always a possibility, even in those not predisposed to this organism, and, thus, stool cultures should be obtained. Joint aspirates are positive for the organism less often than in other cases of bone and joint sepsis (150,153,164). Although this is partly due to the difficulty in entering the joint, even biopsy specimens and pus seem to yield positive culture results less often than would be expected.

In the report by Reilly and colleagues (161), six of ten cultures from aspiration or biopsy of the SI joint were positive; the same yield as obtained from blood cultures. The technique for aspirating the SI joint has been described (166,167).

The author prefers to aspirate only those cases that do not respond promptly to antibiotics, or that exhibit atypical features, for the following reasons:

- Morbidity and expense associated with this procedure, which usually requires general anesthesia, are high
- Blood or stool culture can identify at least 60% of the organisms
- Most organisms are *S. aureus*
- The literature indicates that most of these patients respond to antistaphylococcic antibiotics.

Reports in the literature demonstrate that surgical debridement of pelvic osteomyelitis is usually not necessary (152,153,164). This contradicts reports in the older literature. The ability of this process to resolve with antibiotic therapy alone is probably due to a variety of factors: the large and diffuse blood supply to the bones, which makes sequestrum formation unlikely; the rigid ligament structure around the SI joint, which contains the spread of infection; and negligible long-term morbidity, even when the joint becomes ankylosed (164). Indications for surgery are those for biopsy in the case of suspected tumor, an unusual presentation, or failure to achieve resolution of the symptoms in a reasonable amount of time. Drainage of a large abscess may be necessary, especially in the presence of systemic symptoms.

Initial antibiotic therapy should be with an intravenous semisynthetic penicillin or first-generation cephalosporin, as used in the treatment of AHO (see Table 13-3). If symptoms resolve and the CRP begins to fall, the patient may be switched to oral antibiotics in 5 to 7 days, if adequate

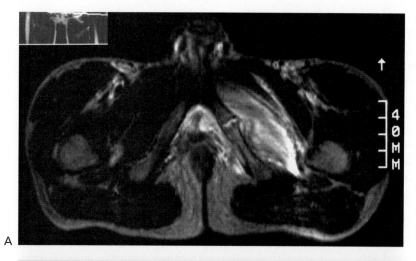

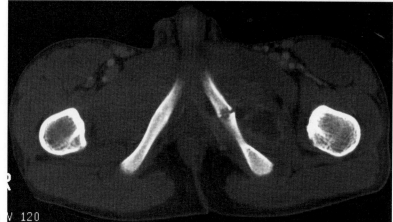

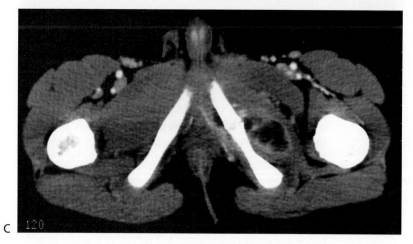

FIGURE 13-13. A: A T2 MR image of a 9-year-old boy with a history of increasing limp and hip pain for 1 week. The edema in the obturator muscle, the increased signal intensity around the ischiopubic synchondrosis, and the suggestion of abscess formation all suggest pelvic osteomyelitis. When the symptoms failed to resolve with intravenous antibiotics, CT-guided needle aspiration of the abscess was performed. **B:** Note the changes in the bone around the ischiopubic synchondrosis seen on the bone windows. **C:** Note the abscess seen on the soft tissue windows. Although MRI might still be the best choice for an initial imaging study in suspected pelvic osteomyelitis because of its ability to detect early changes within the bone, a great deal of information can be obtained from a good CT scan.

blood levels are obtained with oral administration. Initial and subsequent antibiotics should be adjusted to reflect information from blood and stool cultures, in addition to biopsy material, if that has been obtained. Failure of a response suggests that the antibiotic is not effective against the causative organism, a large abscess persists, or the etiology is not infectious.

The Neonate

Both AHO and septic arthritis can occur in the neonatal period. The classic definition of the neonatal period is the first 28 days of life. For the purposes of antibiotic selection in community-acquired infection, however, the physician is well advised to consider this period to extend to the first

8 weeks of life. The pathogenesis, diagnosis, and treatment of bone and joint sepsis differ significantly in the neonate.

The immune system in the neonate is immature. The factors are multiple, with some being specific and others nonspecific, and many of them are incompletely understood (168,169). There are two important effects of this lack of well-developed immunity. First, neonates are susceptible to a wide range of organisms that are less virulent under normal circumstances. Second, because they lack a well-developed immune system, neonates do not have the usual inflammatory response that creates the signs and symptoms so important to early diagnosis.

In most circumstances, the organisms reach the bone or joint by the hematogenous route. In addition to their unusual susceptibility to many organisms that may be considered normal flora, neonates may be subjected to a wider range of organisms and to opportunities for these organisms to gain access to the circulation. This is particularly true of the neonate (especially the premature infant) who is sick and remains in the intensive care unit in the presence of nosocomial pathogens, coupled with invasive monitoring, intravenous feeding, drug administration, and blood sampling. Indwelling vascular catheters, particularly those in the umbilical vessels, have long been recognized as being one of the main sources of infection (170).

There appears to be two types of infection in the neonate: that recognized in the hospital in premature infants, and that which becomes apparent after discharge from the nursery in otherwise healthy, full-term neonates. The type manifest in the hospital usually occurs in premature infants undergoing invasive monitoring. These infants are more likely to have infection caused by *S. aureus* or Gram-negative organisms, to have multiple sites of involvement, and to be systemically ill. More than 40% of affected infants have more than one site of involvement (171,172). The other type is usually manifest between 2 and 4 weeks of life (sometimes as late as 8 weeks), in infants who are not systemically ill, and are developing and feeding normally. These infections are more likely to be due to group B *Streptococcus*, and involve a single site.

Most cases of bone and joint sepsis in the neonate are caused by *S. aureus*, with group B *Streptococcus* being the next most common. Gram-negative organisms probably comprise 10 to 15% of the infections (171–172). *Candida albicans* is not uncommon, but usually occurs along with or after other infection, often in patients on prolonged antibiotic therapy or hyperalimentation (179). It is characterized by an even greater lack of the usual symptoms (e.g., increased warmth, tenderness).

A unique feature of neonatal bone and joint sepsis is the frequent association of contiguous bone and joint involvement and high morbidity due to the subsequent destruction of the growth plate or joint. This association, which has been reported to be as high as 76% (171,172), leads to another important difference between the neonate and the older child, regarding the changing anatomy with growth and maturation. Trueta (31,180) described the changing vascular anatomy of the physis, and particularly the femoral head, during growth. Ogden (181) extensively studied the role that this unique vascular anatomy plays in neonatal osteomyelitis, and Chung (182) beautifully demonstrated this changing anatomy with injected human specimens.

The changing anatomy of the blood supply within the physis has been addressed previously in this chapter. Its importance in neonatal osteomyelitis is that the vascular channels penetrating the physis and the chondroepiphysis (cartilaginous anlage of the epiphysis) permit an early destruction of both, with consequent disturbance of growth and joint congruity. This probably occurs both by lysis of the cartilage, through the direct action of the organisms, and by destruction of the blood vessels (and the consequent avascular changes) by the inflammatory process (181,183).

Ogden's studies led him to conclude that the frequent association of bone and joint involvement was the result of primary bone infection, and was mainly due to the vascular canals traversing the physeal plate and the chondroepiphysis, allowing early abscess formation in the chondroepiphysis, which could rupture into the joint. An additional factor is that the metaphysis in neonates may lie within the capsule of the joint, thus creating septic arthritis when the pus penetrates the metaphysis and elevates the periosteum (181,183). The lesson for the physician is that, when a septic joint is diagnosed in the neonate, a thorough search for osteomyelitis in an adjacent metaphysis or epiphysis is mandatory.

The diagnosis of bone and joint sepsis in the neonate is not easy, largely because of the absence of signs and symptoms secondary to the immature immune system. In one report on the value of bone scintigraphy in detection of neonatal osteomyelitis, the sensitivity for diagnosing focal disease by clinical findings was 20%, radiography 65%, and bone scintigraphy 90%. This illustrates the need for a high index of suspicion and reliance on tests other than examination, for the localization of the disease (184).

The most common presenting findings are swelling, followed by pseudoparalysis and tenderness. The large amount of fat surrounding the limbs of the neonate often makes detection of swelling difficult, whereas the lack of apparent illness often leads the unsuspecting physician to ascribe the lack of motion or apparent pain to some other cause. The diagnosis in the septic premature neonate is often delayed while other causes, such as meningitis or pneumonia, are sought.

Because early diagnosis is so important, the evaluation of the septic infant for osteomyelitis or septic arthritis should be serial, and not sequential. Any neonate with sepsis should be suspected of musculoskeletal sepsis. Any infant who exhibits disuse, discomfort of a joint with motion, or tenderness of a limb should be suspected of having bone or joint sepsis.

Other than possible soft tissue swelling, radiographic changes do not accompany an early diagnosis. The ^{99m}Tc bone scan is useful because it can survey the entire skeleton and detect changes before they are radiographically apparent. Ash and Gilday (185), however, found that only 32% of proved sites of osteomyelitis in 10 neonates were positive on the bone scan. This lack of ability to detect osteomyelitis may be partly due to the lack of inflammatory response to the infection, or because the infectious focus lies adjacent to the active growth plate, and is thus obscured by the uptake of the isotope in the growth plate. Subsequently, Bressler and colleagues (186) reported a more favorable experience, detecting all 25 sites of proved osteomyelitis in 15 affected infants. The improved results appear to be due to higher-resolution equipment and magnification views of all suspected areas.

Routine laboratory evaluation is of little value. The leukocyte count and differential leukocyte count are not reliably elevated. The sedimentation rate is usually elevated, but is a nonspecific finding. The blood cultures are positive in about 50% of patients with proven infection.

Once the area of involvement is identified, aspiration is mandatory. This permits confirmation, either through obtaining pus, a positive Gram-stain, or a positive culture. The author strongly believes that in any neonate with known osteomyelitis or septic arthritis, both hip joints should be aspirated because:

- Multiple sites of involvement are common
- The proximal femur and hip joint are frequently involved
- Symptoms and signs are often subtle or lacking
- The hip is the most difficult joint to examine
- The window of opportunity for effective treatment is small
- The hip joint is the most frequent site of permanent sequelae.

The antibiotic management of the neonate is difficult, and should be undertaken in conjunction with a physician having such experience. The selection of the antibiotic is guided by the probable causative organisms, and modified by positive Gram-staining and culture. The dosage varies, depending on the degree of prematurity and the status of hepatic or renal function. Because penicillinase-resistant forms of *S. aureus*, in addition to Gram-negative enteric organisms, are possible, initial antibiotic selection should cover these organisms, as well as group B *Streptococcus*. Choices may include oxacillin, along with gentamicin or a third-generation cephalosporin such as cefotaxime or ceftazidime. Ceftriaxone (Rocephin) may also be used if there is no jaundice. If methicillin-resistant *S. aureus* is suspected, vancomycin should be considered in the initial therapy.

Some authors have implied that surgical drainage may worsen the result (172), and others have implied success without surgical drainage (174). Such studies suffer from treatment of only the most severe cases with surgery, accep-

tance of a high incidence of complications, and inadequate follow-up to detect the magnitude of growth alteration. It would seem to be even more imperative to treat the neonate with surgical debridement because adequate immune mechanisms are lacking. Therefore, when pus is found its removal is advised. This cannot be adequately accomplished with repeated aspiration, and therefore this form of therapy is not recommended.

Sickle Cell Disease

Sickle cell disease is the result of an autosomal recessive gene that produces abnormal hemoglobin, with numerous effects. Marrow hyperplasia, as a mechanism to compensate for the reduced oxygen-carrying capacity of the erythrocytes, resorbs both trabeculae and cortex, whereas reactive bone formation thickens the existing trabeculae. Susceptibility to infections other than osteomyelitis (e.g., sepsis, pneumonia) is increased, growth and sexual development are retarded, and infarction of bone and other organs is common. This section discusses only those factors relating to bone and joint infection.

The gene responsible for production of the abnormal hemoglobin (hemoglobin S gene) occurs predominantly in those of African descent, but is also present in whites in Greece, Turkey, Italy, and India. It is estimated that between 8 and 30% of African-Americans carry the hemoglobin S gene. About 2.5% of African-Americans are estimated to be homozygous for the gene that produces the clinical picture of sickle cell anemia. Although patients who are homozygous for the sickle cell gene are those most likely to be affected with bone infarction and infection, those who have hemoglobin SC disease, or hemoglobin *S. thalassemia*, are also predisposed. The pathophysiologic effects of the abnormal hemoglobin molecule are discussed in Chapter 11.

Although the orthopaedist is most familiar with the bone manifestations of this disease, it is important to remember that the most serious, common, and important infections result from the *Pneumococcus* organism. This is because those children who are homozygous for the sickle gene have defects in the alternate complement pathway, defects in opsonic activity, and impaired splenic function, which renders them susceptible to infection from pneumococci (187). In addition, these children may have an increased susceptibility to *H. influenzae*. Neither of these organisms play a large role in the bone and joint sepsis seen by the orthopaedist.

The incidence of osteomyelitis in patients with sickle cell anemia is low (particularly in the United States), despite the attention it receives in the literature. In 1971, Specht (188) found only 82 cases in the literature, whereas the few cases reported over several years in other large centers attest to the infrequent occurrence (189,190). This low incidence is even more important to the orthopaedist, when considered relative to the number of admissions for sickle cell crisis, a clinically similar presentation (190).

The presentation of osteomyelitis or sickle cell crisis in patients with sickle cell disease does not differ significantly. Because infection is thought to follow bone infarction, both conditions may coexist. The patient with known sickle cell disease in crisis presents as an uncomfortable child with pain in one or more joints or bones. Mild swelling is often present, joint effusions are not uncommon, and bone tenderness is usual. A late but differentiating feature is that with proper management the pain of infarction is usually markedly diminished by 3 to 5 days, whereas that of infection is not, unless antibiotics are also administered.

The leukocyte count and differential are not helpful in distinguishing infection from infarction. The ESR must be interpreted with caution, because it is elevated in both infarction and infection. In addition, the ESR tends to be falsely low in patients with sickle cell disease. The ESR is more likely to be above 20 mm/h in those with infection (191,192), and significant elevations should raise the suspicion of sepsis.

The initial radiologic manifestations of osteomyelitis in sickle cell disease are indistinguishable from those of bone infarction, and consist of periosteal new bone along the diaphysis. As the infection proceeds, however, a diffuse moth-eaten appearance of the bone occurs, with longitudinal fissuring and increasing periosteal bone formation. This results in the typical radiographic findings of a chronic diaphyseal bone infection with involucrum and sequestrum. Frequently, the other changes of sickle cell disease are seen also—the result of marrow hyperplasia and previous bone infarction (Fig. 13-14).

The role of bone scintigraphy to differentiate marrow infarction from infection has been controversial (190, 193,194). An understanding of the local pathophysiology in both conditions explains the problem and the potential usefulness of this modality. Bone infarction initially produces an area of decreased vascularity, and thus decreased isotope uptake. Once the inflammatory reaction to the in-

farction is established, however, the vascularity around the infarction results in increased isotope uptake. This probably occurs between 3 and 7 days after the infarction. Once it occurs, the scintigraphic appearance is the same as that of infection, which also produces increased vascularity and increased isotope uptake.

Therefore, if bone scintigraphy is to be useful, it must be performed early, preferably within 72 h of the onset of symptoms. Two different scans must be used: a ^{99m}Tc bone scan, followed by a bone marrow scan with a different isotope. Increased uptake on the ^{99m}Tc scan, with decreased uptake on the marrow scan, suggests infection (190,195). Although gallium 67 citrate scanning after ^{99m}Tc scanning has been recommended, it has not been found useful by others (190), and its high radiation dose to the child is an additional factor to consider.

The use of MRI has not proven to be of great value. This is in part because the findings of marrow infarction, as well as those in the soft tissues, are not reliably distinguished from sepsis (196). At the same time, other reports value ultrasonography in the differentiation of osteomyelitis from vasoocclusive crisis by demonstrating subperiosteal fluid and thickening of the periosteum (197,198). The answer as to why ultrasonography was successful when MRI failed lies in the details of these reports. In the reports of ultrasound diagnosis, many other parameters were actually used to arrive at the diagnosis.

A unique manifestation of this disorder is a condition known as sickle cell dactylitis, or hand–foot syndrome (24,199). The condition occurs in infants and young children, usually those younger than 4 years of age. No case of a child older than 7 years of age has been reported. It may precede the diagnosis of sickle cell disease. The actual incidence is probably between 10 and 20% of children with sickle cell disease, and it seems to be more common in Africa. Although it is logical to assume that it is due to infarction, there is also evidence that it may be secondary to acute marrow hyperplasia, because it is not seen once the hands and feet are no longer the site of active hematopoietic production.

Patients present with acute symmetric or asymmetric painful swelling of the hands and feet. Although considered to be a benign condition, obviating further evaluation (199), *Salmonella* osteomyelitis has been associated with this condition (200,201). Laboratory tests do not help in the differential diagnosis. Radiographic findings in the hand–foot syndrome at first demonstrate only soft tissue swelling, followed in 7 to 14 days by the formation of subperiosteal new bone. This is followed by medullary resorption and the appearance of irregular densities, in addition to cortical thinning. The changes revert to normal in weeks to months. Thus, radiographs do not help in the differential diagnosis.

With so few objective findings and tests to help in the differential diagnosis of bone infarction and osteomyelitis, how should the orthopaedist approach the patient in a clini-

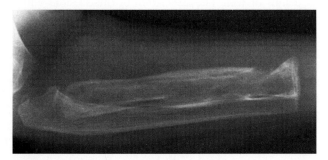

FIGURE 13-14. Lateral radiograph of the forearm in this infant demonstrate the typical changes of sickle cell osteomyelitis: longitudinal fissuring, diaphyseal location of the infection, and developing involucrum. These changes would be expected in any chronic infection of bone, and are not unique to sickle cell osteomyelitis.

cal situation, wherein the diagnosis could be either? Awareness, repeated examination, and blood cultures are basic and important. High fever, an elevated ESR, and a sequential bone scan early in the course of the disease may raise the suspicion of osteomyelitis. Aspiration of the suspected bone, with Gram-staining and culturing of all material, should not be postponed when the orthopaedist or another caring for the child suspects infection. This is the only test that confirms the diagnosis, and allows appropriate early treatment.

In the literature, recommendations for or against surgical debridement are variable: Some believe it to be the best treatment (202), some believe that patients do well without surgery (191,192,203), and others report surgery without specific indications (191,192). A close look at the outcomes and complications of this disease lead the modern orthopaedist to question the treatment of osteomyelitis without surgical drainage. Although in children the diaphyseal infections eventually heal, the contemporary standard of care seeks to avoid the diaphyseal destruction commonly seen, and the morbidity of prolonged hospitalization, intravenous antibiotic administration, and late sequelae. In other words, early diagnosis (not common in reports in the literature) and prompt drainage of an abscess, especially in an area of infarction, may result in outcomes comparable with normal children having the usual course of pyogenic osteomyelitis.

The question of using a tourniquet in patients with sickle cell disease who are undergoing extremity surgery is frequently raised because of the possibility that the ischemia may provoke thrombosis. This does not seem to be a problem; when the patient is properly prepared for surgery, no complications from the use of a tourniquet should result (204,205).

Which organism is the most common cause of osteomyelitis in sickle cell disease: *S. aureus* or *Salmonella?* This is a frequent test question, although it has little relevance in practice because both are so common that antibiotics must be given against both organisms until cultures establish the etiology. In addition, the literature is contradictory on which organism is the most common (191,203,205). A recent article reviewing the world literature since 1959 found *Salmonella* to be the most common (207).

Initial antibiotic choices are cefotaxime (Claforan) or ceftriaxone (Rocephin), each of which covers both *S. aureus* and *Salmonella* species, including those *Salmonella* resistant to ampicillin, chloramphenicol, or trimethoprim-sulfamethoxazole (Bactrim) (Table 13-3).

Arthritis may be seen in various forms in patients with sickle cell disease (208). The most common is an aseptic arthritis, most likely due to the sickle cell disease. It may be seen during crisis, but is more often a transient synovitis, usually involving the knee, which resolves within 5 days (209,210). A second form of aseptic arthritis is that associated with a remote *Salmonella* infection. This may be seen with other organisms, and the exact mechanism is not clear. Finally, the patient with sickle cell disease may have a septic arthritis. When this is the case, *Salmonella* is not the most likely organism. *Salmonella* is a rare organism in septic arthritis (210); when it occurs, it is most often in patients without sickle cell disease. When *Salmonella* septic arthritis occurs in sickle cell patients, it is most often from contiguous spread of osteomyelitis. More likely organisms in septic arthritis are *Staphylococcus* species (202,212). As with osteomyelitis, there is a difference of opinion on the advisability of arthrotomy for drainage (202,212).

Chronic Recurrent Multifocal Osteomyelitis

In 1972, a condition described as "subacute and chronic symmetrical osteomyelitis" was reported in the radiology literature (213). Since then, more than 50 cases of this disorder, which has come to be known as "chronic recurrent multifocal osteomyelitis" (CRMO) have been described. Females are affected in about 70% of the cases (214). This entity is distinct from pyogenic osteomyelitis, and is associated with a variety of other curious disorders of bone and skin. These associations include chronic sclerosing osteomyelitis of Garré, condensing osteitis of the clavicle, sternocostoclavicular hyperostosis, and palmoplantar pustulosis.

The clinical picture is characterized by the insidious onset of pain, often with swelling and occasionally erythema, suggesting infection of the bone. In a retrospective review of 14 patients with CRMO, 86% presented with a single tender swollen periarticular site (215). Patients usually remain ambulatory. Although more often multifocal, the initial presentation may be unifocal, progressing to multifocal. Although arthritis is more common in adults, it may be seen in adolescents (216). This and subsequent attacks are usually associated with symptoms of malaise and occasionally low-grade fever.

A curious, associated condition is palmoplantar pustulosis, a descriptive term for vesicles that may appear on the hands or feet. The association of these lesions with a variety of bone lesions is common, and all of these various conditions, previously described as being associated with palmoplantar pustulosis, are probably the same disease (217). These lesions do not occur in all cases, but seem to recur with recurrence of the bone symptoms. The bone lesions and the clinical course do not seem to differ between patients with and without these skin manifestations.

The subsequent course of resolution, then recurrence months later, is characteristic of this disease. Subsequent flare-ups are associated with the same findings and symptoms of the initial attack. The same or different bones may be involved. Generally, the symptoms recur over a period of 2 years; however, symptoms may recur as many as 5 years later. Growth arrest has been both absent (216) and present (218) in different series.

Laboratory findings are distinct from the usual findings in pyogenic osteomyelitis because the leukocyte count remains normal. The sedimentation rate is elevated, and cultures of bone and blood are negative. It has been noted that the chemotactic activity of the polymorphonuclear cells is increased, whereas in the presence of bacterial infection, this activity is decreased (214).

The descriptions of the pathology in the bony lesions vary in the literature (214,217,218). This variation probably results from sampling differences and the stage of the lesion at the time of the biopsy. It seems that early lesions consist of infiltration predominantly with neutrophils. This is followed by infiltration with fibrovascular tissue and inflam-matory cells (predominantly lymphocytes and plasma cells). Osteoblasts and trabecular thickening follow.

At the time of presentation, the characteristic metaphyseal lesions are usually well developed. These lesions consist of poorly delimited eccentric metaphyseal lucencies along the physeal border. These lesions have been shown to cross into the epiphysis (216,221). The most common sites for these lesions are the distal and proximal metaphyses of the tibia and femur. Other affected sites are the distal radius and ulna, the distal fibula, and the metatarsals (Fig. 13-15). From a review of the literature, it seems that almost every bone has been reported as being involved, including the pelvis.

As healing occurs, sclerosis surrounds the lesion. When the lesion extends into the cortex, periosteal reaction may

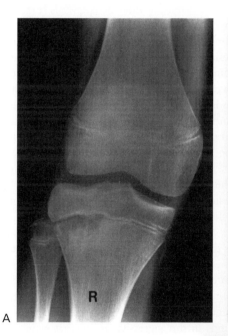

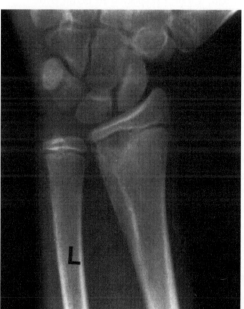

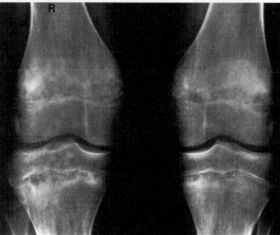

FIGURE 13-15. A 12-year-old girl presented with recurrent limp over a period of 18 months. She complained of pain in the right knee. Examination demonstrated tenderness about the right knee, but no other signs of inflammation. **A:** Radiograph of the right knee showed metaphyseal irregularity of the proximal tibia. **B:** Skeletal survey demonstrated additional similar lesions in the opposite knee, distal tibia, and radius. These lesions were asymptomatic. **C:** Radiographs 1 year later show diffuse metaphyseal changes of the distal femur and proximal tibia of both legs. No antibiotics were administered, and the symptoms resolved over the next several months.

occur. This is more likely to be seen early in the course in the small tubular and flat bones. This picture can be confused with bony neoplasm, such as leukemia, Ewing sarcoma, or eosinophilic granuloma.

The clavicle is frequently involved, presenting as a chronic sclerosing osteomyelitis (220). When present, this starts in the medial end of the clavicle and may present with both lucencies and an onionskin periosteal reaction.

Bone scintigraphy shows increased uptake in radiographically apparent lesions, and also helps to identify lesions that are not apparent on plain radiographs. In one report, bilateral lesions were found in 64% of the patients, and bone scintigraphy was very useful in finding the asymptomatic lesions (215).

It is doubtful that every case needs to undergo biopsy. If the picture is characteristic, little is to be gained. There may well be circumstances wherein the diagnosis is in doubt, in which case biopsy is necessary to rule out a malignancy, or to obtain culture from a lesion suspected of being pyogenic or tuberculous.

The most likely confusion is between subacute osteomyelitis and chronic recurrent multifocal osteomyelitis. Gamble and Rinsky (222) compared groups of patients with each other. From their data, the only helpful initial finding is the presence of multiple bone lesions in patients with chronic recurrent multifocal osteomyelitis. The age, symptoms, and laboratory findings were similar in both groups. Occasionally the periosteal reaction can indicate a more serious bone lesion, such as Ewing sarcoma, when it is the only lesion.

There is no specific treatment for this disorder, and the symptoms resolve without treatment. In most cases, nonsteroidal antiinflammatory medications ameliorate the pain. Antibiotics have not been demonstrated to have any effect on the course of the disorder, and are not indicated.

Subacute Osteomyelitis

In 1965, Harris and Kirkaldy-Willis (223) called attention to a subacute form of pyogenic osteomyelitis in which there had been no acute symptoms and the patient had received no antibiotics. Four years later, King and Mayo (224) reported a similar group of patients. The characteristic presenting features were no previous acute attack to suggest evolution of an acute osteomyelitis to a chronic form, insidious onset of pain, absence of systemic signs, and radiographic presence of a bone lesion at the time of presentation. They found these lesions in both the epiphysis and diaphysis, and described the various radiographic presentations.

Regardless of the location within the bone, the presentation is usually the same: weeks to months of worsening pain that started insidiously, and limp and tenderness with swelling visible, depending on the location. In addition, the laboratory findings are similar in most cases, and are distinct from AHO. The leukocyte count is usually normal or only slightly elevated. The ESR is usually elevated, although usually not as high as in AHO. Blood cultures are usually negative, although curettings from the lesions are frequently culture-positive, usually for *S. aureus*. Histology is compatible with acute and chronic inflammation.

Radiographic lesions are usually seen at the time of presentation. Far from being uniform, these lesions can present in many different locations and with a plethora of radiographic features. This highlights the main problem that faces the treating physician: the differential diagnosis of the lesion. Gledhill's classification (225) was further expanded by Roberts and colleagues (226) (Fig. 13-16). Differentiating some of these lesions from tumor is the most difficult part of the diagnosis (227).

The most common type of subacute osteomyelitis in the pediatric age group is the metaphyseal lesion (types IA and IB) (228). This represents a true Brodie abscess, a localized abscess of bone without previous acute illness. The lesion is located eccentrically in the metaphysis, frequently with visible extension into the epiphysis (Fig. 13-17). The lesion may have a sclerotic border, or may be irregular and ill-defined. The second most common type is the epiphyseal lesion (type V) (229–231). The radiographic appearance is similar to the lesion in the metaphysis; it also may extend across the plate into the metaphysis. The other lesions—erosion of the metaphyseal cortex (type II); localized conical and periosteal reaction (type III); onionskin cortical reaction in the diaphysis (type IV); and those involving the vertebral body (type VI)—are seen less commonly.

Increasingly seen in patients presenting with a limp is the presence of these lesions in the tarsal bones (232). The lesions most often are lytic in the talus and calcaneus, and sclerotic in the other bones.

As mentioned, the differential diagnosis of these lesions is the most important step in correct treatment, and is often the most difficult. In a series of 71 children with subacute osteomyelitis, Ross and Cole (233) divided the lesions into two categories: aggressive lesions (26) and cavities in the region of the metaphysis and epiphysis (45). All of the lesions in the aggressive group that were in the diaphysis or metaphysis demonstrated onionskin periosteal new bone. Two lesions were in the spine. The other lesions were all in the metaphysis or epiphysis, and had the typical radiologic features of type I and V lesions described above. The differential diagnoses of a type V lesion in the epiphysis include chondroblastoma and osteoid osteoma (and osteoblastoma), with eosinophilic granuloma, enchondroma, and chondromyxoid fibroma being less common. Of these, only chondroblastoma produces a periosteal response. The differential diagnoses of the typical type I lesion include eosinophilic granuloma, and perhaps giant cell tumor. Computerized tomography can be useful in the questionable case. The type III metaphyseal lesion, with erosion of the cortex, can be confused with osteosarcoma. A recent report of a characteristic finding on T1-weighted MR images may prove helpful in some cases. While not pathognomonic, the finding

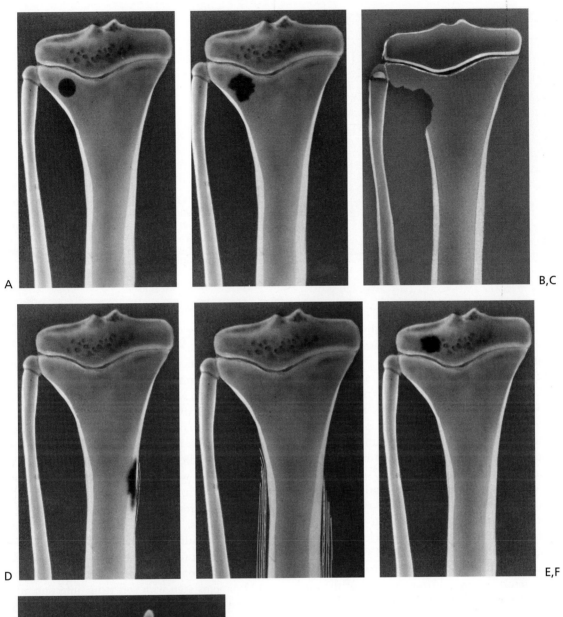

A

B,C

D

E,F

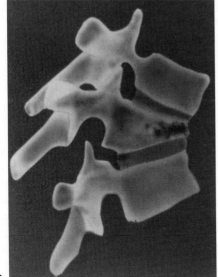

G

FIGURE 13-16. The variety of presentations of subacute hematogenous osteomyelitis in the classification of Roberts and colleagues (226). **A:** Type 1A is a punched-out metaphyseal lesion resembling an eosinophilic granuloma. **B:** Type 1B is similar to type 1A, but has a sclerotic cortex. **C:** Type 2 lesions erode the metaphyseal bone, often including the cortex, and appear as aggressive lesions. **D:** Type 3 lesions are localized cortical and periosteal reactions, simulating osteoid osteoma. **E:** Type 4 lesions produce onionskin–like periosteal reactions in the diaphysis, and resemble Ewing sarcoma. **F:** Type 5 lesions are epiphyseal erosions. **G:** Type 6 lesions involve the vertebral bodies.

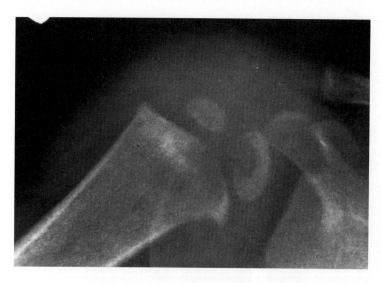

FIGURE 13-17. A 13-month-old girl presented for examination when her mother noted the child experienced discomfort when lifting her arms while her mother changed the child's clothes. *Haemophilus influenzae* was cultured from the lesion. The epiphyseal lesion communicates with the metaphyseal lesion.

of a rim of tissue, which is hyperintense relative to the main cavity, called the "penumbra sign," suggests infection as opposed to tumor (234).

The appearance of the typical lesion of a bone abscess in the epiphysis or metaphysis is so characteristic that Ross and Cole believed that it was diagnostic, and could be treated without biopsy or curettage. For these patients, they recommended 48 h of intravenous semisynthetic penicillin or first-generation cephalosporin, followed by 6 weeks of oral antibiotic. Eighty-seven percent of 37 children were healed with one course of antibiotics. Failure increased with the age of the child, and led to curettage and a further course of antibiotic. The authors do not mention the dosage of oral antibiotic, nor whether adequate serum levels of antibiotic, were verified in these patients. This 13% failure rate may be improved with a longer course of intravenous antibiotic, without resort to surgical treatment. All of the cases of aggressive lesions underwent biopsy and curettage. Hamdy et al. have subsequently reviewed 24 cases treated with antibiotics only, and 20 with surgical debridement and antibiotics, and concluded that there was no difference in the results (235).

Puncture Wounds of the Foot

Since Johanson's 1968 report (236), orthopaedic surgeons have become increasingly aware of the association between puncture wounds of the foot and *Pseudomonas aeruginosa* as the causative organism of deep infections that follow. It was subsequently demonstrated that *Pseudomonas* can be recovered from the inner spongy sole of well-worn tennis shoes (237). *P. aeruginosa* is a Gram-negative aerobic organism with anaerobic tolerance, which is found widely in soil, water, and on the skin. As a human pathogen seen in orthopaedic conditions, it seems to have an affinity for cartilage.

However, despite the common isolation of *Pseudomonas*

from puncture wound of the foot, it is important to remember that *S. aureus* is the most common soft tissue infection following puncture wound. In addition, *Aeromonas hydrophilia* is common when puncture wounds or lacerations occur in fresh water, e.g., ponds (238). Gentamicin or Bactrim are effective against this organism.

Fitzgerald and Cowan (239) identified puncture wounds of the foot as the reason for an emergency room visit in 0.8% of children younger than the age of 15 years. Of the total number with puncture wounds, 8.4% who were seen within the first 24 h after the injury, either had cellulitis at the time of presentation or returned within the first 4 days with cellulitis. Of those presenting 1 to 7 days after the injury, cellulitis was present in 57%. Only 0.6% of those who were not referred to the emergency room for an established infection subsequently developed osteomyelitis. Of 132 patients seen with soft tissue infection after puncture wound of the foot, 112 had a prompt response to soaks, rest, elevation, and antibiotics.

The importance of these data is that most infections after puncture wounds of the foot do not develop osteomyelitis or septic arthritis. This has been confirmed by a more recent report, which found osteomyelitis in only 16% of 44 children admitted to the hospital with puncture wounds of the foot (240). The cases of cellulitis that do not develop osteomyelitis or septic arthritis after puncture wounds of the foot represent the denominator usually not seen by the orthopaedist. Most of these infections respond to nonoperative therapy, such as rest, elevation, and oral antibiotics.

A major dilemma is the initial management of the puncture wound. Suggestions for "debridement and irrigation with loose closure over small irrigation tubes" are impractical, given the number of puncture wounds occurring annually in the United States, and the infrequency of serious infection (236). Similarly, the recommendation that "any deep wounds should be surgically debrided" seems impractical, because the treating physician would not know how deep the puncture wound is without anesthesia and surgical exploration (241).

Given the data on the development of cellulitis and osteomyelitis after puncture wounds, it appears that subsequent development of osteomyelitis and septic arthritis is mostly determined by whether the nail punctures the bone or joint. It is usually impossible for the initial treating physician to know this, although there should be a high degree of suspicion if the wound is over the metatarsal heads, the lateral border of the foot, or the heel—areas where the bone is in close approximation to the skin of the sole of the foot.

A reasonable approach to the initial management of a puncture wound of the foot includes superficial debridement of the skin and inspection for a foreign body, because a foreign body is found in almost 3% of cases (239). Tetanus prophylaxis is important. Because of the possibility of cellulitis developing in the first several days, patients should be advised to return at the first sign of infection. There does not seem to be any solid evidence either for or against the routine use of antibiotics in the initial management. They can be used effectively in the management of cellulitis, and

there is no effective oral antibiotic for *Pseudomonas* osteomyelitis or septic arthritis in the pediatric age group.

The typical course of osteomyelitis or septic arthritis is the onset of pain and swelling 2 to 5 days after the puncture, when the initial symptoms should be gone. At this time, soaks, elevation, and an oral antistaphylococcic antibiotic are prescribed. If the patient has cellulitis, this regimen usually results in a cure. When osteomyelitis or septic arthritis is present the symptoms may improve, but do not disappear. This is probably due to the mixed flora in these infections. Finally, either continued pain and swelling or radiographic changes prompt the correct diagnosis. Good treatment includes close follow-up of those puncture wounds having signs of infection, and appropriate treatment if signs and symptoms of cellulitis do not resolve promptly on oral antibiotic treatment.

Initially, the signs and symptoms of cellulitis and osteomyelitis or septic arthritis can be difficult to differentiate. Pain on motion of a specific metatarsophalangeal joint is usually indicative of a septic arthritis in that joint. Dorsal swelling on the forefoot, or swelling laterally and medially around the heel, is often an additional sign of a serious deep infection (Fig. 13-18). Aspiration is helpful, not only in

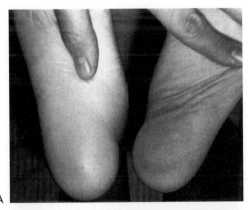

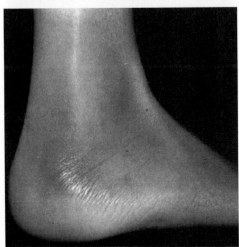

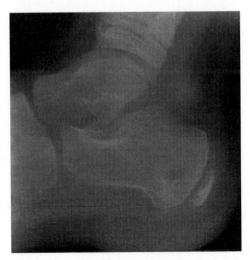

FIGURE 13-18. This patient was seen with pain 2 weeks after a puncture wound of the heel. He returned to the emergency department 3 days after the puncture wound because of increasing pain and swelling. Therapy was begun with a first-generation cephalosporin antibiotic. He experienced temporary improvement, but later the pain became worse. **A:** Note the swelling of the affected heel, when compared with the opposite contralateral heel side. **B:** Because of the dense septated tissue in the heel, osteomyelitis of the calcaneus usually is seen laterally. The swelling and erythema on the lateral side of the heel indicates deep infection. **C:** A radiograph demonstrates a lytic lesion of the heel, in addition to the soft tissue swelling. *Pseudomonas aeruginosa* was cultured from the infected site.

locating pus, but in obtaining material for culture. If no pus is obtained, bone scintigraphy may help in the early differentiation of cellulitis from osteomyelitis or septic arthritis. More recently, it has been suggested that MRI may be a more cost-effective way of diagnosing early osteomyelitis in the foot, following puncture wounds (242).

Pseudomonas infection of a bone or joint is a surgical disease; the failure of antibiotics alone to resolve these infections has been adequately demonstrated (243). The surgical approach may be either dorsal or volar, but must give adequate access to both the bones and joints in the region of the puncture, because *P. aeruginosa* is a cartilage-seeking organism. Some surgeons believe that the volar approach leaves a potentially painful scar. When properly placed, however, this should not be the case. This approach has the advantage of directly exposing the puncture track, which is an essential part of the surgery, because of the high incidence of foreign material found at surgical debridement (239,244). The dorsal approach allows direct access to the joints and bones through a more anatomic and easier-to-extend approach, which is not limited by the considerations of placement on the sole of the foot. This can be combined with a limited debridement of the volar puncture wound. Except in the most extensive cases of destruction of the calcaneus, in which the "cloven hoof" incision can be used, this bone should be approached from a medial or lateral incision, or from both.

Infections due to puncture wounds have two characteristics: They are caused by multiple organisms, and *P. aeruginosa* is usually one of them. For this reason, it makes sense to begin antibiotic therapy with a combination of antibiotics effective against both Gram-positive organisms and Gram-negative organisms, including *P. aeruginosa*. An initial choice may be ceftazidime (Fortaz) and gentamicin or oxacillin and gentamicin (Table 13-3). Jacobs and coworkers (243,244) suggest that 7 days of intravenous antibiotics after adequate surgical debridement are sufficient, although others recommend longer treatment (e.g., 10 days to 2 weeks).

Ciprofloxacin is another antibiotic that is effective against *Pseudomonas*. However, its use in children has been limited by reports of interfering with the growth plate in animal studies. Despite this, it has been used in cystic fibrosis and other serious infections in children, without reports of ill effects on cartilage or growth.

In cases that fail to respond to the above treatment, the fast-growing mycobacteria (e.g., *Mycobacterium chelonae* and *Mycobacterium fortuitum*) should be considered as possible pathogens.

Gonococcal Arthritis

Gonococcal arthritis is usually a sexually transmitted disease caused by the Gram-negative diplococcus, *Neisseria gonorrhoeae*. In the newborn, the disease is contracted from the mother during passage through the birth canal, and results most commonly in conjunctivitis and scalp abscesses. When the disease is noted after the newborn period, before puberty, and in sexually inactive adolescents, sexual abuse should be suspected. Gonococcal infection is most common in women in the second and third decade, and therefore is seen frequently in the adolescent age group. Although gonococcal infection can take many forms, the orthopaedist is most likely to encounter this infection as septic arthritis in the disseminated form of the disease.

In the adolescent, the infection most often results from dissemination of a genitourinary infection, which is frequently asymptomatic. The delay between the genitourinary infection and the arthritis is variable, ranging from a few days to several weeks. In adolescence, the disseminated form of the disease is associated with pregnancy and menstruation, periods of low progesterone activity (245).

The orthopaedist needs to be especially aware of the possibility of sexual abuse in patients with gonococcal arthritis. Sexual abuse may occur in as many as 10% of all abuse cases, and it is estimated that between 5 and 20% of sexually abused children have a sexually transmitted disease, most commonly gonococcal infection (246,247). Children who are identified with or suspected of having a gonococcal infection should have cultures of all mucous membranes, including pharynx, vagina, and rectum, before the administration of antibiotics. These cultures should be handled in a manner that permits them to be used as evidence in court. In addition, reporting of suspected cases is mandated by the Child Abuse Reporting Law. For all of these reasons, the orthopaedist should involve a knowledgeable pediatrician in the evaluation of these patients.

The classic presentation is rash, tenosynovitis, and migratory polyarthralgia. Only about one-third of the cases develop a distinctive, but not pathognomonic rash, which is a result of gonococcal septicemia. The initial lesion is a small erythematous macule. This may disappear or develop a small vesicle, followed by a necrotic center that may form a pustule. The tenosynovitis, when seen, often affects the dorsal surface of the wrist and hand. This finding, like the skin rash, is nonspecific and can be caused by other organisms.

The clinical presentation of the disseminated disease with septic arthritis begins with chills and fever in about three-fourths of the patients. Joint involvement is polyarticular in 80% of cases. The knee is most often affected, but it is important to remember that any joint, large or small, can be involved. The size of the effusion may vary widely, and may even be absent. The involved joints are usually painful. The nature of the arthritis does not appear to have changed over the past several decades, although treatment with antibiotics has resulted in the virtual elimination of joint destruction (248–252). Osteomyelitis still may be seen as an occasional complication (221).

The leukocyte count is elevated in two-thirds of the patients. Culture is the only way to confirm the diagnosis. Culture and Gram-staining of joint fluid, and of the cervix of postpubertal girls and the vagina of prepubertal girls, should be performed. Any urethral or prostatic discharge in the male should also be cultured and examined by Gram-staining. Blood cultures should be routine. The organism may occasionally be isolated from skin lesions, but Gram-staining gives a higher yield.

N. gonorrhoeae is a difficult organism to grow, and special care is needed in the handling of the material for culture. Because the organism is sensitive to cold, material for culture should be plated directly onto a warm medium, whenever possible. Special culture tubes for transport of gonococcal cultures are available, and should be used, in addition to prompt delivery of specimens to the bacteriology laboratory, when direct-plating is not feasible. Cultures from sterile sites (e.g., blood, synovial fluid) are plated on chocolate blood agar. Cultures from nonsterile sites (e.g., the vagina, skin lesions) should be plated on selective media (e.g., Thayer-Martin agar) that contains antibiotics to inhibit the growth of other organisms. Cultures are grown in a 5 to 10% CO_2 atmosphere.

The increasing resistance of *N. gonorrhoeae* to penicillin and tetracycline makes parenteral administration of a third-generation cephalosporin (e.g., ceftriaxone, 50 mg/kg/day, intramuscularly or intravenously, once daily) the initial drug of choice (Table 13-3). If the organism is demonstrated to be sensitive to penicillin, it can be used. Recommendation for drainage of the joints remains variable. In the hip joint, there is no controversy; surgical drainage, as for pyogenic septic arthritis caused by any organism, is required. In other large joints with large amounts of purulent fluid, surgical drainage may be preferable to repeated needle aspiration. If surgical drainage is used, it is wise to leave a closed suction drain in the joint, because the tendency to reaccumulate fluid is greater than with other forms of septic arthritis.

Tuberculosis

Fewer cases of tuberculosis were reported in the United States in 1985 since reporting began in 1953. Between 1985 and 1991, the incidence rose sharply, only to slightly decrease in both 1992 and 1993 for all age groups except those younger than 15 years of age. During this period, the largest increase was reported for patients born outside of the United States and its territories. In 1993, these patients comprised almost 30% of the reported cases. California, New York, and Texas saw the largest increases. The increased incidence has been accompanied by human immunodeficiency virus infection and multi-drug–resistant organisms.

Because extrapulmonary tuberculosis is more common among children, particularly those younger than 5 years of age, the orthopaedic surgeon must again become aware of this possibility when evaluating chronic joint inflammation or chronic bone lesions.

Patients who are exposed to tuberculosis may or may not become infected, and those who are infected may or may not become diseased. There is a time lag between infection and diagnosis of the extrapulmonary disease of about 1 year.

Most patients are infected by human contact because bovine tuberculosis has been eliminated in this country by the pasteurization of milk. The lungs are the most common site of initial infection in children; the kidneys are not. The tubercle bacilli may disseminate to bones or joints during the lymphatic and hematogenous spread of the initial infection. If the initial lung infection remains untreated, involvement of the bones and/or joints occurs in 5 to 10% of children (253). The development of the lesions in bone is time- and location-related. Dactylitis may occur within a few months in younger children. Long-bone involvement may occur in 1 to 3 years.

The initial focus in the bone is usually the epiphysis or metaphysis, and rarely the diaphysis. As the osteomyelitis develops, it enlarges the area of bone destruction in a centrifugal fashion, producing a characteristic round cystic lesion with ill-defined margins. These lesions are filled with an inflammatory granulation tissue, creating a reactive hyperemia, which produces a wide area of osteopenia surrounding the lesion. This process is almost purely destructive or lytic, with little or no bone reaction (Fig. 13-19)—thus, the lack of sclerotic margins and a periosteal response. Because of the chronicity and hyperemia, widening and accelerated growth of the epiphysis may be seen. The physeal plate offers little resistance to the spread of the infection, as it does in other pyogenic infections. Before extraosseous abscess formation the bone lesions may mimic pyogenic infection or tumors such as eosinophilic granuloma.

Most skeletal tuberculosis affects the spine. The infection almost always begins in the vertebral body, usually the anterior one-third. The most frequent site of involvement in the spine is the lower thoracic and upper lumbar spine. Paravertebral abscess formation is characteristic, and calcification developing within the abscess is almost diagnostic of a tuberculous abscess. The discs become involved when two adjacent vertebral bodies are affected. The bone lesions in the vertebral bodies are mainly destructive (Fig. 13-20).

Skeletal tuberculosis outside of the axial skeleton usually affects the major joints, particularly the hip and knee. Isolated joint infections, unusual in childhood, are initially characterized by effusion, in addition to synovial proliferation and thickening. In the early stages there are no radiographic characteristics that separate tuberculous arthritis from any chronic inflammation of the joint. As with the bone lesions, the hyperemia causes widespread osteopenia, and may cause overgrowth of the epiphyses. The infection proceeds both by pannus formation over the articular cartilage and by erosion of the subchondral bone, beginning at the synovial margins (254). The result is joint space narrowing and subchondral cystic erosion. Early in the process, the clinical and radiologic findings may closely resemble

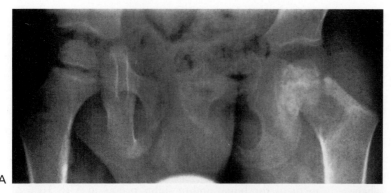

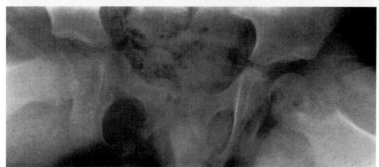

FIGURE 13-19. **A** and **B:** Radiographs of a 3-year-old boy who recently moved to the United States from Mexico. The child had complaints of increasing limp on the left, pain that worsened at night, and no significant limitation of activity. Examination demonstrated limited motion with irritability. Laboratory studies showed a normal complete blood count, erythrocyte sedimentation rate of 25 mm/h, and a positive purified protein derivative test. Open biopsy confirmed the diagnosis of tuberculosis by histology and culture. (Courtesy of Hugh Watts, M.D.)

those of JRA or pigmented villonodular synovitis. Laboratory studies, however, should easily separate these entities.

As the infection continues untreated, large amounts of caseous material and pus accumulate and dissect along normal tissue planes. Eventually, a sinus track to the surface is formed—a hallmark of a long-standing neglected case. The abscess formed by tuberculous infection is called a "cold abscess," because of the lack of any signs of acute inflammation.

Two other presentations occur in childhood. The first, tuberculous dactylitis, may resemble sickle cell dactylitis, with swelling of the phalanges, metacarpals, and metatarsals. Tuberculous dactylitis is usually not very painful, however, and onset is usually consecutive, rather than simultaneous. Before the availability of radiographs, this was called *spina* (Latin for "a short bone") *ventosa* (meaning "inflated with air"). The radiographs show a cyst-like expansion of the tubular bones, with thinning of the cortex (255). A second presentation is with multifocal cystic involvement of the bone. This is characterized by areas of simultaneous destruction in the shafts of long bones and in flat bones, with a strong tendency to symmetry (256).

The first and most important step in the diagnosis of tuberculous infection of the bone or joint is to consider it as a possibility. In addition, when tuberculosis is diagnosed, underlying HIV infection must also be considered. Tuberculosis should be considered whenever a chronic-appearing bone lesion is encountered. Early diagnosis is important to prevent spread to a contiguous joint. The clinical picture

is variable, depending on the location and the stage of the disease. It is characterized by its insidious onset; lack of characteristic inflammatory features, such as erythema; and bone destruction or joint involvement greater than the symptoms would suggest.

Laboratory studies usually show a normal leukocyte count and an elevated ESR. The purified protein derivative skin test usually is positive. Radiographic changes are usually present at the time of presentation. The diagnosis depends on the identification of the organism, *Mycobacterium tuberculosis*. Positive cultures are obtained in 85.5% of patients who have both pulmonary and extrapulmonary disease, in 83.5% of those with only pulmonary disease, and in 76.5% of those who have only extrapulmonary disease (257).

Tuberculosis produces a widespread inflammatory response which may mislead the surgeon in obtaining biopsy material, especially if the synovium is to undergo biopsy. In cases with bone lesions, the granulation tissue filling the cystic bone lesion is the best material for biopsy. In tuberculosis arthritis without bone involvement, the biopsy should be taken from the peripheral junction of the synovium with the bone, or preferably from the junction of the synovium with a cyst (258).

The treatment of skeletal tuberculosis is medical. Surgical debridement of the bone lesions is not necessary for a cure, although drainage of large abscesses often improves the patient's overall constitutional symptoms (256,258,259). In addition, open surgical biopsy is often necessary. Because of the effectiveness of drug therapy, there is little chance

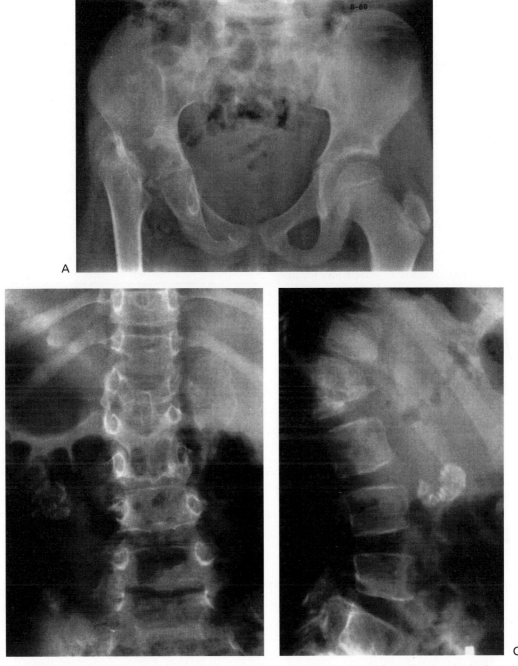

FIGURE 13-20. A: Anteroposterior (AP) radiograph of a 10-year-old girl from Mexico who had a past history of several operations on the right hip for tuberculosis presented with increasing back pain and kyphosis. **B** and **C:** AP and lateral views of the spine show bony destruction of the vertebral body, with relative preservation of the intervertebral disc and the calcified node; both are features of tuberculosis. Open biopsy confirmed the diagnosis of tuberculosis. (Courtesy of Hugh Watts, M.D.)

that surgical biopsy will lead to sinus formation. It is important to always be aware that superinfection with pyogenic organisms can occur, and this may be a reason for apparent treatment failure with antitubercular drugs. This is particularly true when a sinus has formed (259).

Several studies on tuberculous spondylitis demonstrate that surgery is necessary primarily to treat the kyphosis and not the tuberculosis; many cases do well with only medical management (260–262). Indications for surgery remain relative, and include neurologic involvement, spinal instability, and failure of medical treatment. Although patients with neurologic involvement can recover with medical management, they seem to do so faster with surgical management (260). Surgical treatment of the kyphosis produces a higher rate of union and less deformity than regimens without surgical stabilization (261,262). Thus, it appears that with contemporary surgical and anesthetic techniques tuberculous kyphosis is best treated early with anterior surgery for debridement and strut grafting. The treatment of spinal instability, especially that spanning more than two disc spaces, is difficult and probably requires both anterior arthrodesis with strut-grafting and posterior arthrodesis with instrumentation (263).

Although the effectiveness of ambulatory drug treatment has been demonstrated (261,262), there is evidence of an increasing incidence of resistant strains, due most likely to inadequate treatment of the initial infection (257). This emphasizes both the need for constant surveillance for drug resistance and the importance of careful supervision of outpatient oral therapy, to be certain that compliance is optimal.

Initial antimicrobial agent selection depends on the likelihood of drug-resistant organisms, whereas long-term selection should be guided by susceptibility testing. In those who are not at high risk for drug-resistant organisms, various regimens of isoniazid, rifampin, and pyrazinamide are recommended (264). In children who come from areas where antibiotics are sold over the counter, where high rates of drug-resistant tuberculosis occur, and when incomplete treatment may have resulted in multidrug-resistant strains, ethambutol or streptomycin should be added to the standard three-drug regimen. Treatment of bone and joint tuberculosis in children should be continued for 1 year.

References

Bone and Joint Infection

1. Peltola H, Vahvanen V. A comparative study of osteomyelitis and purulent arthritis with special reference to aetiology and recovery. *Infection* 1984;12:75.
2. Morey BF, Peterson HA. Hematogenous pyogenic osteomyelitis in children. *Orthop Clin North Am* 1975;6:935.
3. Morey BF, Bianco AJ Jr, Rhodes KH. Septic arthritis in children. *Orthop Clin North Am* 1975;6:923.
4. Craigen MA, Watters J, Hackett JS. The changing epidemiology of osteomyelitis in children. *J Bone Joint Surg Br* 1992;74:541.
5. Espersen F, Frimodt MN, Thamdrup RV, et al. Changing pattern of bone and joint infections due to *Staphylococcus aureus*: study of cases of bacteremia in Denmark, 1959–1988. *Rev Infect Dis* 1991;13:347.
6. Gillespie WJ. Epidemiology in bone and joint infection. *Infect Dis Clin North Am* 1990;4:361.
7. Gillespie WJ. The epidemiology of acute haematogenous osteomyelitis of childhood. *Int J Epidemiol* 1985;14:600.
8. Gillespie WJ, Nade SML. *Musculoskeletal infections.* Melbourne, Australia: Blackwell Scientific, 1987.
9. Jones NS, Anderson DJ, Stiles PJ. Osteomyelitis in a general hospital. A five-year study showing an increase in subacute osteomyelitis. *J Bone Joint Surg Br* 1987;69:779.
10. Bowerman SG, Green NE, Mencio GA. Decline of bone and joint infections attributable to *Haemophilus influenzae* type b. *Clin Orthop* 1997;341:128.
11. Koch R. Die aetiologie der tuberkulose. *Berl Klin Wochenschr* 1882;19:779.
12. Pasteur L. Del'extension de la theorie des germes a l'etiologie de quelques maladies communes. *Bull Acad Med* 1880;9:435.
13. Rodet A. Etude experimental aur l'osteomyelite infectieuse. Acad Sci 1884;99:569–571. In: Bick EM, ed. *Classics of orthopaedics.* Philadelphia: JB Lippincott, 1976:461.
14. Weaver JB, Tyler MW. Experimental staphylococcaemia and hematogenous osteomyelitis. *J Bone Joint Surg* 1943;25:791.
15. Norden CW. Experimental osteomyelitis. (I) S description of the model. *J Infect Dis* 1970;122:410.
16. Morrissy RT, Haynes DW. Acute hematogenous osteomyelitis: a model with trauma as an etiology. *J Pediatr Orthop* 1989;9:447.
17. Whalen JL, Fitzgerald RHJ, Morrissy RT. A histological study of acute hematogenous osteomyelitis following physeal injuries in rabbits. *J Bone Joint Surg Am* 1988;70:1383.
18. Everett ED, Hirschmann JV. Transient bacteremia and endocarditis prophylaxis: a review. *Medicine* 1977;56:61.
19. Burrows H. *Some factors in the localization of disease in the body.* New York: William Wood, 1932.
20. Dich VQ, Nelson JD, Haltalin KC. Osteomyelitis in infants and children. *Am J Dis Child* 1975;129:1273.
21. Gilmour WN. Acute hematogenous osteomyelitis. *J Bone Joint Surg Br* 1962;44:842.
22. Manche E, Rombouts GV, Rombouts JJ. Acute hematogenous osteomyelitis due to ordinary germs in children with closed injuries. Study of a series of 44 cases. *Acta Orthop Belg* 1991;57:91.
23. Shandling B. Acute hematogenous osteomyelitis: a review of 300 cases treated during 1953–1959. *South Afr Med* 1960;34:520.
24. Watson RJ, Burko H, Megas H, et al. The hand-foot syndrome in sickle cell disease in young children. *Pediatrics* 1963;31:975.
25. Olney BW, Papasian CJ, Jacobs RR. Risk of iatrogenic septic arthritis in the presence of bacteremia: a rabbit study. *J Pediatr Orthop* 1987;7:524.
26. Schurman DJ, Mirra J, Ding A, et al. Experimental *E. coli* arthritis in the rabbit: a model of infectious and post-infectious inflammatory synovitis. *J Rheumatol* 1977;4:118.
27. Hobo T. Zur pathogenese de akuten haematogenen osteomyelitis, mit berucksichtigungder vitalfarbungs leher. *Acta Scolar Med Kioto* 1921;4:1.
28. Schenk RK, Wiener J, Spiro D. Fine structural aspects of vascular invasion of the tibial epiphyseal plate of growing rats. *Acta Anat* 1968;69:1.
29. Speers DJ, Nade SML. Ultrastructural studies of *Staphylococcus aureus* in experimental acute haematogenous osteomyelitis. *Infect Immun* 1985;49:443.
30. Matsushita K, Hamabe M, Matsuoka M, et al. Experimental hematogenous osteomyelitis by *Staphylococcus aureus*. *Clin Orthop* 1997;334:291.
31. Trueta J. The normal vascular anatomy of the human femoral head during growth. *J Bone Joint Surg Br* 1957;39:358.
32. Tiku K, Tiku ML, Skosey JL. Interleukin-1 production by human polymorphonuclear neutrophils. *J Immunol* 1986;136:3677.
33. Dinarello CA, Cannon JG, Mier JW, et al. Multiple biological activities of human recombinant interleukin-1. *J Clin Invest* 1986;77:1734.

34. Malech HL, Gallin JI. Neutrophils in human disease. N Engl J Med 1987;317:687.

35. Johnson AH, Campbell WG, Callahan BC. Infection of rabbit knee joints after intra-articular injection of *Staphylococcus aureus. Am J Pathol* 1970;60:165.

36. Arvidson S, Holme T, Lindholm B. The formation of extracellular proteolytic enzymes by *Staphylococcus aureus. Acta Pathol Microbiol Scand* 1972;80:835.

37. Dingle JT. The role of lysomal enzymes in skeletal tissue. *J Bone Joint Surg Br* 1973;55:87.

38. Harris EDJ, Parker HG, Radin EL, et al. Effects of proteolytic enzymes on structural and mechanical properties of cartilage. *Arthritis Rheum* 1972;15:497.

39. Harris ED, McCroskery PA. The influence of temperature and fibril stability on degradation of cartilage collagen by rheumatoid synovial collagenase. *N Engl J Med* 1974;290:1.

40. Oronsky A, Ignarro L, Perrer R. Release of cartilage mucopolysaccharide-degrading neutral protease from human leukocytes. *J Exp Med* 1973;138:461.

41. Steinberg JJ, Sledge CB. Co-cultivation models of joint destruction. In: Dingle JT, Gordon JL, ed. *Cellular interactions.* Amsterdam: Elsevier/North-Holland, 1981:263.

42. Smith L, Schurman DJ, Kajiyama G, et al. The effect of antibiotics on the destruction of cartilage in experimental infectious arthritis. *J Bone Joint Surg Am* 1987;69:1063.

43. Curtiss PHJ, Klein L. Destruction of articular cartilage in septic arthritis. I. In vitro studies. *J Bone Joint Surg Am* 1963;45:797.

44. Curtiss PHJ, Klein L. Destruction of articular cartilage in septic arthritis. II. In vivo studies. *J Bone Joint Surg Am* 1965;47:1595.

45. Daniel D, Akeson W, Amiel D, et al. Lavage of septic joints in rabbits: effects of chondrolysis. *J Bone Joint Surg Am* 1976; 58:393.

Diagnosis

46. Faden H, Grossi M. Acute osteomyelitis in children. Reassessment of etiologic agents and their clinical characteristics. *Am J Dis Child* 1991;145:65.

47. Scott RJ, Christofersen MR, Robertson WWJ, et al. Acute osteomyelitis in children: a review of 116 cases. *J Pediatr Orthop* 1990;10:649.

48. Griebel M, Nahlen B, Jacobs RF, et al. Group A streptococcal postvaricella osteomyelitis. *J Pediatr Orthop* 1985;5:101.

49. Gabay C, Kushner I. Acute-phase proteins and other systemic responses to inflammation. *New Engl J Med* 1999;340:448.

50. Jaye DL, Waites KB. Clinical applications of C-reactive protein in pediatrics. *Pediatr Infect Dis J* 1997;16:735.

51. Peltola H, Vahvanen V, Aalto K. Fever, C-reactive protein, and erythrocyte sedimentation rate in monitoring recovery from septic arthritis: a preliminary study. *J Pediatr Orthop* 1984;4: 170.

52. Pepys MB. C-reactive protein fifty years on. *Lancet* 1981;1:653.

53. Unkila-Kallio L, Kallio MJT, Eskola J, et al. Serum C-reactive protein, erythrocyte sedimentation rate, and white blood cell count in acute hematogenous osteomyelitis of children. *Pediatrics* 1994;93:59.

54. Tejani N, Chonmaitree T, Rassin DK, et al. Use of C-reactive protein in differentiation between acute bacterial and viral otitis media. *Pediatrics* 1995;95:664.

55. Fink CW, Nelson JD. Septic arthritis and osteomyelitis in children. *Clin Rheum Dis* 1986;12:423.

56. Shmerling RH, Delbanco TL, Tosteson AN, et al. Synovial fluid tests. What should be ordered? *JAMA* 1990;264:1009.

57. Morrissy RT. Septic arthritis. In: Gustilo RB, Genninger RP, Tsukayama DT, eds. *Orthopaedic infection: diagnosis and treatment.* Philadelphia: WB Saunders, 1989.

58. Baldassare AR, Chang F, Zuckner J. Markedly raised synovial fluid leucocyte counts not associated with infectious arthritis in children. *Ann Rheum Dis* 1978;37:404.

59. Wilson NIL, DiPaola M. Acute septic arthritis in infancy and childhood. *J Bone Joint Surg Br* 1986;68:584.

60. Vaughan PA, Newman NM, Rosman MA. Acute hematogenous osteomyelitis in children. *J Pediatr Orthop* 1987;7:652.

61. Kohler RB, Wheat LJ. Rapid diagnosis by the detection of microbial antigens. *Med Microbiol* 1982;1:327.

62. Merritt K, Boyle WE, Dye SK, et al. Counter immunoelectrophoresis in the diagnosis of septic arthritis caused by *Haemophilus influenzae. J Bone Joint Surg Am* 1976;58:414.

63. Hoeffel DP, Hinrichs SH, Garvin KL. Molecular diagnostics for the detection of musculoskeletal infection. *Clin Orthop* 1999;360:37.

64. Capitanio MA, Kirkpatrick JA. Early roentgen observations in acute osteomyelitis. *Am J Roentgenol Radium Ther Nucl Med* 1970;108:488.

65. Brown I. A study of the "capsular" shadow in disorders of the hip in children. *J Bone Joint Surg Br* 1975;57:175.

66. Volberg FM, Sumner TE, Abramson JS, et al. Unreliability of radiographic diagnosis of septic hip in children. *Pediatrics* 1984; 74:118.

67. Cabanela ME, Sim FH, Beabout JW, et al. Osteomyelitis appearing as neoplasms: a diagnostic problem. *Arch Surg* 1974; 109:68.

68. Lindenbaum S, Alexander H. Infections simulating bone tumors. *Clin Orthop* 1984;184:193.

69. Willis RB, Rozencwaig R. Pediatric osteomyelitis masquerading as skeletal neoplasia. *Orthop Clin North Am* 1996;27:625.

70. Francis MD, Fogelman I. 99m Tc diphosphonate uptake mechanism on bone. In: Fogelman I, ed. *Bone scanning in clinical practice.* London: Springer-Verlag, 1987:7.

71. Howie DW, Savage JP, Wilson TG, et al. The technetium phosphate bone scan in the diagnosis of osteomyelitis in childhood. *J Bone Joint Surg Am* 1983;65:431.

72. Sundberg SB, Savage JP Foster, BK. Technetium phosphate bone scan in the diagnosis of septic arthritis in childhood. *J Pediatr Orthop* 1989;9:579.

73. Sullivan DC, Rosenfield NS, Ogden J, et al. Problems in the scintigraphic detection of osteomyelitis in children. *Radiology* 1980;135:731.

74. Sullivan JA, Vasileff T, Leonard JC. An evaluation of nuclear scanning in orthopaedic infections. *J Pediatr Orthop* 1980;1:73.

75. McCoy JR, Morrissy RT, Seibert J. Clinical experience with the technetium-99 scan in children. *Clin Orthop* 1981;154:175.

76. Berkowitz ID, Wenzel W. "Normal" technetium bone scans in patients with acute osteomyelitis. *Am J Dis Child* 1980;134: 828.

77. Trackler RT, Miller KE, Sutherland DH, et al. Childhood pelvic osteomyelitis presenting as a "cold" lesion on bone scan: case report. *J Nucl Med* 1976;17:620.

78. Canale ST, Harkness RM, Thomas PA, et al. Does aspiration of bones and joints affect results of later bone scanning? *J Pediatr Orthop* 1985;5:23.

79. Hernandez RJ, Conway JJ, Poznanski AK, et al. The role of computed tomography and radionuclide scintigraphy in the localization of osteomyelitis in flat bones. *J Pediatr Orthop* 1985; 5:151.

80. Tang JS, Gold RH, Bassett LW, et al. Musculoskeletal infection of the extremities: evaluation with MR imaging. *Radiology* 1988; 166:205.

81. Mazur JM, Ross G, Cummings RJ, et al. Usefulness of magnetic resonance imaging for the diagnosis of acute musculoskeletal infections in children. *J Pediatr Orthop* 1995;15:144.

82. Alexander JE, Seibert JJ, Glasier CM, et al. High-resolution hip ultrasound in the limping child. *J Clin Ultrasound* 1989;17:19.

83. Zawin JK, Hoffer FA, Rand FF, et al. Joint effusion in children with an irritable hip: US diagnosis and aspiration. *Radiology* 1993;187:459.

84. Zieger MM, Dorr U, Schulz RD. Ultrasonography of hip joint effusions. *Skeletal Radiol* 1987;16:607.

85. Dorr U, Zieger M, Hauke H. Ultrasonography of the painful hip. Prospective studies in 204 patients. *Pediatr Radiol* 1988; 19:36.

86. Royle SG. Investigation of the irritable hip. *J Pediatr Orthop* 1992;12:396.

87. Howard CB, Einhorn M, Dagan R, et al. Ultrasound in diagnosis and management of acute haematogenous osteomyelitis in children. *J Bone Joint Surg Br* 1993;75:79.

Differential Diagnosis

88. Hann IM, Gupta S, Palmer MK, et al. The prognostic significance of radiological and symptomatic bone involvement in childhood acute lymphoblastic leukemia. *Med Pediatr Oncol* 1979;6:51.

89. Rogalsky RJ, Black GB, Reed MH. Orthopaedic manifestations of leukemia in children. *J Bone Joint Surg Am* 1986;68:494.

90. Clausen N, Gotze H, Pedersen A, et al. Skeletal scintigraphy and radiography at onset of acute lymphocytic leukemia in children. *Med Pediatr Oncol* 1983;11:291.

91. McCormack LJ, Dockerty MB, Ghormley RK. Ewing's sarcoma. *Cancer* 1952;5:

92. Bell RS, Mankin HJ, Doppelt SH. Osteomyelitis in Gaucher disease. *J Bone Joint Surg Am* 1986;68:1380.

93. Del BMA, Champoux AN, Bockers T, et al. Septic arthritis versus transient synovitis of the hip: the value of screening laboratory tests. *Ann Emerg Med* 1992;21:1418.

94. Kocher MS, Zurakowski D, Kasser JR. Differentiating between septic arthritis and transient synovitis of the hip in children: an evidence-based clinical prediction algorithm. *J Bone Joint Surg Am* 1999;81:1662.

95. Bisno AL. Group A streptococcal infections and acute rheumatic fever. *N Engl J Med* 1991;325:783793.

Treatment

96. Barton LL, Dunkle LM, Habib FH. Septic arthritis in childhood. A 13-year review. *Am J Dis Child* 1987;141:898.

97. Shaw BA, Kasser JR. Acute septic arthritis in infancy and childhood. *Clin Orthop* 1990;257(Aug):21.2

98. Rotbart HA, Glode MP. *Haemophilus influenzae* type b septic arthritis in children: report of 23 cases. *Pediatrics* 1985;75:254.

99. Lundy KW, Kehl DK. Increasing prevalence of *Kingella kingae* in osteoarticular infections in young children. *J Pediatr Orthop* 1998;18:262.

100. Yagupsky P, Dagan R, Howard CW, et al. High prevalence of *Kingella kingae* in joint fluid from children with septic arthritis revealed by the BACTEC blood culture system. *J Clin Microbiol* 1992;30:1278.

101. Gamble JG, Rinsky LA. *Kingella kingae* infection in healthy children. *J Pediatr Orthop* 1988;8:445.

102. Lacour M, Duarte M, Beutler A, et al. Osteoarticular infections due to *Kingella kingae* in children. *Eur J Pediatr* 1991;150:612.

103. Bradley JS, Kaplan SL, Tan TQ, et al. Pediatric pneumococcal bone and joint infections. *Pediatrics* 1998;102:1376.

104. Eisenberg JM, Kitz DS. Savings from outpatient antibiotic therapy for osteomyelitis. Economic analysis of a therapeutic strategy. *JAMA* 1986;255:1584.

105. Bryson YJ, Connor JD, Leuers M, et al. High dose dicloxacillin

106. Kolyvas E, Shronheim G, Marks MI, et al. Oral antibiotic therapy of skeletal infections in children. *Pediatrics* 1980;65:867.

treatment of acute staphylococcal osteomyelitis in children. *J Pediatr* 1979;94:673.

107. Kocher MS, Zurakowski D, Kasser JR. Differentiating between septic arthritis and transient synovitis of the hip in children: an evidence-based clinical prediction algorithm. *J Bone Joint Surg Am* 1999;81:12.

108. Nelson JD, Bucholz RW, Kusmiesz H, et al. Benefits and risks of sequential parenteral-oral cephalosporin therapy for suppurative bone and joint infections. *J Pediatr Orthop* 1982;2:255.

109. Weinstein MP, Stratton CW, Hawley HB, et al. Multicenter collaborative evaluation of a standardized serum bactericidal test as a predictor of therapeutic efficacy in acute and chronic osteomyelitis. *Am J Med* 1987;83:218.

110. Wolfson JS, Swartz MN. Serum bactericidal activity as a monitor of antibiotic therapy. *N Engl J Med* 1985;312:968.

111. MacLowry JD. Perspective: the serum dilution test. *J Infect Dis* 1989;160:624.

112. Straton CW. Serum bactericidal test. *Clin Microbiol Rev* 1988; 1:19.

113. Smith BR, Rolston KV, LeFrock JL, et al. Bone penetration of antibiotics. *Orthopaedics* 1983;6:187.

114. Tetzlaff TR, Howard JB, McCracken GH, et al. Antibiotic concentrations in pus and bone of children with osteomyelitis. *J Pediatr* 1978;92:135.

115. Nelson JD, Howard JB, Shelton S. Oral antibiotic therapy for skeletal infection of children. I. Antibiotic concentration in suppurative synovial joint. *J Pediatr* 1978;92:131.

116. Bryan RE, Hammond D. Interaction of purulent material with antibiotics used to treat pseudomonas infection. *Antimicrob Agents Chemother* 1974;6:700.

117. Bryan LE, Van den Elzen HM. Streptomycin accumulation in susceptible and resistent strains of *Escherichia coli* and *Pseudomonas aeruginosa*. *Antimicrob Agents Chemother* 1976;9:928.

118. Donowitz GR, Mandell GL. Beta-lactam antibiotics. *New Engl J Med* 1988;318:419.

119. Farrar WE, O'Dell NM. Comparative β-lactamase resistance and antistaphylococcal activities of parenterally and orally administered cephalosporins. *J Infect Dis* 1978;137:490.

120. Sabath LD, Garner C, Wilcox C, et al. Effect of inoculum and of beta-lactamase on the anti-staphylococcal activity of thirteen penicillins and cephalosporins. *Antimicrob Agents Chemother* 1975;8:344.

121. Waldvogle FA, Medoff G, Swartz MN. Osteomyelitis: a review of clinical features, therapeutic considerations and unusual aspects. *N Engl J Med* 1970;282:198.

122. Braude AI, Jones JL, Douglas HI. The behavior of *Escherichia coli* endotoxin (somatic antigen) during infectious arthritis. *J Immunol* 1963;90:297.

123. Ginsburg I, Sela MN. The role of leukocytes and their hydrolases in the persistence, degradation, and transport of bacterial constituents in tissues: relation to chronic inflammatory processes in staphylococcal, streptococcal, and mycobacterial infections and in chronic periodontal disease. *CRC Crit Rev Microbiol* 1976;4:249.

124. Ginsburg J, Goultchin A, Stabholtz N, et al. Streptococcal and staphylococcal arthritis. *Agents Actions* 1980;7:260.

125. Green NE, Edwards K. Bone and joint infections in children. *Orthop Clin North Am* 1987;18:555.

126. LaMont RL, Anderson PA, Dajani AS, et al. Acute hematogenous osteomyelitis in children. *J Pediatr Orthop* 1987;7:579.

127. Goldstein WM, Gleason TF, Barmada R. A comparison between arthrotomy and irrigation and multiple aspirations in the treatment of pyogenic arthritis. *Orthopaedics* 1983;6:1309.

128. Letts RM, Wong E. Treatment of acute osteomyelitis in chil-

dren by closed-tube irrigation: a reassessment. *Can J Surg* 1975; 18:60.

129. Patterson DC. Acute suppurative arthritis in infancy and childhood. *J Bone Joint Surg Br* 1970;52:474.
130. Skyhar MJ, Mubarak SJ. Arthroscopic treatment of septic knees in children. *J Pediatr Orthop* 1987;7:647.
131. Stanitski CL, Harvell JC, Fu FH. Arthroscopy in acute septic knees. Management in pediatric patients. *Clin Orthop* 1989; 241:209.

Results

132. Blockey NJ, Watson JT. Acute osteomyelitis in children. *J Bone Joint Surg Br* 1970;52:77.
133. Cole WG, Dalziel RE, Leitl S. Treatment of acute osteomyelitis in childhood. *J Bone Joint Surg Br* 1982;64:218.
134. Molan RAB, Piggot J. Acute osteomyelitis in children. *J Bone Joint Surg Br* 1977;59:2.

Special Conditions

Spine

135. Smith AlDF. A benign form of osteomyelitis of the spine. *JAMA* 1933;101:335.
136. Bremner AE, Neligan GA. Benign form of acute osteitis of the spine in young children. *BMJ* 1953;1:856.
137. Ghormley RK, Bickel WH, Dickson DD. A study of acute infectious lesions of the intervertebral disks. *South Med J* 1940; 33:347.
138. Ring D, Johnston CE, Wenger KR. Pyogenic infectious spondylitis in children: the convergence of discitis and vertebral osteomyelitis. *J Pediatr Orthop* 1995;15:652.
139. Song KS, Ogden JA, Ganey T, et al. Contiguous discitis and osteomyelitis in children. *J Pediatr Orthop* 1997;17:470.
140. Coventry MB, Ghormley RK, Kernohan JW. The intervertebral discitis microscopic anatomy and pathology. Part I. Anatomy, development and physiology. *J Bone Joint Surg* 1945;27:105.
141. Crock HV, Yoshizawa H. *The blood supply of the vertebral column and spinal cord in man.* New York: Springer-Verlag, 1977.
142. Hassler O. The human intervertebral disc: a microangiographical study on its vascular supply at various ages. *Acta Orthop Scand* 1969;40:765.
143. Wiley AM, Trueta J. The vascular anatomy of the spine and its relationship to pyogenic vertebral osteomyelitis. *J Bone Joint Surg Br* 1959;41:796.
144. Rocco HD, Erying EJ. Intervertebral disk infections in children. *Am J Dis Child* 1972;123:448.
145. Spiegel PG, Kengla KW, Isaacson AS, et al. Intervertebral discspace inflammation in children. *J Bone Joint Surg Am* 1972;54: 284.
146. Wenger DR, Bobechko WP, Gilday DL. The spectrum of intervertebral disc-space infection in children. *J Bone Joint Surg Am* 1978;60:100.
147. An HS, Vaccaro AR, Dolinskas CA, et al. Differentiation between spinal tumors and infections with magnetic resonance imaging. *Spine* 1991;16(suppl 8):334.
148. Boston HC, Bianco AJJ, Rhodes KH. Disk space infections in children. *Orthop Clin North Am* 1975;6:953.
149. Menelaus MB. Discitis: an inflammation affecting the intervertebral disc in children. *J Bone Joint Surg Br* 1964;46:16.

Pelvis and Sacroiliac Joint

150. Schaad UB, McCracken GH, Nelson JD. Pyogenic arthritis of the sacroiliac joint in pediatric patients. *Pediatrics* 1980;66:375.

151. Morgan A, Yates A. The diagnosis of acute osteomyelitis of the pelvis. *Postgrad Med J* 1966;42:74.
152. Beaupre A, Carroll N. The three syndromes of iliac osteomyelitis in children. *J Bone Joint Surg Am* 1979;61:1087.
153. Reilly JP, Gross RH, Emans JB, et al. Disorders of the sacroiliac joint in children. *J Bone Joint Surg Am* 1988;70:31.
154. Chung SMK, Borns P. Acute osteomyelitis adjacent to the sacroiliac joint in children. *J Bone Joint Surg Am* 1973;55:630.
155. Edwards MS, Baker CJ, Granberry WM, et al. Pelvic osteomyelitis in children. *Pediatrics* 1978;61:62.
156. Jarvis J, McIntyre W, Udjus K, et al. Osteomyelitis of the ischiopubic synchondrosis. *J Pediatr Orthop* 1985;5:163.
157. Kloiber R, Udjus K, McIntyre W, et al. The scintigraphic and radiographic appearance of the ischiopubic synchondroses in normal children and in osteomyelitis. *Pediatr Radiol* 1988;18: 57.
158. Ailsby RL, Staheli LT. Pyogenic infections of the sacroiliac joint in children. Radioisotope bone scanning as a diagnostic tool. *Clin Orthop* 1974;100:96.
159. Farley T, Conway J, Shulman ST. Hematogenous pelvic osteomyelitis in children. *Am J Dis Child* 1985;139:946.
160. Miller JH, Gates GF. Scintigraphy of sacroiliac pyarthrosis in children. *JAMA* 1977;238:2701.
161. Reilly JP, Gross RH, Emans JB, et al. Disorders of the sacroiliac joint in children. *J Bone Joint Surg Am* 1988;70:31.
162. Morgan JG, Schlegelmilch JG, Spiegel PK. Early diagnosis of septic arthritis of the sacroiliac joint by use of computed tomography. *J Rheumatol* 1981;8:879.
163. Viani RM, Bromberg K, Bradley JS. Obturator internus muscle abscess in children: report of seven cases and review. *Clin Infect Dis* 1999;28:117.
164. Coy JTI, Wolf CR, Brower TD, et al. Pyogenic arthritis of the sacroiliac joint: long-term follow-up. *J Bone Joint Surg Am* 1976; 58:845.
165. Sucato DJ, Gillespie R. *Salmonella* pelvic osteomyelitis in normal children: report of two cases and a review of the literature. *J Pediatr Orthop* 1997;17:463.
166. Hendrix RW, Lin P-J, Kane WJ. Simplified aspiration or injection technique for the sacro-iliac joint. *J Bone Joint Surg Am* 1982;64:1249.
167. Miskew DB, Block RA, Witt PF. Aspiration of infected sacroiliac joints. *J Bone Joint Surg Am* 1979;61:1071.

The Neonate

168. Gotoff SP. Neonatal immunity. *J Pediatrics* 1974;85:149.
169. Kuo KN, Lloyd-Roberts GC, Orme IM, et al. Immunodeficiency and infantile bone and joint infection. *Arch Dis Child* 1975;50:51.
170. Lim MO, Gresham EL, Franken EAJ, et al. Osteomyelitis as a complication of umbilical artery catheterization. *Am J Dis Child* 1977;131:142.
171. Bergdahl S, Ekengren K, Eriksson M. Neonatal hematogenous osteomyelitis: risk factors for long-term sequelae. *J Pediatr Orthop* 1985;5:564.
172. Fox L, Sprunt K. Neonatal osteomyelitis. *Pediatrics* 1978;62: 535.
173. Edwards MS, Baker CJ, Wagner ML, et al. An etiologic shift in infantile osteomyelitis: the emergence of the group B streptococcus. *J Pediatr* 1978;93:578.
174. Ish-Horowicz MR, McIntyre P, Nade S. Bone and joint infections caused by multiply resistant *Staphylococcus aureus* in a neonatal intensive care unit. *Pediatr Infect Dis J* 1992;11:82.
175. Knudsen CJM, Hoffman EB. Neonatal osteomyelitis. *J Bone Joint Surg Br* 1990;72:846.
176. Memon IA, Norman MB, Jacobs NM, et al. Group B strepto-

coccal osteomyelitis and septic arthritis. *Am J Dis Child* 1979; 133:921.

177. Monk PM, Reilly BJ, Ash JM. Osteomyelitis in the neonate. *Radiology* 1982;145:677.

178. Weissberg ED, Smith AL, Smith DH. Clinical features of neonatal osteomyelitis. *Pediatrics* 1974;53:505.

179. Yousefzadeh DK, Jackson JH. Neonatal and infantile candidal arthritis with or without osteomyelitis: a clinical and radiographical review of 21 cases. *Skeletal Radiol* 1980;5:77.

180. Trueta J. The three types of acute haematogenous osteomyelitis. A clinical and vascular study. *J Bone Joint Surg Br* 1959;41:671.

181. Ogden JA. Pediatric osteomyelitis and septic arthritis: the pathology of neonatal disease. *Yale J Biol Med* 1979;52:423.

182. Chung SMK. The arterial supply of the developing proximal end of the human femur. *J Bone Joint Surg Am* 1976;58:961.

183. Kemp HBS, Lloyd-Roberts GC. Avascular necrosis of the capital epiphysis following osteomyelitis of the proximal femoral metaphysis. *J Bone Joint Surg Br* 1974;56:688.

184. Aigner RM, Fueger GF, Ritter G. Results of three-phase bone scintigraphy and radiography in 20 cases of neonatal osteomyelitis. *Nucl Med Commun* 1996;17:20.

185. Ash JM, Gilday DL. The futility of bone scanning in neonatal osteomyelitis: concise communication. *J Nucl Med* 1980;21:417.

186. Bressler EL, Conway JJ, Weiss SC. Neonatal osteomyelitis examined by bone scintigraphy. *Radiology* 1984;152:685.

Sickle Cell Disease

187. Landesman SH, Rao SP, Ahonkhai VI. Infections in children with sickle cell anemia. *Am J Pediatr Hemat Oncol* 1982;4:407.

188. Specht EE. Hemoglobinopathic *salmonella* osteomyelitis. *Clin Orthop* 1971;79:110.

189. Engh CA, Hughes JL, Abrams RC, et al. Osteomyelitis in the patient with sickle-cell disease. *J Bone Joint Surg Am* 1971;53:1.

190. Keely K, Buchanan GR. Acute infarction of long bones in children with sickle cell anemia. *J Pediatr* 1982;101:170.

191. Mallouh A, Talab Y. Bone and joint infection in patients with sickle cell disease. *J Pediatr Orthop* 1985;5:158.

192. Syrogiannopoulos GA, McCracken GHJ, Nelson JD. Osteoarticular infections in children with sickle cell disease. *Pediatrics* 1986;78:1090.

193. Kim HC, Alavi A, Russell MO, et al. Differentiation of bone and bone marrow infarcts from osteomyelitis in sickle cell disorders. *Clin Nucl Med* 1989;14:249.

194. Rao S, Solomon N, Miller S, et al. Scintigraphic differentiation of bone infarction from osteomyelitis in children with sickle cell disease. *Pediatrics* 1985;107:685.

195. Kim HC, Alavi A, Russell MO, et al. Differentiation of bone and bone marrow infarcts from osteomyelitis in sickle cell disorders. *Clin Nuclear Med* 1989;14:249.

196. Frush DP, Heyneman LE, Ware RE, et al. MR features of soft tissue abnormalities due to acute marrow infarction in five children with sickle cell disease. *AJR Am J Roentgenol* 1999;173:989.

197. Sadat-Ali M, al-Umran K, al-Habdan I, et al. Ultrasonography: can it differentiate between vasoocclusive crisis and acute osteomyelitis in sickle cell disease? *J Pediatr Orthop* 1998;18:552.

198. Booz MM, Hariharan V, Aradi AJ, et al. The value of ultrasound and aspiration in differentiating vaso-occlusive crisis and osteomyelitis in sickle cell disease patients. *Clin Radiol* 1999;54:636.

199. Worrel VT, Burera V. Sickle-cell dactylitis. *J Bone Joint Surg Am* 1976;58:1161.

200. Greene WB, McMillan CW. *Salmonella* osteomyelitis and hand-foot syndrome in a child with sickle cell anemia. *J Pediatr Orthop* 1987;7:716.

201. Noonan WJ. *Salmonella osteomyelitis* presenting as "hand-foot syndrome" in sickle-cell disease. *BMJ* 1982;284:1464.

202. Sankaran KM, Sadat AM, Kutty MK. Septic arthritis in sickle cell disease. *Int Orthop* 1988;12:255.

203. Adeyokunnu AA, Hendrickse RG. *Salmonella* osteomyelitis in childhood. *Arch Dis Child* 1980;55:175.

204. Adu-Gyamfi Y, Sankarankutty M, Marwa S. Use of a tourniquet in patients with sickle-cell disease. *Can J Anesth* 1993;40:24.

205. Stein RE, Urbaniak J. Use of the tourniquet during surgery in patients with sickle cell hemoglobinopathies. *Clin Orthop* 1980; 151:231.

206. Sadat-Ali M, Sankaran-Kutty M, Kutty K. Recent observations on osteomyelitis in sickle-cell disease. *Int Orthop* 1985;9:97.

207. Burnett MW, Bass JW, Cook BA. Etiology of osteomyelitis complicating sickle cell disease. *Pediatrics* 1998;10:296.

208. Henderson RC, Rosenstein BD. *Salmonella* septic and aseptic arthritis in sickle-cell disease. A case report. *Clin Orthop* 1989; 248:261.

209. Espinoza LR, Spilberg I, Osterland CK. Joint manifestations of sickle-cell disease. *Medicine* 1974;53:295.

210. Orozoco-Alcala J, Baum J. Arthritis during sickle cell crisis. *N Engl J Med* 1973;288:420.

211. Jackson MA, Nelson JD. Etiology and medical management of acute suppurative bone and joint infections in pediatric patients. *J Pediatr Orthop* 1982;2:313.

212. Ebong WW. Septic arthritis in patients with sickle-cell disease. *Br J Rheumatol* 1987;26:99.

Chronic Recurrent Multifocal Osteomyelitis

213. Giedion A, Holthusen W, Masel LF, et al. Subacute and chronic "symmetrical" osteomyelitis. *Ann Radiol* 1972;15:329.

214. Jurik AG, Helmig O, Ternowitz T, et al. Chronic recurrent multifocal osteomyelitis: a follow-up study. *J Pediatr Orthop* 1988;8:49.

215. Madnell GA, Contreras SJ, Conard K, et al. Bone scintigraphy in the detection of chronic recurrent multifocal osteomyelitis. *J Nucl Med* 1998;39:1778.

216. Carr AJ, Cole WG, Roberton DM, et al. Chronic multifocal osteomyelitis. *J Bone Joint Surg Br* 1993;75:582.

217. Kawai K, Doita M, Tateishi H, et al. Bone and joint lesions associated with pustulosis palmaris et plantaris: a clinical and histological study. *J Bone Joint Surg Br* 1988;70:117.

218. Manson D, Wilmot DM, King S, et al. Physeal involvement in chronic recurrent multifocal osteomyelitis. *Pediatr Radiol* 1989;20:76.

219. Bjorksten B, Boquist L. Histopathological aspects of chronic recurrent multifocal osteomyelitis. *J Bone Joint Surg Br* 1980; 62:376.

220. Jurik AG, Moller BN. Chronic sclerosing osteomyelitis of the clavicle: a manifestation of chronic recurrent multifocal osteomyelitis. *Arch Orthop Trauma Surg* 1987;106:144.

221. Manson D, Wilmot DM, King S, et al. Physeal involvement in chronic recurrent multifocal osteomyelitis [see comments]. *Pediatr Radiol* 1989;20:76.

222. Gamble JG, Rinsky LA. Chronic recurrent multifocal osteomyelitis: a distinct clinical entity. *J Pediatr Orthop* 1986;6:579.

Subacute Osteomyelitis

223. Harris NG, Kirkaldy-Willis WH. Primary subacute pyogenic osteomyelitis. *J Bone Joint Surg Br* 1965;47:526.

224. King DM, Mayo KM. Subacute haematogenous osteomyelitis. *J Bone Joint Surg Br* 1969;51:458.

225. Gledhill RB. Subacute osteomyelitis in children. *Clin Orthop* 1973;96:57.
226. Roberts JM, Drummond DS, Breed AL, et al. Subacute hematogenous osteomyelitis in children: a retrospective study. *J Pediatr Orthop* 1982;2:249.
227. Cottias P, Tomeno B, Anract P, et al. Subacute osteomyelitis presenting as a bone tumour. A review of 21 cases. *Int Orthop* 1997;21:243.
228. Bogoch E, Thompson G, Salter RB. Foci of chronic circumscribed osteomyelitis (Brodie's abscess) that traverse the epiphyseal plate. *J Pediatr Orthop* 1984;4:162.
229. Azouz EM, Greenspan A, Marton D. CT evaluation of primary epiphyseal bone abscesses. *Skeletal Radiol* 1993;22:17.
230. Green NE, Beauchamp RD, Griffin PP. Primary subacute epiphyseal osteomyelitis. *J Bone Joint Surg Am* 1981;63:107.
231. Sorensen TS, Hedeboe J, Christensen ER. Primary epiphyseal osteomyelitis in children. Report of three cases and review of the literature. *J Bone Joint Surg Br* 1988;70:818.
232. Ezra E, Wientroub S. Primary subacute haematogenous osteomyelitis of the tarsal bones in children. *J Bone Joint Surg Br* 1997;79:983.
233. Ross ERS, Cole WG. Treatment of subacute osteomyelitis in childhood. *J Bone Joint Surg Br* 1985;67:443.
234. Grey AC, Davies AM, Mangham DC, et al. The "penumbra sign" on T1-weighted MR imaging in subacute osteomyelitis: frequency, cause and significance. *Clin Radiol* 1998;53:587.
235. Hamdy RC, Lawton L, Carey T, et al. Subacute hematogenous osteomyelitis: are biopsy and surgery always indicated? *J Pediatr Orthop* 1996;16:220.

Puncture Wounds of the Foot
236. Johanson PH. Pseudomonas infections of the foot following puncture wounds. *JAMA* 1968;204:170.
237. Fisher MC, Goldsmith JF, Gilligan PH. Sneakers as a source of *Pseudomonas aeruginsoa* in children with osteomyelitis following puncture wounds. *Pediatrics* 1985;106:607.
238. Weber CA, Wertheimer SJ, Ognjan A. *Aeromonas hydrophilia*—its implications in freshwater injuries. *J Foot Ankle Surg* 1995;34:442.
239. Fitzgerald RH, Cowan JDE. Puncture wounds of the foot. *Orthop Clin North Am* 1975;6:965.
240. Laughlin TJ, Armstrong DG, Caporusso J, et al. Soft tissue and bone infections from puncture wounds in children. *West J Med* 1997;166:126.
241. Reichl M. Septic arthritis following puncture wound of the foot. *Arch Emerg Med* 1989;6:277.
242. Lau LS, Bin G, Jaovisidua S, et al. Cost effectiveness of magnetic resonance imaging in diagnosing *Pseudomonas aeruginosa* infection after puncture wound. *J Foot Ankle Surg* 1997;36:36.
243. Jacobs RF, Adelman L, Sack CM, et al. Management of *Pseudomonas* osteochondritis complicating puncture wounds of the foot. *Pediatrics* 1982;69:432.
244. Jacobs RF, McCarthy RE, Elser JM. *Pseudomonas* osteochondritis complicating puncture wounds of the foot in children: a 10-year evaluation. *J Infect Dis* 1989;160:657.

Gonococcal Arthritis
245. Holmes K, Counts G, Beaty H. Disseminated gonococcal infection. *Ann Intern Med* 1971;74:979.
246. Rimsza M, Niggemann E. Medical evaluation of sexually abused children: a review of 311 cases. *Pediatrics* 1982;69:8.
247. White ST, Loda FA, Ingram DL. Sexually transmitted diseases in sexually abused children. *Pediatrics* 1983;72:16.
248. Cooperman MB. Gonococcus arthritis in infancy. A clinical study of forty-four cases. *Am J Dis Child* 1927;33:932.
249. Cooperman MB. End results of gonorrheal arthritis. A review of seventy cases. *Am J Surg* 1928;5:241.
250. Spink WW, Keefer CS. Gonococcic arthritis: pathogenesis, mechanism of recovery and treatment. *JAMA* 1938;109:1448.
251. Wehrbein HL. Gonococcus arthritis—a study of six hundred cases. *Surg Gyn Obstet* 1929;49:105.
252. Wise CM, Morris CR, Wasilauskas BL, et al. Gonococcal arthritis in an era of increasing penicillin resistance. Presentations and outcomes in 41 recent cases (1985–1991). *Arch Intern Med* 1994;154:2690.

Tuberculosis
253. Smith MJD, Stack KR, Marquis JR. Tuberculosis and opportunistic mycobacterial infections. In: Fegin RO, Cherry JD, eds. *Pediatric infectious diseases*. 3rd ed. Philadelphia: WB Saunders, 1992:1327.
254. Phemister DB, Hatcher CH. Correlation of pathological and roentgenological findings in the diagnosis of tuberculous arthritis. *AJR Am J Roentgenol* 1933;29:736.
255. Hardy JB, Hartmenn JR. Tuberculous dactylitis in childhood. *J Pediatr* 1947;30:146.
256. Shannon BF, Moore M, Houkom JA, et al. Multifocal cystic tuberculosis of bone. *J Bone Joint Surg Am* 1990;72:1089.
257. Jereb JA, Cauthen GM, Kelly GD, et al. The epidemiology of tuberculosis. In: Friedman LN, ed. *Tuberculosis: current concepts and treatment*. Boca Raton, FL: CRC, 1994:17.
258. Versfeld GA, Solomon A. A diagnostic approach to tuberculosis of bones and joints. *J Bone Joint Surg Br* 1982;64:446.
259. Martini M, Adjrad A, Boudjemaa A. Tuberculous osteomyelitis. A review of 125 cases. *Int Orthop* 1986;10:201.
260. Lifeso RM, Weaver P, Harder EH. Tuberculous spondylitis in adults. *J Bone Joint Surg Am* 1985;67:1405.
261. Medical Research Council Working Party on Tuberculosis of the Spine. Five-year assessment of controlled trials of ambulatory treatment, debridement and anterior spinal fusion in the management of tuberculosis of the spine; studies in Bulawayo (Rhodesia) and in Hong Kong. *J Bone Joint Surg Br* 1978;60:163.
262. Medical Research Council Working Party on Tuberculosis of the Spine. Five-year assessment of controlled trials of inpatient and outpatient treatment and of plaster-of-Paris jackets for tuberculosis of the spine in children on standard chemotherapy. Studies in Masan and Pusan, Korea. *J Bone Joint Surg Br* 1976;58:399.
263. Rajasekaran S, Soundarapandian S. Progression of kyphosis in tuberculosis of the spine treated by anterior arthrodesis. *J Bone Joint Surg Am* 1989;71:1314.
264. Pediatrics AAO. Tuberculosis. In: Peter G, ed. *Report of the Committee on Infectious Diseases, 23*. Elk Grove Village, IL: American Academy of Pediatrics, 1994:488.

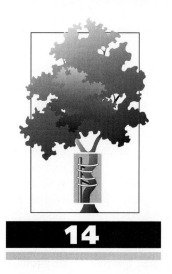

14

BONE AND SOFT TISSUE TUMORS

DEMPSEY S. SPRINGFIELD
MARK C. GEBHARDT

Primary bone and soft tissue tumors in the pediatric age group are uncommon and when they occur, usually benign. There are two primary malignant tumors of bone, osteosarcoma and Ewing sarcoma/peripheral (or primitive) neuroectodermal tumor (PNET), and one soft tissue sarcoma, rhabdomyosarcoma, which occur predominantly in the pediatric patient. The orthopaedist must remain alert because the malignant tumor is an unexpected event, and its infrequency can result in improper or delayed initial management. The orthopaedist who sees pediatric patients, but is not prepared to manage a malignant or aggressive benign musculoskeletal tumor, must be comfortable with evaluating patients with musculoskeletal tumors, and know whom to refer and whom to manage. This chapter reviews the common bone and soft tissue tumors of childhood; it discusses how the patients present, what physical findings to expect, and how the plain radiographs should look; and it suggests additional diagnostic and staging evaluations and treatment. This chapter is not intended to be a definitive text of musculoskeletal pathology, and includes only the more common tumors of childhood.

MOLECULAR BIOLOGY OF TUMORS

Dramatic improvements in the survival of children with previously lethal sarcomas have occurred in the last 30 years from the use of adjuvant chemotherapy. One of the intriguing aspects about childhood sarcomas is that despite similar histologies, stages, and prognostic factors, some patients re-

D. S. Springfield: Leni and Peter W. May Department of Orthopaedics, Mount Sinai School of Medicine; Department of Orthopaedics, Mount Sinai Hospital, New York, New York 10029.

M. C. Gebhardt: Department of Orthopaedic Surgery, Harvard Medical School, Boston, Massachusetts 02115; Orthopaedic Service, Massachusetts General Hospital, Boston, Massachusetts 02114.

spond well to treatment, whereas others seem to be resistant to chemotherapy. To date, patients with good prognoses cannot be distinguished from those with poor prognoses except by crude clinical characteristics, such as the presence of metastatic disease at diagnosis. Recent molecular findings in sarcomas may shed light on the biologic behavior of sarcomas and their response to chemotherapy.

One method of seeking genetic alterations in tumors is to examine the chromosomes by karyotype analysis. The identification of recurrent chromosomal abnormalities provides clues regarding sites of potential gene mutations. Normally, there are 23 pairs of chromosomes in the human cell nucleus. Osteosarcomas in general have multiple, bizarre karyotypic abnormalities: Some chromosomes are missing, some are duplicated, and some are grossly altered. All high-grade osteosarcomas studied to date have complex karyotypes and nonclonal chromosome aberrations superimposed on complex clonal events (1,2). Low-grade parosteal osteosarcoma, on the other hand, is characterized by the presence of a ring chromosome, accompanied by no or few other abnormalities. Although it is usually possible to distinguish high-grade from low-grade osteosarcoma by standard histology, in other tumors the karyotype information can be diagnostically useful. In addition to possibly providing prognostic information, the specific chromosomal aberrations provide clues that assist molecular biologists looking for gene mutations (2).

In contrast to osteosarcoma, Ewing sarcomas, PNETs, and alveolar rhabdomyosarcomas have single chromosomal translocations characteristic of their respective histologies. In these tumors, part of one chromosome is transposed to part of another chromosome through a breakpoint. In these tumors, a novel gene and gene protein product are created that presumably give the cell a growth advantage. The most common translocations for these tumors are listed in Table 14-1.

The demonstration of translocations has been useful in the differential diagnosis of round cell tumors. Under the light microscope, there is little to distinguish one of these tumor types from the other, and although immunohistochemistry helps to an extent, it is at times difficult to be sure of the diagnosis. Demonstration of these characteristic karyotypic findings makes pathologists more secure in their diagnosis, and has helped with the classification of these tumors. To perform a karyotype analysis, short-term cultures and metaphase spreads are necessary, but these are labor-intensive and require fresh tissue (4). More recent techniques, with fluorescent *in situ* hybridization and reverse transcriptase-polymerase chain reaction, allow rapid analysis for the presence of translocations, and these techniques can be performed on frozen and sometimes paraffin-embedded tissue (5,6).

These translocations have import beyond establishing the diagnosis. For several years, the distinction between Ewing sarcoma and PNET was difficult, and clinicians were not sure whether to treat them differently. The observation that both Ewing sarcoma, a poorly differentiated mesenchymal tumor of uncertain cell lineage, and PNET, a tumor believed to be of neural crest origin, shared the same chromosomal translocation led pathologists to believe that both were related neuroectodermal tumors (7,8). There is debate regarding whether one or the other has a better prognosis, but the treatment strategies used today are the same for both tumors (9–11).

More recently, these markers have been used in staging and follow-up of high-risk patients (12). Using reverse transcriptase-polymerase chain reaction technology, one can detect small numbers of tumor cells in a bone marrow or peripheral blood cell population. This makes the interpretation of bone marrow aspirates more precise, and may provide a means of earlier detection of relapses after treatment. It is hoped that the gene products of these translocations can also be used in treatment strategies. Because the novel genes formed from the translocation make a novel protein that normal cells do not make, antibodies or targeted T cells can be generated to specifically kill tumor cells. This is being tried in early-phase trials of relapsed patients with rhabdomyosarcoma and Ewing sarcoma/PNET, and if it works, it may be a way of treating patients who fail standard drug therapy.

Genetic alterations in the DNA of sarcomas have been well demonstrated. Mutations in genes, called "oncogenes," give some evidence relative to the pathogenesis of these tumors, and may have some prognostic and therapeutic import (13,14). Oncogenes are normal cellular genes (*protooncogenes*) that are necessary for the normal development and function of the organism (15). When they are mutated, they may produce a protein capable of inducing the neoplastic state. Oncogenes act through a variety of mechanisms to deregulate cell growth. This is obviously a very complex process and may involve more than one genetic event.

There are two categories of oncogenes: *dominant oncogenes* and *tumor-suppressor genes* (15). The dominant oncogenes encode proteins that are involved in signal transduction, i.e., transmitting an external stimulus from outside the cell to the machinery controlling replication in the cell

TABLE 14-1. CYTOGENETIC FINDINGS IN EWING SARCOMA/PERIPHERAL (OR PRIMITIVE) NEUROECTODERMAL TUMOR AND ALVEOLAR RHABDOMYOSARCOMA

Tumor	Translocation	Genes
Ewing sarcoma/peripheral (or primitive) neuroectodermal tumor	t(11;22)(q24;q12)	EWS-FLI-1
	t(21;22)(q22;q12)	EWS-ERG
Alveolar rhabdomyosarcoma	t(2;13)(q35;q14)	PAX3-FKHR PAX7-FKHR

(From ref. 3, with permission.)

nucleus. Mutant cellular signal transduction genes keep the cell permanently "turned on." The protein products of oncogenes also function as aberrant growth factors, growth factor receptors, or nuclear transcription factors. These types of genes seem to have a lesser role in osteosarcomas.

A second class of genes, the tumor suppressor genes, are genes that encode proteins whose normal role is to restrict cell proliferation (16–20). They act as brakes rather than accelerators of growth. Their normal role is to regulate the cell cycle and keep it in check.

The retinoblastoma gene (*RB1*) was the first gene recognized in this class (21,22). Osteosarcomas are very frequent in patients with hereditary retinoblastoma, both in the orbit and in the extremities, unrelated to irradiation. It was subsequently learned that osteosarcomas in these patients as well as spontaneous osteosarcomas carry mutations or deletions of the *RB1* gene. It was one of the first clues that osteosarcomas had a genetic cause. It is estimated that approximately 60 to 75% of sporadic osteosarcomas have an abnormality of the *RB1* gene, or do not express a functional RB1 product (14). The retinoblastoma gene is located on the long arm of chromosome 13 (13q14), and is 200 kilobases in length. Its product is a 105- to 110-kilodalton nuclear phosphoprotein (pRB) that appears to have a cell cycle regulatory role. The retinoblastoma protein acts as a signal protein to connect the cell cycle with the transcription of genes that mediate the cell cycle. Deactivation of the *RB1* gene or absence of pRB allows cells to enter the cell cycle in an unregulated fashion, a condition that imparts a growth advantage to the affected cell. It should be noted that one copy of the gene is sufficient for a normal phenotype. A child born with a normal and a mutant or absent allele will not manifest retinoblastoma until some event occurs in retinoblasts to alter the normal allele. If both copies thus become deranged, the normal check on the cell cycle disappears and the conditions for the neoplastic state are met.

The second tumor suppressor gene to be identified was the *p53* gene (23–25). Located on the short arm of chromosome 17 (17p), its product is a nuclear phosphoprotein that has a cell cycle regulatory role similar to that of the Rb protein. Like RB, inactivation of p53 gives the cell a growth advantage, probably as a result of loss of cell cycle regulation. p53 may be inactivated by a variety of mutations, including a single base change (point mutation) that increases the half-life of the protein, allelic loss, rearrangements, and deletions of the *p53* gene. Each of these mechanisms can result in tumor formation by loss of growth control. It is estimated that about 25% of osteosarcomas have detectable mutations of the *p53* gene (26).

The *p53 protein* is a transcription factor, meaning that it binds to regions of other genes (DNA), and controls the expression of genes responsible for cell cycle control (cell growth), apoptosis (programmed cell death), and other metabolic functions, such as control of repair of DNA damage. p53 acts in concert with Rb, and a variety of other proteins,

to regulate the cell cycle by a complex cascade of enzymes, of which Rb probably has the central role. Apoptosis has recently become recognized as an important mechanism by which chemotherapy and radiotherapy kill cancer cells. p53 is involved in this process, and appears to arrest cell division after sublethal damage (e.g., by radiation), to give the cell time to repair DNA defects before the next division (27–29). If repair does not take place, the cell undergoes apoptosis and dies. If p53 is not functional, the cell may survive and accumulate genetic defects, leading to malignant transformation. Osteosarcomas have been shown to have a variety of mutations of the *p53* gene (30–39). Preliminary evidence suggests that overexpression of mutant p53 protein, detected by immunohistochemistry or loss of heterozygosity of the *p53* gene, is related to outcome in human osteosarcoma (40,41).

In sarcomas, genetic defects other than p53 and Rb have been detected. One example is a gene called *mdm-2*, which is a zinc finger protein amplified in some sarcomas (23,42–44). It inactivates p53 protein by binding to p53, and prevents its transcription factor activity. Cordon-Cardo et al. (45) studied 211 adult soft tissue sarcomas by immunohistochemistry, using monoclonal antibodies to mdm-2 and p53, and demonstrated a correlation between overexpression of mdm-2/p53 and poor survival. Patients without mutations in either gene (mdm-2/p53 −) had the best survival, those with one mutation (either mdm-2 +/p53 − or mdm-2 −/p53 +) had intermediate survival, and those with mutations in both genes (mdm-2 +/p53 +) had the worst survival.

Not only are genetic mutations found in the tumors of patients with sarcomas, but mutations may also be present in all somatic cells (*germline mutations*) in patients with heritable cancer (46–53). Although such defects do not appear to be common in the general population, germline p53 mutations are present in patients who are part of a familial cancer syndrome. These families have a variety of cancers, often at an early age, and osteosarcomas and soft tissue sarcomas are a fairly common occurrence in these kindreds. Identification of patients with p53 germline mutations can be useful in determining which patients in an affected family are at risk for developing cancers, but much more work is needed in genetic counseling to determine how best to use this information. A recent study showed that germline mutations were present in approximately 3 to 4% of children with osteosarcoma, and that the detection of these mutations was more accurate than family history in predicting family cancer susceptibility (54).

How is this information useful for treatment? One possibility is that p53 mutations may be a potential biologic marker of prognosis and response to treatment (chemotherapy). There is some preliminary evidence that p53 mutations in the tumor may portend a worse prognosis in osteosarcoma. More recently, the association of p53 and apoptosis has suggested possible strategies for chemotherapy, based on the status of the p53 pathway (28,29). Gene therapy (replacing the missing or mutated gene by transfection with viral carriers) is often discussed, but there are major technical hurdles to overcome before this technology can be used to treat cancers in humans. However, it might be possible to make tumor cells more antigenic, or to make them more sensitive to antineoplastic drugs, by gene transfer. Another strategy would be to alter normal cells to make them less sensitive to damage by chemotherapeutic agents. Currently, these techniques pose technical challenges, but they offer realistic promise for the near future.

Another exciting area in the molecular biology of sarcomas is multidrug resistance (MDR). MDR probably explains why some patients respond to chemotherapy and others do not. Drug resistance may be intrinsic (present at diagnosis) or acquired (appearing after treatment of a tumor) (55,56). At least four basic mechanisms of drug resistance are now recognized under the category of the MDR phenotype. They are (a) changes in glutathione metabolism, (b) alterations in topoisomerase II, (c) non–P-glycoprotein (P-gp)-mediated mechanisms, and (d) P-gp-mediated mechanisms (1,2). Recent evidence has suggested that P-gp may be of particular relevance to osteosarcoma.

P-gp is a glycoprotein encoded by the MDR-1 gene on the long arm of chromosome 7 in humans (55,57,58). MDR-1 is one member of the aneurysmal bone cyst (ABC) superfamily of genes that encode membrane transport proteins, which function as unidirectional membrane pumps using adenosine triphosphate hydrolysis to work against a concentration gradient. P-gp is a 170-kilodalton protein located in the cell membrane that functions as an energy (adenosine triphosphate)–requiring pump that excludes certain classes (amphipathic compounds) of drugs from the cell. This physiologic mechanism is believed to be important in certain organ systems, such as the blood–brain barrier, placenta, liver, kidney, and colon for ridding the cell of unwanted toxins, but it is also responsible for actively excluding chemotherapeutic agents, such as *Vinca* alkaloids, anthracyclines, colchicine, etoposides, and taxol (many of which are active in osteosarcoma protocols) from the cancer cell. Another feature of the P-gp mechanism which may have some relevance to therapeutic strategies is that some classes of drugs can reverse the MDR phenotype by blocking the action of the pump. These drugs include verapamil, cyclosporin A, tamoxifen, and others.

Several studies have demonstrated that some (25 to 69%) sarcomas display the MDR phenotype at diagnosis, and that relapsed sarcomas show higher incidence and intensity of MDR expression (59–64). These studies suffer from small numbers of patients and a variety of methods by which MDR was tested, so comparisons of studies and accurate determination of the incidence of MDR expression are difficult to accomplish. In addition, the age of the patient and the sarcoma type appear to be related to the incidence of detectable P-gp at diagnosis. One study showed that osteo-

sarcomas have a higher incidence of MDR than other types of adult sarcomas (65). Serra et al. (61) demonstrated that overexpression of P-gp protein was evident in 23% of primary and 50% of metastatic osteosarcomas.

Recently, Baldini et al. (66) reported on 92 patients with nonmetastatic extremity osteosarcoma treated with chemotherapy and surgery, and related immunohistochemically determined P-gp expression to event-free survival. They found that P-gp expression predicted a decreased probability of remaining event-free, and was more predictive than histologic response to preoperative chemotherapy.

Findings such as these are important in planning future protocols in human osteosarcoma. The drug-resistant tumor is becoming better identified as one that has a poor histologic response to preoperative chemotherapy and that expresses P-gp. Undoubtedly, it is more complex than this, and other mechanisms will pertain. Several caveats exist. One is the complexity of defining the resistant tumor. Preoperative chemotherapy requires 10 to 12 weeks to provide an estimate of histologic necrosis unless ways can be found to accurately predict percentage of necrosis by positron emission tomographic scans, thallium scans, and/or gadolinium-enhanced magnetic resonance imaging. Detection of P-gp at diagnosis is difficult, and no one method has proven superior. It is probably not sufficient to demonstrate the presence of P-gp; also important is whether the pump is functioning to exclude cytotoxic agents from the tumor cell. Ideally, one would like to reverse the action of the P-gp mechanism, but just as there are not new agents to rescue patients who have poor histologic response, the agents currently available to reverse MDR are of limited benefit. They are potentially problematic in that they make the normal cell less tolerant to chemotherapy, and thereby increase toxicity, and in other tumors their use has not proven to be effective (56,58). The future probably lies in developing more effective reversing agents, and in defining other drug-resistant mechanisms.

EVALUATION

The differential diagnosis for patients who present with a bone or soft tissue mass includes neoplasia, infection, and trauma. Infection and trauma are more common than neoplasia, and one of these is usually the explanation of a mass or abnormality seen on a radiograph. Neoplasia should not be forgotten. The consequences of the mismanagement of a patient with a musculoskeletal tumor can be grave (Fig. 14-1).

Chief Complaint

Pain is the most common presenting complaint of a patient with a musculoskeletal tumor. The characteristics of the pain can help determine the diagnosis. Ask the patient:

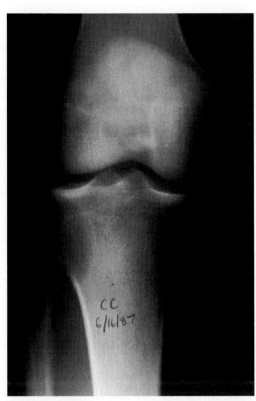

FIGURE 14-1. Anteroposterior radiograph of the knee of a young man who complained of it "giving way." The orthopaedist who saw the patient suspected a derangement, and the patient eventually had arthroscopic surgery. A radiolucent lesion can easily be seen in the lateral aspect of the proximal tibial metaphysis and epiphysis. This giant cell tumor of bone was missed because the physician did not consider this diagnosis when he was examining the patient or the radiograph. By the time the tumor was recognized, it had grown so large that resection and allograft reconstruction were required. Had it been treated when this radiograph was taken, a curettage and bone graft packing, or polymethyl methacrylate packing probably would have been done.

Most children and parents date the onset of symptoms to a traumatic event. The specific nature of the trauma and the relation of the trauma to the current symptoms must be evaluated thoroughly. Trauma without a definitive fracture can be the explanation for an abnormal radiograph but should not be used as the explanation, even for a periosteal reaction, unless the history is perfectly consistent. With the increased level of organized sports for children, there has been an increased incidence of fatigue fractures, and these fractures can be confused with neoplasias. Be cautious about ascribing a lesion to trauma.

The child presenting with a fracture should be questioned about the specifics of the injury that produced the fracture. Most lesions that lead to a pathologic fracture are easily recognized on a plain radiograph, but occasionally they may not be obvious. When the traumatic event seems insignificant, a pathologic fracture should be suspected. The patient should be asked about symptoms, no matter how minimal, before the fracture. Most aggressive benign tumors and malignant tumors produce pain before the bone is weakened enough to fracture. Inactive benign tumors are almost always asymptomatic until the bone breaks.

Medical History

Most children have no significant past medical history, but inquiries should be made. Has the child had a previous fracture? Has the child had other illnesses? Have radiographs been taken previously? Do not assume that the patient or the family will volunteer significant past medical history. Ask specific questions.

Review of Systems

Ask specifically about systemic symptoms of fever, decreased appetite, irritability, and decreased activity. Most patients with musculoskeletal tumors do not have systemic symptoms, and the presence of a systemic illness should alert the physician to the possibility of an underlying generalized disorder or osteomyelitis. Patients with Ewing sarcoma may have elevated temperature, weight loss, and malaise, but this is the exception rather than the rule. Even children with large primary malignant musculoskeletal tumors usually appear healthy. Patients with cancer do not always present with obvious signs of the underlying malignancy.

Most children with a soft tissue mass do not have symptoms. If the patient is younger than 5 years of age, the mass usually is noted first by a parent. The parent is convinced that the mass appeared overnight, but this is rarely the case. Teenagers may report the presence of a mass, but often only after a few weeks or months of waiting for it to resolve spontaneously. Painful soft tissue masses are most often abscesses. The majority of even malignant soft tissue tumors do not produce significant symptoms until they are large. Although most of the soft tissue masses seen in children

Where is the pain? How did it begin? Is it sharp, dull, radiating, or constant? Is it associated with activity? Is there a particular activity that makes the pain worse? What makes the pain better? Does it wake you at night? Is the intensity of the pain increasing, staying the same, or diminishing?

Patients who have active benign tumors (e.g., ABCs, chondroblastoma, and chondromyxofibroma) usually have a mild, dull, slowly progressive pain that is worse at night and aggravated by activity. Patients with malignant musculoskeletal tumors complain of a more rapidly progressive symptom complex, not specifically related to activity, which often awakens them at night. Occasionally, the pain pattern is diagnostic. The pain of an osteoid osteoma is so typical that the diagnosis should be strongly suspected from the history. This pain is a constant intense pain that is worse at night, and it is almost always relieved by aspirin or nonsteroidal antiinflammatory drugs (NSAIDs). The pain caused by a Brodie abscess is similar to that of an osteoid osteoma, but the Brodie abscess pain is rarely relieved by aspirin.

prove to be benign, all soft tissue masses, even those in children, should be considered malignant tumors until proven otherwise. The consequences of mistaking a malignant soft tissue tumor for a benign tumor can be devastating, whereas the consequences of approaching a benign tumor as if it were a malignancy are minimal.

Physical Examination

All patients with musculoskeletal complaints, especially those in the pediatric age group, should have a complete physical examination. Not only can important information be gained about the specific disorder being evaluated, but other significant abnormalities may be found. Café-au-lait lesions of the skin are a clue that the patient has fibrous dysplasia or neurofibromatosis. Numerous hard, nontender, fixed masses near the ends of long bones are diagnostic of multiple osteochondroma. Exophthalmos and otitis media indicate that the patient has Hand-Schüller-Christian disease.

The affected extremity should be examined carefully. The gait pattern should be recorded, muscular atrophy measured, and abnormalities in the vascular supply and motor and sensory innervation noted. The range of motion of the adjacent joint should be measured. If there is a mass present it should be measured, and the presence of erythema, tenderness, pulsations, bruit, or increased temperature should be noted.

Soft, movable, nontender masses, especially those in the subcutaneous tissues, usually are benign. These can be felt best when lubricant is applied on the overlying skin. Firm-to-hard, fixed or tethered, tender masses, especially those deep to the superficial fascia, are more likely to be malignant, but neurofibroma, deep lipoma, and cyst usually are firm to the touch. Transilluminate the mass; if light is transmitted more easily through the mass than through the surrounding tissue, the mass is a fluid-filled cyst.

Plain Radiograph Examination

Patients with musculoskeletal complaints should have at least anteroposterior and lateral plain radiographs. Good-quality plain radiographs (at least two views, preferably at 90 degrees) are necessary. The entire lesion must be observed. The radiograph should be reviewed systematically. Look at the bone, all of it, and every bone on the radiograph. Ask yourself these questions: Is there an area of increased or decreased density? Is there endosteal or periosteal reaction, and if there is, what are the characteristics of the reaction? Is there cortical destruction? Is it localized or are there multiple defects? Is the margin in the tumor well defined or poorly defined? Is there a reactive rim of bone surrounding the lesion? Are there densities within a radiolucent lesion? Is the bone of normal, increased, or decreased overall density? Is the joint normal? Is there loss of articular

cartilage? Is the subchondral bone normal, thick, or thin? Are there abnormalities in the bone on both sides of the joint? Are there intraarticular densities? Is there a soft tissue mass? Are there calcifications or ossifications in the soft tissue? By looking specifically for abnormalities, it is unlikely that an abnormality will be missed. The pelvis and the scapula are exceptions to this rule. Large tumors involving the pelvis or the scapula, even those with marked destruction of bone, can be extremely difficult or impossible to see on a plain radiograph. If there is a suggestion that the patient has a pelvic or a scapular tumor, bone scanning and computed axial tomography (CT) or magnetic resonance imaging (MRI) are recommended.

Enneking (67) teaches that four sets of questions should be asked when looking at plain radiographs of a possible bone tumor.

1. Where is the tumor? This refers to the lesion's anatomic location: long bone or flat bone; epiphyseal, metaphyseal, or diaphyseal; and medullary canal, intracortical, or surface.
2. What is the tumor doing to the bone? Is there erosion of the bone, and if so, what is the pattern?
3. What is the bone doing to the tumor? Is there periosteal or endosteal reaction? Is it well-developed? Is it sharply defined?
4. Are there intrinsic characteristics within the tumor that indicate its histology? Is there bone formation by the tumor? Is there calcification? Is the lesion completely radiolucent?

The examination of a radiograph should not be a casual glance, but a detailed study of all tissue present. Do not forget to specifically examine the soft tissues visible on the radiograph.

Most bone tumors can be diagnosed correctly after obtaining the history, performing a physical examination, and examining the plain radiograph. When the specific diagnosis is made from these examinations, additional studies are requested only if they are necessary for treatment. Specific treatment often can be planned from only the history, physical examination, and plain radiographs. For example, a 16-year-old boy with a hard, fixed mass in the distal femur that has not increased in size for more than 1 year, and has been present for 9 years, complains of pain after direct trauma to this mass. Plain anteroposterior and lateral radiographs confirm the clinically suspected diagnosis of osteochondroma. Further evaluation to make the diagnosis is not necessary, but if surgical resection is elected as the treatment, CT or MRI may be useful in planning the operative procedure.

When the specific diagnosis cannot be made, it should be possible to limit the differential to three or four diagnoses, and appropriate additional evaluations can be requested. CT, MRI, nuclear bone scanning (technetium, gallium, thallium, and indium), and positron emission tomography may reveal findings that are diagnostic, or that provide needed information with which to plan a subsequent biopsy. For example, a 10-year-old boy complains of mild knee pain that has been present for 3 months, has loss of knee flexion, and on the lateral radiograph of the distal femur there is a bone density lesion attached to the posterior femoral cortex. From this information, the lesion is recognized as either a parosteal osteosarcoma or an osteocartilaginous exostosis. A technetium bone scan, with increased activity in the area of the lesion does not distinguish between these two, but both CT and MRI allow one to distinguish between a parosteal osteosarcoma and an osteocartilaginous exostosis. A parosteal osteosarcoma is attached to the cortex of the bone, whereas an osteocartilaginous exostosis arises from the cortex, and has a medullary canal continuous with the medullary canal of the bone. CT or MRI is critical in the evaluation of a patient in this clinical setting.

Additional Diagnostic Studies

Laboratory Examinations

Urine and serum laboratory values in musculoskeletal neoplasia are usually normal. Only a few musculoskeletal disorders are associated with abnormal laboratory values. The erythrocyte sedimentation rate (ESR), or sedimentation rate, is nonspecific but sensitive. Patients with infections or malignant tumors usually have an elevated ESR, but patients with benign disease should have a normal value. A normal ESR value can be used to increase the physician's confidence that a suspected benign, inactive lesion is just that. A markedly elevated value (>180 mm/h) supports a diagnosis of infection, and may be just what is needed to justify an early aspiration of a bone or soft tissue lesion. Patients with active benign or malignant musculoskeletal tumors, particularly those with Ewing sarcoma, often have an elevated ESR, but it is rarely greater than 80 mm/h. C-reactive protein is another serum value that indicates systemic inflammation. It increases and returns to normal more quickly that ESR.

Serum alkaline phosphatase is present in most tissues in body, but the bone and the hepatobiliary system are the predominant sources. In the pediatric age group conventional high-grade osteosarcoma is associated with elevated serum alkaline phosphatase (68). Not all patients with osteosarcoma have elevated serum alkaline phosphatase, and therefore, a normal value does not exclude osteosarcoma from the diagnosis. A minimal elevation can be observed with numerous processes, even a healing fracture. Adults with elevated serum alkaline phosphatase secondary to bone disease are most likely to have Paget disease of bone or diffuse metastatic carcinoma. Patients with a primary liver disorder have elevated serum alkaline phosphatase as well, but they also have elevated serum 5-nucleotidase, elevated leucine aminopeptidase, and glutamyl transpeptidase deficiency. These are not elevated in primary bone tumors.

Serum and urine calcium and phosphorus should be measured, especially if a metabolic bone disorder is suspected. Serum lactic dehydrogenase (LDH) is elevated in some patients with osteosarcoma, and Ewing sarcoma patients with elevated levels have a worse prognosis (69–71). Elevated LDH may also indicate relapse in a patient who has been treated for these tumors. Patients entering chemotherapy treatment protocols will need to have LDH levels determined to stratify them on the protocol. Other laboratory determinations are not helpful, and are not recommended.

Radionuclide Scans

Technetium bone scanning is readily available, safe, and an excellent method to evaluate the activity of the primary lesion (Fig. 14-2). In addition, bone scanning is the most practical method to survey the entire skeleton. Technetium 99 attached to a polyphosphate is injected intravenously, and after a delay of 2 to 4 h the polyphosphate, with its attached technetium, concentrates in the skeleton proportional to the production of new bone. A disorder that is associated with an increase in bone production increases the local concentration of technetium 99 and produces a "hot spot" on the scan. The technetium bone scan can be used to evaluate the activity of a primary lesion, to search for other bone lesions, and to indicate extension of a lesion beyond what is seen on the plain radiograph. The polyphosphate–technetium 99 compound also concentrates in areas of increased blood flow, and soft tissue tumors usually have increased activity compared with normal soft tissues. The technetium scan can be used to evaluate blood flow if images are obtained during the early phases immediately after injection of the technetium. The polyphosphate–technetium 99 is cleared and excreted by the kidneys, so the kidneys and the bladder have more activity than other organs. The technetium scan is sensitive but nonspecific. The principal value of a radionuclide scan is as a means of surveying the entire skeleton for clinically unsuspected lesions. In approximately 25% of cases of Langerhans cell histiocytosis and plasmocytoma, the bone scan is normal, or there is decreased activity at the site of the lesion (72–74).

Gallium 67 imaging is another radionuclide study to evaluate both bone and soft tissue tumors (75). This examination takes longer to perform (24 to 72 h) than technetium 99 scanning (2 h), but it is believed to be useful in the evaluation of musculoskeletal tumors (76) because it can help differentiate a musculoskeletal infection from a neoplasia. Gallium scans are most useful when evaluating a patient suspected of having an occult infection. Scanning should be performed before a surgical procedure, because the operative site has increased uptake on the radionuclide scan.

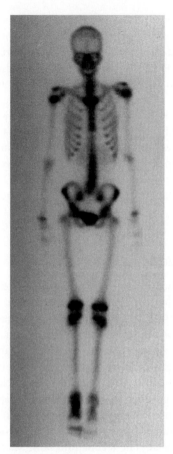

FIGURE 14-2. This is an anterior view of a whole body technetium 99 bone scan. This patient has an osteoid osteoma of her talus, and there is increased activity in the talus. There is also increased activity in the distal tibia, which is thought to be a reaction to the local increased blood flow. Technetium 99 bone scanning is an efficient means of evaluating the entire skeleton of a patient with a bone lesion. It is important to have the entire skeleton scanned, rather than limit the scan to a small part of the skeleton.

Thallium scans have been used to evaluate a tumor's response to therapy before resection (77,78). Because thallium uptake correlates well with the vascular supply of a tumor, decreased thallium uptake after therapy is a reflection of tumor necrosis, which is the best evidence that the chemotherapy is working. Unfortunately, to date the accuracy of thallium scanning is not sufficient for it to be completely reliable.

Positron emission tomography (PET) is being used more frequently in the evaluation of musculoskeletal tumors (79). Fluoro-2-deoxy-D-glucose (FDG) PET is the type of PET used most frequently in the musculoskeletal system. Because there is a differential uptake of FDG between neoplastic tissue and normal tissue (neoplastic tissue has greater uptake), it is possible to identify neoplastic tissue on a PET scan. The role of PET in the evaluation and monitoring of patients with musculoskeletal neoplasia is under investigation.

Computed Axial Tomography

When introduced in the late 1970s, CT dramatically improved the evaluation of bone and soft tissue tumors. Anatomic location and extent could be determined accurately. This improved the accuracy of anatomic localization, so that less radical surgery can be performed safely. Often, a specific diagnosis can be made or a suspected diagnosis can be confirmed after seeing the CT scan. Smaller nodules are seen on whole-lung CT scans than are seen with plain chest radiographs or whole-lung linear tomographs. With CT the abdomen can be evaluated thoroughly without surgical exploration.

The most common error made when requesting CT is not asking specific questions of the radiologist. Radiologists do not know what specific information the orthopaedist wants; only if specific questions are asked is the maximum value of CT realized. A specific differential diagnosis should be made from the presentation and plain radiographs. Only then can a decision be made regarding whether to request CT, MRI, both, or neither. Ask the radiologist to determine the lesion's location and its density and vascularity, and to search for intralesional characteristics that may provide a diagnostic clue. Have the radiologist include the contralateral normal extremity on the CT scan for comparisons.

The density of a bone or soft tissue mass on a CT scan is called its "attenuation coefficient" and is measured in Hounsfield units (HU) (Fig. 14-3). The density of water is 0 HU; tissues more dense than water have a positive value, and tissues less dense than water have a negative value. The vascularity of a lesion can be evaluated by measuring the increase in the attenuation coefficient of a lesion after intravenous infusion of contrast, and comparing this increase to that in an adjacent muscle. Normal muscle has an attenuation coefficient of approximately 60 HU, and increases 5 to 10 HU with a bolus of intravenous contrast. Fat has an attenuation coefficient of approximately −60 HU, and cortical bone usually has a value of more than 1,000 HU.

CT can be performed quickly with the newer "spiral" scanners and is less anxiety-producing, so sedation is less likely to be needed compared with MRI. CT remains most useful in the evaluation of small lesions in or immediately adjacent to the cortex (e.g., osteoid osteoma on the surface) and lesions with fine mineralization or calcifications (e.g., chondroblastoma). Percutaneous biopsies of musculoskeletal lesions can be performed with the assistance of localization obtained with CT. For all other situations, MRI has replaced CT.

Magnetic Resonance Imaging

MRI does not expose the patient to radiation, and has proved to be the most useful tool in the evaluation of musculoskeletal lesions. MRI produces images of the body in

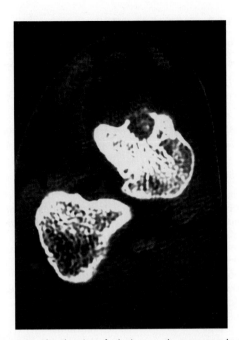

FIGURE 14-3. The density of a lesion can be measured on a computed tomography scan. This cortical bone lesion is an osteoid osteoma. The radiologist can measure the actual density of the lesion and provide information regarding the type of tissue. The measurements are made in Hounsfield units, after a developer of computed tomography. Zero Hounsfield units is the density of water. Negative units are less dense than water (fat measures approximately –70 Hounsfield units), and positive units are more dense than water (cortical bone measures greater than 1,000 Hounsfield units).

all three planes (axial, sagittal, and coronal) as easily as in a single plane, and possesses no known hazards to the patient.

The images are produced by a computer program that converts the reactions of tissue hydrogen ions in a strong magnetic field excited by radio waves. By adjusting excitation variables, images that are T1- and T2-weighted are obtained. A variety of techniques have been used to produce images of improved quality compared with routine T1- and T2-weighted images. The use of gadolinium as an intravascular contrast agent allows one to judge the vascularity of a lesion, providing even more information about the tumor. Fat suppression images with gadolinium enhancement often are especially useful to demonstrate a soft tissue neoplasia. As with CT, it is important for the orthopaedist requesting MRI to discuss the case with the radiologist. The radiologist can then determine the optimal setting to see the lesion.

MRI is the single most important diagnostic test after physical examination and plain radiography for evaluating a musculoskeletal lesion. The ability to view the lesion in three planes, determine its intraosseous extent, see the soft tissue component clearly, and have an idea of the tissue type from one diagnostic test makes MRI a powerful tool (80). Unfortunately, variations in technique mean that it is important that the examination be planned carefully if the

most information possible is to be obtained (see Chapter 3). The radiologist must understand what questions need to be answered from the MRI. As a rule, it is important that the image be reviewed while it is being made, to ensure that the entire lesion is examined. Image the entire bone. T1-weighted (with and without gadolinium), T2-weighted, and fat-suppression techniques are the minimal images needed.

Staging

Patients with neoplasia can be separated into groups based on the extent of their tumor and its potential for metastasis. These groups are called stages. Grouping patients by their stage helps the physician predict a patient's risk of local recurrence and metastasis. This facilitates making treatment decisions about individual patients and helps in the comparison of treatment protocols. Staging systems are based on the histologic grade of the tumor, the tumor's size and location, and the presence of regional or distant metastasis. The presence of a metastasis at the time of presentation is a bad prognostic sign, and, regardless of other findings, puts the patient in the highest-risk stage. For patients without metastasis at presentation, the histologic grade of the tumor is the principle prognostic predictor. Size is next in importance. Higher histologic grade and larger tumors are associated with the worst prognosis.

There are two common staging systems used for musculoskeletal tumors. The task force on malignant bone tumors of the American Joint Commission on Staging and End Result Studies published a staging system for soft tissue tumors in 1977 (81). This system was revised in 1987 (82,83). This staging system is based on the histologic grade (G), local extent or size (T), whether or not there is involvement of nodes (N), and metastases (M). The tumors are separated into three histologic grades (G1, low grade; G2, medium grade; G3, high grade) and two sizes (T1 for less than 5 cm, T2 for equal to or greater than 5 cm). Patients with nodal involvement are designated N1, and those without nodal involvement are designated N0. Patients with metastatic disease are designated M1, and those without metastatic disease are designated M0. There are four stages, with subclasses in each stage. The patient with stage 1 has the best prognosis, and the patient with stage 4 has the worst prognosis (Table 14-2).

Enneking and colleagues (84) also proposed a musculoskeletal staging system. This system is used more often by orthopaedists involved in the management of patients with musculoskeletal tumors. It was designed to be simple, straightforward, and clinically practical. The tumors are separated into only two histologic grades (I, low grade; II, high grade) and two anatomic extents (A, intracompartmental; B, extracompartmental). Patients with metastatic disease in either a regional lymph node or a distant site are grouped together as stage III. Each bone is defined as its own separate

TABLE 14-2. REVISED AMERICAN JOINT COMMISSION STAGING SYSTEM FOR SOFT TISSUE SARCOMA

Stage	Description
Stage I	
IA—G1, T1, N0, M0	Grade 1 tumor, <5 cm in diameter with no regional lymph node or distant metastasis
IB—G1, T2, N0, M0	Grade 1 tumor, ≥5 cm in diameter with no regional lymph node or distant metastasis
Stage II	
IIA—G2, T1, N0, M0	Grade 2 tumor, <5 cm in diameter with no regional lymph node or distant metastasis
IIB—G2, T2, N0, M0	Grade 2 tumor, ≥5 cm in diameter with no regional lymph node or distant metastasis
Stage III	
IIIA—G3, T1, N0, M0	Grade 3 tumor, <5 cm in diameter with no regional lymph node or distant metastasis
IIIB—G3, T2, N0, M0	Grade 3 tumor, ≥5 cm in diameter with no regional lymph node or distant metastasis
Stage IV	
IVA—G1–3, T1–2, N1, M0	Tumor of any grade or size with histologically verified metastasis to regional lymph nodes, but no distant metastasis
IVB—G1–3, T1–2, N0–1	Clinically diagnosed distant metastasis

G1, low grade; G2, medium grade; G3, high grade; T1, <5 cm; T2, ≥5 cm; N0, no nodal involvement; N1, nodal involvement; M0, no metastases; M1, metastases.
(From ref. 82, with permission.)

TABLE 14-3. SURGICAL SITES

Intracompartmental	Extracompartmental
Intraosseous	Extraosseous soft tissue extension
Intraarticular	Extraparticular soft tissue extension
Superficial to deep fascia	Deep fascial extension Intraosseous or extrafascial extension
Paraosseous	
Intrafascial compartments	
Ray of hand or foot	Extrafascial planes or spaces
Posterior calf	Midfoot and hindfoot
Anterolateral leg	Popliteal space
Anterior thigh	Groin-femoral triangle
Medial thigh	Intrapelvic
Posterior thigh	Midhand
Buttocks	Antecubital fossae
Volar forearm	Axilla
Dorsal forearm	Periclavicular
Anterior arm	Paraspinal
Posterior arm	Head and neck
Periscapular	

(From ref. 84, with permission.)

A marginal surgical margin is achieved when a tumor is removed by dissecting between the normal tissue and the tumor's pseudocapsule. This is a surgical margin obtained when a tumor is "shelled out." A wide surgical margin is achieved when the tumor is removed with a surrounding cuff of normal, uninvolved tissue. This is often referred to as *en bloc* resection. A radical surgical margin is achieved when the tumor and the entire compartment (or compartments) are removed together. This usually is accomplished only with an amputation that is proximal to the joint just proximal to the lesion (e.g., an above-knee amputation for a tibial tumor). As a rule, benign lesions can be managed with an intralesional or marginal surgical margin, but malignant tumors require a wide surgical margin. Radical surgical margins are reserved for recurrent tumors and the most infiltrative malignancies.

anatomic compartment. The soft tissue anatomic compartments are defined as muscle groups separated by fascial boundaries (Table 14-3). There are five stages in this system (Table 14-4).

Enneking and colleagues (84) also introduced four terms to indicate the surgical margin of a tumor resection. These terms are commonly used, and provide a means of describing the relation between the histologic extent of the tumor and the resection margin. The surgical margins are defined as intralesional, marginal, wide, and radical. An intralesional margin is the surgical margin achieved when a tumor's pseudocapsule is violated and gross tumor is removed from within the pseudocapsule. An incisional biopsy and a curettage are two common examples of an intralesional margin.

TABLE 14-4. SURGICAL STAGES

Stage	Grade	Site and Size
IA	Low	Intracompartmental (T1)
IB	Low	Extracompartmental (T2)
IIA	High	Intracompartmental (T1)
IIB	High	Extracompartmental (T2)
III	Any grade; regional or distant metastasis	Any site or size

T1, <5 cm; T2, ≥5 cm.
(From ref. 84, with permission.)

Biopsy

Biopsy should be the last step in the evaluation of a patient with a bone or soft tissue tumor, and it should be performed only after careful planning (85–87). Often, biopsy proves unnecessary after the patient has been thoroughly evaluated, the diagnosis having been made by the clinical setting and radiographic findings. When a biopsy is required, the prebiopsy evaluation improves the chance that adequate and representative tissue will be obtained, the least amount of normal tissue will be contaminated, and the pathologist will make an accurate diagnosis. Biopsies performed without an adequate prebiopsy evaluation are more likely to produce unsatisfactory results.

The purpose of the biopsy is to confirm the diagnosis suspected by the physician after the evaluation, or to determine which diagnosis, among a limited differential diagnosis, is correct. In addition to providing confirmation for a specific diagnosis, the tissue obtained must be sufficient for histologic grading. It must be representative of the tumor, and because many musculoskeletal tumors are heterogeneous, the specific site from which the tissue is taken is important. The surgeon who is willing to assume the surgical management of the patient, regardless of the diagnosis, should biopsy the patient's tumor. The biopsy incision and the tissue exposed during the biopsy must be excised with the tumor, if a wide surgical margin resection proves to be necessary. If the surgeon who performs the resection has planned and performed the biopsy, the patient has a better chance of limb salvage and less risk of local recurrence (86). The surgeon should consult with the radiologist and the pathologist before performing the biopsy to get their suggestions of the best tissue to obtain. Discussing the case with the pathologist the day before the biopsy also allows the pathologist to be better prepared when he or she is expected to make a diagnosis from a frozen section.

Needle biopsy and fine-needle aspirate biopsy often are suggested (88–91). Usually, they can be performed without general anesthesia and hospital admission, saving money and the need for general anesthesia. The needle track can be seeded with tumor, and should be excised at the time of the definitive resection. Needle biopsy and fine-needle aspirate biopsy must be planned just as open biopsy is planned, and the responsible surgeon should decide how the biopsy is to be performed. Needle biopsy and fine-needle aspirate biopsy are most useful for lesions whose clinical presentations are diagnostic, and when treatment is either nonsurgical or requires presurgical therapy. Although an experienced pathologist usually can make the correct diagnosis from a well-done needle biopsy or a fine-needle aspirate biopsy, more mistakes are made with these techniques than with open biopsy, and histologic grading can be difficult or impossible without open biopsy (88,89,91).

Plan the biopsy carefully. Think about possible future treatment, especially limb-salvage resection. The skin incision and deep dissection should be made so that they can be resected with the tumor at the time of definitive limb-salvage operation. Longitudinal skin incisions are better than transverse skin incisions. The dissection should be as limited as possible, flaps should not be raised, and neurovascular bundles should not be exposed. The dissection should be through a muscle, not between muscles. The tumor's pseudocapsule and a portion of the tumor should be excised as a block and sent to the pathologist. A frozen section analysis should be done, even when there are no plans for immediate additional surgery. The pathologist should be certain that adequate and diagnostic tissue is available. Only when dense bone is biopsied is it impossible to obtain a frozen section analysis. The pathologist should set aside tissue for subsequent examination with an electron microscope. Some tissue should be kept frozen in the event that immunohistochemistry is required.

A tourniquet can be used during the biopsy, but deflate the tourniquet before closure. The tumor should be manipulated as little as possible, and do not use a compressive bandage to exsanguinate the extremity, but rather elevate the extremity for 3 to 5 min before inflating the tourniquet.

Extra care should be taken to achieve hemostasis before closing the wound. The hematoma from the biopsy may contain tumor cells, and will require resection if surgery is the treatment. The wound can be drained, but the exit site of the drain must be in line with the incision and close to it. The drain track is resected with the tumor and the biopsy incision.

Occasionally an excisional biopsy, rather than an incisional biopsy, is indicated. An excisional biopsy is appropriate when the lesion is small, and can be excised with a cuff of normal tissue. An excisional biopsy may be appropriate even when a major resection is required. If the preoperative evaluation strongly supports the diagnosis of a malignancy, particularly one for which a frozen section analysis will be difficult to do, an excisional biopsy should be considered. The choice between an incisional biopsy and an excisional biopsy usually is easy to make. A clinically obvious exostosis on the proximal tibia should have an excisional biopsy, if it is biopsied at all. A surface osteosarcoma, diagnosed based on the results of plain radiography and CT or MRI, can be excisionally biopsied with a resection. A large aggressive lesion within the distal femur and invading the adjacent soft tissues should be biopsied incisionally. This decision is more difficult when the evaluation reveals a small, active, possibly low-grade malignancy on the proximal humerus or the distal radius. An incisional biopsy exposes uncontaminated tissues to the tumor, and if the tumor proves to be a malignancy, the definitive resection is more complicated. If the lesion can be treated with curettage or a marginal excision, the incisional biopsy leads to the least functional loss. The final decision is made for each patient based not only on the tumor's characteristics, but also on the patient's desires. Some patients want to take the least chances, and are willing to accept the possibility of slight overtreatment, whereas others choose to take one step at a time. It is the surgeon's responsibility to inform the patient so that an informed decision can be made.

An added advantage of the excisional biopsy is that the pathologist is able to examine the entire lesion, improving the accuracy of the pathologic examination. Musculoskeletal tumors often are heterogeneous, and the amount of tissue obtained with an incisional biopsy always is limited. It can be particularly difficult to distinguish active benign cartilage tumors from low-grade chondrosarcomas. When the entire lesion, especially its connection with the adjacent bone and soft tissue, is seen the distinction is made more easily.

A final note of caution is offered with regard to the biopsy: Osteomyelitis is more common than bone tumors, especially in children, and osteomyelitis often mimics neoplasia. The reverse also is true; whenever performing a biopsy, even when the diagnosis seems obvious, culture the tumor and biopsy the infection.

SPECIFIC BONE TUMORS

This text is not designed to be a definitive musculoskeletal pathology text, and only those tumors that are common are discussed. The authors have tried to confine the discussion to pertinent information regarding the tumors, their evaluation, and their treatment.

Bone-forming Tumors

Osteoid Osteoma

Jaffe (92) is credited with the initial description of osteoid osteoma, distinguishing it from a sterile abscess called a Brodie abscess, and from Garré osteomyelitis. It is a benign tumor and accounts for 11% of the benign bone tumors in Dahlin's series from the Mayo Clinic (93). The patient is usually a young boy (males are affected more commonly than females, at a ratio of 3:1; 80% are between 5 and 24 years of age at the time of their initial symptoms) complaining of an intense pain at the site of the lesion.

The pain is an unrelenting, sharp, boring pain, worse at night and, almost without exception, completely relieved by aspirin or NSAIDs. The pain is not related to activity. The pain is thought to be attributable to prostaglandins produced by the nidus. The relief obtained with aspirin and NSAIDs is most likely the result of their ability to block prostaglandin's action. If a patient has the typical pain of an osteoid osteoma, but is not relieved by aspirin, the diagnosis of an osteoid osteoma should be doubted. The patient may have pain before any abnormality appears on the plain radiograph, and often the patient has had an electromyogram, a myelogram, or an arthrogram, before the typical plain radiographic changes are seen. Some patients are sus-

pected of having a psychosomatic disorder before the osteoid osteoma is found.

Osteoid osteomas may arise in any bone, but one-half of them are found in the femur or the tibia, whereas the other half are distributed throughout the rest of the skeleton (Fig. 14-4). The proximal femur is a common site. It is also a site at which it may be difficult to find the lesion. Young patients with persistent pain in the groin, the middle thigh, or the knee should be suspected of having an osteoid osteoma. The other common location of an occult osteoid osteoma is the spine. When osteoid osteoma arises in the spine, usually it is located in the posterior elements (Fig. 14-5). The osteoid osteoma in the spine does not elicit a significant bony reaction, and is very difficult to see on plain radiographs. The patient presents most commonly with a painful scoliosis (94,95). When a patient with scoliosis complains of back pain, osteoid osteoma should be considered. A technetium bone scan is particularly useful when the clinical presentation suggests an osteoid osteoma but the lesion cannot be found on the plain radiograph. It reveals an area of increased uptake, supporting a diagnosis of osteoid osteoma, and shows the lesion's location.

Patients with osteoid osteoma show few abnormalities on physical examination, with the exception of scoliosis in patients with osteoid osteoma of the spine. The child may walk with a limp and have atrophy of the involved extremity. If the bone with the osteoid osteoma can be palpated directly, it will be tender. Local erythema or increased temperature are not seen, and joint motion is normal. Serum and urine laboratory values are normal.

The plain radiographic appearance of an osteoid osteoma is of dense reactive bone, and usually is diagnostic. The lesion itself (the nidus, less than 15 mm in diameter) is radiolucent, but often is not seen on the plain radiograph, because of the density of the intense bone reaction that surrounds it. The nidus may be on the surface of the bone, within the cortex, or on the endosteal surface. Lesions on the endosteal surface have less reaction than lesions within or on the cortex. The lesion and the reaction are associated with increased uptake on the radionuclide study (technetium bone scan) (96). The nidus is best demonstrated by CT (97). The distance between the CT scan sections should be small (1 to 2 mm), so that the nidus is not missed. The window settings of the CT scanner should be adjusted so that the dense reaction around the lesion does not obscure the small, low-density nidus. When the nidus is found, it helps to have the distance from a bony landmark to the nidus measured on the scan, so that the nidus can be found at the time of surgical removal. MRI has been used to examine osteoid osteoma, and the diagnosis may be suspected, but the associated edema and reaction make the diagnosis less specific than with CT.

On gross inspection, the nidus of an osteoid osteoma is red and surrounded by dense white bone. The nidus is small, usually not more than 5 to 10 mm in diameter. A lesion that is identical histologically to the nidus of an osteoid

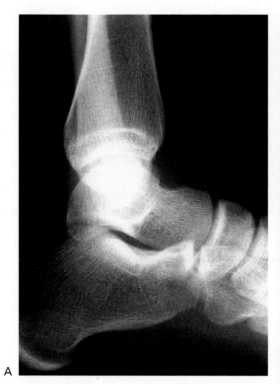

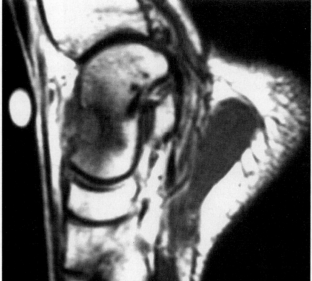

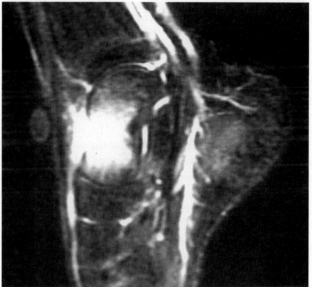

FIGURE 14-4. A: This plain radiograph is a lateral view of an 18-year-old woman's ankle. She complained of severe pain for 6 months, which was totally relieved by aspirin. There is a small erosion in the anterior neck of her talus. (Her computed tomography scan is seen in Fig. 14-3.) **B:** The sagittal view of a T1-weighted magnetic resonance image shows the lesion in her anterior talus. **C:** The T2-weighted magnetic resonance image reveals the extensive edema that is characteristic of osteoid osteoma.

osteoma, but larger than 2 cm, is called an osteoblastoma. The nidus is composed of numerous vascular channels, osteoblasts, and thin, lace-like osteoid seams (Fig. 14-6). Multinucleated giant cells can be seen, but are not common.

The pain of an osteoid osteoma can resolve spontaneously (98). Kneisl and Simon (99) treated 24 patients with osteoid osteoma. Thirteen were operated on immediately, and all had complete relief of pain. Nine were treated with NSAIDs. Three subsequently elected to have surgery, but six eventually became free of pain (an average of 33 months). It is believed that osteoid osteoma is a spontaneously healing lesion that eventually involutes over a period of years, and the nidus completely ossifies. Occasionally, a patient uses aspirin or NSAIDs to control the symptoms

until the pain disappears, but most often the intensity of pain, the time it takes for the lesion to heal spontaneously, and the amount of medication required is not tolerable, and the patient elects to have surgery. Complete removal of the nidus relieves the patient's pain. Partial removal may provide temporary relief, but the pain usually returns (100). Only the nidus needs to be excised, whereas the reactive bone around the nidus does not need to be removed.

There are two surgical methods of removing the nidus. The conventional method is a block resection of the nidus and most of the surrounding reactive bone. The other is a curettage of the nidus. The advantage of the block resection is the greater assurance that all of the nidus is removed, but this technique requires removal of a segment of the cortex,

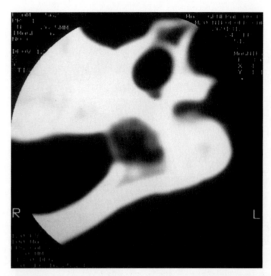

FIGURE 14-5. This is a computed tomography scan cut through a lesion in the pedicle of a teenager with neck pain. The lesion has all of the characteristics of osteoid osteoma. It could not be seen clearly on the plain radiograph, but there was a discrete focus of increased uptake on a technetium 99 bone scan.

operatively, or seen intraoperatively, block excision is preferred. Intraoperative radionuclide scanning and intra-operative tetracycline-fluorescence demonstration have been reported as methods of finding the nidus in the operating room and assuring the surgeon of its complete removal (101–104). The authors have not found these techniques necessary. Preoperative planning and careful localization of the nidus is the most important means of ensuring that the nidus can be found during the operation.

Radiofrequency ablation has become an accepted means of treating osteoid osteoma (105–107). The procedure is performed under general anesthesia, but usually can be done without hospitalization. Using CT to control placement, a needle biopsy is performed to confirm the diagnosis. Then, through the same needle track a radiofrequency electrode with an internal thermistor is placed in the nidus. The patients were not protected, nor were their activities limited after the heat ablation, and there have been no complications. Other closed methods of treatment have been reported (108).

Osteoblastoma

Osteoblastoma is sometimes called "giant osteoid osteoma" because it is histologically identical to osteoid osteoma, but larger. Unlike osteoid osteoma, osteoblastoma is not surrounded by dense reactive bone. Cementoblastoma of the jaw is histologically identical to osteoblastoma. Osteoblastoma is less common than osteoid osteoma, accounting for less than 1% of the primary bone tumors in Dahlin's series (93).

The typical patient is a boy in the second decade of life (50% of the patients are between 10 and 20 years of age, although the age range is from 5 to 35 years of age) complaining of back pain (approximately 50% of the lesions

and produces a marked reduction in the strength of the bone. The defect created by the excision may need to be bone-grafted, and the patient's extremity may need to be protected for an extended period of time. The advantage of the curettage technique is that the bone is not weakened significantly, and bone grafting is not required. However, with curettage it is more difficult to be certain that all of the nidus is removed.

If curettage is the excision technique used, the nidus must be accurately localized preoperatively, and seen intraoperatively. When the nidus cannot be localized accurately pre-

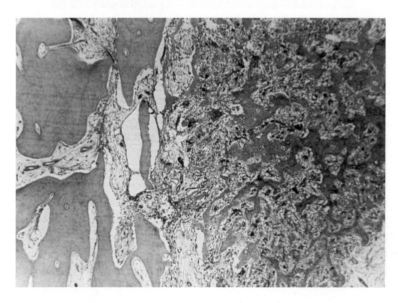

FIGURE 14-6. Histologic appearance of an osteoid osteoma. The bone tissue on the **left** is reactive trabeculae surrounding the nidus (**right**). The nidus is composed of osteoid, multinucleated giant cells, osteoblasts, and vessels. A thorough curettage of the nidus was done, and the patient's pain resolved completely. (Original magnification ×10.)

are in the spine). The pain of an osteoblastoma is not as severe as the pain of an osteoid osteoma, and aspirin or NSAIDs do not have such a dramatic effect. There are no physical findings characteristic of osteoblastoma. When the tumor is in the spine, the patient has decreased motion of the spine in the involved area. Osteoblastomas are tender, and direct palpation often localizes a lesion, even when it cannot be seen on a plain radiograph.

Extremity lesions are usually diaphyseal; the patient often has a limp and mild atrophy, and complains of pain directly over the lesion. Blood and urine laboratory examinations are normal. The appearance of osteoblastoma on a radiograph is variable. It is usually a mixed radiolucent, radiodense lesion, more lucent than dense. There is minimal reaction in the surrounding bone. Lesions in the spine may be difficult or impossible to see when initially examining the plain radiograph, but when located by other studies, the subtle abnormality on the plain radiograph can usually be appreciated.

Clues to look for on the plain radiograph to indicate the location of an osteoblastoma are an irregular cortex, loss of pedicle definition, and enlargement of the spinous process. As with osteoid osteoma, CT is the best method of localization. On the CT scan, the lesion usually "expands the bone" and has intralesional stippled ossifications and a high attenuation coefficient (100 HU or more). Osteoblastoma on the radionuclide scan has increased uptake, and technetium bone scanning is an excellent method of initially screening a patient suspected of having an osteoblastoma. The bone scan localizes the lesion, but it is not specific enough to plan a surgical resection for lesions in the spine.

Osteoblastomas should be excised surgically. They continue to enlarge and damage the bone and adjacent structures if left untreated. A wide surgical resection is preferred when practical, but an extended curettage is sufficient for most cases. As much of the surrounding bone should be removed as possible. Most osteoblastomas are controlled by the extended curettage, but recurrence is not uncommon, and some can be locally aggressive. It is difficult to give a percentage risk of local recurrence, but in the authors' experience, it is less than 10% of cases. Although irradiation has been used in the management of these patients, there is little evidence that it is of benefit.

The histology of an osteoblastoma is identical to the nidus of an osteoid osteoma. There should not be abnormal mitoses, although mitotic activity can be observed. There are osteoblasts, multinucleated giant cells, seams of osteoid, and a rich vascular bed. Schajowicz and Lemos (109) suggested that a subset of osteoblastoma be termed malignant osteoblastoma. They believe that this subset has histologic features that are worse than those of the usual osteoblastoma, is more aggressive locally, and is more likely to recur after limited surgery. A rare osteoblastoma metastasizes but still meets the histologic definitions of a benign tumor, although it probably should be classified as low-grade osteosarcoma.

Osteosarcoma

Osteosarcoma is defined as a tumor in which malignant spindle cells produce bone. There are two major variants that have significantly different clinical presentations and prognoses. The more common osteosarcoma is classic high-grade or conventional, and the other is juxtacortical. Some authors separate juxtacortical osteosarcomas into parosteal and periosteal. Less common variants of osteosarcoma (e.g., intracortical, soft tissue, radiation-induced, Paget) are not discussed in this text.

Classic High-grade Osteosarcoma. The patient is usually a teenager (about 50% of the patients present during the second decade of life; more than 75% are between 8 and 25 years of age) complaining of pain and a mass around the knee (Figs. 14-7 and 14-8). Half of the lesions are located in the distal femur or the proximal tibia. The proximal humerus, proximal femur, and pelvis are the next most common sites. The pain precedes the appreciation of the mass by a few weeks to 2 or 3 months. Boys and girls are affected with equal frequency. The patient does not have systemic symptoms, and usually feels well. The mass is slightly

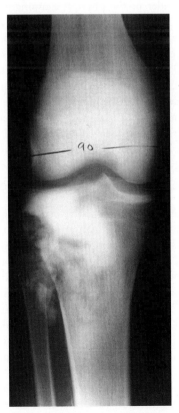

FIGURE 14-7. This is an anteroposterior plain radiograph of an 18-year-old man with an osteosarcoma of his proximal tibia. There is increased density in the proximal tibia associated with cortical destruction and extraosseous bone formation. Biopsy was confirmatory.

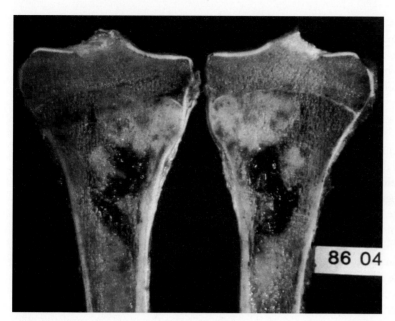

FIGURE 14-8. Classic high-grade osteosarcoma of the proximal tibia. The tibia was bisected for examination. The tumor is composed of an osteoblastic component in the metaphysis, which is up to, and just through, the epiphyseal plate; there also is a more distal cystic component. The tumor has penetrated the cortex, and has a small extracortical component. The patient had not received preoperative chemotherapy, but was treated successfully with limb salvage resection and knee arthrodesis. The patient received postoperative adjuvant chemotherapy, and has been continuously free of disease for 4 years.

tender, firm-to-hard, and fixed to the bone but not inflamed. The adjacent joint usually has restricted motion.

The remainder of the physical examination is normal, except in the rare (less than 1%) patient who presents with metastases or multiple focal osteosarcoma. One-half of all patients have elevated serum alkaline phosphatase (extremely high serum alkaline phosphatase values indicate a worse prognosis), and approximately one-fourth of all patients have elevated serum LDH (an elevated LDH also is associated with a worse prognosis). The remainder of the blood and urine laboratory values are normal.

The plain radiograph of an osteosarcoma is usually diagnostic. The typical lesion is located in the metaphysis, involves the medullary canal, is both lytic (radiolucent) and blastic (radiodense), and has an extraosseous component and a periosteal reaction suggestive of a rapid growth (Codman triangle or sunburst pattern). Many osteosarcomas have a soft tissue component, with a fluffy density suggestive of neoplastic bone, adjacent to the more obvious bone lesion. Those osteosarcomas that consist primarily of cartilage or fibrous tissue are almost purely radiolucent. Telangiectatic osteosarcoma, a histologic variant of classic high-grade osteosarcoma, may be mistaken on a radiograph for an ABC or a giant cell tumor. This will not be a clinical problem for the pathologist if adequate clinical information is provided by the surgeon.

MRI is the method of choice for evaluating suspected osteosarcoma. The lesion's extent is more clearly defined by MRI, especially the intraosseous component. The lesion can be seen in all three planes, and its soft tissue extension is easily appreciated. It is critical that the entire bone be included on at least one plane (usually the coronal view). The tumor should be viewed with a minimum of T1-weighted (with and without gadolinium), T2-weighted, and fat-suppressed images.

Osteosarcomas should be resected with at least a wide surgical margin, and the anatomic extent of the tumor is the principal determinant of what operation will be required. MRI is the best method to determine the anatomic extent of an osteosarcoma. The relation of osteosarcoma to the major neurovascular bundle must be determined. The muscles invaded by the soft tissue component must be identified. Involvement of the adjacent joint must be looked for, the intraosseous extent measured, and the presence of metastasis noted. Talking to the radiologist before MRI is performed helps to ensure that all this information is obtained.

Chest radiography and whole lung CT are performed because of the relatively high incidence of patients presenting with pulmonary metastasis (approximately 10%).

The technetium bone scan shows increased uptake in the area of the tumor. Occasionally it is useful in determining the intraosseous extent, although MRI is more accurate. More importantly, technetium scanning is an excellent screen of the entire skeleton for occult bone lesions. On rare occasions a lung metastasis is seen on the bone scan, but usually a hot spot in the chest on the bone scan is secondary to involvement of a rib.

There are five major histologic types of conventional osteosarcoma, and each is graded for the degree of malignancy. The histologic type is determined by the predominant cell type of the tumor. Although initially it was thought that the different types had distinct prognoses, it is now recognized that if matched for size and histologic grade, all types

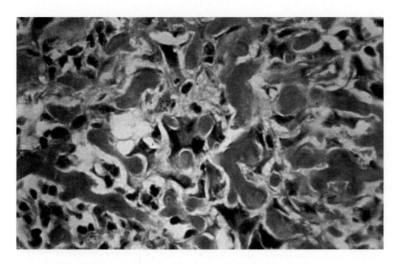

FIGURE 14-9. Histologic appearance of classic high-grade osteosarcoma. The malignant spindle cells are recognized by their abnormal variation in size and shape. No mitotic figures are seen in this photomicrograph, but abnormal mitoses usually are seen in high-grade conventional osteosarcoma. (Original magnification ×40.)

have the same prognosis. Even telangiectatic osteosarcoma, which was originally described as having a particularly poor prognosis, is thought to have the same prognosis as the other classic high-grade osteosarcomas.

The five types are osteoblastic, chondroblastic, fibroblastic, mixed, and telangiectatic osteosarcomas. These tumors are graded on a scale of either 1 to 3 or 1 to 4. The higher the histologic grade, the worse the prognosis. Most osteosarcomas are grade 3 or 4, and of the mixed type. The tumor is composed of a mixture of neoplastic cells, but must have malignant spindle cells making osteoid. Atypical mitoses are common, and small areas of necrosis are usually seen (Fig. 14-9).

Treatment of classic high-grade osteosarcoma includes adjuvant chemotherapy and surgical resection. The standard protocol consists of chemotherapy (neoadjuvant; usually three or four courses of a multidrug regimen), then surgical resection, and finally additional chemotherapy (Fig. 14-10). The entire treatment takes almost 1 year. The surgical resection can almost always be done without an amputation of the extremity, and less radical surgery is being performed now compared with only a few years ago. Recently, Picci and associates suggested that patients whose tumors have more than 90% necrosis after preoperative chemotherapy do not require as wide a surgical margin as patients with less necrosis (110,111). The use of neoadjuvant chemotherapy has not produced increased survival compared with postoperative adjuvant chemotherapy, but it does seem to make surgery easier, and gives the pediatric oncologist a predictor of survival.

The three most important drugs used for osteosarcoma are doxorubicin (Adriamycin), high-dose methotrexate, and cisplatin. The majority of chemotherapy protocols include these three drugs in various dosage schedules, in addition to one or more other drugs. The development of granulocyte-stimulating factor to counteract bone marrow suppression, has allowed increased intensification of the treatment with

fewer complications; granulocyte-stimulating factor is now used routinely. Overall survival has increased to more than 60%, with even better survival for those patients with greater than 90% necrosis after chemotherapy (112–122).

Limb-salvage surgery is being performed for all but the largest of osteosarcomas. Amputation is done in less than

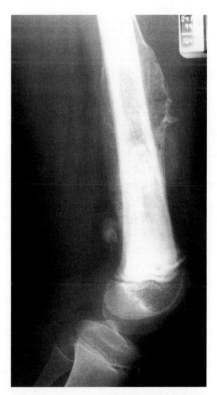

FIGURE 14-10. This plain radiograph is a lateral view of the distal femur of a patient who has had standard preoperative chemotherapy. The original lesion had a large extraosseous component that has been reduced in size, and there has been "maturing" of the periosteal reaction. The patient's pain diminished, and the range of motion in her knee returned to normal.

20% of cases (122–126). The accepted incidence of local recurrence is between 5 and 10%, which does not seem to increase the incidence of death (125). This is an area of concern, however, because it appears that the vast majority of patients with local recurrence die of their disease (123,125). One explanation is that local recurrence is a sign of a more aggressive tumor, not solely the consequence of poor surgery. That being said, however, the insistence on wide margins is paramount. The tumor with a small amount of surrounding normal tissue is resected. This usually means 1 or 2 cm of normal bone proximal and/or distal to the extent of the tumor and a small cuff of muscle directly on the tumor and bone. It is uncommon to perform extraarticular resection unless there is gross extension of tumor into a joint, and increasingly close bone margins are accepted in an attempt to save a young child's growth plate or a patient's articular cartilage.

The management of patients with pathologic fractures is controversial. There is an increased incidence of local recurrence if limb-salvage resection is performed, but this increased incidence of local recurrence does not seem to increase the risk of death (123,127–130). The usual management of a patient with a pathologic fracture and osteosarcoma is to treat the fracture closed, give neoadjuvant chemotherapy, and perform limb salvage if negative surgical margins can be obtained.

The patient younger than 10 or 11 years, whose tumor resection requires the removal of a major growth plate (distal femur, proximal tibia, or proximal humerus), presents a special problem (131–135). Older patients with limb-length inequality can be managed with a combination of initial lengthening, opposite-side growth arrest, and heel lifts. A variety of techniques have been developed to manage the patient who has so much growth left in his or her extremity that these simple methods are insufficient. Some patients will have a conventional amputation, and this remains an excellent method for many patients. There have been advances in prosthetic design during the past decade, and patients with amputations do not require additional operations (as patients with limb salvage do), and remain the most physically active patients. Variations on a conventional amputation (either a rotationplasty or a tibial turn-up) can be done, particularly for the young patient with an osteosarcoma in the femur, to improve function, compared with conventional amputation (136–156). Limb salvage for the patient younger than 10 years is particularly difficult. All methods require repeated operations, and their long-term success has yet to be completely documented. The most common method currently used involves a "growing" endoprosthesis (131,133,157–165). There are a number of methods to make the endoprosthesis grow, but they all require a repeat operation every 8 to 12 months. In addition, as the child grows in length, the bone grows in diameter, and fixation is problematic.

Juxtacortical Osteosarcoma. Osteosarcomas that arise from or are adjacent to the external surface of the bone behave differently than those that arise from within the medullary canal. They are less aggressive locally, have less potential for distant metastasis, and are less common than conventional osteosarcoma. There seem to be two distinct juxtacortical osteosarcomas, parosteal and periosteal, but neither is common, and how distinct they are from one another remains a topic of debate. Parosteal osteosarcoma is most commonly located in the posterior aspect of the distal femur, and is composed of bone and low-grade malignant fibrous tissue. Periosteal osteosarcoma is more often located in the diaphysis, and is composed of bone and cartilage with malignant spindle cells.

Geschickter and Copeland (166) were the first to describe osteosarcoma. They thought that there were two distinct lesions, a benign parosteal bone-forming tumor and a malignant bone-forming tumor, but all osteosarcomas are defined as malignant, and have the potential to metastasize. The patient's age at presentation varies over a greater range (10 to 45 years) than in classic high-grade osteosarcoma, and the median age of presentation tends to be slightly older (167–171). The patient usually complains of a painless mass that blocks motion in the adjacent joint. This is most often knee flexion, because the posterior distal femur is the most common site of a juxtacortical osteosarcoma (93). Occasionally the patient complains of a mild, dull ache in the area of the tumor, but symptoms are minimal. The mass is fixed, hard, and nontender. The adjacent joint may have limited passive and active motion as a result of the mechanical block from the tumor. Inflammation is not observed. The patient's laboratory values are normal.

The plain radiograph is almost always diagnostic, but the findings may be mistaken for osteocartilaginous exostosis (Fig. 14-11). The lesion arises from the cortex, which may be normal or thickened. The juxtacortical osteosarcoma often wraps around the bone, with the periosteum between the tumor and the underlying cortex. This growth pattern (wrapping around the bone) produces the "string sign" on the plain radiograph, with a thin radiolucent line between the lesion and the cortex of the bone. The lesion itself is dense, and has the pattern of bone. There is increased uptake on the technetium bone scan. The appearance of the lesion on a CT scan is characteristic, and distinguishes a juxtacortical osteosarcoma from an exostosis. Juxtacortical osteosarcoma is attached to the cortex growing out into the soft tissue and may invade the cortex, but the normal cortex is intact (167,168,171). An exostosis arises from the cortex, and the cortex of the normal bone becomes the cortex of the exostosis, with the medullary canal of the bone communicating with the medullary canal of the exostosis. Intraosseous extension of the tumor is seen more easily with MRI than with CT.

An incisional biopsy of a juxtacortical osteosarcoma can be difficult to interpret, and based on histology alone, the

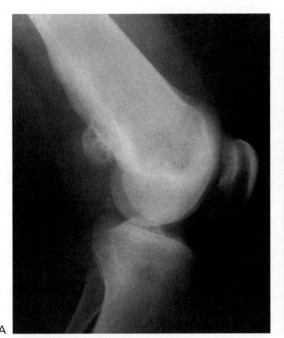 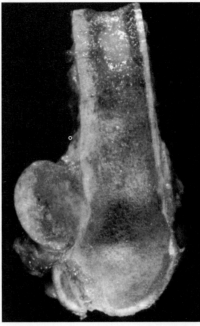

A B

FIGURE 14-11. A: Lateral radiograph of the distal femur and knee of a patient with a parosteal osteosarcoma. The posterior distal femoral cortex is thickened and slightly irregular. The radiodensity adjacent to the posterior cortex is the central portion of the parosteal osteosarcoma. Surrounding this bony mass is a nonossified component of the tumor, composed primarily of fibrous tissue, but with some cartilage. This patient was treated with limb-salvage wide resection of the distal femur, and underwent reconstruction with an osteoarticular allograft. No chemotherapy was used, and the patient has remained free of disease for 5 years. **B:** The parosteal osteosarcoma is larger than it appears on the plain radiograph. The cap of fibrous tissue and cartilage can be seen covering the bony center. The tumor is attached to the cortex, but does not extend through it. This gross relation is similar to that of an exostosis, and may lead to a mistaken histologic diagnosis. The gross difference between an exostosis, and a parosteal osteosarcoma is that the stalk of an exostosis is cortical bone that blends with the cortex of the host bone, and the medullary canal of the stalk and host bone are connected (see Fig. 14-13B). The parosteal osteosarcoma, conversely, is attached to the cortex, but the cortex of host bone is intact, and the medullary canal does not communicate with the parosteal osteosarcoma.

lesion can be mistaken for an exostosis. This is particularly true when juxtacortical osteosarcoma is not suspected by the clinician, or when the pathologist does not examine the radiograph. This lesion, more than most, is diagnosed by its clinical and radiographic presentation, and is confirmed by histology. An excisional biopsy is recommended in most cases. The lesion is composed of regularly arranged bone, with a background of usually bland spindle cells and fibrous tissue. A cartilage cap is often present. Parosteal osteosarcomas are graded histologically on a scale of 1 to 3 (170). Higher-grade lesions, especially those with medullary involvement, have a greater risk of metastasizing (usually to the lung) than those of lower grade without medullary extension (169,173–177).

When the diagnosis can be relatively certain from the preoperative studies, a wide excisional biopsy is recommended. The cortical margin should be generous and the tumor pseudocapsule not disturbed. When a lesion from the posterior distal femur is resected, the neurovascular bundle usually can be freed from the lesion without dissecting the pseudocapsule, but the posterior capsule of the knee and the posterior aspect of the femoral condyle usually must be resected with the tumor. Those lesions that wrap around the bone and have gross invasion of the medullary canal may require a resection that includes the entire end of the bone.

The initial resection is the best opportunity to control the lesion without an amputation. Most patients do not need adjuvant chemotherapy because the cure with surgery alone is approximately 80% (167,168,170,171,178,179). Patients with histologic grade 3 lesions probably should receive adjuvant chemotherapy, especially if the medullary canal has been invaded, although the data are limited (170).

The periosteal osteosarcoma is another type of juxtacortical osteosarcoma (93,180,181). It is most common in the anterior proximal tibia, and it tends to be diaphyseal in location. It has a sunburst appearance on the plain radiograph, and is composed of malignant cartilage and bone (182). A wide surgical resection is recommended (169, 180,181,183). The place of adjuvant chemotherapy is controversial; as with parosteal osteosarcoma, probably only patients with grade 3 lesions should receive it.

Local Control of Extremity Sarcomas. The "gold standard" for achieving local control in patients with bone and soft tissue sarcomas in the extremities is amputation. However, no one wants to lose a limb if it can be prevented, and the authors have learned that sarcomas can be safely resected as long as a cuff of normal tissue can be kept surrounding the resected specimen. This is called "achieving a wide margin of resection." Usually adjuvant therapies such as chemotherapy are used either before or after these resections.

There is a fairly wide experience with limb salvage in adults. Children have the added problems of growth, small size, and (it is hoped) more longevity, which make reconstruction more challenging. The options for limb salvage include osteoarticular and intercalary allografts, metallic prostheses, and vascularized and nonvascularized autograft transplants. All of these are used at various times by the tumor surgeon. Rotationplasty is another option somewhere between limb salvage and amputation; it is occasionally useful in very young patients.

The child must first be a limb-salvage candidate. This means that the tumor is located such that the major nerves and vessels can be preserved, and enough muscle will remain to make the limb functional. MRI is the best imaging test to aid in the decision (80). It shows the extent of the tumor within the medullary cavity, the extent of the soft tissue mass, and the relationship of the mass to the joint, nerves, and vessels. Most of the time the adjacent joint is not involved, but the epiphysis is frequently involved with tumor (184,185). This must be carefully assessed. Usually, the patient will have received chemotherapy preoperatively, which makes the resection easier in tumors without a matrix, such as Ewing sarcoma/PNET, because the mass becomes smaller.

In some locations, such as the fibula and clavicle, no bony reconstruction is necessary. Very young children with bone tumors of the foot and ankle are usually best treated by ray, Syme, or below-knee amputation. Soft tissue sarcomas at these sites may be resectable without amputation, if it is possible to achieve wide margins with or without adjuvant irradiation. A method of using a metatarsal head in the tibial stump to prevent stump overgrowth has been described, and seems to be useful (186,187).

For tumors of the distal femur or proximal tibia, the resection will almost certainly include an epiphyseal center. In children near skeletal maturity, this will not lead to a major limb-length inequality. An allograft or prosthesis 1 to 2 cm longer than the length of bone that is resected can be used, and a contralateral epiphysiodesis can be performed at a later date, if necessary. As long as the predicted discrepancy is less than 2 cm, no special reconstruction is necessary. In younger children, limb length is more of a concern. One option is to reconstruct with an osteoarticular allograft, and

treat the limb-length discrepancy using standard methods of epiphysiodesis, closed femoral shortening, or limb lengthening. The allograft has the advantage of not disturbing the adjacent growth plate. Growth arrest of the adjacent growth plate may occur by placing a prosthetic stem across it. One difficulty with this approach is obtaining a graft of appropriate size. For children older than 10 years, it is usually possible to use a small adult bone. Use of grafts with open growth plates is not advised because they will fracture through the allograft physis. Use of an osteoarticular allograft for the proximal tibia has the advantage of providing a site of attachment for the patellar ligament. The results of allografts for limb salvage in osteosarcoma are reasonable, but the patient should not expect normal limb function (131, 188–194). A good or excellent result, based on a functional evaluation system devised by Mankin et al. (195), can be expected in about 65 to 70% of patients. It should be noted that there are no ideal measures of function after limb salvage (although several have been developed), and this remains an area of investigation. In general, if patients can return to normal walking activities without supports or braces, it is considered to be a good result. Seldom can they return to contact sports or running activities (196). Complications include infection, nonunion, fracture, and joint instability (195,197,198). If the patient survives, he or she may need joint arthroplasty at some time in the future, but by then the patient should be old enough that growth is no longer a consideration. Growth equalization can be achieved by contralateral epiphysiodesis, limb shortening, or ipsilateral lengthening (132,134). The experience with limb lengthening in these patients is limited because limb length is seldom a major issue.

Another option is the use of a metallic prosthesis. Modular prostheses are now available that allow the surgeon to construct an implant of suitable length in the operating room (133,199). Custom implants are seldom necessary. Some prostheses have the ability to be expanded as the child grows (131,133,157,159,160,162–165). There are a variety of types, but perhaps the best is the modular prosthesis that can be lengthened by removing one of the body segments and replacing it with another segment 1 to 2 cm longer (133). This is not a simple operation because the soft tissues form a dense fibrous layer around the implant, which must be resected or released to achieve lengthening. The neurovascular structures are difficult to identify in these lengthening procedures, and are at risk for direct and stretching injury. Usually it is possible to achieve at least 2 cm of length per procedure. In very young patients, this must be repeated every 6 months until maturity, at which point revision to an adult prosthesis may be necessary. There are few data on these prostheses, but at least one report shows that it is possible to gain 2 to 18 cm in length, and to have equal limb lengths at skeletal maturity (162). The issues of prosthetic failure, loosening, wear of polyethylene, and infection remain unresolved. The choice of implant or reconstructive method is up to the surgeon and the family. Prostheses are more functional initially, but their longevity is unknown. Expandable prostheses have a high failure rate (133). More than 80% of these will require revision by 5 years, and the revision rate appears to be higher in uncemented prostheses. Many of these patients will have knee stiffness and the infection rate, especially in the tibia, may be as high as 38%, although this can be improved with the liberal use of gastrocnemius flaps (133). The modular prosthesis has been reported to have a 5-year revision-free and amputation-free survival rate of 75%, presumably because it is mechanically stronger and less complex (133). Function appears better in children who are older than 8 years at the time of the reconstruction. Allografts require more difficult rehabilitation, but they hold the promise of superior longevity. It is very important to tell the patient in either case that the function will not be normal, and that neither reconstruction is meant to return the patient to sports activities. For lower-extremity sarcomas about the knee or hip, it is the authors' feeling that patients older than 8 to 10 years with open growth plates, are best treated with allografts to preserve the adjacent growth center, but that skeletally mature patients may be better served by prostheses because of the easier recovery and rehabilitation. In either case, subsequent revisions or eventual amputation may be necessary.

For diaphyseal lesions, an intercalary resection can be performed that spares the adjacent joints and occasionally the epiphyseal plates. These patients can be reconstructed with intercalary allografts and/or vascularized fibulae (191,192,200). Recently, a method of using an allograft to provide initial stability, augmented by a vascularized fibular graft to achieve quicker union and long-term healing potential, was described (201–203). This technique is especially helpful when only a small segment of the epiphysis remains after the resection.

For lesions of the proximal humerus, intraarticular or extraarticular resection is usually performed (204–207). If the rotator cuff and part of the deltoid can be preserved, reconstruction with an osteoarticular allograft yields good results (208,209). Some surgeons prefer to use an endoprosthesis with the allograft to prevent late joint collapse and fracture (188,210). In either case, the allograft position allows attachment of the rotator cuff, which is an advantage over the use of a prosthesis. For extraarticular resections when both the deltoid and the rotator cuff are sacrificed, arthrodesis, using allograft, vascularized fibula, or both, is indicated (211). It is difficult to achieve an arthrodesis, but when it works, it is very functional. When a formal Tikhoff-Linberg resection, which includes the scapula, is necessary, the reconstruction is more difficult; leaving a flail upper extremity may be the only option (204,207,212,213).

For very young patients with tumors of the distal femur, or older patients who want to be athletically active, rotationplasty is an option (136–140,143,145–147,150,151,

156). In these patients, above-knee amputation would lead to a very short stump with a poor lever arm (214). Rotationplasty, by taking advantage of the tibia and foot, provides a longer lever arm and an active "knee" joint. It also avoids resection of the major nerves, so that phantom pain is not an issue. The physical appearance without the prosthesis is disturbing to some patients, but with a prosthesis they look similar to other amputees and function much better than above-knee amputees (139,142,144,145,152, 215). The technical details are well described elsewhere (143), and the technique has been described for lesions of the proximal tibia and the proximal femur (141,149,153); more recently, similar procedures have been described for the upper extremity (216). It is very important to have frank discussions with the patient and his or her family about the appearance and expected outcome of this reconstruction. Having the patient meet another patient who has undergone rotationplasty, or at least viewing a video and meeting with an experienced physical therapist and prosthetist, can be very helpful. Interestingly, young patients do not view this as an amputation, because the foot is still present, and the long-term psychological outcomes of these patients has been very good.

CHEMOTHERAPY FOR MUSCULOSKELETAL TUMORS

It was not until the 1970s that chemotherapy was believed to be effective for malignant tumors of the musculoskeletal system. The extremely high incidence of metastatic disease in patients with osteosarcoma (more than 80%) and Ewing sarcoma (more than 85%), and some promising results in patients with metastatic sarcoma, prompted the use of adjuvant chemotherapy in patients who did not have documented disease but in whom the risk of having subclinical metastases was high (217). The early results were exciting, and even the use of what was considered minimal amounts of less-than-optimal drugs improved survival. These early studies led to the acceptance of adjuvant chemotherapy for Ewing sarcoma, osteosarcoma, and rhabdomyosarcoma (218–230). There are no chemotherapeutic agents believed to be effective for chondrosarcoma (231), and the use of chemotherapy for soft tissue sarcomas (except rhabdomyosarcoma) remains controversial (232–234).

In the 1980s, preoperative chemotherapy was introduced, and preoperative administration is now standard for the initial chemotherapy for patients with Ewing sarcoma, osteosarcoma, and rhabdomyosarcoma (26,115,116,119, 217,235–248). "Neoadjuvant chemotherapy" is a term used to indicate that the patient receives chemotherapy before the definitive treatment of the primary lesion. This was initially used as a means of treating patients with osteosarcoma who were waiting for the production of a custom prosthesis. The effect of chemotherapy on the tumor was significant and of prognostic significance, leading to the routine use of preoperative chemotherapy.

There are numerous chemotherapeutic protocols for the three skeletal malignancies for which chemotherapy is used (Ewing sarcoma, osteosarcoma, and rhabdomyosarcoma). All use more than one drug, and usually three to five. Most protocols are between 9 and 12 months long. Approximately one-third of the chemotherapy is given preoperatively, and the remainder is given after surgery.

The drugs used for musculoskeletal tumors include:

Doxorubicin (Adriamycin), a cytotoxic anthracycline antibiotic that passively enters the cell to diffuse into the nucleus, where it binds nucleic acids and prohibits DNA synthesis (217). It is cardiotoxic, myelosuppressive, and produces alopecia. It is given intravenously in divided doses over 6 months, with 450 mg/m^2 recommended as the maximum dose.

Methotrexate is an antimetabolite that inhibits dihydrofolic acid reductase. This interferes with DNA synthesis and repair, and alters cellular replication. When administered in high doses (12 mg/m^2 intravenously), leucovorin or citrovorum factor is given to the patient to rescue the normal cells. Leucovorin is a chemically reduced derivative of folic acid and is used by the cells to complete normal cell functions without the need for dihydrofolic acid reductase. Tumor cells seem less able to use leucovorin than normal cells, and this difference allows methotrexate to be effective against malignant tumors. The primary side effects of methotrexate are gastrointestinal, including nausea, vomiting, and loss of appetite.

Cisplatin is a heavy metal that is thought to cause intrastrand cross-links in DNA, and therefore interference with the DNA. It is given intravenously in doses of 75 to 100 mg/m^2 repeatedly over the course of the treatment. The principal side effect of cisplatin is nephrotoxicity.

Cyclophosphamide (Cytoxan) is a synthetic drug chemically related to nitrogen mustard. It cross-links DNA and interferes with DNA functions. It is given intravenously at a dose of 40 to 50 mg/kg in divided doses over 4 to 5 days. The major side effects of cyclophosphamide are gastrointestinal disorders and myelosuppression.

Ifosfamide is a synthetic analog of cyclophosphamide, with similar actions. It is given intravenously at 1.2 g/m^2/day for 5 days.

Vincristine is an alkaloid from the periwinkle plant. It is thought to arrest dividing cells in the metaphase state by inhibiting microtubule formation in the mitotic spindle. It is given intravenously at weekly intervals at doses of 1.4 mg/m^2 in adults and 2.0 mg/m^2 in children. The major side effect of vincristine is peripheral neuropathy.

Bleomycin is a cytotoxic glycopeptide antibiotic from a strain of *Streptomyces verticillus* that inhibits DNA synthesis. It also probably inhibits RNA and protein synthesis. It is given intravenously at 0.25 to 0.50 U/kg once or twice per week. The most serious side effect of bleomycin is a 10% incidence of severe pulmonary fibrosis.

Actinomycin D (dactinomycin) is one of a number of actinomycin antibiotics from *Streptomyces*. It binds to DNA by intercalation with the phenoxazone ring. This inhibits the DNA from being a template for RNA and synthesizing itself. It is given intravenously at 0.5 mg/day for 5 days. Dactinomycin produces nausea and vomiting, and is myelosuppressive.

These drugs are given in various combinations and doses, depending on the specific diagnosis, the protocol, the response of the patient, and the aggressiveness of the medical oncologist.

Cartilaginous Tumors

Cartilaginous tumors include enchondroma, exostosis (osteocartilaginous exostosis, osteochondroma), chondromyxofibroma, periosteal chondroma, chondroblastoma, and chondrosarcoma. The benign tumors are common, especially enchondroma and exostosis, whereas chondrosarcoma is extremely rare in the pediatric age group (93,249,250).

Enchondroma

The origin of enchondroma is debatable, and it probably is not a true neoplasia. It may be the result of epiphyseal growth cartilage that does not remodel and persists in the metaphysis, or it may result from persistence of the original cartilaginous anlage of the bone (251). Both possibilities have been suggested as explanations of the cause of this common benign tumor. The majority of patients with a solitary enchondroma present with either a pathologic fracture through a lesion in the phalanx, which is the most common location (251) (the proximal humerus and the distal femur are the other common locations for enchondroma), or the history that the lesion was an incidental finding on a radiograph taken for another reason (Fig. 14-12). Enchondromas are common lesions that account for 11% of benign bone tumors (93,253). They do not need to be removed. The problem they present is diagnostic. Usually, the diagnosis can be made from the clinical setting and the plain radiograph. Forty percent of enchondromas are found in the bones of the hand or feet—usually a phalanx. An enchondroma should not produce symptoms unless there is a pathologic fracture. There are no associated blood or urine abnormalities. The femur and proximal humerus are the next most common sites. Enchondromas are located in the metaphysis and are central lesions in the medullary canal. The bone may be wider than normal, but this is caused by the lack of remodeling in the metaphysis rather than by expansion of the bone by the tumor. The cortex may be thin or normal; the lesion is radiolucent in the pediatric age group, but later has intralesional calcifications. There should be no periosteal reaction. In the pediatric pa-

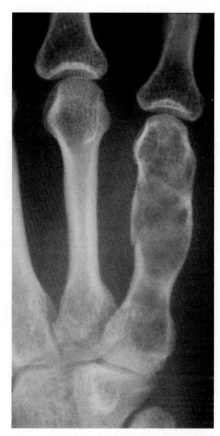

FIGURE 14-12. This enchondroma of the fifth metacarpal is typical. The shaft is enlarged, and the lesion is radiolucent. This patient had been aware of this lesion since she was 10 years of age. She had sustained numerous pathologic fractures, and decided to have it curetted. The curettage was done after the fracture had healed.

tient, unicameral bone cysts have a similar radiographic appearance, but they are most common in the proximal femur and the proximal humerus. The appearance of an enchondroma on MRI is typical. The cartilage matrix has an intermediate signal intensity on the T1-weighted image and a high signal intensity on the T2-weighted image (80, 254–258). It should have a sharp margin with the adjacent bone without peripheral edema.

When the findings are typical for an enchondroma, no biopsy is necessary. Repeat plain radiography and physical examination should be performed in approximately 6 weeks, then every 3 to 6 months for 2 years. Although there are reports of solitary enchondromas differentiating into chondrosarcomas, usually late in adult life, this does not occur frequently enough to justify the removal of all enchondromas. The patient should be advised that after age 30 years if the lesion becomes painful or enlarges, it should be considered a low-grade chondrosarcoma and be surgically resected.

Incisional biopsy usually is contraindicated. Pathologists

have difficulty distinguishing between active enchondroma (most pediatric-age patients have active lesions) and low-grade chondrosarcoma. The clinical course is the best measure of the lesion's significance, and an incisional biopsy alters the status of the lesion and makes subsequent evaluation difficult. If the patient or the patient's parents insist on biopsy, it is best that the entire lesion be removed.

Patients with multiple enchondroma (Ollier disease) are much less common than those with solitary enchondromas. Multiple enchondroma was originally described in the late 1800s by Ollier (259). Most patients with Ollier disease have bilateral involvement, but with unilateral predominance. These patients have growth deformities, both angular and in length. Their extremity deformities should be managed surgically to maintain the function of the limbs without specific regard to the enchondroma. Patients with Ollier disease have an increased risk of developing secondary chondrosarcoma later in life, and should be so advised (260–262). The incidence of secondary chondrosarcoma in patients with Ollier disease is not known, but may be as high as 25%. The pelvis and shoulder girdle are the most common locations of secondary chondrosarcoma.

Maffucci disease consists of multiple enchondroma and soft tissue hemangioma (263). Patients with this disorder have an even greater risk of developing malignant cartilage tumors than patients with Ollier disease; more importantly, they have a great risk of developing carcinoma of an internal organ (264).

Exostosis

The terms "osteochondroma," "osteocartilaginous exostosis," and "exostosis" are used interchangeably. This lesion was first described in the early 1800s. It is common. Although the pathogenesis of this lesion is not known, an abnormality or injury to the periphery of the growth plate has been suggested as the cause (251). It has been shown in an experimental animal study that the periphery of the growth plate can be traumatized and a typical exostosis produced.

The patient with a solitary exostosis usually is brought in by a parent who has just noticed a mass adjacent to a joint. The patient usually has no symptoms. An occasional patient has loss of motion in the adjacent joint, attributable to the size of the mass. The patient often has been aware of the mass for months to years, and reports that it has been slowly enlarging. Some patients have pain resulting from irritation of an overlying muscle, repeated trauma, pressure on an adjacent neurovascular bundle, or inflammation in an overlying bursa. On physical examination, the mass is nontender, hard, and fixed to the bone. The rest of the physical examination is normal.

Exostoses are so characteristic on a plain radiograph that they should be diagnosed from their radiographic appearance alone (Fig. 14-13). The mass is a combination of a radiolucent cartilaginous cap with varying amounts of ossifi-

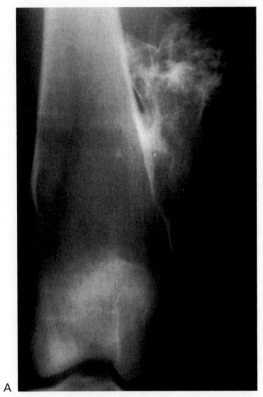

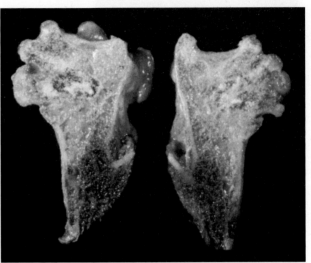

FIGURE 14-13. A: Anteroposterior radiograph of the distal femur with a typical pedunculated exostosis. The cortex of the lesion blends into the cortex of the femur. The exostosis has an irregular proximal end that is covered by a cartilaginous cap. The pathologic material is the cartilage, but what is seen on the radiograph is the bone formed by enchondral ossification of the cartilage. This patient repeatedly hit the mass while playing football, and it was marginally excised. A small rim of the cortex of the femur was removed along with the exostosis because occasionally any residual cartilage that lies at the base of the stalk can lead to a recurrence. **B:** Gross bisected specimen from the same patient. The femoral attachment is inferior, and the cortex of the femur can be seen blending with the cortex of the exostosis. The medullary canal of the femur is filled with hematopoietic marrow, and appears dark. The hematopoietic marrow extends into the base of the exostosis, but most of the marrow of the exostosis is fatty. There is a thin, cartilaginous cap. In a child, a cartilaginous cap more than 1 cm thick is of no concern, but in an adult a cartilaginous cap of more than 1 cm is considered to indicate early malignant degeneration to secondary chondrosarcoma.

cation and calcification. The amount of calcification and bone formation increases with age. The base may be broad (sessile exostosis) or narrow (pedunculated exostosis). In both types, the cortex of the underlying bone opens to join the cortex of the exostosis, so that the medullary canal of the bone is in continuity. This usually can be appreciated on the plain radiograph, but if not, CT or MRI establishes this finding and confirms the diagnosis.

In the pediatric age group exostoses should be expected to grow. They may continue to grow well into the third decade of life. This is not a sign of malignancy. Only after 30 years of age should growth of an exostosis be thought to indicate malignant degeneration. The growth rate is not steady, and occasionally a lesion grows more rapidly than expected. Removal of the lesion in a child is indicated only for those patients who have symptoms attributable to pres-

sure on a neurovascular bundle or irritation of the overlying muscle. Removal in a young child may result in damage to the growth plate and recurrence of the lesion. Malignant degeneration is extremely rare in children and uncommon in adults. Malignant degeneration is more common in lesions of the scapula, the pelvis, and the proximal femur. Although it is often stated that the risk of malignant degeneration is as high as 20%, the real incidence is not known. It is probably less than 5%.

Gross examination of an exostosis reveals a lesion that looks like a cauliflower. It has an irregular surface covered with cartilage. The cartilage is usually less than 1 cm thick, except in the young child, in which it may be 2 or 3 cm thick. In an adult, when the cartilaginous cap is thicker than 1 cm a secondary chondrosarcoma should be suspected (253,257,265–269). Deep in the cartilaginous cap there is a variable amount of calcification, enchondral ossification, and normal bone with a cortex and cancellous marrow cavity. The microscopic appearance of the cartilaginous cap typically is benign hyaline cartilage.

Some patients have multiple exostoses (270–272). A patient may have three or four lesions, but more often there are 10 to 15. Usually, the patient has exostoses of all shapes and sizes. They are concentrated in the metaphysis of the long bones, but may be in the spine, the ribs, the pelvis, and the scapula. On physical examination, they are hard, fixed masses adjacent to joints. Patients with multiple exostoses usually are shorter than average but not below the normal range. They have loss of motion in the affected joints, especially forearm rotation, elbow extension, hip abduction and adduction, and ankle inversion and eversion.

Multiple heritable exostosis is transmitted by an autosomal dominant gene with a variable penetrance, and usually half of the children of an affected parent have clinical manifestations (270,273,274). An extensively involved parent may have a child with minimal involvement, or vice versa. In the majority of patients with multiple heritable exostoses, the radiographic appearance of the proximal femur is diagnostic. The femoral neck is short and broad with multiple bony excrescences.

After the age of 30 years, patients with multiple heritable exostoses have an increased risk of developing secondary chondrosarcoma (266,267,273,275–281). Secondary chondrosarcoma in the pediatric age group is extremely rare (282,283). Occasionally, one or more of the exostoses are removed to relieve the pain related to repeated local trauma, or to improve the motion of the adjacent joint. Those lesions in the pelvis and the spine should be observed closely because they have the greatest risk of undergoing malignant degeneration. The authors do not recommend removing these lesions simply because they are present.

The authors advise patients with exostosis, whether single or multiple, to be examined and to undergo radiography at least yearly. Patients are told to report symptoms or increasing size immediately. Patients older than 30 years of age with an enlarging exostosis should have it removed as if it were a secondary chondrosarcoma, because this usually is the case (284).

Chondromyxofibroma

Chondromyxofibroma is a rare tumor. The patient is usually a male (males are more frequently affected than females at a ratio of 2 to 1) in the second or third decade of life (93,285). The patient complains of a dull, steady pain that is usually worse at night. The only positive physical finding is tenderness over the involved area, and occasionally a deep mass can be appreciated. Approximately one-third of chondromyxoid fibromas occur in the tibia, usually proximally. It is a radiolucent lesion that involves the medullary canal, but is eccentric and erodes the cortex (253,286) (Fig. 14-

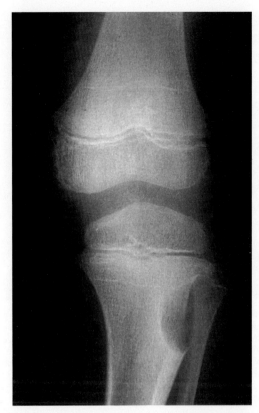

FIGURE 14-14. Anteroposterior radiograph of a chondromyxofibroma of the proximal lateral tibia. The lesion is typically an eccentric, radiolucent abnormality that usually destroys the cortex but is contained by the periosteum. As in this case, the radiographic appearance of chondromyxofibroma is often similar to that of an aneurysmal bone cyst.

14). It may be covered by only periosteum, and is often mistaken for the more common ABC. The solid nature of chondromyxofibroma versus the cystic nature of an ABC, as seen on MRI, is a means of differentiating between these two lesions. The natural history is not known because of infrequency and the fact that surgical treatment is nearly universal. Thorough curettage and bone grafting are recommended.

Chondroblastoma

Chondroblastoma, or Codman tumor, initially was thought to be a variant of giant cell tumor of bone. Codman's detailed description in 1931 was of an "epiphyseal chondromatous giant cell tumor" (287). Jaffe and Lichtenstein in 1942 (288) suggested that it be called "benign chondroblastoma," and separated it from giant cell tumor of bone. Codman was particularly interested in the shoulder, and he thought that this lesion was found principally in the proximal humerus (Fig. 14-15). It has since become clear that chondroblastoma is found in many bones, but the proximal

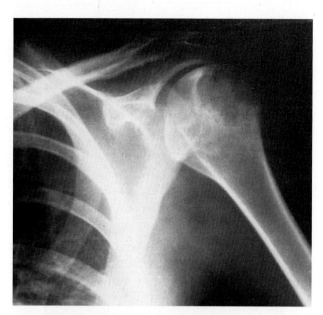

FIGURE 14-15. Radiograph of a chondroblastoma in the proximal humeral epiphysis. This is a typical Codman tumor. The lesion is both epiphyseal and metaphyseal, has an irregular reactive border, and has intralesional calcifications, although these are difficult to see on plain radiographs. Giant cell tumor of bone is similar to chondroblastoma, except that there are no intralesional calcifications. This patient was treated with curettage and bone grafting.

humerus is the most common site (approximately 20%) (93,289–291).

Chondroblastoma accounts for 1% of bone tumors (93). The patient with a chondroblastoma is usually in the second decade of life, with an open growth plate, but it occurs in older patients as well. The initial symptoms are of pain in the joint adjacent to the lesion, and the patient usually presents with joint complaints. The findings on physical examination also may suggest an intraarticular disorder because most patients have an effusion and diminished motion in the adjacent joint. Frequently the patient is believed to have chronic synovitis; he or she does not have other symptoms or abnormal physical findings. The patient's laboratory data are normal.

The lesion arises in the secondary ossification center. In children, it is the most common neoplastic lesion of the secondary ossification center (292), and in adults, only giant cell tumor of bone involves the secondary ossification center more often. (Osteomyelitis is the most common diagnosis in adults to produce a lesion in the secondary ossification center.) On the plain radiograph, the lesion is radiolucent, usually with small foci of calcification (293). The calcification is best seen on a CT scan. There is usually a reactive rim of bone surrounding the lesion, and sometimes metaphyseal periosteal reaction. The edema associated with chondroblastoma can be appreciated on MRI (Fig. 14-16). There is increased uptake on a technetium bone scan. Chest radiog-

raphy or CT should be performed, because chondroblastoma is one of the benign bone tumors that can have lung implants and still be considered benign (294). Chondroblastoma and osteochondritis dissecans can have a similar appearance on plain radiographs, but they should not be confused with one another. Osteochondritis dissecans produces an abnormality in the subchondral bone, but with chondroblastoma the subchondral bone is almost always normal. Patients with chondroblastoma have more of an effusion than patients with osteochondritis dissecans, and their pain is constant and not related to activity as it is in patients with osteochondritis dissecans.

The histologic appearance of chondroblastoma is typical, and this disorder is rarely confused with other diagnoses. It consists of small cuboidal cells (chondroblasts) closely packed together to give the appearance of a cobblestone street (288–291). In addition, there are areas with varying amounts of amorphous matrix that often contains streaks of calcification, and usually there are numerous multinucleated giant cells. Chondroblastoma is not as vascular as osteoblastoma, and there are few, if any, mitoses, and no abnormal mitoses (Fig. 14-17).

Chondroblastomas progress and invade the joint. They should be treated when found. Curettage is the treatment of choice, but it must be a thorough curettage and extend beyond the reactive rim (291). The lesion should be seen adequately at the time of the curettage, which usually means that the joint must be opened. Iatrogenic seeding of a joint is not a significant risk, and intraarticular surgical exposure is recommended if this facilitates visualization. The majority of recurrences are cured with a second curettage, but a rare lesion can be locally aggressive, and requires a wide resection (290). Chondroblastoma of the pelvis frequently behaves more aggressively than that in long bones, and an initial wide excision is recommended.

Most patients are close to skeletal maturity when the diagnosis is made, and the risk of growth disturbance from the tumor or its treatment is minimal. When the patient is younger than 10 years old care should be taken not to damage the growth plate.

Periosteal Chondroma

This is an uncommon lesion that arises from the surface of the cortex, deep in the periosteum (295–297). The patient usually complains of pain at the site of the lesion. More than half of these lesions are found in the proximal humerus, and the others are evenly dispersed through the long bones. The lesion often can be palpated. It is a nontender, hard mass that is fixed to the bone. The plain radiograph is typical (Fig. 14-18). Periosteal chondroma is a scalloped defect on the outer surface of the cortex, occasionally with intralesional calcifications and minimal periosteal reaction. Microscopically, periosteal chondroma is benign cartilage, but it appears more active than enchondroma. It has been mis-

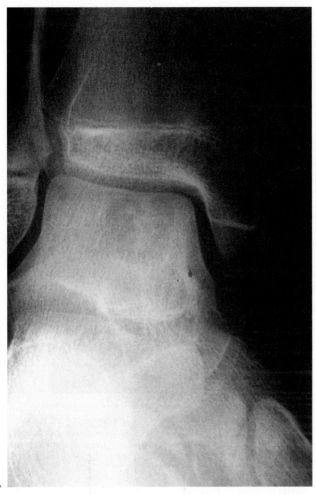

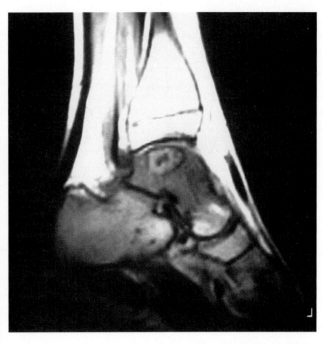

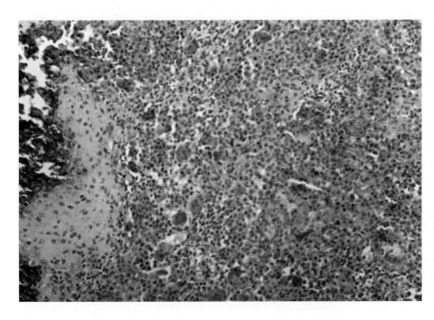

FIGURE 14-16. A: This is an anterior view of a 14-year-old girl's ankle. She complained of pain and swelling, and had limited range of motion in the joint. There is a radiolucent lesion in the talus that is close to the subchondral bone. There are central calcifications. **B:** The sagittal T1-weighted magnetic resonance image reveals the lesion and an associated edema. This lesion is a chondroblastoma, and was treated with curettage.

FIGURE 14-17. Histologic appearance of a chondroblastoma. The tumor consists of cuboidal cells (i.e., chondroblasts), varying amounts of amorphous matrix (some of which is calcified), and multinucleated giant cells. Calcification is seen (**left**). The cuboidal cells fit together in such a manner that they have the appearance of cobblestones. (Original magnification ×10.)

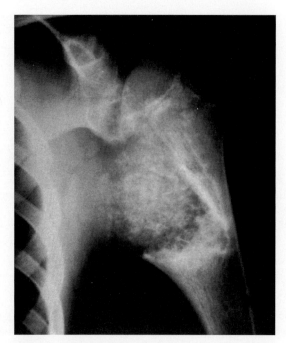

FIGURE 14-18. Radiograph of the shoulder of a 12-year-old boy. The large periosteal chondroma involves the medial aspect of the metaphysis. Most such tumors are smaller. This patient had no symptoms; the lesion was found by the boy's pediatrician on routine physical examination, and an incisional biopsy confirmed the diagnosis. The lesion was only partially removed. The tumor did not change appreciably during 2 years of follow-up.

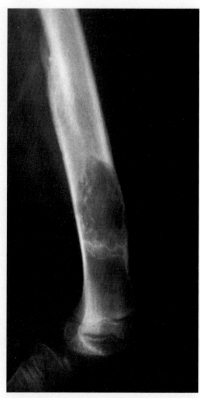

FIGURE 14-19. Lateral radiograph of the distal femur with a large nonossifying fibroma (NOF). The patient had sustained a pathologic fracture that had healed, but the lesion persisted. NOF is usually a metaphyseal, radiolucent, irregular lesion surrounded by a reactive rim of bone. As is often the case, the cortex surrounding a large NOF is thin and appears to be expanded. Although this lesion eventually heals spontaneously, its large size and persistence after pathologic fracture indicated that curettage and bone grafting were necessary. NOFs that replace more than half of the bone should be curetted and grafted.

taken for chondrosarcoma. Because local recurrence is a risk, a wide excision, including the underlying cortex, is the treatment of choice.

Lesions of Fibrous Origin

Nonossifying Fibroma

Nonossifying fibroma, which is also known as fibroma of bone, nonosteogenic fibroma, metaphyseal fibrous defect, and fibrous cortical defect, is probably the most common lesion of bone (298–302). Up to 40% of children have this lesion, which is found most often between the ages of 4 and 8 years (303). Ninety percent are in the distal femur. These are asymptomatic lesions that are found only if a radiograph is taken for another reason or when the patient has a pathologic fracture. The patient has no abnormal physical findings, and the serum and urine chemistries are normal.

Nonossifying fibroma should be recognized based on the clinical presentation and plain radiographic findings (298). Biopsy for diagnosis is rarely necessary. Two radiographic appearances are seen. The more common fibroma is a small (less than 0.5 cm) radiolucent lesion within the cortex, with a sharply defined border. Most authors call this lesion a "fibrous cortical defect" (93). There is little or no increased uptake on the technetium bone scan.

The other appearance is that of a metaphyseal lesion eccentrically located (Fig. 14-19). This lesion probably started out as a fibrous cortical defect, but continued to enlarge. It appears to have arisen from within the cortex, expanding into the medullary cavity and raising the periosteum. The lesion is surrounded by a well-defined thin rim of reactive bone. There should be no acute periosteal reaction unless there has been a fracture. There may be slightly increased uptake on the technetium bone scan. Multiple nonossifying fibromas occur in approximately 20% of patients. Usually they are found in the lower extremities, so investigators suggest obtaining plain radiographs of both lower extremities, whenever a nonossifying fibroma is found.

Both lesions consist of benign, spindle, fibroblastic cells arranged in a storiform pattern (298,299) (Fig. 14-20). Multinucleated giant cells are common, and areas of large, lipid-laden macrophages often can be seen. Hemosiderin within the fibroblastic stromal cells and multinucleated giant cells is usual. There is no bone formation within the lesion, and mitoses are not seen.

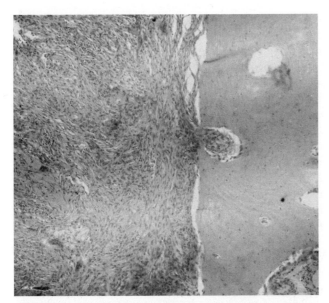

FIGURE 14-20. Low-power histologic view of a typical nonossifying fibroma. The fibroma is composed of benign fibrous tissue and multinucleated giant cells. Hemosiderin is often present. The nonossifying fibroma is invading cortical bone (**right**). (Original magnification ×10.)

The small cortical lesion (fibrous cortical defect) needs no treatment, but should be observed. Repeat radiographs at 3- to 6-month intervals for 1 to 2 years are suggested. These lesions should heal spontaneously. Nonossifying fibroma may need surgery. Nonossifying fibromas that are less than 50% of the diameter of the bone can be merely observed, but curettage and packing with bone graft should be considered if they enlarge (304–306). Patients who present with nonossifying fibromas that are more than 50% of the diameter of the bone should consider having the lesions curetted and packed with bone graft. According to Arata and colleagues (306), these patients have an increased risk of developing pathologic fractures. Many patients with these large nonossifying fibromas elect not to have surgery, and reduce their activity instead. This is an alternative treatment.

Patients who present with pathologic fractures should have the fractures treated nonoperatively if possible. The fracture should heal without difficulty in a normal length of time. There is no evidence that the healing of the fracture increases the chances of spontaneous healing of a nonossifying fibroma, or of any other benign lesion. Nonossifying fibroma usually heals spontaneously, which may happen after the fracture, but usually the fracture callus obscures the radiolucent lesion and the physician is fooled into thinking that the lesion is healing. When the callus has remodeled and the cortices become distinct on the radiograph, the lesion can be seen again. Patients with pathologic fractures must be followed until the callus has remodeled sufficiently so that a final determination can be made about the status of the underlying nonossifying fibroma. If it per-

sists after the fracture has healed, curettage and bone grafting are suggested.

Fibrous Dysplasia

Fibrous dysplasia may not be a true neoplasia, but a developmental abnormality caused by a somatic mutation with a defect in the formation of bone (see Chapter 7). It is a common disorder that produces a variety of complaints and physical findings. The majority of patients (approximately 85%) have a single skeletal lesion (monostotic fibrous dysplasia), whereas the remainder have numerous lesions (polyostotic fibrous dysplasia). The patients with polyostotic fibrous dysplasia may have only two or three small areas of involvement, or may have extensive skeletal abnormalities with grossly deformed bones.

The patient with monostotic fibrous dysplasia usually presents without symptoms, and the lesion is found when a radiograph is taken for unrelated reasons (307–310). Occasionally the child presents with a pathologic fracture or angular deformity. A rib is the most common location of monostotic fibrous dysplasia, but any bone can be involved. There are no physical findings associated with monostotic fibrous dysplasia, and the café-au-lait lesions and endocrine abnormalities sometimes found in patients with polyostotic fibrous dysplasia, do not occur in patients with the monostotic variant. Serum and urine chemistries are normal in patients with fibrous dysplasia.

The plain radiograph is often diagnostic, although the radiographic appearance of fibrous dysplasia is variable (Fig. 14-21A). It is a medullary process that typically produces a ground-glass appearance on the radiograph. The lesion is usually diaphyseal. The diaphysis is larger than normal, and the ground-glass appearance of the medullary canal blends into the thinned cortex so that it is difficult to define the border between the medullary canal and the cortex. When typical-appearing lesions are seen in a single bone or in a single limb, the diagnosis is almost certain. There may be an angular deformity in the bone, especially when the lesion is large. The lesions may mature with age and become radiodense or cystic. Fibrous dysplasia shows excessive uptake on a technetium bone scan out of proportion to what one might predict from the plain radiographic appearance.

The patient with polyostotic fibrous dysplasia usually presents around the age of 10 years, complaining of an angular deformity of a bone (307,311–314). The most common deformity is varus of the proximal femur, or shepherd's crook deformity. The light brown skin lesions with irregular borders are called "coast of Maine" café-au-lait spots. The lesions with smooth borders associated with neurofibromatosis are called "coast of California" café-au-lait spots.

Hyperthyroidism and diabetes mellitus have been reported as associated endocrinopathies, and vascular tumors have been seen in association with fibrous dysplasia (313,315–318). Albright syndrome is a triad of fibrous dys-

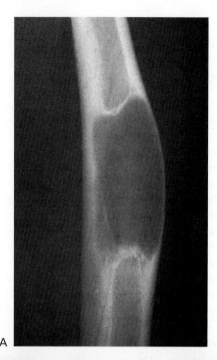

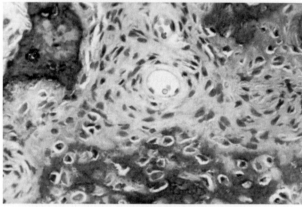

FIGURE 14-21. **A:** Radiograph of a fibrous dysplasia in the diaphysis of a long bone. The ground-glass appearance, the thin cortex, and the angular deformity of the bone are all typical features of fibrous dysplasia. Because this lesion was large and the patient had an angular deformity, a cortical bone graft was placed within the cortex to increase the strength of the bone. Curettage of the lesion probably does not increase local control, but should be performed if it can be carried out easily. Fibrous dysplastic bone is structurally weak, and cortical grafts are more likely to improve the strength of the bone and not be resorbed by the host. **B:** Histologic appearance of fibrous dysplasia. The tumor is mostly fibrous tissue composed of collagen and fibroblast. Small bits of bone and osteoid, often having a "C" or an "O" shape, seem to have been sprinkled on the fibrous tissue. Osteoblasts are not seen, and the bone seems to be produced by the fibroblastic cells. (Original magnification ×40.)

plasia, café-au-lait spots, and precocious puberty (315). The lesions in polyostotic fibrous dysplasia tend to be more unilateral than bilateral. The radiographic appearance of the lesion is the same as in patients with monostotic disease. The structural strength of bones with fibrous dysplasia is

reduced as a result of the poorly organized trabecular pattern and the thinned cortex. The weakness of the bones leads to the deformities that are usually present.

Microscopically, fibrous dysplasia, both the monostotic and polyostotic forms, is composed of fibrous tissue with normal-appearing nuclei and irregularly shaped strands of osteoid and bone (Fig. 14-21B). There are few if any osteoblasts present, and the osteoid and bone seem to arise directly from the background fibrous stoma. The bone is irregularly organized, and often has a "C" or an "O" shape. Multinucleated giant cells are rare in fibrous dysplasia, and there should be few mitoses, and none of these cells should be abnormal. Nodules of cartilage may be present in typical fibrous dysplasia.

Monostotic fibrous dysplasia usually does not need surgical treatment. Occasionally, a solitary lesion will be painful and curettage with grafting is required. Small lesions can be packed with cortical cancellous bone graft (autogenous or allogenic), whereas large lesions are probably better treated with cortical bone grafts. A special circumstance is a lesion in the femoral neck. These lesions seem to have a risk of developing fatigue fractures, and cortical bone grafting is recommended (319). Resorption of the bone graft with recurrence of fibrous dysplasia can occur, and the patient should be seen in follow-up for up to 5 years. Occasionally it is necessary to augment the bone with long-term or permanent internal fixation to prevent repeated fractures and relieve pain. Progressive bone deformity is unusual in patients with monostotic fibrous dysplasia. Patients with polyostotic fibrous dysplasia are more often in need of surgical therapy. Bone deformity is the most common indication. The proximal femur is the most challenging bone to manage. Once a varus deformity develops, it is important not only to bone graft (preferably cortical bone), but to correct the angular deformity with a valgus osteotomy. Rigid internal fixation is recommended (307,320–328).

Osteofibrous Dysplasia

Kempson (329) described the osteofibrous dysplasia lesion, which is found in the mandible and the anterior cortex of the tibia of children. It is benign, but may be locally aggressive. It is *not* a healing nonossifying fibroma. The patients usually do not have symptoms, and usually are brought to the physician's attention by a parent who has noticed an anterior bowing or mass in the tibia. The lesion is almost always located within the anterior cortex of the tibia, and is best seen on the lateral radiograph (Fig. 14-22). There are usually numerous radiolucent lesions with a rim of reactive bone. There is increased uptake on the technetium bone scan in the area of the lesion.

Although Kempson (329) suggested the name "ossifying fibroma," the more commonly used term is "osteofibrous dysplasia" (330–334). Some authors believe that osteofibrous dysplasia is a type of fibrous dysplasia, but this is

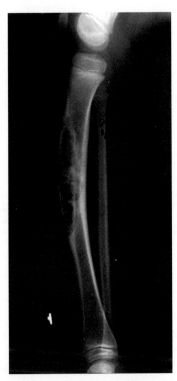

FIGURE 14-22. Lateral radiograph of the leg of a patient with osteofibrous dysplasia. Found almost exclusively in the tibia, this lesion involves the anterior cortex, and can extend into the medullary canal. The tibia commonly has an anterior bow.

controversial. Fibrous dysplasia has numerous characteristics that osteofibrous dysplasia does not have. Fibrous dysplasia arises from the medullary canal, and rarely produces bowing of the tibia. It rarely recurs after curettage, and is not an aggressive lesion unless the patient has polyostotic disease. Osteofibrous dysplasia, on the other hand, arises from the cortex and involves the medullary canal late in the disease process. It usually is associated with a bowed tibia, and quickly recurs if curetted. Usually it requires a resection for control. There have been few studies of patients with osteofibrous dysplasia with adequate follow-up, but many of these lesions slowly progress, and are eventually resected.

The authors recommend observation of the lesion when it is found in a patient younger than 10 years of age. Incisional biopsy is not necessary in most cases, because the clinical presentation is diagnostic. In addition, the biopsy reveals only a small portion of the lesion, and does not change the initial management. Bracing may not prevent progressive bowing, but can be tried if there is an angular deformity. If the lesion progresses before closure of the growth plate, biopsy and resection are suggested. If the patient presents after closure of the growth plate, especially if the lesion is large (more than 3 or 4 cm in diameter) or has aggressive features on plain radiographs, a biopsy is suggested. If an adamantinoma is found a wide resection is recommended. If the biopsy reveals osteofibrous dysplasia, it is best to excise the entire lesion for a complete histologic examination to rule out the possibility of there being a focus of adamantinoma. If the lesion is small (less than approximately 3 cm) and the patient has no symptoms, continued observation is suggested.

Adamantinoma has a clinical presentation similar to osteofibrous dysplasia. In adamantinoma, however, usually the patient is older (third decade of life), and the lesion appears more aggressive on the radiographs (e.g., soft tissue extension, acute periosteal reaction, large size, involvement of the medullary canal), but this is not always the case. It has been suggested that there is another type of adamantinoma that looks extremely similar to osteofibrous dysplasia, even with histologic examination. One must be suspicious of the diagnosis of osteofibrous dysplasia, especially in a progressive lesion in a patient older than 10 years of age (335,336).

If a lesion suspected of being an osteofibrous dysplasia is going to be observed, the patient should undergo radiography at least every 6 months until the lesion heals or is resected. Typical adamantinoma has a risk of metastasizing, but it is not known if the adamantinoma that looks like osteofibrous dysplasia can metastasize (333).

Miscellaneous Lesions

Langerhans Cell Histiocytosis

"Langerhans cell histiocytosis" is the name selected to refer to what we once called "histiocytosis X," and includes the syndromes eosinophilic granuloma, Hand-Schüller-Christian disease, and Letterer-Siwe disease (337,338). In 1941 Farber suggested that eosinophilic granuloma, Hand-Schüller-Christian disease, and Letterer-Siwe disease were related (339). Later, Lichtenstein published an article agreeing with Farber, and suggested the term "histiocytosis X" (340). This is a disorder of the Langerhans histiocytes, and although eosinophils are a common component of the lesion, they are not necessary for the diagnosis (Fig. 14-23).

Eosinophilic granuloma usually occurs in patients between the ages of 5 and 15 years. The skull is the most commonly involved site (341) (Fig. 14-24). Many of the skull lesions probably are not diagnosed because the only abnormality is a painless, small, spontaneously resolving lump in the scalp. The vertebral bodies and the ilium are the next most common sites of involvement (342–344). Those lesions in long bones may weaken the bone sufficiently that the patient presents with activity-related pain suggestive of a fatigue fracture, or with a pathologic fracture. The lesion is a radiolucent abnormality with sharp borders of transition and often no reaction by the host bone. An apparent central sequestrum of bone may be seen. Eosinophilic granuloma usually results in increased uptake on a technetium bone scan, but as many as 25% of lesions will

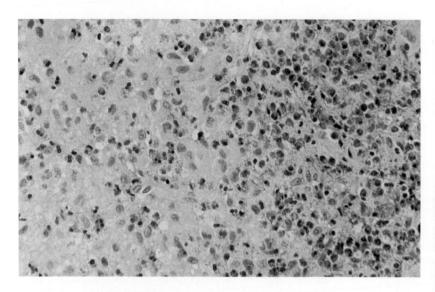

FIGURE 14-23. Low-power view of an eosinophilic granuloma (Langerhans granuloma). The eosinophils are numerous, but it is the presence of histiocytes that defines this tumor. The histiocytes are large cells with a clear, folded nucleus and a prominent nucleolus. (Original magnification ×10.)

not be associated with abnormal bone scans (72,73, 345–350) (Fig. 14-25).

Patients with eosinophilic granuloma do not progress to Hand-Schüller-Christian disease, but should be evaluated on presentation to exclude the presence of that syndrome.

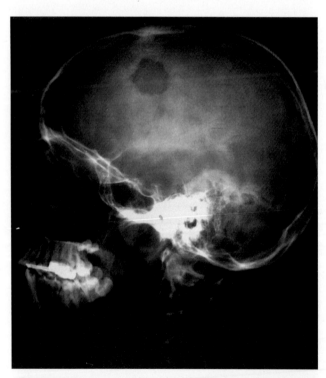

FIGURE 14-24. This is a lateral plain radiograph of the skull of a patient with a solitary Langerhans cell histiocytosis (eosinophilic granuloma). The skull is the single most common site of involvement for eosinophilic granuloma. Plain radiographs of the skull are recommended when eosinophilic granuloma is suspected. These lesions rarely require treatment.

Obtaining a lateral skull film to observe the size of the sella turcica, and a first voided urine specimen after overnight fluid restriction to prove that the patient can concentrate his or her urine, is the easiest way to evaluate the patient for diabetes insipidus. Liver enzymes should be determined. A skeletal survey also should be done to look for other lesions. Multiple lesions can be seen in eosinophilic granuloma. If any of these parameters are abnormal, the patient should be referred to a pediatric hematologist. The authors routinely seek a consultation from a pediatric hematologist for all patients with Langerhans cell histiocytosis.

It was believed that eosinophilic granuloma needed to be treated, and many children underwent irradiation, curettage, or excision. At present, it is believed that the majority of these lesions are self-healing, and that no specific treatment is necessary (338). Intralesional injection of corticosteroids has been recommended by some physicians (351–353).

Hand-Schüller-Christian disease is a combination of bone lesion, exophthalmos, and diabetes insipidus. Patients with this disorder should be treated with systemic corticosteroids or chemotherapy (354–357).

Letterer-Siwe disease is a malignant form of Langerhans cell histiocytosis. Most patients present before 3 years of age with skin, visceral, and brain lesions, and they may or may not have bone lesions. They require aggressive chemotherapy (341,358–360).

Unicameral Bone Cysts

Unicameral bone cysts are not always unicameral. They also are called "simple bone cysts," but they may not be simple to treat. These common lesions usually are found when the patient sustains a pathologic fracture. Their radiographic appearance is so typical that most can be diagnosed without

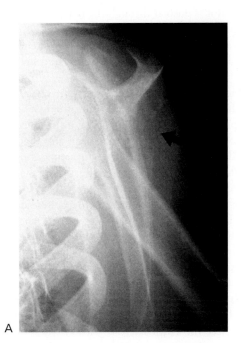

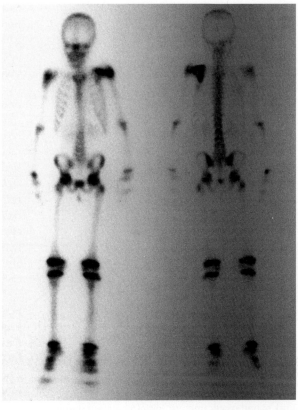

Anterior   Posterior   B

A

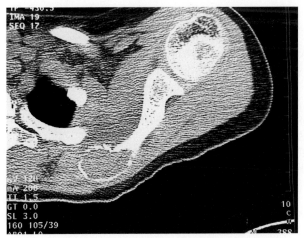

FIGURE 14-25. A: This plain radiograph is an oblique view of an 8-year-old girl's scapula. The *arrow* points to a subtle area of cortical erosion. The patient complained of pain, and there was a tender mass over the scapula. **B:** On the anterior view of the same patient's technetium 99 bone scan, the increased uptake in the scapula is easily seen. This patient has a solitary Langerhans cell histiocytosis (eosinophilic granuloma), but her lesion is associated with increased uptake. This is true in the majority of cases. **C:** On the computed tomography scan, a lesion is seen in the medial border of the scapula. After biopsy, curettage without graft was curative.

a biopsy (Fig. 14-26). The proximal humerus and the proximal femur account for 90% of unicameral bone cysts (361–365). The cysts seem to arise from the epiphyseal plate, and are immediately adjacent to the plate extending into the metaphysis (366–369). The metaphyseal bone does not remodel and the metaphysis is broader than normal, but not broader than the width of the epiphyseal plate. A thin rim of bone borders the unicameral bone cyst. The surrounding bone is not reactive, and there is no acute periosteal reaction. When the cyst becomes mature (latent), usually after the patient reaches the age of 10 years, the epiphysis grows away from the lesion. The unicameral bone cyst eventually heals spontaneously and fills in with bone. No evidence of its previous existence is seen.

Treatment is to prevent a pathologic fracture. Some lesions remain small and do not present a significant risk to the patient. Other lesions are large (e.g., proximal humeral lesions), are in high-stress anatomic sites (e.g., the femoral

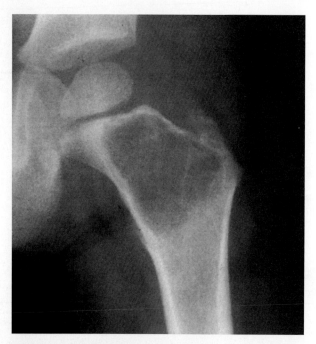

FIGURE 14-26. Anteroposterior radiograph of a proximal femoral unicameral bone cyst (UBC). UBCs are radiolucent lesions immediately adjacent to the growth plate that extend into the metaphysis. This UBC is considered active because it is immediately adjacent to the growth plate and the patient is younger than 10 years old. Large lesions in the proximal femur should be treated because of the risk of pathologic fracture. Initial treatment should be a corticosteroid injection.

neck), or persist after the patient has become a young adult, and in these cases treatment is indicated. Only those patients who have unicameral bone cysts that are at risk for pathologic fracture should be treated (370–375). Injection is recommended rather than an operative procedure because the results of injection are equal to those of curettage and bone grafting, whereas the risk, recovery, and cost are less. Intracystic injection of corticosteroids is the treatment of choice as an initial means of stimulating the cyst to heal (376,377). Before the common use of corticosteroid injections, curettage and autogenous bone grafting had been the most common treatment. Operative treatment with curettage and autogenous bone grafting is reserved for those lesions that do not respond to repeated injections of corticosteroid (361,376,378–380). The number of injections that should be tried before deciding to operate is not agreed upon. The authors give at least three injections approximately 1 month apart before resorting to an open operative procedure. The injection of autogenous bone marrow is a technique advocated by some (381). In a study of ten patients whose unicameral bone cysts were treated with autogenous marrow, all were free of pain within 2 weeks of the injection, and all healed completely within 1 year.

The injection of corticosteroid was introduced by Scaglietti and colleagues (377,382). It has been used extensively

and is an established method of treatment of a unicameral bone cyst. It should be performed with anesthesia (usually general anesthesia), and with the aid of fluoroscopic visualization. An 18- or 20-gauge spinal needle is passed percutaneously into the cyst. The wall of the cyst is penetrated easily by an 18-gauge needle with the stylet in place. Rotating the needle as it is pushed through the bone often helps it penetrate the cortex. Clear yellow or slightly bloody fluid should be obtained. If no fluid is aspirated, the diagnosis of unicameral bone cyst should be questioned and the lesion biopsied.

Once the fluid has been withdrawn a second needle is introduced into the cyst as far from the first as possible. A radiopaque dye (usually Renografin 60) is injected into the cyst to confirm that it is unicameral, and that all parts fill with dye. Frequently the draining veins are seen shortly after the cyst is injected. If the cyst has more than one cavity, each one should be injected.

It is not known if the type of corticosteroid used is important, but methylprednisolone acetate (Depo-Medrol) is probably the most commonly used steroid. There is no standard amount of corticosteroid. Usually, 80 mg is sufficient for a small cyst, and up to 160 mg may be used for large cysts. There are two techniques for corticosteroid injection. One is to inject the corticosteroid under pressure, with the second needle occluded, to rupture the cyst wall. The other is to inject the corticosteroid without pressure, using the second needle as a vent. It is unclear which method is better. A repeat radiograph is taken in 1 month, and if there is no evidence of early healing (e.g., increased thickness of the reactive wall), a repeat injection is done. Repeated injections are often needed, but more than three to five probably are not beneficial.

The rare unicameral bone cyst that requires operative treatment should be curetted and packed with bone graft. When the cyst is adjacent to the growth plate, care should be taken not to damage the epiphyseal cartilage during curettage (383). Autogenous bone or allograft cortical cancellous bone can be used to pack the cavity (361,378,384,385). Freeze-dried cortical cancellous allograft is particularly advantageous because it is associated with an excellent healing rate and little, if any, incidence of complications, and no secondary incision is required to obtain the autogenous bone graft. Calcium sulfate tablets are an alternative material that can be used to fill the cavity (386,387).

Aneurysmal Bone Cysts

An ABC is a controversial lesion (361,363,388–391). Some investigators believe that this lesion occurs only in association with another bone tumor, whereas others recognize ABCs as a primary diagnosis (389,392,393). ABCs often occur in association with a number of benign tumors (e.g., giant cell tumor, chondroblastoma, osteoblastoma), or with osteosarcoma (389). When it is a secondary lesion, the primary lesion usually is obvious, and the ABC component is limited to only a small portion of the tumor. Secondary ABCs are classified with their underlying diagnosis. The presence of a secondary ABC does not change the therapy or prognosis of the underlying primary tumor.

A primary ABC occurs most commonly in teenagers (80%). More than 50% of these cysts arise in large tubular bones, and almost 30% occur in the spine. The patient usually complains of a mild, dull pain, and only rarely is there a clinically apparent pathologic fracture. The patient's physical examination is usually normal, and there are no abnormal laboratory findings associated with ABC.

On the plain radiograph an ABC is a radiolucent lesion arising eccentrically within the medullary canal of the metaphysis (Fig. 14-27). It resorbs the cortex and elevates the periosteum, generally making the bone wider than the epiphyseal plate. Usually, there is a thin shell of reactive periosteal bone, but occasionally this bone cannot be seen. When ABC arises in a long bone, it is metaphyseal. When it arises in the spine, it originates in the posterior elements but it

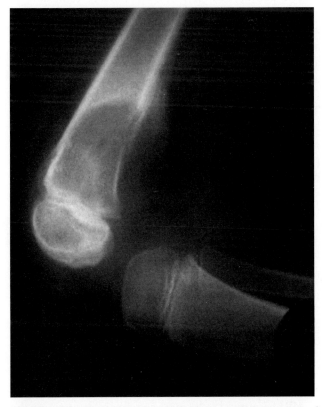

FIGURE 14-27. Radiograph of a distal femur with an aneurysmal bone cyst involving the distal metaphysis, and extending through the posterior cortex. As in this patient, an aneurysmal bone cyst may have the appearance of an aggressive tumor. When the cyst erodes through the cortex it usually is contained by the periosteum, which reacts and produces bone. The differential diagnosis should include aneurysmal bone cyst, osteosarcoma (telangiectatic variant), Ewing sarcoma, and osteomyelitis. This patient was successfully treated with curettage and bone grafting.

may extend into the body, and not uncommonly will extend to an adjacent vertebral body or rib. Giant cell tumor of the bone and telangiectatic osteosarcoma may have identical radiographic appearances as an ABC (379,389). The periosteal reaction has an aggressive appearance, and the lesion may be mistaken for an aggressive or malignant tumor (363). ABCs may arise in the cortex and elevate the periosteum with or without involving the medullary canal.

The CT scan is helpful in making the diagnosis of ABC. The lesion should have a density of approximately 20 HU, and this does not increase with intravenous contrast injection. When the patient lies still for 20 to 30 min, the cells in the fluid within the cyst cavity settle, and a fluid/fluid level can be seen (394). Similar findings can be seen on MRI. Fluid/fluid level was originally described in ABC but has subsequently been seen in a number of other lesions. It cannot be considered diagnostic of ABC. An ABC has an increased uptake of technetium on the bone scan, but often the scan has a central area of decreased uptake (395).

ABCs should be biopsied to establish the diagnosis, then curetted and packed with bone graft. The pathologist should be advised in advance, and the possibility of a telangiectatic osteosarcoma should be discussed. It is uncommon for the histologic appearance of an ABC to be confused with that of a telangiectatic osteosarcoma, although the radiographic and gross appearances can be identical. On gross inspection, an ABC is a cavitary lesion with a villous lining. Microscopic examination reveals the lining to be composed of hemosiderin-laden macrophages, multinucleated giant cells, a fibrous stroma, and usually small amounts of woven bone (Fig. 14-28). The microscopic appearance of the lining of the ABC is similar to that of a giant cell tumor of bone.

The majority of ABCs are treated successfully with curettage and packing of bone graft. The first recurrence can be recuretted and grafted. Embolization has been used to decrease blood loss during surgery, and has been associated with fewer recurrences (396,397). Whether embolization is necessary or of help is debatable. Cryosurgery has also been reported (361,388,398). Cryosurgery has associated complications, and it is not considered necessary in most cases. It may play a role in the treatment of recurrent lesions. Definitive resection can be performed when the consequences of the resection are minimal, but it is absolutely necessary only when the lesion has a particularly aggressive clinical growth pattern.

An ABC of the spine (approximately 30% of cases) can present a particularly challenging problem. The lesion always involves the posterior elements, but can also involve the vertebral body. The patients complain initially of pain at the site of the lesion, but the ABC often is not found until the patient has nerve root or cord compression. Radiotherapy has been used in the management of patients with ABC of the spine, but surgery is recommended for all patients as the initial means of treatment. Most cases are controlled with simple curettage. Usually the posterior ele-

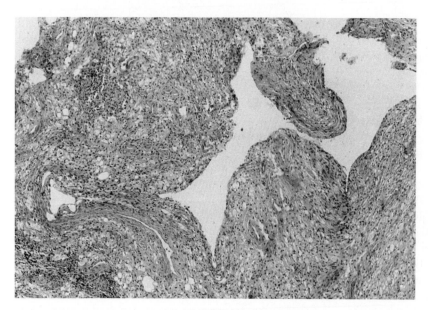

FIGURE 14-28. Low-power view of the tissue lining an aneurysmal bone cyst. The lining is composed of fibrous tissue with multinucleated giant cells, foamy histiocytes, hemosiderin, and, often, spicules of immature bone (not seen). The fronds and spaces are typical. (Original magnification ×10.)

ments are resected, and involvement of the pedicles or the body is curetted. If complete laminectomy is performed, a short posterior fusion is advised. Radiotherapy can be used in the postoperative period, but usually this is reserved for the rare case of rapid recurrence with soft tissue infiltration. Postoperative MRI or CT is recommended as a baseline study with which to compare any later scans.

Ewing Sarcoma/Peripheral Neuroectodermal Tumor

Ewing sarcoma and peripheral (or primitive) neuroectodermal tumor (EWS/PNET) are discussed together because they are closely related (247,399). Both have the same chromosomal translocation between chromosomes 11 and 22, similar presentations, identical treatments, and almost identical histologic characteristics. PNET is also called Askin tumor, and was originally identified from tumors classified as Ewing sarcoma. EWS/PNETs are thought to arise from the neural crest. At least 90% have a characteristic chromosomal translocation [t(11:22)(q24:q12)]. This translocation leads to a novel fusion protein called EWS-FLI1 (400,401).

EWS/PNET was the most lethal of all primary bone tumors before the routine use of adjuvant chemotherapy, with a 5-year survival of approximately 15% (402). Before the use of adjuvant chemotherapy, most patients were treated with irradiation alone. With improved survival associated with adjuvant chemotherapy the role of surgery has been reevaluated, and there is evidence, albeit only from retrospective studies, that surgical resection combined with chemotherapy produces improved survival compared with survival after irradiation and chemotherapy (239,402–413).

The patient with EWS/PNET initially complains of pain. Some have generalized symptoms of fever, weight loss, and malaise, but this is not the usual presentation. Males are affected at a 3:2 ratio over females, and most patients are between the ages of 5 and 30 years. Any bone may be affected. The femur is the most common site of origin (20%); the pelvis and the humerus are also common sites. There is usually a soft tissue mass associated with the bone lesion, and on physical examination this mass often can be palpated. The mass is warm, firm, and tender, and it may be pulsatile. There are no specific abnormal laboratory values diagnostic of EWS/PNET, but the sedimentation rate often is increased. Elevated LDH is a poor prognostic sign (247,399).

The typical plain radiograph of a EWS/PNET reveals diffuse destruction of the bone, extension of the tumor through the cortex, a soft tissue component, and a periosteal reaction (414) (Fig. 14-29). The periosteal reaction may produce a Codman triangle, an "onionskin" appearance, or a sunburst appearance. These suggest an aggressive lesion that has rapidly penetrated the cortex and elevated the periosteum. The extraosseous soft tissue mass and medullary canal involvement can be seen on CT and MRI scans, and usually are more extensive than what was expected from the plain radiograph (80,415,416).

MRI has proved to be more accurate in determining the intramedullary extent of EWS than CT. The inflammation around the tumor is seen with MRI more easily than with other studies, and its extent is often more than expected from the other tests. The technetium bone scan is most useful in finding occult bone metastasis. Approximately 5% of these patients present with pulmonary metastasis.

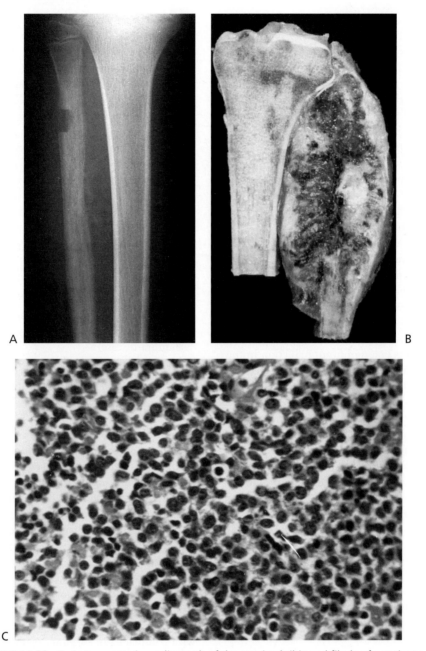

FIGURE 14-29. **A:** Anteroposterior radiograph of the proximal tibia and fibula of a patient with Ewing sarcoma involving the proximal fibula. The fibular cortical detail is lost, and erosion of the medial surface, soft tissue mass, and periosteal reaction—all typical findings of Ewing sarcoma—are present. The combination of these findings is indicative of an aggressive process. Acute osteomyelitis may have this appearance, but the patient usually has other signs of infection. The defect in the lateral aspect of the fibula is attributable to an incisional biopsy of the bone. The bone should not be biopsied if there is sufficient soft tissue extension. This will lessen the chance of pathologic fracture. In addition, the extraosseous tumor is usually more easily cut, and the histologic appearance is better. **B:** Gross specimen of Ewing sarcoma of the proximal fibula, similar to the case in **A**. The tumor has replaced the proximal fibula, and there is a large soft tissue mass, with invasion of surrounding muscles and no involvement of the tibia. This patient chose to have an immediate amputation, although this is not standard treatment. **C:** Histologic appearance of Ewing sarcoma. The nuclei are easily seen, and there are nucleoli within each nucleus. The cells are small and round, with very little variation in nuclear appearance. Mitoses are rare. The cytoplasm is faint and difficult to see, and the cytoplasmic borders are poorly defined. (Original magnification ×10.)

The histologic appearance of EWS/PNET is that of a small, round, cell tumor. The EWS/PNET cell has a distinct nucleus with minimal cytoplasm and an indistinct cytoplasmic border (7,417–419). The cells are similar and mitoses are uncommon. Necrotic areas usually are seen. There are glycogen granules in the cytoplasm, and these produce the positive periodic acid Schiff (PAS) stain on routine histologic examination. The intracellular glycogen granules are diastase positive (i.e., exposure to diastase will break the glycogen down, eliminating PAS staining). The glycogen can be seen as dense cytoplasmic granules with the electron microscope. Increasingly, genetic analysis is being done for EWS/PNET to identify the 11:22 translocation as a means of establishing the diagnosis.

Treatment of EWS/PNET is a combination of chemotherapy and either irradiation or surgery (245,412, 420–432). The drugs commonly used include vincristine, doxorubicin, cyclophosphamide, ifosfamide, and etoposide. Actinomycin D, a drug used previously, is currently used less often. Most protocols begin with two to four courses of chemotherapy before deciding how to manage the primary tumor. This usually results in a significant reduction in the size of the primary tumor. Surgical resection is recommended if the functional consequences of the resection are acceptable (406–408,433–435). If the margins are close and viable tumor is present in the resected specimen, postoperative irradiation is recommended. If the primary tumor cannot be resected without undue morbidity, irradiation alone can be used (223,224,423,436–445). The total dosage should be kept as low as possible, usually around 50 gray (Gy), and certainly less than 60 Gy, because dosages of more than 60 Gy are associated with an unacceptable incidence of later irradiation-associated sarcomas (446–453).

Current survival statistics for patients presenting without metastasis reveal a 5-year disease-free survival of greater than 65% (444). Patients who present with metastasis have less chance of being cured but should be treated aggressively because some will survive.

Soft Tissue Tumors

The majority of soft tissue tumors in children are benign (454). Only rhabdomyosarcoma in the younger age group and synovial cell sarcoma in teenagers and older patients occur with any frequency, and they are both rare tumors (455). Hemangioma, the fibromatoses, neurilemoma, and neurofibroma are more common. The physician must be aware of the possibility of malignant soft tissue tumor in the child and evaluate any lump carefully (456).

Hemangioma

Hemangioma may be a true neoplasia, a hamartoma, or an arteriovenous malformation. Its origin is controversial. It is important that the abnormality be recognized as a benign lesion that in certain circumstances regresses spontaneously, and in others infiltrates the muscle and occasionally bone. Hemangiomas are the most common tumors in infancy and childhood, and account for 7% of benign soft tissue tumors in all age groups. They are most common in the head and neck regions, but also may be found in internal organs, especially the liver. Often an intrahepatic hemangioma can be seen on a CT scan of the abdomen taken for another reason, and its existence is of little concern.

Enzinger and Weiss (457) provide a classification of vascular tumors of soft tissue. The borderline malignant and malignant vascular tumors are not pertinent to this discussion; therefore, only the benign tumors are included:

- localized hemangioma
- capillary hemangioma (including juvenile type)
- cavernous hemangioma
- venous hemangioma
- arteriovenous hemangioma (racemose hemangioma)
- epithelioid hemangioma (angiolymphoid hyperplasia, Kimura disease)
- hemangioma of granulation tissue type (pyogenic granuloma)
- miscellaneous hemangiomas of deep soft tissue (synovial, intramuscular, neural)
- angiomatosis (diffuse hemangioma)

Capillary hemangioma constitutes the largest group of benign vascular tumors. The juvenile hemangioma variant of capillary hemangioma occurs in 1 of every 200 live births. They may be cutaneous or deep, and usually are seen within the first few weeks of life, often enlarging for the first 6 months but then regressing and becoming 75 to 95% involute by the age of 7 years. Capillary hemangiomas do not require treatment.

Cavernous hemangiomas are not as common as the capillary type, but do not spontaneously regress and may require treatment. They most commonly arise within muscle, and invade tissue planes extensively. The patient often presents with complaints of swelling, tenderness, and inflammation secondary to thrombophlebitis within the hemangioma. This inflammation resolves within a few days, and can be treated with local heat and oral aspirin. The noninflamed hemangioma is soft and ill defined. The patient may have no symptoms or the sensation of heaviness or a tight feeling in the extremity. On the plain radiograph there are often small, smooth, round calcifications called "phleboliths." The appearance of hemangiomas on MRI is virtually diagnostic, because they are composed of smooth, regular blood vessels and normal fat.

The cavernous hemangiomas have an indirect communication with the major vascular tree, and are not easily filled with contrast for angiography or venography; they are better visualized with MRI. Occasionally a tourniquet proximal to the hemangioma permits filling of the tumor veins at the time of venography or angiography (Fig. 14-30). If an intravenous injection does not demonstrate the hemangioma, the dye can be injected directly into the hemangioma. CT, particularly if performed with intravenous contrast, is almost always diagnostic. The hemangioma has varying densities with multiple dye-filled areas. Biopsy is performed only to confirm the diagnosis, and resection is not necessary unless the patient has repeated bouts of inflammation or complaints of discomfort (usually a full or tight feeling), or the parents are anxious about the mass.

Surgical excision usually is not required. When surgery is performed the hemangioma often recurs unless the entire muscle (or muscles) involved is resected. These lesions are probably best considered congenital abnormalities that involve most of the veins in the extremity. When the grossly involved veins are resected the surrounding vessels dilate, resulting in clinical recurrence. Hemangiomas do not undergo malignant degeneration, and although they can produce significant abnormalities in the extremity surgical resection is rarely curative, although it may reduce the symptoms. Irradiation has been used with varying benefit. Embolization also has been used for patients who have severe pain.

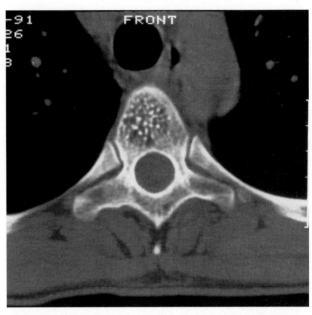

FIGURE 14-31. Computed tomography scan of a typical hemangioma of the vertebral body. The small foci of increased density are thickened trabeculae of bone, and the low-density areas are filled with the hemangiomatous tissue.

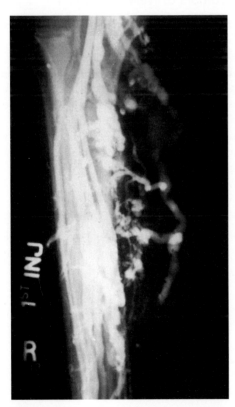

FIGURE 14-30. Venogram of a patient with hemangioma of the calf. The hemangioma communicated with the deep venous system and was easily filled when normal veins were injected with contrast; this is not always the case. This patient had two pulmonary emboli, and the hemangioma was confined to the gastrocnemius muscle. Therefore, the entire gastrocnemius muscle was resected.

Direct injections have been used, but there are few data regarding the results, and published reports of this management have not been found.

Hemangioma of bone, either solitary or diffuse, is a hamartoma, and not a true neoplasia. The solitary lesions are more frequent, especially in the vertebral bodies where they are most often found (Fig. 14-31). Solitary lesions may occur in any bone, but the skull is the second most common site. These lesions do not produce symptoms, and usually are found when a radiograph is taken for another reason. The radiograph and CT scan are diagnostic. The bone has a honeycomb appearance, with increased trabecular markings around radiolucencies.

Patients with multiple lesions are more likely to present during the first or second decade of life, with either mild discomfort or pathologic fracture. These patients can have involvement of their viscera and skin. When multiple sites are involved they are usually the long bones of the extremities and the short bones of the hands and feet. Treatment should be symptomatic, with curettage and bone grafting for lesions that weaken the bone. Lesions that do not produce symptoms, or that are not at risk for fracture should be observed. They should resolve with time.

Fibromatoses

Benign fibrous lesions in children are relatively common and rarely malignant. Extraabdominal desmoid, or aggressive fibromatosis, is the most common benign fibrous lesion seen in children (458). The less common lesions are not discussed in this text. Enzinger and Weiss (457) discuss these elsewhere.

Extraabdominal desmoid or aggressive fibromatosis is the most common benign fibrous tumor seen in patients older than 10 years of age (459). The patient presents with mild pain and a slowly enlarging mass. The mass is deep, firm, and slightly tender, but it is not inflamed. The adjacent joint is normal. A soft tissue mass can be seen on a plain radiograph, but there are no distinguishing features. Calcifications within the mass are not expected.

There is usually increased activity in the lesion on the technetium bone scan, although some large masses will not display increased uptake. Often, even when the lesion is immediately adjacent to the bone, there is no increased uptake of technetium. The mass has a density similar to that of muscle on the CT scan, but usually it is more vascular and can be distinguished best from the surrounding tissue by performing CT while the patient is infused with intravenous contrast. The classic collagen bundles produce a relative signal void (dark on T1- and T2-weighted images) on MRI, but because the cellularity varies, fibromatoses may have an appearance on MRI similar to any soft tissue neoplasia (460,461).

Histologically, fibromatosis has the appearance of scar tissue (457,462). It is composed of dense bundles of collagen with evenly dispersed benign cells (Fig. 14-32). The cell of origin is believed to be the myofibroblast. The histologic appearance and cell of origin of fibromatosis are identical to those of plantar fibromatosis and Dupuytren contracture, but the latter conditions are not as clinically aggressive as fibromatosis. Although they recur, they do not extend proximally out of the feet or hands as seen in aggressive fibromatosis.

Aggressive fibromatosis is an infiltrative lesion, and local excision rarely removes the entire tumor. Often what in the operating room appears to be the extent of the tumor is found to have microscopic tumor when examined by the pathologist. Fortunately, the presence of a positive margin at the initial resection does not always lead to a local recurrence, and it is recommended to observe the patient for a local recurrence. Approximately half of the patients will develop recurrent disease regardless of the histologic margin. Those patients whose lesions recur must be widely excised if local control is to be expected. Patients younger than 10 years of age have a greater risk of developing a local recurrence than older patients. When a wide surgical margin is accomplished with the resection of the recurrence, local control is usually achieved. When the second surgical margin is microscopically positive, irradiation is recommended (459). The majority of a patient's lesions will be controlled with this combination. Low-dose methotrexate and vinblastine (355,463) have been used to treat some patients with aggressive fibromatosis, and the initial reports have been encouraging, but the effect of this treatment is unpredictable. Fibromatosis has a variable clinical course, and the treatment needs to be individualized for each patient.

Benign Tumors of Nerve Origin

There are two common benign tumors that arise from nerves: neurilemoma and neurofibroma (457,462). Neurilemomas, or schwannomas, arise from the nerve sheath. They occur most often in early adulthood, and usually are solitary and slow-growing. The patient usually presents with a painless mass, and has a Tinel sign when the mass is tapped. The mass may be from any nerve, but it is often in the superficial tissue arising from a small sensory nerve. When arising from a spinal nerve root, the foramen may be enlarged because of the pressure of the tumor on the

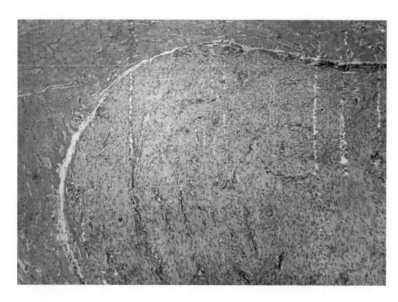

FIGURE 14-32. Histologic appearance of fibromatosis. The lesion infiltrates a muscle, and is more cellular than the typical fibromatosis. A wide resection was attempted, but this patient had a microscopically positive margin. One year later, the patient had not had a recurrence. (Original magnification ×10.)

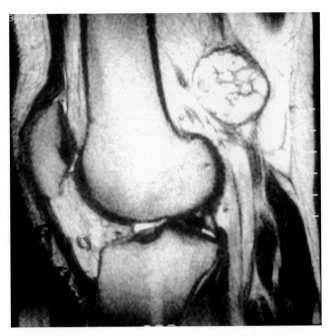

FIGURE 14-33. This is a sagittal view of a T1-weighted magnetic resonance image. The round, well-circumscribed mass posterior to the femur is within the peroneal nerve. It proved to be a schwannoma. Schwannomas have a typical appearance on magnetic resonance images. If they arise from a major nerve, as is the case in this patient, the nerve can usually be traced into the lesion. The schwannoma is smooth, slightly oblong, and has both bright and intermediate signals.

bone. Nerve dysfunction is uncommon, and is seen only when the nerve is compressed between the tumor and an adjacent rigid structure. Patients with superficial nerve lesions usually present early with small tumors, but deep-seated lesions may be large before they are discovered (Fig.

14-33). Neurilemoma rarely is seen in patients with von Recklinghausen disease because neurofibroma is the common type in these patients. Neurilemomas are nodular masses with a distinct capsule, and are easily separated from the nerve of origin. Their microscopic appearance is a combination of a cellular area (Antoni A) and a myxoid area (Antoni B). The Antoni A area is composed of benign spindle cells that tend to have their nuclei stacked with intervening cytoplasm (Fig. 14-34). The nuclear stacking is called a "palisaded appearance," and the arrangement of alternating nuclei and cytoplasm is called a "Verocay body." The Antoni B area is composed of myxomatous tissue with less cellularity than the Antoni A area. Neurilemomas are treated by marginal excision without sacrificing the affected nerve. Neurilemomas should not recur.

Neurofibromas may arise as a solitary lesion or multiple lesions. The majority, maybe as many as 90%, are solitary and are not characteristic of von Recklinghausen disease. They may arise in the skin or be associated with a recognizable peripheral nerve. Like neurilemomas, they usually present as a painless mass with a Tinel sign. Unlike neurilemomas, they tend to be intimately associated with the nerve fibers. Fortunately, most arise from small cutaneous nerves and can be removed without loss of nerve function. Histologically, neurofibromas are not encapsulated and invade the nerve fibers and, rarely, the adjacent soft tissue. The cells are elongated, wavy, and have dark-staining nuclei. There is a collagen matrix composed of stringy-appearing fibers. Neurites usually are seen within the lesion. Surgical resection is recommended for those lesions that are solitary and not associated with a major nerve. Lesions arising from a major nerve can be resected, but the nerve fascicles must be split and the neurofibroma removed from between them. Neither solitary neurilemoma nor neurofibroma has a sig-

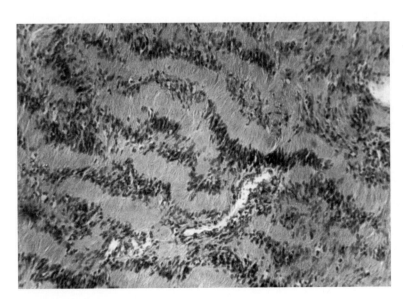

FIGURE 14-34. Histologic appearance of a neurilemoma (Antoni A area). The nuclei are stacked, giving the lesion a palisaded appearance. (Original magnification ×10.)

nificant incidence of malignant degeneration, although patients with neurofibromatosis have a small risk of developing neurofibrosarcoma.

Rhabdomyosarcoma

Rhabdomyosarcoma is a malignant tumor of muscle (3,246,464–466). It was once thought to occur in adults and children with almost equal frequency, but, since the middle 1970s, most of the adult tumors once called rhabdomyosarcoma have been reclassified as malignant fibrous histiocytoma. Rhabdomyosarcoma is believed to be extremely rare in adults, but it is the most common malignant soft tissue tumor in patients younger than 15 years of age. It accounts for approximately 3.5% of children's malignancies, and there are approximately 350 new cases per year in the United States (246,467). There are four histologic patterns: embryonal, botryoid-type, alveolar, and pleomorphic (468–470).

Botryoid-type rhabdomyosarcoma is histologically identical to the embryonal pattern, but is considered a separate entity because of its gross appearance. A botryoid rhabdomyosarcoma is an embryonal cell type that involves a hollow viscus. Pleomorphic rhabdomyosarcoma is a histologic type seen in adults, and is the least common. Embryonal rhabdomyosarcoma is the most common type, and usually arises in the head, the neck, the genitourinary tract, and the retroperitoneum. It is rare in the extremities. Botryoid rhabdomyosarcoma tends to occur in the first decade of life. The current treatment is a combination of chemotherapy, surgery, and, if not totally excised, irradiation. When chemotherapy is given preoperatively, the surgery required is less radical, and adequate surgical margins are more easily achieved.

Alveolar rhabdomyosarcoma is more common in the extremities than in the trunk, and is seen in older children and young adults usually between 10 and 25 years of age (227,246,471–476). The patient presents with a rapidly growing, painless mass deep within the muscle. This occurs with equal frequency in the upper and lower extremities. There are no clinical or laboratory findings that distinguish rhabdomyosarcoma from other soft tissue tumors.

Characteristic chromosomal abnormalities have been identified in the alveolar subtype (5,477–479). Approximately 70% of the tumors will have a translocation between chromosome 13 and chromosome 2, whereas another 30% will have the translocation between chromosome 13 and chromosome 1. Prognostic variables include histologic subtype, size of the tumor, site of the tumor, and age of the patient (480–483). Alveolar subtype, larger tumors, patients older than 10 years of age, and extremity location are associated with a poor prognosis. Therefore, the patients that the orthopaedist treats tend to do worse than those treated by the urologist and the otolaryngologist. Alveolar rhabdomyosarcoma, like the other subtypes, is treated with

a combination of chemotherapy and surgery (226,227, 246,484–488). Irradiation can be used if total surgical resection cannot be achieved without excessive morbidity. If the lesion is small it should be totally resected initially. Unlike in rhabdomyosarcoma at other sites, preoperative chemotherapy should be considered, because this often makes total resection of an extremity lesion possible when it was not possible before chemotherapy. A wide surgical margin is recommended (230,487,489–491). Unless the patient has palpable regional lymph node enlargement, biopsy of the lymph nodes is not necessary. Preoperative irradiation is reserved for lesions that would require an amputation to obtain a wide margin. Postoperative irradiation is used when no preoperative irradiation was given and the surgical margins are positive for tumor (486,492–494). Survival is related to stage, but the overall survival for a patient with extremity rhabdomyosarcoma is approximately 60% (3,464,481,485,486,495,496).

The histologic appearance of embryonal rhabdomyosarcoma can vary (473,475). This lesion consists of poorly differentiated rhabdomyoblasts with limited collagen matrix. The rhabdomyoblasts are small, round-to-oval cells with dark-staining nuclei and limited amounts of eosinophilic cytoplasm. Cross-striations are not seen regularly. Alveolar rhabdomyosarcoma is composed of small, round-to-oval tumor cells loosely arranged together in groups by dense collagen bundles. This arrangement of cells in groups produces an alveolar appearance; hence the name.

The Intergroup Rhabdomyosarcoma Committee, with representation from both the Pediatric Oncology Group and the Children's Cancer Study Group, has been the dominant group treating rhabdomyosarcoma in the United States. Their management and cooperative efforts have resulted in major advances in the management of this malignancy (230). Their staging system for patients with rhabdomyosarcoma is currently in use (474,476,483,497) (Table 14-5).

Synovial Cell Sarcoma

Synovial cell sarcoma is a malignant tumor of soft tissue whose cellular characteristics suggest that the tumor arises from primitive synovial cells, but it rarely occurs within a joint (233,457). Unlike other soft tissue sarcomas, synovial cell sarcomas occur frequently in the hand and foot (498). They usually are in the deep soft tissues near a joint. These tumors account for 10% of all soft tissue sarcomas (457). Most patients are between 15 and 35 years of age, and males predominate slightly. Patients with synovial cell sarcoma often complain of pain before they have palpable masses, and many patients give a history of having complained of pain for 2 to 4 years before the lesion was found. Synovial cell sarcoma, although rare, may be the explanation for persistent pain in a young patient (454,499–502).

The usual physical finding is the firm, slightly tender

TABLE 14-5. INTERGROUP RHABDOMYOSARCOMA STAGING SYSTEM

Stage	Site	Size	Nodes	Metastases
1	Orbit Head and neck Genitourinary (not bladder or prostate)	Any	Any	None
2	Bladder and prostate Extremity Cranial parameningeal Other	≤5 cm	None or unknown	None
3	Bladder and prostate Extremity Cranial parameningeal Other	≤5 cm ≥5 cm	Clinically involved Any	None None
4	All	Any	Any	Present

mass. Up to 25% of these patients have metastasis to regional lymph nodes, and the lymph nodes should be examined carefully (503). The patient's blood and urine laboratory values are normal.

The lesion occurs in all parts of the body. The head, the neck, and the trunk account for approximately 15% of the lesions, whereas the upper and lower extremities account for more than 50% of them. Almost 10% of the lesions arise in the hands or feet.

Synovial cell sarcomas may have calcifications or ossifications within the tumor, and these often are seen on plain radiographs. The radiodensities are usually very small. Small, irregular calcific foci, or irregular ossification within a soft tissue tumor should suggest the diagnosis of synovial cell sarcoma. The CT scan demonstrates a soft tissue mass, with these calcified densities deep within the tumor. Although the small foci of calcification or mineralization are not seen as well with MRI as with CT, MRI is preferred over CT as the staging test (504). This is true for all soft tissue masses. Neurofibrosarcoma and fibrosarcoma also can have intralesional calcification, but synovial cell sarcoma is the most common tumor with intralesional densities.

The characteristic histologic findings are of a biphasic tumor with areas of epithelioid or glandular appearance mixed with areas having spindle cell appearance (457). Usually the spindle cell component predominates (Fig. 14-35). Some synovial cell sarcomas have only the spindle cell component and are called monophasic synovial cell sarcomas. There seem to be no clinically significant differences between the two types. Mitoses are usually present, but the tumor is more difficult to grade histologically than other soft tissue sarcomas. Synovial cell sarcoma is almost always a high-grade soft tissue sarcoma.

Surgical resection is, and has been, the principal treatment of synovial cell sarcoma (499–502,505–510). Adju-

vant chemotherapy is used, but the data regarding the efficacy in synovial cell sarcoma are equivocal at best (500, 509,511,512). In adults and older children with synovial cell sarcoma, as in those with other soft tissue sarcomas, preoperative radiotherapy is used in conjunction with nonradical surgery in an attempt to salvage more extremities. Approximately 15% of synovial sarcomas occur in the feet (498). It was believed that the scarring from irradiation precluded its use in the feet and hands, but with modern techniques adjuvant irradiation and marginal resection can be performed in the majority of sarcomas of the feet or hands with preservation of a functioning extremity. Preoperative irradiation and surgery are recommended for most soft tissue sarcomas of the feet. This has been successful in saving extremities and controlling the disease locally, but the incidence of metastatic disease remains high, at slightly more than 50% (233,455,500,501,505,508,512,513).

Benign Synovial Tumors

There are only two neoplasias that arise from the synovial lining of a joint. Synovial cell sarcoma has been reported to have arisen from within a joint, but this is decidedly rare, and the majority of synovial sarcomas arise within periarticular soft tissues and do not invade joints. Synovial chondromatosis and pigmented villonodular synovitis arise from synovial tissue and are found in joints, bursa, and tendon sheaths. They are the only two neoplasias that commonly occur in the joint.

Synovial Chondromatosis. Synovial chondromatosis is a disorder of the synovial tissues (457). It is most common in the knee but can arise in any joint, tendon sheath, or bursa. Its cause is unknown, and it has no recognized familial pattern of occurrence. The subliminal lining of the joint

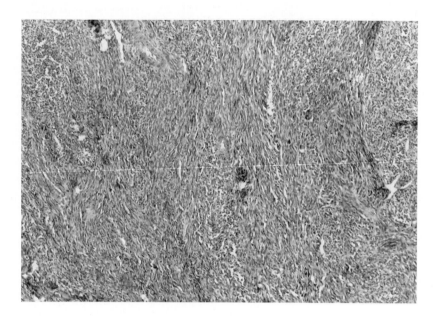

FIGURE 14-35. Low-power view of the spindle component of a synovial cell sarcoma. This lesion is composed of malignant spindle cells with a minimal amount of matrix. At a higher power, mitotic figures are seen. Other areas of this tumor have a glandular appearance, which is the reason that this synovial cell sarcoma is a biphasic tumor. (Original magnification ×10.)

produces small nodules of hyaline-appearing cartilage that are extruded from the synovial lining to become loose bodies within the joint (Fig. 14-36). The cartilage may become necrotic if they become large, or they may undergo enchondral ossification if they have a blood supply. In both cases, they can be seen on plain radiographs. Without the calcification or the ossification, the cartilage is radiolucent and not visible on routine radiographs.

The disease is rare in children, and presents most commonly between the ages of 20 and 50 years. The most common joint involved is the knee, with the elbow next in frequency, and the hip third. The patient usually presents with mild discomfort, minimal loss of motion, and a joint effusion. There may be a history of locking. The knee may appear normal on examination, but usually there is a moderate-to-large effusion, limited motion, and a boggy synovium. The plain radiographs show nothing abnormal or small intraarticular calcified bodies. The arthrogram is diagnostic with an irregular synovial surface and normal-to-thinned synovial fluid. The MRI scan is usually diagnostic.

Most patients have sufficient symptoms and require removal of loose bodies. Usually synovectomy is performed, but recurrence is common as the synovial lining is regenerated (514). The process seems to have a limited natural

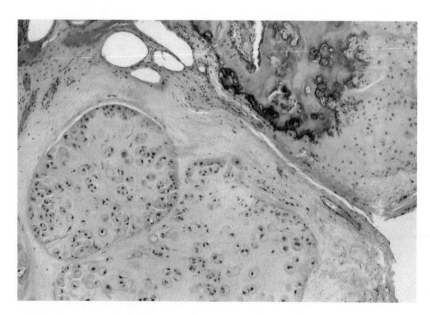

FIGURE 14-36. Low-power view of synovial chondromatosis. The nodules of cartilage are formed within the synovial lining and extruded into the joint to produce loose bodies. The nodules can undergo enchondral ossification if they have a blood supply **(top right)**.

history, and the production of new loose bodies ceases after 1 or 2 years.

Pigmented Villonodular Synovitis. Pigmented villonodular synovitis (PVNS) is a rare disorder of the synovial tissues that may be a true neoplasia, although it has been suggested that it is caused by an infectious process (457,515). The synovial lining becomes proliferative and hypertrophic. It can involve a joint (most commonly the knee) or a tendon sheath. When tendon sheaths are involved, PVNS usually occurs in the hand or the foot. The patient presents with a swollen joint that is usually painless. The synovial tissue is boggy on examination. The joint fluid has old, dark blood in it, and it is common for the diagnosis to be suspected first when the joint is aspirated just before the injection of contrast material for arthrography. The arthrogram or MRI scan is diagnostic, with a thickened shaggy lining and demonstration of dark pigment signal on MRI (516).

The majority of the patients with PVNS are between 20 and 40 years of age (515). The plain radiograph is usually normal except for the soft tissue swelling, but occasionally the proliferative synovial tissues invade the bones adjacent to the joint. This happens most frequently when the hip joint is involved. MRI is the best radiographic method to evaluate the extent of the lesion. Bone invasion can be appreciated, as can the extent of enlargement of the synovial cavity. Synovectomy is the treatment of choice, but there is a high incidence of recurrence (approximately 50%) (515). Intraarticular injection of radioactive materials (dysprosium or yttrium) has been used successfully as a means of controlling recurrent disease. Some patients have minimal symptoms with their recurrence and accept the chronic swelling. As long as the bones remain uninvolved, there is no absolute indication for surgical removal. Patients are followed with clinical examination and plain radiography. For patients with diffuse involvement, recurrence is common (more than 75%), but most have no or little progression or symptoms and do not need treatment.

References

Molecular Biology of Tumors

1. Fletcher JA, Gebhardt MC, Kozakewich HP. Cytogenetic aberrations in osteosarcomas: nonrandom deletions, rings, and double-minute chromosomes. *Cancer Genet Cytogenet* 1994;77:81.
2. Bridge JA, Nelson M, McComb E, et al. Cytogenetic findings in 73 osteosarcoma specimens and a review of the literature. *Cancer Genet Cytogenet* 1997;95:74.
3. Arndt CA, Crist WM. Common musculoskeletal tumors of childhood and adolescence. *N Engl J Med* 1999;341:342.
4. Fletcher JA, Kozakewich HP, Hoffer FA, et al. Diagnostic relevance of clonal cytogenetic aberrations in malignant soft-tissue tumors. *N Engl J Med* 1991;324:436.
5. Barr FG, Chatten J, D'Cruz CM, et al. Molecular assays for chromosomal translocations in the diagnosis of pediatric soft tissue sarcomas. *JAMA* 1995;273:553.
6. Kumar S, Pack S, Kumar D, et al. Detection of EWS-FLI-1 fusion in Ewing's sarcoma/peripheral primitive neuroectodermal tumor by fluorescence in situ hybridization using formalin-fixed paraffin-embedded tissue. *Hum Pathol* 1999;30:324.
7. Dehner LP. Primitive neuroectodermal tumor and Ewing's sarcoma. *Am J Surg Pathol* 1993;17:1.
8. Navarro S, Cavazzana AO, Llombart-Bosch A, et al. Comparison of Ewing's sarcoma of bone and peripheral neuroepithelioma: an immunocytochemical and ultrastructural analysis of two primitive neuroectodermal neoplasms. *Arch Pathol Lab Med* 1994;118:608.
9. Schmidt D, Herrmann C, Jurgens H, et al. Malignant peripheral neuroectodermal tumor and its necessary distinction from Ewing's sarcoma: a report from the Kiel Pediatric Tumor Registry. *Cancer* 1991;68:2251.
10. Terrier P, Henry-Amar M, Triche TJ, et al. Is neuro-ectodermal differentiation of Ewing's sarcoma of bone associated with an unfavourable prognosis? *Eur J Cancer* 1995;31A:307.
11. Hartman KR, Triche TJ, Kinsella TJ, et al. Prognostic value of histopathology in Ewing's sarcoma: long-term follow-up of distal extremity primary tumors. *Cancer* 1991;67:163.
12. West DC, Grier HE, Swallow MM, et al. Detection of circulating tumor cells in patients with Ewing's sarcoma and peripheral primitive neuroectodermal tumor. *J Clin Oncol* 1997;15:583.
13. Gebhardt MC. Molecular biology of sarcomas. *Orthop Clin North Am* 1996;27:421.
14. Hansen MF. Molecular genetic considerations in osteosarcoma. *Clin Orthop* 1991:237.
15. Varmus J, Weinberg R. *Genes and the biology of cancer.* New York: Scientific American Library, 1993:67.
16. Cavenee WK, Koufos A, Hansen MF. Recessive mutant genes predisposing to human cancer. *Mutat Res* 1986;168:3.
17. Hatakeyama M, Herrera RA, Makela T, et al. The cancer cell and the cell cycle clock. *Cold Spring Harbor Symp Quant Biol* 1994;59:1.
18. Hinds PW, Weinberg RA. Tumor suppressor genes. *Curr Opin Genet Dev* 1994;4:135.
19. Weinberg RA. Tumor suppressor genes. *Science* 1991;254:1138.
20. Weinberg RA. The molecular basis of oncogenes and tumor suppressor genes. *Ann NY Acad Sci* 1995;758:331.
21. Dryja TP, Friend S, Weinberg RA. Genetic sequences that predispose to retinoblastoma and osteosarcoma. *Symp Fundam Cancer Res* 1986;39:115.
22. Friend SH, Bernards R, Rogelj S, et al. A human DNA segment with properties of the gene that predisposes to retinoblastoma and osteosarcoma. *Nature* 1986;323:643.
23. Hung J, Anderson R. p53: functions, mutations and sarcomas. *Acta Orthop Scand Suppl* 1997;273:68.
24. Lane DP. Cancer: p53, guardian of the genome. *Nature* 1992; 358:15.
25. Miller C, Koeffler HP. P53 mutations in human cancer. *Leukemia* 1993;7(Suppl 2):S18.
26. Link M, Eilber F. Osteosarcoma. In: Pizzo P, Poplack D, eds. *Principles and practice of pediatric oncology.* Philadelphia: JB Lippincott, 1997:889.
27. Ding HF, Fisher DE. Mechanisms of p53-mediated apoptosis. *Crit Rev Oncol* 1998;9:83.
28. Fisher DE. Apoptosis in cancer therapy: crossing the threshold. *Cell* 1994;78:539.
29. Lowe SW, Bodis S, Bardeesy N, et al. Apoptosis and the prognostic significance of p53 mutation. *Cold Spring Harbor Symp Quant Biol* 1994;59:419.
30. Ueda Y, Dockhorn-Dworniczak B, Blasius S, et al. Analysis of mutant P53 protein in osteosarcomas and other malignant and benign lesions of bone. *J Cancer Res Clin Oncol* 1993;119:172.
31. Andreassen A, Oyjord T, Hovig E, et al. p53 abnormalities in different subtypes of human sarcomas. *Cancer Res* 1993;53:468.

32. Lonardo F, Ueda T, Huvos AG, et al. p53 and MDM2 alterations in osteosarcomas: correlation with clinicopathologic features and proliferative rate. *Cancer* 1997;79:1541.

33. Smith-Sorensen B, Gebhardt MC, Kloen P, et al. Screening for TP53 mutations in osteosarcomas using constant denaturant gel electrophoresis (CDGE). *Hum Mutat* 1993;2:274.

34. Diller L, Kassel J, Nelson CE, et al. p53 functions as a cell cycle control protein in osteosarcomas. *Mol Cell Biol* 1990;10:5772.

35. Toguchida J, Yamaguchi T, Ritchie B, et al. Mutation spectrum of the p53 gene in bone and soft tissue sarcomas. *Cancer Res* 1992;52:6194.

36. Miller CW, Aslo A, Won A, et al. Alterations of the p53, Rb and MDM2 genes in osteosarcoma. *J Cancer Res Clin Oncol* 1996;122:559.

37. Miller CW, Aslo A, Tsay C, et al. Frequency and structure of p53 rearrangements in human osteosarcoma. *Cancer Res* 1990; 50:7950.

38. Masuda H, Miller C, Koeffler HP, et al. Rearrangement of the p53 gene in human osteogenic sarcomas. *Proc Natl Acad Sci USA* 1987;84:7716.

39. Mulligan LM, Matlashewski GJ, Scrable HJ, et al. Mechanisms of p53 loss in human sarcomas. *Proc Natl Acad Sci USA* 1990; 87:5863.

40. Abudu A, Mangham DC, Reynolds GM, et al. Overexpression of p53 protein in primary Ewing's sarcoma of bone: relationship to tumour stage, response and prognosis. *Br J Cancer* 1999;79: 1185.

41. Yamaguchi T, Toguchida J, Yamamuro T, et al. Allelotype analysis in osteosarcomas: frequent allele loss on 3q, 13q, 17p, and 18q. *Cancer Res* 1992;52:2419.

42. Chen J, Lin J, Levine AJ. Regulation of transcription functions of the p53 tumor suppressor by the mdm-2 oncogene. *Mol Med* 1995;1:142.

43. Chen J, Wu X, Lin J, et al. mdm-2 inhibits the G1 arrest and apoptosis functions of the p53 tumor suppressor protein. *Mol Cell Biol* 1996;16:2445.

44. Ladanyi M, Cha C, Lewis R, et al. MDM2 gene amplification in metastatic osteosarcoma. *Cancer Res* 1993;53:16.

45. Cordon-Cardo C, Latres E, Drobnjak M, et al. Molecular abnormalities of mdm2 and p53 genes in adult soft tissue sarcomas. *Cancer Res* 1994;54:794.

46. Porter DE, Holden ST, Steel CM, et al. A significant proportion of patients with osteosarcoma may belong to Li-Fraumeni cancer families. *J Bone Joint Surg Br* 1992;74:883.

47. Birch JM, Hartley AL, Blair V, et al. Cancer in the families of children with soft tissue sarcoma. *Cancer* 1990;66:2239.

48. Toguchida J, Yamaguchi T, Dayton SH, et al. Prevalence and spectrum of germline mutations of the p53 gene among patients with sarcoma. *N Engl J Med* 1992;326:1301.

49. Diller L, Sexsmith E, Gottlieb A, et al. Germline p53 mutations are frequently detected in young children with rhabdomyosarcoma. *J Clin Invest* 1995;95:1606.

50. Li FP, Fraumeni JF Jr. Prospective study of a family cancer syndrome. *JAMA* 1982;247:2692.

51. Malkin D. p53 and the Li-Fraumeni syndrome. *Cancer Genet Cytogenet* 1993;66:83.

52. Malkin D, Li FP, Strong LC, et al. Germ line p53 mutations in a familial syndrome of breast cancer, sarcomas, and other neoplasms. *Science* 1990;250:1233.

53. Knudson AG. Antiongenes and human cancer. *Proc Natl Acad Sci USA* 1993;90:10914.

54. McIntyre JF, Smith-Sorensen B, Friend SH, et al. Germline mutations of the p53 tumor suppressor gene in children with osteosarcoma. *J Clin Oncol* 1994;12:925.

55. Kartner N, Ling V. Multidrug resistance in cancer. *Sci Am* 1989; 260:44.

56. Kuttesch JF Jr. Multidrug resistance in pediatric oncology. *Invest New Drugs* 1996;14:55.

57. Chan HS, Grogan TM, Haddad G, et al. P-glycoprotein expression: critical determinant in the response to osteosarcoma chemotherapy. *J Natl Cancer Inst* 1997;89:1706.

58. Chan HS, Grogan TM, DeBoer G, et al. Diagnosis and reversal of multidrug resistance in paediatric cancers. *Eur J Cancer* 1996; 32A:1051.

59. Vergier B, Cany L, Bonnet F, et al. Expression of MDR1/P glycoprotein in human sarcomas. *Br J Cancer* 1993;68:1221.

60. Kusuzaki K, Hirata M, Takeshita H, et al. Relationship between P-glycoprotein positivity, doxorubicin binding ability and histologic response to chemotherapy in osteosarcomas. *Cancer Lett* 1999;138:203.

61. Serra M, Scotlandi K, Manara MC, et al. Analysis of P-glycoprotein expression in osteosarcoma. *Eur J Cancer* 1995;31A:1998.

62. Suto R, Abe Y, Nakamura M, et al. Multidrug resistance mediated by overexpression of P-glycoprotein in human osteosarcoma *in vivo*. *Int J Oncol* 1998;12:287.

63. Scotlandi K, Serra M, Nicoletti G, et al. Multidrug resistance and malignancy in human osteosarcoma. *Cancer Res* 1996;56: 2434.

64. Stein U, Walther W, Wunderlich V. Point mutations in the mdr1 promoter of human osteosarcomas are associated with *in vitro* responsiveness to multidrug resistance relevant drugs. *Eur J Cancer* 1994;30A:1541.

65. Stein U, Wunderlich V, Haensch W, et al. Expression of the mdr1 gene in bone and soft tissue sarcomas of adult patients. *Eur J Cancer* 1993;29A:1979.

66. Baldini N, Scotlandi K, Barbanti-Brodano G, et al. Expression of P-glycoprotein in high-grade osteosarcomas in relation to clinical outcome. *N Engl J Med* 1995;333:1380.

Evaluation

67. Enneking W. *Musculoskeletal tumor surgery.* New York: Churchill Livingstone, 1983.

68. Bacci G, Dallari D, Battistini A, et al. The prognostic value of serum alkaline phosphatase in osteosarcoma of the limbs. *Chir Organi Mov* 1992;77:171.

69. Link MP, Goorin AM, Horowitz M, et al. Adjuvant chemotherapy of high grade osteosarcoma of the extremity. *Clin Orthop Relat Res* 1991;270:8.

70. Luksch R, Sampietro G, Collini P, et al. Prognostic value of clinicopathologic characteristics including neuroectodermal differentiation in osseous Ewing's sarcoma family of tumors in children. *Tumori* 1999;85:101.

71. Glaubiger DL, Makuch RW, Schwarz J. Influence of prognostic factors on survival in Ewing's sarcoma. *Natl Cancer Inst Monogr* 1981:285.

72. Parker BR, Pinckney L, Etcubanas E. Relative efficacy of radiographic and radionuclide bone surveys in the detection of the skeletal lesions of histiocytosis X. *Radiology* 1980;134:377.

73. Siddiqui AR, Tashjian JH, Lazarus K, et al. Nuclear medicine studies in evaluation of skeletal lesions in children with histiocytosis X. *Radiology* 1981;140:787.

74. Woolfenden JM, Pitt MJ, Durie BG, et al. Comparison of bone scintigraphy and radiography in multiple myeloma. *Radiology* 1980;134:723.

75. Kirchner PT, Simon MA. The clinical value of bone and gallium scintigraphy for soft-tissue sarcomas of the extremities. *J Bone Joint Surg Am* 1984;66:319.

76. Simon MA, Kirchner PT. Scintigraphic evaluation of primary bone tumors: comparison of technetium-99m phosphonate and gallium citrate imaging. *J Bone Joint Surg Am* 1980;62:758.

77. Imbriaco M, Yeh SD, Yeung H, et al. Thallium-201 scintigra-

phy for the evaluation of tumor response to preoperative chemotherapy in patients with osteosarcoma. *Cancer* 1997;80:1507.

78. Ramanna L, Waxman A, Binney G, et al. Thallium-201 scintigraphy in bone sarcoma: comparison with gallium-67 and technetium-MDP in the evaluation of chemotherapeutic response. *J Nucl Med* 1990;31:567.

79. Leskinen S, Lapela M, Lindholm P, et al. Metabolic imaging by positron emission tomography in oncology. *Ann Med* 1997;29:271.

80. Jaramillo D, Laor T, Gebhardt MC. Pediatric musculoskeletal neoplasms: evaluation with MR imaging. *Magn Reson Imaging Clin North Am* 1996;4:749.

81. Russell WO, Cohen J, Enzinger F, et al. A clinical and pathological staging system for soft tissue sarcomas. *Cancer* 1977;40:1562.

82. Suit HD, Mankin HJ, Wood WC, et al. Treatment of the patient with stage M0 soft tissue sarcoma. *J Clin Oncol* 1988;6:854.

83. Peabody TD, Gibbs CP Jr, Simon MA. Evaluation and staging of musculoskeletal neoplasms. *J Bone Joint Surg Am* 1998;80:1204.

84. Enneking WF, Spanier SS, Goodman MA. A system for the surgical staging of musculoskeletal sarcoma. *Clin Orthop Relat Res* 1980;153:106.

85. Mankin HJ, Lange TA, Spanier S. The hazards of biopsy in patients with malignant primary bone and soft-tissue tumors. *J Bone Joint Surg Am* 1982;64:1121.

86. Mankin HJ, Mankin CJ, Simon MA. The hazards of the biopsy, revisited. Members of the Musculoskeletal Tumor Society. *J Bone Joint Surg Am* 1996;78:656.

87. Simon MA, Biermann JS. Biopsy of bone and soft-tissue lesions. *J Bone Joint Surg Am* 1993;75:616.

88. Akerman M, Rydholm A, Persson BM. Aspiration cytology of soft-tissue tumors: the 10-year experience at an orthopedic oncology center. *Acta Orthop Scand* 1985;56:407.

89. Ball AB, Fisher C, Pittam M, et al. Diagnosis of soft tissue tumours by Tru-Cut biopsy. *Br J Surg* 1990;77:756.

90. Ghelman B, Lospinuso MF, Levine DB, et al. Percutaneous computed-tomography-guided biopsy of the thoracic and lumbar spine. *Spine* 1991;16:736.

91. Kissin MW, Fisher C, Carter RL, et al. Value of Tru-Cut biopsy in the diagnosis of soft tissue tumours. *Br J Surg* 1986;73:742.

Specific Bone Tumors

92. Jaffe H. "Osteoid osteoma": a benign osteoblastic tumor composed of osteoid and atypical bone. *Arch Surg* 1935;31:709.

93. Unni K. *Dahlin's bone tumors: general aspects and data on 11,087 cases.* Philadelphia: Lippincott-Raven, 1996:143.

94. Keim HA, Reina EG. Osteoid-osteoma as a cause of scoliosis. *J Bone Joint Surg Am* 1975;57:159.

95. Freiberger R. Osteoid osteoma of the spine: a cause of backache and scoliosis in children. *Radiology* 1960;75:232.

96. Smith FW, Gilday DL. Scintigraphic appearances of osteoid osteoma. *Radiology* 1980;137:191.

97. Herrlin K, Ekelund L, Lovdahl R, et al. Computed tomography in suspected osteoid osteomas of tubular bones. *Skeletal Radiol* 1982;9:92.

98. Golding J. The natural history of osteoma with a report of twenty cases. *J Bone Joint Surg Br* 1954;36:218.

99. Kneisl JS, Simon MA. Medical management compared with operative treatment for osteoid-osteoma. *J Bone Joint Surg Am* 1992;74:179.

100. Norman A. Persistence or recurrence of pain: a sign of surgical failure in osteoid-osteoma. *Clin Orthop* 1978:263.

101. Ayala AG, Murray JA, Erling MA, et al. Osteoid-osteoma: intra-operative tetracycline-fluorescence demonstration of the nidus. *J Bone Joint Surg Am* 1986;68:747.

102. Ghelman B, Thompson FM, Arnold WD. Intraoperative radioactive localization of an osteoid-osteoma: case report. *J Bone Joint Surg Am* 1981;63:826.

103. Gore DR, Mueller HA. Osteoid-osteoma of the spine with localization aided by 99 mTc-polyphosphate bone scan: case report. *Clin Orthop* 1975:132.

104. Rinsky LA, Goris M, Bleck EE, et al. Intraoperative skeletal scintigraphy for localization of osteoid-osteoma in the spine: case report. *J Bone Joint Surg Am* 1980;62:143.

105. Tillotson CL, Rosenberg AE, Rosenthal DI. Controlled thermal injury of bone: report of a percutaneous technique using radiofrequency electrode and generator. *Invest Radiol* 1989;24:888.

106. Rosenthal DI, Alexander A, Rosenberg AE, et al. Ablation of osteoid osteomas with a percutaneously placed electrode: a new procedure. *Radiology* 1992;183:29.

107. Rosenthal DI, Hornicek FJ, Wolfe MW, et al. Percutaneous radiofrequency coagulation of osteoid osteoma compared with operative treatment. *J Bone Joint Surg Am* 1998;80:815.

108. Voto SJ, Cook AJ, Weiner DS, et al. Treatment of osteoid osteoma by computed tomography guided excision in the pediatric patient. *J Pediatr Orthop* 1990;10:510.

109. Schajowicz F, Lemos C. Malignant osteoblastoma. *J Bone Joint Surg Br* 1976;58:202.

110. Picci P, Sangiorgi L, Rougraff BT, et al. Relationship of chemotherapy-induced necrosis and surgical margins to local recurrence in osteosarcoma. *J Clin Oncol* 1994;12:2699.

111. Picci P, Bohling T, Bacci G, et al. Chemotherapy-induced tumor necrosis as a prognostic factor in localized Ewing's sarcoma of the extremities. *J Clin Oncol* 1997;15:1553.

112. Souhami RL, Craft AW, Van der Eijken JW, et al. Randomized trial of two regimens of chemotherapy in operable osteosarcoma: a study of the European Osteosarcoma Intergroup. *Lancet* 1997;350:911.

113. Bramwell VH. The role of chemotherapy in the management of non-metastatic operable extremity osteosarcoma. *Semin Oncol* 1997;24:561.

114. Provisor AJ, Ettinger LJ, Nachman JB, et al. Treatment of non-metastatic osteosarcoma of the extremity with preoperative and postoperative chemotherapy: a report from the Children's Cancer Group. *J Clin Oncol* 1997;15:76.

115. Bacci G, Ferrari S, Mercuri M, et al. Neoadjuvant chemotherapy for extremity osteosarcoma: preliminary results of the Rizzoli's 4th study. *Acta Oncol* 1998;37:41.

116. Bacci G, Ferrari S, Donati D, et al. Neoadjuvant chemotherapy for osteosarcoma of the extremity in patients in the fourth and fifth decade of life. *Oncol Rep* 1998;5:1259.

117. Link MP, Goorin AM, Horowitz M, et al. Adjuvant chemotherapy of high-grade osteosarcoma of the extremity: updated results of the Multi-Institutional Osteosarcoma Study. *Clin Orthop* 1991:8.

118. Link MP, Goorin AM, Miser AW, et al. The effect of adjuvant chemotherapy on relapse-free survival in patients with osteosarcoma of the extremity. *N Engl J Med* 1986;314:1600.

119. Uchida A, Myoui A, Araki N, et al. Neoadjuvant chemotherapy for pediatric osteosarcoma patients. *Cancer* 1997;79:411.

120. Eilber F, Giuliano A, Eckardt J, et al. Adjuvant chemotherapy for osteosarcoma: a randomized prospective trial. *J Clin Oncol* 1987;5:21.

121. Goorin AM, Andersen JW. Experience with multiagent chemotherapy for osteosarcoma: improved outcome. *Clin Orthop* 1991:22.

122. Meyer WH, Malawer MM. Osteosarcoma: clinical features and evolving surgical and chemotherapeutic strategies. *Pediatr Clin North Am* 1991;38:317.

123. Bacci G, Ferrari S, Mercuri M, et al. Predictive factors for local recurrence in osteosarcoma: 540 patients with extremity tumors followed for minimum 2.5 years after neoadjuvant chemotherapy. *Acta Orthop Scand* 1998;69:230.

124. Gherlinzoni F, Picci P, Bacci G, et al. Limb sparing versus amputation in osteosarcoma: correlation between local control, surgical margins and tumor necrosis. Istituto Rizzoli experience. *Ann Oncol* 1992;3(Suppl 2):S23.

125. Rougraff BT, Simon MA, Kneisl JS, et al. Limb salvage compared with amputation for osteosarcoma of the distal end of the femur: a long-term oncological, functional, and quality-of-life study. *J Bone Joint Surg Am* 1994;76:649.

126. Springfield DS, Schmidt R, Graham-Pole J, et al. Surgical treatment for osteosarcoma. *J Bone Joint Surg Am* 1988;70:1124.

127. Scully SP, Temple HT, O'Keefe RJ, et al. The surgical treatment of patients with osteosarcoma who sustain a pathologic fracture. *Clin Orthop* 1996:227.

128. Jaffe N, Spears R, Eftekari F. Pathological fracture in osteosarcoma: impact of chemotherapy on primary tumor and survival. *Cancer* 1987;59:701.

129. Abudu A, Sferopoulos NK, Tillman RM, et al. The surgical treatment and outcome of pathological fractures in localised osteosarcoma. *J Bone Joint Surg Br* 1996;78:694.

130. Pochanugool L, Subhadharaphandou T, Dhanachai M, et al. Prognostic factors among 130 patients with osteosarcoma. *Clin Orthop* 1997:206.

131. Finn HA, Simon MA. Limb-salvage surgery in the treatment of osteosarcoma in skeletally immature individuals. *Clin Orthop* 1991:108.

132. Gonzalez-Herranz P, Burgos-Flores J, Ocete-Guzman JG, et al. The management of limb-length discrepancies in children after treatment of osteosarcoma and Ewing's sarcoma. *J Pediatr Orthop* 1995;15:561.

133. Ward WG, Yang RS, Eckardt JJ. Endoprosthetic bone reconstruction following malignant tumor resection in skeletally immature patients. *Orthop Clin North Am* 1996;27:493.

134. Moseley CF. Management of leg-length disparities after tumor surgery (Editorial). *J Pediatr Orthop* 1995;15:559.

135. Rao BN, Champion JE, Pratt CB, et al. Limb salvage procedures for children with osteosarcoma: an alternative to amputation. *J Pediatr Surg* 1983;18:901.

136. Hanlon M, Krajbich JI. Rotationplasty in skeletally immature patients: long-term followup results. *Clin Orthop* 1999:75.

137. Merkel KD, Gebhardt M, Springfield DS. Rotationplasty as a reconstructive operation after tumor resection. *Clin Orthop* 1991:231.

138. Kotz R. Rotationplasty. *Semin Surg Oncol* 1997;13:34.

139. Steenhoff JR, Daanen HA, Taminiau AH. Functional analysis of patients who have had a modified Van Nes rotationplasty. *J Bone Joint Surg Am* 1993;75:1451.

140. Gottsauner-Wolf F, Kotz R, Knahr K, et al. Rotationplasty for limb salvage in the treatment of malignant tumors at the knee: a follow-up study of seventy patients. *J Bone Joint Surg Am* 1991;73:1365.

141. Winkelmann WW. Hip rotationplasty for malignant tumors of the proximal part of the femur. *J Bone Joint Surg Am* 1986;68:362.

142. Murray MP, Jacobs PA, Gore DR, et al. Functional performance after tibial rotationplasty. *J Bone Joint Surg Am* 1985;67:392.

143. Kotz R, Salzer M. Rotation-plasty for childhood osteosarcoma of the distal part of the femur. *J Bone Joint Surg Am* 1982;64:959.

144. Catani F, Capanna R, Benedetti MG, et al. Gait analysis in patients after Van Nes rotationplasty. *Clin Orthop* 1993:270.

145. Cammisa FP Jr, Glasser DB, Otis JC, et al. The Van Nes tibial rotationplasty: a functionally viable reconstructive procedure in children who have a tumor of the distal end of the femur. *J Bone Joint Surg Am* 1990;72:1541.

146. Heeg M, Torode IP. Rotationplasty of the lower limb for childhood osteosarcoma of the femur. *Aust NZ J Surg* 1998;68:643.

147. Badhwar R, Agarwal M. Rotationplasty as a limb salvage procedure for malignant bone tumours. *Int Orthop* 1998;22:122.

148. Merkel KD, Reinus WR, Miller G, et al. Modification of the Van Nes rotationplasty: report of a case. *Clin Orthop* 1997:195.

149. Winkelmann WW. Rotationplasty. *Orthop Clin North Am* 1996;27:503.

150. Kawai A, Hamada M, Sugihara S, et al. Rotationplasty for patients with osteosarcoma around the knee joint. *Acta Med Okayama* 1995;49:221.

151. Capanna R, Del Ben M, Campanacci DA, et al. Rotationplasty in segmental resections of the femur. *Chir Organi Mov* 1992;77:135.

152. van der Windt DA, Pieterson I, van der Eijken JW, et al. Energy expenditure during walking in subjects with tibial rotationplasty, above-knee amputation, or hip disarticulation. *Arch Phys Med Rehabil* 1992;73:1174.

153. Krajbich JI. Modified Van Nes rotationplasty in the treatment of malignant neoplasms in the lower extremities of children. *Clin Orthop* 1991:74.

154. de Bari A, Krajbich JI, Langer F, et al. Modified Van Nes rotationplasty for osteosarcoma of the proximal tibia in children. *J Bone Joint Surg Br* 1990;72:1065.

155. Krajbich JI, Carroll NC. Van Nes rotationplasty with segmental limb resection. *Clin Orthop* 1990:7.

156. Schwartz HS, Frassica FJ, Sim FH. Rotationplasty: an option for limb salvage in childhood osteosarcoma. *Orthopedics* 1989;12:257.

157. Kenan S, Bloom N, Lewis MM. Limb-sparing surgery in skeletally immature patients with osteosarcoma. *Clin Orthop Relat Res* 1991;270:223.

158. Unwin PS, Walker PS. Extendible endoprosthesis for the skeletally immature. *Clin Orthop Relat Res* 1966;322:179.

159. Kenan S, Lewis MM. Limb salvage in pediatric surgery: the use of the expandable prosthesis. *Orthop Clin North Am* 1991;22:121.

160. Cool WP, Grimer RJ, Carter SR, et al. Longitudinal growth following a growing endoprosthesis replacement of the distal femur in the skeletally immature. In: *Eighth International Symposium on Limb Salvage (ISOLS), Florence, Italy, 1995*.

161. Schindler OS, Cannon SR, Briggs TW, et al. Use of extendable total femoral replacements in children with malignant bone tumors. *Clin Orthop* 1998:157.

162. Schiller C, Windhager R, Fellinger EJ, et al. Extendable tumour endoprostheses for the leg in children. *J Bone Joint Surg Br* 1995;77:608.

163. Schindler OS, Cannon SR, Briggs TW, et al. Stanmore custom-made extendible distal femoral replacements: clinical experience in children with primary malignant bone tumours. *J Bone Joint Surg Br* 1997;79:927; erratum 1998;80:562.

164. Verkerke GJ, Schraffordt Koops H, Veth RP, et al. First clinical experience with a noninvasive extendable endoprosthesis: a limb-saving procedure in children suffering from a malignant bone tumor. *Artif Organs* 1997;21:413.

165. Eckardt JJ, Safran MR, Eilber FR, et al. Expandable endoprosthetic reconstruction of the skeletally immature after malignant bone tumor resection. *Clin Orthop* 1993:188.

166. Geschickter C, Copeland M. Parosteal osteoma of bone: a new entity. *Ann Surg* 1951;133:790.

167. Campanacci M, Picci P, Gherlinzoni F, et al. Parosteal osteosarcoma. *J Bone Joint Surg Br* 1984;66:313.

168. Okada K, Frassica FJ, Sim FH, et al. Parosteal osteosarcoma: a clinicopathological study. *J Bone Joint Surg Am* 1994;76:366.

169. Schajowicz F, McGuire MH, Santini Araujo E, et al. Osteosarcomas arising on the surfaces of long bones. *J Bone Joint Surg Am* 1988;70:555.

170. Ahuja SC, Villacin AB, Smith J, et al. Juxtacortical (parosteal) osteogenic sarcoma: histological grading and prognosis. *J Bone Joint Surg Am* 1977;59:632.

171. Unni KK, Dahlin DC, Beabout JW, et al. Parosteal osteogenic sarcoma. *Cancer* 1976;37:2644.

172. Hudson TM, Springfield DS, Benjamin M, et al. Computed tomography of parosteal osteosarcoma. *Am J Roentgenol* 1985; 144:961.

173. Bertoni F, Present D, Hudson T, et al. The meaning of radiolucencies in parosteal osteosarcoma. *J Bone Joint Surg Am* 1985; 67:901.

174. Wold LE, Unni KK, Beabout JW, et al. Dedifferentiated parosteal osteosarcoma. *J Bone Joint Surg Am* 1984;66:53.

175. Shuhaibar H, Friedman L. Dedifferentiated parosteal osteosarcoma with high-grade osteoclast-rich osteogenic sarcoma at presentation. *Skeletal Radiol* 1998;27:574.

176. Wold LE, Unni KK, Beabout JW, et al. High-grade surface osteosarcomas. *Am J Surg Pathol* 1984;8:181.

177. Picci P, Campanacci M, Bacci G, et al. Medullary involvement in parosteal osteosarcoma: a case report. *J Bone Joint Surg Am* 1987;69:131.

178. Enneking WF, Springfield D, Gross M. The surgical treatment of parosteal osteosarcoma in long bones. *J Bone Joint Surg Am* 1985;67:125.

179. Sheth DS, Yasko AW, Raymond AK, et al. Conventional and dedifferentiated parosteal osteosarcoma: diagnosis, treatment, and outcome. *Cancer* 1996;78:2136.

180. Hall RB, Robinson LH, Malawar MM, et al. Periosteal osteosarcoma. *Cancer* 1985;55:165.

181. Ritts GD, Pritchard DJ, Unni KK, et al. Periosteal osteosarcoma. *Clin Orthop* 1987:299.

182. deSantos LA, Murray JA, Finklestein JB, et al. The radiographic spectrum of periosteal osteosarcoma. *Radiology* 1978;127:123.

183. Unni KK, Dahlin DC, Beabout JW. Periosteal osteogenic sarcoma. *Cancer* 1976;37:2476.

184. Simon MA, Bos GD. Epiphyseal extension of metaphyseal osteosarcoma in skeletally immature individuals. *J Bone Joint Surg Am* 1980;62:195.

185. Enneking WF, Kagan AD. Transepiphyseal extension of osteosarcoma: incidence, mechanism, and implications. *Cancer* 1978; 41:1526.

186. O'Neal ML, Bahner R, Ganey TM, et al. Osseous overgrowth after amputation in adolescents and children. *J Pediatr Orthop* 1996;16:78.

187. Benevenia J, Makley JT, Leeson MC, et al. Primary epiphyseal transplants and bone overgrowth in childhood amputations. *J Pediatr Orthop* 1992;12:746.

188. Dick HM, Malinin TI, Mnaymneh WA. Massive allograft implantation following radical resection of high-grade tumors requiring adjuvant chemotherapy treatment. *Clin Orthop* 1985: 88.

189. Mnaymneh W, Malinin TI, Makley JT, et al. Massive osteoarticular allografts in the reconstruction of extremities following resection of tumors not requiring chemotherapy and radiation. *Clin Orthop* 1985:76.

190. Dick HM, Strauch RJ. Infection of massive bone allografts. *Clin Orthop* 1994:46.

191. Gebhardt MC, Flugstad DI, Springfield DS, et al. The use of bone allografts for limb salvage in high-grade extremity osteosarcoma. *Clin Orthop* 1991:181.

192. Alman BA, De Bari A, Krajbich JI. Massive allografts in the

193. treatment of osteosarcoma and Ewing sarcoma in children and adolescents. *J Bone Joint Surg Am* 1995;77:54.

193. Hornicek FJ Jr, Mnaymneh W, Lackman RD, et al. Limb salvage with osteoarticular allografts after resection of proximal tibia bone tumors. *Clin Orthop* 1998:179.

194. Gitelis S, Piasecki P. Allograft prosthetic composite arthroplasty for osteosarcoma and other aggressive bone tumors. *Clin Orthop Relat Res* 1991;270:197.

195. Mankin HJ, Gebhardt MC, Jennings LC, et al. Long-term results of allograft replacement in the management of bone tumors. *Clin Orthop* 1996:86.

196. Enneking WF, Dunham W, Gebhardt MC, et al. A system for the functional evaluation of reconstructive procedures after surgical treatment of tumors of the musculoskeletal system. *Clin Orthop* 1993:241.

197. Berrey BH Jr, Lord CF, Gebhardt MC, et al. Fractures of allografts: frequency, treatment, and end-results. *J Bone Joint Surg Am* 1990;72:825.

198. Lord CF, Gebhardt MC, Tomford WW, et al. Infection in bone allografts: incidence, nature, and treatment. *J Bone Joint Surg Am* 1988;70:369.

199. Freedman EL, Eckardt JJ. A modular endoprosthetic system for tumor and non-tumor reconstruction: preliminary experience. *Orthopedics* 1997;20:27.

200. Ortiz-Cruz E, Gebhardt MC, Jennings LC, et al. The results of transplantation of intercalary allografts after resection of tumors: a long-term follow-up study. *J Bone Joint Surg Am* 1997; 79:97.

201. Manfrini M, Gasbarrini A, Malaguti C, et al. Intraepiphyseal resection of the proximal tibia and its impact on lower limb growth. *Clin Orthop* 1999:111.

202. Innocenti M, Ceruso M, Manfrini M, et al. Free vascularized growth-plate transfer after bone tumor resection in children. *J Reconstr Microsurg* 1998;14:137.

203. Capanna R, Manfrini M, Ceruso M, et al. A new reconstruction for metadiaphyseal resections: a combined graft (allograft shell plus vascularized fibula). Preliminary results. In: Brown KLB, ed. *Complications of limb salvage: prevention, management and outcome.* Montreal: International Symposium of Limb Salvage, 1991:319.

204. Capanna R, van Horn JR, Biagini R, et al. The Tikhoff-Linberg procedure for bone tumors of the proximal humerus: the classical extensive technique versus a modified transglenoid resection. *Arch Orthop Trauma Surg* 1990;109:63.

205. Malawer MM. Tumors of the shoulder girdle: technique of resection and description of a surgical classification. *Orthop Clin North Am* 1991;22:7.

206. Cheng EY, Gebhardt MC. Allograft reconstructions of the shoulder after bone tumor resections. *Orthop Clin North Am* 1991;22:37.

207. Voggenreiter G, Assenmacher S, Schmit-Neuerburg KP. Tikhoff-Linberg procedure for bone and soft tissue tumors of the shoulder girdle. *Arch Surg* 1999;134:252.

208. O'Connor MI, Sim FH, Chao EY. Limb salvage for neoplasms of the shoulder girdle: intermediate reconstructive and functional results. *J Bone Joint Surg Am* 1996;78:1872.

209. Gebhardt MC, Roth YF, Mankin HJ. Osteoarticular allografts for reconstruction in the proximal part of the humerus after excision of a musculoskeletal tumor. *J Bone Joint Surg Am* 1990; 72:334.

210. Jensen KL, Johnston JO. Proximal humeral reconstruction after excision of a primary sarcoma. *Clin Orthop* 1995:164.

211. Scarborough MT, Helmstedter CS. Arthrodesis after resection of bone tumors. *Semin Surg Oncol* 1997;13:25.

212. Kumar VP, Satku SK, Mitra AK, et al. Function following limb

salvage for primary tumors of the shoulder girdle: 10 patients followed 4 (1–11) years. *Acta Orthop Scand* 1994;65:55.

213. Malawer MM, Sugarbaker PH, Lampert M, et al. The Tikhoff-Linberg procedure: report of ten patients and presentation of a modified technique for tumors of the proximal humerus. *Surgery* 1985;97:518.

214. Jacobs PA. Limb salvage and rotationplasty for osteosarcoma in children. *Clin Orthop* 1984:217.

215. McClenaghan BA, Krajbich JI, Pirone AM, et al. Comparative assessment of gait after limb-salvage procedures. *J Bone Joint Surg Am* 1989;71:1178.

216. Windhager R, Millesi H, Kotz R. Resection-replantation for primary malignant tumours of the arm: an alternative to forequarter amputation. *J Bone Joint Surg Br* 1995;77:176.

Chemotherapy for Musculoskeletal Tumors

217. Balis F, Holcenberg J, Poplack D. General principles of chemotherapy. In: Pizzo P, Poplack D, eds. *Principles and practice of pediatric oncology*. Philadelphia: JB Lippincott, 1997:215.

218. Sutow WW, Sullivan MP, Fernbach DJ, et al. Adjuvant chemotherapy in primary treatment of osteogenic sarcoma: a Southwestern Oncology Group study. *Cancer* 1975;36:1598.

219. Jaffe N, Frei EI, Traggis D, et al. Adjuvant methotrexate and citrovorum-factor treatment of osteogenic sarcoma. *N Engl J Med* 1974;291:994.

220. Rosenberg SA, Cabner BA, Young RC, et al. Treatment of osteogenic sarcoma. I. Effect of adjuvant high-dose methotrexate after amputation. *Cancer Treat Rep* 1979;63:739.

221. Rosen G, Murphy ML, Huvos AG, et al. Chemotherapy, en bloc resection, and prosthetic bone replacement in the treatment of osteogenic sarcoma. *Cancer* 1976;37:1.

222. Tepper J, Glaubiger D, Lichter A, et al. Local control of Ewing's sarcoma of bone with radiotherapy and combination chemotherapy. *Cancer* 1980;46:1969.

223. Graham-Pole J. Ewing sarcoma: treatment with high dose radiation and adjuvant chemotherapy. *Med Pediatr Oncol* 1979;7:1.

224. Tefft M, Razek A, Perez C, et al. Local control and survival related to radiation dose and volume and to chemotherapy in non-metastatic Ewing's sarcoma of pelvic bones. *Int J Radiat Oncol Biol Phys* 1978;4:367.

225. Jaffe N, Paed D, Traggis D, et al. Improved outlook for Ewing's sarcoma with combination chemotherapy (vincristine, actinomycin D and cyclophosphamide) and radiation therapy. *Cancer* 1976;38:1925.

226. Maurer HM, Moon T, Donaldson M, et al. The Intergroup Rhabdomyosarcoma Study: a preliminary report. *Cancer* 1977; 40:2015.

227. Hays DM, Soule EH, Lawrence W Jr, et al. Extremity lesions in the Intergroup Rhabdomyosarcoma Study (IRS-I): a preliminary report. *Cancer* 1982;49:1.

228. Hays DM, Sutow WW, Lawrence W Jr, et al. Rhabdomyosarcoma: surgical therapy in extremity lesions in children. *Orthop Clin North Am* 1977;8:883.

229. Frei ED, Jaffe N, Gero M, et al. Adjuvant chemotherapy of osteogenic sarcoma: progress and perspectives. *J Natl Cancer Inst* 1978;60:3.

230. Lawrence W Jr, Hays DM, Heyn R, et al. Surgical lessons from the Intergroup Rhabdomyosarcoma Study (IRS) pertaining to extremity tumors. *World J Surg* 1988;12:676.

231. Eriksson AI, Schiller A, Mankin HJ. The management of chondrosarcoma of bone. *Clin Orthop* 1980:44.

232. McCoy DM, Levine EA, Ferrer K, et al. Pediatric soft tissue sarcomas of nonmyogenic origin. *J Surg Oncol* 1993;53:149.

233. Miser J, Triche T, Kinsella T, et al Other soft tissue sarcomas

234. Donaldson SS. The value of adjuvant chemotherapy in the management of sarcomas in children. *Cancer* 1985;55:2184.

235. Winkler K, Beron G, Delling G, et al. Neoadjuvant chemotherapy of osteosarcoma: results of a randomized cooperative trial (COSS-82) with salvage chemotherapy based on histological tumor response. *J Clin Oncol* 1988;6:329.

236. Pignatti G, Bacci G, Picci P, et al. Telangiectatic osteogenic sarcoma of the extremities: results in 17 patients treated with neoadjuvant chemotherapy. *Clin Orthop Relat Res* 1991;270: 99.

237. Winkler K, Bieling P, Bielack S, et al. Local control and survival from the Cooperative Osteosarcoma Study Group studies of the German Society of Pediatric Oncology and the Vienna Bone Tumor Registry. *Clin Orthop Relat Res* 1991;270:79.

238. Bacci G, Picci P, Ruggieri P, et al. Neoadjuvant chemotherapy for the treatment of osteosarcoma of the limbs: preliminary results in 100 patients treated preoperatively with high doses of methotrexate i.v. followed by cisplatin (i.a.) and adriamycin. *Chir Organi Mov* 1991;76:1.

239. Aparicio J, Munarriz B, Pastor M, et al. Long-term follow-up and prognostic factors in Ewing's sarcoma: a multivariate analysis of 116 patients from a single institution. *Oncology* 1998;55: 20.

240. Ferrari S, Mercuri M, Rosito P, et al. Ifosfamide and actinomycin-D, added in the induction phase to vincristine, cyclophosphamide and doxorubicin, improve histologic response and prognosis in patients with non metastatic Ewing's sarcoma of the extremity. *J Chemother* 1998;10:484.

241. Bacci G, Picci P, Mercuri M, et al. Predictive factors of histological response to primary chemotherapy in Ewing's sarcoma. *Acta Oncol* 1998;37:671.

242. Bacci G, Picci P, Ferrari S, et al. Primary chemotherapy and delayed surgery for nonmetastatic osteosarcoma of the extremities: results in 164 patients preoperatively treated with high doses of methotrexate followed by cisplatin and doxorubicin. *Cancer* 1993;72:3227.

243. Bacci G, Picci P, Pignatti G, et al. Neoadjuvant chemotherapy for nonmetastatic osteosarcoma of the extremities. *Clin Orthop* 1991:87.

244. Juergens H, Kosloff C, Nirenberg A, et al. Prognostic factors in the response of primary osteogenic sarcoma to preoperative chemotherapy (high-dose methotrexate with citrovorum factor). *Natl Cancer Inst Monogr* 1981:221.

245. Bacci G, Picci P, Ferrari S, et al. Neoadjuvant chemotherapy for Ewing's sarcoma of bone: no benefit observed after adding ifosfamide and etoposide to vincristine, actinomycin, cyclophosphamide, and doxorubicin in the maintenance phase. Results of two sequential studies. *Cancer* 1998;82:1174.

246. Wexler L, Helman L. Rhabdomyosarcoma and the undifferentiated sarcomas. In: Pizzo PA, Poplack D, eds. *Principles and practice of pediatric oncology*. Philadelphia: JB Lippincott, 1997: 799.

247. Horowitz M, Malawer M, Woo S, et al. Ewing's sarcoma family of tumors: Ewing's sarcoma of bone and soft tissue and the peripheral primitive neuroectodermal tumors. In: Pizzo P, Poplack D, eds. *Principles and practice of pediatric oncology*. Philadelphia: JB Lippincott, 1997:831.

248. Winkler K, Beron G, Kotz R, et al. Neoadjuvant chemotherapy for osteogenic sarcoma: results of a cooperative German/Austrian study. *J Clin Oncol* 1984;2:617.

Cartilaginous Tumors

249. Campanacci M. *Bone and soft tissue tumors*. New York: Springer-Verlag, 1990:433.

of childhood. In: Pizzo P, Poplack D, eds. *Principles and practice of pediatric oncology*. Philadelphia: JB Lippincott, 1997:865.

250. Schajowicz F. *Tumors and tumorlike lesions of bone.* Berlin: Springer-Verlag, 1994:71.

251. Milgram JW. The origins of osteochondromas and enchondromas: a histopathologic study. *Clin Orthop* 1983:264.

252. Noble J, Lamb DW. Enchondromata of bones of the hand: a review of 40 cases. *Hand* 1974;6:275.

253. Giudici MA, Moser RP Jr, Kransdorf MJ. Cartilaginous bone tumors. *Radiol Clin North Am* 1993;31:237.

254. van der Woude HJ, Bloem JL, Pope TL Jr. Magnetic resonance imaging of the musculoskeletal system. Part 9. Primary tumors. *Clin Orthop* 1998:272.

255. Geirnaerdt MJ, Bloem JL, Eulderink F, et al. Cartilaginous tumors: correlation of gadolinium-enhanced MR imaging and histopathologic findings. *Radiology* 1993;186:813.

256. Golfieri R, Baddeley H, Pringle JS, et al. Primary bone tumors: MR morphologic appearance correlated with pathologic examinations. *Acta Radiol* 1991;32:290.

257. Masciocchi C, Sparvoli L, Barile A. Diagnostic imaging of malignant cartilage tumors. *Eur J Radiol* 1998;27(Suppl 1):S86.

258. Bohndorf K, Reiser M, Lochner B, et al. Magnetic resonance imaging of primary tumours and tumour-like lesions of bone. *Skeletal Radiol* 1986;15:511.

259. Ollier M. Exostoses osteogeniques multiples. *Lyon Med* 1898; 88:484.

260. Cowan WK. Malignant change and multiple metastases in Ollier's disease. *J Clin Pathol* 1965;18:650.

261. Schwartz HS, Zimmerman NB, Simon MA, et al. The malignant potential of enchondromatosis. *J Bone Joint Surg Am* 1987; 69:269.

262. Cannon SR, Sweetnam DR. Multiple chondrosarcomas in dyschondroplasia (Ollier's disease). *Cancer* 1985;55:836.

263. Bean W. Dyschondroplasia and hemangiomata (Maffucci's syndrome). *Arch Intern Med* 1955;95:767.

264. Lewis RJ, Ketcham AS. Maffucci's syndrome: functional and neoplastic significance. Case report and review of the literature. *J Bone Joint Surg Am* 1973;55:1465.

265. Norman A, Sissons HA. Radiographic hallmarks of peripheral chondrosarcoma. *Radiology* 1984;151:589.

266. Garrison RC, Unni KK, McLeod RA, et al. Chondrosarcoma arising in osteochondroma. *Cancer* 1982;49:1890.

267. Canella P, Gardini F, Boriani S. Exostosis: development, evolution and relationship to malignant degeneration. *Ital J Orthop Traumatol* 1981;7:293.

268. Lee JK, Yao L, Wirth CR. MR imaging of solitary osteochondromas: report of eight cases. *Am J Roentgenol* 1987;149:557.

269. Lange RH, Lange TA, Rao BK. Correlative radiographic, scintigraphic, and histological evaluation of exostoses. *J Bone Joint Surg Am* 1984;66:1454.

270. Solomon L. Hereditary multiple exostosis. *J Bone Joint Surg Am* 1963;45:292.

271. Jaffe H. Hereditary multiple exostosis. *Arch Pathol* 1943;36: 335.

272. Shapiro F, Simon S, Glimcher MJ. Hereditary multiple exostoses: anthropometric, roentgenographic, and clinical aspects. *J Bone Joint Surg Am* 1979;61:815.

273. Schmale GA, Conrad EU 3rd, Raskind WH. The natural history of hereditary multiple exostoses. *J Bone Joint Surg Am* 1994; 76:986.

274. Peterson HA. Multiple hereditary osteochondromata. *Clin Orthop* 1989:222.

275. Merchan EC, Sanchez-Herrera S, Gonzalez JM. Secondary chondrosarcoma: four cases and review of the literature. *Acta Orthop Belg* 1993;59:76.

276. Saunders C, Szabo RM, Mora S. Chondrosarcoma of the hand arising in a young patient with multiple hereditary exostoses. *J Hand Surg Br* 1997;22:237.

277. Du YK, Shih HN, Wang JM, et al. Dedifferentiated chondrosarcoma arising from osteochondromatosis: a case report. *Chang Keng I Hsueh* 1991;14:130.

278. Solomon L. Chondrosarcoma in hereditary multiple exostosis. *S Afr Med J* 1974;48:671.

279. Wuisman PI, Jutte PC, Ozaki T. Secondary chondrosarcoma in osteochondromas: medullary extension in 15 of 45 cases. *Acta Orthop Scand* 1997;68:396.

280. Kilpatrick SE, Pike EJ, Ward WG, et al. Dedifferentiated chondrosarcoma in patients with multiple osteochondromatosis: report of a case and review of the literature. *Skeletal Radiol* 1997; 26:370.

281. Sharma SR, Chandra P, Gadekar NG. Sarcomatous-change in diaphysial aclasis (report of two cases). *Indian J Cancer* 1967; 4:95.

282. Aprin H, Riseborough EJ, Hall JE. Chondrosarcoma in children and adolescents. *Clin Orthop* 1982:226.

283. Young CL, Sim FH, Unni KK, et al. Chondrosarcoma of bone in children. *Cancer* 1990;66:1641.

284. Hudson T. *Radiographic-pathologic correlation of musculoskeletal lesions.* Baltimore: Williams & Wilkins, 1987.

285. Rahimi A, Beabout JW, Ivins JC, et al. Chondromyxoid fibroma: a clinicopathologic study of 76 cases. *Cancer* 1972;30: 726.

286. Bertoni F, Bacchini P. Classification of bone tumors. *Eur J Radiol* 1998;27(Suppl 1):S74.

287. Codman E. Epiphyseal chondromatous giant cell tumor of the upper end of the humerus. *Surg Gynecol Obstet* 1931;52:543.

288. Jaffe H, Lichtenstein L. Benign chondroblastoma of bone: a reinterpretation of the so-called calcifying or chondromatous giant cell tumor. *Am J Pathol* 1942;18:969.

289. Dahlin DC, Ivins JC. Benign chondroblastoma: a study of 125 cases. *Cancer* 1972;30:401.

290. Huvos AG, Marcove RC. Chondroblastoma of bone: a critical review. *Clin Orthop* 1973;95:300.

291. Springfield DS, Capanna R, Gherlinzoni F, et al. Chondroblastoma: a review of seventy cases. *J Bone Joint Surg Am* 1985;67: 748.

292. Gardner DJ, Azouz EM. Solitary lucent epiphyseal lesions in children. *Skeletal Radiol* 1988;17:497.

293. McLeod RA, Beabout JW. The roentgenographic features of chondroblastoma. *Am J Roentgenol* 1973;118:464.

294. Green P, Whittaker RP. Benign chondroblastoma: case report with pulmonary metastasis. *J Bone Joint Surg Am* 1975;57:418.

295. Boriani S, Bacchini P, Bertoni F, et al. Periosteal chondroma: a review of twenty cases. *J Bone Joint Surg Am* 1983;65:205.

296. Lichtenstein L, Hall J. Periosteal chondroma: a distinctive benign cartilage tumor. *J Bone Joint Surg Am* 1952;34:691.

297. Rockwell MA, Saiter ET, Enneking WF. Periosteal chondroma. *J Bone Joint Surg Am* 1972;54:102.

Lesions of Fibrous Origin

298. Friedland JA, Reinus WR, Fisher AJ, et al. Quantitative analysis of the plain radiographic appearance of nonossifying fibroma. *Invest Radiol* 1995;30:474.

299. Bullough PG, Walley J. Fibrous cortical defect and non-ossifying fibroma. *Postgrad Med J* 1965;41:672.

300. Hudson TM, Stiles RG, Monson DK. Fibrous lesions of bone. *Radiol Clin North Am* 1993;31:279.

301. Marks KE, Bauer TW. Fibrous tumors of bone. *Orthop Clin North Am* 1989;20:377.

302. Brower AC, Culver JE Jr, Keats TE. Histological nature of

the cortical irregularity of the medial posterior distal femoral metaphysis in children. *Radiology* 1971;99:389.

303. Caffe J. On fibrous defects in cortical walls of growing tubular bones. In: Levine S, ed. *Advances in pediatrics*, vol 7. Chicago: Year Book, 1955:13.

304. Easley ME, Kneisl JS. Pathologic fractures through nonossifying fibromas: is prophylactic treatment warranted? *J Pediatr Orthop* 1997;17:808.

305. Peterson HA, Fitzgerald EM. Fractures through nonossifying fibromata in children. *Minn Med* 1980;63:139.

306. Arata MA, Peterson HA, Dahlin DC. Pathological fractures through non-ossifying fibromas: review of the Mayo Clinic experience. *J Bone Joint Surg Am* 1981;63:980.

307. Grabias SL, Campbell CJ. Fibrous dysplasia. *Orthop Clin North Am* 1977;8:771.

308. Henry A. Monostotic fibrous dysplasia. *J Bone Joint Surg Br* 1969;51:300.

309. Stanton RP, Montgomery BE. Fibrous dysplasia. *Orthopedics* 1996;19:679.

310. Steward M, Gilmer W, Edmunson A. Fibrous dysplasia of bone. *J Bone Joint Surg Am* 1962;44:302.

311. Lichtenstein L. Polyostotic fibrous dysplasia. *Arch Surg* 1938; 36:874.

312. Gurler T, Alper M, Gencosmanoglu R, et al. McCune-Albright syndrome progressing with severe fibrous dysplasia. *J Craniofac Surg* 1998;9:79.

313. Lee PA, Van Dop C, Migeon CJ. McCune-Albright syndrome: long-term follow-up. *JAMA* 1986;256:2980.

314. Harris W, Dudley H, Barry R. The natural history of fibrous dysplasia: an orthopaedic, pathological, and roentgenographic study. *J Bone Joint Surg Am* 1962;44:207.

315. Albright F, Butler A, Hampton A, et al. Syndrome characterized by osteitis fibrosa disseminata, area of pigmentation and endocrine dysfunction, with precocious puberty in females. *N Engl J Med* 1937;216:727.

316. Danon M, Robboy SJ, Kim S, et al. Cushing syndrome, sexual precocity, and polyostotic fibrous dysplasia (Albright syndrome) in infancy. *J Pediatr* 1975;87:917.

317. Mauras N, Blizzard RM. The McCune-Albright syndrome. *Acta Endocrinol Suppl* 1986;279:207.

318. MacMahon HE. Albright's syndrome: thirty years later. (Polyostotic fibrous dysplasia.) *Pathol Annu* 1971;6:81.

319. Enneking WF, Gearen PF. Fibrous dysplasia of the femoral neck: treatment by cortical bone-grafting. *J Bone Joint Surg Am* 1986;68:1415.

320. Breck LW. Treatment of fibrous dysplasia of bone by total femoral plating and hip nailing: a case report. *Clin Orthop* 1972; 82:82.

321. Bryant DDD, Grant RE, Tang D. Fibular strut grafting for fibrous dysplasia of the femoral neck. *J Natl Med Assoc* 1992; 84:893.

322. Connolly JF. Shepherd's crook deformities of polyostotic fibrous dysplasia treated by osteotomy and Zickel nail fixation. *Clin Orthop* 1977:22.

323. DePalma AF, Ahmad I. Fibrous dysplasia associated with Shepherd's crook deformity of the humerus. *Clin Orthop* 1973;97: 38.

324. Funk FJ Jr, Wells RE. Hip problems in fibrous dysplasia. *Clin Orthop* 1973;90:77.

325. Freeman BH, Bray EWD, Meyer LC. Multiple osteotomies with Zickel nail fixation for polyostotic fibrous dysplasia involving the proximal part of the femur. *J Bone Joint Surg Am* 1987; 69:691.

326. Guille JT, Kumar SJ, MacEwen GD. Fibrous dysplasia of the proximal part of the femur: long-term results of curettage and bone-grafting and mechanical realignment. *J Bone Joint Surg Am* 1998;80:648.

327. Jaffe KA, Dunham WK. Treatment of benign lesions of the femoral head and neck. *Clin Orthop* 1990:134.

328. Shih HN, Chen YJ, Huang TJ, et al. Treatment of fibrous dysplasia involving the proximal femur. *Orthopedics* 1998;21: 1263.

329. Kempson R. Ossifying fibroma of long bones. *Arch Pathol* 1966; 82:218.

330. Campanacci M, Laus M. Osteofibrous dysplasia of the tibia and fibula. *J Bone Joint Surg Am* 1981;63:367.

331. Campbell CJ, Hawk T. A variant of fibrous dysplasia (osteofibrous dysplasia). *J Bone Joint Surg Am* 1982;64:231.

332. Kotzot D, Stoss H, Wagner H, et al. Jaffe-Campanacci syndrome: case report and review of literature. *Clin Dysmorphol* 1994;3:328.

333. Springfield DS, Rosenberg AE, Mankin HJ, et al. Relationship between osteofibrous dysplasia and adamantinoma. *Clin Orthop* 1994:234.

334. Wang JW, Shih CH, Chen WJ. Osteofibrous dysplasia (ossifying fibroma of long bones): a report of four cases and review of the literature. *Clin Orthop* 1992:235.

335. Schajowicz F, Santini-Araujo E. Adamantinoma of the tibia masked by fibrous dysplasia: report of three cases. *Clin Orthop* 1989:294.

336. Hazelbag HM, Taminiau AH, Fleuren GJ, et al. Adamantinoma of the long bones: a clinicopathological study of thirty-two patients with emphasis on histological subtype, precursor lesion, and biological behavior. *J Bone Joint Surg Am* 1994;76:1482.

Miscellaneous Lesions

337. Stull MA, Kransdorf MJ, Devaney KO. Langerhans cell histiocytosis of bone. *Radiographics* 1992;12:801.

338. Sessa S, Sommelet D, Lascombes P, et al. Treatment of Langerhans-cell histiocytosis in children: experience at the Children's Hospital of Nancy. *J Bone Joint Surg Am* 1994;76:1513.

339. Farber S. The nature of "solitary or eosinophilic granuloma" of bone. *Am J Pathol* 1941;17:625.

340. Lichtenstein L. Histiocytosis X: integration of eosinophilic granuloma of bone, "Letterer-Siwe disease," and "Schuller-Christian disease" as related manifestations of a single nosologic entity. *Arch Pathol* 1953;56:84.

341. Kilpatrick SE, Wenger DE, Gilchrist GS, et al. Langerhans' cell histiocytosis (histiocytosis X) of bone: a clinicopathologic analysis of 263 pediatric and adult cases. *Cancer* 1995;76:2471.

342. Levine SE, Dormans JP, Meyer JS, et al. Langerhans' cell histiocytosis of the spine in children. *Clin Orthop* 1996:288.

343. Ippolito E, Farsetti P, Tudisco C. Vertebra plana: long-term follow-up in five patients. *J Bone Joint Surg Am* 1984;66:1364.

344. O'Donnell J, Brown L, Herkowitz H. Vertebra plana–like lesions in children: case report with special emphasis on the differential diagnosis and indications for biopsy. *J Spinal Disord* 1991; 4:480.

345. Crone-Munzebrock W, Brassow F. A comparison of radiographic and bone scan findings in histiocytosis X. *Skeletal Radiol* 1983;9:170.

346. Dogan AS, Conway JJ, Miller JH, et al. Detection of bone lesions in Langerhans cell histiocytosis: complementary roles of scintigraphy and conventional radiography. *J Pediatr Hematol Oncol* 1996;18:51.

347. Howarth DM, Mullan BP, Wiseman GA, et al. Bone scintigraphy evaluated in diagnosing and staging Langerhans' cell histiocytosis and related disorders. *J Nucl Med* 1996;37:1456.

348. Schaub T, Eissner D, Hahn K, et al. Bone scanning in the

detection and follow-up of skeletal lesions in histiocytosis X. *Ann Radiol* 1983;26:407.

349. Van Nieuwenhuyse JP, Clapuyt P, Malghem J, et al. Radiographic skeletal survey and radionuclide bone scan in Langerhans cell histiocytosis of bone. *Pediatr Radiol* 1996;26:734.

350. Westra SJ, van Woerden H, Postma A, et al. Radionuclide bone scintigraphy in patients with histiocytosis X. *Eur J Nucl Med* 1983;8:303.

351. Egeler RM, Thompson RC Jr, Voute PA, et al. Intralesional infiltration of corticosteroids in localized Langerhans' cell histiocytosis. *J Pediatr Orthop* 1992;12:811.

352. Schreuder HW, Pruszczynski M, Lemmens JA, et al. Eosinophilic granuloma of bone: results of treatment with curettage, cryosurgery, and bone grafting. *J Pediatr Orthop B* 1998;7:253.

353. Bernstrand C, Bjork O, Ahstrom L, et al. Intralesional steroids in Langerhans cell histiocytosis of bone. *Acta Paediatr* 1996;85:502.

354. Raney RB Jr, D'Angio GJ. Langerhans' cell histiocytosis (histiocytosis X): experience at the Children's Hospital of Philadelphia, 1970–1984. *Med Pediatr Oncol* 1989;17:20.

355. Raney RB Jr. Chemotherapy for children with aggressive fibromatosis and Langerhans' cell histiocytosis. *Clin Orthop* 1991:58.

356. West WO. Velban as treatment for disseminated eosinophilic granuloma of bone: follow-up note after seventeen years. *J Bone Joint Surg Am* 1984;66:1128.

357. Womer RB, Raney RB Jr, D'Angio GJ. Healing rates of treated and untreated bone lesions in histiocytosis X. *Pediatrics* 1985;76:286.

358. Nezelof C, Basset F. Langerhans cell histiocytosis research: past, present, and future. *Hematol Oncol Clin North Am* 1998;12:385.

359. Conter V, Reciputo A, Arrigo C, et al. Bone marrow transplantation for refractory Langerhans' cell histiocytosis. *Haematologica* 1996;81:468.

360. Morgan G. Myeloablative therapy and bone marrow transplantation for Langerhans' cell histiocytosis. *Br J Cancer Suppl* 1994;23:S52.

361. Campanacci M, Capanna R, Picci P. Unicameral and aneurysmal bone cysts. *Clin Orthop* 1986:25.

362. Baker DM. Benign unicameral bone cyst: a study of forty-five cases with long-term follow up. *Clin Orthop* 1970;71:140.

363. Capanna R, Campanacci DA, Manfrini M. Unicameral and aneurysmal bone cysts. *Orthop Clin North Am* 1996;27:605.

364. Neer C, Francis K, Marcove R, et al. Treatment of unicameral bone cyst: a follow-up study of one hundred seventy-five cases. *J Bone Joint Surg Am* 1966;48:731.

365. Makley JT, Joyce MJ. Unicameral bone cyst (simple bone cyst). *Orthop Clin North Am* 1989;20:407.

366. Cohen J. Unicameral bone cysts: a current synthesis of reported cases. *Orthop Clin North Am* 1977;8:715.

367. Chigira M, Maehara S, Arita S, et al. The aetiology and treatment of simple bone cysts. *J Bone Joint Surg Br* 1983;65:633.

368. Cohen J. Etiology of simple bone cyst. *J Bone Joint Surg Am* 1970;52:1493.

369. Lokiec F, Wientroub S. Simple bone cyst: etiology, classification, pathology, and treatment modalities. *J Pediatr Orthop B* 1998;7:262.

370. Kruls HJ. Pathological fractures in children due to solitary bone cysts. *Reconstr Surg Traumatol* 1979;17:113.

371. Lee JH, Reinus WR, Wilson AJ. Quantitative analysis of the plain radiographic appearance of unicameral bone cysts. *Invest Radiol* 1999;34:28.

372. Ahn JI, Park JS. Pathological fractures secondary to unicameral bone cysts. *Int Orthop* 1994;18:20.

373. Kaelin AJ, MacEwen GD. Unicameral bone cysts: natural history and the risk of fracture. *Int Orthop* 1989;13:275.

374. McGlynn FJ, Mickelson MR, El-Khoury GY. The fallen fragment sign in unicameral bone cyst. *Clin Orthop* 1981:157.

375. Reynolds J. The "fallen fragment sign" in the diagnosis of unicameral bone cysts. *Radiology* 1969;92:949.

376. Oppenheim WL, Galleno H. Operative treatment versus steroid injection in the management of unicameral bone cysts. *J Pediatr Orthop* 1984;4:1.

377. Scaglietti O, Marchetti PG, Bartolozzi P. Final results obtained in the treatment of bone cysts with methylprednisolone acetate (Depo-Medrol) and a discussion of results achieved in other bone lesions. *Clin Orthop* 1982:33.

378. Farber JM, Stanton RP. Treatment options in unicameral bone cysts. *Orthopedics* 1990;13:25.

379. Hecht AC, Gebhardt MC. Diagnosis and treatment of unicameral and aneurysmal bone cysts in children. *Curr Opin Pediatr* 1998;10:87.

380. Spence KF Jr, Bright RW, Fitzgerald SP, et al. Solitary unicameral bone cyst: treatment with freeze-dried crushed cortical-bone allograft. A review of one hundred and forty-four cases. *J Bone Joint Surg Am* 1976;58:636.

381. Yandow SM, Lundeen GA, Scott SM, et al. Autogenic bone marrow injections as a treatment for simple bone cyst. *J Pediatr Orthop* 1998;18:616.

382. Scaglietti O, Marchetti PG, Bartolozzi P. The effects of methylprednisolone acetate in the treatment of bone cysts: results of three years follow-up. *J Bone Joint Surg Br* 1979;61:200.

383. Stanton RP, Abdel-Mota'al MM. Growth arrest resulting from unicameral bone cyst. *J Pediatr Orthop* 1998;18:198.

384. Spence KF, Sell KW, Brown RH. Solitary bone cyst: treatment with freeze-dried cancellous bone allograft. A study of one hundred seventy-seven cases. *J Bone Joint Surg Am* 1969;51:87.

385. Neer CS, Francis KC, Johnston AD, et al. Current concepts on the treatment of solitary unicameral bone cyst. *Clin Orthop* 1973;97:40.

386. Altermatt S, Schwobel M, Pochon JP. Operative treatment of solitary bone cysts with tricalcium phosphate ceramic: a 1 to 7 year follow-up. *Eur J Pediatr Surg* 1992;2:180.

387. Peltier LF, Jones RH. Treatment of unicameral bone cysts by curettage and packing with plaster-of-Paris pellets. *J Bone Joint Surg Am* 1978;60:820.

388. Biesecker JL, Marcove RC, Huvos AG, et al. Aneurysmal bone cysts: a clinicopathologic study of 66 cases. *Cancer* 1970;26:615.

389. Martinez V, Sissons HA. Aneurysmal bone cyst: a review of 123 cases including primary lesions and those secondary to other bone pathology. *Cancer* 1988;61:2291.

390. Tillman BP, Dahlin DC, Lipscomb PR, et al. Aneurysmal bone cyst: an analysis of ninety-five cases. *Mayo Clin Proc* 1968;43:478.

391. Lichtenstein L. Aneurysmal bone cysts. *Cancer* 1950;3:279.

392. Nguyen BD, Lugo-Olivieri CH, McCarthy EF, et al. Fibrous dysplasia with secondary aneurysmal bone cyst. *Skeletal Radiol* 1996;25:88.

393. Szendroi M, Arato G, Ezzati A, et al. Aneurysmal bone cyst: its pathogenesis based on angiographic, immunohistochemical and electron microscopic studies. *Pathol Oncol Res* 1998;4:277.

394. Hudson TM. Fluid levels in aneurysmal bone cysts: a CT feature. *Am J Roentgenol* 1984;142:1001.

395. Hudson TM. Scintigraphy of aneurysmal bone cysts. *Am J Roentgenol* 1984;142:761.

396. Green JA, Bellemore MC, Marsden FW. Embolization in the treatment of aneurysmal bone cysts. *J Pediatr Orthop* 1997;17:440.

397. DeRosa GP, Graziano GP, Scott J. Arterial embolization of

aneurysmal bone cyst of the lumbar spine: a report of two cases. *J Bone Joint Surg Am* 1990;72:777.

398. Marcove RC, Sheth DS, Takemoto S, et al. The treatment of aneurysmal bone cyst. *Clin Orthop* 1995:157.

399. Grier HE. The Ewing family of tumors: Ewing's sarcoma and primitive neuroectodermal tumors. *Pediatr Clin North Am* 1997;44:991.

400. Delattre O, Zucman J, Melot T, et al. The Ewing family of tumors: a subgroup of small-round-cell tumors defined by specific chimeric transcripts. *N Engl J Med* 1994;331:294.

401. Meier VS, Kuhne T, Jundt G, et al. Molecular diagnosis of Ewing tumors: improved detection of EWS-FLI-1 and EWS-ERG chimeric transcripts and rapid determination of exon combinations. *Diagn Mol Pathol* 1998;7:29.

402. Pritchard DJ, Dahlin DC, Dauphine RT, et al. Ewing's sarcoma: a clinicopathological and statistical analysis of patients surviving five years or longer. *J Bone Joint Surg Am* 1975;57:10.

403. Damron TA, Sim FH, O'Connor MI, et al. Ewing's sarcoma of the proximal femur. *Clin Orthop* 1996:232.

404. Li WK, Lane JM, Rosen G, et al. Pelvic Ewing's sarcoma: advances in treatment. *J Bone Joint Surg Am* 1983;65:738.

405. Terek RM, Brien EW, Marcove RC, et al. Treatment of femoral Ewing's sarcoma. *Cancer* 1996;78:70.

406. Horowitz ME, Neff JR, Kun LE. Ewing's sarcoma: radiotherapy versus surgery for local control. *Pediatr Clin North Am* 1991;38:365.

407. Sudanese A, Toni A, Ciaroni D, et al. The role of surgery in the treatment of localized Ewing's sarcoma. *Chir Organi Mov* 1990;75:217.

408. Toni A, Sudanese A, Ciaroni D, et al. The role of surgery in the local treatment of Ewing's sarcoma of the extremities. *Chir Organi Mov* 1990;75:262.

409. Wilkins RM, Pritchard DJ, Burgert EO Jr, et al. Ewing's sarcoma of bone: experience with 140 patients. *Cancer* 1986;58:2551.

410. Pritchard DJ. Surgical experience in the management of Ewing's sarcoma of bone. *Natl Cancer Inst Monogr* 1981:169.

411. Sailer SL, Harmon DC, Mankin HJ, et al. Ewing's sarcoma: surgical resection as a prognostic factor. *Int J Radiat Oncol Biol Phys* 1988;15:43.

412. Bacci G, Toni A, Avella M, et al. Long-term results in 144 localized Ewing's sarcoma patients treated with combined therapy. *Cancer* 1989;63:1477.

413. O'Connor MI, Pritchard DJ. Ewing's sarcoma: prognostic factors, disease control, and the reemerging role of surgical treatment. *Clin Orthop* 1991:78.

414. Gebhardt MC. Bone tumors in children: differential characteristics and treatment. *Postgrad Med* 1984;76:87.

415. Hudson TM, Hamlin DJ, Enneking WF, et al. Magnetic resonance imaging of bone and soft tissue tumors: early experience in 31 patients compared with computed tomography. *Skeletal Radiol* 1985;13:134.

416. Rosenthal DI. Computed tomography of orthopedic neoplasms. *Orthop Clin North Am* 1985;16:461.

417. Terrier P, Llombart-Bosch A, Contesso G. Small round blue cell tumors in bone: prognostic factors correlated to Ewing's sarcoma and neuroectodermal tumors. *Semin Diagn Pathol* 1996;13:250.

418. Brinkhuis M, Wijnaendts LC, van der Linden JC, et al. Peripheral primitive neuroectodermal tumour and extra-osseous Ewing's sarcoma: a histological, immunohistochemical and DNA flow cytometric study. *Virchows Arch* 1995;425:611.

419. Shimada H, Newton WA Jr, Soule EH, et al. Pathologic features of extraosseous Ewing's sarcoma: a report from the Intergroup Rhabdomyosarcoma Study. *Hum Pathol* 1988;19:442.

420. Gururangan S, Marina NM, Luo X, et al. Treatment of children with peripheral primitive neuroectodermal tumor or extraosseous Ewing's tumor with Ewing's-directed therapy. *J Pediatr Hematol Oncol* 1998;20:55.

421. Raney RB, Asmar L, Newton WA Jr, et al. Ewing's sarcoma of soft tissues in childhood: a report from the Intergroup Rhabdomyosarcoma Study, 1972 to 1991. *J Clin Oncol* 1997;15:574.

422. Bacci G, Ferrari S, Avella M, et al. Non-metastatic Ewing's sarcoma: results in 98 patients treated with neoadjuvant chemotherapy. *Ital J Orthop Traumatol* 1991;17:449.

423. Goldman A. Ewing's sarcoma: treatment with high-dose radiation and adjuvant chemotherapy. *Recent Results Cancer Res* 1982;80:115.

424. Rosen G, Caparros B, Nirenberg A, et al. Ewing's sarcoma: ten-year experience with adjuvant chemotherapy. *Cancer* 1981;47:2204.

425. Vietti TJ, Gehan EA, Nesbit ME Jr, et al. Multimodal therapy in metastatic Ewing's sarcoma: an intergroup study. *Natl Cancer Inst Monogr* 1981:279.

426. Nesbit ME Jr, Perez CA, Tefft M, et al. Multimodal therapy for the management of primary, nonmetastatic Ewing's sarcoma of bone: an intergroup study. *Natl Cancer Inst Monogr* 1981:255.

427. Craft A, Cotterill S, Malcolm A, et al. Ifosfamide-containing chemotherapy in Ewing's sarcoma. The Second United Kingdom Children's Cancer Study Group and the Medical Research Council Ewing's Tumor Study. *J Clin Oncol* 1998;16:3628.

428. Craft AW, Cotterill SJ, Bullimore JA, et al. Long-term results from the first UKCCSG Ewing's Tumour Study (ET-1). United Kingdom Children's Cancer Study Group (UKCCSG) and the Medical Research Council Bone Sarcoma Working Party. *Eur J Cancer* 1997;33:1061.

429. Wexler LH, DeLaney TF, Tsokos M, et al. Ifosfamide and etoposide plus vincristine, doxorubicin, and cyclophosphamide for newly diagnosed Ewing's sarcoma family of tumors. *Cancer* 1996;78:901; erratum 1997;79:867.

430. Antman K, Crowley J, Balcerzak SP, et al. A Southwest Oncology Group and Cancer and Leukemia Group B phase II study of doxorubicin, dacarbazine, ifosfamide, and mesna in adults with advanced osteosarcoma, Ewing's sarcoma, and rhabdomyosarcoma. *Cancer* 1998;82:1288.

431. Ahrens S, Hoffmann C, Jabar S, et al. Evaluation of prognostic factors in a tumor volume-adapted treatment strategy for localized Ewing sarcoma of bone: the CESS 86 experience. Cooperative Ewing Sarcoma Study. *Med Pediatr Oncol* 1999;32:186.

432. Sauer R, Jurgens H, Burgers JM, et al. Prognostic factors in the treatment of Ewing's sarcoma. The Ewing's Sarcoma Study Group of the German Society of Paediatric Oncology CESS 81. *Radiother Oncol* 1987;10:101.

433. Frieden RA, Ryniker D, Kenan S, et al. Assessment of patient function after limb-sparing surgery. *Arch Phys Med Rehabil* 1993;74:38.

434. Kimber C, Michalski A, Spitz L, et al. Primitive neuroectodermal tumours: anatomic location, extent of surgery, and outcome. *J Pediatr Surg* 1998;33:39.

435. Givens SS, Woo SY, Huang LY, et al. Non-metastatic Ewing's sarcoma: twenty years of experience suggests that surgery is a prime factor for successful multimodality therapy. *Int J Oncol* 1999;14:1039.

436. Arai Y, Kun LE, Brooks MT, et al. Ewing's sarcoma: local tumor control and patterns of failure following limited-volume radiation therapy. *Int J Radiat Oncol Biol Phys* 1991;21:1501.

437. Perez CA, Tefft M, Nesbit ME Jr, et al. Radiation therapy in the multimodal management of Ewing's sarcoma of bone: report of the Intergroup Ewing's Sarcoma Study. *Natl Cancer Inst Monogr* 1981:263.

438. Tefft M. Treatment of Ewing's sarcoma with radiation therapy. *Int J Radiat Oncol Biol Phys* 1981;7:277.

439. Razek A, Perez CA, Tefft M, et al. Intergroup Ewing's Sarcoma Study: local control related to radiation dose, volume, and site of primary lesion in Ewing's sarcoma. *Cancer* 1980;46:516.

440. Lewis RJ, Marcove RC, Rosen G. Ewing's sarcoma: functional effects of radiation therapy. *J Bone Joint Surg Am* 1977;59:325.

441. Tefft M, Chabora BM, Rosen G. Radiation in bone sarcomas: a re-evaluation in the era of intensive systemic chemotherapy. *Cancer* 1977;39:806.

442. Dunst J, Sauer R, Burgers JM, et al. Radiation therapy as local treatment in Ewing's sarcoma: results of the Cooperative Ewing's Sarcoma Studies CESS 81 and CESS 86. *Cancer* 1991;67:2818.

443. Perez CA, Tefft M, Nesbit M, et al. The role of radiation therapy in the management of non-metastatic Ewing's sarcoma of bone: report of the Intergroup Ewing's Sarcoma Study. *Int J Radiat Oncol Biol Phys* 1981;7:141.

444. Dunst J, Jurgens H, Sauer R, et al. Radiation therapy in Ewing's sarcoma: an update of the CESS 86 trial. *Int J Radiat Oncol Biol Phys* 1995;32:919.

445. Donaldson SS, Torrey M, Link MP, et al. A multidisciplinary study investigating radiotherapy in Ewing's sarcoma: end results of POG #8346. Pediatric Oncology Group. *Int J Radiat Oncol Biol Phys* 1998;42:125.

446. Tucker MA, D'Angio GJ, Boice JD Jr, et al. Bone sarcomas linked to radiotherapy and chemotherapy in children. *N Engl J Med* 1987;317:588.

447. Greene MH, Glaubiger DL, Mead GD, et al. Subsequent cancer in patients with Ewing's sarcoma. *Cancer Treat Rep* 1979;63:2043.

448. Smith LM, Cox RS, Donaldson SS. Second cancers in long-term survivors of Ewing's sarcoma. *Clin Orthop* 1992;275.

449. Freeman CR, Gledhill R, Chevalier LM, et al. Osteogenic sarcoma following treatment with megavoltage radiation and chemotherapy for bone tumors in children. *Med Pediatr Oncol* 1980;8:375.

450. Kuttesch JF Jr, Wexler LH, Marcus RB, et al. Second malignancies after Ewing's sarcoma: radiation dose-dependency of secondary sarcomas. *J Clin Oncol* 1996;14:2818.

451. Smith LM, Donaldson SS. Incidence and management of secondary malignancies in patients with retinoblastoma and Ewing's sarcoma. *Oncology* 1991;5:135; discussion 142, 147.

452. Bechler JR, Robertson WW Jr, Meadows AT, et al. Osteosarcoma as a second malignant neoplasm in children. *J Bone Joint Surg Am* 1992;74:1079.

453. Le Vu B, de Vathaire F, Shamsaldin A, et al. Radiation dose, chemotherapy and risk of osteosarcoma after solid tumours during childhood. *Int J Cancer* 1998;77:370.

Soft Tissue Tumors

454. Smith JT, Yandow SM. Benign soft-tissue lesions in children. *Orthop Clin North Am* 1996;27:645.

455. Pappo AS, Pratt CB. Soft tissue sarcomas in children. *Cancer Treat Res* 1997;91:205.

456. Meyer JS, Dormans JP. Differential diagnosis of pediatric musculoskeletal masses. *Magn Reson Imaging Clin North Am* 1998;6:561.

457. Enzinger F, Weiss S. *Soft tissue tumors.* New York: CV Mosby, 1993.

458. Jaffe H. *Tumors and tumorous conditions of the bones and joints.* Philadelphia: Lea & Febiger, 1968:256.

459. Faulkner LB, Hajdu SI, Kher U, et al. Pediatric desmoid tumor: retrospective analysis of 63 cases. *J Clin Oncol* 1995;13:2813.

460. Eich GF, Hoeffel JC, Tschappeler H, et al. Fibrous tumours in children: imaging features of a heterogeneous group of disorders. *Pediatr Radiol* 1998;28:500.

461. Sundaram M, McGuire MH, Herbold DR. Magnetic resonance imaging of soft tissue masses: an evaluation of fifty-three histologically proven tumors. *Magn Reson Imaging* 1988;6:237.

462. Hajdu S. *Pathology of soft tissue tumors.* Philadelphia: Lea & Febiger, 1979.

463. Weiss AJ, Lackman RD. Low-dose chemotherapy of desmoid tumors. *Cancer* 1989;64:1192.

464. Dagher R, Helman L. Rhabdomyosarcoma: an overview. *Oncologist* 1999;4:34.

465. Malogolowkin MH, Ortega JA. Rhabdomyosarcoma of childhood. *Pediatr Ann* 1988;17:251, 254.

466. Maurer HM. Rhabdomyosarcoma in childhood and adolescence. *Curr Probl Cancer* 1978;2:1.

467. Stiller CA, Parkin DM. International variations in the incidence of childhood soft-tissue sarcomas. *Paediatr Perinat Epidemiol* 1994;8:107.

468. Pappo AS. Rhabdomyosarcoma and other soft tissue sarcomas of childhood. *Curr Opin Oncol* 1995;7:361.

469. Pappo AS, Shapiro DN, Crist WM, et al. Biology and therapy of pediatric rhabdomyosarcoma. *J Clin Oncol* 1995;13:2123.

470. Pappo AS, Shapiro DN, Crist WM. Rhabdomyosarcoma: biology and treatment. *Pediatr Clin North Am* 1997;44:953.

471. Triche TJ. Diagnosis of small round cell tumors of childhood. *Bull Cancer* 1988;75:297.

472. LaQuaglia MP. Extremity rhabdomyosarcoma: biological principles, staging, and treatment. *Semin Surg Oncol* 1993;9:510.

473. Dodd S, Malone M, McCulloch W. Rhabdomyosarcoma in children: a histological and immunohistochemical study of 59 cases. *J Pathol* 1989;158:13.

474. Tsokos M. The diagnosis and classification of childhood rhabdomyosarcoma. *Semin Diagn Pathol* 1994;11:26.

475. Newton WA Jr, Soule EH, Hamoudi AB, et al. Histopathology of childhood sarcomas: Intergroup Rhabdomyosarcoma Studies I and II. Clinicopathologic correlation. *J Clin Oncol* 1988;6:67.

476. Andrassy RJ, Corpron CA, Hays D, et al. Extremity sarcomas: an analysis of prognostic factors from the Intergroup Rhabdomyosarcoma Study III. *J Pediatr Surg* 1996;31:191.

477. Noguera R. Cytogenetics and tissue culture of small round cell tumors of bone and soft tissue. *Semin Diagn Pathol* 1996;13:171.

478. Scrable H, Witte D, Shimada H, et al. Molecular differential pathology of rhabdomyosarcoma. *Genes Chromosomes Cancer* 1989;1:23.

479. Barr FG. Molecular genetics and pathogenesis of rhabdomyosarcoma. *J Pediatr Hematol Oncol* 1997;19:483.

480. Ghavimi F, Mandell LR, Heller G, et al. Prognosis in childhood rhabdomyosarcoma of the extremity. *Cancer* 1989;64:2233.

481. Crist WM, Garnsey L, Beltangady MS, et al. Prognosis in children with rhabdomyosarcoma: a report of the Intergroup Rhabdomyosarcoma Studies I and II. Intergroup Rhabdomyosarcoma Committee. *J Clin Oncol* 1990;8:443.

482. Raney RB Jr, Crist WM, Maurer HM, et al. Prognosis of children with soft tissue sarcoma who relapse after achieving a complete response: a report from the Intergroup Rhabdomyosarcoma Study I. *Cancer* 1983;52:44.

483. Tsokos M, Webber BL, Parham DM, et al. Rhabdomyosarcoma: a new classification scheme related to prognosis. *Arch Pathol Lab Med* 1992;116:847.

484. Antman K, Crowley J, Balcerzak SP, et al. An intergroup phase III randomized study of doxorubicin and dacarbazine with or without ifosfamide and mesna in advanced soft tissue and bone sarcomas. *J Clin Oncol* 1993;11:1276.

485. Maurer HM, Gehan EA, Beltangady M, et al. The Intergroup Rhabdomyosarcoma Study-II. *Cancer* 1993;71:1904.

486. Crist W, Gehan EA, Ragab AH, et al. The Third Intergroup Rhabdomyosarcoma Study. *J Clin Oncol* 1995;13:610.

487. Hays DM, Raney RB, Crist WM, et al. Secondary surgical procedures to evaluate primary tumor status in patients with chemotherapy-responsive stage III and IV sarcomas: a report from the Intergroup Rhabdomyosarcoma Study. *J Pediatr Surg* 1990;25:1100.

488. Pratt CB, Hustu HO, Kumar AP, et al. Treatment of childhood rhabdomyosarcoma at St. Jude Children's Research Hospital, 1962–78. *Natl Cancer Inst Monogr* 1981:93.

489. LaQuaglia MP, Ghavimi F, Penenberg D, et al. Factors predictive of mortality in pediatric extremity rhabdomyosarcoma. *J Pediatr Surg* 1990;25:238; discussion 243.

490. Johnson DG. Trends in surgery for childhood rhabdomyosarcoma. *Cancer* 1975;35:916.

491. Corpron CA, Andrassy RJ. Surgical management of rhabdomyosarcoma in children. *Curr Opin Pediatr* 1996;8:283.

492. Wharam MD, Hanfelt JJ, Tefft MC, et al. Radiation therapy for rhabdomyosarcoma: local failure risk for clinical group III patients on Intergroup Rhabdomyosarcoma Study II. *Int J Radiat Oncol Biol Phys* 1997;38:797.

493. Raney RB Jr, Gehan EA, Hays DM, et al. Primary chemotherapy with or without radiation therapy and/or surgery for children with localized sarcoma of the bladder, prostate, vagina, uterus, and cervix: a comparison of the results in Intergroup Rhabdomyosarcoma Studies I and II. *Cancer* 1990;66:2072.

494. Ransom JL, Pratt CB, Shanks E. Childhood rhabdomyosarcoma of the extremity: results of combined modality therapy. *Cancer* 1977;40:2810.

495. Pedrick TJ, Donaldson SS, Cox RS. Rhabdomyosarcoma: the Stanford experience using a TNM staging system. *J Clin Oncol* 1986;4:370.

496. Hays DM. Rhabdomyosarcoma. *Clin Orthop* 1993:36.

497. Lawrence W Jr, Gehan EA, Hays DM, et al. Prognostic significance of staging factors of the UICC staging system in childhood rhabdomyosarcoma: a report from the Intergroup Rhabdomyosarcoma Study (IRS-II). *J Clin Oncol* 1987;5:46.

498. Gross E, Rao BN, Bowman L, et al. Outcome of treatment for pediatric sarcoma of the foot: a retrospective review over a 20-year period. *J Pediatr Surg* 1997;32:1181.

499. Henderson SA, Davis R, Nixon JR. Synovial sarcoma: a clinicopathological review. *Int Orthop* 1991;15:251.

500. Marcus KC, Grier HE, Shamberger RC, et al. Childhood soft tissue sarcoma: a 20-year experience. *J Pediatr* 1997;131:603.

501. Pappo AS, Fontanesi J, Luo X, et al. Synovial sarcoma in children and adolescents: the St. Jude Children's Research Hospital experience. *J Clin Oncol* 1994;12:2360.

502. Schmidt D, Thum P, Harms D, et al. Synovial sarcoma in children and adolescents: a report from the Kiel Pediatric Tumor Registry. *Cancer* 1991;67:1667.

503. Gaakeer HA, Albus-Lutter CE, Gortzak E, et al. Regional lymph node metastases in patients with soft tissue sarcomas of the extremities: what are the therapeutic consequences? *Eur J Surg Oncol* 1988;14:151.

504. Morton MJ, Berquist TH, McLeod RA, et al. MR imaging of synovial sarcoma. *Am J Roentgenol* 1991;156:337.

505. Horowitz ME, Pratt CB, Webber BL, et al. Therapy for childhood soft-tissue sarcomas other than rhabdomyosarcoma: a review of 62 cases treated at a single institution. *J Clin Oncol* 1986;4:559.

506. Ladenstein R, Treuner J, Koscielniak E, et al. Synovial sarcoma of childhood and adolescence: report of the German CWS-81 study. *Cancer* 1993;71:3647.

507. Ferrari A, Casanova M, Massimino M, et al. Synovial sarcoma: report of a series of 25 consecutive children from a single institution. *Med Pediatr Oncol* 1999;32:32.

508. Lee SM, Hajdu SI, Exelby PR. Synovial sarcoma in children. *Surg Gynecol Obstet* 1974;138:701.

509. Blakely ML, Spurbeck WW, Pappo AS, et al. The impact of margin of resection on outcome in pediatric nonrhabdomyosarcoma soft tissue sarcoma. *J Pediatr Surg* 1999;34:672.

510. Philippe PG, Rao BN, Rogers DA, et al. Sarcomas of the flexor fossae in children: is amputation necessary? *J Pediatr Surg* 1992;27:964.

511. Marcus RB Jr. Current controversies in pediatric radiation oncology. *Orthop Clin North Am* 1996;27:551.

512. Fontanesi J, Pappo AS, Parham DM, et al. Role of irradiation in management of synovial sarcoma: St. Jude Children's Research Hospital experience. *Med Pediatr Oncol* 1996;26:264.

513. Ryan JR, Baker LH, Benjamin RS. The natural history of metastatic synovial sarcoma: experience of the Southwest Oncology Group. *Clin Orthop* 1982:257.

514. Shpitzer T, Ganel A, Engelberg S. Surgery for synovial chondromatosis: 26 cases followed up for 6 years. *Acta Orthop Scand* 1990;61:567.

515. Goldman AB, DiCarlo EF. Pigmented villonodular synovitis: diagnosis and differential diagnosis. *Radiol Clin North Am* 1988;26:1327.

516. Steinbach LS, Neumann CH, Stoller DW, et al. MRI of the knee in diffuse pigmented villonodular synovitis. *Clin Imaging* 1989;13:305.

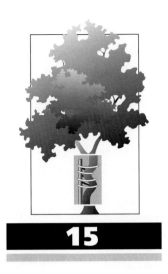

15

CEREBRAL PALSY

THOMAS S. RENSHAW

Cerebral palsy is a generic term used to describe certain clinical syndromes whose common feature is the abnormal control of motor function by the brain. The abnormal control results in a nonprogressive disorder of movement and/or posture, but the manifestations can change with growth, development, and maturation. Often, sensory and other brain functions are involved.

The etiologic agents of cerebral palsy afflict the immature brain to produce neuropathologic lesions that do not worsen. Although some parts of brain development continue throughout childhood, Gage has defined the "immature brain" as being younger than age 2 years. Accepting this definition, one may classify and code a brain lesion occurring thereafter as producing static encephalopathy, with a specific cause, instead of cerebral palsy, which may be coded without a known causative agent (1). In general, this differentiation does not affect the prognosis, and most clinicians refer to both as cerebral palsy.

BASIC BRAIN DEVELOPMENT

An excellent overview of brain development has been provided by Goldberg (2). During the first trimester of embryonic life, the brain differentiates into a grossly recognizable cerebrum, cerebellum, and other structures. An insult dur-

T. S. Renshaw: Department of Orthopaedic Surgery, Yale University, New Haven, Connecticut 06520; Department of Orthopaedic Surgery, Yale–New Haven Hospital, New Haven, Connecticut 06510.

ing this period usually produces a structural lesion that is detectable by magnetic resonance imaging (MRI).

Neurons begin to develop early in the second trimester, originating in the periventricular regions and migrating toward the surface of the cerebral cortex. By the fifteenth week of gestation fetal reflex movements can be detected. At the end of the second trimester all neurons have been formed and any damage or loss cannot be replaced.

Synaptic connections begin to be established early in the third trimester and intensify after birth. Glialization, which begins in the second trimester, occurs at least until age 2 years (3). Myelination in the brain does not begin until late in the third trimester, but continues into adolescence in a well-defined pattern. As more pathways become myelinated, primative reflexes drop out, mostly during the first 6 months of life, and normal postural reflexes appear. As myelination continues pathology in the brain becomes apparent. Brain morphologic maturation, as detectable by MRI, has been reported to continue through at least age 10 years (4).

As Goldberg points out, only after the neuronal pathways from brain lesions have become myelinated and can be tested and found to be abnormal can such lesions be detected. Because different pathways are myelinated at different times, spastic diplegia usually is not detected until at least 8 to 10 months of age, hemiplegia usually at about 20 to 24 months, and athetosis usually after 24 months (2).

ETIOLOGY

In most cases of cerebral palsy only risk factors can be identified, and not specific causes. The etiology is not necessarily the result of a brain insult that occurred in the prenatal or perinatal period. Only approximately 10 to 15% of patients in one large group had documented perinatal hypoxia or other problems (5). Cerebral palsy is not solely the result of prematurity because 60 to 65% of afflicted children were born at full term (1). Although only approximately 10% of cerebral palsy patients weigh less than 1,500 grams at birth, in this low birth weight group the risk of having cerebral palsy is 90 per 1,000, compared with 3 per 1,000 if weighing more than 2,500 grams and appropriate for gestational age (1,5,6). Low birth weight for gestational age and prematurity are commonly associated with the development of spastic diplegia (6).

Maternal risk factors in the prenatal period include infection, drug or alcohol abuse, epilepsy, mental retardation, hyperthyroidism, severe toxemia, an incompetent cervix, and third-trimester bleeding (4). Genetic abnormalities, teratologic agents, or congenital malformations of the child's brain may play a causative role, and in some patients, there may be multiple contributing agents (7–9).

Risk factors in the perinatal period include trauma; kernicterus; vaginal bleeding at the time of admission; placental complications such as abruptio, premature rupture of membranes, and chorionitis; and hypoxia or anoxia. It has been suggested that four questions must have positive answers in order to establish birth asphyxia as the probable cause of cerebral palsy (10):

1. Was there evidence of marked and prolonged intrapartum asphyxia?
2. Did the newborn exhibit signs of moderate or severe hypoxic-ischemic encephalopathy?
3. Is the neurologic condition one that intrapartum asphyxia could explain?
4. Has the clinical evaluation been extensive enough to exclude other conditions?

Oxytocin augmentation, cord prolapse, and breech presentation also have been associated with increased risk for cerebral palsy, but only if accompanied by low apgar scores (1).

Postnatally, an insult can come from head trauma (11); vascular accidents in the brain; central nervous system infections; kernicterus; hypoxia or anoxia from such causes as near drowning, suffocation, and cardiac arrest; and other problems. The long-term manifestations of cerebral palsy, caused by different specific agents, have not been extensively studied, but there is evidence that postnatal infectious causes commonly produce more severe orthopaedic deformities than do many other agents (12).

The brain lesion is permanent and nonprogressive, but the natural history of cerebral palsy is not static. Growth and maturation of not only the central nervous system but other systems as well often result in changing musculoskeletal problems in the child.

PREVALENCE

Cerebral palsy is found in from 1 to 7 per 1,000 children throughout most of the world, theoretically being more common in geographic regions where prenatal maternal and perinatal infant care are poor (3,13). In regions where sophisticated neonatal intensive care units exist, the risk of brain damage may be reduced by early treatment of certain problems, but also the lives of very premature infants and those with other life-threatening problems are often saved. In this latter group, the incidence of cerebral palsy is higher than in the general population. The result is that the incidence of cerebral palsy is only slightly reduced by preventing some cases, while saving others who have cerebral palsy who would not have survived (3). Twin pregnancies result in a child with cerebral palsy about 12 times more commonly than do single pregnancies. This is largely related to low birth weight (14). The prevalence of the neuropathic types and anatomic patterns of cerebral palsy varies greatly in many reports because of the widely differing populations studied. For example, a study containing the residents of state institutions shows many more severely involved individuals than does a study derived from a large private medical practice.

CLASSIFICATION

Cerebral palsy is classified by the neuropathic type of motor dysfunction and by the anatomic region of involvement.

Neuropathic Types

Spastic

This is the most common type of motor dysfunction. In cerebral palsy spasticity is an upper motor neuron syndrome caused by a lesion of the pyramidal system of the brain. The manifestations are a velocity-dependent increase in muscle tone and hyperexcitable tonic stretch reflexes. Spasticity is usually accompanied by weakness, loss of muscle control or dexterity, interference with balance, fatigability, and often the simultaneous contracting of antagonistic muscles (15). Severe spasticity is often referred to as rigidity. Joint contractures are common in spastic cerebral palsy.

Athetoid

Athetosis is a type of dyskinesia (abnormal movement) caused by an extrapyramidal brain lesion. It is characterized by purposeless writhing movements which become intensified when the child is frightened or excited. With pure athetosis, joint contractures are uncommon and muscle tone may not be increased. Tendon lengthenings in children with athetosis are often unpredictable, and may result in the creation of an opposite deformity that is more difficult to treat. Decades ago athetosis comprised about 25% of the cases of cerebral palsy because a major cause, Rh incompatibility with resulting kernicterus, was not so easily detected and prevented as is now the case. Dystonia, a phenomenon of increased general muscle tone, distorted postures, and abnormal positions that are induced by voluntary movements can occur together with athetosis.

Ataxic

Ataxic cerebral palsy is uncommon. It is a disturbance of coordinated movement, most noticed when walking, and is usually the result of cerebellar dysfunction. A mild intention tremor may be present, contractures are rare, and except for the treatment of scoliosis and hip dysplasia, surgery is rarely necessary.

Mixed

Children with mixed cerebral palsy have both pyramidal and extrapyramidal motor control abnormalities. Variable amounts of spasticity, athetosis, and/or ataxia occur together in this form. Sometimes the athetoid component is barely detectable, but it may nevertheless make surgical treatment less predictable.

Hypotonic

Generalized hypotonia may last for 2 or 3 years, and is most often a stage through which an infant passes before developing overt spasticity or ataxia. The brain lesion is present but masked by lack of myelination of the pathways that will carry its abnormal messages. Occasionally, mentally retarded children are erroneously referred to as having hypotonic cerebral palsy.

Anatomic Patterns

Quadriplegia

Quadriplegia, also known as tetraplegia, implies involvement of all four limbs. Many of these children have global involvement with mental retardation; bulbar dysfunction, manifested by drooling, dysarthria, and dysphagia; and seizures. The usual cause is severe hypoxia. After initially presenting as a floppy baby, the child shows delayed developmental milestones. The spectrum of severity is variable, from having no sitting ability or head control to being able to walk independently.

Diplegia

With diplegia, both lower extremities are always involved to a greater extent than the upper extremities, which are affected to some degree. A substantial percentage of diplegia results from prematurity. There has often been associated periventricular hemorrhage in and/or around the third ventricle, producing the characteristic lesion of diplegia (periventricular leukomalacia) in the motor fibers to the lower extremities before they enter the internal capsule (1). Intelligence is usually normal.

Hemiplegia

In hemiplegia, one side of the body is involved, the upper limb being more affected than the lower. The diagnosis is not often made until after walking has begun or fine motor hand control is noted to be deficient. A focal traumatic, vascular, or asymmetric infectious lesion is likely to be the cause of hemiplegia.

Seizure disorders are most frequently seen in this type of involvement, probably because of the focal brain lesion (4). The seizures usually begin in the first 2 years of life (16). Children with hemiplegia are also more likely to have homonymous hemianopsia and stereognostic deficits than are those with other types of involvement (4). Asymmetry of upper and lower limb growth, with the involved side being smaller, is also a common finding and probably is related to the trophic factor of sensory loss (17).

Other Types

Anatomic patterns of involvement are not always clear-cut, and some patients do not fit these common types. Blair and Stanley found only 55% intraobserver agreement in a cerebral palsy classification study (18).

Double hemiplegia refers to bilateral, usually symmetric involvement, with the upper extremities being more afflicted than the lower extremities. Triplegia implies difficulty with any three limbs, usually both lower and one upper. Monoplegia means only one limb is affected.

Paraplegia is used to describe involvement of the lower extremities only. This is a rare occurrence as the result of a brain injury, and such a pattern of motor dysfunction should alert the physician to the possibility of pathology in the spinal cord or canal.

ASSOCIATED PROBLEMS IN OTHER SYSTEMS

Central Nervous System

Other central nervous system problems occur as the result of global brain involvement, but the spinal cord usually is spared. Seizures afflict about 30% of children with cerebral palsy, and are most often seen with patients who have hemiplegia and quadriplegia, with mental retardation, or in postnatally acquired syndromes (19).

Mental retardation, defined as IQ less than 50, occurs in 30 to 65% of children with cerebral palsy (19). It is most prevalent in those with spastic quadriplegia. Other problems include behavioral and emotional difficulties; perceptual disorders; learning disorders; bulbar involvement with drooling, difficulty swallowing, and speech impairment; sensory deafness (which is most often seen in those with extrapyramidal involvement); and visual difficulties, such as perceptual problems, strabismus, nystagmus, and cortical blindness. Visual problems affect about 50% of children with cerebral palsy (1), so visual screening examinations are important for young children.

Gastrointestinal System

Problems with this system are particularly common in more severely involved children. Constipation and fecal impaction are common problems in children with global involvement. Impaired swallowing, vomiting, esophageal reflux, and hiatal hernia can cause aspiration and the risk of severe pneumonia, epigastric pain, profound feeding problems, and poor nutrition (20). Children with cerebral palsy who are malnourished have soft tissue wasting and interference with growth (21,22). When they undergo surgery they are at higher risk for postoperative infections (23).

Assessment of nutrition includes composition of the diet, especially regarding calorie and protein intake, and the feeding history. Can the child feed him- or herself, and if not, who is the feeder? Is the swallowing competent or does frequent aspiration occur? A radiologic contrast study of swallowing and to rule out gastroesophageal reflux may be helpful. Nutritional status can be poor despite obesity, and therefore studies such as total serum proteins and albumin; iron, iron-binding capacity, and transferrin levels; hemoglobin and erythrocyte mean corpuscular volume; and total lymphocyte count may be helpful to assess nutritional status (24,25). This is routinely done preoperatively with patients who will undergo extensive spinal surgery, but is not necessary for all preoperative workups. Keep in mind, however, that no single study is an absolute indicator of malnutrition.

Correction of malnutrition is best accomplished by enteric feeding augmentation, if possible. If swallowing is impaired, a tube-feeding program should be considered. When oral or tube-feeding supplementation is not feasible, the child should be referred to an appropriate surgeon for consideration for a feeding gastrostomy or jejunostomy. Gastroesophageal reflux sometimes can be managed successfully by medical means, but may require surgical fundoplication.

Genitourinary System

Bladder dysfunction and urinary incontinence are common in severely afflicted children. They also have a higher incidence of urinary tract infections than the normal population. This may relate to bladder dysfunction and retrograde colonization from frequent diaper soiling, or to urolithiasis, probably caused by dehydration and urinary stasis.

McNeal and colleagues, in a study of cerebral palsy patients, noted that 28% complained of enuresis, 26% had stress incontinence, 18% had urgency, and 36% had more than one symptom (26).

DIAGNOSIS

The diagnosis usually is established by a pediatrician or a neurologist before the child has had occasion to visit the orthopaedic surgeon. In some instances, however, an unexplained abnormal posturing, limp, toe walking, limb asymmetry, joint tightness, developmental delay, or other finding enables the orthopaedist to make the diagnosis of cerebral palsy.

History

Except for familial spastic paraparesis and congenital ataxia which are inherited conditions, cerebral palsy is not a genetic disease. The medical history begins with a search for possible causes and risk factors, including environmental agents, abnormal events during the pregnancy, the details of the birth, and assessment of the neonatal and infantile periods. Next, it is important to assess some benchmark physical developmental milestones, such as sitting, crawling, cruising, and walking (Table 15-1). These may be normal with hemiplegia. The review of systems should be thorough to detect any of the commonly related problems. A history of previous treatment, including surgery, is essential.

Physical Examination

The main goals of the physical examination are:

- to determine the grades of muscle strength and selective control;
- to evaluate the muscle tone and determine whether it is normal, hypotonic, spastic, athetoid, or mixed;
- to assess reflexes and sensory function;
- to evaluate the degree of deformity or muscle contracture at each of the major joints;
- to assess linear, angular, and torsional deformation of the spine and long bones, and fixed hand or foot deformities;
- to appraise balance, equilibrium, and standing or walking postures.

Physical assessment begins with observation of the child while taking the history. Next, as a dynamic examination evaluate the head control, sitting balance, the ability to crawl, the ability to pull up to stand, standing posture and balance, and the ability to walk. Observational gait assessment is imperative in those who can walk. The remainder of the examination is performed on the examining table, or, better yet, on the parent's lap, if the child is age 4 or 5 years or younger. The primitive neurologic reflexes, tendon reflexes, sensation, muscle strength, muscle tone, joint range of motion, contractures, torsional abnormalities, and spine should be assessed (1,27,28). Remember that motor dysfunction in the extremities can also be a manifestation of a brain or spinal cord tumor, infection, or other problem.

At the end of the initial history and physical examination formulate a functional assessment of the patient for documentation at that time and for communicating with other health care professionals. The following is an example of such an assessment: "The patient is a 5-year-old boy with spastic quadriplegic cerebral palsy. He is the product of a 32-week uncomplicated pregnancy, and was delivered by emergency cesarean section because of uncontrolled uterine bleeding. He has fair head control, poor sitting balance, and has never pulled to stand, or walked. He is able to communicate discomfort only, and does not participate in any activities of daily living."

Other Tests

Specialized gait analysis, valuable in the management of certain patients with cerebral palsy, is rarely necessary for diagnostic purposes. It may be useful in differentiating between idiopathic toe walking and mild spastic diplegia (29–31).

The diagnosis of conditions such as dysmorphic syndromes or congenital metabolic, neurologic, and muscular diseases, usually can be differentiated from global involvement with cerebral palsy, by clinical examination, and, if necessary, chromosomal analysis. Special imaging techniques, including MRI, positron emission tomography (PET), and computed tomography (CT), are useful in the evaluation of intracranial pathology.

Plain radiographs may be important. If there is any sign of a spinal deformity, radiographs in the coronal or sagittal planes, or both, document the degree, and sometimes the cause (e.g., a congenital vertebral anomaly), of the deformity. It can be argued that a periodic (every 12 months) coronal plane radiograph of the pelvis is necessary for the early detection of hip pathology, such as acetabular dysplasia or subluxation, in children with spastic diplegia or quadriplegia who are not walking (Fig. 15-1). These problems may not be clinically detectable, and are more easily managed and have better outcomes if treated early. Weight-bearing radiographs of the feet and ankles in the anteroposterior and maximally dorsiflexed lateral projections document the status of foot deformities when surgical intervention is being considered.

TABLE 15-1. SIMPLE DEVELOPMENTAL MILESTONES

Milestone	Average Age Achieved (mo)	95th Percentile
Head control	3	6
Independent sitting	6	9
Crawling	8	Some never do
Pull up to stand	8	12
Independent walking	12	17

(From ref. 3, with permission.)

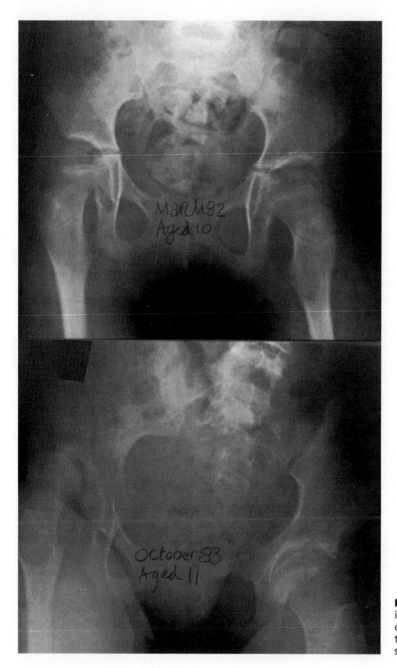

FIGURE 15-1. Radiographs showing substantial changes in the right hip, including dislocation, which developed over a few months at age 10 years. Annual hip evaluations, including radiographs, are important in detecting such problems.

COMMON TYPES OF CEREBRAL PALSY AND THEIR MANAGEMENT

The remainder of this chapter uses the formats of spastic quadriplegia, diplegia, and hemiplegia; athetoid cerebral palsy; and the upper extremity, to discuss the principles and techniques of management of common problems.

Many centers have developed cerebral palsy management programs conducted by teams of knowledgeable specialists. Team members usually include a pediatrician, orthopaedic surgeon, neurologist, consultant neurosurgeon, clinical nurse specialist, physical therapist, occupational therapist, speech–language specialist, social worker, educator, and psychologist (4). It is especially important for the team members to frequently communicate and confirm that they are in agreement, at least substantially, so that the family does not receive mixed or conflicting messages about their child's problems or care. The family is the most important member of the team.

Assessment of Treatment Results. Unfortunately, most treatment methods in cerebral palsy are not grounded in databased research, but rather are based on empiricism, opinions, and experience, as the best that can be done. Fortunately, physicians now recognize that treatment must be measured in terms of technical outcomes, functional health assessments, and patient satisfaction (2). Many measurement instruments now have been developed and validated (32). These include gait analysis, the Gross Motor Function Measure, the Pediatric Orthopaedic Society of North America's Health Status Questionnaire (33), the Gillette Children's Specialty Healthcare Normalcy Index and Functional Assessment Questionnaire, and the WeeFIM. In time, these and others should provide the needed data to base clinical care on reliable critical pathways.

Spastic Quadriplegia

An example for spastic quadriplegia is a patient with global involvement who is unable to walk and who requires nearly total care. Of paramount importance are the priorities of such a person which are, in order of importance:

- communication with others;
- the ability to take care of activities of daily living, especially personal hygiene;
- mobility in the environment; and
- walking (29).

Only about 20% of children with spastic quadriplegia will eventually walk. Realistic goals for nonambulatory orthopaedic care are directed toward maintaining balanced, comfortable sitting. The specific objectives are achievement and maintenance of:

- a straight spine and a level pelvis;
- located, mobile, painless hips that flex to at least 90 degrees for comfortable sitting, and extend to at least 30 degrees of flexion, to accomplish pivot transfers;
- mobile knees that flex for sitting, and can extend enough (to <20 degrees or less of flexion) to be controlled by orthoses for transfers;
- plantigrade feet for wearing shoes and for comfort on the footplates of wheelchairs;
- an appropriate wheelchair;
- management of problems in the other systems.

It is important to understand that it is in the wheelchair that the patient with spastic quadriplegia will spend most waking hours. The chair should be considered a total body orthosis, to be fitted and maintained by an expert (Fig. 15-2). The ability to independently transfer in and out of a wheelchair greatly facilitates the ability to live in a group-home setting for an adult with spastic quadriplegia. It is beneficial for all concerned to have a physical therapist experienced with patients in wheelchairs collaborate in developing the wheelchair prescription. The following should be considered in wheelchair design:

Foot rests:
   should be long enough for the shoes,
   either should support the entire foot in a plantigrade

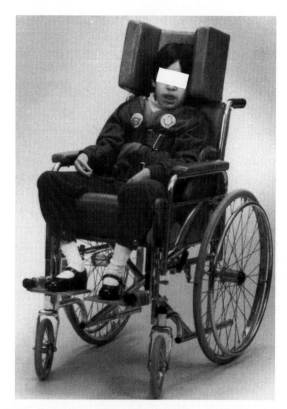

FIGURE 15-2. An appropriately fitted wheelchair provides proper body positioning, including head control.

position or be removed to allow free dangling of fixed deformities, such as severe equinus, to avoid increased pressure over a small area of contact,
   should be able to swing out of the way for entering and exiting the chair, and
   should accommodate foot restraint straps if needed.
Seat:
   height must allow the feet to correctly contact the foot rests,
   depth should entirely support each of the thighs, which may not be of equal lengths, but not compress the popliteal area,
   width should not compress the trochanters, but also should not allow lateral shifting or excessive tilting of the pelvis,
   firmness should be as much as tolerated by the patient to provide maximum pelvic stability without creating excessive skin pressure over bony prominences,
   contour should be incorporated, if necessary, for comfort.
Chairback:
   height should support the patient's trunk from the pelvis to the midscapular region,
   width should accommodate the trunk and any needed thoracic support pads,
   firmness should be as firm as is comfortable to aid in preventing collapsing kyphosis,

contouring should be incorporated, if necessary, to accommodate scoliosis,

reclining may be a necessary feature.

Restraint components:

may be necessary for foot, leg, pelvic, trunk, arm, or head control.

Portability:

is necessary if transportation in the community is desired.

Propulsion method:

the patient's arms,

an attendant,

motorization.

Because the child's waking activities are performed while sitting, the spine and hips are of prime importance, and are often the site of major problems in spastic quadriplegia. Other lower extremity problems specific to the ambulatory patient with spastic quadriplegia are addressed in the section on spastic diplegia.

Hyperlordosis

Increased lordosis in the lumbar spine is almost never a primary deformity in cerebral palsy. It is usually secondary to hip flexion contractures, and it responds to appropriate correction of those contractures by such means as stretching exercises or surgical lengthening of the psoas tendon. Hyperlordosis can also be a compensatory deformity below a rigid thoracic hyperkyphosis, and it usually responds to correction of the primary problem. When surgical spinal fusion is necessary to correct severe scoliosis, it is essential to consider the sagittal plane spinal balance and to preserve adequate lumbar lordosis by avoiding overdistraction across the lumbar spine.

Hyperkyphosis

Hyperkyphosis is most commonly seen in the young child with cerebral palsy who has weak spinal extensor musculature and a resultant long, C-shaped kyphotic posturing of the entire spine. This is almost always flexible, correcting fully on prone lying. It is best controlled by proper seating adaptation such as restraint straps on the wheelchair, slight reclining of the back, or, less often, by a thoracolumbosacral orthosis to provide sitting support. There is debate regarding whether increasing sitting support inhibits the function in the spinal extensor muscles and weakens them further, and whether physical therapy or muscle stimulation is helpful in maintaining or enhancing spinal extensor muscle strength.

Kyphosis occasionally occurs in the lumbar spine as the result of overly tight hamstring muscles. This kyphosis disappears with proximal lengthening of the hamstrings.

Children with cerebral palsy are not immune to the spinal deformities that afflict other children, so thoracic hyperkyphosis as the result of the Scheuermann condition, or postural juvenile kyphosis may also occur. Indications for orthotic treatment in these kyphotic conditions are similar to those in other children, but spinal orthotics are not likely to be as well tolerated.

Scoliosis

Scoliosis is more prevalent in all types of cerebral palsy compared with the general population, and varies directly with the severity of motor involvement. With patients who have mild hemiplegia, scoliosis occurs in fewer than 5%; with patients with severe spastic quadriplegia, its occurrence is much greater; in all cerebral palsy patients, it is about 25%. Specific increased risk factors for curve progression are quadriplegia, younger age, poor sitting balance, pelvic obliquity, and the presence of multiple curves.

Scoliosis in cerebral palsy is different from idiopathic scoliosis. It develops earlier; is more likely to be progressive; progresses beyond skeletal maturity, especially when the curve exceeds 40 degrees; is markedly less responsive to orthotic control; and is more likely to require surgical treatment.

As with idiopathic or other types of scoliosis, there are only three appropriate options for management. These are observation with documentation, orthotic treatment, or surgical stabilization. Observation alone is indicated for a curve that is of insufficient magnitude to require treatment (25–30 degrees), or is present in a patient whose best interests may not be served by active surgical intervention. The latter category is difficult to define: It would include the most severely involved individuals who are unable to perceive or interact with their environment in any meaningful fashion, based on severe and global compromise of their cognitive and sensory perceptual abilities. Only careful study by members of the cerebral palsy team and the patient's family can lead to this assessment. In such cases, the overall management goals are the patient's safety and comfort.

The orthotic treatment of scoliosis in quadriplegic cerebral palsy was based mostly on hope and empiricism until two studies showed that it rarely succeeds in controlling a curve (34,35). Most quadriplegic patients from each center did not experience any meaningful curve control from orthotic treatment. In some cases, however, an orthosis may slow curve progression, particularly in curves of 30 to 60 degrees, allowing beneficial growth in an immature spine before definitive surgical stabilization. At best no more than 15% of brace-treated curves stop progressing, and this may simply reflect the natural history of some cases of scoliosis in cerebral palsy (35). Ambulatory patients with spastic diplegia may develop idiopathic-type scoliotic curves. In these milder cases of cerebral palsy, brace control may be successful. Orthoses and other types of external devices for trunk support may be of value in improving sitting balance, particularly for those patients in whom surgery is not indicated. If the patient can tolerate a total-contact low-profile orthosis, this is the most effective and economical means of providing improved trunk support, even if it is a relatively soft orthosis (36). This is often not the case, however, and a custom-molded trunk or total-body–supporting wheelchair insert is required. These devices are difficult to fit properly, often quickly outgrown, and expensive. They must provide adequate pelvic alignment, trunk control, and head support (37). Nevertheless, the ability to sit as erectly and comfortably as possible is essential for a totally involved patient. Good sitting improves the patient's mental outlook, communication ability, respiratory function, ease of feeding, gastrointestinal function, hand usage, and mobility in the environment (38).

Surgical stabilization of progressing scoliosis is the only way to stop such a curve, in most cases (39,40). The benefit of a procedure of this magnitude and expense has been questioned by some (41), but most orthopaedic surgeons strongly believe that the surgery is worthwhile particularly in preventing loss of the ability to sit (Figure 15-3). Postoperative patients with reasonably balanced nonprogressive scoliosis have much better endurance for sitting; this greatly improves their quality of life when they can sit up comfortably for several hours, or even all day, and not have frequent substantial back pain that requires recumbency most of their waking hours. According to their caregivers they also are

much easier to feed, dress, and transport than those with severe untreated scoliosis. Most likely, after fusion they have less back discomfort, better pulmonary function, and less decubitus skin ulceration than similarly involved patients with severe untreated scoliosis (but this has not been proven) (42).

Once a curve exceeds 40 to 45 degrees magnitude it is likely to continue progressing, and surgery is usually indicated. Posterior internal fixation with a segmental system, such as double rods with cross-links connected to the spine by multiple hooks; sublaminar wires; interspinous wires; pedicle screws; or combinations of these techniques and an adequate posterior fusion mass is usually employed[➡2.6]. This is needed to achieve a balanced spine over a reasonably level pelvis, the objective of such surgery (42–45). Whenever possible, a larger and more rigid rod is preferable to provide better correction, resist deforming forces, and promote a solid arthrodesis. It is essential to achieve spinal balance in both the coronal and sagittal planes to maximize sitting balance. An abundance of allograft bone or an effective bone graft substitute should be available to generate the strong fusion mass.

Fusion limits are usually from the upper thoracic region

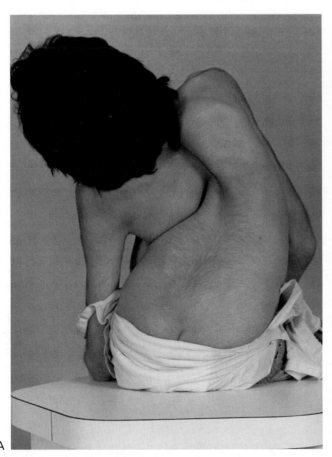

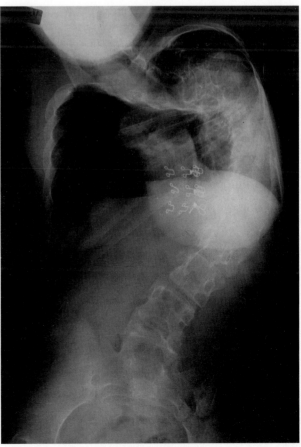

A   B

FIGURE 15-3. Clinical (**A**) and radiographic (**B**) images of a girl with cerebral palsy who has severe, untreated scoliosis. She is unable to sit for more than a few minutes.

(T1–T3) to L5, or more commonly, to the pelvis. When the fusion does not extend to the upper thoracic region there is an increased risk of developing a substantial junctional kyphosis cephalad to it. This may interfere with the ability of the patient to see at or above the horizontal, or may require constant and eventually painful neck hyperextension to do so. No matter how cephalad the upper fusion level or what type the fixation, some patients still develop a junctional kyphosis. Although applying a bilateral two-level clawed-hook configuration at the cephalad end of the rods (Fig. 15-4) with preservation of the uppermost posterior ligaments may help to prevent a junctional kyphosis, this has not been consistently successful.

Fusions should include the pelvis, if pelvic obliquity exceeds 10 degrees from the intercrestal iliac line to the top of L5 or L4, when measured on a sitting anteroposterior radiograph. Otherwise, pelvic obliquity may continue to progress and make sitting more difficult. Various techniques for pelvic fixation are available, including hooks, rods, and screws anchored to various bones, but none have withstood the test of time better than the Galveston technique [➥2.6–2.7] (46).

Routine anterior spinal surgery is not necessary in cerebral palsy. The most common indication for anterior spinal surgery in this condition is to improve curve correctability. Increased correction may be needed:

- to level the pelvis when pelvic obliquity is rigid and severe;
- to balance the spine in large, rigid curves that do not correct to less than 50 or 60 degrees during supine bending or maximum traction radiographs;
- to release the anterior tether of a kyphos; or
- to attempt to improve respiratory function or decrease the likelihood of the development of a pseudarthrosis in severe curves.

In such cases, a release of the deforming structures is accomplished by dividing the anterior longitudinal ligament, excising the annulus fibrosis, and removing all of the disc material and endplate cartilage back to the posterior annulus and posterior longitudinal ligament, and packing bone graft into the disc spaces. This may be done via an open thoracotomy, or, perhaps with less morbidity, by an endoscopic technique. Anterior internal fixation is rarely necessary when strong, rigid posterior fixation is performed. The anterior and the posterior operations are accomplished at the same surgical setting rather than staging them by several days or weeks (27).

There are several other important considerations when managing a spinal deformity by surgical means in a patient with cerebral palsy. One-third of the patients are malnourished (47) and may have gastroesphageal reflux, as discussed earlier. Detecting and correcting these conditions preoperatively helps prevent postoperative wound infection and healing problems by improving the patient's nutritional status (48). Determination of the serum transferrin level, albumin level, and total lymphocyte count are commonly used to assess nutritional status. An index using transferrin and albumin levels to identify malnourished patients has been developed (49).

Intraoperative blood loss should be calculated carefully, expressed in terms of percentage of blood volume, and appropriately replaced to avoid hypovolemia or dangerous coagulopathies, especially when blood loss nears 50% of the blood volume. With this method preoperative blood volume must be accurately estimated, and suctioned blood loss plus blood in weighed sponges should be carefully measured. Another means of monitoring blood loss and replacement is by calculating erythrocyte mass and considering hematocrit measurements in the lost blood as well as in the replacement source.

Postoperative pulmonary problems, such as hypoventilation, atelectasis, aspiration pneumonia, and the adult respiratory distress syndrome may occur, and every preventive effort, including rapid mobilization of the patient, must be enlisted.

Spondylolysis and Spondylolisthesis

Although spondylolysis and spondylolisthesis do not occur in nonambulatory patients, they have been reported in ambulatory patients with cerebral palsy with an incidence similar to that in the general population. No increased severity of symptoms or relation to hip flexion contractures has been noted (50). Treatment is similar to that recommended for children who do not have cerebral palsy.

Hip Problems

About 70 to 90% of the hip problems in cerebral palsy occur with spastic quadriplegia. The common problems are contractures, hip at risk, subluxation, and dislocation. Causative factors of hip problems are probably combinations of muscle imbalance, acetabular dysplasia, pelvic obliquity, excessive femoral anteversion, increased femoral neck valgus, lack of weightbearing, and maldirected resultant force vectors across the hip joint. Femoral anteversion is greater at all age levels in children with cerebral palsy than in the normal population. It does not change significantly after age 6 years (51), and is greater in ambulatory children than in nonwalkers (52).

Because of increased muscle tone and some contracture, it can be difficult to detect even substantial hip abnormalities by routine physical examination. For this reason it may be wise to obtain an annual screening supine anteroposterior radiograph of the hips in children with spastic quadriplegia, and in patients with spastic diplegia who do not walk.

In all but the most severely involved children, hip dislocation should be prevented. Hip subluxation or dislocation, although more common before the age of 6 years, may occur at any age. Hips at risk and hips that are subluxated rarely

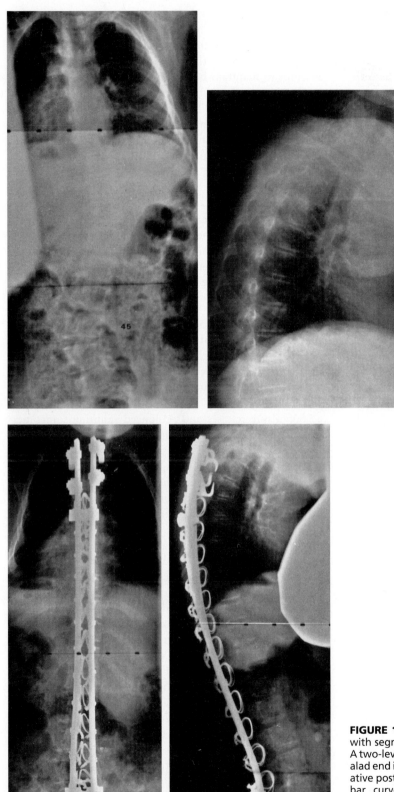

FIGURE 15-4. Treatment of scoliosis by posterior spinal fusion with segmental instrumentation, using mostly sublaminar wires. A two-level, transverse process, pedicle claw was used at the cephalad end in an attempt to prevent junctional kyphosis. **A:** Preoperative posteroanterior radiograph demonstrates a 45-degree lumbar curve. **B:** Preoperative lateral radiograph demonstrates associated thoracic kyphosis. **C:** Postoperative posteroanterior radiograph. **D:** Postoperative lateral radiograph demonstrates the cephalad claw configuration of the hooks.

cause discomfort, but dislocation can lead to pain. Studies have reported pain in approximately 50% of cerebral palsy patients with dislocated hips (53,54), and the associated increased contractures may make care more difficult and worsen sitting balance. One study, however, found that surgical reduction of dislocated hips did not improve pain or sitting ability (55). Until more studies with longer follow-up are available regarding treatment of dislocated hips in cerebral palsy, most surgeons follow the management described in the following section.

Hip Management

Hip at Risk. The hip at risk has increased valgus and anteversion and a shallow acetabulum, but no subluxation. Tightness and contractures in the adductor and flexor muscles are usually present. Without treatment, hips at risk often progress to subluxation or dislocation, particularly if there is less than 30 degrees of abduction in flexion or extension, and/or with hip flexion contractures of greater than 20 degrees. Such progression may be very slow (months to years) or occur much more rapidly. Because the literature lacks valid data regarding the likelihood of such hips worsening, it is not possible to predict the natural history of every hip at risk in cerebral palsy. That leaves the surgeon with the options of closely following hips at risk or intervening. Unless the patient is so cerebrally compromised as to preclude surgical treatment most surgeons will intervene, realizing that at least in some cases the hip pathology would not have been progressive. The use of stretching exercises alone as treatment for hips at risk is rarely, if ever, successful. In young children with hips at risk and mild or absent muscle tightness, night splinting, in an attempt to improve acetabular depth, is an option that some surgeons might choose. That night splinting can reliably increase acetabular depth, however, has not been confirmed by a well-controlled study.

Surgical treatment of the hip at risk consists of lengthening and weakening of the tight adductors and flexors [➡**3.17**] (56–58). The adductor longus may be all that needs releasing, especially in those who walk, but the gracilis, and occasionally part of the adductor brevis muscles also, may require release in order to gain abduction to at least 45 degrees for each extended hip and 60 degrees abduction for each hip in flexion. The issue of whether to release or transfer the adductors is discussed in the section on spastic diplegia. Tenotomy or elongation of the psoas tendon, sparing the iliacus fibers, should be performed. Psoas tenotomy, in a nonambulatory patient with spastic quadriplegia, may be performed either at the pelvic brim or at the lesser trochanter. Tenotomy at the more caudal site may produce more hip flexor weakness, a situation of no consequence to a nonwalker, but one that may be detrimental to an ambulatory patient who needs adequate hip flexor power to lift the limb for step climbing (2). Psoas tenotomy at the pelvic brim is performed in the manner

described by Sutherland et al. (59). On rare occasions the psoas may not be tendinous at that level, and the tenotomy must be done more distally. Then it is wise to suture the proximal cut end of the tendon to the hip capsule in an attempt to maintain better hip flexor strength.

Postoperatively, some surgeons use abduction splinting for several months. This is applied at night, and always within the child's range of comfortable abduction. The value of such splinting is questionable. Postoperatively, physical therapy is begun as soon as the second postoperative day (60). In the past, anterior branch, or even complete, obturator neurectomy has been performed to denervate the adductor muscles, in addition to lengthening them. Now this is rarely done because most surgeons believe it to be unnecessary when an adequate adductor release (i.e., allowing 60 degrees of passive abduction) has been performed. If the child has an athetoid component, in addition to spasticity, obturator neurectomy should never be done. That can result in a severe, disabling abduction contracture.

Subluxation. Hip subluxation is defined as uncovering of more than one-third of the femoral head and a break in the Shenton line, but with the femoral head maintaining at least some contact with the acetabulum (45,61). Surgical treatment of a subluxation can prevent subsequent dislocation (62,63).

Soft tissue releases and prolonged splinting sometimes can be successful in very young children. When only soft tissue surgery is deemed necessary to treat unilateral subluxation and the patient is younger than 9 years, bilateral releases may be best because the contralateral hip is usually at least somewhat abnormal or likely to become so, if only unilateral surgery is done (64).

The subluxated hip most often has increased femoral valgus, anteversion, or both, and requires corrective proximal femoral osteotomy (63,65–67). To stabilize the hip joint, varus of the femoral neck is usually reduced to about 115 degrees in an ambulatory child, or even less in a nonambulator [➡**4.1–4.3, 4.6**]. In addition to appropriate tendon releases, derotation of the excessive femoral anteversion to approximately 10 to 20 degrees (or 30 to 45 degrees of passive internal hip rotation) is performed to prevent posterior subluxation (68,69) (Fig. 15-5). The younger the patient, the more likely is the valgus and anteversion to recur postoperatively, especially if the child is under age 4 years (70). If the magnitude of the subluxation exceeds 50%, an open reduction and capsulorrhaphy will improve the result (71).

If bony surgery (a varus rotational osteotomy with or without a pelvic osteotomy) is required, prophylactic surgery on a well-covered contralateral hip with adequate abduction is not necessary, regardless of the age or ambulatory status of the patient (72).

If acetabular dysplasia is present (acetabular index >25 degrees) (73), it almost always should be corrected surgically. An exception might be a child younger than 4 or 5 years with very mild dysplasia and recently fully corrected abnor-

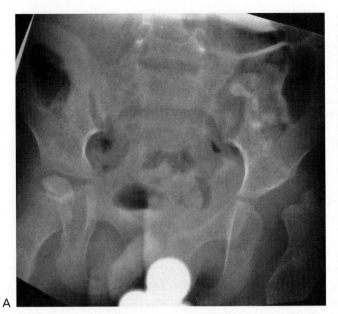 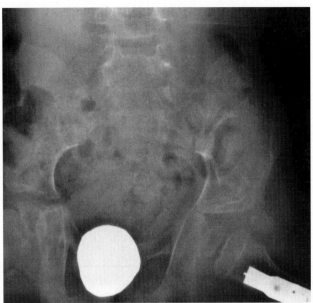

FIGURE 15-5. Dislocation of the left hip in this patient with spastic quadriplegia was treated by varization-derotation osteotomy and innominate osteotomy. **A:** Complete dislocation of left hip. **B:** Status, post-open reduction and femoral and pelvic osteotomies.

mal valgus and anteversion. In this situation acetabular remodeling may occur from the stimulation of redirecting the force vector across the hip joint from the lateral actebular rim to the center of the acetabulum. Older children have much less potential for biologic remodeling to normalize the acetabulum after femoral varization and rotation osteotomies.

The dysplastic acetabulum in cerebral palsy is shallow. In nonambulators, the acetabular deficit is superior, posterior, and usually more severe than in ambulatory patients. It is almost always associated with an increase in the femoral neck-shaft angle and femoral anteversion. The femoral anteversion is greater in ambulators (52).

Acetabular dysplasia is corrected surgically by choosing the appropriate pelvic osteotomy and being certain that its prerequisites are met. Arthrographic evaluation and, if necessary to define the pathoanatomy, three-dimensional reformatted CT scanning images can be helpful in the decision-making process (52,74).

The Salter, Steel, Sutherland, Pemberton, pericapsular, Dega (75), and Chiari osteotomies, and shelf augmentation of the acetabular rim, all have been successful in cerebral palsy when appropriate indications are met [➡3.7–3.12] (45,76–82). If the acetabulum is found to be deficient superiorly and anteriorly, or purely superiorly, an anterolateral rotational osteotomy, such as a Salter, Steel, or Sutherland procedure, or a Pemberton osteotomy, is appropriate. Often, there is superior and posterior deficiency, in which case, restoration of lateral and posterior coverage by a shelf-augmentation procedure, an Albee shelf, a Dega procedure (83), or a pericapsular osteotomy (68,73) may

be more appropriate. The Chiari osteotomy can be performed if the superior acetabular rim has not been so proximally eroded that the cut will enter the sacroiliac joint.

Dislocation. Hip dislocation may be addressed by relocation procedures (84), by accepting the dislocation, by proximal femoral resection (85), or, less commonly, by hip arthrodesis or total hip replacement arthroplasty (86,87). If the dislocation occurred within 1 year, and/or if the anatomy does not appear excessively distorted, most surgeons elect to perform anterior open reduction and capsulorrhaphy, combined with appropriate soft tissue releases (usually adductors and psoas tendon) and a proximal femoral shortening, varization, and rotation osteotomy. Often, a degree of acetabular dysplasia is associated with the dislocation, and it is wise to correct this at the same time. The pelvic procedure should be tailored to the situation, as described in the previous discussion of the subluxated hip.

If the hip has been dislocated for longer than 1 year, achieving a painless, mobile, stable hip from open reduction and other surgery is less likely because of joint incongruity and eroded articular cartilage on the femoral head. When such a hip is painless, no treatment is required. When the hip is painful, proximal femoral resection with muscle interposition, as described by Castle and Schneider, has a high success rate [➡3.16] (85,88). This resection is performed at the subtrochanteric level, the thickened capsule and gluteus medius muscle are sewn over the acetabular inlet, and a muscle cuff of vastus lateralis is sewn over the beveled femoral stump (Fig. 15-6). It is critical to carefully save as much vastus lateralis as possible during the initial dissec-

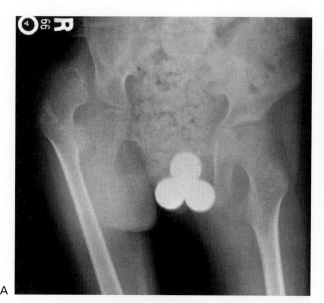
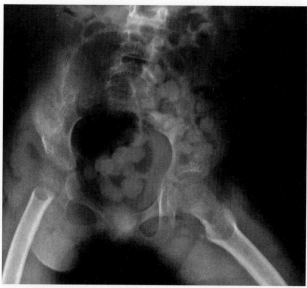

FIGURE 15-6. This nonambulatory child's painful dislocated right hip was treated by resection of the proximal femur just distal to the lesser trochanter and oversewing muscle flaps. This is known as the Castle procedure. His pain was relieved. **A:** Preoperative anteroposterior radiograph shows the dislocated right hip with femoral head deformity and acetabular dysplasia. **B:** Postoperative radiograph. The proximal femur has been resected at the distal end of the lesser trochanter.

tion, and to provide a good, thick muscle covering over the femoral stump. Postoperative management should consist of a bilateral pantaloon or a one-and-a-half–hip spica cast for about 3 to 4 weeks, then comfortable but effective exercises to assure maintenance of the desired range of hip motion. This range is the minimal flexion contracture: at least 100 degrees of flexion, neutral rotation, and abduction to at least 20 degrees. Postoperative traction or external fixators are rarely necessary. The result is usually good motion and good pain relief, but definite thigh-shortening, which must be accommodated in the seat of the wheelchair. Following proximal femoral resection, it is very common to have spasm and discomfort for several days, weeks, or even months. This usually will eventually resolve, but analgesics and antispasmodic medications may be necessary for a prolonged time. A successful trial of an intrathecal baclofen injection may indicate the use of a baclofen pump during this period. Heterotopic ossification about the hip is almost universally seen after proximal femoral resection, and single-dose radiation therapy should be considered to minimize its magnitude.

Femoral head resection, combined with subtrochanteric valgus pelvic support osteotomy, has been successful in relieving the pain of chronic hip dislocation (89,90).

The Girdlestone intertrochanteric resection has been tried for the painful dislocated hip. The likelihood of continuing postoperative pain from femoral-iliac impingement has caused most surgeons to abandon this procedure.

Arthrodesis is another option, but may be difficult to accomplish in nonambulatory patients with severe spasticity. When enough flexion is provided to make sitting comfortable, it may limit the ability to comfortably lie supine. Arthrodesis, therefore, is not often performed.

The reported experience is small with replacement arthroplasty for painful dislocated hips (89). This procedure is indicated most often for the ambulatory adult with mild to moderate spasticity and severe degenerative arthritis of the hip.

Osteoarthritis. The located osteoarthritic hip in cerebral palsy need not be treated surgically, unless it is painful and nonsurgical methods have failed. In that case, arthrodesis and replacement arthroplasty have both been successful, the latter being preferred because of less postoperative morbidity and easier management (91). Arthrodesis **[→3.13]** is usually performed in a position appropriate for walking, sitting, and lying: 30 degrees of flexion, 5 to 10 degrees abduction, and neutral rotation for an ambulatory patient, and 45 degrees of flexion for a nonambulator. Leg-length equalization should be considered in walking patients because it may defer the development of back pain (92).

Extension Contracture. Extension contracture of the hip occasionally occurs in the severely spastic child with quadriplegia. The probable cause is tightly contracted hamstrings, which are hip extensors, as well as knee flexors. Often it is seen with extensor thrust, a rigid and sustained hip extension that can greatly interfere with comfortable sitting, because the extension contracture does not allow adequate hip flexion. When severe it can literally push and slide the child out of the wheelchair. The treatment options for mild extension contracture are proximal lengthening of the hamstrings [➡**3.19**] or injections into the hamstrings of neuromotor blocking agents, such as botulinum A toxin or alcohol. For more than mild extension contractures, lengthening of the proximal hamstrings is indicated (21,42). If this is not adequate, posterior capsulotomy of the hip and release of the external rotator muscles may also be necessary. Unfortunately, recurrence of extension contractures is common and often rapid following proximal hamstring lengthening.

Extension Plus Abduction Contracture. Extension plus abduction contracture of the hip is not common. It most often occurs after injudicious release of the flexors and adductors in patients who have athetosis, and is also seen after aggressive flexor and adductor releases in patients who have severe spasticity or rigidity and previously undetected cospasticity in the hip extensor and abductor muscles. Cospasticity can be difficult to detect even by careful physical examination, but both flexion and extension of the joint are substantially limited, as are abduction and adduction. Gait analysis may detect cospasticity in ambulatory patients.

Because of their writhing movements patients who have athetosis rarely develop contractures that require surgical releasing. The problem is with the mixed spastic–athetoid patient with tightness, in whom the surgeon cannot determine precisely just how much to weaken the spastic muscle. It is definitely better to err on the side of underrelease.

The treatment of mild cases of extension plus abduction contracture of the hip consists of stretching exercises and proper seating in the wheelchair. Data regarding the use of tone-reducing measures in this situation are currently lacking, but a trial of intrathecal baclofen may be useful. With more severe involvement, surgical treatment is necessary. This involves release of the proximal hamstrings, the femoral and iliotibial band insertions of the gluteus maximus, the external rotator muscles, and even posterior capsulotomy of the hip joint, if necessary. In long-standing severe contractures, femoral shortening may be necessary to prevent overstretching of the sciatic nerve (93).

Spastic Diplegia

Most children with spastic diplegia walk, although late walking is the rule, and it is not unusual for a diplegic child not to begin ambulation until age 4 years or even later (94). Motor improvement often reaches a plateau at about age 7 years, so that if a child is not walking by then there is little likelihood that he or she will walk (27,95). The severity of lower extremity involvement is the most important factor in walking ability. A seizure disorder, marked flaccidity, persistent abnormal primitive reflexes, or a dislocated hip are deterrents to walking, whereas intelligence, upper extremity severity index, or birth weight do not correlate closely with walking prognosis (95). Mental retardation has little or no effect on walking ability (27,96).

TABLE 15-2. BLECK'S WALKING PROGNOSIS CRITERIA

1. Asymmetric tonic neck reflex (ATNR)
2. Neck-righting reflex (NRR)
3. Moro reflex (MR)
4. Symmetric tonic neck reflex (STNR)
5. Parachute reaction (PR)
6. Foot-placement reaction (FPR)
7. Extensor thrust (ET)

These tests are performed in order on nonambulatory children after the age of 12 months. When one of the following is present (ATNR, NRR, MR, STNR, ET) or absent (PR, FPR), one point is given. A score of zero gives a good prognosis for walking; patients with one point have a guarded prognosis; and two or more points indicates a poor prognosis.

(From ref. 27, with permission.)

Bleck (Table 15-2) and Beals (Table 15-3) have described criteria for predicting the likelihood of walking in children with cerebral palsy (95,97–99), and Campos da Paz studied 272 children with cerebral palsy and found that achievement of head balance before age 9 months, independent sitting by 24 months, and crawling by 30 months were good prognostic indicators for walking, whereas lack of head control by age 20 months indicated a poor prognosis (100). Conversely, Molnar and Gordon, in a study of 233 children with cerebral palsy, found that in children younger than age 2 years, independent sitting was not a good predictor for walking ability, but that after age 4 years inability to sit predicted nonambulation (96).

Hoffer and colleagues classified ambulation for meningomyelocele into four functional levels. This classification is also appropriate for use in children with cerebral palsy:

1. Community ambulators: These patients walk indoors and outdoors for most of their activities, and may need crutches, braces, or both. They use a wheelchair only for long trips out of the community.
2. Household ambulators: These patients walk only indoors and with apparatus. They are able to get in and out of the chair and bed with little or no assistance. They may use the wheelchair for some indoor activities at home and school, and for all activities in the community.

TABLE 15-3. BEALS' WALKING PROGNOSIS CRITERIA

Severity Index*	Walking Prognosis
>18	Free walking by age 3 years
12–18	Free walking by age 7 years
10–11	Free or crutch walking by age 6 years
0–9	Crutch or no walking

* The severity index is defined as the motor age in months at the chronologic age of 3 years.
(From ref. 27, with permission.)

3. Nonfunctional ambulators: Walking for these patients is a therapeutic exercise at home, in school, or in the hospital. Afterward, they use their wheelchairs to get from place to place and to satisfy all their needs for transportation.
4. Nonambulators: These patients are wheelchair-bound, but usually can transfer from chair to bed (101).

Children with spastic diplegia are less-often afflicted with scoliosis, seizures, speech impediments, and major problems in other systems than are those with quadriplegia. Hip dislocation is also less likely, but excessive valgus and anteversion of the proximal femur, acetabular dysplasia, and hips at risk or subluxated are not uncommon.

The majority of children with cerebral palsy have problems with balance. In diplegia, posterior equilibrium is most often affected, but this does not obviate walking or require the use of cane or crutches. Crutches are necessary if anterior balance is defective. If lateral balance is significantly involved, a walker will be needed. Severe lateral equilibrium disturbances usually preclude any walking.

Gait Analysis. Gait analysis in cerebral palsy is an objective and well-established method of documentation that allows the careful study of the various components of pathologic gait, the energy expended (102), and the outcomes of treatment protocols. Gait analysis is discussed in Chapter 5 of this textbook, and in others devoted exclusively to the subject (1).

A recent study indicates that when experienced physicians added gait analysis data to their own clinical evaluations, they changed their surgical recommendations about half the time, with more decreases than increases in procedures (103). Whether this will improve surgical outcomes and reduce costs has not been studied. Although preoperative gait analysis is theoretically desirable, it is neither possible nor necessary for every child who undergoes surgery. Nevertheless, every surgeon who treats children with cerebral palsy should have a good knowledge of normal and pathologic human gait, and understand gait analysis and pattern recognition (104) (Fig. 15-7). The application of his or her observational gait assessment then will be more accurate.

The prerequisites for normal gait are:

- stability of the foot and entire lower extremity in stance phase;
- clearance of the ground by the foot in swing phase;
- appropriate prepositioning of the foot at the end of swing phase;
- adequate step length; and
- maximization of energy conservation (1).

Observational gait analysis is done by watching the child walk repeatedly while viewing the gait from the front, back, and side. Study only one component at a time (e.g., cadence, stride length, the foot, the knee, the hip, lower-extremity

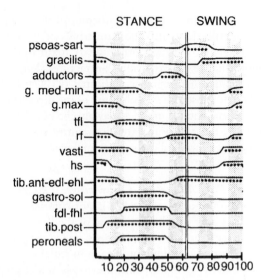

FIGURE 15-7. Chart of normal muscle-firing patterns (*dotted lines*) for the lower extremities. The patterns of a child with cerebral palsy are compared with these normal data.

rotational alignment, the pelvis, the trunk), recognizing that often there are differences between the sides. Gage has described observational gait analysis in detail (1). For a given child, intraobserver observations are more accurate than interobserver observations (105). In either situation, the opportunity to study a videotape of the gait from the front, back, and sides, with zoom capability for the feet, increases accuracy.

Pattern recognition allows the surgeon to observe the gait cycles of the walking child, look for the priorities of gait and deviations from normal, and correlate this information to the findings on static physical examination. If all this information is consistent with a recognized standard pattern (e.g., one of the types of hemiplegia or a diplegic gait with equinovalgus feet, tight hamstrings, tight hip flexors and adductors, and increased femoral anteversion) there is a strong likelihood of success after applying the proper surgical procedures to address each problem.

It would be ideal to review a high-tech gait analysis on every ambulatory cerebral palsy patient preoperatively if cost and accessibility to sophisticated gait labs were not a problem. In reality, surgeons will be most comfortable without gait analysis with those patients who have apparently straightforward patterns of gait pathology (Fig. 15-8). Nevertheless, gait analysis provides a more precise definition of the gait abnormality in more complex cases, such as those with severe diplegia and those who have had previous surgery with little success.

Treatment Methods

The treatment categories for patients with spastic diplegia are modulation of spasticity (oral medications, intramuscu-

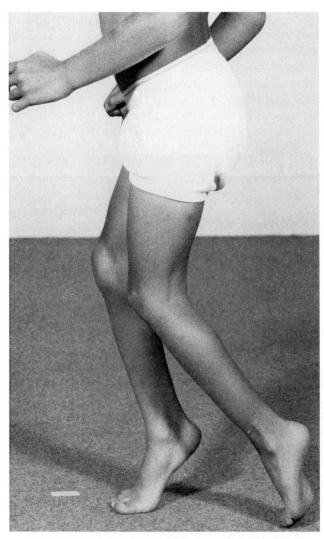

FIGURE 15-8. An example of a common spastic diplegic gait pattern. Note the ankle equinus, knee flexion, hip flexion, internal rotation of the entire limb, and compensatory lumbar lordosis.

lar injections, intrathecal injections, selective dorsal rhizotomy), physical therapy, orthotics and/or manipulation and casting, and musculoskeletal surgery. These modalities are discussed in this section.

Oral Medications. Ideally, an orally administered medication would appropriately temper spasticity and allow nearly normal voluntary muscle control to occur over the long term. Unfortunately, such an agent does not exist. Many types of muscle relaxants, antispasmodics, and neuroinhibitory medications have been tried to little or no avail, mostly because therapeutic doses are so large that the substantial accompanying drowsiness is unacceptable (106). Oral pharmacotherapy, widely accepted as effective for problems in cerebral palsy, has been limited to anticonvulsants for seizures and diazepam for superimposed postoperative myo-

spasms, by its probable effect of increasing presynaptic inhibition (107), and perhaps for its tranquilizing effect on pain perception.

Intramuscular Injections. The purposes of injecting various substances into muscles or around nerves are:

- to weaken a muscle and improve the balance of forces across a joint in order to assess whether this will improve function. This is a temporary effect, but in some cases it may be of value to allow a stretching and strengthening physical therapy program to perhaps avoid or, more likely, defer the need for surgery;
- to separate severe spasticity from fixed-joint contracture;
- to determine which muscle is the major contributor to an abnormal posture; and
- to assess the performance of antagonistic muscles (108).

The most common lower-extremity muscle injected is the gastrocnemius to reduce equinus deformity. Other common sites are the hamstrings and hip adductors. Repeated injections may be necessary to achieve the desired effect, and injecting some substances can be painful unless general anesthesia is used.

The shortest-acting drug is a local anesthetic agent, injected in the immediate vicinity of a specific nerve to block its fibers and allow the physician to observe the effect. If the effect is beneficial, then repeating the injection with another longer-acting agent should reproduce the effect (109). If the goal is to make the effect permanent, phenol is used to destroy the nerve fibers.

Another means of weakening the muscle is to inject 45% alcohol into its fibers in a more regional distribution to inhibit nerve transmission and, thereby, muscle contraction. This is painful and requires general anesthesia. When successful, the effect of alcohol injection lasts for a variable period, but usually approximately 6 weeks (27,110).

Botulinum-A Toxin. A newer agent for intramuscular injection is botulinum-A toxin (BTX), a neurotoxin produced by *Clostridia* bacteria. It is delivered into or near sites of nerve arborization, and blocks the release of acetylcholine from presynaptic vesicles at the myoneural junction. Recovery of tone results from the sprouting of new nerve terminals, which peaks at about 60 days (111,112). The agent is injected using a 23- or 25-gauge needle, usually without local or general anesthesia, but topical anesthesia will prevent the discomfort that rarely lasts more than 5 minutes. The muscles are located by palpation. To reach muscles that are deep or difficult to localize, electromyographic guidance and electrical stimulation have been used (113). BTX diffuses readily, so the injection should be placed in the muscle belly (114).

BTX is quite expensive, and optimal dosage regimens have not been agreed upon. It has been shown to be a safe technique, whose effects on muscles begin in 12 to 72 h, and usually last for 3 to 6 months or longer (115–117). Injections may be repeated after 2 or more weeks, and up to six injections may be given at a site, until the desired response in muscle tone reduction has been achieved. This treatment is contraindicated in the presence of fixed joint contractures. It is most useful in very young patients when a limited number of muscles are involved (117), and the surgeon wishes to defer surgical intervention until the child is older, has a stabilized gait pattern, or other components of the child's problem can be more precisely identified and addressed. A double-blind trial in 12 patients with equinovarus or equinovalgus foot deformities showed improvement in five of six treated patients, and improvement in two of six placebo-injected patients (118). A report of 14 children who had BTX treatment for equinus showed marked improvement (mean 6.7 months) in six, mild improvement in three, and no improvement in five (119). Other studies have found it to be longer-lasting with fewer side effects, and equally, or more efficient, at improving equinus gait than serial casting (110,120), but combining the two may be beneficial (121). In the upper extremity BTX has shown beneficial effects, particularly in relieving tight elbow flexors and thumb flexors. This has improved hygiene and cosmesis, but not fine motor function (122). Independent of motor function, BTX is usually effective in relieving pain from muscle spasms (119). Unanswered but essential questions are:

- whether or not the expensive and temporary tone reduction will allow physical therapy efforts to succeed in avoiding, rather than just delaying, the need for surgery;
- what is the optimal dosage protocol;
- when and what are the effects of BTX antibody formation; and
- what aberrations and their controlling muscles are most appropriate for this treatment?

Intrathecal Injections. Baclofen (Lioresal) is an agonist of the neuroinhibitor gamma-aminobutyric acid which interferes with release of excitatory transmitters that cause spasticity (107). When injected intrathecally, it acts on the spinal cord synaptic reflexes to broadly decrease lower-extremity spasticity for about 8 h (1). In the upper extremity, there is a lesser reduction of tone, about equal to that achieved by selective posterior rhizotomy, but no change in joint range of motion (123). It has poor lipid solubility and does not cross the blood–brain barrier very effectively, so when given orally large doses are required, and excessive lethargy is the result. Beneficial long-term effects are realized when administered intrathecally by a refillable, subcutaneously implanted pump. This provides a ten-times greater concentration in the spinal fluid than does comparable oral dosing (124). Problems and complications from using the pump are decreasing as experience improves, and include

infection, catheter breakage, fistula, equipment malfunction, and the need for frequent refilling with the medication.

Large long-term outcome studies are not yet available. It appears that this treatment may be most helpful for patients with dystonia and spasticity who have hygiene problems or difficulty with sitting (121). Another group of patients may be those who are ambulatory and have underlying weakness. This second group cannot tolerate the additional weakness imposed by selective dorsal rhizotomy. Recognizing that adequate data on which to base a recommendation for its use in specific patients is weak or lacking, it appears that intrathecal baclofen is of definite benefit in about one-half the patients in studies thus far reported (124–126). It also may be of some aid in assessing the potential benefit of selective posterior rhizotomy. In the doses used to treat spasticity, baclofen has no effect on athetosis (127).

Selective Posterior Rhizotomy. This procedure has been employed for several decades (128), but only in the past 15 years has it been widely used in North America (129,130). Unlike earlier attempts to surgically or electrically alter the central nervous system beneficially (e.g., cerebellar stimulation) (131), it has met with growing acceptance. The principle of selective posterior rhizotomy is to reduce spasticity and balance muscle tone by altering the control exhibited by the anterior horn cells in the spinal cord. The normal inhibitory influences on the gamma efferent system, produced by higher centers in the brain and carried to the anterior horn cell by long intraspinal tracts are deficient in cerebral palsy, as is the ability to coordinate movement as mediated through the extrafusal fibers from the alpha motor neurons. Selective posterior rhizotomy attempts to limit the stimulatory inputs from the muscle spindles in the lower limbs that arrive by the afferent fibers in the dorsal roots. This is done by sectioning only those dorsal rootlets whose impulses exert excessive faciliatory influence on the anterior horn cell, and thus better balance these influences.

The operation is performed under general anesthesia without relaxants. The lumbar laminae and the intervening ligaments are removed as an en bloc laminoplasty from L1 to S1, preserving the facet joints. Then, individual posterior rootlets from the L1 to S1 posterior roots are carefully dissected out and electrically stimulated. The electromyographic and physical responses are noted, and those rootlets that supply the offending muscles are surgically divided. Rootlets are spared if they show decremental and squared-type electromyographic responses. They are divided if the responses are incremental, clonic, multiphasic, sustained, or contralateral, although this determination is not always easy. In most cases, up to 70 rootlets per root are stimulated, and 25 to 50% are sectioned. The laminae and ligament complex are then replaced. The theoretical advantages of laminoplasty compared to laminectomies, at each level, are that it is faster, may result in less scarring in the spinal canal, and replacement of the intact laminae may prevent some cases of lumbar instability or deformity.

The patient best served by selective posterior rhizotomy is the young child (age 3–8 years) with:

- spastic diplegic involvement;
- voluntary motor control;
- reasonable intelligence and motivation;
- no fixed contractures;
- good trunk control;
- the ability to walk with good underlying strength and balance; and who has
- severe, pure spasticity; and was
- preterm or of low birth weight (132).

Full-term children are more likely to have rigidity plus spasticity, and therefore may not respond as favorably to selective posterior rhizotomy (1,128). Availability for, and cooperation with, postoperative physical therapy are prerequisites for the procedure because therapy may be required three or four times per week for as long as a year to regain strength. The procedure is not indicated in children with athetosis, ataxia, rigidity, dystonia, antigravity muscle and truncal weakness or hypotonia, overlengthened tendons, and severe fixed contractures. Information regarding any benefits in those with spastic quadriplegia is limited (133). The results of unilateral rhizotomy in spastic hemiplegia are not available, but at least one source does not recommend it (128).

In the early postoperative period, the patient is weaker than before surgery and requires intensive physical therapy, but once the acute rehabilitation are complete, improvement in the lower extremities may be dramatic and perhaps lasting. Sometimes even improvements in upper-extremity function, seizure control, bladder function, swallowing, speech, and personality are seen after an overall reduction in muscle tone (134). Results thus far show lasting reduction in spasticity; increased hip, knee, and ankle range of motion; often a plantigrade foot in stance; increased stride length and walking speed; and no increase in sensory deficits (128,134–138). Three randomized trials comparing rhizotomy with physical therapy have now been published (139–141). These indicate that rhizotomy is more successful at reducing muscle tone, and often at improving motor function.

Although this procedure reduces spasticity and tone, it does not affect joint contractures or the overly contracted musculotendinous unit. These must be treated by orthopaedic surgical procedures after rehabilitation from the rhizotomy. It is estimated that up to 65% of patients require additional procedures, with those older than 4 years at the time of rhizotomy requiring more orthopaedic procedures (129,142,143).

Selective posterior rhizotomy can be beneficial, but it is not a miracle procedure, nor does it cure cerebral palsy. The patient will still have poor motor control and balance, muscle weakness, contractures, sensory involvement, and/ or persisting primitive reflexes if he or she did so preoperatively.

As with virtually everything else in medicine, there are some caveats. An occasional patient develops rapid and severe hip subluxation or dysplasia after this type of rhizotomy (144). Heterotopic ossification around the hip has been reported to occur after varus derotation osteotomy of the proximal femur, with patients who have spastic quadriplegia who have previously had selective posterior rhizotomy (145). Patients with preexisting lumbar lordosis of more than 60 degrees on a sitting lateral radiograph are at risk for the development of postoperative lumbar hyperlordosis (146,147). Spondylolysis and spondylolisthesis have also been reported (148). Another study noted that after rhizotomy, its only consistent negative effect is some increase in sagittal plane anterior pelvic tilt in independent ambulators (137). Perhaps the most common problem after rhizotomy, other than weakness, is the development of planovalgus foot deformities reported in up to 50% of cases (143,149). The deformity is often severe enough to require surgical correction.

Long-term results with many patients followed over several decades are not yet available, but thus far an increased risk of developing scoliosis or kyphosis has not been reported. Another question remaining to be answered is whether late neuropathic arthropathy will occur, but this seems unlikely.

Selective posterior rhizotomy is a demanding procedure for the patient, the family, and the professional staff. Although there is little risk involved, it is expensive, long-term results are not known, and careful patient selection and surgical technique are mandatory. Nevertheless, it can be of substantial benefit to many children.

Physical Therapy. There are several possible roles for physical therapy in cerebral palsy, some generally well accepted and some not. The brain lesion impacts on motor function in four major ways, with individual variation in the involvement of each. These are:

- loss of selective motor control and dependence on primitive reflexes;
- abnormal muscle tone that is influenced by posture, position, or movement;
- muscle imbalance between agonists and antagonists; and
- impaired body-balance mechanisms.

Numerous attempts to modify the central nervous system, and to alter substantial motor dysfunction by external physical means, have been employed exhaustively over the past several decades. The goal is to produce major improvement in voluntary control, tone, and muscle and body balance. In general, most therapists work in a cephalocaudal sequence to try to establish head control, trunk balance for sitting, then reciprocal lower-extremity mobility for crawling, pulling to stand, and, hopefully, functional walking.

The treatment methods include neurodevelopmental therapy, sensory integration therapy, patterning, conductive education, pressure-point stimulation, bracing, and stretching, and many recreation-based therapies (150). For any of these techniques to succeed, the brain probably has to be modified or reprogrammed to make new connections that function almost as well as those it originally made (2), and this may not be possible.

The results and benefits of most of these methods continue to be debated (151–155). There is considerable difference of opinion regarding which modalities should be employed, at what age, how often (from once per week to virtually continuous therapy for 18 h a day), by whom, and how the results are to be measured, documented, and assessed. Some published studies suggest that certain physical therapy programs can improve a cerebral palsy child's joint contractures, motor status, and social motivation (4,156,157), whereas others suggest that they do not (153). Significant problems with the literature include small heterogenous samples, nonrandomized treatment, lack of controlled data, and patient attrition from many studies (153). In many instances it is difficult or impossible to determine whether the therapy was of benefit, or if improvement in motor skills was the result of the child's obligatory neurologic maturation and the learning of substitution patterns and coping methods completely independent from any restructuring of neurocentral control patterns. For some children, certain therapy programs may make a difference. In this regard, it is important that motor function be documented periodically by the therapist during the child's early growth years. This can be done using such systems as the Movement Analysis of Infants, the Gross Motor Performance Measure, Pediatric Evaluation of Disability Inventory, and WeeFIM (158,159).

Much less controversial is that during the first 3 years of life a program that focuses on compensation techniques, showing parents how positioning can facilitate mobility, maintaining joint range of motion, and educating parents about cerebral palsy is helpful. A major source of psychological stress in mothers of handicapped children is the dependency of the child on the mother for accomplishing the activities of daily living. A therapy program that teaches mothers easier ways to work with their child is of great value (160).

Whenever possible, it is beneficial that a parent perform much of the physical therapy, and not rely totally on the physical therapist (4). This saves professional fees, minimizes trips to the therapist and interference with school time, and positively involves parents and even siblings with the child. Many parents, however, decline such involvement because of other family or career demands, or simply because they are too tired to commit the time and effort necessary.

Frequent sessions and protracted therapy programs are expensive and time-consuming, and generate hopes and expectations for all involved. If not of benefit, or if ineffective modalities are employed, the therapy process can raise false hopes, increase frustrations for the child and the family, waste large sums of money, and sometimes unbalance interactions among the members of the family unit (4,151).

There is general agreement that postoperative rehabilitative physical therapy is not only helpful but it is usually essential to maximize the benefits of most types of orthopaedic surgery in cerebral palsy. The patient and the therapist are the ones who will overcome the early postoperative weakness, stiffness, and discomfort. The goals are to maintain or improve joint range of motion, regain preoperative muscle strength, maximize ambulation, and improve function, if possible. How long should the postoperative therapy continue, and how frequently should it be done? This varies with the magnitude of the surgery performed. It may be necessary for as little as 1 or 2 weeks, or as long as several months. The family may be able to provide the treatments on a daily basis. If all treatments must be provided by the therapist, two or three times per week is standard.

Another potential benefit of physical therapy is the prevention of joint contractures by the supervision of a daily range of motion program for those who lack the motor strength and voluntary control to maintain their own ranges. This type of program can be done by a parent, an aide, or a caretaker, and does not require the services of a physical therapist, other than to develop and monitor the program. As previously noted, however, data proving the benefit of such a program are lacking. In some severely involved children, it is impossible to prevent contractures no matter how aggressive the treatment.

An unresolved issue is the duration of maintenance physical therapy. Although some parents want and even demand therapy two or three times a week for the life of their child, there is no evidence that any type of physical therapy can have a beneficial, lasting effect on motor function beyond early-to-middle childhood (age 4–8 years). Children older than this no doubt benefit more by devoting their time (and their families' and society's resources) to the development of communication, cognitive, and recreational skills, instead of endless therapy sessions.

It is irrefutable that the physical therapist can be of great benefit to the child and family. She or he is a resource, and sometimes a case manager for:

- adaptive and therapeutic equipment, including seating systems;
- fabricating some types of splints and basic orthotics;
- educating the family about cerebral palsy and the child's deficits and potential;
- advising the family regarding modifications in the home using community resources;
- acting as liaison with the school; and
- as a realistic, supportive health care professional (161).

Of great importance is a good two-way communication pathway between the therapist and the physician. The therapist is often the primary person who documents the child's neuromotor status, monitors progress, and may recommend surgery or other treatments.

A different therapy approach, described in a pilot study, is that of using low-intensity transcutaneous electric stimulation in an attempt to strengthen weaker antagonistic lower-extremity muscles. The treatment is applied only at night. In a small group of patients, some motor improvement was noted, but was lost after the stimulation was withdrawn (162). More investigation of this approach is necessary before its clinical relevance is determined.

Orthotics. Orthotic devices are classically used to prevent deformity, to improve function by substituting for a weakened muscle, or to protect a weakened part. In cerebral palsy, they are most commonly used to:

- stabilize feet, ankles, and knees;
- maintain nighttime hip abduction to prevent subluxation;
- possibly slow the progression of spinal deformity, to obtain beneficial growth or improve sitting balance; and
- as night splints to prevent hand and wrist deformity.

Progress has been made in understanding the biomechanics of the lower extremities in cerebral palsy, and developing strong, lightweight, comfortable new materials for the orthoses. Lower-extremity orthotics almost never will have to extend above the knee with patients who have spastic diplegia (163). For foot control, the UCBL (University of California Biomechanics Laboratory) orthosis is most popular. This can maintain forefoot, hindfoot, and subtalar alignment in a supple, not rigid, foot, but cannot control the ankle.

Various types of ankle–foot orthoses (AFOs) include the solid-ankle type, to control the entire foot, provide mediolateral ankle stability, and maintain the ankle in a rigid plantigrade position to preserve the plantar flexion–knee extension couple. The solid-ankle AFO is the best choice for the spastic foot, and can be used in almost any instance. Modifications to the solid-ankle AFO have been made to improve foot and ankle function. An example is the posterior leaf-spring AFO, which does not provide mediolateral ankle stability, but allows some plantar flexion and dorsiflexion from neutral, while preventing footdrop. This type is used when spasticity is minimal. It stores minimal kinetic energy during dorsiflexion, and gives back minimal energy at push-off. Articulated AFOs have hinged ankles and plantar flexion stops, which prevent equinus and excessive extensor thrust while allowing free dorsiflexion during gait. They also allow more tibialis anterior muscle function. Although articulated AFOs better allow dorsiflexion activities, such as bending over and stair climbing, they provide less ankle support, are bulky, and do not fit into shoes well, and are more likely to cause heel irritation. They may also prevent a needed plantar flexion–knee extension couple, and may

allow triggering of the gastrocnemius stretch reflex, causing the patient to fight the brace (158). Another type of AFO is the floor-reaction type, of which there are several varieties. It uses the plantar flexion–knee extension couple to prevent knee-flexion crouch and gain appropriate stance-phase knee extension during gait, provided that the foot is plantigrade, no significant knee flexion contracture is present (<10 degrees), hip extension is full, and no major rotational malalignments are present in the limb. This approach has essentially eliminated the need to ever prescribe a KAFO (knee-ankle-foot orthosis) in an ambulatory child with cerebral palsy. The main indication for KAFOs is to brace the lower limbs for ease of transfer in a nonambulatory patient.

Manipulation and Casting. Obtaining beneficial elongation of tight or contracted musculotendinous units or joint capsules can sometimes be accomplished by gentle, nonpainful, repeated passive stretching, followed by maintaining the correction with casts, splints, or adjustable orthotic devices. This treatment method has the potential to cause pain to the child, and to raise false hopes for improvement when applied to more than mild spasticity, tightness, or contractures, or when used in patients who are unable to accurately communicate their discomfort.

With properly selected patients, manipulation and casting can sometimes improve, at least temporarily, contractures of the ankle, knee, elbow, wrist, or hand (164). The process may be repeated from every few days to a week, and various casting materials, dropout casts, removable splints, and orthotics with dial-lock or ratchet hinges may be used. The use of nerve or muscle blocks as an adjunct may sometimes be worthwhile.

Another method, known as "inhibition casting," has been employed for several years. This treatment is applied to the lower-extremities by carefully molding bilateral plaster below-knee casts in an attempt to inhibit certain normal tonic plantar reflexes, especially grasp, and thus reduce overall lower-extremity tone. A probable added benefit is stabilization of the foot and ankle by the well-molded cast. The casts are either left in place or changed weekly for 3 or 4 weeks, during which time intensive physical therapy is performed. Hinged AFOs are then substituted for the casts. This method has reportedly been successful in some hands (165–169), but because the noted improvement may not be maintained for more than a few months, others have not considered it to be of value (170).

Orthopaedic Surgery. Surgical treatment is a rapid and dramatic means of altering the structure and function of the musculoskeletal system in children with cerebral palsy. It is almost always the only effective means when fixed myostatic contracture exists. Lengthening a muscle also weakens it. This may help to gain muscle balance about a joint, but strengthening an antagonist may still be desirable, and difficult or impossible. In most cases, the muscles that contract eccentrically, producing deceleration and shock absorption, are the most appropriate for lengthening, and loss of function rarely occurs. Concentric or accelerator muscles initiate, rather than modulate, movement, and may be substantially weakened by lengthening. In these situations, such as with the iliopsoas muscle, it may be better to intramuscularly lengthen the tendinous portion and accept some residual contracture in exchange for preserving needed strength. What follows are recommendations for the treatment of the most common problems and deformities in an ambulatory child who has spastic diplegia.

Treatment of Specific Problems

In most cases, the patient has several abnormal elements in the disturbed gait. Best results are obtained from surgery if all of the abnormalities are identified preoperatively and corrected during the same surgical setting (171,172), requiring only one rehabilitation period. Little or no benefit is derived by simply performing one procedure, such as a triceps surae lengthening, and waiting to assess its effect on other abnormal elements of the child's gait before proceeding to correct them. This strategy does not improve the final result, and inflicts unnecessary discomfort, hospitalization, and rehabilitation on the child.

The best age to perform the surgery varies with the patient and the problems. Ideally it would be after the gait pattern has stabilized, which is about age 4 or 5 years in nonafflicted children, and then or later in children with cerebral palsy, but before age 8 years. Certainly, surgery can be successful in older children and adults. In cases in which the hips are at risk for dislocation, or when there is progressive or substantial acetabular dysplasia, surgery should not be delayed, regardless of age.

In the immediate postoperative period, the major concerns related to the orthopaedic surgical procedures are pain management, relief of superimposed myospasms, and minimization of the child's anxiety. Giving the analgesic medication through the existing intravenous access line, using patient-controlled analgesia when possible, routinely administering diazepam for 48 to 72 h to lessen myospasms, providing continuous caudal analgesia through a small catheter, and the presence of kind, supportive personnel, are most helpful to the child.

Overall, the postoperative management is aimed at restoration of joint motion, muscle strength, and improved gait as rapidly as possible. During this period, it may be beneficial to use night splints for comfort, and to prevent joint positioning that could contribute to recurrent contractures. Such splinting should never exceed the comfort tolerance of the child. In this regard, it is sometimes necessary to alternate control of one ankle and the opposite knee on successive nights, or use splinting only during the day, when it can be effectively monitored. The value of night splinting is not universally accepted, and valid well-controlled studies proving its efficacy are lacking. It is expensive and can be burdensome and uncomfortable for the patient because of malfitting splints, the frustration of substantially restricted mobility, or maintenance of a continuous overstretch on muscles.

When only soft tissue surgery has been done, ambulation may begin within a few days postoperatively. If osteotomies or subtalar arthrodeses were performed, partial weightbearing may begin as soon as 3 weeks postoperatively, assuming that the internal fixation is adequate. Full, unrestricted weightbearing should probably be deferred until radiographic evidence of adequate early bony healing is seen, usually by about 6 weeks. It may take at least 3 months, and sometimes longer, to regain the preoperative level of strength after most multiple lower-extremity surgical procedures with patients who have spastic diplegia.

Hallux Valgus. Hallux valgus and bunions occur commonly in cerebral palsy, most likely because of a combination of muscle imbalance with adductor hallucis overactivity and externally applied forces, such as inadequate clearance resulting from equinovalgus deformity of the foot and ankle, forcing the phalanges of the great toe into valgus (173,174). Equinus, and particularly valgus, of the foot must be corrected first to achieve a lasting good result from hallux valgus surgery in cerebral palsy.

Indications for surgery in this condition are pain and difficulty with proper shoeing; rarely is cosmesis alone an indication. There are myriad operations for the correction of hallux valgus, and most have been used with varying degrees of success in cerebral palsy [➡7.12–7.14]. When spasticity is mild, such procedures as ostectomy, capsulorrhaphy, adductor hallucis release or transfer, and proximal or distal first metatarsal osteotomy can be successful (175–179). With recurrence, or with patients who have more severe spasticity, the McKeever metatarsophalangeal arthrodesis (180), with the joint in a few degrees of valgus and 10 degrees of dorsiflexion relative to the floor, is an excellent procedure (174).

Ankle Equinus. Pure equinus of the ankle, without associated valgus or varus, is not common. It is the result of overactivity or contracture of the triceps surae group, which is normally six times stronger than the ankle dorsiflexors (181). Most of the overactivity is in the gastrocnemius muscle. The soleus is usually not the major problem. The equinus deformity can be treated by serial manipulation and casting, which is most successful with patients who are young, have less spasticity, and whose equinus in mild. Recurrence of the equinus deformity after several months is not uncommon after manipulation and casting.

Another nonsurgical method is the intramuscular injection of botulinum-A toxin into the gastrocnemius. This will not help in fixed myostatic contracture, but can improve or correct equinus temporarily in mild cases. Mostly, it simply delays the need for surgery. Further study is necessary to determine if patients who will realize permanent correction can be identified.

Lasting correction most often requires surgical elongation of the gastrocnemius unit, which, if performed as an isolated procedure, usually can be done as outpatient surgery (173,183). Elongation is most commonly done by lengthening the Achilles tendon (which also lengthens the soleus), by either multiple partial tenotomies, the Hoke triple-cut (184), or White double-cut (185,186) techniques (either percutaneously or open), or by an open step-cut lengthening [➥7.16–7.17]. When percutaneous techniques are employed, care should be taken to avoid completely dividing the Achilles tendon. Some surgeons have advocated methods of attempting to quantify the exact amount of lengthening necessary (187,188). These methods have not gained wide acceptance.

Some authors advocate the Baker (189,190) or Vulpius (191,192) fascial division type of lengthening of the gastrocnemius aponeurosis alone. This method has the advantage of not only preserving, but actually generating more soleus strength for pushoff (193). Whether it results in a higher recurrence rate is debatable (194). Similar results have been reported in studies comparing tendon lengthening with muscle lengthening in the treatment of equinus deformity (195,196).

A less popular method is Achilles tendon advancement anteriorly (i.e., closer to the talus) on the calcaneus to decrease its power by decreasing its lever arm (197–199). This procedure is more complex than the tendon lengthenings, and has not been demonstrated to be superior. Its best results occur when it is combined with other procedures (195).

Regardless of the surgical technique selected, the result is usually good (200). Recurrence rates are inversely proportional to the age of the child at the time of surgery; lower rates are seen in older children. Before age 4 years, the recurrence rate is about 25%, whereas it approaches zero when the surgery is done after age 8 years (201,202). After surgical lengthening, some believe it is beneficial to control the ankle with a night splint and an orthosis to prevent recurrent deformity and improve function (203). Others have shown that orthotics do not prevent recurrent deformity (204). A reasonable approach is to use an AFO to improve functional stability or control weakness in those who need it, and to reserve night splinting for those who show signs of early recurrent tightness. If the patient has voluntary active foot dorsiflexion to more than 10 degrees, there is a good likelihood that an AFO will not be necessary.

The patient is treated with a below-knee cast for 2 to 3 weeks if only the gastrocnemius aponeurosis has been lengthened or an incomplete Achilles tenotomy (e.g., the Hoke technique) has been done. The below-knee cast is left in place for 4 to 6 weeks after step-cut lengthening of the Achilles tendon.

A problem to be avoided is the postoperative develop-

ment of a calcaneus deformity from overlengthening the heel cord, particularly in a patient with athetosis. Treatment for an overlengthened heel cord is difficult, but some have had success with shortening the Achilles tendon by surgical reattachment or imbrication, and Tardieu and Tardieu suggest a period of casting the ankle in plantar flexion, followed by orthotic control at plantigrade during the day and in equinus at night (204).

Foot and Ankle Equinovarus. Ankle equinus, varus of the hindfoot, and, often, varus and supination of the forefoot are present in this deformity. It is most often seen in hemiplegia, but also may occur in children with diplegia and quadriplegia. The hindfoot varus is most likely caused by overactivity of the tibialis posterior muscle, whereas varus and supination of the forefoot are more likely the result of overactivity of the tibialis anterior, which may also contribute to hindfoot varus. Peroneal muscle weakness may also be a factor.

For treatment of hindfoot equinovarus, correction of the equinus, as described above, must be combined with lengthening or split transfer of the tibialis posterior tendon [➥7.18]. Lengthening may be by the step-cut method or by intramuscular tenotomy cephalad to the musculotendinous junction, which is also known as the "Frost procedure" (163,205). Some surgeons prefer to split the tendon and transfer the lateral half to the peroneus brevis tendon (206,207) in order not to weaken the muscle as much as would a lengthening. Others believe that some weakening is desirable. There are several reports of good results with the split transfer, and many indicate that preoperative gait analysis is not necessary for a successful outcome (208).

Although anterior transfer of the tibialis posterior tendon through the interosseous membrane to the dorsum of the foot has been advocated (150,209), it should not be done in cerebral palsy patients. This transfer can result in a calcaneovalgus deformity that is very difficult to correct (210).

In varus and supination foot deformities caused by overactivity of the tibialis anterior muscle, a split transfer of the lateral half of its tendon to the cuboid bone usually successfully balances the foot (211). DeGnore and Greene use hindfoot varus, which occurs in the swing phase of gait, and a positive confusion test as their indication for split anterior tibialis tendon transfer (212). The validity of the confusion test, however, has been questioned because it does not predict ankle kinematics in the swing phase of gait (213).

Nonrigid varus of the hindfoot often occurs with varus and supination of the forefoot. In this situation, split anterior tibialis tendon transfer, combined with posterior tibialis tendon lengthening, is appropriate.

When the hindfoot varus is rigid, bony surgery, in addition to addressing the triceps surae and tibialis posterior units, is necessary to correct the deformity (214). This can be accomplished by a laterally based, closing-wedge osteotomy of the calcaneus with staple or screw fixation, which is technically difficult to reduce and adequately fix. Easier and very effective is obliquely dividing the calcaneus in the coronal plane, posterior and parallel to the peroneal tendons, sliding the posterior fragment laterally, and fixing it with a cannulated or cancellous screw or pins. Assuming adequate internal fixation with either procedure, a below-knee cast is necessary until bony healing has occurred (usually 6–8 weeks). Subsequent orthotic control of the foot and ankle may or may not be necessary.

Foot and Ankle Equinovalgus. This is the most common situation with patients who have diplegia, followed by equinovarus and calcaneus with about equal prevalence (215). Its cause is probably muscle imbalance, with triceps surae overactivity and weakness of the tibialis posterior muscle, with relative overpull of the peroneal musculature (216). The equinus is addressed as described above. It should not be assumed that the valgus originates at the subtalar joint. It may be coming from the ankle, so weightbearing radiographs of the ankle should be studied as part of the surgical planning. If the ankle valgus is really in the distal tibia, it may be corrected by osteotomy, or, in some cases, by hemiepiphyseodesis, screw fixation, or stapling of the medial side of the physis, if sufficient growth remains.

Subtalar valgus, which is mild and supple, can be controlled by an orthosis, either an AFO or a UCBL type. The orthosis may be augmented by intramuscular lengthening of the peroneus brevis tendon which decreases the power of the muscle by one grade (217). The peroneus longus tendon should not be lengthened because a varus deformity may ensue. Transfer of the peroneus brevis to the tibialis

posterior tendon has been performed, but published series with evaluations of results are lacking (216).

With more severe valgus that is passively correctable, surgery is usually required, because orthotic control rarely succeeds. This is particularly true if there has been failure of an orthosis to control the hindfoot valgus, such that painful calluses and blisters result on the medial side of the foot.

Most surgeons prefer either an Evans or modified Evans lateral opening-wedge lengthening osteotomy of the distal calcaneus (218), or a subtalar arthrodesis using internal fixation and bone grafting [➡7.4, 7.10, 7.11] (219) (Fig. 15-9). Calcaneal lengthening restores support of the talus, and does not involve fusion of a joint. It should be combined with medial plication and peroneal lengthening, as described by Mosca (220). Subtalar fusion with internal fixation rigidly fixes the subtalar joint, and yields a higher fusion rate than the classic Grice procedure or modifications thereof, which rely on bone graft alone (221–225).

Stabilization also may be accomplished by arthroereisis, using a staple or an inert plastic block (226). This technique may be effective in some very young children, but it is not widely accepted. Multiple series with adequate long-term follow-up are lacking.

Another method of correcting a supple valgus hindfoot deformity is by medial displacement of an oblique osteotomy of the calcaneus with screw or pin fixation. Although limited experience with this procedure has been reported, the osteotomy heals rapidly, preserves subtalar motion, and is easy to perform (227).

When rigid, nonreducible hindfoot valgus is present the options are a sliding medial-displacement calcaneal osteotomy (228), a lateral opening-wedge or medial closing-wedge

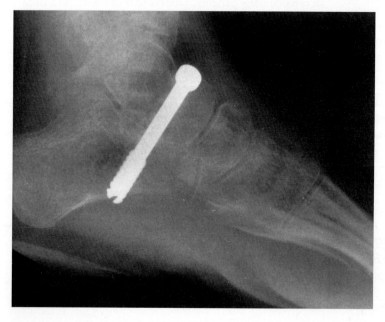

FIGURE 15-9. Postoperative lateral radiograph of a subtalar arthrodesis stabilized by a cannulated screw and augmented by iliac autograft bone.

osteotomy of the proximal calcaneus, a combined calcaneal-cuboid–cuneiform osteotomy (229) or a triple arthrodesis. Triple arthrodesis provides correction (230), but is best avoided in very young patients in whom growth of the foot will be substantially inhibited. For this reason, it probably should not be performed on a child who is not within about 2 years of the end of growth. Triple arthrodesis [➡**7.9**] appears to be successful over the long term with patients who have mild involvement and are community ambulators. It has been reported not to increase the risk of later development of midfoot and ankle osteoarthritis as the result of abnormal mechanical forces being transferred to those joints over a long period (231). It is always important to achieve the best possible muscle balance at the foot and ankle; otherwise, even a triple arthrodesis may deform in time.

External Tibial Torsion. External (lateral) tibial torsion is usually associated with excessive femoral anteversion and pes planovalgus. Inadequate foot clearance may also be a factor.

Profound external tibial torsion substantially shortens the lever-arm effect of the foot in generating the plantar flexion–knee extension couple, which facilitates knee extension in the midstance and late stance phases of gait and helps to prevent crouch. Stance phase is often shortened, the base of support is unstable, and pushoff power is compromised. The solution to this problem is distal derotational osteotomies of the tibia and fibula at the supramalleolar level to align the ankle and foot progression angle with the direction of gait and the axis of the knee [➡**6.8**]. The fibula is divided transversely just proximal to the syndesmosis, and the tibia is divided about 2.5 cm above the physis. In younger children fixation by crossed smooth Steinmann pins, cut and bent extracutaneously, and an above-knee cast is adequate. The pins are removed, and the cast changed to below-knee at 6 weeks. In older children, the surgeon may choose to use a T-plate and screws and a short-leg cast. As with any surgical procedure near to an open physis, care must be taken to avoid inadvertent damage to the growth plate.

Knee-flexion Deformity. Knee-flexion deformity may be a true flexion contracture, but is more often simply caused by spastic and tight hamstring muscles, without fixed capsular contracture (232). The medial hamstrings usually are the major problem (233). Very often there is an associated hip flexion contracture and a crouched gait. Rarely, knee flexion may be a coping mechanism for calcaneus deformity (hyperdorsiflexion) at the ankle. More often, the ankle is neutral or in equinus. Equinus must be corrected when hamstrings are lengthened or genu recurvatum may result. It is essential to assess and address all factors to appropriately manage a crouched gait.

As a general rule, the hamstrings require lengthening when straight-leg raising cannot exceed 70 degrees above the horizontal, or when the popliteal angle (i.e., the sagittal femorotibial angle with maximum knee extension, the patient supine, and the hip first flexed to 90 degrees) is less than 135 degrees (i.e., 45 degrees short of full extension). Lengthening the medial hamstrings is performed by incising the fascial aponeurosis of the semimembranosis muscle at a minimum of two levels, and step-cut lengthening or tenotomizing the semitendinosis and gracilis tendons [➡**4.23**]. If after these procedures the lateral hamstrings are still tight (popliteal angle less than 160 degrees), they may also require aponeurotic lengthening (234,235).

Postoperatively, hamstring lengthenings with or without distal rectus femoris transfers are managed in removable knee-immobilizer splints, which can easily fit over a below-knee cast. Passive range of motion exercises may begin on the second or third postoperative day. If no bony surgery has been performed walking training may begin as early as the fifth postoperative day. When adequate quadriceps strength has been regained, usually by the fourth postoperative week, the knee immobilizers may be discarded or used as night splints. Between physical therapy sessions sitting should be done with the knees alternately in extension and flexion.

Good results at the knee can sometimes be obtained by lengthening the hamstrings proximally (236) [➡**3.19**]. It has been found, however, that lumbar lordosis may increase after this procedure because of the overactive hip flexors; also, the desired effect on the distal hamstring tightness may not be achieved (237). It must be remembered that the hamstrings are also hip extensors, sometimes contributing up to a one-third of the extensor torque (238,239). Hip extensor power is somewhat lessened by hamstring lengthening, especially proximal hamstring lengthening. Therefore, this procedure may increase a preexisting hip flexion contracture, as well as increase the lumbar lordosis, if the iliopsoas unit is not addressed concomitantly. Gait analysis has shown that in some patients with a crouch gait, the hamstrings may be of normal or even excessive length. This is seen with simultaneous hyperflexion of the hip. In this situation hamstring lengthening alone may further weaken hip extensor power and increase the already severe hip-flexion deformity. To preserve some of the hip extensor power of the hamstrings, Gage has recommended transfer of the distal semitendinosis to the lateral femoral metaphysis. This may minimally augment external rotation at the hip (1).

Rectus Femoris Transfer. A finding commonly associated with knee-flexion deformity is cospasticity of the rectus femoris muscle and the hamstrings. The rectus may be firing continuously throughout the gait cycle, or mostly during swing phase, but the result often is a stiff-knee gait with less than 80% of normal knee motion. In this situation when the hamstrings alone are lengthened, a stiff, extended-knee gait frequently results. There is lack of adequate knee flexion in swing phase, and that interferes with foot clearance so that circumduction or vaulting may be necessary to compensate (240). The stiff-knee gait may be prevented by transferring the distal rectus femoris tendon medially and posteriorly [➡4.24]. The transfer does not affect gait abnormalities in the transverse plane (i.e., intoeing or out-toeing), and it makes no difference whether the transfer is attached to the sartorius, gracilis, semitendinosus, or iliotibial band (241,242). This transfer is successful in restoring adequate (60 degrees) knee flexion in the swing phase of gait. It has been shown that transfer is necessary to accomplish this, not just tenotomy of the distal rectus femoris tendon (242,243). The indication for distal rectus femoris transfer is a preoperative range of knee motion during gait of less than 80% of normal (less than 45 to 50 degrees) and hamstring–rectus femoris cospasticity, with nonphasic activity of the rectus during the swing phase of gait (243–245).

Unfortunately the static assessment of hamstring tightness by straight-leg raising or by measuring the popliteal angle, does not correlate with the dynamic range of knee motion during gait (246).

Without gait analysis, one is left to assess knee motion during gait either by clinical observation or the study of a videotape of gait. Recent work also suggests that a positive Duncan-Ely test does not predict abnormal EMG activity, and neither the type of abnormal EMG activity in the rectus nor the magnitude of the restricted preoperative knee range of motion are significant variables in determining the success of the transfer (242). The beneficial effects of rectus transfer (increased velocity, stride length, and knee range of motion) may diminish significantly over time (247).

Hip Adduction Contracture.

Tightness in the hip adductors can result in a scissoring type of gait pattern, and predisposes the patient to hip dysplasia or subluxation. Generally, when the hips cannot be abducted beyond 30 degrees in flexion or extension, adductor release or transfer (either posteriorly to the ischial tuberosity, which has its advocates [87,248] or posteriorly and distally to the gracilis [249]) is indicated [➡3.18]. There seems to be little difference in the results from release or transfer (250,251), but one study reports a high incidence of pelvic obliquity and hip subluxation after adductor transfer to the ischium (252). Neurectomy of the anterior branch of the obturator nerve is rarely indicated in diplegic patients who can walk, because it excessively weakens the adductor brevis muscle and can result in a wide-based gait with hyperabduction of the hips (253). The hip adductors function to stabilize the hip against excessive abduction during gait, running, and in activities such as skiing, skating, and horseback riding. The gait stability they provide allows more effective hip flexor and extensor activity. Thus, it is important not to "go for broke" and overlengthen or overweaken the adductors in ambulatory patients.

Release of the tight adductors [➡3.17] is performed with the patient supine, through either a longitudinal or trans-

verse incision, depending on the preference of the surgeon. The adductor longus is always completely divided. Often, this is adequate to accomplish the objective of adductor release for most surgeons. This is at least 60 degrees of passive abduction on each side, with the hip and knee flexed to 90 degrees, or at least 45 degrees of passive abduction with the hip and knee extended (the medial hamstrings are also hip adductors). At times, some of the adductor brevis may also need to be released, and it may be necessary to divide the gracilis muscle to achieve the desired abduction.

Hip Flexion Contracture.

A hip flexion contracture is best detected by the Thomas test, the prone extension test, or both (254). When the contracture exceeds about 20 to 25 degrees it should be released. Most contractures are caused by a spastic, contracted iliopsoas unit, and often hamstring lengthenings and rectus femoris transfers are necessary, and are combined with psoas recessions. This combination of procedures has very little or no significant effect on pelvic tilt (255).

In ambulatory children release of the iliopsoas tendon by tenotomy at the lesser trochanter weakens hip flexor power excessively, and may prohibit enough hip flexion strength to lift the limb in climbing stairs (256). Ambulatory children should have tenotomy of the psoas tendon alone, not the iliacus fibers, performed over the brim of the pelvis (257). Care must be exercised to differentiate the psoas tendon from the femoral nerve. Occasionally, the psoas is not tendinous at this level. Then a recession to the anterior hip capsule is performed via an adductor approach.

Hip flexor releases are treated postoperatively by lying prone several times per day. Painful muscle spasms are particularly common in the first few days after hip surgery, and may be treated with diazepam and analgesics. It is desirable to begin gentle passive range of motion exercises by the second or third day after flexor or adductor releases, and gait training may begin 5 to 7 days postoperatively. After 3 weeks, more vigorous muscle strengthening exercises are tolerated.

Lumbar Hyperlordosis.

Hyperlordosis is usually the result of compensation for bilateral hip flexion contractures. Correcting the contractures corrects the excessive lordosis. It should be remembered that other conditions, such as compensation for a rigid thoracic kyphosis, also produce lumbar hyperlordosis.

Intoeing.

Intoeing is most commonly the result of excessive femoral anteversion (frequently measuring 60 to 70 degrees), but occasionally is caused by increased spasticity in the internal rotator muscles of the hip (the medial hamstrings or the anterior fibers of the gluteus medius and tensor fascia lata) (233). Excessive femoral anteversion, causing intoeing, rarely exists as an isolated finding in spastic diplegia.

It is usually accompanied by lower-extremity musculotendinous tightness or contractures that also require correction.

Derotational osteotomy of the femur is the treatment for increased femoral anteversion. The appropriate age for the osteotomy is whenever other lower-extremity surgery is being done. This usually means after age 4 years. The derotation may be at the supracondylar region [➡4.18] in younger children with mild to moderate spasticity, and may be secured either by crossed Steinmann pins (42) and a hip spica cast, or by an external fixator. In older children, and at any age with substantial spasticity, it is best to perform the osteotomy at the intertrochanteric level [➡4.6] and to preserve the attachment of the iliopsoas. Fixation with a strong blade-plate or screw-plate may avoid the need for a postoperative spica cast and allow early hip motion with patients who have adequate bone stock. Such strong internal fixation obviates the problems of loss of fixation and malunion, which occasionally occur after the pin and cast fixation of distal femoral osteotomies. The proximal osteotomy is facilitated by placing the patient in the prone position and using the approach described by Root and Siegal (258). If subluxation and/or coxa valga are present, varus can be added to the osteotomy. Another option for derotation in children older than age 10 years is in the subtrochanteric region with fixation by a locked intramedullary rod, but this cannot be combined with varization.

Femoral derotational osteotomies to correct excessive anteversion require external rotation of the distal segment, which tightens the medial hamstrings. To prevent this increased medial hamstring tightness, which may actually increase internal rotation, these hamstrings usually need to be lengthened when femoral derotation is performed.

Other methods of treating intoeing gait in children with cerebral palsy have been advocated. Two of these are transfer of the semitendinosus tendon to the distal lateral femur (1) and posteromedial transfer of the distal tendon of the rectus femoris. These techniques have not been shown to be effective for intoeing (241). It should be remembered that transfer of the distal tendon of the rectus femoris, either medially or laterally, does improve knee flexion for foot clearance during the swing phase of gait (241). Another reported technique is transfer of the greater trochanter [➡4.9], with its attached gluteus medius muscle to the anterior proximal femur, so that it may function as an external rotator, as well as an abductor (259). This abductor transfer, although sometimes successful, can produce an abductor weakness type of gait and has not been widely adopted (42).

Spastic Hemiplegia

Children afflicted with spastic hemiplegia have involvement of one side of the body, with the arm and hand more severely involved than the lower extremity. On closer evaluation, very mild involvement on the contralateral side is often found, especially in those with more severe affliction (1).

The hemiplegia type comprises about 30% of all cerebral palsy cases. About 1 in 3 patients have a seizure disorder, and almost one-half have some degree of mental retardation (3). More common than mental retardation is an attention deficit, learning, or behavioral disorder (260). A history of head trauma or intracranial hemorrhage is frequently found in spastic hemiplegia. Virtually all patients are community ambulators, although only about half can walk by 18 months of age (3). Some limb-length inequality and a difference in foot size are the rule, but rarely require any treatment.

The stereotyped concept of the patient with hemiplegia includes equinovarus at the foot and ankle, flexion at the knee and hip, internal rotation of the lower limb, internal rotation at the shoulder, flexion at the elbow, pronation of the forearm, flexion and ulnar deviation at the wrist, and thumb-in-palm with finger flexion in the hand. Actually, the degree of involvement with spastic hemiplegia is a spectrum, which has been separated into four subtypes (155). It is essential in planning treatment to quantify the involvement. Surgical results should be predictably good.

Type I hemiplegia is characterized by weakness of the tibialis anterior muscle, and the triceps surae group is not tight. This type is manifest as a footdrop and a steppage gait, with plantar flexion disappearing during stance phase. It is easily treated with an appropriate AFO. A posterior leaf spring or an articulated ankle type is usually superior to a solid-ankle AFO in this condition (261). The most difficult part of management is to get the child to wear the orthosis if he or she has no other noticeable variation from normality. One reported surgical approach to this type of hemiplegic problem has been transfer of the flexor digitorum longus and flexor hallucis longus tendons to the dorsum of the foot (262). Experience with this technique is limited, and meaningful long-term results are not available.

Type II hemiplegia has tibialis anterior muscle weakness plus spasticity in the triceps surae group, and usually in the tibialis posterior muscle. This produces an equinovarus deformity of the foot and ankle, which persists throughout all phases of gait, and can produce some knee hyperextension late in stance phase. The problem is addressed by lengthening the gastrocnemius aponeurosis or the Achilles tendon, lengthening or performing a split transfer of the tibialis posterior tendon (206,207), and providing an AFO if needed. Split posterior tibial tendon transfer is useful for correction of the varus heel in stance phase when there is no fixed deformity and the muscle is firing in phase (during stance). Often the tibialis posterior is active throughout the gait cycle. In that case it is better to lengthen its tendon rather than perform the split transfer (3). Rarely, the tibialis anterior muscle, instead of being weak, is overactive during the swing phase of gait. Then, a split anterior tibialis tendon transfer can be effective in achieving transverse plane balance of the foot (211). This is usually combined with tibialis posterior tendon-lengthening.

Postopoeratively, an AFO may be needed to assist a weak tibialis anterior, or to aid in preventing recurrent equinus deformity. Some children are orthosis-free after the surgery. The risk of recurrence of the equinus deformity in hemiplegia decreases as the child grows older, being reported at about 25% below the age of 4 years and 12% thereafter (3).

In type III hemiplegia, not only are the triceps surae and tibialis posterior muscles spastic and usually contracted, but hamstring involvement is also present, often with cospasticity of the rectus femoris. This produces a stiff, flexed knee gait with equinovarus foot and ankle deformity. Successful treatment includes the tendon surgery discussed for type II and the addition of medial hamstring lengthenings, often combined with a distal rectus femoris tendon transfer, as described in the section on spastic diplegia. Again, the appropriate AFO may be necessary postoperatively, sometimes temporarily, and sometimes permanently.

Type IV hemiplegia has the features of type III, with the addition of hip flexor and adductor spasticity or contracture. Iliopsoas lengthening, by release of the psoas tendon over the pelvic brim, and appropriate adductor releases are added to the treatment recommended for those with type III involvement.

This classification is helpful in the management of most patients with spastic hemiplegia. It is not infallible, however, and patients occasionally are encountered who have profound equinus with little or no varus; who have increased ipsilateral femoral anteversion, in addition to type IV involvement; or who have other abnormalities.

Athetoid Cerebral Palsy

Children with athetoid cerebral palsy have abnormal muscle tension and tone, which may increase with voluntary activity. Their resting state often includes limb movements that are purposeless, involuntary, and almost continuously changing. The movements are coarse and irregular, often give the child the appearance of squirming or writhing, and extensor tone predominance is the rule. The movements disappear during sleep (263).

The muscle tension often changes with the emotional state. The athetoid movements are greater in the more distal parts of the limbs, and often rapidly flow from flexion to extension, adduction to abduction, and pronation to supination. Because of the almost constant motion, most of the joints are put through a full range of motion, and contractures are not common unless there is an asymmetric component of mixed spasticity present.

Most children with substantial athetosis are not able to walk. Their mobility is by power wheelchair, often with an adapted steering mechanism. The therapeutic focuses for these children should be on communication methods, on facilitating their control over activities of daily living, and on wheelchair mobility (264).

The gait pattern of those few patients with athetosis who can walk is random, inconsistent, and influenced by many external stimuli. Without a consistent baseline, the results of soft tissue surgery are unpredictable. Tenotomies and muscle releases should be done infrequently, and then very carefully with patients who have significant athetosis, because often the result is a severe, almost untreatable deformity opposite the one originally addressed.

Scoliosis is not uncommon in athetoid patients, and responds well to the internal fixation and spinal fusion techniques described earlier. Adult athetoid patients may develop profoundly painful degenerative spondylosis and myelopathy in the cervical spine, sometimes with upper-extremity weakness and even instability. One study identified two-thirds of athetoid patients by age 44 years, and all patients older than age 55 years, with moderate or severe cervical disc degeneration (265). The most common motion segment is C5–C6. This usually responds well to anterior cervical fusion (266), but severe athetosis and dystonia can make postoperative immobilization very difficult. In this situation, the use of BTX injections into the neck muscles can be extremely beneficial in eliminating involuntary neck motions (267).

UPPER EXTREMITY INVOLVEMENT

Most upper-extremity involvement occurs with patients who have spastic hemiplegia and quadriplegia. When considering treatment, it is essential to consider the function of the entire upper limb, and of the child to whom it is attached. It has long been reported that the problems of spasticity, weakness, poor motor control, poor proprioception and stereognosis, and joint contractures, reduce or eliminate the possible benefits of tendon lengthenings, transfers, or other surgical treatment in most cases. Patients with hemiplegia have been reported to have better results than do patients who have quadriplegia, and postoperative function is usually better with right hemiplegia than with left (268). Mental retardation, visual deficits, behavioral problems, and particularly dyskinetic involvement also may contraindicate upper extremity surgery. Fewer than 5% of patients are appropriate candidates for such surgery (269). Nevertheless, a recent report of 718 procedures in 134 patients over a 25-year period indicates that only high motivation and fair-to-good motor control affect upper-extremity surgical outcome, and mentation, sensibility, and the type of cerebral palsy do not influence the surgical result (270).

Patients with hemiplegic involvement often have functional improvement after upper-extremity surgery. Substantial cosmetic improvement or facilitation of care, such as dressing and gloving, can be achieved in severely involved patients. Patients who are most likely to benefit from upper-extremity surgery in cerebral palsy are those with:

- spasticity, not athetosis;
- reasonable intelligence and good motivation;
- stable trunk and body position;

- good hand proprioception, stereognosis, touch, and other sensations;
- no fixed contractures and adequate passive range of motion of all upper-extremity joints;
- reasonable hand function, with good hand placement capability and voluntary control; and
- age between 5 and 20 years (111,271).

In some instances, the use of preoperative dynamic electromyographic studies aids in decision-making regarding lengthening or transferring musculotendinous units (272–274).

An important indication for surgical correction of wrist and elbow contractures can be cosmesis. Older children and adolescents with reasonable intelligence who function well in public may have a negative body image, with a rigid, contracted wrist and elbow. This may also have a negative effect on peer group acceptance. In such cases, correction of those deformities, although having no benefit for upper-extremity function, can be of immense psychological value to the patient.

Nonsurgical Treatment

Traditional nonsurgical treatment modalities include passive range of motion exercises and passive night splinting to attempt to prevent contractures and serial casting, or judiciously applied dynamic splinting to attempt correction of mild contractures in the absence of much spasticity. The daytime use of splints in attempts to improve function almost always meets with failure in hands with poor sensation and control, and may actually increase spasticity. Outcome studies of splinting are lacking. It is doubtful that the satisfaction of "doing something" alone justifies the cost.

Recently, BTX injections have shown promise in selected upper-extremity muscles, but the effects are temporary unless a stretching program or another means of lengthening the muscles succeeds during the temporary period. BTX will probably most help a hemiplegic child with spasticity, no joint contractures, and reasonable hand function. The best early results have involved blocking the biceps, pronator teres, flexor carpi ulnaris, and thumb flexors and adductors (114,122). Whether surgery is merely deferred or can sometimes be avoided with BTX treatment is not yet known.

Surgical Treatment

Before undertaking an upper-extremity surgery program it is essential for patients and families to understand that realistic goals are improved function and appearance. Normality is not a possible result, and any improvement will require careful evaluation and planning. As with the lower extremity, it is wise to perform all needed procedures at one operative setting. It is certainly possible to have different surgical teams operating on the upper and lower extremities at the same time. Some common upper-extremity surgical procedures and their indications in spastic patients follow. Those patients with athetosis almost never have enough voluntary control to benefit from upper-extremity surgery.

Shoulder

Although it is rarely necessary to operate on the shoulder with severe spasticity, adduction and internal rotation contractures may develop, caused by tightness of the subscapularis and pectoralis major muscles. If hand function is reasonable but the ability to position the hand in space is compromised, correction of shoulder contractures is appropriate. This is accomplished by releasing the tendon of the subscapularis and lengthening the tendon of the pectoralis major. If this does not provide the needed correction, a proximal humeral derotational osteotomy, fixed with a compression plate, usually solves the problem (269,271).

An uncommon problem for people with hemiplegia is shoulder abduction when running, caused by deltoid muscle spasticity. This may be relieved by musculotendinous lengthening of the deltoid (114).

Elbow

The elbow is prone to develop flexion and pronation contractures in children with substantial spasticity. The flexion contracture is caused by the spasticity of the biceps, brachialis, and brachioradialis. Serial casting, dropout casts (long-arm casts with the posterior plaster above the elbow removed to allow further extension while blocking further flexion), dynamic splints, and BTX have been discussed already.

Surgery is usually necessary to gain lasting correction. The indications are to improve the ability to position a functional hand in space, to improve hygiene or prevent skin breakdown, and to improve appearance. Most flexion contractures of the elbow can be corrected by resecting the lacertus fibrosus, and by fractional lengthening of the brachialis and the biceps, plus release of the brachioradialis origin (114). Occasionally, step-cut lengthening of the biceps and anterior capsulotomy of the elbow is necessary (269).

Pronation deformity of the elbow is the result of overactivity of the pronator teres, perhaps the pronator quadratus, and weakness of supination. When combined with a flexion contracture in a young child, dislocation of the radial head may occur. The pronation component forces the dorsum of the hand or forearm to assist in bimanual tasks. Correcting the contracture to permit supination allows use of the hand. Surgical treatment of pronation contracture consists either of distal release or transfer of the pronator teres muscle (269). If passive supination is full, some advocate transfer of the pronator teres tendon through the interosseous membrane (114) or posterior to the radius to an anterolateral insertion so that it can function as a supinator (268). Results of this transfer are not always good, and a fixed supination deformity is a larger problem than a pronation deformity (268). Release of the pronator alone is usually successful, and is preferred by most surgeons.

Wrist

Prior to operating across the wrist, the status of the finger flexors and extensors must be determined. Flexion deformity or contracture with some ulnar deviation is the usual finding at the wrist in spastic upper extremities. This is usually associated with pronation of the forearm and weakness of the wrist extensor muscles. If flexor spasticity is minimal and finger extension is good, simply lengthening the flexor carpi ulnaris or the flexor carpi radialis, but not both, may be helpful. Another usually effective means of weakening spastic wrist and finger flexors is the flexor and pronator release procedure (271,276). The disadvantage of this operation is that it is nonselective, releasing all wrist and finger flexors and the pronator teres from the medial epicondyle of the distal humerus (42).

Flexor spasticity often is very severe, and extensor weakness is profound. In such cases, flexor carpi ulnaris transfer is recommended [➥1.7] (276,277). Before transfer an electromyogram can be performed to determine the phase of the muscle if that cannot be determined by clinical examination. Transfer of the flexor carpi ulnaris tendon around the ulnar border of the wrist and into the extensor carpi radialis brevis, is indicated if the transferred muscle is active during grasp, and the patient has poor wrist extension and poor grasp but can actively extend the fingers with the wrist in neutral or dorsiflexion (8,278) (Fig. 15-10). If the flexor carpi ulnaris muscle is active during release and there is adequate grasp but poor release, it is transferred to the extensor digitorum comminus tendons. At least one long-term follow-up study has indicated that transfer to the wrist extensor is less predictable than transfer to the finger extensors (279). Regardless of the site of transfer, the flexor carpi radialis tendon should not be lengthened in association with flexor carpi ulnaris transfer because that risks overly weakening wrist flexion.

Wrist arthrodesis eliminates any useful compensatory or functional motion of the wrist, and prevents the wrist from any helpful participation in grasp and release by a tenodesis effect of the extrinsic muscles. It is indicated most often for the markedly deformed carpus in severely involved patients for hygienic or cosmetic reasons, such as putting the hand through a sleeve or into a pocket or a mitten.

Ulnar deviation of the wrist may be caused by overactivity in the extensor carpi ulnaris muscle with volar displacement of its tendon. Split transfer of its tendon to the extensor carpi radialis brevis has been recommended (271).

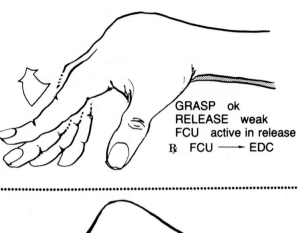

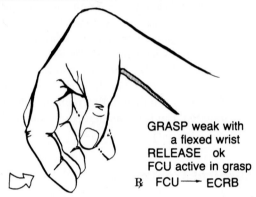

FIGURE 15-10. The spastic hemiplegic hand. The hand at top will benefit from transfer of the flexor carpi ulnaris (FCU) to augment the extensor digitorum communis (EDC). At the bottom, the hand needs augmentation of wrist extension by transferring the flexor carpi ulnaris to the extensor carpi radialis brevis (ECRB).

Hand

The common hand deformities are:

- flexion and adduction of the thumb; and
- either clawing with hyperextension of the finger metacarpophalangeal joints, with flexion contractures of the distal finger joints; or
- full flexion at all finger joints; or
- swan-neck deformities of the fingers.

Thumb-in-palm deformities are complex, and require careful assessment before the appropriate treatment can be recommended. In most cases, the adductor pollicis and first dorsal interosseus muscles overpower the abductor pollicis longus and the extensor pollicis longus and brevis muscles. Common patterns of deformity are:

- metacarpal adduction contracture;
- metacarpal adduction contracture with metacarpophalangeal (MCP) flexion contracture;
- metacarpal adduction contracture with MCP hyperextension contracture; and
- metacarpal adduction contracture with MCP and interphalangeal joint flexion contractures.

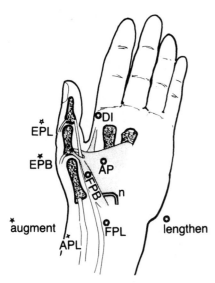

FIGURE 15-11. The repertoire of operations for the thumb-in-palm deformity. Shortened muscles should be lengthened, and weak long muscles should be shortened and augmented. An unstable metacarpophalangeal joint should be stabilized. *AP*, adductor pollicis; *APL*, abductor pollicis longus; *DI*, first dorsal interosseous; *EPB*, extensor pollicis brevis; *EPL*, extensor pollicis longus; *FPB*, flexor pollicis brevis; *FPL*, flexor pollicis longus.

In all types, there are contractures of the skin of the first web and tight fascial bands in the first dorsal interosseous and adductor aponeuroses (114). There are different ways to surgically treat these deformities, but in principle all involve release of contractures of the skin, joints, and spastic muscles; joint stabilization; and augmentation of the weakened muscles [➡1.8] (269,271,280) (Fig. 15-11).

Often the problem in the claw hand with wrist flexion and metacarpophalangeal hyperextension is imbalance between the wrist flexors and extensors. This is usually addressed by transferring either the flexor carpi radialis or the flexor carpi ulnaris to the extensor carpi radialis brevis (271).

If finger flexion deformity is a mild but functional problem, fractionally lengthening the flexor digitorum sublimis and profundus muscles is of benefit. This is done by complete transverse circumferential release of their aponeuroses in the proximal third of the forearm. In tightly flexed fingers that cannot be extended, even with the wrist flexed, an effective treatment is tenotomies of the flexor digitorum profundus and sublimis tendons at different levels in the distal forearm. With the fingers extended the proximal ends of the sublimis tendons are then sutured to the distal ends of the profundus tendons (sublimis to profundus transfers). Tenotomies of the wrist flexors usually are also necessary. With more severe involvement proximal row carpectomy can be used to gain additional length in the soft tissues, or wrist arthrodesis may be necessary to stabilize the hand for assisting.

The often seen swan-neck deformities of the fingers result from intrinsic muscle spasticity and extrinsic extensor overpull, partly caused by the wrist-flexion deformity, by compensation for weak wrist extensors, or by both, with resultant overpull on the central slip of the extensor mechanism. With time the volar plate becomes incompetent and the proximal interphalangeal joint may subluxate and become fixed. In the latter situation it is unlikely that function can be improved with surgery. With early or mild deformities correction of the wrist flexion alone may suffice, and splinting may be added if the deformities are <40 degrees. With more severe deformities the surgical treatment is much more complex (114,269,271).

Appropriate postoperative care, especially after tendon transfers, is essential to the success of hand and upper extremity surgery in cerebral palsy. Recommended treatment for most patients is 4 weeks of complete immobilization, then an intensive exercise program with emphasis on reach, grasp, and release. Removable splints are used for several months during the day, and often at night, for several years (269). Although it is realized that only a small percentage of children with spastic cerebral palsy benefit from upper-extremity surgery, such reconstruction can be of substantial benefit for the appropriate patient.

References

1. Gage JR. *Gait analysis in cerebral palsy.* London: MacKeith, 1991.

Basic Brain Development

2. Goldberg MJ. Measuring outcomes in cerebral palsy. *J Pediatr Orthop* 1991;11:682.
3. Rang M. Cerebral palsy. In: Morrissy RT, ed. *Lovell and Winter's pediatric orthopaedics.* 3rd ed. Philadelphia: JB Lippincott, 1990.
4. Russman BS, Gage JR. Cerebral palsy. *Curr Probl Pediatr* 1989; 19:65.

Etiology

5. Nelson KB, Ellenberg JH. Antecedents of cerebral palsy II. Multivariate analysis of risk. *N Engl J Med* 1986;315:81.
6. Atkinson S, Stanley FJ. Spastic diplegia among children of low and normal birthweight. *Dev Med Child Neurol* 1983;25:693.
7. Delong MR. Possible involvement of central pacemakers in clinical disorders of movement. *Fed Proc* 1978;37:2171.
8. *Orthopaedic Knowledge Update 3.* Park Ridge, IL: American Academy of Orthopaedic Surgeons, 1990:286.
9. Weindling AM, Rochefort MJ, Claverty SA, et al. Development of cerebral palsy after ultrasonographic detection of periventricular cysts in the newborn. *Dev Med Child Neurol* 1985;27:800.
10. Freeman JM, Nelson KB. Intrapartum asphyxia and cerebral palsy. *Pediatrics* 1988;82:240.
11. Diamond LJ, Jaudes PK. Child abuse in a cerebral palsied population. *Dev Med Child Neurol* 1983;25:169.
12. Loder RT. Orthopaedic aspects of children with infectious (central nervous system) postnatal cerebral palsy. *J Pediatr Orthop* 1992;12:527.

Prevalence

13. Nelson KB, Ellenberg JH. Epidemiology of cerebral palsy. In: Schoenberg BS, ed. *Advances in neurology*, vol. 19. New York: Raven, 1978:421.
14. Grether JK, Nelson KB, Cummins SK. Twinning and cerebral palsy: experience in four northern California counties, births 1983 through 1985. *Pediatrics* 1993;92:854.

Classification

15. Young RR, Wiegner AW. Spasticity. *Clin Orthop* 1987;219:50.
16. Cohen ME, Duffner PK. Prognostic indicators in hemiparetic cerebral palsy. *Ann Neurol* 1981;9:953.
17. Aram DM, Ekelman BL, Satz P. Trophic changes following early unilateral injury to the brain. *Dev Med Child Neurol* 1986; 28:165.
18. Blair E, Stanley FJ. An epidemiologic study of cerebral palsy in Western Australia 1956–1975. III: postnatal aetiology. *Dev Med Child Neurol* 1982;27:615.

Associated Problems in Other Systems

19. Gibbs FA, Gibbs EL, Perstein MA, Rich CL. Electroencephalographic and clinical aspects of cerebral palsy. *Pediatrics* 1963; 32:73.
20. Cadman D, Richards J, Feldman W. Gastro-esophageal reflux in severely retarded children. *Dev Med Child Neurol* 1978;20: 95.
21. Elmer E, Wenger DR, Mubarak SJ, et al. Proximal hamstring lengthening in the sitting cerebral palsy patient. *J Pediatr Orthop* 1992;12:329.
22. Patrick J, Boland M, Stoski D, Burray GE. Rapid correction of wasting in children with CP. *Dev Med Child Neurol* 1986; 28:734.
23. Jevsevar DS, Karlin LI. The relationship between preoperative nutritional status and complications after an operation for scoliosis in patients who have cerebral palsy. *J Bone Joint Surg Am* 1993;75:880.
24. Jensen JE, Jensen TG, Smith TK, et al. Nutrition in orthopaedic surgery. *J Bone Joint Surg Am* 1982;64:1263.
25. Lonstein JE. Cerebral palsy. In: Weinstein SL, ed. *The pediatric spine—principles and practice*. New York: Raven, 1994.
26. McNeal DM, Hawtrey CE, Wolraich MG. Symptomatic neurogenic bladder in a cerebral palsied population. *Dev Med Child Neurol* 1983;25:612.

Diagnosis

27. Bleck EE. *Orthopaedic management of cerebral palsy.* Philadelphia: WB Saunders, 1979.
28. Thompson G, Rubin I, Bilenker R. *Comprehensive management of cerebral palsy.* New York: Grune & Stratton, 1983.
29. Hicks R, Durinick N, Gage JR. Differentiation of idiopathic toe-walking and cerebral palsy. *J Pediatr Orthop* 1988;8:160.
30. Kalen V, Adler N, Bleck EE. Electromyography of idiopathic toe walking. *J Pediatr Orthop* 1986;6:31.
31. Pape KE, Kirsch SE, Galil A, et al. Neuromuscular approach to the motor deficits of cerebral palsy: a pilot study. *J Pediatr Orthop* 1993;13:628.

Common Types of Cerebral Palsy and Their Management

32. Campbell SK. Quantifying the effects of interventions for movement disorders resulting from cerebral palsy. *J Child Neurol* 1997;11S:S61.

33. Daltroy LH, Liang MH, Fossel AH, et al. The POSNA Pediatric Musculoskeletal Functional Health Questionnaire: Report on Reliability, Validity, and Sensitivity to Change. *J Pediatr Orthop* 1998;18:561.
34. Olafsson Y, Saraste H, Al-Dabbagh Z. Brace treatment in neuromuscular spine deformity. *J Pediatr Orthop* 1999;19:376.
35. Renshaw TS, Larkin J. Results of orthotic treatment of scoliosis in cerebral palsy (abstract). *Orthop Trans* 1987;11:38.
36. Letts RM, Rathbone MD, Yamashita T, et al. Soft Boston orthosis in management of neuromuscular scoliosis: a preliminary report. *J Pediatr Orthop* 1992;12:470.
37. Rang M, Douglas G, Benner GC, Koreska J. Seating for children with cerebral palsy. *J Pediatr Orthop* 1981;1:279.
38. Nwaobi OM, Smith PD. Effect of adaptive seating on pulmonary function of children with CP. *Dev Med Child Neurol* 1986; 28:351.
39. Gersoff W, Renshaw TS. Treatment of scoliosis in CP by posterior spinal fusion with Luque-rod segmental instrumentation. *J Bone Joint Surg Am* 1988;70:41.
40. Thometz JG, Simon SR. Progression of scoliosis after skeletal maturity in institutionalized adults who have cerebral palsy. *J Bone Joint Surg Am* 1988;70:1290.
41. Kalen V, Conklin M, Sherman F. Untreated scoliosis in severe cerebral palsy. *J Pediatr Orthop* 1992;12:337.
42. Green NE. Cerebral palsy. In: Canale ST, Beaty JH, eds. *Operative pediatric orthopaedics*. St. Louis: Mosby-Year Book, 1991: 611.
43. Allen BL, Ferguson RL. Technique: L-rod instrumentation for scoliosis in cerebral palsy. *J Pediatr Orthop* 1982;2:87.
44. Lonstein JE, Akbarnia BA. Operative treatment of spinal deformities in patients with cerebral palsy or mental retardation. *J Bone Joint Surg Am* 1983;65:43.
45. Sponseller PD, Whiffen JR, Drummond DS. Interspinous process segmental spinal instrumentation for scoliosis in cerebral palsy. *J Pediatr Orthop* 1986;6:559.
46. Allen BL, Ferguson RL. The Galveston technique for L-rod instrumentation of the scoliotic spine. *Spine* 1982;7:276.
47. Tredwell SJ. Complications of Spinal Surgery. In: Weinstein SL, ed. *The pediatric spine*. New York: Raven, 1994;1761.
48. Drvaric DM, Roberts JM, Burke SW, et al. Gastroesophageal evaluation in totally involved cerebral palsy patients. *J Pediatr Orthop* 1987;7:187.
49. Rainey-Macdonald CG, Holiday RL, Wells GA, et al. Validity of a two-variable nutritional index for use in selecting candidates for nutritional support. *JPEN* 1983;7:15.
50. Hennrikus WL, Rosenthal RK, Kasser JR. Incidence of spondylolisthesis in ambulatory cerebral palsy patients. *J Pediatr Orthop* 1993;13:37.
51. Laplaza FJ, Root L, Tassanawipas A, Glasser DB. Femoral torsion and neck-shaft angles in cerebral palsy. *J Pediatr Orthop* 1993;13:192.
52. Abel MF, Wenger DR, Mubarak SJ, Sutherland DH. Quantitative analysis of hip dysplasia in cerebral palsy: a study of radiographs and 3-D reformatted images. *J Pediatr Orthop* 1994;14: 283.
53. Cooperman DR, Bartucci E, Dietrick E, Millar EA. Hip dislocation in spastic cerebral palsy: long term consequences. *J Pediatr Orthop* 1987;7:268.
54. Moreau MJ, Drummond DS, Rogala E, et al. Natural history of the dislocated hip in spastic cerebral palsy. *Dev Med Child Neurol* 1979;21:749.
55. Pritchett JW. Treated and urtreated unstable hips in severe cerebral palsy. *Dev Med Child Neurol* 1990;32:3.
56. Onimus M, Allamel G, Manyone P, Laurain JM. Prevention of hip dislocation in cerebral palsy by early psoas and adductors tenotomies. *J Pediatr Orthop* 1991;11:432.

57. Phelps W. Prevention of acquired dislocation of the hip in cerebral palsy. *J Bone Joint Surg Am* 1959;41:440.

58. Silver RL, Rang M, Chan J, et al. Adductor release in non ambulant children with cerebral palsy. *J Pediatr Orthop* 1985; 5:672.

59. Sutherland DH, Zilberfarb JL, Kaufman KR, et al. Psoas release at the pelvic brim in ambulatory patients with cerebral palsy: operative technique and functional outcome. *J Pediatr Orthop* 1997;17:563.

60. Miller F, Dias RC, Dabney KW, et al. Soft-tissue release for spastic hip subluxation in cerebral palsy. *J Pediatr Orthop* 1997; 17:571.

61. Sharrard WJW, Allen MH, Heany SH, et al. Surgical prophylaxis of subluxation and dislocation of the hip in cerebral palsy. *J Bone Joint Surg Am* 1975;57:160.

62. Bagg MR, Farber J, Miller F. Long-term follow-up of hip subluxation in cerebral palsy patients. *J Pediatr Orthop* 1993;13: 32.

63. Hoffer MM, Stein GA, Koffman M, Prietto M. Femoral varus-derotation osteotomy in spastic cerebral palsy. *J Bone Joint Surg Am* 1985;67:1229.

64. Carr C, Gage JR. The fate of the non operated hip in cerebral palsy. *J Pediatr Orthop* 1987;7:262.

65. Houkom JA, Roach JW, Wenger DR, et al. Treatment of acquired hip subluxation in CP. *J Pediatr Orthop* 1986;6:285.

66. Kalen V, Bleck EE. Prevention of spastic paralytic dislocation of the hip. *Dev Med Child Neurol* 1985;27:17.

67. Lonstein JE, Beck K. Hip dislocation and subluxation in CP. *J Pediatr Orthop* 1986;6:521.

68. Bleck EE. I. Cerebral palsy hip deformities: is there a consensus? (editorial). *J Pediatr Orthop* 1994;14:281.

69. Brunner R, Baumann JU. Clinical benefit of reconstruction of dislocated or subluxated hip joints in patients with spastic cerebral palsy. *J Pediatr Orthop* 1994;14:290.

70. Brunner R, Baumann JU. Long-term effects of intertrochanteric varus-derotation osteotomy on femur and acetabulum in spastic cerebral palsy: an 11 to 18 year follow-up study. *J Pediatr Orthop* 1997;17:585.

71. Mubarak SJ, McNerney NP, Wenger DR. Pericapsular acetabuloplasty for treatment of the dysplastic hip in cerebral palsy: results and complications in one hundred and four patients. Lake Buena Vista, FL: Presented at the Pediatric Orthopaedic Society of North America, 1999.

72. Gordon JE, Parry SA, Capelli AM, et al. The effect of unilateral varus rotational osteotomy with or without pelvic osteotomy on the contralateral hip in patients with perinatal static encephalopathy. *J Pediatr Orthop* 1998;18:734.

73. Mubarak SJ, Valencia FG, Wenger DR. One-stage correction of the spastic dislocated hip. *J Bone Joint Surg Am* 1992;74: 1347.

74. Heinrich S, MacEwen GD, Zembo M. Hip dysplasia, subluxation, and dislocation in cerebral palsy: an arthrographic analysis. *J Pediatr Orthop* 1991;11:488.

75. Morrissy RT. *Atlas of pediatric orthopaedic surgery.* 2nd ed. Philadelphia: Lippincott-Raven, 1996.

76. Chiari K. Medial displacement osteotomy of the pelvis. *Clin Orthop* 1974;98:55.

77. Osterkamp J, Caillouette JT, Hoffer MM. Chiari osteotomy in cerebral palsy. *J Pediatr Orthop* 1988;8:274.

78. Pemberton PA. Pericapsular osteotomy for congenital dislocation of the hip. *J Bone Joint Surg Am* 1965;47:65.

79. Staheli LT. Technique: slotted acetabular augmentation. *J Pediatr Orthop* 1981;1:321.

80. Steel HH. Triple osteotomy of the innominate bone. *Clin Orthop* 1977;122:116.

81. Sutherland DH, Greenfield R. Double innominate osteotomy. *J Bone Joint Surg Am* 1977;59:1082.

82. Zuckerman JD, Staheli LT, McLaughlin JF. Acetabular augmentation for progressive hip subluxation in CP. *J Pediatr Orthop* 1984;4:436.

83. Dega W. Osteotomia trans-iliakalne w leczeniu wrodzonej dysplazji biodra. *Chir Narz Ruchu Ortop Polska* 1974;39:601.

84. Gross MS, Ibrahim K, Wehner J, et al. Combined surgical procedure for treatment of hip dislocation in CP (abstract). *Dev Med Child Neurol* 1984;26:255.

85. Castle ME, Schneider C. Proximal femoral resection-interposition arthroplasty. *J Bone Joint Surg Am* 1978;60:1051.

86. Koffman M. Proximal femoral resection or THR in severely disabled cerebral spastic patients. *Orthop Clin North Am* 1981; 12:91.

87. Root L, Spero C. Hip adductor transfer compared with adductor tenotomy in cerebral palsy. *J Bone Joint Surg Am* 1981;63: 767.

88. McCarthy RE, Simon S, Zawacky R, Reese N. Proximal femoral resection to allow adults who have severe cerebral palsy to sit. *J Bone Joint Surg Am* 1988;70:1011.

89. McHale KA, Bagg M, Nason SS. Treatment of the chronically dislocated hip in adolescents with cerebral palsy with femoral head resection and subtrochanteric valgus osteotomy. *J Pediatr Orthop* 1990;10:504.

90. Segal LS, Reighard C. Subtrochanteric valgus osteotomy and femoral head resection for chronic painful dislocated hips in patients with cerebral palsy. Lake Buena Vista, FL: Presented at the Pediatric Orthopaedic Society of North America, 1999.

91. Root L, Goss JR, Mendes J. The treatment of the painful hip in cerebral palsy by total hip replacement or hip arthrodesis. *J Bone Joint Surg Am* 1986;68:590.

92. Benaroch TE, Richards BS, Haideri N, et al. Intermediate follow-up of a simple method of hip arthrodesis in adolescent patients. *J Pediatr Orthop* 1996;16:30.

Extension Plus Abduction Contracture

93. Szalay EA, Roach JW, Houkom JA, et al. Extension-abduction contracture of the spastic hip. *J Pediatr Orthop* 1986;6:1.

94. Norlin R, Odenrick P. Development of gait in spastic children with CP. *J Pediatr Orthop* 1986;6:674.

95. Beals R. Spastic paraplegia and diplegia: an evaluation of the non-surgical and surgical factors influencing the prognosis for ambulation. *J Bone Joint Surg Am* 1966;48:827.

96. Molnar GE, Gordon SV. Predictive value of clinical signs for early prognostication of motor function in cerebral palsy. *Arch Phys Med* 1976;57:153.

97. Bleck EE. Locomotor prognosis in cerebral palsy. *Dev Med Child Neurol* 1975;17:18.

98. Bleck EE. Orthopaedic management in cerebral palsy. *Clin Dev Med* 1987;99/100:17.

99. Renshaw TS, Green NE, Griffin PP, et al. Cerebral palsy: orthopaedic management. *Instr Course Lect* 1996;45:475.

100. Campos da Paz A Jr. Walking prognosis in cerebral palsy: a 22-year retrospective. Sun Valley, ID: Presented at the American Orthopaedic Association 107th Annual Meeting, June 1994.

101. Hoffer MM, Felwell E, Perry R, et al. Functional ambulation in patients with myelomeningocele. *J Bone Joint Surg Am* 1973; 55:137.

102. Rose J, Medeiros JM, Parker R. Energy cost index as an estimate of anergy expenditure of CP children during assisted ambulation. *Dev Med Child Neurol* 1985;27:485.

103. DeLuca PA, Davis RB, Ounpuu S, et al. Alterations in surgical decision making in patients with cerebral palsy based on thrii-dimensional gait analysis. *J Pediatr Orthop* 1997;17:608.

104. Sutherland DH, Oishen R, Cooper L, Woo SL-Y. The development of mature gait. *J Bone Joint Surg Am* 1980;62:336.
105. Krebs DE, Edelstein JE, Fishman S. Reliability of observational kinematic gait analysis. *Phys Ther* 1985;65:1027.
106. Pransatelli MR. Oral pharmacology for the movement disorders of cerebral palsy. *J Child Neurol* 1996;11S:13S.
107. Wright T, Nicholson J. Physiotherapy for the spastic child: an evaluation. *Dev Med Child Neurol* 1973;15:146.
108. Gracies JM, Elovic E, McGuire J, et al. Traditional pharmacological treatments for spasticity. Part I: local treatments. *Muscle Nerve Suppl* 1997;6:S61.
109. Carpenter EB. Role of nerve blocks in the foot and ankle in cerebral palsy: therapeutic and diagnostic. *Foot Ankle* 1983;4:164.
110. Carpenter EB, Seltz DB. Intramuscular alcohol as an aid in management of spastic cerebral palsy. *Dev Med Child Neurol* 1980;22:497.
111. Cosgrove AP, Corr TS, Graham HK, et al. Botulinum toxin in the management of the lower limb in cerebral palsy. *Dev Med Child Neurol* 1994; 36:386.
112. Lagueny A, Burbaud P. Mechanism of action, clinical indication and results of treatment of botulinum toxin. *Neurophysiol Clin* 1996;26:216.
113. O'Brien CF. Injection techniques for botulinum toxin using electromyography and electrical stimulation. *Muscle Nerve Suppl* 1997;6:S176.
114. Waters PM, Van Heest A. Spastic hemiplegia of the upper extremity in children. *Hand Clin* 1998;14:119.
115. Cosgrove AP, Graham HK. Botulinum toxin-A in the management of children with cerebral palsy (abstract). *Orthop Trans* 1993;16:625.
116. Koman LA, Mooney JF, Smith B, Goodman A, Mulvaney T. Management of cerebral palsy with botulinum-A toxin: preliminary investigation. *J Pediatr Orthop* 1993;13:489.
117. Pullman SL, Greene P, Fahn S, et al. Approach to the treatment of limb disorders with botulinum toxin A. Experience with 187 patients. *Arch Neurol* 1996;53:617.
118. Koman LA, Mooney JF, Smith B, et al. Management of cerebral palsy with botulinum-A toxin: preliminary investigation. *J Pediatr Orthop* 1993;13:489.
119. Zelnik N, Giladi N, Goikhman I, et al. The role of botulinum toxin in the treatment of lower limb spasticity in children with cerebral palsy—a pilot study. *Isr J Med Sci* 1997;33:129.
120. Corry IS, Cosgrove AP, Duffy CM, et al. Botulinum toxin A compared with stretching casts in the treatment of spastic equinus: a randomised prospective trial. *J Pediatr Orthop* 1998;18:304.
121. Sanchez-Carpintero R, Narbona J. Botulinum toxin in spastic infantile cerebral palsy: results in 27 cases during one year. *Rev Neurol* 1997;25:531.
122. Corry IS, Cosgrove AP, Walsh EG, et al. Botulinum toxin A in the hemiplegic upper limb: a double-blind trial. *Dev Med Child Neurol* 1997;39:185.
123. Albright AL, Barry MJ, Fasick MP, et al. Effects of continuous intrathecal baclofen infusion and selective posterior rhizotomy on upper extremity spasticity. *Pediatr Neurosurg* 1995;23:82.
124. Armstrong RW. Intrathecally administered baclofen for treatment of children with spasticity of cerebral origin. *J Neurosurg* 1997;87:409.
125. Gerszten PC, Albright AL, Barry MJ. Effect on ambulation of continuous intrathecal baclofen infusion. *Pediatr Neurosurg* 1997;27:40.
126. Gerszten PC, Albright AL, Johnstone GF. Intrathecal baclofen infusion and subsequent orthopedic surgery in patients with spastic cerebral palsy. *J Neurosurg* 1998;88:1009.
127. Albright AL, Cervi A, Singletary J. Intrathecal baclofen for spasticity in cerebral palsy. *JAMA* 1991;265:1418.
128. Oppenheim WL, Peacock WJ. Selective dorsal rhizotomy (abstract). *J Pediatr Orthop* 1991;11:690.
129. Peacock WJ, Arlens L, Berman B. CP spasticity: selective posterior rhizotomy. *Pediatr Neurosci* 1987;13:61.
130. Peacock WJ, Staudt LA. Functional outcomes following selective posterior rhizotomy in children with cerebral palsy. *J Neurosurg* 1991;74:380.
131. Davis R, Schulman J, Delahanty A. Cerebellar stimulation for cerebral palsy: double blind study. *Acta Neurochir Suppl* 1987; 39:126.
132. Staudt LA, Peacock WJ. Selective posterior rhizotomy for the treatment of spastic cerebral palsy. In: Long T, ed. *Pediatric physical therapy*, vol. 1. Baltimore: Williams & Wilkins, 1989.
133. Bretas CT, Dias LS, Gaebler-Spira D. Selective posterior rhizotomy in spastic quadriplegia: results (abstract). *Orthop Trans* 1993;16:627.
134. Oppenheim WL. Selective posterior rhizotomy for spastic cerebral palsy—a review. *Clin Orthop* 1990;253:20.
135. Berman B, Peacock WJ, Vaughan CL, et al. Assessment of patients with spastic cerebral palsy before and after rhizotomy (abstract). *Dev Med Child Neurol* 1987;55(suppl):24.
136. Boscarino LF, Ounpuu S, Davis RB III, et al. Effects of selective dorsal rhizotomy on gait in children with cerebral palsy. *J Pediatr Orthop* 1993;13:174.
137. Perry J, Adams J, Cahan LD. Foot-floor contact patterns following selective dorsal rhizotomy (abstract). *Dev Med Child Neurol Suppl* 1989;31:19.
138. Tippets RH, Walker ML, Liddell KL. Long-term follow-up of selective dorsal rhizotomy for relief of spasticity in cerebral-palsied children (abstract). *Dev Med Child Neurol Suppl* 1989; 31:19.
139. Steinbok P, Reiner AM, Beauchamp R, et al. A randomized clinical trial to compare selective posterior rhizotomy plus physiotherapy with physiotherapy alone in children with spastic diplegic cerebral palsy. *Dev Med Child Neurol* 1997;39:178.
140. McLaughlin JF, Bkornson KF. Selective dorsal rhizotomy. *Dev Med Child Neurol* 1998;40:220.
141. Wright FV. Evaluation of selective dorsal rhizotomy. *Dev Med Child Neurol* 1998;40:227.
142. Chicoine MR, Park TS, Vogler GP, et al. Predictors of ability to walk after selective dorsal rhizotomy in children with cerebral palsy. *Neurosurgery* 1996;38:711.
143. Carroll KL, Moore KR, Stevens PM. Orthopedic procedures after rhizotomy. *J Pediatr Orthop* 1998;18:69.
144. Greene WB, Dietz FR, Goldberg MJ, et al. Rapid progression of hip subluxation in cerebral palsy after selective posterior rhizotomy. *J Pediatr Orthop* 1991;11:494.
145. Payne LZ, DeLuca PA. Heterotopic ossification after rhizotomy and femoral osteotomy. *J Pediatr Orthop* 1993;13:733.
146. Crawford K, Karol LA, Herring JA. Severe lumbar lordosis after dorsal rhizotomy. *J Pediatr Orthop* 1996;16:336.
147. Millis MB. Rapidly progressive lumbar hyperlordosis following selective posterior rhizotomy for spastic quadriplegia (abstract). *Orthop Trans* 1993;16:10.
148. Peter IC, Hoffman EB, Arens L, et al. Spondylolysis and spondylolisthesis after five-level lumbosacral laminectomy for selective posterior rhizotomy in cerebral palsy. *Child's Nervous Sys* 1993;9:285.
149. Arens L, Peacock W, Peter J. Selective posterior rhizotomy: a long-term follow-up study. *Child Nerv Syst* 1989;5:148.
150. Root L, Miller SR, Kirz P. Posterior tibial tendon transfer in patients with cerebral palsy. *J Bone Joint Surg Am* 1987;69:1133.
151. Herndon WA, Troup P, Yngve DA, et al. Effects of neurodevel-

opmental treatment on movement patterns of children with cerebral palsy. *J Pediatr Orthop* 1987;7:395.

152. Kanda T, Yuge M, Yamori Y, et al. Early physiotherapy in the treatment of spastic diplegia. *Dev Med Child Neurol* 1984;26:438.

153. Palmer FB, Shapiro BK, Wachtel RC, et al. The effects of physical therapy on cerebral palsy: a controlled trial in infants with spastic diplegia. *N Engl J Med* 1988;318:803.

154. Piper MC, Kumos VI, Willis DM, et al. Early physical therapy effects on the high risk infant: a randomized control trial. *Pediatrics* 1986;78:216.

155. Winters TF, Gage JR, Hicks R. Gait patterns in spastic hemiplegia in children and young adults. *J Bone Joint Surg Am* 1987;69:437.

156. Paine RS. On the treatment of cerebral palsy: the outcome of 177 patients, 74 totally untreated. *Pediatrics* 1962;29:605.

157. Scherzer AL, Mike V, Ilson J. Physical therapy as a determinant of change in the cerebral palsied infant. *Pediatrics* 1976;58:47.

158. Loder RT. The ambulatory child with cerebral palsy. *Orthopaedic knowledge update pediatrics*. Rosemont: American Academy of Orthopaedic Surgeons, 1996:19.

159. Young NL, Wright JG. Measuring pediatric physical function. *J Pediatr Orthop* 1995;15:244.

160. Breslaw N, Starvich KS, Mortimer EA. Psychological stress in mothers of disabled children. *Am J Dis Child* 1982;136:682.

161. Sussman MD. Role of the physical therapist in treatment of children with cerebral palsy (abstract). *J Pediatr Orthop* 1991;11:688.

162. Papariello SG, Skinner SR. Dynamic electromyography analysis of habitual toe walkers. *J Pediatr Orthop* 1985;5:171.

163. Ruda R, Frost HM. Cerebral palsy: spastic varus and forefoot adductus treated by intramuscular posterior tibial tendon lengthening. *Clin Orthop* 1971;79:61.

164. Bleck EE. Management of the lower extremities in children who have cerebral palsy. *J Bone Joint Surg Am* 1990;72:140.

165. Cusick B, Sussman M. Short leg casts: their role in the management of cerebral palsy. *Phys Occup Ther Pediatr* 1982;2:93.

166. Duncan W, Mott D. Foot reflexes and the use of the "inhibitive cast." *Foot Ankle* 1983;4:145.

167. Otis JC, Root L, Kroll MA. Measurement of plantar flexor spasticity during treatment with tone-reducing casts. *J Pediatr Orthop* 1985;5:682.

168. Sussman MD. Casting as an adjunct to neurodevelopmental therapy in cerebral palsy. *Dev Med Child Neurol* 1983;25:804.

169. Sussman MD, Cusick B. The role of short-leg, tone reducing casts as an adjunct to physical therapy of patients with cerebral palsy. *Johns Hopkins Med Bull* 1979;145:112.

170. Watt J, Sims D, Harckham F, et al. A prospective study of inhibitive casting as an adjunct to physiotherapy for cerebral palsied children. *Dev Med Child Neurol* 1986;28:480.

171. Browne AO, McManus F. One-session surgery for bilateral correction of lower limb deformities in spastic diplegia. *J Pediatr Orthop* 1987;7:259.

172. Norlin R, Tkaczuk H. One-session surgery for correction of lower extremity deformities in children with cerebral palsy. *J Pediatr Orthop* 1985;5:208.

173. Holstein A. Hallux valgus: an acquired deformity of the foot in cerebral palsy. *Foot Ankle* 1980;1:33.

174. Renshaw TS, Sirkin RB, Drennan JC. The management of hallux valgus in cerebral palsy. *Dev Med Child Neurol* 1979;21:202.

175. Ball J, Sullivan JA. Treatment of the juvenile bunion by Mitchell osteotomy. *Orthopedics* 1985;10:1249.

176. Bleck EE. Forefoot problems in cerebral palsy—diagnosis and management. *Foot Ankle* 1984;4:188.

177. Helal B. Surgery for adolescent hallux valgus. *Clin Orthop* 1981;157:50.

178. Luba R, Rosman M. Bunions in children—treatment with a modified Mitchell osteotomy. *J Periatr Orthop* 1984;4:44.

179. Scranton PE, Zuckerman JD. Bunion surgery in adolescents—results of surgical treatment. *J Pediatr Orthop* 1984;4:39.

180. McKeever DC. Arthrodesis of the first metatarsophalangeal joint for hallux valgus, hallux rigidus, and metatarsus primus varus. *J Bone Joint Surg Am* 1952;34:129.

181. Silver RL, de la Garza J, Rang M. The myth of muscle imbalance: a study of relative strengths and excursions of normal muscles about the foot and ankle. *J Bone Joint Surg Br* 1985;67:432.

182. Greene WB. Achilles tendon lengthening in cerebral palsy: comparison of inpatient versus ambulatory surgery. *J Pediatr Orthop* 1987;7:256.

183. Moreau MJ, Lake DM. Outpatient percutaneous heel cord lengthening in children. *J Pediatr Orthop* 1987;7:253.

184. Hoke M. An operation for stabilizing paralytic feet. *J Orthop Surg* 1921;3:494.

185. Graham HK, Fixsen JA. Lengthening of the calcaneal tendon in spastic hemiplegia by the White technique: a long term review. *J Bone Joint Surg Br* 1988;70:472.

186. White JW. Torsion of the Achilles tendon: its surgical significance. *Arch Surg* 1943;46:784.

187. Gaines RW, Ford TB. A systematic approach to the amount of Achilles tendon lengthening in CP. *J Pediatr Orthop* 1985;4:448.

188. Garbarino JL, Clancy M. A geometric method of calculating tendo Achillis lengthening. *J Pediatr Orthop* 1985;5:573.

189. Baker LD, Hill LM. Foot alignment in the cerebral palsy patient. *J Bone Joint Surg Am* 1964;46:1.

190. Baker LD. A rational approach to the surgical needs of the cerebral palsy patient. *J Bone Joint Surg Am* 1956;38:313.

191. Javors JR, Klaaren HE. The Vulpius procedure for correction for equinus deformity in CP. *J Pediatr Orthop* 1987;7:191.

192. Vulpius O, Stoffel A. *Orthopaedische Operationslehre*. Stuttgart: Ferdinand Enke, 1913.

193. Rose SA, DeLuca PA, Davis RB III, et al. Kinematic and kinetic evaluation of the ankle after lengthening of the gastrocnemius fascia in children with cerebral palsy. *J Pediatr Orthop* 1993;13:727.

194. Olney BW, Williams PF, Menelaus MB. Treatment of spastic equinus by aponeurosis lengthening. *J Pediatr Orthop* 1988;8:422.

195. Etnyre B, Chambers CS, Scarborough NH, Cain TE. Preoperative and postoperative assessment of surgical intervention for equinus gait in children with cerebral palsy. *J Pediatr Orthop* 1993;13:24.

196. Sharrard WJW, Bernstein S. Equinus deformity in cerebral palsy: a comparison between elongation of the tendo calcaneus and gastrocnemius recession. *J Bone Joint Surg Br* 1972;54:272.

197. Stevens DB, Opfell AR, Stanley N, Walker JL. Heel cord advancement for treatment of spastic equinus deformity in children (abstract). *Orthop Trans* 1993;16:625.

198. Strecker WB, Via MW, Oliver SK, Schoenecker PL. Heel cord advancement for treatment of equinus deformity in cerebral palsy. *J Pediatr Orthop* 1990;10:105.

199. Throop FB, DeRosa GP, Reeck C, Waterman S. Correction of equinus in cerebral palsy by the Murphy procedure of tendo calcaneus advancement: a preliminary communication. *Dev Med Child Neurol* 1975;17:182.

200. Grant AD, Feldman R, Lehman WB. Equinus deformity in CP. A retrospective analysis of treatment and function in 39 cases. *J Pediatr Orthop* 1985;5:678.

201. Rattey TE, Leahey L, Hyndman J, et al. Recurrence after Achil-

les tendon lengthening in cerebral palsy. *J Pediatr Orthop* 1993; 13:184.

202. Taussig G, Pilliard D. Triceps lengthening in children with cerebral palsy performed before the age of six years. Results at the end of growth. *Rev Chir Orthop* 1988;74:79.

203. Banks HH. Equinus and cerebral palsy—its management. *Foot Ankle* 1983;4:149.

204. Tardieu G, Tardieu C. Cerebral palsy: mechanical evaluation and conservation correction of limb joint contractures. *Clin Orthop* 1987;219:63.

205. Majestro TC, Ruda R, Frost HM. Intramuscular lengthening of the posterior tibialis tendon. *Clin Orthop* 1963;79:59.

206. Green NE, Griffin PP, Shiavi R. Split posterior tibial tendon transfer in spastic cerebral palsy. *J Bone Joint Surg Am* 1983; 65:748.

207. Kling TF, Kaufer HA, Hensinger RN. Split posterior tibial tendon transfers in children with cerebral spastic paralysis and equinovarus deformity. *J Bone Joint Surg Am* 1985;67:186.

208. Snyder M, Kumar SJ, Stecyk MD. Split tibialis posterior tendon transfer and tendo-Achilles lengthening for spastic equinovarus feet. *J Pediatr Orthop* 1993;13:20.

209. Bisia RS, Louis HJ, Albano P. Transfer of tibialis posterior tendon in cerebral palsy. *J Bone Joint Surg Am* 1976;58:497.

210. Schneider M, Balon K. Deformity of the foot following anterior transfer of the posterior tibial tendon and lengthening of the Achilles tendon for spastic equinovarus. *Clin Orthop* 1977;125: 113.

211. Hoffer MM, Barakat G, Koffman M. 10 year follow-up of split anterior tibial tendon transfer in cerebral palsied patients with spastic equinovarus deformity. *J Pediatr Orthop* 1985;5:432.

212. DeGnore LT, Greene WB. Split anterior tibialis tendon transfer in cerebral palsy (abstract). *Orthop Trans* 1993;16:785.

213. Davids JR, Holland WC, Sutherland DH. Significance of the confusion test in cerebral palsy. *J Pediatr Orthop* 1993;13:717.

214. Silver CM, Simon SD, Lichtman HM. Long-term follow-up observations on calcaneal osteotomy. *Clin Orthop* 1974;99:181.

215. O'Connell PA, D'Souza L, Dudeney S, et al. Foot deformities in children with cerebral palsy. *J Pediatr Orthop* 1998;18:743.

216. Bennet GC, Rang M, Jones D. Varus and valgus deformities of the foot in cerebral palsy. *Dev Med Child Neurol* 1982;24: 499.

217. Nather A, Fulford GE, Stewart K. Treatment of valgus hindfoot in cerebral palsy by peroneus brevis lengthening. *Dev Med Child Neurol* 1984;26:335.

218. Evans D. Calcaneo-valgus deformity. *J Bone Joint Surg Br* 1975; 57:270.

219. Dennyson WG, Fulford GE. Subtalar arthrodesis by cancellous grafts and metallic internal fixation. *J Bone Joint Surg Br* 1976; 58:507.

220. Mosca VS. Calcaneal lengthening for valgus deformity of the hindfoot. *J Bone Joint Surg Am* 1995;78:500.

221. Barrasso JA, Wile PB, Gage JR. Extra-articular subtalar arthrodesis with internal fixation. *J Pediatr Orthop* 1984;4:555.

222. Grice DS. The role of subtalar fusion in the treatment of valgus deformities of the feet. *AAOS Instr Course Lect* 1959;16:127.

223. McCall RE, Lillich JS, Harris JR, Johnston FA. The Grice extra-articular arthrodesis: a clinical review. *J Pediatr Orthop* 1985; 5:442.

224. Moreland JR, Westin WG. Further experience with Grice subtalar arthrodesis. *Clin Orthop* 1986;207:113.

225. Scott SM, Janes PC, Stevens PM. Grice subtalar arthrodesis followed to skeletal maturity. *J Pediatr Orthop* 1988;8:176.

226. Crawford AH, Kucharzuk D, Roy DR, Blibo J. Subtalar stabilization of the planovalgus foot by staple arthroereisis in young children who have neuromuscular problems. *J Bone Joint Surg Am* 1990;72:840.

227. Koman LA, Mooney JF, Goodman A. Management of valgus hindfoot deformity in pediatric cerebral palsy patients by medial displacement osteotomy. *J Pediatr Orthop* 1993;13:180.

228. Schwend RM, Millis MB, Hall JE. Calcaneal displacement osteotomy for correction of hindfoot deformities. San Francisco, CA: Presented at the American Academy of Orthopaedic Surgeons 60th Annual Meeting, 1993.

229. Rathjen KE, Mubarak SJ. Cancaneal-cuboid-cuneiform osteotomy for the correction of valgus foot deformities in children. *J Pediatr Orthop* 1998;18:775.

230. Tenuta J, Shelton YA, Miller F. Long-term follow-up of triple arthrodesis in patients with cerebral palsy. *J Pediatr Orthop* 1993;13:713.

231. Aiona M. Triple arthrodesis in cerebral palsy: long-term results (abstract). *Orthop Trans* 1993;16:626.

232. Damron T, Breed A, Roecker E. Hamstring tenotomies in cerebral palsy: long-term retrospective analysis. *J Pediatr Orthop* 1991;11:514.

233. Sutherland DH, Schottstaedt ER, Larsen LJ, et al. Clinical and EMG study of seven spastic children with internal rotation gait. *J Bone Joint Surg Am* 1969;51:1070.

234. Hsu L, Helena L. Distal hamstring elongation in the management of spastic cerebral palsy. *J Pediatr Orthop* 1990;10:378.

235. Relmers J. Contracture of the hamstrings in spastic cerebral palsy. A study of three methods of operative correction. *J Bone Joint Surg Br* 1974;56:102.

236. Sharps CH, Clancy M, Steel HH. A long term retrospective study of proximal hamstring release for hamstring contracture. *J Pediatr Orthop* 1984;4:443.

237. Drummond DS, Rogala E, Templeton J, Cruess R. Proximal hamstring release for knee flexion and crouched gait in cerebral palsy. *J Bone Joint Surg Am* 1974;56:1598.

238. Hoffinger SA, Rab GT, Abou-Ghaida H. Hamstrings in cerebral palsy crouch gait. *J Pediatr Orthop* 1993;13:722.

239. Waters RL, Perry J, McDaniels JM, House K. The relative strength of the hamstrings during hip extension. *J Bone Joint Surg Am* 1974;56:1592.

240. Perry J. Distal rectus femoris transfer. *Dev Med Child Neurol* 1987;29:153.

241. Ounpuu S, Mulk E, Davis RB III, et al. Rectus femoris surgery in children with cerebral palsy. Part I: the effect of rectus femoris transfer location on knee motion. *J Pediatr Orthop* 1993;13: 325.

242. Chambers H, Lauer AL, Kaufmen K, et al. Prediction of outcome after rectus femoris surgery in cerebral palsy: the role of cocontraction of the rectus femoris and vastus lateralis. *J Pediatr Orthop* 1998;18:703.

243. Ounpuu S, Mulk E, Davis RB III, et al. Rectus femoris surgery in children with cerebral palsy. Part II: a comparison between the effect of transfer and release of the distal rectus femoris on knee motion. *J Pediatr Orthop* 1993;13:331.

244. Gage JR, Perry J, Hicks RR, et al. Rectus femoris transfer to improve knee function of children with cerebral palsy. *Dev Med Child Neurol* 1987;29:159.

245. Sutherland DH, Santi M, Abel MF. Treatment of stiff-kneed gait in cerebral palsy: a comparison by gait analysis of distal rectus femoris transfer versus proximal rectus release. *J Pediatr Orthop* 1990;10:433.

246. Ferguson RL, Gulliford PT, McMulkin M, et al. Clinical correlation between static straight leg raise and popliteal angular measurements vs. dynamic gait lab measurements of knee extension. Lake Buena Vista, FL: Presented at the Pediatric Orthopaedic Society of North America, 1999.

247. Bruno RJ, Sirirungruangsarn Y, Berzins A, et al. Gait analysis after rectus femoris transfer in children with cerebral palsy. Lake

Buena Vista, FL: Presented at the Pediatric Orthopaedic Society of North America, 1999.

248. Baumann J, Meyer E, Schurmann E. Hip adductor transfer to the ischial tuberosity in spastic and paralytic hip disorders. *Arch Orthop Trauma Surg* 1978;92:107.

249. Beals TC, Thompson, NE, Beals RK. Modified adductor muscle transfer in cerebral palsy. *J Pediatr Orthop* 1998;18:522.

250. Griffin PP, Wheelhouse WW, Shiavi R. Adductor transfer for adductor spasticity: clinical and EMG gait analysis. *Dev Med Child Neurol* 1979;19:783.

251. Reimers J, Poulsen S. Adductor transfer versus tenotomy for stability of the hip in spastic cererbral palsy. *J Pediatr Orthop* 1984;4:52.

252. Scott A, Chambers C, Cain TE, et al. Adductor transfers in cerebral palsy: long-term results studied be gait analysis (abstract). *Orthop Trans* 1993;16:626.

253. Matsuo T, Tada S, Hajime T. Insufficiency of the hip adductor after anterior obturator neurectomy in 42 children with cerebral palsy. *J Pediatr Orthop* 1986;6:686.

254. Staheli LT. The prone hip extension test. *Clin Orthop* 1977;123:12.

255. DeLuca PA, Ounpuu S, Davis RB, et al. Effect of hamstring and psoas lengthening of pelvic tilt in patients with spastic diplegic cerebral palsy. *J Pediatr Orthop* 1998;18:712.

256. Matsuo T, Hara H, Tada S. Selective lengthening of the psoas and rectus femoris and preservation of the illacus for flexion deformity of the hip in cerebral palsy patients. *J Pediatr Orthop* 1987;7:690.

257. Sutherland DH, Zilberfarb JL, Kaufman KR, et al. Psoas release at the pelvic brim in ambulatory patients with cerebral palsy: operative technique and functional outcome. *J Pediatr Orthop* 1997;17:563.

258. Root L, Siegal T. Osteotomy of the hip in children: posterior approach. *J Bone Joint Surg Am* 1980;62:571.

259. Steel HH. Gluteus medius and minimus insertion advancement for correction of internal rotation gait in cerebral palsy. *J Bone Joint Surg Am* 1980;62:919.

260. Silver LB. Controversial approaches to treating learning disabilities and attention deficit disorders. *Am J Dis Child* 1986;140:1045.

261. Brunner R, Meier G, Ruepp T. Comparison of a stiff and a spring-type ankle-foot orthosis to improve gair in spastic hemiplegic children. *J Pediatr Orthop* 1998;18:719.

262. Hiroshima K, Hamada S, Shimizu N, et al. Anterior transfer of the long toe flexors for the treatment of spastic equinovarus and equinus foot in cerebral palsy. *J Pediatr Orthop* 1988; 8:164.

263. DeJong RN. *The neurologic examination.* New York: Hoeber-Harper, 1958.

264. Butler C. Effects of powered mobility on self initiated behaviors of very young children with locomotor disability. *Dev Med Child Neurol* 1986;28:325.

265. Harada T, Ebara S, Kajiura I, et al. Cervical spondylosis in patients with athetoid cerebral palsy (abstract*). Orthop Trans* 1993;16:790.

266. Samilson RL. Orthopaedic aspects of cerebral palsy. *Clin Dev Med* 1975;52/53:142.

267. Racette BA, Lauryssen C, Perlmutter JS. Preoperative treatment with botulinum toxin to facilitate cervical fusion in dystonic cerebral palsy. Report of two cases. *J Neurosurg* 1998;88:328.

Upper Extremity Involvement

268. *Orthopaedic knowledge update 2.* Park Ridge, IL: American Academy of Orthopaedic Surgeons, 1987:191.

269. Skoff H, Woodbury DF. Current concepts review: management of the upper extremity in cerebral palsy. *J Bone Joint Surg Am* 1985;67:500.

270. Van Heest AE, House JH, Cariello C. Upper extremity surgical treatment of cerebral palsy. *J Hand Surg* 1999;24A:323.

271. Mital MA, Sakellarides HT. Surgery of the upper extremity in the retarded individual with spastic cerebral palsy. *Orthop Clin North Am* 1981;12:127.

272. Hoffer MM, Perry J, Melkonian G. Dynamic EMG and decision-making for surgery in the upper extremity of patients with cerebral palsy. *J Hand Surg* 1979;4:424.

273. Mowery CA, Gelberman RH, Rhoades C. Upper extremity tendon transfers in cerebral palsy: electromyographic and functional analysis. *J Pediatr Orthop* 1985;5:69.

274. Perry J, Hoffer MM. Preoperative and postoperative dynamic EMG as an aid in planning tendon transfers in children with cerebral palsy. *J Bone Joint Surg Am* 1977;59:531.

275. Inglis AE, Cooper W. Release of the flexor-pronator origin for flexion deformities of the hand and wrist in spastic paralysis. *J Bone Joint Surg Am* 1966;48:847.

276. Ono CM, Lipp EB. Green-Banks flexor carpi ulnaris transfer to wrist extensors for spastic cerebral palsy (abstract). *Orthop Trans* 1993;16:325.

277. Thometz JG, Tachdjian MO. Long term follow-up of the flexor carpi ulnaris transfer in spastic hemiplegia children. *J Pediatr Orthop* 1988;8:407.

278. Beach W, Strecker WB, Coe J, et al. Use of the Green transfer in treatment of patients with spastic cerebral palsy: 17 year experience. *J Pediatr Orthop* 1991;11:731.

279. Hoffer MM, Lehman M, Mitani M. Long-term follow-up on tendon transfers to the extensors of the wrist and fingers in patients with cerebral palsy. *J Hand Surg* 1986;11:836.

280. House J, Gwathmey G, Fidler M. A dynamic approach to the thumb-in-palm deformity in cerebral palsy. *J Bone Joint Surg Am* 1981;63:216.

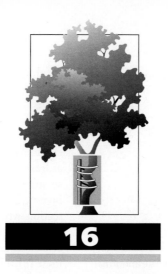

16

MYELOMENINGOCELE

RICHARD E. LINDSETH

Myelomeningocele is the most complex treatable congenital malformation of the central nervous system. Its effect on the child, the parents, and the medical community may be devastating. The initial treatment, which consists of closure of the meningocele and insertion of a ventriculoperitoneal shunt, is straightforward and well within the capability of most neurosurgeons. The child is then referred to the orthopaedist for rehabilitation.

The orthopaedic care of these patients is strongly influenced by factors beyond an orthopaedist's control, including changes in the neurologic system, urologic abnormalities, societal pressures, education, and the availability of medical resources. It is almost impossible to carry out the necessary treatment program without a coordinated interdisciplinary team consisting of a neurosurgeon, an orthopaedist, a urolo-

gist, a social worker, physical and occupational therapists, educators, a pediatrician, and a nurse specialist. If these services cannot be provided, the child should be referred to a clinic that can provide them.

CLASSIFICATION AND PATHOLOGY

The pathologic description of spina bifida and associated neurologic abnormalities was made by von Recklinghausen in 1886 (1). His observations remain current, and only recently have we begun to understand the pathologic processes that lead to the formation of myelomeningocele and other associated diseases.

Neural tube defects are grouped together under the generic terms "myelodysplasia," "spinal dysraphia," and "spina bifida aperta." These are not to be confused with "spina bifida occulta," which is a common radiographic finding of a lack of fusion of the spinous process of the lower lumbar and sacral spine without neurologic abnormalities. Neural tube defects

Richard E. Lindseth: Department of Orthopaedic Surgery, Indiana University School of Medicine, Indianapolis, Indiana 46202.

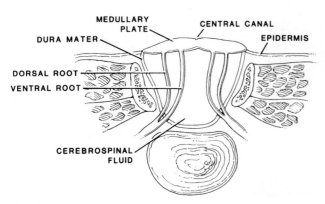

FIGURE 16-1. Cross-section of myelomeningocele. The abnormal cord is part of the sac, and is elevated out of the canal.

can be divided into four subtypes: meningocele, myelomeningocele, lipomeningocele, and rachischisis.

A cyst involving only the meninges but not any neural elements is called a "meningocele." It often requires surgical excision and closure by a neurosurgeon. However, it does not cause neurologic or orthopaedic abnormalities, and further treatment is not needed.

A myelomeningocele includes the abnormal neural elements as a part of the sac (Fig. 16-1). The sac may assume any size, form, or location along the spine. It is less likely to be epithelialized than a meningocele sac. The neural elements are abnormal, and pronounced peripheral neurologic deficits are common. Central nervous system abnormalities, including Arnold-Chiari deformity and hydrocephalus, are common.

A "lipomeningocele" is a lesion in which the sac contains a lipoma that is intimately involved with the sacral nerves. These lesions often are epithelialized at birth. Children with lipomeningocele may not have hydrocephaly or other central nervous system abnormalities. Neurologic function, which is almost normal at birth, may become impaired with growth. This abnormality is similar to other abnormalities of the spine, including dermoid sinus, dermoid cyst, and diastematomyelia. When paralysis occurs, it rarely extends above the lumbosacral area. Progressive neurologic loss should be the major concern in the treatment of these children.

"Rachischisis" is a complete absence of the skin and sac, with exposure of the muscle and the presence of a dysplastic spinal cord without evidence of a covering. Occasionally even the bone is exposed, but usually there is a thin covering of muscle.

The embryologic development of myelomeningocele is unknown. There are two opposing schools of thought that have existed since the initial description of the disease (1): von Recklinghausen's hypothesis that the defect was caused by lack of closure of the spine, and Morgagni's proposal that it was caused by a rupture of a previously closed neural tube (2–7). Proponents of each theory have gained prominence.

The formation of the myelomeningocele occurs early in life, probably between the third and fourth weeks of gestation. This has two implications. The first is that if myelo-

meningocele is to be prevented by eliminating teratogenic factors and providing a nutritional supplement it must be done very early—preconception—if possible. The second implication is that the lesion has occurred before limb bud development, yet most often the limb bud of the lower extremity is essentially normal. This seems to suggest that at least initially neurologic function is normal and remains so until late in prenatal development. This has led some investigators to evaluate the benefit of delivery by cesarean section when maturity of the lungs permits, avoiding the trauma to the neural plate caused by the decrease in amniotic fluid as maturity progresses, and by the birth process itself (8). However, the studies are inconclusive.

The roof of the myelomeningocele is composed of the spinal cord. It is open from the central canal posteriorly through the dorsal columns (Fig. 16-1). The anterior roots are intact, whereas the posterior roots to the dorsal cord are more likely to be involved in the pathologic process. The central canal of the cord is open and communicates with the fourth ventricle of the brain; this allows the cerebral spinal fluid to flow to the outside. Because of the probable involvement of the posterior columns, sensory and proprioception abnormalities probably are worse than the motor abnormalities. This abnormality of sensory feedback and crossing nerve fibers around the central cord may explain the lack of coordinated reciprocal functioning and the presence of spasticity frequently observed in children with myelomeningocele.

The attachment of the spinal cord to the meningocele sac prevents the normal upward migration of the spinal cord with growth. This produces the tethered cord. Even with surgical release of the spinal cord from all adhesions at the time of sac closure, there is a likelihood of reattachment of the cord during the healing process with recurrence of tethered cord syndrome later in life. The incidence of symptomatic retethering is unknown. However, it seems that the more it is looked for the more common it becomes.

Because of tethered cord, brain development, or hydrocephaly, almost all children with myelomeningocele have displacement of the brain stem through the foramen magnum into the cervical neural canal, known as Arnold-Chiari type II malformation. The extent of the displacement determines the type of deformity. Type I malformation has minimal deformity; type II deformity consists of the displacement of the medulla oblongata and the spinal cord to the extent that the cervical nerve roots must take an upward course to reach their outlet foramina (Fig. 16-2). This is the most common deformity in myelomeningocele. The type III deformity is more severe in displacement and includes part of the cerebellum.

The final pathologic abnormality is hydrocephaly, which consists of excessive cerebral spinal fluid in the ventricles of the brain. Almost 90% of children with myelomeningocele develop hydrocephaly, which communicates to a persistently open central canal of the cord, which in turn communicates with the meningocele sac. This open communication of the central canal and the fourth ventricle permits the

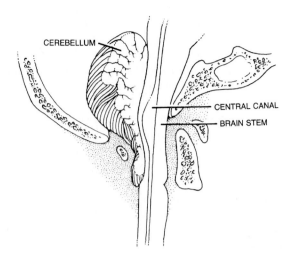

FIGURE 16-2. Arnold-Chiari type II malformation of the brain stem. This is the most common type of malformation seen in myelomeningocele. The medulla oblongata is displaced distally through the foramen magnum into the cervical neural canal. The ventricle communicates with the still-open central canal of the cord.

outflow of the cerebral spinal fluid, decompresses the ventricular pressure, and relieves the hydrocephaly. However, at the time of sac closure the fluid flow from the central canal is stopped and hydrocephaly returns. If hydrocephaly is not shunted, the fluid pressure increases in the brain and the spinal cord, which causes brain atrophy, hydromyelia, and eventually syringomyelia.

NEUROLOGIC ABNORMALITY

The neurologic abnormality defies simple classification (9) because of the complex abnormalities of the central nervous system, which include hydrocephaly, Arnold-Chiari deformity, hydrosyringomyelia, tethered cord, and injury to the posterior column of the spinal cord. Attempts to classify the level of paralysis by muscle function as though the defect is similar to a spinal cord injury seen in vertebral fractures are unsuccessful. Sharrard and Grosfield (10) initially formulated the classification by lumbar segmental levels based on motor segmental innervation using the level of the anterior horn cells in the spinal cord. This classification does not match the clinical observation of function in the lower extremities. For example, there is confusion in the literature about what is an L4 versus an L5 level of paralysis. The problem is using muscle activity to describe the level of paralysis when central nervous system dysfunction is common. If sensation, the most severely damaged nerve function, is used to describe the level of paralysis the classification better describes what is seen clinically. Muscles that can communicate with the brain through sensory feedback are functional. Muscles that cannot do this may be ignored by the brain and become flaccid or spastic, and function only by reflex. The author recommends that classification of function be made by sensory level, rather than motor level, because it will be more consistent between patients and between different observers. Another area of confusion is whether the level of paralysis is based on which muscles are working or upon which muscles are paralyzed.

Another confounding variable is abnormality of coordinated muscle function due to brain stem abnormalities. On manual testing the muscles contract to simple commands, such as "Extend (or flex) the knee." However, on complex coordinated activities such as walking, the leg muscles do not contract as expected, but contract and relax simultaneously in a co-contraction rather than sequentially, as seen in normal gait (Fig. 16-3). This dynamic co-contraction is

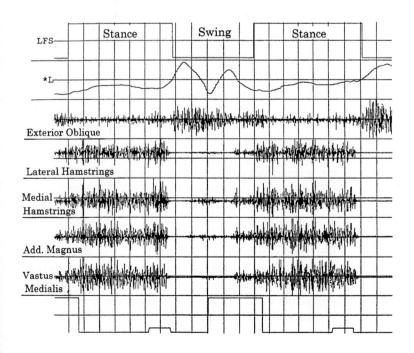

FIGURE 16-3. Dynamic electromyograms taken during a gait assessment analysis of a 5-year-old child with an L4 level of paraplegia and a type II Arnold-Chiari malformation. Surface electrodes were used during this analysis. The external oblique muscle is a swing phase muscle. The medial and lateral hamstrings, the adductor magnus, and the vastus medialis contract simultaneously throughout the stance phase. This observation has been checked using fine-wire electrodes, which show that the simultaneous contraction is not caused by crosstalk between the surface electrodes.

very common in the L3 to L5 level of paralysis, and may explain the knee flexion contractures in these patients, despite normal quadriceps strength. The author observed this phenomenon in a child with hydrocephalus and Arnold-Chiari deformity without myelomeningocele. This may suggest that it is related to the brain stem rather than to the meningocele itself.

Other common neurologic defects that are not well understood, are decreased perceptual motor function of the hands and attention deficit disorder manifested by short attention span at school (11).

GENETICS, ETIOLOGY, AND PRENATAL DIAGNOSIS

Approxiamtely 6,000 infants in the United States are born each year with neural tube defects. This includes anencephaly, myelomeningocele, and related abnormalities. Gradual decrease in incidence worldwide has occurred over the last 30 years (12). The reason for this fluctuation is not clear, and probably involves both genetic and environmental factors.

Most neural tube defects occur as isolated malformations caused by a variety of factors, both inherited and acquired (13,14). This pattern is known as "multifactorial inheritance." In the United States, the overall incidence of neural tube defects is 0.15% among whites and 0.04% among African-Americans. After the birth of one affected child, the risk of a second affected child is higher (15,16). In the United States the occurrence of a neural tube defect in first-degree relatives of an affected member was 3.2%, in second-degree relatives, 0.5%, and in third-degree relatives, 0.17% (14).

Not all neural tube defects are multifactorially inherited; some are caused by chromosome abnormalities, and others are caused by single-gene abnormalities. Usually, children with chromosomal or single-gene abnormalities have other birth defects. Some cases of spina bifida and anencephaly are entirely produced environmentally. These abnormalities are caused by exposure during pregnancy to teratogenic agents such as valproic acid taken for seizure control (17).

Yates and colleagues (11) have shown an association between susceptibility of offspring with neural tube defects and depressed red cell folate levels which cannot be attributed entirely to low dietary intake of folate. They postulate that a factor that predisposes a person to the current neural tube defect is an inherent disorder of folate metabolism. This theory is supported by a study by Sellar and Nevin (18) in which a decreased incidence of neural tube defects was found in children of mothers taking periconceptional vitamin supplementation. The FDA recommends that all women of child-bearing age receive 0.4 mg folate before conception and during early pregnancy. The Centers for Disease Control and Prevention (17) recommends that women who fall into the high-risk group of bearing a child with a neural tube defect because of giving birth to a prior affected child, or having a first-degree relative with a neural tube defect, receive a larger dose of folate, 4.0 mg/day.

Prenatal diagnosis of a neural tube defect allows the family, in consultation with the medical community, to make informed decisions about its child. These decisions range from termination of pregnancy to attempts to improve the outcome of pregnancy by improved perinatal care in institutions medically prepared to provide optimal care for the child. The aim of any prenatal screen for open neural tube defect is to be able to pinpoint women with a sufficiently high risk of having an affected infant to justify carrying out special diagnostic procedures such as amniocentesis for amniotic fluid, alpha-fetoprotein and acetylcholinesterase determinations, and detailed ultrasonography for examination of the fetus (19). Women who have had an infant with a neural tube defect carry enough risk of having another affected child to justify undergoing amniocentesis. Longitudinal ultrasound examination of the fetal spine provides vital information about the presence or absence of neural tube defect. The sensitivity of ultrasound examination is excellent for studying women at high risk for carrying a fetus with neural tube defect. In almost all fetuses with anencephaly, and in at least 80% of fetuses with open spina bifida, diagnoses are correct. When no abnormalities are found on detailed ultrasound examination, amniocentesis is recommended for evaluation for alpha-fetoprotein and acetylcholinesterase (20).

NATURAL HISTORY

Most children born with myelomeningocele die in early infancy if left untreated. This has been documented in several series of untreated children in the late 1950s and early 1960s. The mortality rates range from 90 to 100% (21,22). The cause of death in most infants is meningoventriculitis. Surgical treatment is not necessary for survival if antibiotics are administered and nutrition is maintained. However, the surviving children are disabled further by a high level of paralysis and increased mental retardation resulting from the continued trauma to the spinal cord and the uncontrolled hydrocephaly, which would not have been present if surgical treatment had been carried out.

During the 1970s, there was an attempt to select patients for treatment according to the criteria suggested by Lorber (22). However, most neurosurgeons have had great difficulty in withholding all forms of treatment from selected infants with myelomeningocele. They are performing initial sac closure and ventriculoperitoneal shunts on most infants with myelomeningocele.

Because most patients are treated with initial closure and ventriculoperitoneal shunt, a new and different natural history of the disease following this early treatment is being studied and documented. Studies conducted in the 1960s cannot be equated with the disease course of the children of this decade. An important discovery about the nature of myelomeningocele during the last 15 years is that the disease is not static but may undergo progressive neurologic degeneration, manifested by increasing levels of paralysis and decreasing upper-extremity function (23–25). Neurologic deterioration can be sudden and dramatic, or very slow and insidious. It is extremely important that the orthopaedist carry out a detailed neurologic evaluation including upper and lower extremities and motor function at each clinic visit, and any change in function requires a referral to the neurosurgeon for appropriate diagnosis and treatment. Three major areas of deterioration of the central nervous system have been found: hydrocephaly and associated hydrosyringomyelia, Arnold-Chiari deformity, and tethered cord syndrome.

Hydrocephaly

Hydrocephaly is a common disabling abnormality found in myelomeningocele due to obstruction of fluid movement by complex deformities of the posterior fossa and brain stem. In 1974, Lorber showed that, of patients *without* hydrocephaly, 30% had IQs above 100, 50% had IQs between 80 and 99, 12% had IQs between 60 and 79, and 8% had IQs under 60. In contrast, of patients *with* hydrocephaly, only 20% had IQs above 100, 30% had IQs between 80 and 99, 30% had IQs between 60 and 79, and 20% had IQs under 60 (22). Perceptual motor abnormalities appeared to be the biggest factor in intellectual function. Most of these children perform well in their verbal scores but are considerably below average in their perceptual motor and hand function scores.

Although, in some children with myelomeningocele the hydrocephaly becomes arrested in infancy without evidence of increasing head size or symptoms of acute intracranial pressure, most children require a ventriculoperitoneal or ventriculoatrial shunt (26). Considerable improvements in the design and construction of the shunt have been achieved; however, it is still an unsophisticated device for controlling the right amount of ventricular pressure. Shunt failure can occur at any age, and must be evaluated at each clinic visit.

In the young child shunt failure is accompanied by the typical symptoms of hydrocephaly. However, in the older age groups shunt malfunction rarely is associated with signs of acute hydrocephaly, such as nausea, vomiting, and severe headache, except first thing in the morning (24,26,27).

Because of the communication of the fourth ventricle with the persistent central canal of the cord, increased hydrocephaly results in fluid entering the central canal, causing dilation and pressure in the cord when the child is upright (6). If left unresolved, this eventually causes the formation of hydrosyringomyelia. Three problems have been shown to result from hydrosyringomyelia. The first problem is increasing paralysis of the lower extremities, occasionally associated with increased spasticity and, to a lesser extent, back pain. This problem is seen usually when the child is in his or her early school-age years. The second problem is progressive scoliosis which may occur as early as 5 years of age, but is more likely to be seen in the 7-to-10-year-old group (26,27). The third problem is weakness of the hands and upper extremity (24). This occurs when the child is in the teenage years. Most of these symptoms are resolved by early correction of the hydrocephalus by shunt replacement.

Arnold-Chiari Deformity

Associated with hydrocephaly is the Arnold-Chiari deformity, which is classified into three types according to the degree of displacement of the brain stem and hindbrain through the foramen magnum. Most of these affected children have a type II anomaly, which is characterized by displacement of the medulla oblongata into the cervical neural canal through the foramen magnum, requiring the cervical roots to take an upward course to reach their outlet foramina (Fig. 16-2).

The symptoms of an Arnold-Chiari type II deformity in infants includes periodic apnea, stridor, nystagmus, weak or absent cry, and upper-extremity spasm and weakness. Symptoms come in episodes between which the infant may show minimal involvement. The cause of the episodic nature of the symptoms is not determined. During childhood symptoms include spastic weakness of the upper extremities and, occasionally, leg involvement. Children also have nystagmus, stridor, difficulties in swallowing, and depressed or absent cough reflex. Symptoms in older patients still are being determined, and probably include scoliosis, decreased upper-extremity function, neck pain, and decreased respiratory function. The most serious difficulties appear to be present in infancy and decrease as the child matures.

In many children, following initial placement of the ventriculoperitoneal shunt to control hydrocephalus brain stem symptoms usually resolve on their own and do not require surgical decompression procedures. In a few infants and children in whom the brain stem compressive symptoms persist or progress, the posterior fossa and upper spinal region are decompressed surgically. The effect of aggressive treatment of Arnold-Chiari deformity on overall survival and function has yet to be determined.

Tethered Cord Syndrome

Tethered cord syndrome is another major cause of decreased nerve function (28). During the formation of the myelomeningocele, the open neural elements are attached to the ectoderm at its periphery. This prevents it from migrating cephalad during the growth of the fetus. Consequently, all children with myelomeningocele have a degree of tethered cord at the time of birth. During closure of the sac, the everted spinal cord is dissected from the skin and allowed to fall back inside the neural canal. If any dermal elements are left attached to the spinal cord, dermoid cysts may develop and eventually cause decreasing function in the lumbosacral roots by direct pressure on the nerve elements.

After sac closure there still is a tendency for the spinal cord to become adherent to the meningocele repair. As the child grows this adherence again produces a tethered cord and prevents the spinal cord from migrating cephalad during growth. Although many children have a tethering of their spinal cord, only a few actually have symptoms of the condition and require surgical release. Because the posterior part of the spinal cord is adherent to the meningocele repair, and the cord proximal to the meningocele is held posteriorly where it is compressed by the posterior neural arch in the area of the lumbar lordosis, most symptoms are associated with posterior column abnormalities.

Pain appears to be a prominent symptom of the tethered cord syndrome and may occur in the lower lumbar spine, in the area of the myelomeningocele, or the sacral roots, with pain in the buttock and the posterior thigh. The pain is also activity-related, and becomes worse after walking long distances. In addition, increasing spasticity and decreasing function of the lower extremities are frequently present. Occasionally there is an associated progressive scoliosis associated with marked lordosis. Changes in dermatomal somatosensory-evoked potentials are present, and are helpful in making the diagnosis if serial examinations have been made (29). Changes in bladder function are common. The diagnosis of tethered cord syndrome is made on clinical evaluation, not by the presence or absence of a tethered cord on radiographic MRI study. The MRI describes the nature of the tether and confirms the diagnosis. The diagnosis of tethered cord syndrome in thoracic level paraplegics is rare, and becomes more common the lower the level of paralysis. In the author's experience surgical release of the tethered cord rarely provides complete return of lost function. The diagnosis must be made early, and appropriate care must be provided before major loss occurs.

Latex Hypersensitivity

During the past 10 years there have been increasing reports of severe immediate-type allergic reactions to latex exposure (30). Although anyone may become sensitized to latex, three groups appear to have a high risk: children with myelomeningocele, health care workers, and workers in the latex industry. The reported incidence is as high as 34% in myelomeningocele children, and may increase in the future (31).

All patients should be questioned about a history of latex allergy. A history suggesting sensitivity includes swelling or itching of the lips from blowing up balloons or after dental examinations, and swelling or itching of the skin after contact with any rubber products. Other information that may suggest increased risk of latex allergy includes hand eczema; oral itching after eating bananas, chestnuts, or avocados; and multiple surgical procedures in infancy.

There is no standard test for latex allergy. Skin testing with a latex extract or glove extract may be the best test available. However, anaphylaxis has occurred in spina bifida patients during skin testing. In vitro tests may not be sensitive enough to detect all persons who may be at risk for latex contact.

Because of the high incidence of latex allergy in myelomeningocele it is recommended that all patients, regardless of history, should have their surgery performed in a latex-free environment. There have been several lists published of latex-containing items. However, they are being revised almost daily, and no list should be considered complete. Some things that are labeled "latex," such as latex paint, are not latex based. It is best to ask the manufacturer if there is any question. If the child is known to be allergic, the parents will be able to tell what things need to be avoided in the hospital environment. However, in surgery, it must be assumed that the child is sensitive to all latex material. A latex-free environment is one in which no latex gloves are used by any personnel in the operating room, and there should be no latex accessories (e.g., catheters, adhesives, tourniquets, anesthesia equipment) that come into direct contact with the patient.

EFFECT OF MYELOMENINGOCELE ON DEVELOPMENTAL SEQUENCE

The normal child undergoes a sequential development of fine motor, gross motor, personal, social, language, and cognitive skills, which are the result of the child's physical abilities and his or her interaction with the environment (11). Three major areas that interfere with normal development of the myelomeningocele child are residual physical deformity, iatrogenic factors, and restrictions by society.

Medical treatment of children with myelomeningocele contributes greatly to their delayed development. Prolonged and frequent hospitalization during the first years of life, although often necessary, considerably interferes with the learning experiences of the child. Hoppenfield (32) pointed out that because of this environmental deprivation a 1-month-old infant with myelomeningocele frequently cannot follow a light to a midline, fix both eyes on the light, and respond to the sound of a rattle.

Along with the frequent shunt malfunctions and repeated hospitalizations the child also is placed in casts and splints to treat physical deformity, which further interferes with mobility and physical contact with parents, and prevents parent–child bonding. As the child becomes older, individuality often is denied as he or she is treated as a disease entity rather than a person. In the clinic the children frequently are undressed to their diapers then paraded before members of the clinic without regard for their embarrassment. The tendency is to treat them as asexual beings. If it is necessary to present a physical function abnormality to a group for discussion or education, a picture or a video recording should be used.

The last impediment to normal development is the resistance of society to accept and accommodate handicapped persons. Although there have been considerable improvements in treatment of children with myelomeningocele during the last 10 years, there still are considerable societal barriers to these children. For example, access to schools, playgrounds, amusement parks, sporting events, movie theaters, and private homes are limited to some extent. Also, acceptance of handicapped people in the employment market is restricted.

Although many previously mentioned factors are beyond control, these myelomeningocele patients can be helped to overcome their handicap. Hospitalization and treatment programs must be planned to interfere as little as possible with the normal developmental sequence, particularly in infancy. We must work within the clinics, schools, and to a larger extent, society, to promote acceptance of these patients as individuals, and help them carry out the four principle tasks of childhood and adolescence: establishment of a stable self-image, acceptance of an adult sexual role, development of independence, and choice of a career (33).

Development of a positive self-image and adult sexuality is a difficult task. Because of the physical impairment of children with myelomeningocele, personal interactions among peers is severely restricted, beginning in early childhood and extending into adolescence. The child with myelomeningocele looks different because of braces, orthopaedic shoes, wheelchairs, and deformities; these are barriers to peer acceptance. These feelings of being different may never be erased, even if the cause of these feelings is eliminated (34). Sexual information for these patients often is avoided or erroneous. Shurtleff et al. (8) showed that many adults with myelomeningocele could have sexual relationships, including procreation; however, knowledge about the specific problems in myelomeningocele is meager, and a local resource person may be difficult to find.

Development of independence is a complex issue between the parents and their dependent, handicapped child. The parents are often overprotective of the child. This protective attitude is also present in school and in society at large, especially if the child is confined to a wheelchair.

The choice of a career is also difficult. High school counselors are not trained to advise disadvantaged children, especially those with perceptual motor abnormalities of the hands. Government programs are not available until the patient is 18 years old or has graduated from high school. This is too late. Employment opportunities also are limited by the lack of ability to get health insurance.

TREATMENT

Treatment of children with myelomeningocele is not a matter of what can be done, but what should be done for each child. The decision-making may begin prenatally if the diagnosis is made by alpha-fetoprotein testing or ultrasound examination. The option to continue or terminate the pregnancy can be made at this time. If it is continued, decisions must be made on how to improve the prognosis of the child. These include referral, before delivery, to a center experienced in the care of these children so that adequate planning and preparation for the family can be carried out. If the diagnosis is made after birth then the next decision is whether the meningocele should be closed and the child treated. Most children are treated unless there are other deformities present that are not compatible with life, such as anencephaly, congenital heart disease, pulmonary insufficiency, and other congenital malformations. In some cases, the lesion may be surgically untreatable.

Orthopaedic treatment is intertwined with the neurosurgical treatment. It is also tied in with urologic treatment. Almost all of these children have urologic abnormalities that require bladder drainage by conduits or intermittent catheterization. Frequent infection may spread to orthopaedic surgical areas, and the orthopaedic treatment of spine deformity influences the ability of the patient for self-catheterization.

Orthopaedic treatment of myelomeningocele has three major goals. The first goal is to provide for maximal use of residual ability to maintain range of motion and stability of the spine and extremities. The second is to provide for mobility by means of a wheelchair and other wheeled devices or by ambulation. The third goal is to prevent deterioration of neurologic function. Although it is true that the actual treatment of the central nervous system is performed by the neurosurgeon, the diagnosis of decreased function is made from observations of the spine and extremities by the orthopaedist. It cannot be assumed, because these patients are being seen and followed-up by neurosurgeons, that subtle changes in function are going to be observed. Teamwork is essential in treatment of children with myelomeningocele.

The ability to walk is important and often necessary in our society, despite recent advances in wheelchair design and wheelchair accessibility in the community. It also is the desire of every child with spina bifida. Although it is possible for most paraplegic children to walk to some degree during preschool and school age, many adults are not able to continue walking. Abnormalities of the spine and legs are often the cause for this inability. There are four necessary requirements of walking: alignment of trunk and legs; range of motion; control of the hip, knee, and ankle joints; and power to provide forward motion.

The alignment of the spine and the legs must be such that the center of gravity passes through the joints of the pelvis, the hip, the knee, and the foot. Deformities of the spine, such as scoliosis, kyphosis, and pelvic obliquity, prevent the center of gravity from passing through the center of the hip joint. Contractures of the hip or knee also will prevent stable weightbearing.

Motion of the lumbosacral spine and the hip are essential for functional walking. Motion of the knee is less important, and is useful only in clearing the swing leg. Mobility of the spine must allow the center of gravity to be shifted from side to side over the stance leg. Motion of the hip is the most important part of walking. Analysis of spina bifida children who maintain walking ability has shown normal flexion/extension of the hip. Thirty degrees of motion is necessary for forward progression. If there is less motion than this, then pelvic motion must help compensate for this decreased motion.

The child must be able to control the position of the trunk and hip, knee, and ankle joints, during the gait cycle. If this cannot be performed by muscle activity then it must be provided by an orthotic device. The determination of available muscles to control the joints is dependent on the level of paralysis.

The thoracic-level paraplegic has no active muscle contraction across the hip joint, and no feeling below the groin or in the hip. The child has no control of the hip, and the hip is unstable, even though it may be reduced and appear stable on radiograph examination. Stability for walking can only be provided by an orthosis that crosses the hip joint.

The upper lumbar paraplegic child has several muscles crossing the hip joint. These muscles include the hip flexors and the hip adductors. These children have some sensation crossing the hip joint. Contraction of the hip flexors causes the hip to flex, pitching the child forward. In order to keep from falling it is necessary to place most of his or her weight on the arms and crutches or walker. This is not a useful posture for walking and must be corrected. There is no way of surgically providing stability to this hip, and, similar to the thoracic-level paraplegic, the stability must be provided by an orthosis.

The middle and lower lumbar paraplegic child has hip flexors and adductors, knee extensors, and weak knee flexors. These children do not have normal hip extension or hip abduction, which are the most important muscles for standing and walking. Their weak hamstring muscles have a tendency to extend the hip and make these children walk without the need for orthotic control of the hip. The result of this is knee-flexion contracture. The force imbalance around the hip results in eventual hip dislocation. A decrease in the force imbalance, and increase of the control of the hip, can be obtained only by moving muscles to a more functional position or by adding muscles to the hip. Muscles available for transfer include the iliopsoas, the abdominal muscles, and the adductor muscles. Control of the hip and knee can be achieved by muscle activity; however, the ankle requires an orthosis.

The sacral-level paraplegic child has sufficient muscle control around the hip, the knee, and the ankle to provide the necessary stability.

The force necessary to move forward is beyond the muscle contraction needed to control the joint. In normal individuals it is provided by the calf muscle, which pushes people forward into their next step, and the hip extensors, which pull forward after the foot hits the floor. Both of these muscles have sacral level innervation and are paralyzed in almost all spina bifida children. In the thoracic and upper-lumbar levels of paraplegia the arms become the power producers to move forward. The arms are not designed for this activity and are inefficient. Weight gain is also a problem because many of these patients become obese. Consequently, it takes increased energy to walk and the walking pace is much slower than normal. Eventually, most thoracic and upper lumbar–level paraplegic people discover that the wheelchair is a much more efficient means of transportation.

The middle and lower lumbar–level paraplegics substitute trunk shift and sway to produce the forward motion. Much of the motion is from side to side, rather than forward. This also is an inefficient method of walking, and some children abandon it for a wheelchair when they become adults. The use of muscle transfers to increase hip extension does aid in the efficiency of walking and may keep the patient walking longer.

Spine

Spine deformity is so common in myelomeningocele that it should be considered part of the disease complex (35). The spine deformities usually are progressive and may cause severe disability, interfere with rehabilitation, and negate previous treatment to maintain ambulation.

The most obvious and consistent abnormality of myelomeningocele spinal deformity is the incomplete posterior arch in the lumbosacral spine. This abnormality affects many aspects of scoliosis and kyphosis treatment. Other congenital malformations also may be present (36). Hemivertebrae and diastematomyelia may occur at any level along the spine. Similarly, unsegmented bars may occur at any level. They are particularly difficult to identify and evaluate if they occur in the area of the spina bifida, where the facet joints, lamina, and spinous processes are difficult to identify on standard radiographs.

The spinal curvature often appears at a younger age than that typical for most developmental abnormalities. It may be present by 2 to 3 years of age, becoming severe by age 7. Because of the early onset of the deformity, treatment plans need to anticipate growth of the spine. However, the projections for growth in children with myelomeningocele are different from those for children with normal growth potential. Children with myelomeningocele may have slow growth due to growth hormone deficiency, and mature earlier than usual, often by 9 to 10 years of age in girls and 11 to 12 years in boys. The cause of the hormonal abnormalities has not been discerned, but they are treatable if it is necessary for the overall management of the child.

Another factor that needs to be considered in the surgical treatment of these patients is the high infection rate (35,37–39). These patients are subject to frequent septicemias due to urinary tract infections. Most of these children have chronic contamination of the urinary tract, which always has the potential to progress into an infection. During surgical procedures adequate drainage of the bladder and appropriate antibiotics should be a routine part of the surgical management. The skin in the area of the meningocele repair is often of poor quality, and gives minimal coverage to the instrumentation.

These children also have deformity of the pelvis and hips that affects spine balance. For example, asymmetric hip contractures may cause lumbar scoliosis, pelvic obliquity, and abnormal lordosis in the standing or sitting position. Similarly, correction of the spine in the treatment of scoliosis can position the legs in a way that prevents functional sitting or standing.

As with all children with spinal deformities, the goals of treatment are the prevention of further deformity and the creation of a stable, balanced spine. Children with myelomeningocele, however, require more precise correction of the deformities. Residual deformity may prevent them from sitting, standing, or walking. Pressure sores are likely to develop if pelvic obliquity remains, and their sagittal plane alignment must allow them to perform intermittent self-catheterization.

Scoliosis and Lordosis

Scoliosis occurs in almost 100% of patients with thoracic-level paraplegia (40). Eighty-five percent of these curves are greater than 45 degrees. As the paralysis level lowers, so does the incidence of scoliosis. At the fourth lumbar level of paraplegia the instance of curvature decreases to about 60%, with only 40% requiring surgical intervention (40) (Fig. 16-4). Lordosis without concurrent scoliosis is rare, and usually is caused by hip-flexion contractures. Historically it has been seen after spinal–peritoneal shunting for hydrocephalus; however, this procedure is rarely performed.

Several causes for the scoliosis have been identified. A C-shaped scoliosis is usually caused by muscle weakness associated with high-level paraplegia. It also may be associated with asymmetric levels of paralysis or a spastic hemiplegia due to the hydrocephalus. This type of scoliosis may be associated with kyphosis rather than lordosis. Typically, this curve pattern occurs at a young age, often in infancy, and is usually progressive. If severe spasticity is present an intraspinal rhizotomy or cordectomy may be necessary (42).

Hydromyelia, or hydrosyringomyelia associated with uncompensated hydrocephalus, can cause scoliosis (24–27). The scoliosis is usually in the thoracic or the thoracolumbar region, and it is typically S-shaped. Because of stiffness in the area of the myelomeningocele in the lumbar spine, the compensation for the major curve may be incomplete and associated with pelvic obliquity. Scoliosis may be the only

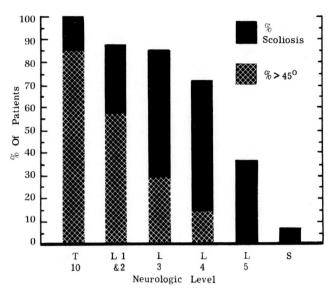

FIGURE 16-4. Incidence and severity of scoliosis, based on the level of paraplegia. (From ref. 41, with permission.)

clinical sign of shunt malfunction or progressive hydromyelia, and may occur at any age, even early in childhood. Headache, nausea, vomiting, and vision changes—the usual signs of hydrocephalus—may be absent. Other symptoms of hydromyelia are back pain, weakness of the upper extremities, and increasing paralysis of the legs. It has been shown that reinserting a functional shunt may decrease the scoliosis if it is less than 50 degrees (27).

Another cause of scoliosis is the tethered cord syndrome (23,28,43). This abnormality is caused by attachment of the spinal cord to the area of the myelomeningocele, preventing its upward migration with growth. This syndrome may be associated with other intraspinal pathologies, such as dermoid tumors, lipomas, and diastematomyelia. The scoliosis is usually in the dorsal lumbar or lumbar spine with a marked increase in lumbar lordosis. Results of releasing the tethered cord are variable, but frequently curve progression is stopped; in a few cases, it improves. If the curve is more than 50 degrees, the scoliosis should be corrected and stabilized with spine fusion.

Congenital malformations, including the lack of formation and the lack of segmentation (36,44), may exist in combination with hydromyelia, tethered cord, or muscle paralysis. When evaluating a child with scoliosis the physician must consider each component of the scoliosis in the treatment program. Because of the high number of neurologic abnormalities associated with scoliosis a referral to a neurosurgeon should be made at the first sign of increasing scoliosis. It may be necessary to reinsert the shunt, untether the spinal cord, and treat the congenital scoliosis, if all are present.

Diagnostic Studies. At each visit a thorough neurologic examination of muscle strength, levels of sensation, and reflex activity of the upper and lower extremities should be carefully documented. If scoliosis is developing, the documented changes in neurologic function are of major diagnostic importance to the etiology of the scoliosis.

Radiographic evaluation should be carried out annually from the age of 1 year. These radiographs should be taken while the child is sitting, when the child can do so. This eliminates the problems related to hip flexion contracture and asymmetric abduction and adduction. If there is documented progressive scoliosis, additional radiographic examination is indicated. Magnetic resonance imaging (MRI) probably gives the most information without requiring invasive studies (45). MRI of the head and cervical spine evaluates the hydrocephalus and the degree of Arnold-Chiari malformation. The cervical, thoracic, and lumbar spine also should be scanned. The cervical and thoracic spine are evaluated for the appearance of syrinx or hydromyelia. The scan of the lumbar spine provides information on the posterior displacement of the conus and the presence of intraspinal tumors, such as lipoma or dermoid cysts. The MRI studies must be interpreted in association with the clinical findings to determine the cause of the scoliosis. The presence of a tethered cord is common, and it alone may not be the cause of the deformity. In the author's experience the scoliosis is in the lumbar spine with the apex at the last intact neural arch; the lordosis is in excess of 90 degrees; and other signs of tethered cord, such as changes in bladder function and neurologic function of the legs, are present.

Computed tomography (CT) also can be used. However, to get the maximum benefit from the study contrast material is usually necessary for evaluation of the spinal cord. Both MRI and CT studies usually require sedation or anesthesia in young children.

Treatment. If the scoliosis continues to progress after neurologic problems have been corrected, orthopaedic treatment is indicated. If the spine is balanced and the curve is 30 degrees or less, observation probably is indicated. However, if the curve is unbalanced or greater than 30 degrees the center of gravity falls outside of the pelvic base of support, the spine will become unstable, and progression of the deformity is almost assured. A trial of bracing is indicated in children younger than the age of 7 years if the curve is supple and can be corrected easily. However, because bracing in paralytic scoliosis is passive, the brace tends to deform the rib cage and produce pressure sores in the area of insensate skin. In infants special care is needed to avoid abdominal compression, which may make it difficult for the child to breathe and eat. Although the use of a brace is only temporary, it may delay the necessity of surgery until the child is 8 or 9 years old, when many of these children are beginning adolescence (36,46).

The most effective spinal orthosis is a two-piece, polypropylene, bivalved, molded body jacket. This design allows the brace to be expanded or contracted throughout the day, to allow for eating, and allows some adjustability for growth.

Meticulous care is required because pressure sores are frequent, and once they develop, it is almost impossible to continue using the brace for control of the curve. In general, the child begins orthosis wear slowly, starting at 1 h intervals, after which the skin should be inspected. If any redness does not disappear within 4 h, the orthosis must be modified. The time in the brace is gradually increased over 2 to 3 weeks until the child is wearing it throughout the day except for naps and nighttime. If the family or caregivers are unable to provide this degree of care an orthosis is probably not indicated.

Most of these children require surgical correction and spinal fusion. Levels of fusion depend on the age of the child, the location of the curve, the level of paralysis, and the ambulatory status. As with all children with spinal deformities, the goals of treatment are the prevention of further deformity and the creation of a stable, balanced spine. Children with myelomeningocele, however, require more precise correction of their deformities; because of their paralysis, they are unable to compensate for any residual deformity, which may prevent them from sitting or from standing and walking. Pressure sores are likely to develop if pelvic obliquity remains, and their sagittal plane alignment must allow them to perform intermittent self-catheterization.

The treatment of the tethered cord, even if it is not symptomatic when correction of the scoliosis is performed, is an unsettled issue. Correction of the scoliosis lengthens the posterior spine, and puts the tethered cord on stretch. This may produce neurologic changes, even if they were absent before. Therefore, the neurosurgeons at the author's clinic believe that the tethered cord should be released either before or during the scoliosis surgery. If it is done before, the time between release and the spine surgery should probably be no more than 6 months because of the frequent retethering.

Generally, the same guidelines for instrumentation and fusion of idiopathic scoliosis are applicable to the myelomeningocele spine. The fusion should go from neutral vertebra to neutral vertebra, and the end vertebra should be located within the stable zone. This holds true for thoracic and thoracolumbar curves. However, in double curves, uncompensated curves, and primary lumbar curves, the decision becomes more difficult. The guidelines for fusion and instrumentation in these cases differ from those for idiopathic scoliosis. In general, it is a mistake to fuse short; if there is a question, fuse long. A compensatory thoracic curve should be fused for its entire length, and the fusion should not end in the middle of a sagittal curve or at a junctional kyphosis.

The selection of the level at the distal end usually is complicated by the open vertebral arch, which prevents attachment of the instrumentation to the end vertebra. Lumbar hyperlordosis usually is present, compounding the problem of deciding on the distal level of fusion. In the past, the instrumentation was extended to the pelvis because of the difficulty of getting a firm attachment to the lower lumbar vertebrae [➡2.5, 2.6] (47). With the newer methods of pedicle fixation it may be possible to control some curves without fusing the lumbosacral joint. The indications for extending the fusion mass to the sacrum are not well established. Lumbosacral arthrodesis is difficult to obtain because of the lack of posterior vertebral arch to fuse [➥2.6–2.8]. Consequently, pseudoarthroses and instrumentation failures are common (39). Attempts to correct these problems require repeated surgical procedures and have an uncertain outcome. If a successful fusion to the sacrum is obtained it may deprive ambulatory patients of the ability to walk (48). In wheelchair-bound patients a lumbosacral fusion may cause difficulty because of increased occurrence of pressure sores if the residual pelvic obliquity is 15 degrees or greater. Movement in the lumbosacral spine absorbs much of the angular and rotational movements of the trunk during wheelchair activities. If the lumbosacral spine is fused, these torsional movements are transmitted to the pelvis, creating increased shear between the pelvis, the skin, and the wheelchair seat.

If the lumbosacral joint is not fused, the scoliosis tends to increase, unless the lumbar scoliosis can be corrected to less than 20 degrees and the pelvic obliquity to less than 15 degrees. Therefore, it is important to treat the scoliosis while the curve is small and can be corrected to less than a 20-degree lumbar curve and a 15-degree pelvic obliquity, whether fusion to the sacrum is planned or not. The delay of surgical correction of the scoliosis to allow the spine to grow may lead to an unsatisfactory correction. After spine correction residual pelvic obliquity greater than 15 degrees and less than 35 degrees can be corrected by a bilateral posterior iliac osteotomy, with transfer of a wedge of bone from the long side to the short side. The correction of the pelvic obliquity is necessary if there is difficulty sitting or an ischial ulcer develops (49).

Children with a thoracic or upper lumbar level of paraplegia should be fused to the sacrum (Fig. 16-5). In children with low lumbar and sacral levels of paraplegia, the lumbo-

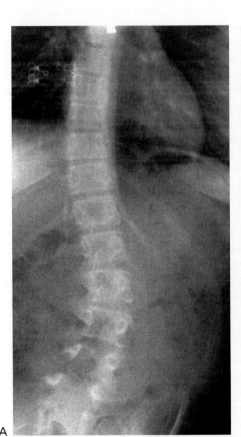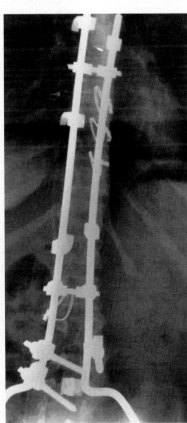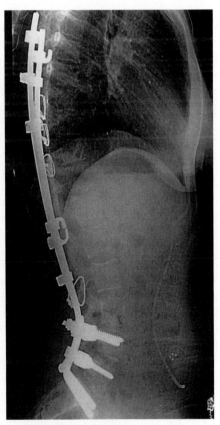

A   B,C

FIGURE 16-5. A 13-year-old girl has an L3-level paraplegia, but is not ambulatory. She is obese and has a progressive lumbar scoliosis and pelvic obliquity. A tethered spinal cord previously was released. **A:** Anteroposterior radiograph shows a 50-degree uncompensated lumbar scoliosis resulting in 35-degrees of pelvic obliquity. There is excessive lumbar lordosis. **B:** Postoperative anteroposterior radiograph shows complete correction of the scoliosis. The sacrum was included in the fusion because the lumbar scoliosis included the first sacral vertebra and the child was not ambulatory. Pedicle screws were used to secure the segmental instrumentation to L4 and L5. Anterior interbody fusion was performed from T10 to the sacrum. **C:** Postoperative radiograph shows restoration of normal sagittal alignment. Lumbar lordosis now measures 55 degrees. The patient has full extension of her hips, and is able to perform intermittent self-catheterization. (From ref. 59, with permission.)

sacral joint should be spared if they are walkers, and the spine can be aligned satisfactorily (Fig. 16-6).

The sagittal deformity also must be evaluated because increased lumbar lordosis is a common deformity. Assessment of sitting, supine, and standing posture must be made before correcting the lumbar lordosis. These children often require a greater degree of lordosis than normal. Restoring the lumbar lordosis to the normal range may uncover a hip-flexion contracture and prevent the child from standing or walking. If too much lordosis is fused into the lumbar spine of a female patient she may not be able to carry out intermittent self-catheterization. The degree of lordosis left in the spine after fusion needs to be tailored to each patient. It is best to treat the hip contractures before correcting the spine. If the hip deformity is not corrected first, positioning of the spine on the operating table will be difficult and torque the spine postoperatively, leading to instrument failure and pseudarthrosis.

Ischial pressure sores also should be treated before spinal fusion to lessen the chance of infection. This is often difficult to do because the pelvic obliquity is a major cause of the ulceration and unless it is corrected, pressure cannot be relieved from the ulcer. In this circumstance, a gluteus maximus myocutaneous flap can be used to promote primary healing. The patient is maintained on an air mattress bed until the spinal correction can be performed. This may seem extreme, but is much less of a problem than an infected spinal fusion that requires instrument removal.

The age of the child at the time of surgery is an important consideration. If the child has not yet reached adolescence, as determined by the beginning of the appearance of pubic hair and a Risser sign of I, there is an almost 100% assurance that the curve will continue to progress despite posterior fusion unless the anterior spine is fused to the same level. The lumbar spine usually is fused anteriorly as well as posteriorly because of the deficient posterior vertebral arch, but if the posterior fusion extends up into the thoracic spine, it must be fused anteriorly as well.

In a child with a progressive curve that cannot be controlled by a brace and who is younger than 8 years old, the preferred treatment is extraperiosteal segmental Luque instrumentation without spinal fusion. Distal fixation of the rods in the area of the open spine is difficult. The author prefers use of the first sacral foramen as the anchor point. The "S" rod attached to the ala is also a possibility. The ilium is also a possibility, although the author has experienced loosening of the rod in the ilium with loss of fixation and erosion of the rod through the skin. Postoperative brace treatment is still indicated, and complications from this approach include rod breakage, wire breakage, and spontaneous fusion. To provide a definitive solution, reoperation is often necessary when the child reaches maturity.

Instrumentation. Spinal fusion is still the most important part of surgical treatment of scoliosis despite the recent ad-

vances in spinal instrumentation. The role of the instrumentation is to improve spinal alignment and the fusion rate, and reduce the need for recumbency or postoperative immobilization. Whatever the instrumentation used, the degree of correctability of the curve is limited. It is important to carry out an early fusion when the deformity is manageable. The amount of correction that is possible is probably limited to about 60 degrees, despite the size of the curve. Occasionally it is possible to produce amazing degrees of correction, but this is not the rule. It is better to correct completely a 60-degree curve than to correct a 120-degree curve to 60 degrees.

It is agreed that anterior and posterior fusion is necessary in the area of the lumbar spine (40,50–52). However, there is no agreement about whether the anterior spine needs to be instrumented. The more severe the deformity to be corrected the greater the indication for using anterior instrumentation. However, there is still a great risk of producing kyphosis of the lumbar spine or at least flattening the normal lumbar lordosis, although some of the newer devices using thicker rods may control the sagittal alignment of the lumbar spine. Anterior instrumentation to the sacrum is difficult, and it is questionable whether an anterior interbody fusion of L5-S1 is necessary. Normally this is a very stable joint, and adequate posterior fusion can be obtained by grafting from the lamina and transverse process of L5 to the sacral ala. However, if the anterior longitudinal ligament is destroyed along with the annulus fibrosis, instability and severe deformity of this joint may occur if the child develops a pseudarthrosis of the lumbosacral joint. Because repair of this deformity and pseudarthrosis can be difficult, it is preferable to end the anterior instrumentation at L4 [➡2.11] in those patients who have a dorsal lumbar curve that ends or is stable at L3-L4. If it is necessary to extend the fusion down to the pelvis, perform an anterior fusion only down to L5, and posteriorly to the pelvis.

Posterior instrumentation has evolved considerably over the last 20 years. Initially, Harrington instrumentation was used [➡2.2–2.4], but because of the lack of posterior vertebral arch, distal fixation of the fusion was difficult unless the instrumentation was extended down to the sacral ala. The alar hooks frequently became displaced, and the pseudarthrosis and complication rates were unacceptably high (52). The child also required postoperative immobilization which increased the occurrence of pressure sores.

Luque instrumentation has become the standard instrumentation for these children (47). Because of the segmental fixation to each vertebra, there is much better control over the spine and postoperative immobilization is not required [➡2.5]. However, it does not fix the length of the spine as a rod with hooks does; therefore, the spine may settle or collapse along the rod, with loss of some correction in the immediate postoperative period. If the rod is contoured to maintain a normal sagittal alignment there is a tendency for the rod to twist into the coronal plane deformity with

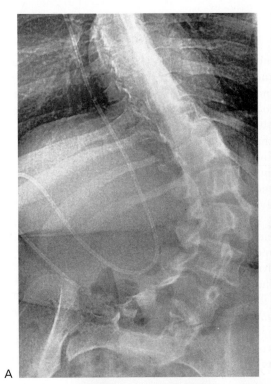
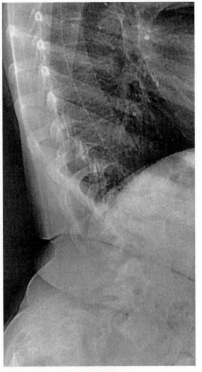

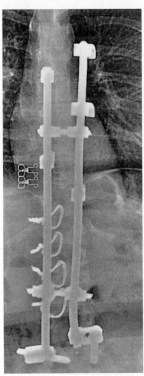
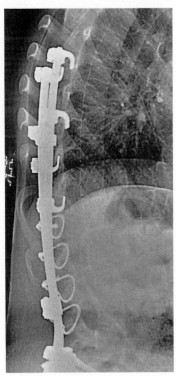

FIGURE 16-6. A mature 12-year-old girl with progressive lumbar scoliosis is an L4-level paraplegic, and is a community walker with ankle–foot orthoses and crutches. **A:** Anteroposterior radiograph shows 55-degree lumbar scoliosis from T10 to L3. There is a 20-degree compensatory curve from L4 to the sacrum. There is residual 30-degree pelvic obliquity. The last intact vertebral arch is L2. **B:** Lateral radiograph shows severe 120-degree lordosis, which is typical of the deformity associated with tethered cord. **C:** Anteroposterior radiograph shows correction of the scoliosis and pelvic obliquity. Pelvic screws are used to fix the distal end vertebrae at L5. The lumbosacral joint was left unfused to allow the patient enough pelvic mobility to continue walking. Release of the tethered cord was performed at the same time as the spine fusion. An anterior interbody fusion was performed from T9 to L5, without instrumentation. **D:** Lateral radiograph shows correction of the lordosis to 45 degrees and the achievement of a normal sagittal alignment. (From ref. 59, with permission.)

loss of correction. This is lessened by the use of the unit rod or multiple transverse rod connectors. Fixation to the open posterior spine in the lumbar area by wires around the pedicle is weak, and extension of the instrumentation to the ilium is usually necessary. Even this distal attachment of the Luque rods is weak because there may be significant osteoporosis of the pelvis. Loosening of the instrumentation and pseudarthrosis of the lumbosacral joint is frequent. Although this is not usually symptomatic, the author has observed increased scoliosis, pelvic obliquity, and pressure sores.

The development of instrumentation that allows segmental fixation [➥2.9], distraction, and compression on the same rod, along with the use of pedicle screws [➥2.8], may solve many problems of instrumentation of the distal spine. The pedicle screws allow the end vertebra to be positioned in three planes, and provide stable segmental instrumentation. This instrumentation may lessen the desirability of anterior instrumentation. Long-term studies have not yet been performed, but early experience indicates that satisfactory results can be obtained (Figs. 16-5 and 16-6).

Whatever the instrumentation used posteriorly, it should be low-profile in design. In the area of the meningocele sac there is poor skin and soft tissue coverage. Prominence of hardware invariably leads to ulceration over the hardware, eventual infection, and the need to remove the instrumentation.

Congenital Scoliosis

Congenital scoliosis may occur anywhere along the spine, including the cervical, the thoracic, and the lumbosacral spines. Congenital malformations may be caused by the lack of formation or segmentation, or a combination of the two. If the malformation occurs in the lumbosacral area the progression of deformity is usually rapid and uncompensated, causing severe pelvic obliquity. Nonoperative methods of treatment do not correct congenital scoliosis, or even prevent it from worsening. These children, because of their neurologic abnormalities, are unable to tolerate an unbalanced spine. Therefore, it is important that treatment be carried out in infancy when the deformity is small, rather than waiting until the child is older and heroic measures are needed to obtain satisfactory alignment.

Posterior fusion of the malformation is rarely successful in preventing progression. Anterior and posterior fusion is the procedure of choice, and it should be performed when a diagnosis of progressive scoliosis is made, usually at 1 year of age. The spine may be approached in staged or separate anterior and posterior procedures, or anterior and posterior interbody fusions may be performed through a posterior approach, using the pedicle as the access conduit to the anterior spine (53) The posterior approach is useful when the malformation is in the upper thoracic spine, where the anterior approach is difficult. If the lumbar curve is already so severe that the pelvic obliquity is greater than 15 degrees,

an osteotomy of the spine to correct the deformity should be considered. Another possibility in a child over 10 years of age is to perform a bilateral posterior iliac osteotomy to balance the pelvis after the spine has been fused (49).

Kyphosis

Lumbar kyphosis is a major deformity that occurs in 8 to 15% of patients with myelomeningocele (32,38,54–57). It often measures 80 degrees or more at birth, and usually progresses with growth. Children with extensive kyphosis are unable to wear braces, have trouble sitting in a wheelchair, and often have ulcerations over the prominent kyphos. Progression of the kyphosis may lead to breathing difficulty because the abdominal contents are crowded into the chest cavity by increasing upward pressure on the diaphragm. These children also have difficulty eating because of loss of abdominal size, which results in a failure to thrive. They are underweight and short in stature. The increased flexion of the trunk also may interfere with drainage of urine if the child has a urethrostomy, a vesicotomy, or an ileostomy.

Kyphosis is almost always progressive, and attempts to delay definitive treatment until the child is older leads to a more severe deformity (7,58). The aorta and the vena cava do not follow the anterior border of the spine across the kyphosis (59); they take the short route, like a bowstring, limiting the amount of surgical correctability. Therefore, it is important to carry out treatment early, even though it may be only a temporizing procedure. A more definitive procedure can be performed later.

The goals of treatment is to increase abdominal height, to allow more room for the abdominal contents, and relieve pressure on the diaphragm and the lungs. In addition, the kyphosis must be minimized to lessen the incidence of pressure sores and move the center of gravity posteriorly to center it over the ischium. This improves the child's ability to sit without using the arms for support.

The kyphosis deformity can be divided into two types (60) (Fig. 16-7). The first type is a collapsing kyphosis; it is often C-shaped and supple, at least during the initial stages. The apex may occur anywhere from the lower dorsal spine to the lumbosacral joint. The second type is a rigid S-shaped lumbar kyphosis with a proximal dorsal lordosis. The kyphosis is usually centered at L2 and the proximal rigid lordosis at about T10. This is the most common variety in the older child because the C-shaped curve often progresses to the S-shaped curve with time.

Collapsing Kyphosis. Conservative treatment, which consists of observation, is usually futile. The curve progresses rapidly, and it is not unusual to see a 2- or 3-year-old child with a kyphosis greater than 100 degrees. In those few instances in which the collapsing curve does not progress rapidly and is less than 20 to 30 degrees, an initial period of

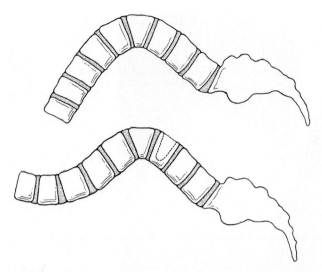

FIGURE 16-7. Two types of lumbar kyphosis: the C-shaped collapsing curve (**top**) and the S-shaped curve (**bottom**). (From ref. 59, with permission.)

observation may be worthwhile. If the curve is supple and the skin is in excellent condition, a brace can be tried. However, because any orthotic device must push over the apical vertebra posteriorly and against the protuberant abdomen anteriorly, it may lead to pressure sores over the gibbus and increased pressure on the abdominal contents. The kyphosis almost always requires surgical correction; this should not be delayed if brace treatment is unsatisfactory.

Collapsing scoliosis in the immature child is difficult to treat surgically. Posterior spinal fusion without instrumentation usually fails because of tension forces in the fusion mass. When instrumentation is used instrument failure is common. Attempts to provide stability by anterior strut fusion with a strut graft also tend to fail in young patients. The fusion creates an anterior unsegmented bar, with growth potential remaining posteriorly. As the child grows, the kyphosis increases. If the surgeon waits until the child is older to carry out anteroposterior fusion with instrumentation along the dorsal lumbar spine, the curve is often so severe that satisfactory correction is difficult if not impossible to obtain. If the anteroposterior fusion is carried out in infancy the resulting spine is too short to allow sufficient room for abdominal volume and respiratory sufficiency.

The anterior structures, including the abdominal wall, the aorta, and the vena cava, are of insufficient length to allow correction to occur without shortening the spine to remove tension from these structures (61,62). Many different procedures have been described to shorten the posterior spine to allow the spine to be straightened and put into more normal sagittal alignment (55–57,63–66). Most of these techniques require fusion of the spine to maintain correction, and therefore should be performed only in an

adolescent child; otherwise, the lumbar spine will be too short.

A method used to shorten the spine which does not require spinal fusion is to remove the ossific nuclei from the vertebrae above and below the apical vertebra, which is left intact (Fig. 16-8A,B). The pedicle and posterior arch are removed from these two vertebrae. The apical vertebra is pushed forward, correcting the kyphosis (60) (Fig. 16-8C). Approximately 100 degrees of kyphosis can be corrected. Because the vertebral body growth centers are left intact the growth of the spine continues, often producing a gradual increase in the lordosis. The spine is not fused so the procedure can be performed in children of any age, even in newborns. It is also possible to perform this surgery without mobilizing the spinal cord or dividing any of the nerve roots. Therefore, it can be performed when nerve function is intact below the level of the kyphosis. If the child is younger than 1 year old, tension-band wiring between the pedicles of the apical vertebra and the vertebrae above and below the osteotomy appears to be sufficient. If the child is older than 1 year Luque instrumentation, placed extraperiosteal and

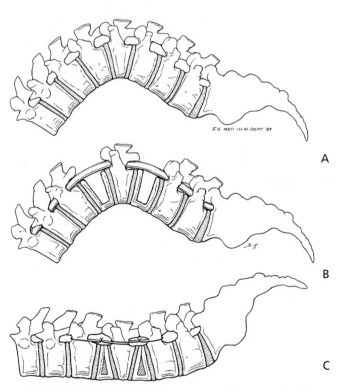

FIGURE 16-8. The C-shaped curve is corrected by removing the ossific nucleus of the vertebrae above and below the apical vertebrae. **A:** The C-shaped kyphosis before removal of the ossific nucleus from the vertebrae. **B:** Spinous processes, laminae, pedicles, and ossific nucleus have been removed from the vertebrae above and below the apical vertebra. The growth plate, disc, and anterior cortex are left intact. **C:** The deformity is reduced by pushing the apical vertebrae forward. Tension band wiring around the pedicles maintains the reduction. (From ref. 67, with permission.)

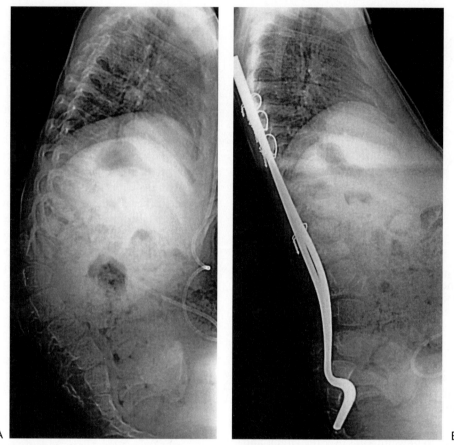

FIGURE 16-9. A 2-year-old child with 65 degrees of progressive kyphosis. **A:** After excision of the ossific nucleus above and below the apical vertebrae the correction is held with a specially modified Luque rod which is inserted into the first sacral foramen.

modified to attach to the sacrum without fusion, should be performed (68) [➥**2.7**]. At least three sublaminar wires on each rod superior to the kyphosis are needed to provide sufficient support (Fig. 16-9). If the child is an adolescent, posterior spinal fusion can be added to the instrumentation.

Skin coverage is often a problem. If the skin is exceedingly scarred or ulcerated over the kyphosis wound breakdown and infection are likely. The problem with skin coverage should be addressed prior to the spinal correction. A myocutaneous flap should be planned and prepared beforehand (69).

Rigid S-shaped Kyphosis. Treatment of the rigid form of upper lumbar kyphosis is difficult and controversial. Conservative nonoperative treatment invariably leads to an increased deformity and difficulty in later correction. In 1968, Sharrard (57) first described resection of the apical vertebral body for the treatment of kyphosis; since then, most authors have recommended vertebral excision as a part of the operative treatment (69). Most of these reports also showed that excision of the apical vertebra may lead to initial correction

of the deformity. However, the deformity has a tendency to recur, often to a worse degree than the initial kyphosis (56), leading to feelings of futility and frustration.

Treatment of the rigid form of kyphosis requires a different approach. Because both the kyphosis and the proximal lordosis are rigid it is necessary to correct both deformities at the same time. This can be accomplished by excising the vertebra(e) (usually two) between the kyphosis and lordosis (56,62,64) (Fig. 16-10) and fusing the apical vertebra to the distal end of the thoracic spine at the level of the resection. In a young child, this is the only area fused, and the osteotomy is held in position by tension-band wiring around the pedicle above and below the resected vertebrae (55,62) (Fig. 16-11). It is important that the paraspinous muscles be sutured behind the area of the spine in order to add a corrective force, decreasing the likelihood of recurrence of the deformity. The correction can also be held by use of rods anchored in the first sacral foramen distally and sublaminal wires proximally, similar to the fixation used in the collapsing kyphosis. If the child is Risser sign I or above, the spine may be fused along the length of the instrumentation.

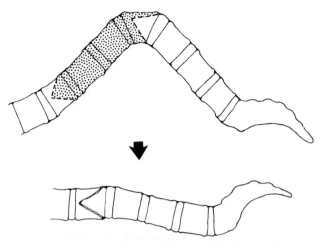

FIGURE 16-10. Bone is removed for correction of a rigid dorsal kyphosis (*shaded area*). The area removed usually includes one or two vertebrae proximal to the apical vertebrae in the area of the fixed lordosis. The vertebrae proximal to the resection and the apical vertebrae are shaped to receive each other in a tongue-and-groove joint to provide stability until bony union is achieved.

Hip

The function of the hip joint depends on neurologic level. The treatment program therefore is based on the level of sensory and motor paralysis (70–72). In a large proportion of myelomeningocele patients, the hips are reduced at birth, with the exception of those children who are breech position

(Fig. 16-12). Following birth, normal hips may become dislocated or dysplastic because of the position of the infant following closure of the back. If the infant is laid on his or her side, continued adduction of the superior hip eventually leads to dislocation. However, if the child can be placed in the prone position with the hips in the "human position" of flexion and 60 degrees of abduction, the hips can be maintained in the reduced position while the spine heals without being soiled by urine or feces (Fig. 16-13). This position also does not preclude placement of a shunt and the therapist can have access to the feet and knees. If abduction splinting is maintained during nap time and night-time after discharge from the hospital most children survive the first year of life with their hips reduced. Generally, the author does not maintain the splinting after the first 3 months of life; however, in other medical centers splints are maintained throughout the first year.

Thoracic Paraplegia

The thoracic-level paraplegic child does not have sensation or muscle control over the lower extremities. Surgery cannot provide stability; it must be provided by an orthosis. Without sensation and motor control reduction of the hip is not necessary for sitting and walking using orthotic aids (74). However, the child needs a functional range of motion without contracture (51). Surgical procedures should be used to provide range of motion so that the child can sit satisfactor-

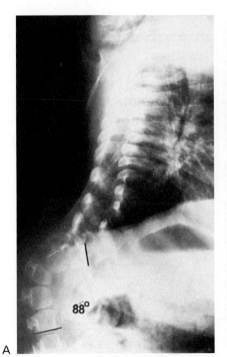
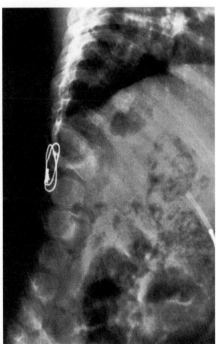
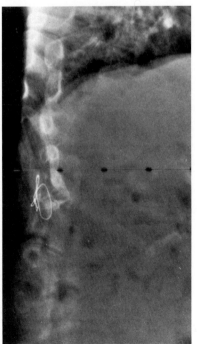

A

B,C

FIGURE 16-11. **A:** A 1-year, 10-month-old child with an 88-degree kyphosis. **B:** Two years after surgery, the kyphosis is at 13 degrees, and the lumbar spine has increased in height from 6.1 to 9 cm. **C:** Twelve years after surgery, the kyphosis is unchanged, and the spine height has increased to 14 cm.

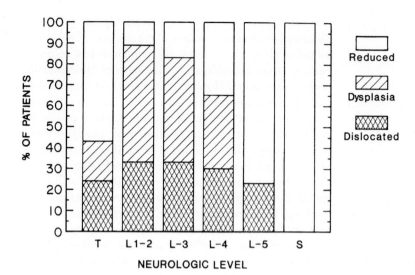

FIGURE 16-12. An evaluation of 100 consecutive infants with myelomeningocele who had not received treatment for their hips.

ily in a wheelchair, lie comfortably in bed, and use orthoses for standing and walking, if indicated.

Treating hip contractures in paraplegics is often frustrating because many contractures return promptly, often to a worse degree than before surgical release. A simple sectioning of tight tendons and release of tight ligamentous structures does not appear to be sufficient. The use of a free fat graft to fill the dead space formed by the release of tendon and capsule has helped prevent the recurrence of contracture

in a few of the author's patients. It is important that prolonged bracing and physical therapy be used to maintain whatever motion has been obtained by surgery.

Fortunately, dislocation of the hip is not usually found in the thoracic-level paraplegic person because of the lack of muscle function. If a hip is becoming dysplastic or is dislocating the cause should be found and treated. Increased muscle tone or spasticity should be treated by muscle release, or perhaps by neurectomy. Pelvic obliquity caused by devel-

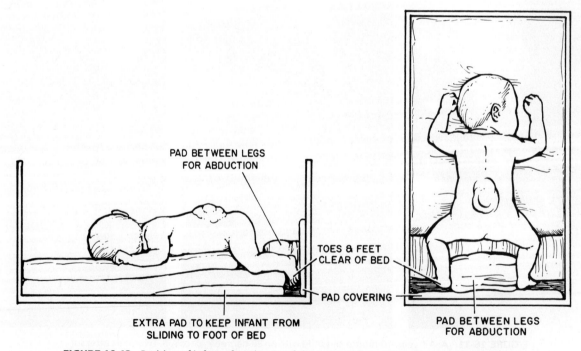

FIGURE 16-13. Position of infant after closure of the spine. This position allows gentle abduction of the hips in the neonatal period. (From ref. 73, with permission.)

oping scoliosis should be treated. Attempts to reduce a dislocated hip are difficult and often unsuccessful. The principal risk of surgically reducing the hip is stiffness. Multiple surgical procedures should be avoided because the risk of stiffness increases with each surgical procedure. It is better to have a supple dislocated hip than a stiff located hip.

The limitation of motion from a dislocated hip usually does not interfere with the overall function of the child. Even in unilateral dislocation, a dislocated hip does not prevent standing in an orthosis, sitting, or lying down, unless an associated adduction contracture is present.

The increased incidence of pressure sores, because of unilateral or bilateral hip dislocation in the absence of contractures or pelvic obliquity, has not been documented. Because of the loss of the greater trochanter as a pressure-accepting area, more pressure is placed on the ischium and sacrum. This would seem to increase the possibility of ulceration. In the presence of hip dislocation, special attention must be made to wheelchair seating.

The orthosis must provide pelvic, hip, knee, ankle, and foot stability. The standing frame, the parapodium, the swivel walker, and hip control orthosis all provide stability (75). At approximately 18 to 24 months of age, if the child has developed head control and sitting balance, a standing orthosis is prescribed. Orthotic devices are needed to provide stability to the lower extremity. The child usually finds these devices to be confining because they are too slow, they require too much energy, and they are too difficult to apply. Consequently, most of these children give up walking by the time they are 8 or 9 years of age, and use a wheelchair for their mobility (72).

Two designs in orthotic devices may change this prognosis for walking. The first is a *reciprocating orthosis* that allows controlled flexion and extension of the hip during walking (76). This decreases the energy requirement and increases walking speed (77). However, this orthosis allows for almost no contractures of the hips or knee, and orthotic breakage may be a frequent occurrence. The second development is a *hip guidance orthosis*, which allows for limited hip motion, while still providing stability (78). These braces may be tried after the age of 3 years and the child is large enough to fit into the smallest size of the orthosis. However, these devices are quite expensive and need to be replaced frequently.

Upper Lumbar Paraplegia

The upper lumbar paraplegic (L1–L2) has sensation in the anterior hip joint and thigh. Motor function includes the iliopsoas and the adductors producing hip flexion and adduction. Flexion adduction contracture of the hip, because of the unrestricted contraction of the hip flexors and adductors, is typical. There is a high incidence of hip dislocation. Attempts to reduce the hip without correcting the muscle imbalance are doomed to failure, and severe ankylosis of

the hips often results. Although providing hip stability for the child without the use of orthosis is possible, up to the present surgical attempts have been unsuccessful. Iliopsoas transfer is contraindicated in children with upper lumbar paraplegia, and often leads to severe extension contractures and increased disability (79,80).

The preferred treatment of children with upper lumbar paraplegia is obtaining range of motion by release of the contracture, including the iliopsoas and adductor tendons, then treating the child in a manner similar to that done for a thoracic-level paraplegic. If range of motion can be obtained, the dislocated hip does not cause disability for either walking or sitting (74,80). Because of the intact sensation across the hip joint, the reciprocating brace and the hip guidance orthosis are useful, and often succeed in continued walking as a mode of mobility into young adulthood (77,78).

Middle and Lower Lumbar Paraplegia

The middle to lower lumbar paraplegic (L3–L5) patient has sensation to below the knee. Muscle function includes hip flexion and adduction, knee extension, and weak knee flexion. Foot dorsiflexion and eversion also may be present. These patients have the potential for control of the hip and knee, and therefore the potential for independent walking.

Gait studies show almost normal sagittal plane motion of the hip, which is responsible for the movement of the child forward. There is an associated increase in hip rotation and abduction and adduction more than normal. This indicates that range of motion and control of the hip are probably the most important factors in walking for these children.

The hip in the middle to lower lumbar-level paraplegic is also a major source of deformity and disability. The natural history of the hip is to undergo progressive dysplasia and dislocation associated with hip-flexion contracture, which becomes evident when the child begins to walk. Muscle imbalance is caused by strong hip flexors, adductors, and absent or weak hip abductors and extensors. This muscle imbalance is exaggerated by the forces of walking when the hip flexors and adductors are used to stabilize the hip during the stance phase of walking, instead of during their typical function in the swing phase. The contraction of the hip flexors and adductors during the stance phase of gait causes the hip to flex and adduct, which produces a shear force across the acetabulum. It is not unusual for these paraplegic children to survive infancy with hips that are not dislocated, then to have them become dislocated at age 3 or 4 years. Attempts to reduce the hip and correct the progressive deformity are unsuccessful unless there is correction of the forces around the hip.

Historically, muscle balance has been obtained at the hip by performing muscle releases. However, taking the muscle control away from the hip does not increase its stability although the hip stays reduced, but increases its instability because of weakness, and requires the use of an orthosis to stabilize the hip for walking (74). This conclusion is not surprising, considering the severely weakened hip made unstable by surgical procedures.

Sharrard initiated another approach to hip instability by transferring the iliopsoas tendon to the greater trochanter, a modification of procedures suggested by Garceau and Mustard to treat instability of the hip following poliomyelitis (81,82,84). The purpose of the tendon transfer was to produce an abduction force across the hip joint during the stance phase of walking, and thereby eliminate the deforming hip flexion force of the iliopsoas. Long-term studies have shown that this transfer is successful in maintaining hip reduction and decreasing the hip-flexion contracture (79,81,83). However, the iliopsoas is transferred out of phase to normal walking, and may decrease the necessary sagittal plane motion necessary for walking, stepping up on a curb, or climbing stairs. The weakness of the hip flexion requires the child to use the rectus femoris and sartorius muscles to flex the hip. This in turn results in extension of the knee, which also makes stair climbing difficult. Because the iliopsoas normally is used as a hip flexor, it continues to contract during the flexion activity of the hip, and also may prevent the hip from flexing, leading to an extension contracture.

Bunch and Hakala (79) have shown that with careful selection of patients preservation of the nerve to the sartorius muscle and intensive physical therapy, stair climbing can be achieved. In many instances, in the lower lumbar-level paraplegic person without pelvic or hip deformity, without spasticity, and with good knee control, gait can be improved to the point that patients may be able to "cruise the mall" using their braces, crutches, or walker, rather than a wheelchair (85).

Transfer of the external oblique muscle from the abdomen to the greater trochanter; posterior transfer of the adductor longus, brevis, and gracilis to the ischium [➡3.18]; and transfer of the tensor fascia lata muscle posteriorly on the ilium and to the tendon of the gluteus maximus, have been used to control the hip (86–88). Studies have shown a maintenance of hip reduction and improvement in the acetabular index and the cente–edge angle after those muscle transfers, similar to the results obtained with Sharrard iliopsoas transfer (Fig. 16-14). In addition, after the three muscle transfers children with L3–L5 paraplegia have shown marked improvement in their walking ability, 70% of whom demonstrated a marked increase in endurance and walking speed. They also have required less bracing. Fifty percent of these children have developed enough stability around their hip to learn to walk independently

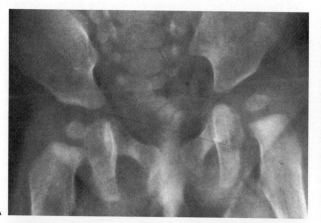

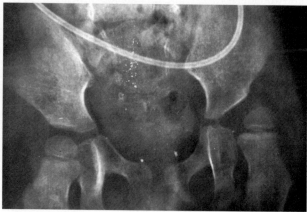

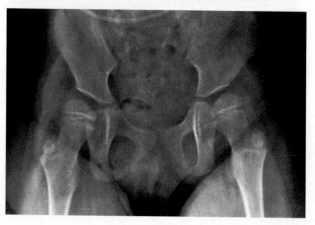

FIGURE 16-14. A: A 2-year-old child with L4 paraplegia begins to walk with ankle–foot orthoses and a walker. The hips are reduced. **B:** One year later, the left hip becomes dysplastic. **C:** Two years after bilateral transfer of the external oblique and adductor muscles the hips are reduced, and the child remains ambulatory.

without crutches or a walker (86). These muscle transfers are performed after the child has reached 2 years of age and learned to walk.

Although improvement in the hip indices can be produced by muscle transfers around the hip, they are not sufficiently forceful to correct major anatomic deformities. It is therefore necessary to reduce the hip and correct femoral and acetabular deformity at the time of, or prior to, the muscle transfer. Continued radiographic evaluation must be made following the reconstruction because recurrent dysplasia is possible.

If the hip is dislocated at birth the author prefers to wait until the child is 1 year of age before carrying out hip reduction to avoid interfering with motor development. If the child is between 1 and 6 years of age an open reduction and capsular plication are carried out to provide stability [➡3.2]. If there is deformity of the femoral neck, a varus femoral shortening osteotomy is indicated [➡4.1–4.3]. Pelvic osteotomy is indicated for severe acetabular dysplasia (89). The type of pelvic osteotomy performed depends on the deformity and the surgeon's preference [➡3.7–3.12]. An arthrogram and a CT scan may help to establish the area of acetabular insufficiency so that a correct procedure can be selected. The muscle transfers are then performed to help maintain reduction. The muscle transfers work better on a reduced hip than a dislocated one. Therefore, the author reduces the hips, even bilateral dislocations, before the age of 4 years. After that age the dysplasia is so great that the success rate is poor and the hips are left dislocated.

Sacral-level paraplegics have intrinsic stability to their hip with sensation and motor control. Dislocation of the hip in these children is rare; however, when it occurs it should be treated as a developmental dislocation of the hip.

Knee

The function of the knee is important to a child with myelomeningocele. Function of the knee is dependent on both the absence of deformity and the presence of stability. It must be stable during stance to accept the weight of the child without buckling, and flex sufficiently during swing to clear the foot. However, it is possible to walk with a stiff knee, and stability is more important than motion. The three deformities that may seriously diminish the ambulatory ability are extension or hyperextension contractures, flexion contractures, and valgus rotational deformities.

In a study of 16 patients with residual hyperextension contractures of the knee, only three were able to walk (72). These children also had difficulty sitting. Fortunately, the incidence of extension contractures is relatively low. There are several causes of extension contractures. One of the most common causes is seen in a child born with a breech presentation and with hyperflexed hips, hyperextended knees, and clubfoot. In these infants, the hamstring tendons usually have displaced anterior to the knee axis perpetuating the hyperextension deformity, although the child may be an L4

or L5 level paraplegic. The next most common cause appears in the middle lumbar level paraplegic person in which the child has quadriceps function, but no perceptible knee flexors. The least-common cause is seen in high-level paraplegic people in whom there is spasticity of the quadriceps muscle. Most of these cases can be treated by passive range of motion and splinting during the neonatal period of life. Although normal range of motion is rarely achieved, 60 to 70 degrees of flexion is common.

For those paraplegic children who do not respond to physical therapy, surgical treatment is indicated. If the child has voluntary function of the quadriceps, a modification of the V-Y plasty of the quadriceps tendons should be performed (Fig. 16-15). This procedure is modified by detaching the vastus medialis and the vastus lateralis from the medial and lateral hamstrings, which slide posterior to the knee axis. This approach often restores the hamstring function, and the child develops both active flexion and exten-

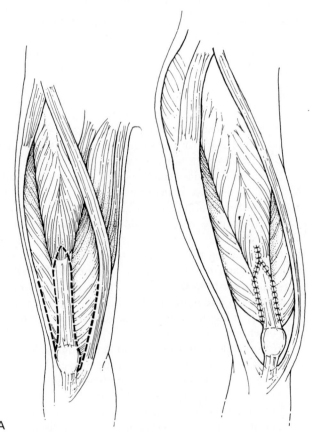

A | | B

FIGURE 16-15. The V-Y quadricepsplasty for hyperextension contracture of the knee. **A:** In addition to the detachment of the rectus femoris tendon from the muscle of the rectus femoris, the vastus medialis, and the vastus lateralis muscles, the vastus medialis and lateralis muscles are separated from the iliotibial band, the lateral hamstrings, the medial hamstrings, and the sartorius muscles. **B:** When the knee is flexed, the hamstring muscles and tensor fascia lata slip posterior to the knee axis, restoring their normal function. The quadriceps muscles are then repaired in the lengthened position. (From ref. 90, with permission.)

sion of the knee. If the quadriceps are not under voluntary control and are spastic, use sectioning of the patellar tendon and the retinaculum.

Flexion deformities are common in these children, even in the face of normal quadriceps function (91). A small degree of contracture, below 20 degrees, seems to be tolerated well, but contraction greater than 30 degrees decreases the likelihood that the child will continue to walk. Contractures over 20 degrees in the adult have a high incidence of patellofemoral pain (92).

The cause of the flexion contracture is not always apparent. In some children spasticity of the hamstrings or gastrocnemius can be implicated. In most middle and low lumbar paraplegic people, the cause appears to be a co-contraction of the hamstring and the quadriceps during the entire stance phase of gait. This lack of coordinated activity occurs only during walking and may not be present during manual testing of muscle activity during the neurologic examination. It appears to be related to brain stem abnormalities. The result of the tug of war between the knee flexors and extensors is persistent knee flexion during stance and decreased knee flexion during swing. A gait study, including EMGs, may be helpful in deciding the cause and treatment of the contracture. However, in most cases, the gait study is for research purposes and the treatment decision is made on clinical evaluation.

In the neonatal period and in infancy, physical therapy may be helpful in decreasing the flexion contracture. In those children who do not respond to physical therapy by 18 months to 2 years of age, surgical correction is indicated.

If the child with flexion contractures has some voluntary function of the medial hamstrings, the hamstrings should be lengthened rather than sectioned. The biceps femoris and the posterior part of the iliotibial band can be sectioned. The gastrocnemius origin should be resected. Almost all children with this deformity need to have a posterior capsulotomy extending from the posterior aspect of the medial collateral ligament to the posterior aspect of the lateral collateral ligament [➡4.23]. In most patients, the anterior cruciate ligament also needs to be partially, if not completely, resected to allow the tibia to slide forward on the femur into extension.

In most children functioning at the low lumbar level the hamstring muscles contract at the same time as the quadriceps muscle throughout the stance phase of walking (Fig. 16-3). For these children the author transfers the insertion of the biceps femoris and the semimembranosus muscles to the cut end of the gastrocnemius muscle on the distal femur. This transfer will assist in extension without flexing the knee. The transfer can be performed at any age because the attachment to the distal femoral epiphysis will allow for future growth. By removing two of the hamstring muscles from the knee flexion, the quadriceps usually will be able to maintain knee extension during stance.

Postoperatively, the patient must wear an above-the-knee orthosis for a prolonged period to prevent the development

of knee instability. In the child older than 6 or 7 years, sufficient deformity may have developed in the femoral condyles to preclude satisfactory soft tissue correction of the contracture, and a distal femoral osteotomy is needed. The osteotomy must be as close to the knee as possible to prevent an anteriorly offset knee joint. There is a tendency for recurrence of deformity with growth, and repeat surgery may be necessary.

Valgus and rotational deformities of the knee primarily are caused by tightness of the iliotibial band and the forces of ambulation. During the Trendelenburg gait pattern, the shift of weight lateral to the hip joint, along with contraction of the adductors and fixed position of the foot to the floor, produce a valgus thrust to the knee. The young child is best treated by muscle transfers to the hip to stabilize his or her gait pattern; by sectioning of the distal iliotibial band if it is contracted; and by placing the child in a knee-ankle-foot orthosis to resist the valgus thrust to the knee. If the deformity becomes fixed, a distal femoral osteotomy [➡4.17] is required to realign the knee.

Stability for the knee in thoracic and upper lumbar paraplegics is provided by an orthosis. Sufficient sensation and motor control of the knee is not present unless the child has functioning of the L4–L5 nerve roots. Without a good quadriceps, some medial hamstring function, and sensation to the tibial tubercle, the child cannot control the knee adequately. Attempts to stabilize the thoracic upper and middle lumbar-level paraplegic patients with a below-the-knee orthosis by means of equinus positioning or with other types of foot positioning should be avoided. Because the child is unable to raise his or her center of gravity to vault over a plantar flexed foot the knee must hyperextend or externally rotate, producing degenerative changes because of a lack of protective sensation (Fig. 16-16).

Foot

The function of the foot of a child paralyzed by myelomeningocele is significantly impaired (120). The severe deformity of the leg and foot, limited ankle and subtalar motion, absent weak or spastic muscles, and the lack of sensation make it almost impossible for the foot to function normally by providing shock absorption, control of floor reaction forces, and the transfer of weight that is necessary for gait (93). Almost all of the myelomeningocele children require treatment of their feet. Even nonambulatory children require adequate positioning of the foot to accept shoe wear, placement on wheelchair foot rests, and prevent pressure sores. Ambulatory children require an accurate correction of deformity. They are unable to compensate for malposition of the foot because of weakness of the trunk, the hip, and the knee, which causes the weightbearing line and the floor reaction force to fall outside the zone of stability of the hip, the knee, and the ankle. For example, a foot that has residual inward rotation produces a varus deformity at

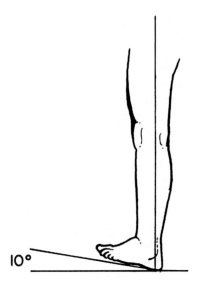

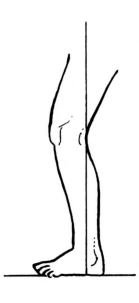

FIGURE 16-16. A 10-degree dorsiflexion of the foot is needed for the leg to progress beyond midstance. If the foot is held in neutral or plantar flexion the tibia cannot progress beyond the vertical without raising of the body—a difficult activity for a paraplegic. Dorsiflexion can be provided by manufacturing the orthosis in dorsiflexion or by elevating the heel of the shoe.

the knee and inward rotation of the leg during the stance phase of gait. Outward rotation of the foot causes a valgus deformity to the knee and an exaggerated outward rotation of the leg during stance. Residual equinus deformity causes hyperextension of the knee and the inability of the child to move the center of gravity beyond midstance. On the other hand, calcaneus deformity allows the tibia to fall forward during midstance, producing knee flexion and a crouched gait. The foot must also be able to compensate for deformity of the knee. For example, a knee-flexion contracture requires the ability of the ankle to dorsiflex so that the heel will contact the floor.

The correction of the deformity by itself is not sufficient. Muscle balance must be achieved in the foot as well. If this muscle imbalance is left uncorrected when the alignment of the foot is obtained the deformity will recur. There are only two choices available to correct the muscle imbalance: removing the muscle force by excising the tendon or transferring the force to another location by tendon transfer. The preservation or removal of muscle activity must be considered carefully in relation to the function of the foot during walking. If the child needs an orthosis to walk then muscle control of the foot is of little importance, and the deforming forces should be eliminated; however, if the child has enough muscular control and sensation to walk without an orthosis, the muscle balance must be obtained by performing the appropriate tendon transfer.

The goals of treatment are to align the foot to allow transfer of the floor reaction force through the center of the ankle and to produce stability of the knee and hip during the stance phase of gait. The motion of the joints in the foot should be preserved which allows preservation of the shock-absorptive capacity of the foot and lessens the possibility of joint degenerations. A rigid foot also has a high incidence of ulceration even if the deformity has been corrected

by subtalar arthrodesis or triple arthrodesis (94). It is also important to avoid bony prominences in the weightbearing area to lessen the likelihood of pressure sores (25).

Talipes Equinovarus Deformity

Talipes equinovarus, or clubfoot, is the most common deformity in these children and occurs in well over 50% (10). It is present in all levels of paraplegia, but the treatment differs at each level as a result of the muscle function that may be present. The correction of the equinovarus deformity in myelomeningocele patients is rarely accomplished by nonoperative means. An attempt to manipulate the foot and cast the deformity during the newborn period is worth a try if the foot is reasonably supple, and can be manipulated into a satisfactory position prior to the casting (1). However, most of these feet are rigid and the success rate with manipulation and casting has been poor. The cast cannot be used to obtain correction because pressure sores will develop. Occasionally after cast treatment the foot appears to be in satisfactory position; however, evaluation of the foot–thigh axis shows that the foot is still internally rotated approximately 45 degrees. This is the result of the severe deformity of the neck of the talus. As the foot is manipulated into the proper relation to the axis of the leg the calcaneus is moved laterally from underneath the talus, depriving it of its support and allowing the talar head to drop plantarward, producing a foot that resembles a congenital vertical talus. If this occurs then further attempts at nonoperative treatment should be abandoned. If satisfactory correction has been achieved then the child must be placed in splints to prevent recurrence of deformity. The splints must be worn continuously until the age of standing. If the foot has not achieved satisfactory correction by the time the infant is 3 months of age the author abandons conservative treatment and recommends surgical correction when the child is 1 year old. This interim period between nonoperative and surgical treatment allows for normal development of the child without the problem of constant cast change and braces. The advantage of performing surgery at the time the child is ready to stand is that weightbearing can be used to maintain the correction along with the orthosis used for ambulation.

The surgical correction of the clubfoot [➡7.1] rarely is accomplished by limited surgery. A radical complete circumferential subtalar release is necessary in order to allow the calcaneus to rotate sufficiently underneath the talus to align the axis of the foot to the axis of the ankle and knee (95). Because of the deformity of the neck of the talus it is then necessary to displace the calcaneus medially beneath the talus so that the posterior facet and the anterior facets are reduced, in order to prevent the talar head from sagging or falling into a vertical position. It is important to repair the tibial calcaneal ligaments with nonabsorbable suture to prevent lateral migration of the calcaneus into valgus. A plantar release and capsulotomy of the calcaneal cuboid joint is usually necessary as well.

Unless the child has a sacral level of paralysis all of the contracted tendons should be resected rather than lengthened because they are spastic and nonfunctional. A simple cutting of the tendons often results in the tendon being caught in the scar, then acting as a tether as the foot grows. This causes recurrence of the deformity. In the L5-level paraplegic person, the anterior tibialis and peroneal tendons also should be released. Leaving them intact often results in a calcaneal valgus deformity. It is better to have a flaccid braceable foot than a deformed foot with muscle activity that is inappropriate for standing. This aggressive treatment gives a satisfactory result in the majority of patients (96).

A major problem during surgical correction of the deformity is skin coverage for the posteromedial aspect of the foot. Many incisions have been tried, but no one incision is free of complications. For the relatively mild deformity, a Cincinnati incision gives adequate results (97). It provides excellent exposure to the medial and lateral side of the subtalar joint. The drawback to this incision is exposure of the heel cord; however, in most of these children, the tendon is sectioned rather than lengthened, and lack of exposure is not critical. The medial and lateral calcaneal vessels must be carefully preserved to provide circulation to the heel. Other incisions, such as the Turco or the two incisions described by Carroll, are equally effective (91,98,99).

With severe deformity, the Cincinnati incision does not appear to be sufficient. The axis of the foot often must rotate almost 90 degrees in relation to its ankle at the time of surgery. The skin on the medial aspect of the foot is insufficient to allow this degree of correction. If the skin is closed with excessive tension it will slough and heal by scar. This scar then contracts as the foot grows and causes recurrent deformity. On the other hand, if the deformity

is not completely corrected in order to allow skin closure, then a satisfactory position of the foot is not obtained. The author now uses a modified posterior medial incision (Fig 16-17). It starts posterolaterally, approximately 5 cm above the ankle at the posterior edge of the fibula. It curves obliquely downward to 1 cm below the medial malleolus. It then curves distally along the medial border of the foot to the first cuneiform, where it curves dorsally over the dorsum of the foot to a point just in front of the lateral malleolus. The incision over the dorsal aspect of the foot is only through the skin, preserving the dorsal veins and nerves of the foot. After the foot has been positioned and pinned in the corrected position an assessment is made about the integrity of the medial skin. If the skin is excessively tight, the incision is extended across the dorsum of the foot. The proximal flap is freed by blunt dissection from the fascia for a distance of 2 cm. There is no subcutaneous dissection of the distal skin. The skin is then allowed to find its normal position without tension. This permits the skin of the proximal flap to keep its normal relation with the leg while the foot rotates underneath it. The incision is then closed with interrupted subcutaneous sutures and a running dermal stitch. This incision relieves the tension on the medial side of the incision and decreases the redundant skin on the lateral aspect of the foot.

Another approach to obtain skin coverage is to insert a subcutaneous balloon (i.e., tissue expander), well before the planned correction of the foot (100). The balloon is gradually expanded by the injection of saline, stretching the skin and subcutaneous tissue. At the time of correction of the foot deformity the balloon is removed and the redundant skin is used to close the incision without tension.

It is rarely possible to correct the metatarsus adductus at the same time as the correction of the hindfoot. The author prefers to do this as a separate procedure when the child is 3 or 4 years of age. Although not always necessary, it needs to be done more often than in idiopathic clubfoot. Soft tissue release is rarely effective in achieving a permanent correction of the metatarsus adductus. A closing-wedge osteotomy of the cuboid and an opening osteotomy of the first cuneiform, with transfer of the wedge of bone from the cuboid to the first cuneiform, is preferred (101,102). The metatarsals II and III are then osteotomized at their base [➡7.6]. The correction is held with multiple pins that are removed in 1 month. The child is held in a walking cast for 1 additional month then placed in suitable orthoses, as needed, for ambulation.

Recurrent equinovarus deformity may be treated by talectomy; however, the deformity has a tendency to recur, and its short distance from the medial malleolus in the plantar aspect of the foot makes it difficult to fit with an orthotic device (95). Another problem with brace wear is that the pressure in the plantar surface of the foot is not distributed evenly, although the foot appears plantigrade. These areas of high pressure may predispose these patients to ulcerations

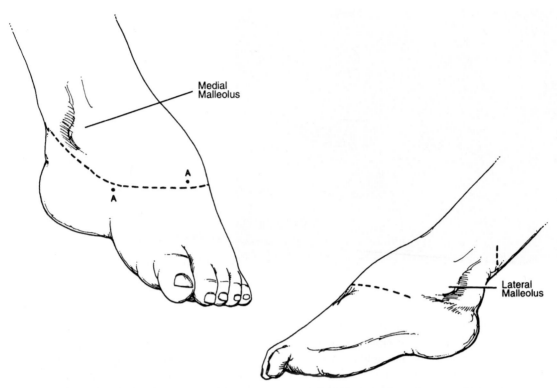

FIGURE 16-17. The incision begins posterolaterally, approximately 5 cm above the ankle at the posterior edge of the fibula. It extends obliquely downward to 1 cm below the medial malleolus. It then curves distally along the medial border of the foot to a point 1 cm distal to the anterior border of the medial malleolus. After the correction of the foot deformity the incision is extended to the first cuneiform, where it curves dorsally over the dorsum of the foot to a point at the anterior edge of the lateral malleolus. The incision over the dorsum of the foot is only through the skin, preserving the dorsal veins and nerves of the foot. The proximal flap is freed by blunt dissection from the fascia for a distance of 2 cm. There is no dissection of the distal skin. The skin is then allowed to find its position relative to the tibia and foot without tension. Usually the two points marked "A" will come together.

(103–105). Persistent wear of an orthosis is essential despite the difficult fit. In the older child severe residual deformity may be corrected by a triple arthrodesis (106). This procedure should be limited to only the extreme cases because of the danger of joint degeneration and skin ulceration caused by the stiffness of the foot. Less severe deformities may be managed by a tarsal metatarsal osteotomy to correct the midfoot deformity and a calcaneal osteotomy to correct the varus deformity of the heel (99).

Calcaneus Deformity

Calcaneal deformities of the foot in the newborn are primarily due to the unopposed contraction of the anterior tibial muscle, the toe extensor muscles, or the peroneal muscles (107). There is flaccid paralysis of the triceps surae. The deformity may be calcaneal valgus, calcaneus, or calcaneal varus, depending on the predominant muscle activity. The deformity is usually progressive, and the calcaneus eventually becomes positioned vertically underneath the talus (Fig.

16-18). The deformity prevents the forefoot from contacting the floor, interfering with balance, preventing the floor reaction force from stabilizing the knee, and causing the child to walk in a flexed-knee or crouched gait. Because of the lack of sensation this deformity leads to heel ulcerations in the teenage years.

Nonoperative treatment is rarely successful. Manipulations of the foot in the newborn period, and bracing as the child becomes older, may provide satisfactory position. However, in most cases the muscles continue to shorten, making brace and shoe wear difficult. In the child younger than 5 years of age with a minor deformity, which includes vertical alignment of the calcaneus, the anterior tibial tendon should be transferred through the interosseous membrane and attached to the calcaneus or released if the deformity is not severe. The decision to transfer or release is made by the strength of the toe extensors. If they are strong, transfer the anterior tibial tendon. At the time of surgery the deformity can be fully corrected; often the anterior tibial tendon is sectioned; then the tendon is not transferred. The

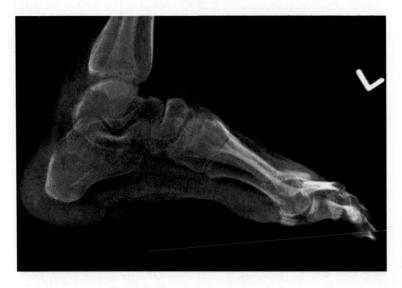

FIGURE 16-18. Lateral radiograph of an L5 paraplegic patient shows the vertical position of the os calcis. Note the hypertrophy of the heel pad.

remaining tight anterior structures should be released so that the foot can be brought into satisfactory position for bracing (108,109). The purpose of the anterior tendon transfer is to relieve a deforming force and to counteract the function of the toe extensors. The transfer is insufficient in power to substitute for the gastrocnemius soleus muscles. Although these patients may learn to walk without an orthosis following the tendon transfer, gait studies have shown they walk better with, than without, the orthosis (110).

In children older than 5 years of age soft tissue procedures rarely are sufficient. These patients also require osteotomy of the calcaneus with posterior displacement of the posterior fragment (111).

If the child has already developed ulceration underneath the calcaneus the treatment must provide correction of the foot deformity, followed by removal of the prominent part of the calcaneus, excision of the ulcer, and primary closure by means of a local flap. To allow the ulcer to heal by secondary intention will not provide reconstitution of the normal weightbearing fat pad. Repeat ulcerations are common. The weightbearing skin and fat pad must be restored in order to prevent recurrence of the ulceration. Posthealing orthotic wear is essential.

Valgus Deformity in the Newborn

Valgus deformities usually are associated with contracture of the lateral musculature of the foot, equinus deformity of the calcaneus, and a lateral displacement of the calcaneus from beneath the talus (112,113). The external appearance of the foot resembles that of a congenital vertical talus, but usually it is less rigid. Nonoperative treatment is rarely successful, despite the observation that the foot often can be manipulated back into a satisfactory position by plantar flexing the foot and rotating the calcaneus beneath the talus.

The lack of active function of the posterior tibial muscle and the spastic activity of the peroneal muscles cause frequent recurrence. Occasionally a rigid form of congenital vertical talus may be found in myelodysplasia (103).

If the foot cannot be manipulated passively into the correct deformity and held with an orthosis, then an aggressive surgical approach is needed at about 1 year of age. The author prefers an extensive subtalar release to allow reduction of the calcaneus beneath the talus. This may require resection of the Achilles tendon and the peroneal tendons. The posterior ankle capsule is divided along with the fibular calcaneal ligaments. The anterior tibial tendon can be resected or transferred back to the neck of the talus. The author prefers to resect the tendon and do the subtalar arthrodesis. The function of the anterior tibial muscle is difficult to determine and it may not perform as expected. In most cases an extraarticular subtalar arthrodesis is needed (31,114,115).

Valgus Deformity in the Older Child

Valgus deformity is common in the ambulatory child and frequently is associated with outward rotation deformity of the foot and the ankle (112,116). The cause of the deformity is undetermined, but is probably related to the floor reaction force during stance without the appropriate muscle control of the posterior tibial muscle. There usually is a lateral tilt to the ankle mortis with shortening of the fibula. The subtalar joint may be deformed as well. The location of the deformity can be determined by standing anteroposterior radiographs of the ankle mortis and foot. The outward rotation of the ankle axis in relation to the knee should be assessed. It may exceed 60 degrees. Pressure sores caused by shoes and orthotic devices are common.

Nonoperative care, including casts, manipulation, and orthoses, will not correct or prevent the deformity. Most children will require surgical correction. The deformity in the tibia and fibula can be corrected by supramalleolar osteotomy that corrects both the valgus and rotation [➡6.8]. If there is minimal outward rotation of the ankle the valgus deformity of the ankle mortis can be treated by a medial tibial epiphysiodesis (117). If the child is young then staples can be used, so they can be removed later after the correction has been obtained. If the valgus deformity is mild and associated with a calcaneus deformity and a minimal outward tibial rotation, a calcaneal fibular tendo Achilles tenodesis can prevent progression of the deformity in about 70% of the patients (117,118). However, stretching of the tenodesis is a major problem, and Shafer and Dias recommend the addition of an anterior tibial tendon transfer to the calcaneus (25). If there is subtalar valgus the foot should be treated like the valgus deformity in the newborn.

Cavus Deformity

Cavus deformity of the foot usually is accompanied with claw toe deformity, and is seen in the sacral-level paraplegic child. These children have normal strength of the anterior tibial and toe extensor muscles, which pull up the midfoot at the base of the first metatarsal and dorsiflex or hyperextend the metatarsal phalangeal joints. The normal functioning peroneus longus plantar flexes the first metatarsal. The paralysis of the gastrocnemius soleus muscles leave the hindfoot in calcaneus position. Active toe flexors flex the interphalangeal joints, and with paralysis the foot intrinsic muscles cannot flex the metacarpal phalangeal joints or extend the interphalangeal joints. These children have enough sensation and muscle control to walk without an orthosis, but frequently develop progressive deformity and ulcerations under their toes, their metatarsal heads, and their heels. Their gait is also abnormal, because of the lack of sufficient power in the gastrocnemius soleus muscles. The cavus deformity is often progressive and may be associated with secondary varus deformity of the foot as the child attempts to use flexor hallucis and digitorum longus muscles to compensate for paralysis of the gastrocnemius soleus muscles.

Conservative treatment by means of an ankle–foot orthosis often provides a temporary solution; however, once the child can walk without the brace, it is difficult to get him or her to wear it again. Therefore, most of these children come to surgical correction.

Surgical treatment must include correction of the bone deformity and soft tissue contracture and restoration of the muscle imbalance. In the young child with mild deformation a plantar fascia release, followed by an ankle–foot orthosis, may provide satisfactory correction of the deformity. Rigid cavus, due to midfoot deformity, can be corrected by a tarsal metatarsal osteotomy associated with plantar release [➡7.7, 7.8]. If the deformity is due to a dorsiflexion deformity of the calcaneus, a calcaneal osteotomy is necessary (119). The calcaneus is moved backward or laterally, as needed, to correct the cavus or cavovarus deformities. Muscle-balancing procedures must consider the phase of the muscle during gait, the power of the muscle available, and the required muscle power necessary for walking (120,121). The primary goal is to have a plantigrade braceable foot without recurrent deformity or pressure sores. If the residual muscle power in the foot is in the poor-to-fair range, then the foot cannot be made functional by muscle transfers, and it is best to lengthen or resect the tendon of the deforming muscle and brace the foot. However, if there is sensation on the sole of the foot and the strength of the toe flexor is good-to-normal, it may be possible to transfer the muscles to the heel to achieve force balance and a satisfactory brace-free gait.

The anterior tibial muscle is a swing-phase muscle, and cannot be made into a stance-phase muscle to substitute for the gastrocnemius soleus muscle unless electromyelogram gait studies show the contrary. In most circumstances it is better to lengthen the tendon and preserve its necessary function of foot clearance during swing. If the foot is in varus, then transfer of its anterior tibial tendon to the midfoot may be useful. Muscle imbalance of the toes can be helped by transfer of the long extensor tendons to the metatarsal heads, with fusion of the interphalangeal joints. This transfer helps elevate the metatarsal heads and prevent recurrent cavus. When the foot is in cavovalgus deformity, the peroneus brevis also can be transferred to the calcaneus.

Charcot Arthropathy

Charcot, or neurotrophic, arthropathy is a progressive degeneration of a joint caused by a lack of protective sensation. This is a problem that primarily affects ambulatory young adult patients who have decreased sensation of the knee, the ankle, and the foot. Because of the pathologic anatomy of the myelomeningocele, the sensory level is usually higher than the motor level. Consequently, these patients often are able to stand and walk, but do not have protective sensation. The patient with paralysis at the L4–L5 level appears to be the most vulnerable (Fig. 16-19). The pathologic process begins following an initial traumatic episode. The initial episode may follow a minor fall that the patient does not consider to be a major injury-producing event. Following this initial traumatic episode, there usually is a considerable amount of swelling and redness around the joint. The appearance of the joint resembles an infection and cellulitis. There may be some minor discomfort but usually no severe pain. Because of the lack of pain the patient often does not seek medical advice and continues to walk on the joint, causing further microfractures to occur. Even if the patient obtains medical consultation the initial radiographs often are unremarkable and the patient is often given antibiotics for the mistaken diagnosis of infection. Once the joint degeneration has become evident on radiograph the joint has been destroyed, and satisfactory outcome is difficult to achieve.

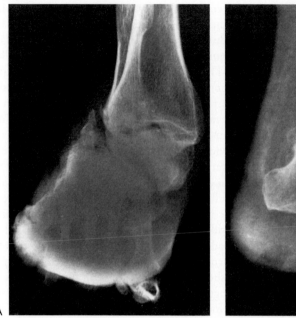
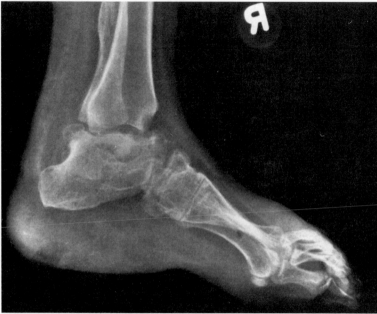

FIGURE 16-19. This Charcot degeneration occurred in a 16-year-old, L5 paraplegic girl who refused to wear her ankle–foot orthosis.

Treatment of the Charcot arthropathy must be instituted early and based on suspicion rather than waiting for radiographic confirmation. The best treatment is a vigorous protection of the joint following the initial episode before additional injury occurs. This may be accomplished by a splint or a cast and by nonweightbearing. If the early treatment has been successful radiographic changes may never be identified. Typically the swelling and erythema subside after 1 or 2 weeks. If they recur after the beginning of weight bearing, then the protection must be resumed for a longer time. The healing usually takes 6 to 8 weeks. However, if the diagnosis and treatment are delayed until the radiograph becomes positive for joint deformity or degeneration, prolonged immobilization and protection must be provided until the process has run its course. This may take 6 to 8 months or longer. The joint protection should be maintained until there is radiographic evidence of healing of the avascular segment of the joint and all swelling and erythema has disappeared. Continued orthotic protection of the foot and ankle or knee is essential.

Orthotic Devices

The goal of treatment of the myelomeningocele foot is a braceable plantigrade foot. Only the sacral-level paraplegic has sufficient sensation and muscle control to gain stability of the foot and ankle without orthotic support. The orthosis must provide stability to the foot and ankle, and ideally should be lightweight and cosmetically acceptable. It should limit all unwanted motion of the foot and ankle, and trans-

mit the floor reaction force to the anterior shin where the child has sensation. The ideal orthosis has not been developed. The closest we can come is a brace made of polypropylene that controls and limits the ankle motion (122). If the ankle is in valgus, or if there is instability of the subtalar joint, the brace can be modified with a supramalleolar strap which uses the principle of the T-strap of the double upright style of orthosis (123). This helps release the pressure on the medial malleolus and the head of the talus.

The author prefers the floor reaction force ankle–foot orthosis that is closed anteriorly over the tibial tubercle so that the floor reaction force can be transmitted directly to the area of intact sensation (Fig. 16-20). It also gives a firm support to the tibia to help extend the knee during midstance (124). Because the orthosis is in part a cylinder, it is much more resistant to rotation and valgus deformation during walking than the more common posterior polypropylene ankle–foot orthosis. Because the ankle is rigid the heel of the shoe must act as the shock absorber at heel strike, and should be of a relatively soft, shock-absorbing material. The foot also must be allowed to simulate 10 degrees of dorsiflexion in order to get the tibia beyond midstance to take the next step (125) (Fig. 16-16). This can be adjusted by the height of the heel or the position of the foot when the mold is made for the brace. The drawback to the floor reaction orthosis is that it is difficult to make and requires a skilled orthotist. There is little margin of error permitted, or maximum gait cannot be achieved.

The downside to an ankle–foot orthosis is that the ankle–foot joint complex cannot absorb the transverse plane

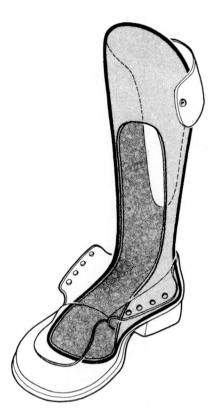

FIGURE 16-20. An ankle–foot orthosis made of a polypropylene shell with a Plastizote lining. The orthosis is closed anteriorly over the tibial tubercle so that the floor reaction force can be transmitted directly to the area of intact sensation. (From ref. 117, with permission.)

forces of gait. The forces are consequently transferred to the knee which is not designed to accept them. A recent study showed that in the S1–2-level paraplegic the brace may be more detrimental to the knee than a benefit to the gait pattern (96).

Shoe inserts and modifications are rarely successful in providing correction of alignment and position deformities of the foot. Most of these children do not have the muscle control or the sensation to take advantage of these devices. They may be helpful in protecting the foot of an S1 level paraplegic.

Fractures of the Femur and Tibia

Fractures of the femur and tibia occur commonly in children with myelomeningocele (66,125). The trauma needed to produce the fracture is often minimal, particularly after cast immobilization. The fractures are usually epiphyseal or metaphyseal (126–129). The peak incidence of fracture appears to be between the ages of 3 and 7 years, but fracture may occur at any age. Fracture is related to the level of paralysis and postoperative immobilization. Metabolic abnormalities have been investigated and found not to be present (130).

Diagnosis of fracture often is missed because of the minimal trauma. If the fracture is not diaphyseal, no instability of the leg may be present, which aids in the diagnosis. The local and systemic response to the fracture also is exaggerated, and consists of swelling of the leg, local warmth, erythema, and fever (131). These signs and symptoms often are misdiagnosed as cellulitis or osteomyelitis. Any unexplained fever in these children in association with a swollen warm leg that appears to be cellulitis should be treated as a fracture until radiographs prove otherwise.

Fracture following postoperative cast immobilization is common, and several studies have reported an incidence of 18 to 45%. Prevention of fractures in the postoperative period include starting the child on weightbearing as soon as possible, and keeping the plaster immobilization time to a minimum. After the cast has been removed extreme caution must be exercised for at least 1 week. Once a fracture has occurred it is best to carry out minimal immobilization and begin weightbearing as soon as possible. If these children are treated with the usual routine of plaster cast and inactivity the osteopenia increases, and repeated fractures are more likely to occur.

In most instances the author prefers a soft cast made of cast padding about 1 inch thick, followed by an elastic bandage and, if necessary, a single lightweight plaster splint. The swelling decreases rapidly, and the soft cast has to be reapplied within 2 or 3 days. The family rewraps the elastic bandage daily. Usually, there is sufficient callus to begin weightbearing in 2 or 3 weeks after casting. If a plaster cast is used weightbearing should be started as soon as possible. If the fracture is close to the hip internal fixation may be necessary to obtain early mobility.

References

Classification and Pathology

1. Walker G. The early management of varus feet in myelomeningocele. *J Bone Joint Surg Br* 1971;53:462.
2. Gardner WJ. Anatomic features common to the Arnold-Chiari and the Dandy-Walker malformations suggest a common origin. *Cleve Clin Q* 1959;26:206.
3. Gardner WJ. Myelocele—rupture of the neural tube? *Clin Neurosurg* 1968;15:57.
4. Gardner WJ. Embryologic origin of spinal malformations. *Acta Radiol (Stockh)* 1966;5:1012.
5. Gardner WJ. Diastematomyelia and the Klippel-Feil syndrome. *Cleve Clin Q* 1964;31:19.
6. Gardner WJ. Myelomeningocele—the result of rupture of the embryonic neural tube. *Cleve Clin Q* 1960;27:88.
7. Morgagni JB. *The seats and causes of diseases investigated by anatomy.* vol. 3. London: A Millar & T Cadell, 1797.
8. Shurtleff DB, Lutly DA, Benedetti TJ, et al. The outcome of pregnancies diagnosed as having a fetus with myelomeningocele. *Kinderchir* 1987;42(suppl):50.

Neurologic Abnormality

9. McDonald CM, Jaffe KM, Shurtleff DB, et al. Modifications to the traditional description of neurosegmental innervation in myelomeningocele. *Dev Med Child Neurol* 1991;33:473.

10. Sharrard WJ, Grosfield I. The management of deformity and paralysis of the foot in myelomeningocele. *J Bone Joint Surg Br* 1968;50:456.

11. Wolfe PH. Development and motivational concepts in Piaget's sensory-motor theory of intelligence. *J Am Acad Child Adolesc Psychiatry* 1963;2:225.

Genetics, Etiology, and Prenatal Diagnosis

12. Stein SC, Feldman JG, Friedlander M, et al. Is myelomeningocele a disappearing disease? *Pediatrics* 1982;69:511.

13. Carter CO. Spina bifida and anencephaly—a problem in genetic-environmental interaction. *J Biosoc Sci* 1969;1:71.

14. Toriello HV, Higgins JV. Occurrence of neural tube defects among first, second, and third degree relatives of proband—results of a USA study. *Am J Med Genet* 1987;15:601.

15. Carter CO, Roberts JA. The risk of recurrence after two children with central nervous system malformations. *Lancet* 1967;1:306.

16. Lawrence KM. Clinical and ethical considerations on alpha-fetoprotein estimated for early prenatal diagnosis of neural tube malformations. *Dev Med Child Neurol* 1974;16(suppl 32):117.

17. Centers for Disease Control and Prevention. Recommendations for the use of folic acid to reduce the number of cases of spina bifida and other neural tube defects. *MMWR Morb Mortal Wkly Rep* 1992;RR-14:41.

18. Seller MJ, Nevin NC. Periconceptional vitamin supplementation and the prevention of neural tube defects in southeast England and North Ireland. *J Med Genet* 1984;21:325.

19. Alan LD, Donald I, Gibson AA, et al. Amniotic fluid alpha-fetoprotein in the antenatal diagnosis of spina bifida. *Lancet* 1973;2:522.

20. Lawrence KM. The recurrence risk in spina bifida cystica and anencephaly. *Dev Med Child Neurol* 1969;11(suppl 20):23.

21. Hide DW, Williams HP, Ellis HL. The outlook for the child with a myelomeningocele for whom early surgery was considered inadvisable. *Dev Med Child Neurol* 1972;14:304.

Natural History

22. Lorber J. Selective treatment of myelomeningocele—to treat or not to treat? *Pediatrics* 1974;53:307.

23. Bunch WH, Scarff TB, Dvonch VM. Progressive loss in myelomeningocele patients. *Orthop Trans* 1983;7:185.

24. Hall PV, Campbell RH, Kalsbeck JE. Myelomeningocele and progressive hydromyelia—progressive paresis in myelodysplasia. *J Neurosurg* 1975;43:457.

25. Schafer MF, Dias LS. *Myelomeningocele—orthopaedic treatment.* Baltimore: Williams & Wilkins, 1983:168.

26. Hall PV, Lindseth RE, Campbell RH, et al. Scoliosis and hydrocephalus in myelocele patients. The effect of ventricular shunting. *J Neurosurg* 1979;50:174.

27. Hall PV, Lindseth RE, Campbell RL, et al. Myelodysplasia and developmental scoliosis. *Spine* 1976;1:48.

28. Heinz ER, Rosenbaum AE, Scarff TB, et al. Tethered spinal cord following myelomeningocele repair. *Radiology* 1979;131:153.

29. Scarff TB, Toleikis JR, Bunch WH, et al. Dermatosomal somatosensory evoked potentials in children with myelomeningocele. *Z Kinderchir Grenzgeb* 1979;28:384.

30. Tosi LL, Slater JE, Shaer C, et al. Latex allergy in spina bifida patients—prevalence and surgical implications. *J Pediatr Orthop* 1993;13:709.

31. Aronson DD, Middleton DL. Extra-articular subtalar arthrodesis with cancellous bone graft and internal fixation for children with myelomeningocele. *Dev Med Child Neurol* 1991;33:232.

Effect of Myelomeningocele on Developmental Sequence

32. Hoppenfeld S. Congenital kyphosis in myelomeningocele. *J Bone Joint Surg Br* 1967;49:276.

33. Hammar SL. The approach to the adolescent patient. *Pediatr Clin North Am* 1973;20:799.

34. Johnson WR. Sex education of the mentally retarded. In: Curz F, Levic GD, eds. *Human sexuality and the mentally retarded.* New York: Brunner Mazel, 1973:57.

Treatment

35. Hull WJ, Moe JN, Winter RB. Spinal deformity in myelomeningocele—natural history, evaluation, treatment. *J Bone Joint Surg Am* 1974;56:1767.

36. Bunch WH. Treatment of the myelomeningocele spine. *Instr Course Lect* 1976;25:93.

37. Drummond DS, Moreau M, Cruess RL. The results and complications of surgery for the paralytic hip and spine in myelomeningocele. *J Bone Joint Surg Br* 1980;62:49.

38. Raycroft JE, Curtis BH. *Spinal curvature in myelomeningocele: natural history and etiology.* St. Louis: CV Mosby, 1972.

39. Sriram K, Bobrtchko WT, Hall JE. Surgical management of spinal deformities in spina bifida. *J Bone Joint Surg Br* 1972;54:666.

40. Mackel JL, Lindseth RE. Scoliosis in myelodysplasia. *J Bone Joint Surg Am* 1975;57:1031.

41. Lindseth RE. Scoliosis etiology and conservative treatment. In: McLaurin RL, et al., eds. *Spina bifida: a multidisciplinary approach.* New York: Praeger, 1986:439.

42. McLaughlin TP, Banta JV, Gahm NH, Raycroft JF. Intraspinal rhizotomy and distal cordectomy in patients with myelomeningocele. *J Bone Joint Surg Am* 1986;68:88.

43. McLone DG, Herman JM, Gabrieli AP, et al. Tethered cord as a cause of scoliosis in children with a myelomeningocele. *Pediatr Neurosurg* 1990;16:8.

44. Winter RB, Moe JN, Eilers VE. Congenital scoliosis. A study of 234 patients treated and untreated. Part I. Natural history. Part II. Treatment. *J Bone Joint Surg Am* 1968;50:1.

45. Breningstall GN, Marker SM, Tubman DE. Hydrosyringomyelia and diastematomyelia detected by MRI in myelomeningocele. *Pediatr Neurol* 1992;8:267.

46. Bunch WH. The Milwaukee brace in paralytic scoliosis. *Clin Orthop* 1975;110:63.

47. Allen BL Jr. The operative treatment of myelomeningocele spinal deformity. *Orthop Clin North Am* 1979;10:845.

48. Mazur JM, Menelaus MB, Dicksen DR, et al. Efficacy of surgical management for scoliosis in myelomeningocele—correction of deformity and alteration of functional status. *J Pediatr Orthop* 1986;6:568.

49. Lindseth RE. Posterior iliac osteotomy for fixed pelvic obliquity. *J Bone Joint Surg Am* 1978;60:17.

50. Banta JV. Combined anterior and posterior fusion for spinal deformity in myelomeningocele. *Spine* 1990;15:946.

51. Menelaus MB. Progress in the management of the paralytic hip in myelomeningocele. *Orthop Clin North Am* 1980;11:17.

52. Osebold WR, Mayfield JK, Winter RB, et al. Surgical treatment of the paralytic scoliosis associated with myelomeningocele. *J Bone Joint Surg Am* 1982;64:841.

53. Lindseth RE, Graziano GP. One-stage anterior transpedicular and unilateral fusion for congenital scoliosis. *Orthop Trans* 1988;12:184.

54. Drennan JC. The role of muscles in the development of human lumbar kyphosis. *Dev Med Child Neurol* 1970;12:33.

55. Eyring EJ, Wanken JJ, Sayers MP. Spinal osteotomy for kyphosis in myelomeningocele. *Clin Orthop* 1972;88:24.

56. Lindseth RE, Selzer L. Vertebral excision for kyphosis in children with myelomeningocele. *J Bone Joint Surg Am* 1979;61:699.

57. Sharrard WJ, Drennan JC. Osteotomy-excision of the spine for lumbar kyphosis in older children with myelomeningocele. *J Bone Joint Surg Br* 1972;54:50.

58. Banta JV, Hamanda JS. Natural history of the kyphotic deformity in myelomeningocele. *J Bone Joint Surg Am* 1976;58:279.

59. Loder RT, Shapiro P, Towbin R, et al. Aortic anatomy in children with myelomeningocele and congenital lumbar kyphosis. *J Pediatr Orthop* 1991;11:31.

60. Lindseth RE. Myelomeningocele spine. In: Weinstein SL, ed. *The pediatric spine: principles and practice.* New York: Raven, 1994.

61. Fromm B, Carstens C, Niethard FU, et al. Aortography in children with myelomeningocele and lumbar kyphosis. *J Bone Joint Surg Br* 1992;74:691.

62. Lintner SA, Lindseth RE. The long-term follow up after proximal resection in children with myelomeningocele and a kyphos deformity. *Orthop Trans* 1993;17:123.

63. Dunn HK. Kyphosis of myelodysplasia—operative treatment based on pathophysiology. *Orthop Trans* 1983;7:19.

64. Hall JE, Poitra B. The management of kyphosis in patients with myelomeningocele. *Clin Orthop* 1977;128:33.

65. Lubicky JP, Fredrickson BE. The combined use of kyphectomy, spinal cord resection, Luque instrumentation, and myocutaneous flaps for severe kyphosis in the myelomeningocele. *Orthop Trans* 1985;9:495.

66. Warner WC Jr, Fackler CD. Comparison of two instrumentation techniques in treatment of lumbar kyphosis in myelodysplasia. *J Pediatr Orthop* 1993;13:704.

67. Lindseth RE. Spine deformity in myelomeningocele. *Inst Course Lect* 1991;40:276.

68. Weisl H. Coxa vara in spina bifida. *J Bone Joint Surg Br* 1983;65:128.

69. Heydermann JS, Gillespie R. Management of myelomeningocele kyphosis in the older child by kyphectomy and segmental spinal instrumentation. *Spine* 1987;12:37.

70. Asher M, Olson J. Factors affecting the ambulatory status of patients with spina bifida cystica. *J Bone Joint Surg Am* 1983;65:350.

71. Lee EH, Carroll NC. Hip stability and ambulatory status in myelomeningocele. *J Pediatr Orthop* 1985;5:522.

72. Lindseth RE. Treatment of the lower extremity in children paralyzed by myelomeningocele. *Instr Course Lect* 1976;25:76.

73. Passo SD. Positioning infants with myelomeningocele. *Am J Nurs* 1974;74:165.

74. Feiwell E, Sakar D, Blatt T. The effect of hip reduction on function in patients with myelomeningocele—potential gains and hazards of surgical care. *J Bone Joint Surg Am* 1978;60:169.

75. Lough LK, Nielsen DH. Ambulation of children with myelomeningocele—parapodium versus parapodium with Orlau swivel modification. *Dev Med Child Neurol* 1986;28:489.

76. McCall RE, Schmidt WT. Clinical experience with the reciprocal gait orthosis in myelodysplasia. *J Pediatr Orthop* 1986;6:157.

77. Yngve DA, Douglas R, Roberts JM. The reciprocating gait orthosis in myelomeningocele. *J Pediatr Orthop* 1984;4:304.

78. Rose GK, Sankarankutt M, Stallard J. A clinical review of the orthotic treatment of myelomeningocele patients. *J Bone Joint Surg Br* 1983;65:242.

79. Bunch WH, Hakala MW. Iliopsoas transfers in children with myelomeningocele. *J Bone Joint Surg Am* 1984;66:224.

80. Hoffer MM, Feiwell E, Perry R, et al. Functional ambulation in patients with myelomeningocele. *J Bone Joint Surg Am* 1973;55:137.

81. Carroll NC, Sharrard WJ. Long term follow up of posterior iliopsoas transplantation for paralytic dislocation of the hip. *J Bone Joint Surg Am* 1972;54:551.

82. Garceau GJ, Kinzel JW. Transplantation of the iliacus muscle for loss of hip abduction power. *Q Bull Indiana Univ Med Center* 1951;13:27.

83. Stillwell A, Menelaus MB. Walking ability after transplantation of the iliopsoas—a long term follow up. *J Bone Joint Surg Br* 1984;66:656.

84. Mustard WT. Iliopsoas transfer for weakness of hip abduction. *J Bone Joint Surg Am* 1952;34:647.

85. Raycroft TF. Posterior iliopsoas transfer—long-term results in patients treated at Newington Children's Hospital. *Orthop Trans* 1987;11:454.

86. Phillips DP, Lindseth RE. Ambulation after transfer of adductors, external oblique, and tensor fascia lata in myelomeningocele. *J Pediatr Orthop* 1992;12712.

87. Thomas LI, Thompson TC, Strub LR. Transplantation of the external oblique muscle for adductor paralysis. *J Bone Joint Surg Am* 1950;32:207.

88. Yngve DA, Lindseth RE. Effectiveness of muscular transfer in myelomeningocele hips measured by radiographic indices. *J Pediatr Orthop* 1982;2:121.

89. Canale TS, Hammond NL III, Cotler JM, et al. Pelvic displacement osteotomy for chronic hip dislocation in myelodysplasia. *J Bone Joint Surg Am* 1975;57:177.

90. Lindseth RE. Extension contracture of the knee. In: McLaurin RL, Oppenheimer S, Dias L, et al., eds. *Spina bifida: a multidisciplinary approach.* New York: Praeger, 1986:40.

91. Dias LS. Surgical management of knee contractures in myelomeningocele. *J Pediatr Orthop* 1982;2:127.

92. Williams JJ, Graham GP, Dunne KB, et al. Late knee problems in myelomeningocele. *J Pediatr Orthop* 1993;13:701.

93. Turco VJ. Surgical correction of the resistant clubfoot: one stage posteromedial release with internal fixation: a preliminary report. *J Bone Joint Surg Am* 1971;53:477.

94. Burke SW, Weinse LS, Maynard MJ. Neuropathic foot ulcers in myelodysplasia. *Orthop Trans* 1991;15:102.

95. Menelaus MB. Talectomy for equinovarus deformity in arthrogryposis and spina bifida. *J Bone Joint Surg Br* 1971;53:468.

96. de Carvallo Neto J, Dias LS, Gabrieli AP. Congenital talipes equinovarus in spina bifida: treatment and results. *J Pediatr Orthop* 1996;16:782.

97. Crawford AH, Marxen JL, Osterfield DL. The Cincinnati Incision—a comprehensive approach for surgical procedures of the foot and ankle in childhood. *J Bone Joint Surg Am* 1982;64:1355.

98. Carroll NC. Pathoanatomy and surgical treatment of the resistant clubfoot. *Instr Course Lect* 1988;37:93.

99. Trieshmann H, Millis M, Hall J, et al. Sliding calcaneal osteotomy for treatment of hindfoot deformity. *Orthop Trans* 1980;4:305.

100. Grant AD, Silver L, Lehman WB, Altar D. The use of tissue expander in clubfoot surgery. Presented at: Pediatric Orthopaedic Society of North America Meeting, May 7, 1990; San Francisco, CA.

101. Kling TF Jr, Schmidt TL, Conklin, MJ. Open wedge osteotomy of the first cuneiform for severe metatarsus adductus. Presented at: Pediatric Orthopaedic Society of North America Meeting, May 7, 1990; San Francisco, CA.

102. McKay DW. New concept of and approach to clubfoot treatment. Section II. Correction of the clubfoot. *J Pediatr Orthop* 1983;3:10.

103. Dias LS, Stern LS. Talectomy in the treatment of resistant tali-

pes equinovarus deformity in myelomeningocele and arthrogryposis. *J Pediatr Orthop* 1987;7:39.

104. Sherk HH, Ames MD. Talectomy in the treatment of the myelomeningocele patient. *Clin Orthop* 1975;75:218.

105. Sherk HH, Marchinski LJ, Clancy M, et al. Ground reaction forces on the plantar surface of the foot after talectomy in the myelomeningocele. *J Pediatr Orthop* 1989;9:269.

106. Duncan JW, Lovell WW. Hoke triple arthrodesis. *J Bone Joint Surg Am* 1978;60:795.

107. Fraser RK, Hoffman EB. Calcaneus deformity in the ambulant patient with myelomeningocele. *J Bone Joint Surg Br* 1991;73:994.

108. Bliss DG, Menelaus MB. The results of transfer of the tibialis anterior to the heel in patients who have a myelomeningocele. *J Bone Joint Surg Am* 1986;68:1258.

109. Rodrigues RC, Dias LS. Calcaneus deformity in spina bifida—results of anterolateral release. *J Pediatr Orthop* 1992;12:461.

110. Banta JV, Sutherland DH, Wyatt M. Anterior tibial transfer to the os calcis with Achilles tenodesis for calcaneal deformity in myelomeningocele. *J Pediatr Orthop* 1982;1:125.

111. Coleman SS. *Complex foot deformities in children.* Philadelphia: Lea & Febiger, 1983:147.

112. Dias LS, Jasty MJ, Collins P. Rotational deformities of the lower limb in myelomeningocele—evaluation and treatment. *J Bone Joint Surg Am* 1984;66:215.

113. Menelaus MB. Pes plano-valgus. In: McLaurin RL, Oppenheimer S, Dias L, et al., eds. *Spina bifida—a multidisciplinary approach.* New York: Prager, 1986:431.

114. Diamond L. Dowel type subtalar arthrodesis in children. *J Bone Joint Surg Am* 1976;58:725.

115. Lee YF, Grogan TJ, Moseley CF. Extra-articular subtalar arthrodesis in myelodysplasia. *Orthop Trans* 1990;14:590.

116. Malhotra D, Puri R, Owen R. Valgus deformity of the ankle in children with spina bifida aperta. *J Bone Joint Surg Br* 1984;66:381.

117. Burkus JK, Moore DW, Raycroft JF. Valgus deformity of the ankle in myelodysplastic patients. Correction of stapling of the medial part of the distal tibial physis. *J Bone Joint Surg Am* 1983;65:1157.

118. Stevens PM, Toomey E. Fibular-Achilles tenodesis for paralytic ankle valgus. *J Pediatr Orthop* 1988;8:169.

119. Bradley GW, Coleman SS. The treatment of the calcaneocavus foot deformity. *J Bone Joint Surg Am* 1981;63:1159.

120. Sutherland DH. *Gait disorders in childhood and adolescence.* Baltimore: Williams & Wilkins, 1984:631.

121. Sutherland DH. An electromyographic study of the plantar flexors of the ankle in normal walking on the level. *J Bone Joint Surg Am* 1966;48:66.

122. Glancy JC, Lindseth RE. The polypropylene solid-ankle orthosis. *Orthot Prosth* 1972;26:16.

123. Lin RS. Application of varus T-strap principle to the polypropylene ankle—foot orthosis. *Orthot Prosthet* 1982;36:67.

124. Lindseth RE. Myelomeningocele. In: Drennan JC, ed. *The child's foot and ankle.* New York: Raven, 1992.

125. Hullin MG, Robb JE, Loudon IR. Ankle–foot orthosis function in low level myelomeningocele. *J Pediatr Orthop* 1992;12:518.

126. Cuxart A, Iborra J, Melendez M, et al. Physeal injuries in myelomeningocele patients. *Paraplegia* 1992;30:791.

127. Edvardsen P. Physeo-epiphyseal injuries of lower extremities in myelomeningocele. *Acta Orthop Scand* 1972;43:550.

128. Korhonen BJ. Fractures in myelodysplasia. *Clin Orthop* 1971;79:145.

129. Kumar SJ, Cowell HR, Townsend P. Physeal, metaphyseal, and diaphyseal injuries of the lower extremities in children with myelomeningocele. *J Pediatr Orthop* 1984;4:25.

130. Repasky D, Richard K, Lindseth RE. Ascorbic acid and fractures in children with myelomeningocele. *J Am Diet Assoc* 1976;69:511.

131. Drummond DS, Moreau M, Cruess RL. Postoperative neuropathic fractures in patients with myelomeningocele. *Dev Med Child Neurol* 1981;23:147.

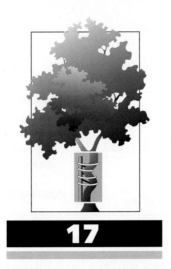

17

OTHER NEUROMUSCULAR DISORDERS

GEORGE H. THOMPSON
FRANK R. BERENSON

G. H. Thompson: Department of Orthopaedic Surgery and Pediatrics, Case Western Reserve University; Pediatric Orthopaedics, Rainbow Babies and Children's Hospital, Cleveland, Ohio 44106.
F. R. Berenson: Department of Pediatrics, Mercer University, Macon, Georgia 31207; Department of Pediatrics, Children's Healthcare of Atlanta at Scottish Rite, Atlanta, Georgia 30342.

Neuromuscular disorders other than cerebral palsy and myelodysplasia are less common, but nevertheless appear in pediatric orthopaedic and neuromuscular clinics. These disorders include the muscular dystrophies and congenital myopathies, spinal muscular atrophy, Friedreich ataxia, hereditary motor sensory neuropathies (HMSN), and poliomyelitis. It is important that an accurate diagnosis be established so that an effective treatment program can be planned and initiated. Delaying the diagnosis may lead to inappropriate treatment and perhaps further pregnancies with involved children in the presence of genetic diseases (1). Accurate diagnosis requires a careful history, physical examination, and appropriate diagnostic studies (2).

HISTORY

The history should include the details of pregnancy, delivery, and growth and development of the involved child. Questions regarding *in utero* activity, complications of delivery, birth weight, Apgar score, problems during the neonatal period, age at achievement of developmental motor milestones, age at onset of the current symptoms, and information regarding whether the condition is static or progressive should be asked. Systemic symptoms, such as cardiac disease, cataracts, seizures, or other abnormalities, should also be ascertained.

The family history is important in diagnosis because these disorders, with the exception of poliomyelitis, are genetic in origin. Family members of an involved child or adolescent may need to be examined for subtle expressions of the same disorder. These same family members may also require hematologic or other studies to arrive at an accurate diagnosis.

PHYSICAL EXAMINATION

Most children who present for evaluation of a suspected neuromuscular disorder have either a delay in developmental milestones, abnormal gait, or foot deformity. There usually is a history of progression. Physical examination consists of a thorough musculoskeletal and neurologic evaluation. Observing the child walking and performing simple tasks, such as arising from a sitting position on the floor, can be beneficial. Observing the gait may reveal decreased arm swing, circumduction of the legs, scissoring, or short cadence. Standing posture may reveal increased lumbar lordosis or wide base position for balance. Also, in the standing position the appearance of the feet should be observed. Pes cavus or cavovarus deformities are common physical findings in many of these disorders. Having the child walk on the heels and toes gives a gross assessment of motor strength, whereas having the child run may reveal an increase in muscle tone or ataxia.

Inspection of the skin should be performed for evidence of skin rashes or other abnormalities. Typical facies of the patient with spinal muscular atrophy and congenital myotonic dystrophy should become familiar to orthopaedic surgeons. The tongue should be examined to detect evidence of fasciculation suggestive of anterior horn cell diseases. Excessive drooling is common in both cerebral palsy and congenital myotonic dystrophy. In the latter, nasal speech may also be present. A thorough ophthalmologic examination is necessary to elicit external ophthalmoplegia or retinitis pigmentosa. Cataracts may develop during adolescence in myotonic dystrophy.

Muscle testing should be carefully performed. Generally, myopathic disorders selectively affect proximal limb muscles before distal muscles. They also demonstrate proportionally greater weakness than the degree of atrophy early in the disease process. The converse is true in neuropathies.

A careful neurologic evaluation usually completes the musculoskeletal examination. Sensory responses must be checked individually and recorded. Decreased vibratory sensation may be present in HMSN, such as Charcot-Marie-Tooth disease. In spinal muscular atrophy the deep tendon reflexes may be absent, but they are increased in cerebral palsy. A positive Babinski sign confirms upper motor neuron disease. Abnormalities in the Romberg test and rapid alternating movements may indicate cerebellar involvement. Mental function evaluation may be necessary, because organic mental deterioration may be part of some neurologic syndromes. In many cases the assistance of a pediatric neurologist can be invaluable in performing a careful neurologic and mental evaluation because minor subtleties may be a clue to diagnosis.

DIAGNOSTIC STUDIES

Appropriate diagnostic studies are imperative in the accurate diagnosis of the myopathic and neuropathic disorders (3–6). These can be divided into hematologic studies, electromyography (EMG) with both nerve conduction studies and needle electrode exam, muscle biopsy, and nerve biopsy. Molecular diagnostic studies have become available for several disorders, such as Duchenne and Becker muscular dystrophies.

Hematologic Studies

The measurement of serum creatine phosphokinase (CPK) is the most sensitive test for demonstrating abnormalities of striated muscle function (7,8). The level of elevation parallels the rate and amount of muscle necrosis and decreases with time as the muscle is replaced by fat and fibrous tissue. The highest CPK levels are typically seen in the earliest stages of Duchenne or Becker muscular dystrophy in which increases of 20 to 200 times normal may be found (4). The level of elevation does not correlate with the severity or rate of progression of the disorder. The highest levels are usually found in Duchenne muscular dystrophy. Umbilical cord blood CPK levels should be obtained in all male infants who are suspected of having this disorder (9). Birth trauma may elevate the CPK in umbilical cord blood, but in the normal child this elevation disappears promptly. The enzyme level remains elevated in true muscular dystrophy. Serum CPK may be mildly or moderately elevated in other dystrophic disorders, such as fascioscapulohumeral muscular dystrophy, Emery-Dreifuss muscular dystrophy, and spinal muscular atrophy. It is also mildly elevated in female carriers of Duchenne muscular dystrophy, although they are asymptomatic. In congenital myopathies and peripheral neuropathies, the CPK levels are usually normal to only mildly elevated. In other neuromuscular disorders that do not directly affect striated muscle, the CPK levels are normal. Serum enzymes, such as aldolase and serum glutamic oxaloacetic transaminase (SGOT), are also important in the study of striated muscle function. Aldolase levels correlate well with the CPK levels (6).

Electromyography

EMG can differentiate between a myopathic and neuropathic process but is rarely helpful in establishing a definitive diagnosis. Characteristics of neuropathic disorders include the presence of fibrillation potentials, increased insertional activity, and high amplitude and increased-duration motor unit potentials (4). The fibrillation potential represents denervated individual muscle fibers firing spontaneously.

Myopathic EMG is characterized by low-voltage, short-duration polyphasic motor unit potentials (4). Myopathies rarely demonstrate EMG changes characteristic of a neuropathy, although in an inflammatory muscle disease with significant muscle breakdown there may be prominent fibrillations. The use of an experienced electromyographer is imperative in the accurate performance and interpretation of EMG data.

Nerve Conduction Studies

Nerve conduction studies are important in the establishment of the diagnosis of peripheral neuropathy in children. Nerve conduction velocities are normal in children with anterior horn cell diseases, nerve root diseases, and myopathies. The normal value in the child older than 5 years of age is 45 to 65 m/s. In infants and younger children, the velocity is lower because myelinization is incomplete.

Motor conduction velocity may be lowered in HMSN (e.g., Charcot-Marie-Tooth disease) before clinical deficits are present. The nerve conduction studies can help determine whether the neuropathy involves an isolated nerve or is a disseminated process.

Muscle Biopsy

Muscle biopsy is the most important test in determining the diagnosis of a neuromuscular disorder (10,11). Muscle biopsy material is usually examined by routine histology, special histochemical stains, and electron microscopy. The criterion for selecting the muscle for biopsy is clinical evidence of muscle weakness. Muscles that are involved but are functioning are selected in chronic diseases such as Duchenne muscular dystrophy because they demonstrate the greatest diagnostic changes. A more severely involved muscle may be chosen in an acute illness because the process has not had sufficient time to progress to extensive destruction. In patients who have proximal lower extremity muscle weakness biopsy of the vastus lateralis is performed, whereas in those with distal weakness the gastrocnemius is biopsied. Biopsy of the deltoid, biceps, or triceps is performed for shoulder girdle or proximal upper extremity weakness.

Muscle biopsies can be performed as an open procedure (10,12) or by percutaneous needle (13). The open technique as described by Banker is preferred (10). The biopsies are obtained under general anesthesia, spinal anesthetic, regional nerve block, or with a field block surrounding the area of incision. It is important that local anesthetic not be infiltrated into the muscle because this may alter the morphology of the muscle. The vastus lateralis is the most common muscle chosen. A 4-cm incision is made and the underlying fascia is incised longitudinally. The muscle is looked at directly to avoid including normal fibrous septae in the specimens. Muscle clamps are used to obtain three specimens. The clamps are oriented in the direction of the muscle fibers. A 2- to 3-mm piece of muscle is grasped in each end of the clamp. The muscle is cut at the outside edge of each clamp and a cylinder of muscle excised. Using a muscle clamp keeps the muscle at its resting length and minimizes artifact. One specimen is quickly frozen in liquid nitrogen ($-160°$C) to prevent loss of soluble enzymes. This specimen is used for light microscopy with a variety of special preparations. The other specimens are used for routine histology and electron microscopy. The wound is subsequently closed in layers. Electrocautery may be used during the closure. If it is used before the biopsy, it may inadvertently damage the specimens and alter the morphology.

Nerve Biopsy

Occasionally biopsy of a peripheral nerve is helpful in demyelinating disorders. Usually the sural nerve is selected for biopsy because of its distal location and lack of autogenous zone of innervation. The patient notices no sensory change or only a mild diminution after excision of the 3- to 4-cm segment of the nerve. Hurley et al. (12) reported a single incision for combined muscle and sural nerve biopsy. An incision over the posterolateral aspect of the calf allows access to the nerve and either the soleus or the peroneal muscles. This avoids the necessity for two incisions. This technique was demonstrated to be accurate in diagnosing disorders in which both a muscle and nerve biopsy may be necessary.

Other Studies

Other studies that may be beneficial in establishing the diagnosis of a neuromuscular disorder include electrocardiogram (ECG), pulmonary function studies, magnetic resonance imaging (MRI), ophthalmologic evaluation, amniocentesis, and pediatric neurology evaluation.

Duchenne muscular dystrophy, Friedreich ataxia, and myotonic dystrophy demonstrate ECG abnormalities. Duchenne muscular dystrophy frequently has mitral valve prolapse secondary to papillary muscle involvement (14,15). Arrhythmias under anesthesia have been reported with both Duchenne and Emery-Dreifuss muscular dystrophies (16,17).

Pulmonary function studies demonstrate involvement of respiratory muscles but do not establish the diagnosis. If respiratory muscle involvement is present the rate of deterioration can be followed with periodic studies. This is important if surgery is contemplated in children or adolescents with muscular dystrophy, spinal muscular atrophy, or

Friedreich ataxia. The forced vital capacity (FVC) is the most important study after arterial blood gas measurements (18).

MRI has been demonstrated to distinguish muscles in neuropathic and myopathic disorders (19). Imaging estimates of the disease severity by degree of muscle involvement correlate well with clinical staging. MRI may also be important in selecting appropriate muscles for biopsy.

Ophthalmologic evaluation may demonstrate subtle or more obvious ocular changes associated with specific disorders.

GENETIC AND MOLECULAR BIOLOGY STUDIES

Genetic research through molecular biologic techniques has tremendously enhanced our understanding of the genetic aspects of many of these disorders (20,21). The exact location of chromosomal and gene defects has led to the possibility of genetic engineering with correction of these disorders. In each of the various disorders, the current status of genetic and molecular biology research, if any, is discussed.

MUSCULAR DYSTROPHIES

The muscular dystrophies are a group of noninflammatory inherited disorders with progressive degeneration and weakness of skeletal muscle without apparent cause in the peripheral or central nervous system. These have been divided by clinical distribution, severity of muscle weakness, and pattern of genetic inheritance (Table 17-1). An accurate diagnosis is important, both for prognosis and management of the individual patient and for identification of genetic factors that may be crucial in planning for subsequent children by the involved family.

TABLE 17-1. CLASSIFICATION OF MUSCULAR DYSTROPHIES

Sex-linked Muscular Dystrophy
  Duchenne
  Becker
  Emery-Dreifuss

Autosomal Recessive Muscular Dystrophy
  Limb-girdle
  Infantile fascioscapulohumeral

Autosomal Dominant Muscular Dystrophy
  Fascioscapulohumeral
  Distal
  Ocular
  Oculopharyngeal

SEX-LINKED MUSCULAR DYSTROPHIES

Duchenne Muscular Dystrophy

Duchenne muscular dystrophy is the most common form of muscular dystrophy. Transmission is by an X-linked recessive trait. A single gene defect is found in the short arm of the X chromosome. The disease is characterized by its occurrence in males, except for rare cases associated with Turner syndrome. In this rare event, the XO karyotype who carries the defective gene may demonstrate the phenotype found in involved males (4). This disorder has a high mutation rate, and a positive family history is present in approximately 65% of cases. Duchenne muscular dystrophy occurs in about 1 in 3,500 live male births, with about one-third of involved children having the disease based on a new mutation.

Becker muscular dystrophy is a similar but less common and less severe form of muscular dystrophy. It occurs in about 1 in 30,000 live male births, becomes apparent later in childhood, and has a more protracted and variable course than Duchenne muscular dystrophy. This disorder is discussed later but is introduced here because of the similar inheritance pattern and molecular biology abnormality.

Clinical Features

Duchenne muscular dystrophy is generally clinically evident when the child is between 3 and 6 years of age. Earlier onset may also occur. The family may have observed that the child's ability to achieve independent ambulation was delayed or that he has become a toe walker. Children 3 years of age or older may demonstrate frequent episodes of tripping and falling, in addition to difficulty in reciprocal motion, such as running or climbing stairs. Inability to hop and jump normally is commonly present.

In Duchenne muscular dystrophy there is progressive weakness in the proximal muscle groups which descends symmetrically in both lower extremities, particularly the gluteus maximus, gluteus medius, quadriceps, and tibialis anterior muscles. The abdominal muscles are involved. Involvement of the shoulder girdle muscles (i.e., trapezius, deltoid, and pectoralis major muscles) and lower facial muscles occurs later. Pseudohypertrophy of the calf muscles caused by the accumulation of fat is common but not invariably present. Most patients have cardiac involvement, most commonly a sinus tachycardia and right ventricular hypertrophy. Life-threatening dysrhythmia or heart failure ultimately develops in about 10% of patients. Many also have a static encephalopathy, with mild or moderate mental retardation (22). Death from pulmonary failure and occasionally from cardiac failure occurs during the second or third decades of life.

During gait the child's cadence is slow and he or she develops compensatory changes in gait and stance as weakness progresses. Sutherland et al. (23,24) documented disease progression by measuring the gait variables of cadence, swing phase, ankle dorsiflexion, and anterior pelvic tilt. The hip extensors, primarily the gluteus maximus, are the first muscle group to be involved. Initially the patient compensates by carrying the head and shoulders behind the pelvis, maintaining the weight line posterior to the hip joint and center of gravity (Fig. 17-1). This produces an anterior pelvic tilt and increases lumbar lordosis. Cadence and swing-phase ankle dorsiflexion decrease, and the patient develops a waddling, wide-based gait with shoulder sway to compensate for gluteus medius weakness. Muscle weakness requires that the force line remain behind the hip joint and in front of the knee joint throughout single limb support (23–25), and hip abductors and quadriceps muscles force the patient to circumduct during the swing phase of gait, while at the same time shifting the weight directly over the hip joint. The generalized pelvic weakness requires considerable forward motion to be generated by the spine for the patient to advance. Ankle plantar flexion becomes fixed and the stance phase is reduced to the forefoot, resulting in even more difficulty with balance and cadence. Foot inversion develops as peroneal strength diminishes. The tibialis posterior muscle, which is one of the last muscles to be involved, is responsible for the inversion or varus deformity of the foot.

Weakness in the shoulder girdle, which occurs 3 to 5 years later, precludes crutch usage to aid in ambulation. It also makes it difficult to lift the patient from under the arms. This tendency for the child to slip a truncal grasp has been termed "Meyeron sign." As the weakness in the upper extremities increases, the child becomes unable to move his or her arms. Although the hands retain strength longer than the arms, use of the hands is limited because of weakness of the arms.

Clinical diagnosis of Duchenne muscular dystrophy is established by physical examination, including gait and specific muscle weakness, and by the absence of sensory deficits. The upper extremity and knee deep-tendon reflexes are lost early in the disease, whereas the ankle reflexes remain positive until the terminal phase. A valuable clinical sign is the Gower sign. The patient is placed prone or in the sitting position on the floor and asked to rise. This is usually difficult, and the patient may require the use of a chair for assistance. The patient is then asked to use his or her hands to grasp the lower legs and force the knees into extension. The patient then walks his or her hands up their extremities to compensate for the quadriceps and gluteus maximum weakness. This sign may also be found in congenital myopathies and spinal muscular atrophy. Appreciation of the contracture of the iliotibial band can be measured by the Ober test. To perform this test, the child is placed on his or her side with both hips flexed. The superior leg is then abducted and extended and allowed to fall into adduction. The degree of abduction contracture can be measured by the number

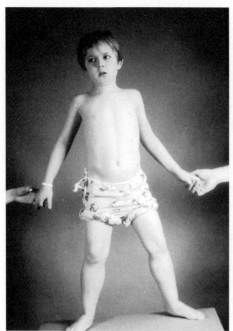
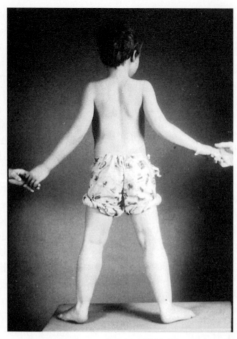
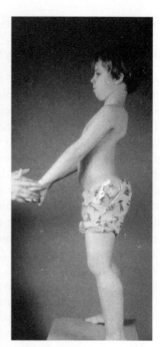

A,B   C

FIGURE 17-1. A: A 7-year-old boy with Duchenne muscular dystrophy demonstrates precarious stance due to mild hip abduction contractures. Observe the pseudohypertrophy of the calves. **B:** Posterior view demonstrates mild ankle equinus in addition to the calf pseudohypertrophy. **C:** Side view shows an anterior tilt to the pelvis and increased lumbar lordosis, and the head and the shoulders are aligned posterior to the pelvis. This characteristic posture maintains the weight line posterior to the pelvis and center of gravity, compensates for the muscle weakness, and helps maintain balance.

of degrees the leg lacks in coming to the neutral position. Tendo Achillis contractures also occur. Contracture of the tendo Achillis and the iliotibial band are the most consistent deformities noted during the physical examination. Macroglossia is also a common finding.

Duchenne muscular dystrophy progresses slowly but continuously. A rapid deterioration may be noted after immobilization in bed, even for short periods after respiratory infections or perhaps extremity fractures. Every effort should be made to maintain a daily ambulatory program. Children are usually unable to ambulate effectively by 10 years of age in the absence of treatment (3,26–28). With loss of standing ability, the child becomes wheelchair-dependent. This results in a loss of the accentuated lumbar lordosis, which protects the child from kyphoscoliosis (28). As a consequence most develop a progressive spinal deformity.

Myocardial deterioration is also a constant finding. ECG changes are present in more than 90% of children with Duchenne muscular dystrophy. The average intelligence quotient of these patients has been shown to be about 80 (22).

Hematologic Studies

The serum CPK is markedly elevated in the early stages of Duchenne muscular dystrophy. This may be 200 to 300 times normal, but decreases as the disease progresses and muscle mass is reduced. CPK levels are also elevated in female carriers, although not as high as in affected boys (two to three times that in normal women and girls). There is an 80% accuracy when the CPK level is repeated at three consecutive monthly intervals (30). Aldolase and SGOT levels also may be elevated, but the elevations are not unique to striated muscle disease.

Electromyography

EMG shows characteristic myopathic changes with reduced amplitude, short duration, and polyphasic motor action potentials (4).

Muscle Biopsy

The muscle biopsy specimen reveals degeneration with subsequent loss of fiber, variation in fiber size, proliferation of connective tissue, and subsequently, of adipose tissue (10,11). Increased cellularity with occasional internal migration of the sarcolemmal nuclei is present. Histochemical loss of clear-cut subdivisions to fiber types, especially with adenosine triphosphatase reaction and tendency toward type I fiber predominance, are also seen.

Genetic and Molecular Biology Studies

A single gene defect in the short arm of the X chromosome has been identified as being responsible for both Duchenne and Becker muscular dystrophies (31,32). The status of genetic and molecular biology in Duchenne muscular dystrophy has been summarized by Shapiro and Specht (4). The gene is located at the Xp21.2 region and spans 2 million base pairs (20,23). It includes 65 exons (i.e., coding regions) and encodes the 400-kd protein dystrophin (33,34). The large size of the gene correlates with the high rate of spontaneous mutation. Dystrophin is a component of cell membrane cytoskeleton and represents 0.01% of skeletal muscle protein. Its distribution within skeletal, smooth, and cardiac muscle and within the brain correlates well with the clinical features in Duchenne and Becker muscular dystrophies. A structural role for the dystrophin protein is suggested by studies demonstrating concentration of the protein in a lattice organization in the cytoplasmic membrane of skeletal muscle fibers (35,36). Demonstrable mutations, deletions, or duplications of dystrophin are found in 70 to 80% of involved males (33,34,37,38). The reading frame hypothesis defines which mutations correlate with the more severe Duchenne muscular dystrophy or with the less severe Becker muscular dystrophy. Mutations that disrupt the translational reading frame or the promoter (i.e., the specific DNA sequence that signals where RNA synthesis should begin) result in a presumably unstable protein, which correlates with Duchenne muscular dystrophy. In contrast, mutations that do not disrupt the translational reading frame or the promoter have a lower molecular weight and semifunctional dystrophin, which correlates with the less severe Becker muscular dystrophy (33,39).

Dystrophin testing (dystrophin immunoblotting), DNA mutation analysis (polymerase chain reaction or DHA [Southern] blot analysis), or both provide an aid to differentiate between Duchenne and Becker muscular dystrophies, and other initially similar disorders, such as dermatomyositis, limb-girdle muscular dystrophy, Emery-Dreifuss muscular dystrophy, and congenital muscular dystrophy (38,40,41). In the latter disorders the dystrophin is normal. In patients with Duchenne muscular dystrophy there is a complete absence of dystrophin, whereas in Becker muscular dystrophy, dystrophin is present but is altered in size, decreased in amount, or both. Nicholson et al. (42) reported a positive relation between the amount of dystrophin and the age at loss of independent ambulation in 30 patients with Duchenne muscular dystrophy and 6 patients with Becker muscular dystrophy. They found that even low concentrations of dystrophin in Duchenne muscular dystrophy may have functional significance and may explain the variability of age when ambulation ceases. The presence of partially functional dystrophin protein is sufficient for minimizing the phenotypic expression leading to the milder disorder of Becker muscular dystrophy (33,37,40). The same tests can be used to improve detection of female carriers (38,41). Based on smaller-than-normal dystrophin protein, two atypical forms of Becker muscular dystrophy have been recognized. These include myalgia without weakness in male patients similar to metabolic myopathy, and cardiomyopathy in male patients with little or no weakness (43).

Research involves the possibility of dystrophin replacement in diseased muscles. This involves the implantation of myoblasts, or muscle precursor cells, into the muscles of patients with Duchenne muscular dystrophy (44). This has been successful in producing dystrophin in the murine mdx model of Duchenne muscular dystrophy (45). Unfortunately, the results in involved males has been disappointing (46–50).

Several forms of experimental treatment of Duchenne muscular dystrophy are being investigated. Prednisone has been demonstrated to have short-term benefits in slowing the progressive weakness for at least 3 years (51,52). However, the associated side effects of weight gain, osteoporosis and myopathy limit its usefulness (53–55). Azathioprine has also been evaluated in Duchenne muscular dystrophy, but has not shown beneficial effects (56).

Treatment

The orthopaedic problems in children with Duchenne muscular dystrophy include decreasing ambulatory ability, soft tissue contractures, and spinal deformity (2–4,57). The goals of treatment should be designed to improve or maintain the functional capacity of the involved child or adolescent.

The treatment modalities in Duchenne muscular dystrophy have been outlined by Drennan (58) and include physical therapy, functional testing, orthoses, fracture management, surgery, wheelchair, cardiopulmonary management, and genetic and psychologic counseling.

Physical Therapy. Physical therapy is directed toward prolongation of functional muscle strength, prevention or correction of contractures by passive stretching, gait training with orthoses and transfer techniques, ongoing assessment of muscle strength and functional capacity, and wheelchair and equipment measurements.

After the diagnosis of Duchenne muscular dystrophy has been established and before muscle strength has deteriorated, a program of maximum-resistance exercises performed several times daily, should be instituted (5,59). This may help prolong strength and delay the onset of soft tissue contractures. Contractures are more effectively delayed or prevented than corrected by physical therapy. Contractures develop in the ambulatory patient because muscle weakness progression results in development of adaptive posturing to maintain lower extremity joint stability. A home exercise program can be effective in minimizing hip and ankle soft tissue contractures. Drennan recommended that exercises be performed twice daily on a firm surface and should include stretching of the tensor fascia lata, hamstrings, knee flexors, and ankle plantar flexors (58). Occasionally serial casting may be useful to correct existing deformities before physical therapy. Knee flexion contractures of less than 30 degrees may benefit by serial or wedge casting. This enhances the use of knee-ankle-foot orthoses (KAFOs). Unless orthoses are used after casting and in conjunction with physical therapy, these contractures rapidly recur.

Functional Testing. Functional testing predominantly involves periodic muscle testing. Muscle strength is tested by measurement of the active range of motion of a joint against gravity. This type of testing allows assessment of the rate of deterioration as well as the functional capacity of the individual.

Orthoses. Lightweight molded plastic ankle-foot orthoses (AFOs) or KAFOs are used in independently ambulatory patients when gait becomes precarious, when early soft tissue contractures of the knees and ankle are developing, and after surgical correction of these deformities (60–63). KAFOs usually are supplemented with a walker because of the excessive weight and the fear of falling. Important prescription components include partial ischial weightbearing support, posterior thigh cuff, and a spring-loaded, drop-lock knee joint with an ankle joint set at a right angle. Ambulation may be extended for up to 3 years by the combined use of surgery and orthoses. The maintenance of a straight lower extremity also enables the nonwalking patient to stand with support and thereby assist in transfers.

Spinal orthoses are usually of no value in progressive spinal deformities, but wheelchair-bound patients, especially those with severe cardiopulmonary compromise and severe scoliosis, may benefit from the use of a custom wheelchair, a thoracic suspension orthosis, or custom thoracic-lumbar spinal orthosis (TLSO) (52). A mobile arm support orthosis attached to the wheelchair may benefit the patient in performing personal hygiene tasks and self-feeding activities (64,65).

Fracture Management. Fractures of the lower extremities occur frequently in children with Duchenne muscular dystrophy. This occurs predominantly after ambulation has ceased and the child is wheelchair-bound. These fractures are best treated by closed reduction and cast immobilization. Occasionally open reduction and internal fixation may be needed. In children who are still ambulatory, it is important that they be placed on a program of early mobilization to allow weightbearing. This may require the use of an electrically powered circle bed. Once early healing is present, the child can be returned to the KAFO to decrease weight and enhance mobility.

Surgery. Contractures of the lower extremities and progressive weakness impair ambulation. Surgery is indicated when independent ambulation becomes precarious and when contractures are painful or interfere with essential daily activities. The major contractures amenable to surgical intervention include equinus and equinovarus contractures of the ankle and foot, knee flexion contractures, and hip flexion and abduction contractures. In thin individuals, these contractures may be released by percutaneous techniques (57,66,67). Orthotic measurements for ambulatory patients should be obtained before surgery. This allows them to be applied shortly after surgery to assist in rapid restoration of ambulation. Correction of contractures and the use of orthoses can prolong effective ambulation by 1 to 3 years (3,25,60–63,67–74). Hsu and Furumasu (25) reported a mean prolongation of walking of 3.3 years in 24 patients with Duchenne muscular dystrophy, ranging in age from 8 to 12 years at the time of surgery. It is usually not possible to restore functional ambulation once the patient has been unable to walk for more than 3 to 6 months (60,68,70). Each patient must be individually assessed to determine the functional needs and the best procedures. Common contraindications for correction of lower extremity contractures include obesity, rapidly progressive muscle weakness, or poor motivation in those who prefer to use a wheelchair rather than attempt ambulation (4).

Foot and Ankle. Equinus contractures occur first, then equinovarus contractures. This is due to a combination of tendo Achillis contracture and muscle imbalance induced by the stronger tibialis posterior muscle. This latter muscle retains good function despite the progression of muscle weakness in other areas. These equinovarus deformities can be managed by a combination of tendo Achillis lengthening (percutaneous open tenotomy [57,60,62,63,69,71] **[➡7.17]**, with or without resection [70]; Vulpius [3,75]; or open Z-lengthening [68,74] **[➡7.16]**) and tibialis posterior lengthening, tenotomy, or transfer through the interosseous membrane to the dorsum of the foot **[➡7.19]** (3,5,28,57,61–63,68–71,76–78). Tibialis posterior transfer prevents recurrence of equinovarus deformities and maintains active dorsiflexion of the foot. Some authors, however, have questioned the necessity of a transfer because it is a more extensive procedure and they prefer tenotomy, recession, or lengthening (5,57,61,69). Postoperative gait analysis has shown that the transferred tibialis posterior muscle is electrically silent (79). Greene (76) has reported that tibialis posterior myotendinous junction recession in 6 patients (12 feet) had an increased recurrence rate when compared with transfer in 9 patients (18 feet), which made the former a less desirable procedure. Percutaneous tendo Achillis lengthening under local anesthesia has been reserved for nonambulatory patients who have a typically equinus deformity and cannot wear shoes. The nonambulatory patient with a moderately severe equinovarus deformity may require open tenotomies of the tendo Achillis, the tibialis posterior, and long toe flexors. Severe equinovarus contractures have been managed effectively by talectomy.

Knee. Knee flexion contractures coexist with hip flexion contractures and develop rapidly when the patient is wheelchair-bound. These contractures limit proper positioning in bed and may lead to the development of hamstring spasm, causing considerable discomfort when the patient attempts to transfer. A Yount procedure (80), (release of the distal aspect of the tensor fascia lata and iliotibial band) is the most common procedure used in correcting knee flexion contractures (57,61–63). Hamstring tenotomies (68), recession or Vulpius-type lengthening (75), and formal Z-lengthening may also be necessary [➡4.23]. These procedures enhance quadriceps power and function as well as relieve symptoms. Postoperatively KAFOs are necessary to prevent recurrence.

Hip. Hip flexion and abduction contractures increase lumbar lordosis and interfere with the ability to stand and to lay comfortably supine. Patients with hip flexion contractures may complain of low back pain. Correction of flexion contractures involves release of the tight anterior muscles, including the sartorius, rectus femoris, and tensor fascia femoris (4,57). Abduction contractures are improved by release of the tensor fasciae lata proximally with use of the Ober procedure (81), modified Soutter release (82), the Yount procedure distally (80), or by complete resection of the entire iliotibial band (28,72).

Upper Extremity. Upper extremity contractures are common in adolescents with Duchenne muscular dystrophy but usually do not require treatment. These contractures include shoulder adduction, elbow flexion, forearm pronation, wrist flexion, metacarpophalangeal and proximal interphalangeal joint flexion, and others. These usually do not preclude the use of wheelchairs. Muscle weakness is the most devastating aspect of upper extremity involvement. Wagner et al. (83) demonstrated wrist ulnar deviation and flexion contractures in addition to contractures of the extrinsic and intrinsic muscles of the fingers, producing boutonniere and swan-neck deformities and hyperextension of the distal interphalangeal joints in adolescents with Duchenne muscular dystrophy. The treatment of upper extremity contractures involves physical therapy with daily passive range of motion exercises. When passive wrist dorsiflexion is limited to neutral, a nighttime extension orthosis may be beneficial. Surgery for these contractures is rarely indicated.

Spinal Deformity. Approximately 95% of patients with Duchenne muscular dystrophy develop progressive scoliosis (29,72,84–91). This typically begins to occur when ambulation ceases, and it is rapidly progressive. About 25% of older ambulating patients, however, have mild scoliosis (26,92). Prolongation of ambulation by appropriate soft tissue releases of the lower extremity contractures, which maintains accentuated lumbar lordosis, can delay the onset of scoliosis (73). The curves are usually thoracolumbar, associated with kyphosis, and lead to pelvic obliquity. Scoliosis cannot be controlled by orthoses or wheelchair seating systems (72,84,93–97). Orthotic management, although it may slow curve progression, does not slow the systemic manifestations of Duchenne muscular dystrophy (e.g., decreasing pulmonary function and cardiomyopathy). These may complicate spinal surgery at a later time. As the scoliosis progresses, it can result in a loss of sitting balance, produce abnormal pressure, and occasionally cause the patient to become bedridden (98). Heller et al. (99) reported improved sitting support with an orthosis in 28 patients who either refused surgery or who were felt to be inoperable.

Surgical correction of scoliosis both improves sitting balance and minimizes pelvic obliquity (84,85,96–98,100, 101). It is usually recommended that a posterior spinal fusion be performed once the curve is greater than 20 degrees (84,85,95–98,101–104). Fusion extends from the upper thoracic spine (T2 or T4) to L5 or the pelvis. It is important to center the patient's head over the pelvis in both the coronal and sagittal planes. This usually allows complete or almost complete correction of the deformity. This maintains sitting balance, improves head control, and allows more independent hand function. Although autogenous bone grafting is used in most patients, there appears to be no difference in fusion rates when allograft bone is used (105–108). Segmental spinal instrumentation techniques using Luque rod instrumentation are most commonly used [➡2.5,2.6] (57,84,85,88,95,100,101,105,106,109–112). Other segmental instrumentation systems, such as Cotrel-Dubousset, TSRH, Isola, and others, can also be used (105,106,110,113). These allow sufficient fixation, so that postoperative immobilization is not necessary (Fig. 17-2). Fixation to the pelvis is achieved using the Galveston or other techniques (102,105,109,110,112,113,115). The latter is felt to maintain better correction of pelvic obliquity. Some authors believe that fusion to L5 is sufficient and that there will be no spinopelvic deformity throughout the remainder of the patient's life (55,107,116,117). However, a postoperative spinopelvic deformity can occur and progress and most authors recommend fusion to the pelvis. Mubarak et al. (88,116) recommend fusion to L5 if the curve is greater than 20 degrees, the FVC is greater than 40%, and the patient is using a wheelchair full time, except for occasional standing. If the patient's curve is greater than 40 degrees or if there is pelvic obliquity greater than 10 degrees, then fusion to the sacropelvis is recommended.

Careful preoperative evaluation, including pulmonary function studies and cardiology consultation, is mandatory because of the associated pulmonary and cardiac abnormalities and the risk for malignant hyperthermia (98,118–121). Children with Duchenne muscular dystrophy have a decreased FVC beginning when they are about 10 years of age due to weakness of the intercostal muscles and associated contractures. There is a linear decrease over time (18,85,91,98,101,104,118). Kurz et al. (18) observed a 4% decrease in percentage of FVC for each year of age or each 10 degrees of scoliosis. It stabilizes at about 25% of normal

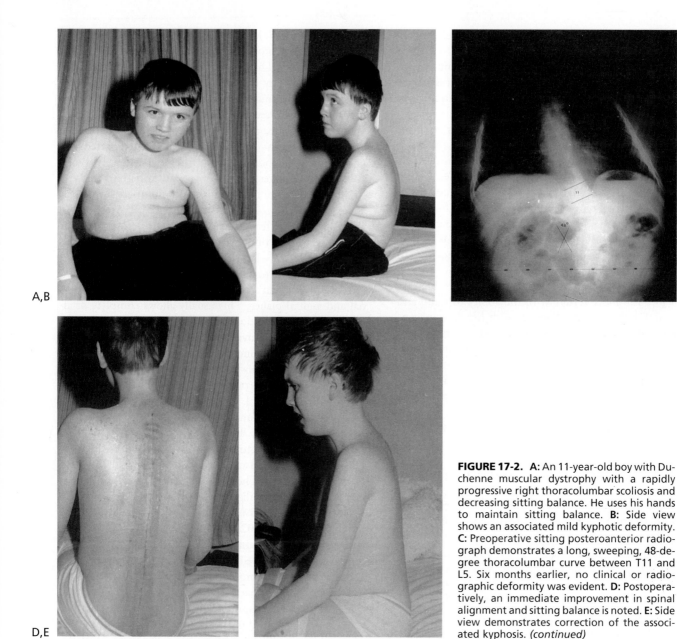

FIGURE 17-2. **A:** An 11-year-old boy with Duchenne muscular dystrophy with a rapidly progressive right thoracolumbar scoliosis and decreasing sitting balance. He uses his hands to maintain sitting balance. **B:** Side view shows an associated mild kyphotic deformity. **C:** Preoperative sitting posteroanterior radiograph demonstrates a long, sweeping, 48-degree thoracolumbar curve between T11 and L5. Six months earlier, no clinical or radiographic deformity was evident. **D:** Postoperatively, an immediate improvement in spinal alignment and sitting balance is noted. **E:** Side view demonstrates correction of the associated kyphosis. *(continued)*

until death. The presence of severe scoliosis may increase the rate of decline in the FVC. Jenkins et al. reported that when the FVC is 30% or less there is an increasing risk for postoperative complication, such as pneumonia and respiratory failure (118). Other authors have made similar observations (18,98,101). Smith et al. (91) found that most patients with curves of more than 35 degrees had FVC less than 40% of predicted normal values, and therefore recommended that spinal arthrodesis be considered for all patients with Duchenne muscular dystrophy when they can no longer walk. Nevertheless, successful surgery can be performed in many patients with FVC as low as 20% of predicted normal valves (106).

It is debated whether spinal stabilization increases the quantity of life, although it definitely increases the quality of the remaining life (85,106,109). In a study of 55 patients with Duchenne muscular dystrophy, of which 32 underwent spinal fusion and 23 did not, Galasko et al. (85) found that FVC remained stable in the operated group for 36 months postoperatively and then fell slightly. In the nonoperated group it progressively declined. The survival data showed that a significantly higher mortality rate was seen in the nonoperated group. This study indicated that spinal stabilization can increase survival for several years if it is done early before significant progression has occurred. Other studies, however, have shown that posterior spinal

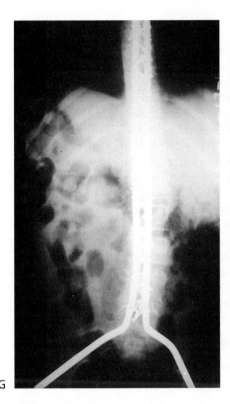
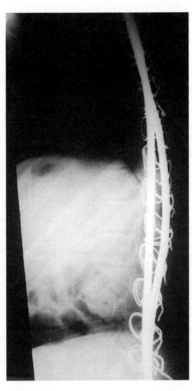

F,G

FIGURE 17-2. *(continued)* **F:** Postoperative sitting radiograph after posterior spinal fusion and Luque rod instrumentation from T4 to the sacrum. The Galveston technique, with insertion of the Luque rod into the wing of the ilium, was used for pelvic fixation. Almost complete correction of his spinal deformity was achieved. **G:** Postoperative lateral radiograph shows improved sagittal alignment.

fusion has no effect on the steady decline in pulmonary function when compared with unoperated patients (103,106,122–124). In addition to correction and stabilization of the spine, patients experience improved quality of life measures, such as function, self image, and cosmesis (103,109,110,125). Parents also reported improved ability to provide care to their child.

Complications are common during and following surgery (85,95–97,103,110,116). These include excessive intraoperative blood loss, neurologic injury, cardiopulmonary compromise, postoperative infection, wound healing, curve progression, hardware problems, and late pseudarthrosis. With respect to intraoperative blood loss, this can be minimized by early surgery and the use of hypotensive anesthesia (107). The increased intraoperative blood loss in patients with Duchenne muscular dystrophy appears to be due to the lack of dystrophin in the smooth muscle, which inhibits normal vasocontraction (126).

The role of intraoperative spinal cord monitoring in children with Duchenne muscular dystrophy is controversial. Noordeen et al. reported that a 50% decrease in amplitude was suggestive of neurologic impairment (127).

Wheelchair. A wheelchair is necessary for patients who are no longer capable of independent ambulation. This is typically a motorized wheelchair to allow the patient to be independent of parents or aides, especially while attending school. The wheelchair may be fitted with a balanced mobile arm orthosis for the purpose of facilitating personal hygiene and feeding (64,65).

Cardiopulmonary Management. Respiratory failure in Duchenne muscular dystrophy is a constant threat and is the most common cause of death early in the third decade of life. Kurz et al. (18) found the vital capacity peaks at the age when standing ceases, then declines rapidly thereafter. The development of scoliosis compounds the problems and leads to further diminution of the vital capacity (123). The complication rate in spinal surgery increases when the FVC is less than 30% of expected. Programs of vigorous respiratory therapy and the use of home negative-pressure and positive-pressure ventilators may allow patients with Duchenne muscular dystrophy to survive into the third and fourth decades of life (128–131).

Cardiac failure may also occur in the second decade of life. After initially responding to digitalis and diuretics, the involved cardiac muscle becomes flabby and the patient goes into congestive heart failure. Myocardial infarction has been reported in boys as young as 10 years of age. There is no correlation between the severity of pulmonary dysfunction and cardiac function or between age and cardiac function (132). The cardiomyopathy of Duchenne muscular dystrophy exists clinically as a separate entity.

Genetic and Psychologic Counseling

Proper diagnosis and early genetic counseling may help prevent birth of additional male infants with Duchenne muscular dystrophy. It must be remembered that approximately 20% of families have already conceived and delivered a second involved male infant before the diagnosis is made in the first (63,133). Genetic counseling with parents and family groups is important in the management of psychological problems arising when the genetic nature of the diagnosis becomes known.

Becker Muscular Dystrophy

Becker muscular dystrophy is similar to Duchenne muscular dystrophy in clinical appearance and distribution of weakness, but it is less severe (134,135). Onset is generally after the age of 7 years and the rate of progression is slower. The patients usually remain ambulatory until adolescence or early adult years. The Gower maneuver may occur as the weakness progresses (Fig. 17-3). Pseudohypertrophy of the calf is common, and eventually equinus and cavus foot deformities develop (Fig. 17-4). Cardiac involvement is frequent. There may be a family history of atypical muscular dystrophy. Pulmonary problems are less severe and the patient's life expectancy is longer.

Treatment

The treatment of the musculoskeletal deformities associated with Becker muscular dystrophy is essentially the same as with Duchenne muscular dystrophy. Ankle and forefoot equinus occur commonly. Shapiro and Specht (4) have reported good success with the Vulpius tendo Achillis lengthening in patients with equinus contractures. A tibialis posterior tendon transfer is performed if necessary [➥**7.19**]. Forefoot equinus may require a plantar release and possibly a midfoot dorsal-wedge osteotomy for correction. The use of orthotics is also beneficial because the rate of progression is slower and the remaining muscle strength greater than in Duchenne muscular dystrophy. The incidence of scoliosis is high, especially in those adolescents who have ceased walking. These patients require careful evaluation and periodic spinal radiographs. Posterior spinal fusion and segmental instrumentation, usually Luque, are beneficial when progression occurs [➥**2.5,2.6**] (134).

Emery-Dreifuss Muscular Dystrophy

Emery-Dreifuss muscular dystrophy is an uncommon sex-linked recessive disorder characterized by early contractures and cardiomyopathy (16). The typical phenotype is seen only in males, although milder or partial phenotypes have been reported in female carriers (137–140). Involved males

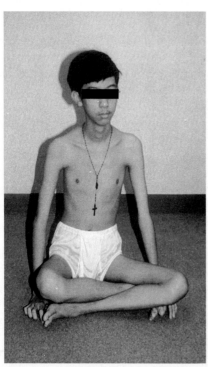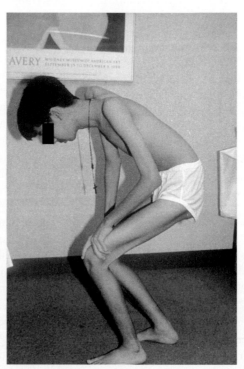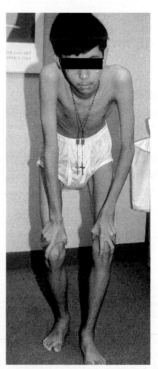

A,B   C

FIGURE 17-3. A: A 13-year-old boy with suspected Becker muscular dystrophy uses the Gower maneuver to stand from a sitting position. **B:** Manually assisted knee extension is necessary to achieve upright stance. **C:** Front view.

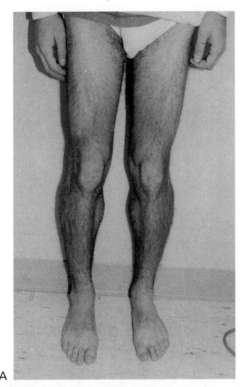 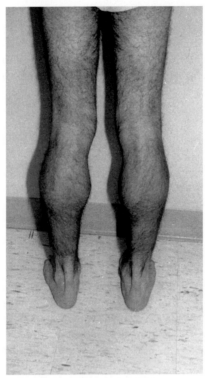

FIGURE 17-4. A: Pseudohypertrophy of the calves in an 18-year-old man with Becker muscular dystrophy. He is a brace-free ambulator. **B:** Posterior view.

show mild muscle weakness in the first 10 years of life and a tendency for toe walking. The Gower maneuver may be present in young children. The distinctive clinical criteria occur in late childhood or early adolescence. These include tendo Achillis contractures, elbow flexion contractures, neck extension contracture, tightness of the lumbar paravertebral muscles, and cardiac abnormalities involving brachycardia and first-degree, and eventually complete, heart block (139–141). The muscle weakness is slowly progressive but there may be some stabilization in adulthood. Most patients are able to ambulate into the fifth and sixth decades of life. Obesity and untreated equinus contractures can lead to the loss of ambulatory ability at an earlier age (4).

The CPK level in patients with Emery-Dreifuss muscular dystrophy is only mildly or moderately elevated. EMG and muscle biopsy are myopathic. The diagnosis of this form of muscular dystrophy should be considered in patients with a myopathic phenotype after Duchenne and Becker muscular dystrophies have been ruled out, usually by dystrophin testing (4). The condition must also be distinguished from scapuloperoneal muscular dystrophy and the rigid spine syndrome (142).

Genetic and Molecular Biology Studies

The gene locus for Emery-Dreifuss muscular dystrophy has been localized to the long arm of the X chromosome at Xq28 in linkage studies (143,144).

Treatment

The treatment of Emery-Dreifuss muscular dystrophy is similar to that used for other forms of muscular dystrophy. The goals are to prevent or correct deformities and maximize function. Treatment modalities include physical therapy, correction of soft tissue contractures, spinal stabilization, and cardiologic intervention.

Physical Therapy. This can be useful in the management of neck extension contractures, elbow flexion contractures, and the tightness of the lumbar paravertebral muscles. Decreased neck flexion, which is characteristic of this disorder, can begin as early as the first decade, but usually is not present until the second decade. This is due to contracture of the extensor muscles and the ligamentum nuchae. According to Shapiro and Specht (4), this does not progress past neutral. Lateral bending and rotation of the neck also become limited as the extensor contractures progress. Physical therapy can be beneficial in maintaining limited flexion of the neck.

Soft Tissue Contractures. Tendo Achillis lengthening and posterior ankle capsulotomy combined with anterior transfer of the tibialis posterior tendon can be beneficial in providing long-term stabilization of the foot and ankle [➟**7.1,7.16,7.19**] (4,139). Elbow flexion contractures usually do not require treatment. These contractures can be as severe as 90 degrees, although most do not exceed 35 degrees (4,98). Full flexion from this position and normal forearm pronation and supination are preserved. Physical therapy may be beneficial to slow the progress of the elbow flexion contractures. Surgery has not been shown to be beneficial.

Spinal Stabilization. Scoliosis is common in this form of muscular dystrophy, but it has a lower incidence of progression. This has been attributed to contractures at the lumbar and ultimately the thoracic paravertebral muscles, which seem to prevent progression (4,139). Those patients with scoliosis need to be followed closely, but most do not require treatment. Curves that progress beyond 40 degrees may require surgical stabilization.

Cardiologic Intervention. Sudden death due to severe bradycardia caused by complete heart block has been a major cause of death in these patients. Most do not have cardiac symptoms preceding death. Merlini et al. (141) reported that 30 of 73 patients with Emery-Dreifuss muscular dystrophy died suddenly, and only four were symptomatic. It is recommended that a cardiac pacemaker be inserted shortly after confirmation of the diagnosis (141,145).

AUTOSOMAL RECESSIVE MUSCULAR DYSTROPHIES

Limb-girdle Muscular Dystrophy

Limb-girdle muscular dystrophy is common and may be more benign than the other forms of muscular dystrophy. It is a rather heterogeneous group of disorders with various classifications proposed for it over the years. The age of onset and rate of progression of muscle weakness are variable. It usually begins in the second or third decade of life. It is transmitted as an autosomal recessive trait, but an autosomal dominant pattern of inheritance has been reported in some families (146,147).

The symptoms of limb-girdle muscular dystrophy are similar to fascioscapulohumeral muscular dystrophy, except that the facial muscles are not involved. The initial muscle weakness involves either the pelvic or shoulder girdle. The rate of progression is usually slow, with soft tissue contractures and disability developing 20 years or more after the onset. The patients remain ambulatory for many years.

The distribution of weakness is similar to that seen in Duchenne and Becker muscular dystrophies. The iliopsoas, gluteus maximus, and quadriceps muscles are involved early in the disease process. Usually, shoulder girdle involvement occurs at about the same time. The serratus anterior, trapezius, rhomboid, latissimus dorsi, and sternal portions of pectoralis major muscles are affected most often. The disease

later spreads to involve other muscles, such as the biceps brachia and the clavicular portion of the pectoralis major. Deltoid involvement may occur but is usually late. Weakness may involve the distal muscles of the limbs, such as the wrist and finger flexors and extensors, in the more severely involved individuals.

Two forms of limb-girdle muscular dystrophy include a more common pelvic-girdle type and a scapulohumeral form. The latter is rare, with symptoms involving primarily the shoulder girdle. Involvement of the pelvic girdle may not occur for many years. In the pelvic-girdle type, there is weakness of the hip extensors and abductors, resulting in accentuated lumbar lordosis, gait abnormalities, and hip instability.

The CPK level is moderately elevated in patients with limb girdle muscular dystrophy. The clinical characteristics are indistinguishable from those of sporadic Becker muscular dystrophy, carriers of Duchenne or Becker muscular dystrophies, and those of childhood acid-maltase deficiency (4). Thus, a dystrophin assay is essential in establishing the diagnosis.

Treatment of limb-girdle muscular dystrophy is similar to that for Duchenne and Becker muscular dystrophies. Significant scoliosis rarely occurs because of the late onset of the disease process. When present, it usually is mild and does not require treatment (136). Involved individuals usually succumb to their disease process before 40 years of age.

Genetic and Molecular Biology Studies

The autosomal recessive form has been linked to chromosome 15q and the autosomal dominant form to 5q (148,149).

Infantile Fascioscapulohumeral Muscular Dystrophy

Infantile fascioscapulohumeral muscular dystrophy (IFSH MD) has been recognized with increasing frequency. It is a more severe variant of the more common later-onset fascioscapulohumeral muscular dystrophy (150–153). It appears to be autosomal recessive, but the affected gene has not been identified. Facial diplegia is noted in infancy, followed by sensorineural hearing loss in childhood (mean age, 5 years). A Möbius type of facial weakness may also be present and progress asymptomatically at a relatively slow pace (154). Ambulation begins at a normal age, but because of progressive muscle weakness, most patients become wheelchair-bound during the second decade of life. Weakness causes the child to walk with the hands and forearms folded across the upper buttocks to provide support for the weak gluteus maximus muscles (4,150,153). This marked lumbar lordosis is progressive and is almost pathognomonic for IFSH

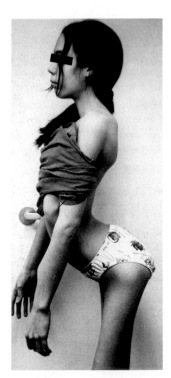

FIGURE 17-5. Marked lumbar lordosis in a 15-year-old girl with infantile fascioscapulohumeral muscular dystrophy. She is still ambulatory but having increasing back pain.

MD (Fig. 17-5). The lordosis leads to fixed hip flexion contractures after the patient is wheelchair-dependent. Equinus or equinovarus deformities and scoliosis occur less frequently.

Treatment

The treatment of patients with IFSH MD is individualized because most patients do not have significant orthopaedic deformities. These patients usually have severely compromised pulmonary functions and succumb in early adolescence. Shapiro et al. outlined the possible treatment modalities for children with IFSH MD. Flexible equinus and equinovarus deformities respond well to AFOs (153). Occasionally, a Vulpius-type tendo Achillis lengthening may be necessary (75). Hip flexion contractures usually do not require treatment in ambulatory patients and it may decrease function. Spinal orthoses control the lordosis but do not provide correction because the spine remains flexible early in the course of the disorder. Because an orthosis interferes with ambulation it is usually not employed. When wheelchair use is full-time, a modified wheelchair with an orthosis may be beneficial, or perhaps a posterior spinal fusion and segmental instrumentation, depending on the severity of the deformity (88). Scapulothoracic stabilization is not necessary because the severity of dysfunction is so severe that

minimal or no improvement in shoulder function can be achieved.

AUTOSOMAL DOMINANT MUSCULAR DYSTROPHIES

Fascioscapulohumeral Muscular Dystrophy

Fascioscapulohumeral muscular dystrophy is an autosomal dominant disorder having variable expression (155). The disease is manifest by muscular weakness of the face, shoulder girdle, and upper arm. It is caused by a gene defect, *FRG1,* on chromosome 4q35 (156,157). There is selective sparing of the deltoid, the distal part of the pectoralis major muscle, and the erector spinae muscles. This results in decreased scapulothoracic motion, with scapular winging and a marked decrease in shoulder flexion and abduction. Glenohumeral motion is usually preserved. The onset may occur at any age but is most common in late childhood or early adulthood. It occurs in both genders but is more common in females. Abortive or mild cases are common. Progression is insidious and periods of apparent arrest may occur. Cardiac involvement and central nervous system involvement are absent. Life expectancy is relatively good.

Initially, the face and shoulder girdle muscles are involved but they may be affected only mildly for many years. Facial signs, which may be present at infancy, include lack of mobility, incomplete eye closure, pouting lips with a transverse smile, and absence of eye and forehead wrinkles. It tends to produce a "popeye" appearance. The shoulder girdle weakness leads to scapular winging. The weight of the upper extremities, together with the weakness of the trapezius, permits the clavicles to assume a more horizontal position. It also leads to a forward-sloping appearance of the shoulders. As the disease progresses, pelvic girdle and tibialis anterior muscle involvement may also occur (150). Scoliosis is rare because of the late onset of the disease process (5).

The CPK levels in patients with fascioscapulohumeral muscular dystrophy are usually normal. The diagnosis is made by physical examination and muscle biopsy (158).

Treatment

The winging of the scapula, with weakness of shoulder flexion and abduction, is the major orthopaedic problem in fascioscapulohumeral muscular dystrophy. The deltoid, supraspinatus, and intraspinatus muscles are usually normal, however, or minimally involved. Posterior scapulocostal fusion or stabilization (scapuloplexy) by a variety of techniques can be beneficial in restoring mechanical advantage of the deltoid and rotator cuff muscles (159–165). This can result in increased active abduction and forward flexion of the shoulder and improved function, as well as cosmesis. Jakab and Gledhill (162) reported the results of a simplified technique for scapulocostal fusion. The technique involves wiring of the medial border of the scapula to ribs three through seven. Internal fixation is achieved with 16-gauge wire. The wires ensure firm fixation and eliminate the need for postoperative immobilization and subsequent rehabilitation. The child uses a sling for 3 to 4 days postoperatively, then begins a physical therapy program. They found that shoulder flexion increased 28 degrees (range, 20–40 degrees) and abduction 27 degrees (range, 20–35 degrees) at a mean follow-up of 2.9 years. This allowed all patients to raise their arms and hands above their heads, conferring a greater mechanical advantage. The beneficial effects do not seem to deteriorate with time (159–161,165).

Distal Muscular Dystrophy

This is a rare form of muscular dystrophy. It is also known as Gower muscular dystrophy. It typically begins after 45 years of age. It is transmitted as an autosomal dominant trait. The initial involvement is in the intrinsic muscles of the hand. The disease process spreads proximally. In the lower extremities the calves and tibialis anterior are first involved. The absence of sensory, especially vibratory, abnormalities differentiates this from Charcot-Marie-Tooth disease.

Ocular Muscular Dystrophy

Ocular muscular dystrophy, also known as "progressive external ophthalmoplegia," is another rare form of muscular dystrophy. It typically begins in the adolescent years. The extraocular muscles are affected, resulting in diplopia and ptosis. This is followed by limitation of ocular movement (166). The upper facial muscles are often affected. The disease is slowly progressive and may involve the proximal upper extremities. The pelvis can be involved late in the disease process. Most patients with this disorder have an identifiable mitochondrial myopathy (167).

Oculopharyngeal Muscular Dystrophy

This form of muscular dystrophy begins in the third decade of life and is particularly common in French Canadians (168,169). Pharyngeal muscle involvement results in dysarthria and dysphasia, which leads to repetitive regurgitation and weight loss. This condition necessitates cricopharyngeal myotomy, which does not alter pharyngeal function (170,171). Ptosis develops in middle life. This disorder is inherited in an autosomal dominant pattern with complete penetrance (168).

MYOTONIA

Myotonia is a group of disorders characterized by the inability of skeletal muscle to relax after a strong contraction from either voluntary movement or mechanical stimulation. This is best demonstrated by a slow relaxation of a clenched fist. The most common myotonias include myotonic dystrophy, congenital myotonic dystrophy, and myotonia congenita. These are all rare disorders that are transmitted by autosomal dominant inheritance (4,20).

Myotonic Dystrophy

Myotonic dystrophy is a systemic disorder characterized by myotonia, progressive muscle weakness, gonadal atrophy, cataracts, frontal baldness, heart disease, and dementia (172). The genetic defect is located on chromosome 19q (19,173). The distal musculature is affected first and the myotonia begins to disappear as muscle weakness progresses. Onset is usually in late adolescence or early adulthood. In women the diagnosis is frequently made only after they have given birth to a child who is more severely involved. The disease spreads slowly proximally and involves the quadriceps, hamstrings, and eventually the hip extensors. The lower extremities are more involved than the upper extremities. The most common presenting symptoms are weakness of the hands and difficulty in walking. Patients may be unable to relax the fingers after shaking hands and may need to palmar flex the hand to open the fingers. Muscles of the face, mandible, eyes, neck, and distal limbs may also be affected. The levels of serum enzymes are normal. Muscle biopsies show type I atrophy of the muscle fibers and the presence of some internal nuclei (11). These are nonspecific findings. The "dive-bomber" pattern on EMG is diagnostic (4).

Examination reveals an expressionless face, ptosis, and a fish mouth that is difficult to close. There is marked wasting of the temporal, masseter, and sternocleidomastoid muscles. Deep tendon reflexes are diminished or lost. Slit lamp examination of the eyes reveals that most patients have lenticular opacities, cataracts, and retinopathy. Cardiac involvement is also common and includes mitral valve prolapse and arrhythmias (174). Organic brain deterioration may also occur. Frontal baldness in men and glaucoma in both genders occurs in midadult life. The course of the disease is one of steady deterioration. Most patients lose the ability to ambulate within 15 to 20 years of onset of symptoms (174). There are no characteristic orthopaedic deformities, although a slight tendency toward increased hindfoot varus has been observed (4). Life span is shortened, and death is usually caused by pneumonia or cardiac failure.

Treatment of myotonic dystrophy is primarily orthotic because the onset is usually after skeletal maturity. An AFO may be beneficial in patients with a drop foot due to weakness of the tibialis anterior and peroneal muscles.

Congenital Myotonic Dystrophy

This is a relatively common muscle disorder of variable expression that occurs most frequently with a mother who has either a forme fruste or mild clinical involvement (175–178). Although it has autosomal dominant transmission, it is predominantly transmitted maternally (177). This is an exception in autosomal dominant disorders and indicates additional maternal factors. Approximately 40% of patients have severe involvement or die in infancy, whereas 60% will be affected later (179). The child may have an expressionless, long, narrow face; hypotonia; delayed developmental milestones; facial diplegia; difficulty feeding due to pharyngolaryngeal palsy; respiratory failure; and mild mental retardation (180). Swallowing improves with growth but the hypotonia persists. Examination shows diffuse weakness and absent deep tendon reflexes. It can appear to be similar to spinal muscular atrophy. Ambulation is usually delayed. If the mother is the carrier, there may be other organic disorders later in life (180). Cataracts usually occur after 14 years of age.

The defective gene has been localized to chromosome 19, and a test for prenatal diagnosis is available (181). There appears to be an expansion of a highly repeated sequence of three nucleotides: cytosine, thymine, and guanine. The trinucleotide repeat is at the 3′ end of a protein kinase gene on chromosome 19, which lengthens as it passed from one generation to another. The length of the sequence correlates with the severity of the disorder.

Orthopaedic problems in congenital myotonia dystrophy include congenital hip dislocation and talipes equinovarus (i.e., clubfeet). There is a tendency to develop soft tissue contractures of other major joints of the lower extremities. Clubfeet may behave like those in arthrogryposis multiplex congenita (182). Serial casting may be tried, but most require surgery, such as an extensive, complete release [➡7.1]. If this fails, a talectomy or Verebelyi-Ogston procedure may be useful (183). Scoliosis is also common and may require orthotic or surgical intervention (136). Because life expectancy is at least to the early adult years, aggressive orthopaedic management improves the quality of life.

Myotonia Congenita

Myotonia congenita is usually present at birth, but does not become clinically apparent until after 10 years of age. In some cases it may present as low back pain or impaired athletic ability (184–186). The severity of the myotonia varies considerably. The distribution is widespread, although it is more marked in the lower extremities than the upper extremities (187). Myotonia is most evident with initial movement. Repetitive movement decreases the myotonia and facilitates later movements. Usually, within 3 to 4 minutes stiffness disappears and normal activities including running are possible. Some patients appear herculean be-

cause of generalized muscle hypertrophy, particularly in the buttocks, thighs, and calves. Children with myotonia congenita have no associated weakness and no other endocrine or systemic abnormalities. The disease is compatible with a normal life span. A patient's disability is not great when the limits of the disease have been accepted. Procainamide and diphenylhydantoin (Dilantin) have been used with some success to decrease the myotonia, but they should be used only in severe cases (188). There are no characteristic orthopaedic deformities (4). The disorder, a chloride channelopathy, is caused by various mutations in the skeletal muscle voltage-gated chloride channel gene *ClC-1* (189,190).

CONGENITAL MYOPATHIES AND CONGENITAL MUSCULAR DYSTROPHY

Congenital myopathies and congenital muscular dystrophy present as a hypotonic or floppy baby at birth or in early infancy. When these conditions occur in an older child, they can present as muscle weakness (191–194). These disorders are not well understood clinically or at the molecular level. The diagnostic categorization is not uniform or predictive. They are defined histologically from muscle biopsies (4,10,11,192,194–196). When the biopsy findings are abnormal but not dystrophic, the patient is diagnosed as having a nonspecific myopathy (4). When considerable fibrosis is present along with necrotic fibers, congenital muscular dystrophy may be diagnosed (194).

CONGENITAL MYOPATHIES

The congenital myopathies include: central core disease, nemaline myopathy (rod-body myopathy), myotubular myopathy (centronuclear), congenital fiber-type disproportion and metabolic myopathies. Differentiation between these types can be accomplished through histochemical analysis and electron microscopy of muscle biopsy specimens (4,10,11,194–196).

Central Core Disease

Central core disease is a nonprogressive autosomal dominant congenital myopathy that frequently presents in infancy with hypotonia or in young children with delayed motor developmental milestones (10,192,195–198). Independent ambulation may not be achieved until 4 years of age. The distribution of muscle involvement is similar to that found in Duchenne muscular dystrophy, with the trunk and lower extremities being more involved than upper extremities and the proximal muscles more than the distal muscle groups. The pelvic girdle is more involved than the shoulder. Use of the Gower maneuver is common. No deterioration in strength occurs with time, sensation is normal, and the deep tendon reflexes are either deceased or absent. Muscle wasting is a common finding, but progression of muscle weakness is rare. Muscle biopsies show mostly type I fibers containing central round or oval regions that are devoid of oxidative enzymes, adenosine triphosphate activity, and mitochondria. Serum CPK and nerve conduction studies are normal, whereas EMGs show myopathic abnormalities. Scoliosis, soft tissue contractures, congenital hip subluxation and dislocation, talipes equinovarus, pes planus, and hypermobility of joints (especially the patella) are the most common musculoskeletal problems and can require treatment (197–201). Scoliotic deformities have patterns similar to those of idiopathic scoliosis, progress rapidly, and tend to be rigid. Posterior spinal fusion and segmental instrumentation yields satisfactory results [➡2.9] (200). Soft tissue contractures about the hip and knee may need to be released. Clubfeet require extensive soft tissue releases to achieve correction [➡7.1]. Congenital dislocation of the hip can be treated by open or closed reduction techniques, but the recurrence rate is high and may require osseous procedures, such as pelvic or proximal femoral osteotomies (201). Central core disease is one of the disorders in which patients are susceptible to malignant hyperthermia. This association with malignant hyperthermia has led to linkage of both disorders to the long arm of chromosome 19 (202,203).

Nemaline Myopathy

Nemaline, or rod-body myopathy, is a variable congenital myopathy that usually begins in infancy or early childhood, with hypotonia affecting all skeletal muscles (4,10, 194–196,204–206). There is no involvement of cardiac muscle. Elongated facies, with a high-arched palette and a nasal, high-pitched voice, frequently are noted. Skeletal changes may resemble those seen in arachnodactyly. Martinez and Lake, in a review of the literature regarding 99 patients, recognized these forms: neonatal (severe), congenital (moderate), and adult onset (204). The neonatal form is characterized by severe hypotonia, with 90% mortality in the first 3 years of life due to respiratory insufficiency. The mean survival after birth was 16 months. The moderate congenital form, which is the most common and prototypic, is diagnosed during or after the neonatal period and has mild or moderate hypotonia, weakness, and delayed developmental milestones. Most patients begin to walk at 2 to 4 years of age, and the weakness is usually nonprogressive or only slowly progressive. The mortality rate is about 5%. Those who die are usually neonates. Death is typically from severe involvement of the pharyngeal and respiratory muscles (207–209). The adult-onset form is characterized by proximal weakness that occasionally progresses acutely. There is no correlation between the number of rods and the phenotype in nemaline myopathy (205).

Soft tissue contractures are uncommon in nemaline myopathy. The major musculoskeletal problems are scoliosis and lumbar lordosis. Posterior spinal fusion and segmental instrumentation [➡2.9] may be indicated in progressive scoliotic deformities (4). Lower extremity orthoses can be beneficial in providing joint stability and aiding ambulation. Because of diminished pulmonary function and a risk for malignant hyperthermia, patients undergoing surgery require careful administration of anesthesia and monitoring (210).

Centronuclear Myopathy

Centronuclear (i.e., myotubular) myopathy is a disorder of considerable variability (10,195,196,211). Muscle biopsies demonstrate persistent myotubes of fetal life (212,213). There are X-linked recessive, autosomal recessive, and autosomal dominant forms (211,214). The defect in the X-linked recessive form is at the locus Xq28. Children have varying degrees of weakness, generally noted in infancy. Patients with X-linked recessive forms are usually severely involved and die in infancy. The autosomal recessive form is hypotonic at birth, but is not progressive and may improve with time. Most of these children are able to walk. They may have a myopathic facies, high-arched palate, and proximal muscle weakness. There is an increased incidence of cavovarus foot deformities, scoliosis, lumbar lordosis, and scapular winging (10). By late adolescence or early adult life, some patients lose their ability to ambulate.

Congenital Fiber-type Disproportion

Congenital fiber-type disproportion is characterized by generalized hypotonia at or shortly after birth. The histologic criteria from muscle biopsies to diagnose this disorder include a predominance in number and a reduction in size of type I fibers and relatively large type II fibers (10,11). It is recognized as a nonspecific pathologic change that occurs in many patients and has a myopathic, neuropathic, or central nervous system origin (10,215). The degree of weakness is variable, and sequential examinations determine the prognosis. Most patients become ambulatory. The most serious problem is life-threatening respiratory infections during the first years of life. Proximal muscle weakness is frequently associated with acetabular dysplasia (215,216). To prevent postural contractures from developing an appropriate lower extremity splint should be used until the patient achieves ambulation. Severe, rigid scoliosis can occur. Orthoses are usually ineffective, and early spinal arthrodesis may be necessary (4).

Metabolic Myopathies

These myopathies represent a broad spectrum of metabolic abnormalities that are generally clinically evident in the first two decades of life (217). These include disorders of glycogenesis and mitochondrial dysfunction. Myopathies caused by metabolic error in the first step of glycolysis are clinically associated with exercise intolerance, in which there are myophosphorylase and phosphofructokinase deficiencies, or with progressive muscle weakness and wasting, in which there are acid maltase or debrancher enzyme deficiencies (218). Defects in the second step of glycogenesis are associated with exercise intolerance. Myopathies caused by deficiencies in mitochondrial enzymes are less well defined and may be associated with severe benign exercise intolerance and progressive myopathic syndromes (218–220).

CONGENITAL MUSCULAR DYSTROPHY

Congenital muscular dystrophy is a rare disorder that generally presents as a floppy baby during infancy, with generalized muscle weakness with involvement of respiratory and facial muscles (221). It is a muscle disorder in which the muscle biopsy demonstrates dystrophic features characterized by considerable perimysial and endomysial fibrosis (194). It is different from Duchenne muscular dystrophy and Becker muscular dystrophy because it affects both males and females, is not associated with massively elevated levels of CPK, does not involve abnormalities of the dystrophin gene or protein, and is associated with a more variable prognosis (4). There are several forms of congenital muscular dystrophy. In one, the infant is weak at birth. Many have severe stiffness of joints, whereas others do not. A few infants have rapid progression and do not survive after the first year of life. Most, however, stabilize and survive into adulthood (222). Another type is seen in Japanese infants and has been termed "Fukuyama congenital muscular dystrophy." It is characterized by a marked developmental defect in the central nervous system (223,224). There is progressive muscle degeneration and mental retardation. Severe joint contractures develop, and many involved children die in the first decade of life. Merosin-deficient congenital muscular dystrophy is associated with white matter changes on brain MRI, and has been linked to chromosome 6q2 (225,226).

Common orthopaedic problems include congenital hip dislocation and subluxation, tendo Achillis contractures, and talipes equinovarus (Fig. 17-6). Because most survive, aggressive orthopaedic management is warranted. This may include physical therapy, orthoses, soft tissue releases, and perhaps osteotomy (4,227). Early physical therapy may be beneficial in the prevention of soft tissue contractures. Soft

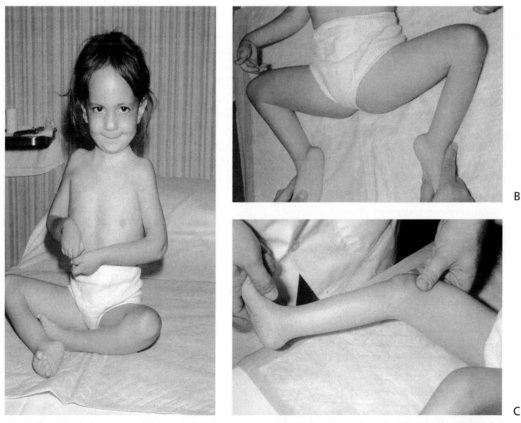

FIGURE 17-6. A: Clinical photograph of a 3-year-old girl with congenital muscular dystrophy. Observe the position of the upper and lower extremities. **B:** The hips are flexed, abducted, and externally rotated. **C:** Moderate knee flexion contractures are present.

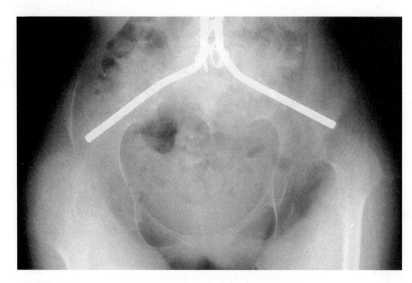

FIGURE 17-7. Pelvic radiograph of an 11-year-old girl with congenital muscular dystrophy, 3 years after posterior spinal fusion and Luque rod instrumentation, including the Galveston technique. She is wheelchair-dependent and has developed bilateral asymptomatic hip dislocations despite extensive soft tissue releases in early childhood.

tissue releases in the treatment of congenital dislocation of the hip are characterized by a high incidence of recurrent dislocation (Fig. 17-7) (227). Progressive scoliosis may be initially treated by an orthosis, although most require surgical stabilization similar to other forms of muscular dystrophy.

SPINAL MUSCULAR ATROPHY

Spinal muscular atrophy is a group of disorders characterized by degeneration of the anterior horn cells of the spinal cord and occasionally the neurons of the lower bulbar motor nuclei, resulting in muscle weakness and atrophy (228–232). They are autosomal recessive disorders that occur in about 1 in 20,000 live births (233). The loss of anterior horn cells is considered to be an acute event without progression. The neurologic deterioration may stabilize and remain unchanged for long periods (234,235). The progression of muscle weakness is a reflection of normal growth that exceeds muscle reserve. Respiratory function is compromised, and atelectasis and pneumonia are the usual causes of death.

Clinical Classification

The clinical features of spinal muscular atrophy vary widely and are based on the age at onset and the functional capacity of the child at the time of diagnosis. This has led to the disorder being classified into three types. These include type I (severe), or acute Werdnig-Hoffman disease; type II (intermediate), or chronic Werdnig-Hoffman disease; and type III (mild), or Kugelberg-Welander disease (236,237). All three are a spectrum of the same disorder, but each has specific diagnostic criteria and prognosis. There is a considerable overlap between these three disorders, however, and most authors consider them to be a single disorder—spinal muscular atrophy (238). Generally, the earlier the onset, the worse the prognosis.

Type I, Acute Werdnig-Hoffman Disease

The Type I spinal muscular atrophy is characterized by clinical onset between birth and 6 months of age. These children typically have severe involvement with marked weakness and hypotonia. They usually die from respiratory failure between 1 and 24 months of age. Because of their young age and severe involvement, they usually do not require orthopaedic intervention. Pathologic multiple fractures may occur due to *in utero* osteoporosis secondary to decreased movement at birth and suggest osteogenesis imperfecta (239). These fractures heal rapidly with immobilization.

Type II, Chronic Werdnig-Hoffman Disease

The clinical onset of type II spinal muscular atrophy varies between 6 and 24 months of age. These children are less involved than those with type I spinal muscular atrophy, but are never able to walk. They may, however, live into the fourth and fifth decades.

Type III, Kugelberg-Welander Disease

The clinical onset of type III spinal muscular atrophy occurs after 2 years of age and usually before age 10 years. Walking is usually possible until late childhood or early adolescence. These patients usually are not able to run. Their motor capacity decreases with time, however, and they have difficulty rising from the floor because of weakness of the pelvic-girdle muscles; this is known as the Gower sign. There is atrophy of the lower limbs, with pseudohypertrophy of the calves. Cranial nerve muscles are usually not affected. They have normal intelligence and may function effectively in society. Both the quality and quantity of life may be extended in type II and type III spinal muscular atrophy by the use of nighttime or full-time assisted ventilation (240).

Functional Classification

Evans et al. (241) have developed a four-group functional classification that may be useful prognostically.

Group I

Children never sit independently, have poor head control, and develop early progressive scoliosis.

Group II

Children have head control and the ability to sit if placed in a sitting position but are unable to stand or walk, even with orthotics.

Group III

Children have the ability to pull to stand and to walk with external support, such as orthoses.

Group IV

Children have the ability to walk and run independently.

Other studies have supported the use of this classification (230,235,237,242).

Genetic and Molecular Biology Studies

Linkage studies have established that the genetic homogeneity for the three types of spinal muscular atrophy occur at the same locus on chromosome 5q (19,228,233,243–245). Two genes have been found to be associated with disease, the survival motor neuron gene (*SMN*) and the neuronal apoptosis inhibitory protein gene (*NAIP*) (229,246,247). The presence of large-scale deletions involving both genes corresponds to a more severe phenotype. Prenatal diagnosis is available with the use of polymerase chain reaction amplification assays. No specific gene therapy is available.

Clinical Features

The clinical features of spinal muscular atrophy vary according to the clinical classification. The clinical characteristics common to all groups are relatively symmetric limb and trunk weakness and muscle atrophy that affects the lower extremities more than the upper extremities and the proxi-

mal muscles more than the distal muscles. Hypotonia and areflexia are present. Sensation and intelligence are normal. In infants, gross fasciculations of the tongue and fine tremors of the fingers are commonly present (234,248). The only muscles not involved are the diaphragm, sternothyroid, sternohyoid, and the involuntary muscles of the intestine, bladder, heart, and sphincters (228,237).

Diagnostic Studies

The studies used in the initial diagnosis of spinal muscular atrophy include laboratory studies, EMG, nerve conduction studies, and muscle biopsies. Hematologic studies in spinal muscular atrophy are not particularly useful (232). The CPK and aldolase levels are normal to only slightly elevated. Electrophysiologic studies, such as EMG, in patients with spinal muscular atrophy show typical neuropathic changes, such as increased amplitude and duration of response (232). Nerve conduction studies in spinal muscular atrophy are typically normal. Muscle biopsies are usually diagnostic, demonstrating muscle fiber degeneration and atrophy of fiber groups (232). However, with the recent advent of genetic testing for this disorder muscle biopsy is usually not necessary.

Radiographic Evaluation

There are no specific radiographic characteristics that are useful in making the diagnosis of spinal muscular atrophy. The most common radiographic abnormalities are nonspecific and include hip subluxation or dislocation and progressive spinal deformity (232). Bowen and Forlin (249) recommended that spinal radiographs, posteroanterior and lateral, be obtained in the sitting position to avoid the compensation seen in the standing and supine positions.

Treatment

The major orthopaedic abnormalities associated with spinal muscular atrophy include the presence of soft tissue contractures of the lower extremities, hip subluxation and dislocation, and spinal deformity (231,232,235).

Lower Extremity Soft Tissue Contractures

Soft tissue contractures of the lower extremities are the result of progressive muscle degeneration and replacement with fibrous tissue. Ambulation may be promoted and soft tissue contractures delayed by the use of orthoses, such as KAFOs (250). Contractures tend to occur most frequently after the child becomes wheelchair-bound. The prolonged sitting posture enhances hip and knee flexion contractures. Hip soft tissue contractures may also result in abnormal growth of the proximal femur and predisposes the patient to coxa valga and progressive hip subluxation. Soft tissue contractures without an associated osseous deformity usually do not require treatment. Even when they are released, the sitting posture of the child enhances their recurrence.

Hip Subluxation and Dislocation

Progressive hip subluxation leading to dislocation occurs predominantly in spinal muscular atrophy types II and III. It is important that this be prevented to provide comfort, sitting balance, and maintain pelvic alignment. A comfortable sitting posture is important if the adolescent or young adult is to function in society. Periodic anteroposterior radiographs of the pelvis, beginning in midchildhood to late childhood, are important to allow early recognition of coxa valga and subluxation. Once diagnosed, it is usually progressive because of the continued muscle weakness and soft tissue contractures. Procedures that have been used with some success in the past include soft tissue releases, such as adductor tenotomy, iliopsoas recession, and medial hamstring lengthening [➡**3.17,3.18**]. This restores some balance to the proximal musculature. Most children will benefit by varus derotation osteotomy if the hip is severely subluxated [➡**4.2,4.3**] (232). If the hip is dislocated, an open reduction with capsulorrhaphy [➡**3.2**] and pelvic osteotomy of the Chiari type may be beneficial [➡**3.11**]. The usual rotation osteotomies (e.g., Salter, Sutherland, Steel) sacrifice posterior coverage to gain lateral (superior) and anterior coverage. In the child who will be predominantly in a sitting position, this lack of posterior coverage may predispose the patient to a posterior subluxation. Therefore, the pelvic osteotomy method chosen must allow improved posterior coverage. This is usually accomplished with the Chiari osteotomy [➡**3.11**] or perhaps a shelf procedure [➡**3.12**]. Even after satisfactory alignment of the hip, resubluxation and dislocation can occur due to the progressive degeneration of the proximal muscles (251). These children require annual clinical and radiographic evaluation to assess the hips postoperatively. Thompson and Larsen (251) reported four cases of recurrent hip dislocation after corrective surgery. Two patients had second operations followed by recurrent dislocation. They questioned the advisability of treatment of hip dislocations in patients with spinal muscular atrophy.

Spinal Deformity

Most children who survive into adolescence develop a progressive spinal deformity. This occurs in 100% of the spinal muscular atrophy children and adolescents with type II and most of those with type III, especially when they lose their ability to walk (235,241,249,252–255). As in other neuromuscular disorders, as the curve progresses there is an adverse effect on pulmonary function (249,255).

The deformity typically begins in the first decade due to severe truncal weakness. Once the deformity begins, it is steadily progressive and can reach severe magnitude unless appropriately managed. The thoracolumbar paralytic C-shaped and single thoracic patterns, usually curved to the right, are most common. About 30% of children also have an associated kyphosis, which is also progressive (253,256). In type II spinal muscular atrophy, the mean expected increase in scoliosis is 8.3 degrees per year, whereas in type III it is 2.9 degrees per year.

Orthotic Management. Bracing is ineffective in preventing or halting the progression of scoliosis or kyphosis in children with spinal muscular atrophy (231,235,241,242, 253, 254, 256–260). However, it can be effective in improving sitting balance and slowing the rate of progression in young ambulatory children (249,260). This has the advantage of allowing them to reach an older, more suitable age for undergoing surgical intervention. Bowen and Forlin (249) recommended orthotic treatment to help maintain posture or slow curve progression in a child 9 years of age or younger with a deformity between 20 and 40 degrees. The thoracolumbar spinal orthosis (TLSO) is the most common orthosis used in children with spinal muscular atrophy. This orthosis must be carefully molded to distribute the forces over a large surface area to prevent skin irritation and breakdown, a major problem for children with neuromuscular diseases. Furumasu et al. (261) found that orthoses decreased function because of less spinal flexibility.

Occasionally, wheelchair modifications can also be effective in controlling truncal alignment and improving sitting posture (232). This also may be beneficial in slowing the rate of curve progression.

Surgery. The criteria for surgical spinal stabilization in spinal muscular atrophy include curve magnitude greater than 40 degrees, satisfactory flexibility on supine lateral bending radiographs, and an FVC greater than 40% of normal (232). When these criteria are met, a posterior spinal fusion using segmental spinal instrumentation techniques, such as Luque rod instrumentation and sublaminar wires [➡**2.5,2.6**], is used (Fig. 17-8) (100,109,111,112,231,235, 242,249,252–254,257–259,261,263,264). Other segmental systems, such as Cotrel-Dubousset, TSRH, Isola, and others, can also be utilized. These, however, do not usually distribute the forces of instrumentation throughout the spine as well as the Luque rods with sublaminar wiring. The spine is usually osteopenic, and there is a risk for bone failure unless the forces of instrumentation are minimized through extensive distribution. Fixation to the pelvis using the Galveston technique (113,114) or other techniques is common (115,263). In most children who are nonambulatory and have pelvic obliquity, fusion to the pelvis provides improved spinopelvic stability and alignment. Anterior spinal fusion and instrumentation are rarely indicated because of the compromised pulmonary status of these children. This may predispose the patient to pulmonary complications postoperatively (242,257). Anterior fusions alone are also too short and do not ade-

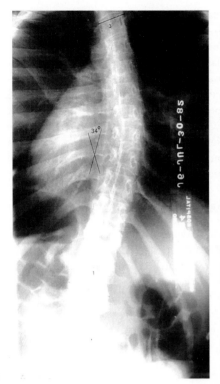
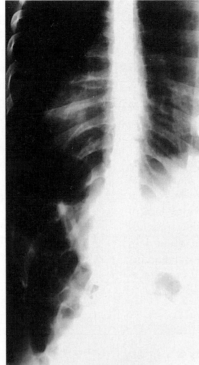
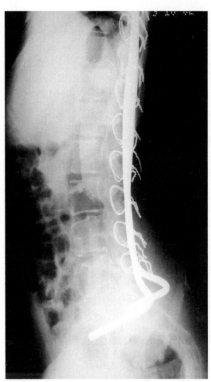
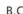

A

B,C

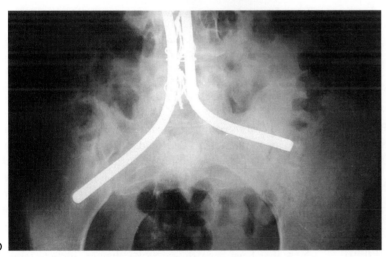

D

FIGURE 17-8. **A:** Sitting posteroanterior spinal radiograph of an 18-year-old woman with spinal muscular atrophy. A slowly progressive scoliosis has affected her wheelchair sitting balance. **B:** Postoperative radiograph after posterior spinal fusion and Luque rod instrumentation using the Galveston technique provided almost complete correction of the spinal deformity. Thirteen years postoperatively she functions independently despite the subsequent need for a tracheostomy and ventilator support. **C:** Lateral view demonstrates preservation of lumbar lordosis, which is important for proper sitting balance. **D:** Anteroposterior view of the pelvis shows proper positioning of the Luque rods in the ilium. They should penetrate as far into the ilium as possible for maximum strength.

quately stabilize the entire spine. When performed, it is combined with a simultaneous or staged posterior spinal fusion, usually with Luque rod instrumentation (100,249). Whatever posterior instrumentation system is used, it is important that no postoperative immobilization be necessary; this enhances sitting balance and pulmonary status and makes transfers easier.

Decreased function has been observed after spine fusion (252,261). Although spinal alignment and sitting balance are improved, the loss of spinal mobility decreases the function of the upper extremities and activities of daily living, such as performing transfers and personal hygiene. Askin et al. (262) recommended early surgery to preserve function.

They too found that patient function may not improve following surgery, but the cosmetic results were gratifying, and there may be improved caregiver ability. However, Bridwell et al. (109) reported improved function, self-image, cosmesis, and caregiver ability in 21 patients with spinal muscular atrophy followed for a mean of 7.8 years postoperatively (range 2 to 12.6 years).

Operative complications are similar to other neuromuscular disorders. These include excessive blood loss, pulmonary complications, neurologic injury, wound infection, loss of fixation due to osteopenia, pseudarthrosis, and death (100,111,127,252,254,256,257,259,263). The use of segmental spinal instrumentation techniques and aggressive preoperative and postoperative respiratory therapy can result in decreased complications. Hypotensive anesthesia and intraoperative spinal cord monitoring may be beneficial in decreasing intraoperative blood loss and neurologic injury. Noordeen et al. reported that a 50% decrease in amplitude may be indicative of an impending neurologic injury (127).

FRIEDREICH ATAXIA

Spinocerebellar degenerative diseases are a group of relatively uncommon disorders that are hereditary and progressive. Friedreich ataxia is the most common form and has orthopaedic implications because of its high incidence of scoliosis. Friedreich ataxia is characterized by slow, progressive spinocerebellar degeneration. It occurs in about 1 in 50,000 live births (265). It is autosomal recessive and occurs most commonly in North America in people of French Canadian heritage. Males and females are affected equally.

Clinical Features

Friedreich ataxia is characterized by a clinical triad consisting of ataxia (which is usually the presenting symptom), areflexia of the knees and ankles, and a positive plantar response, or the Babinski sign (232,266). Geoffroy et al. (267) established strict criteria for the clinical diagnosis of typical Friedreich ataxia. This has been modified by Harding (268). The primary symptoms and signs that occur in all involved patients include onset before the age of 25 years; progressive ataxia of limbs and gait; absent knee and ankle deep tendon reflexes; positive plantar response; decreased nerve conduction velocities in the upper extremities, with small or absent sensory action potentials; and dysarthria. The secondary symptoms and signs that are present in more than 90% of cases include scoliosis, pyramidal weakness in the lower extremities, absent reflexes in the upper extremities, loss of position and vibratory sense in the lower extremities, and an abnormal ECG. Accessory symptoms and signs present in fewer than 50% of cases include optic atrophy, nystagmus, distal weakness and wasting, partial deafness, pes cavus, and diabetes mellitus.

The mean age at onset is between 7 and 15 years, although the range is wide, from 4 years to as late as 25 years of age (232,266–271). Most involved individuals lose their ability to walk and are wheelchair-bound by the second or third decade. Labelle et al. (272) demonstrated that the muscle weakness is always symmetric, initially proximal rather than distal, more severe in the lower extremities, and rapidly progressive when the patients become nonambulatory. The first muscle to be involved is the hip extensor (gluteus maximus). They also demonstrated that muscle weakness is not the primary cause of loss of ambulatory function. Ataxia and other factors also play a role. Death usually occurs in the fourth or fifth decade, due to progressive hypertrophic cardiomyopathy, pneumonia, or aspiration (266,268,273).

Nerve conduction studies show decreased or absent sensory action potentials in the digital and sural nerves. Conduction velocity in the motor and sensory fibers of the median and tibial nerves are moderately slowed. An EMG shows a loss of motor units and an increase in polyphasic potentials. The ECG in adults typically shows a progressive hypertrophic cardiomyopathy. Hematologic tests such as CPK are normal, but there is increased incidence of clinical and chemical diabetes mellitus.

Genetic and Molecular Biology Studies

Chamberlain et al. have demonstrated that individuals with Friedreich ataxia have a defect on chromosome 9q13 (274). Additional studies have identified two loci on chromosome 9 (*D9S5* and *D9S15*) that are linked to Friedreich ataxia (265). It is now known that Friedreich is due to a trinucleotide repeat of GAA, which results in loss of expression of the frataxin protein. There is an inverse relationship between number of trinucleotide repeats and age of onset of the disease (275).

Treatment

The major orthopaedic problems in Friedreich ataxia are pes cavovarus, spinal deformity, and painful muscle spasms (232,266).

Pes Cavovarus

Pes cavovarus is common in patients with Friedreich ataxia. It is slowly progressive and tends to become rigid. When combined with ataxia, it can result in decreased ability to stand and walk. Orthotic management is usually ineffective in preventing the deformity, but an AFO can be used after surgery to stabilize the foot and ankle and to prevent recurrent deformity. Surgical procedures can be used in ambulatory patients to improve balance and walking ability. Procedures that have been shown to be effective include tendo Achillis lengthening and tibialis posterior tenotomy, lengthening, or anterior transfer to the dorsum of the foot [➡7.16,7.19] (232,266). The tibialis anterior muscle may also be involved and may require either tenotomy, lengthening, or centralization to the dorsum of the foot to prevent recurrence. In fixed, rigid deformities, a triple arthrodesis [➡7.9] may be necessary to achieve a plantigrade foot.

Spinal Deformity

Scoliosis occurs in essentially all patients with Friedreich ataxia (266,268,269,271,276,277). The age at onset is variable and usually begins while the patient is still ambulatory. The incidence of curve progression has been shown to correlate to the age at clinical onset of the disease process. Labelle et al. (277) demonstrated that when disease onset is before 10 years of age and scoliosis occurs before 15 years of age, most patient curves progress to greater than 60 degrees and require surgical intervention. When the disease onset is after 10 years of age and the scoliosis occurs after 15 years of age, curve progression is not as severe; most do not reach 40 degrees by skeletal maturity or progress thereafter. There was no correlation between curve progression, degree of muscle weakness, level of ambulatory function, and duration of the disease process. The patterns of scoliosis in patients with Friedreich ataxia are similar to those of adolescent idiopathic scoliosis, rather than to those of neuromuscular scoliosis. The pathogenesis of scoliosis in Friedreich ataxia appears to be not muscle weakness but the ataxia that causes a disturbance of equilibrium and postural reflexes. Double major (i.e., thoracic and lumbar) and single thoracic or thoracolumbar curves are the most common curve patterns (269,270,277,278). Only a few patients have lumbar or long C-shaped thoracolumbar curves. About two-thirds of patients with Friedreich ataxia develop an associated kyphosis greater than 40 degrees (270,277). The treatment of scoliosis in Friedreich ataxia can be either by orthotic or surgical methods.

Orthoses. A thoracolumbar spinal orthosis may be tried in ambulatory patients having 25- to 40-degree curves. It is usually not well tolerated, but it may slow the rate of progression, although rarely does it stabilize the curve (266,269,278). In ambulatory patients, an orthosis may interfere with walking because it prevents compensatory truncal movement necessary for balance and movement.

Surgery. In progressive curves greater than 60 degrees, especially in older adolescents confined to a wheelchair, a single-stage posterior spinal fusion stabilizes the curve and yields moderate correction. Curves between 40 and 60 degrees can be either observed or treated surgically, depending on the patient's age at clinical onset, the age when scoliosis was first recognized, and evidence of curve progression. Posterior segmental instrumentation using Harrington rods and sublaminar wires [➥2.3] or Luque rod instrumentation [➥2.5] has been demonstrated to be effective in achieving correction and a solid arthrodesis (100,111,269,270,276,278). Other segmental systems (e.g., Cotrel-Dubousset, Isola, TSRH) should also be effective [➥2.9]. Fusions are typically from the upper thoracic (T2 or T3) to lower lumbar regions. Fusion to the sacrum is usually unnecessary, except in C-shaped thoracolumbar curves with associated pelvic obliquity (270,278). Autogenous bone supplemented with banked bone, when necessary, usually produces a solid fusion. Anterior surgery, with or without instrumentation, usually followed by a posterior spinal fusion and instrumentation is limited to rigid curves greater than 60 degrees associated with poor sitting balance (278). Surgery is performed only after a thorough cardiopulmo-

nary evaluation and under careful intraoperative and postoperative monitoring. Postoperative immobilization should be avoided. Vertebral osteopenia and spinal stenosis is not a problem in Friedreich ataxia.

Painful Muscle Spasms

Painful muscle spasms occur in some patients with Friedreich ataxia (232). They usually begin in the late adolescent or early adult years and worsen with time. The spasms are characterized by a sudden onset and short duration. The hip adductors and the knee extensors are commonly involved. Initial treatment is usually by massage, heat, and perhaps muscle relaxants, such as diazepam and baclofen. In adults, if the adductor or quadriceps spasms are interfering with perineal care or sitting balance, the patient may benefit by tenotomies. This is rarely necessary.

HEREDITARY MOTOR SENSORY NEUROPATHIES

HMSNs are a large group of variously inherited neuropathic disorders (232,266,279). Charcot-Marie-Tooth disease is the prototype, but there are other disorders with similar but different manifestations.

Classification

The classification system for HMSN is presented in Table 17-2. HMSN types I, II, and III are encountered predominantly in pediatric orthopaedic and neuromuscular clinics, whereas HMSN types IV, V, VI, and VII tend to be late-onset and occur in adults (232).

HMSN type I is an autosomal dominant disorder and includes disorders referred to as peroneal atrophy, Charcot-

TABLE 17-2. CLASSIFICATION OF HEREDITARY MOTOR SENSORY NEUROPATHIES

Type	Terminology	Inheritance
I	Charcot-Marie-Tooth syndrome (hypertrophic form) or Roussy-Levy syndrome (areflexic dystaxia)	Autosomal dominant
II	Charcot-Marie-Tooth syndrome (neuronal form)	Variable
III	Dejerine-Sottas disease	Autosomal recessive
IV	Refsum disease	
V	Neuropathy with spastic paraplegia	
VI	Optic atrophy with peroneal muscle atrophy	
VII	Retinitis pigmentosa with distal muscle weakness and atrophy	

Marie-Tooth disease (hypertrophic form), or Roussy-Levy syndrome. It is a demyelinating disorder that is characterized by peroneal muscle weakness, absent deep tendon reflexes, and slow nerve conduction velocities. HMSN type II is the neuronal form of Charcot-Marie-Tooth disease. It is characterized by persistently normal reflexes, sensory and motor nerve conduction times that are only mildly abnormal, and variable inheritance patterns (232). These two types are clinically similar, although HMSN type II often causes less severe weakness and has a later onset than HMSN type I. HMSN type III is the autosomal recessive disorder, Dejerine-Sottas disease. This disorder begins in infancy and is characterized by more severe alterations in nerve conduction and by sensory disturbances that are more extensive than in HMSN types I and II. The HMSN types I and III are due to demyelinization of peripheral nerves. These are characterized by muscle weakness in the feet and hands, absent deep tendon reflexes, and diminution of distal sensory capabilities, particularly light touch position and vibratory sensation (232).

The four additional types are late onset and rarely seen by pediatric orthopaedists or in pediatric neuromuscular clinics: HMSN type IV, Refsum disease, is characterized by excessive phytanic acid; HMSN type V is an inherited spastic paraplegia, with distal weakness in the limbs presenting in the second decade of life with an awkward gait and equinus foot deformities; HMSN type VI is characterized by optic atrophy in association with peroneal muscle atrophy; and HMSN type VII has retinitis pigmentosa, with distal weakness in the limbs and muscle atrophy.

Diagnostic Studies

Diagnosis of HMSN is made by physical examination in combination with EMG with nerve conduction studies and genetic testing. The EMG findings in HMSN show typical neuropathic changes, with increased amplitude and duration of response. Nerve conduction studies show marked slowing of the rate of impulse conduction in the involved muscles. A biopsy specimen of muscles such as the gastrocnemius demonstrates typical neuropathic findings, including atrophy of the fiber group, with all of the fibers in an abnormal group having uniformly small diameter. A biopsy specimen of a peripheral nerve, usually the sural nerve, shows typical demyelinization, confirming the diagnosis of peripheral neuropathy.

Genetic and Molecular Biology Studies

Many individuals with the HMSN type I have a DNA duplication of a portion of the short arm of chromosome 17 in the region of p 11.2 to p 12 (20,280–282). Additional studies have shown a human peripheral myelin protein-22 gene to be contained within the duplication (283–285). It is thought that the abnormality in the peripheral myelin

protein-22 gene, which encodes the myelin protein, has a causative role in Charcot-Marie-Tooth disease. Either a point mutation in peripheral myelin protein-22 or duplication of the region that contains the peripheral myelin protein-22 gene can result in the disorder (286).

Treatment

Children with HMSN typically present with gait disturbance or foot deformities. The severity of involvement is variable. In severe involvement, there may be proximal muscle weakness. The major orthopaedic problems include pes cavovarus, hip dysplasia, spinal deformity, and hand and upper extremity dysfunction.

Pes Cavovarus

The pathogenesis of cavovarus deformities in children with HMSN and other neuromuscular disorders is becoming better understood (287–292). The components of the pes cavovarus deformity include claw toes; plantar flexed first metatarsal with adduction and inversion of the remaining metatarsals; midfoot malposition of the navicular, cuboid and cuneiforms, leading to a high arch (cavus); and hindfoot varus malposition between the talus and calcaneus (Fig. 17-9). Initially HMSNs affect the more distal muscles. The mildest cases affect the toes and forefoot, whereas the midfoot and hindfoot are progressively affected with progression of the disease process. In a computed tomography study of 26 patients with HMSN I, II, or III, Price et al. (293) found that the interossei and lumbrical muscles of the feet demonstrated earlier and more severe involvement compared with the extrinsic muscles. These intrinsic muscles have the most distal innervation. Even with minimal weakness the invertor muscles, such as the tibialis anterior and tibialis posterior muscles, are stronger than the evertors, such as the peroneus longus; this relation favors the development of adduction and varus deformities.

Pes cavovarus deformities are progressive, but the rate is variable, even among involved family members. Initially, the deformity is flexible but later becomes rigid. Shapiro and Specht point to the plantar flexed first metatarsal as the key finding (232). As the first metatarsal becomes increasingly plantar flexed, this is followed by increasing hindfoot varus and forefoot and midfoot supination and cavus. The block test is useful in defining the mobility of the remainder of the foot in children with a rigid plantar flexed first metatarsal (291).

The goals in the treatment of foot deformities in children with HMSN include maintenance of a straight, plantigrade, and relatively flexible foot during growth (288). This maximizes function and minimizes the development of osseous deformities that may require more extensive surgery in adolescence and early adult years, such as triple arthrodesis.

The treatment options for the management of foot de-

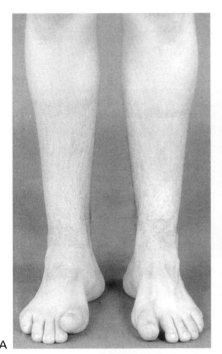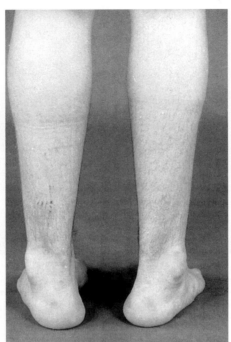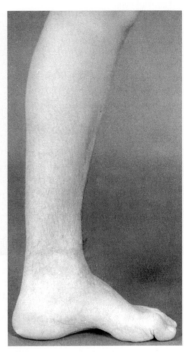

A   B,C

FIGURE 17-9. A: Front view of the lower legs and feet of a 16-year-old boy with hereditary motor sensory neuropathy type I (i.e., Charcot-Marie-Tooth disease). His calves are thin, and he has mildly symptomatic cavus feet. Clawing of the toes is minimal. **B:** Posterior view demonstrates moderate heel varus. **C:** The cavus foot deformity is most apparent when viewed from the medial side. A mild flexion deformity of the great toe interphalangeal joint is present.

formities include: plantar release, plantar-medial release, tendon transfers, calcaneal osteotomy, midtarsal osteotomy, triple arthrodesis, and correction of toe deformities.

Plantar Release. In children younger than 10 years of age who have a mild cavovarus deformity, a plantar release may be beneficial in correcting the plantar flexed first metatarsal and providing correction of the associated flexible hindfoot and midfoot deformities (294). In the radical plantar release described by Paulos et al. (291), selective Z-lengthening of the long toe flexor tendons and tibialis posterior tendon is performed if there is a bowstring effect after plantar release.

Plantar-medial Release. If the hindfoot deformity in the child younger than 10 years of age is rigid, leading to fixed varus deformity, the plantar release may be combined with a medial release (291). The medial structures to be released include the ligamentous and capsular structures between the talus and calcaneus **[➡7.1]** (except the posterior talocalcaneal ligament), and the capsule of the talonavicular joints. The navicular is then reduced onto the head of the talus and secured with a smooth Steinmann pin. The posterior ankle and subtalar joint ligaments and the tendo Achillis are not disturbed because they are necessary for counter-resistance during postoperative serial casting. Once the incision has healed a series of corrective weightbearing casts

are applied. Excellent correction of the entire foot has been reported after this technique.

Tendon Transfers. In children and adolescents who have a flexible cavovarus deformity in which active inversion is associated with relative weakness of the evertor muscles, a transfer of the tibialis anterior tendon to the dorsum of the midtarsal region in line with the third metatarsal may be helpful (295). The transfer is designed to balance strength, but the foot must be aligned initially by a plantar release and perhaps the plantar-medial release.

Other tendinous procedures that may be used depend on the individual needs of the patient. These may include tendo Achillis lengthening **[➡7.16]**, anterior transfer at the tibialis posterior tendon **[➡7.19]**, long toe extensors to the metatarsals or midfoot, and flexor-to-extensor tendon transfers for claw toes (288,291,295,296). Tendo Achillis lengthening is rarely necessary, as the equinus is due to the plantar flexed first metatarsal and forefoot. The hindfoot is typically in a calcaneus position.

Calcaneal Osteotomy. In children who are younger than 10 years of age and who have mild but fixed deformity, a calcaneal osteotomy may be beneficial in correcting the varus deformity of the hindfoot (232). This osteotomy does not interfere with growth because it is not made through

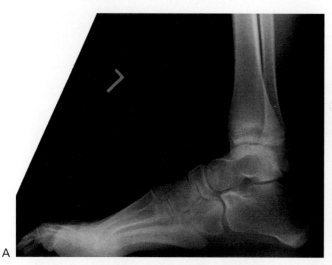
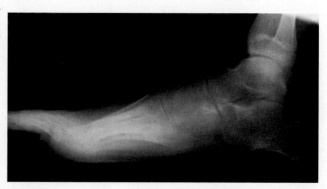

FIGURE 17-10. A: Moderate cavovarus deformity of the left foot in a 14-year-old male with Charcot-Marie-Tooth disease. He was managed by a closing wedge valgus osteotomy at the calcaneus, an opening wedge, plantar-based osteotomy of the medial cuneiform, and soft tissue balancing. **B:** Postoperatively, the cavovarus deformity has been improved. He is a brace-free ambulator due to restoration of muscle balance.

a cartilaginous growth area. To allow lateral translation, the osteotomy is cut slightly obliquely, passing from a superior position on the lateral surface to a more inferior position on the medial surface. It is possible to translate the distal fragment as much as one-third of its transverse diameter, thus allowing conversion of weightbearing from varus to slight valgus. In patients who are older than 10 years of age or who are more severely affected, a lateral closing-wedge calcaneal osteotomy, with lateral translation of the distal and posterior fragments, is performed (Fig.17-10) (232). In both procedures the osteotomy is stabilized with staples or Steinmann pins.

Midtarsal Osteotomy. The midtarsal osteotomy provides correction by removal of a dorsal and slightly laterally based wedge, with the proximal osteotomy cut through the navicular and cuboid bones and the distal cut through the cuboid and three cuneiforms (296). Moderate deformities can be corrected satisfactorily with this procedure, especially if it is augmented with a plantar release, calcaneal osteotomy, and perhaps an anterior transfer of the tibialis anterior tendon. Equinus deformities of the midfoot and varus deformities of the forefoot can be corrected with appropriate wedge resections. Growth retardation and limitation of mobility are minimal compared with after a triple arthrodesis.

Triple Arthrodesis. In adolescents who have reached skeletal maturity and have a severe deformity, walk with difficulty, and cannot run, a triple arthrodesis **[➥7.9]** may be performed. Every attempt should be made to avoid this procedure because of the associated complications of undercorrection, overcorrection, pseudarthrosis of the talo-

navicular joint, and degenerative changes in the ankle and midfoot joints (297–301).

Wetmore and Drennan (300) reported unsatisfactory results in 23 of 30 feet (16 patients) at a mean follow-up at 21 years. The progressive muscle imbalance resulted in recurrent pes cavovarus deformities. There was also an increased incidence of degenerative osteoarthritis of the ankle as a consequence to the deformity and the loss of subtalar joint motion. They felt triple arthrodesis should be limited to patients with severe, rigid deformities. Saltzman et al. reported similar results in 67 feet in 57 patients, including 6 feet in patients with Charcot-Marie-Tooth disease at 25 and 44 years of mean follow-up (302). However, 95% of the patients were satisfied with their clinical results. Ghanem et al. also reported long-term satisfactory results in children who had a triple arthrodesis (288).

The Ryerson triple arthrodesis is preferred because the joint surfaces of the talocalcaneal, talonavicular, and calcaneal cuboid joints are removed, along with appropriate-sized wedges to correct the various components of the hindfoot and midfoot deformities (Fig. 17-11) (296). In patients who have marked equinus of the midfoot and forefoot in relation to a relatively well-positioned hindfoot, the Lambrinudi triple arthrodesis may be performed (296,303). Once an arthrodesis has been performed to straighten the foot, tendon transfers to balance muscle power are of great importance.

Toe deformities in adolescents or after a triple arthrodesis may be corrected by proximal and distal interphalangeal fusion or flexor-to-extensor tendon transfer (304). The great toe may require an interphalangeal joint fusion and transfer of the extensor hallucis longus from the proximal phalanx

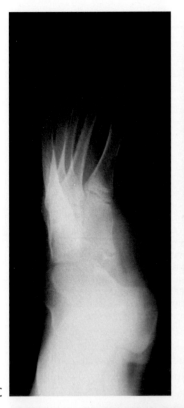
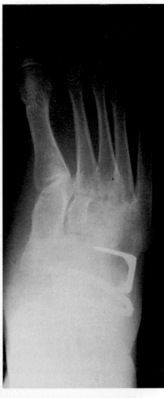

A,C

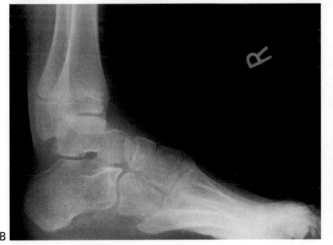

B

FIGURE 17-11. A: Standing anteroposterior radiograph of severe cavovarus deformity of the right foot in a 14-year-old male with Charcot-Marie-Tooth disease. **B:** Lateral radiograph demonstrates a varus hindfoot and midfoot, and a plantar flexed first metatarsal. **C:** Postoperative standing anteroposterior radiograph following a Ryerson triple arthrodesis, soft tissue balancing, and correction of his claw toe deformities. **D:** Lateral radiographs show markedly improved alignment.

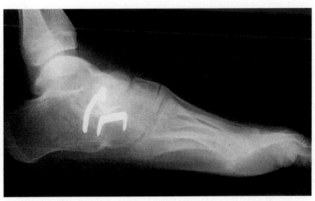

D

to the neck of the first metatarsal (Jones procedure). The latter then serves as a foot dorsiflexor.

Hip Dysplasia

Hip dysplasia in HMSN occurs in about 6 to 8% of involved children (305,306). Occasionally, hips may be dislocatable at birth, although the neuropathy does not become apparent for several years. It is more likely to occur in HMSN type I than HMSN type II because of the more severe neurologic involvement in the former. Walker et al. (306) thought that the slight muscle weakness about the

hip in growing children with HMSN may be sufficient to distort growth and development, leading to dysplasia. Usually, hip dysplasia is diagnosed between 5 and 15 years of age because of mild discomfort (305,306,308). Dysplasia may be present in asymptomatic patients, however (Fig. 17-12). Annual anteroposterior radiographs of the pelvis have been recommended to allow early diagnosis and treatment. Typical radiographic findings include acetabular dysplasia, coxa valga, and subluxation. The treatment of HMSN hip dysplasia includes soft tissue releases to correct contractures and restore muscle balance and pelvic or proximal femoral varus derotation osteotomies or both to stabilize and ade-

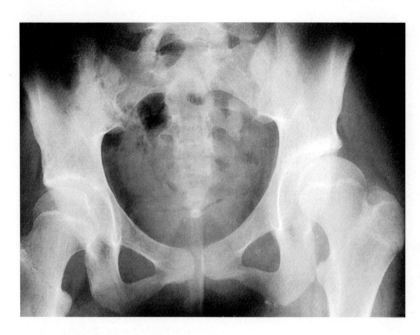

FIGURE 17-12. Anteroposterior pelvic radiograph of a 15-year-old girl with Charcot-Marie-Tooth disease. Asymptomatic acetabular dysplasia of the left hip is visible. The medial joint is slightly widened. The Shenton line is disrupted, and the center-edge angle is 16 degrees. This condition was first observed 6 years previously and did not progress.

quately realign the hip (305,307–310). The type of pelvic osteotomy is determined by the patient's age and severity of the dysplasia. Rotational osteotomies (Salter, Steel) [➡3.5,3.10] are useful in many children with mild dysplasia, while periacetabular osteotomies are useful in adolescents and young adults, and the Chiari osteotomy [➡3.11] when there is severe dysplasia.

Spinal Deformity

Scoliosis was initially thought to occur in about 10% of children with HMSN (311,312). These children were usually ambulatory, with age of onset of spinal deformity of about 10 years. A study by Walker et al. (313) found a 37% incidence of scoliosis or kyphoscoliosis in involved children. The incidence increases to 50% in those who were skeletally mature. Spinal deformity is more common in girls and HMSN type I. Curve progression requiring orthoses or surgery is uncommon. The curve patterns and management are similar to those for idiopathic adolescent scoliosis, except for an increased incidence of kyphosis. As a consequence, orthotic management can be effective in arresting progression of the deformity. If progression reaches 45 to 50 degrees, a posterior spinal fusion and segmental spinal instrumentation can effectively stabilize and partially correct the deformity [➡2.9] (311,312). Intraoperative spinal cord monitoring with somatosensory cortical evoked potentials may show no signal transmission. This is due to the demyelination of the peripheral nerves and perhaps to degeneration of the dorsal root ganglion and dorsal column of the spinal cord (314). A wake-up test may need to be performed.

Hand and Upper Extremity Dysfunction

The upper extremities are involved in about two-thirds of individuals with HMSN (315,316). The involvement tends to be milder, however, and does not appear until a later age. Intrinsic muscle weakness with decreased stability is a relatively common finding. In a study of 68 patients with Charcot-Marie-Tooth disease, the mean age at onset of symptoms in the hands and upper extremities was 19 years. Intrinsic muscle function was initially impaired, and patients became aware of motor weakness and a lack of dexterity. Sensory changes such as numbness are usually present concomitantly. Physical and occupational therapy may be helpful. In some patients operative intervention, such as transfer of the flexor digitorum sublimis to restore opposition, nerve compression releases, soft tissue contracture releases, and joint arthrodeses, may be effective in improving function. Preoperative EMG has been shown to aid in selecting optimal forearm muscles for tendon transfers to the hand (317).

POLIOMYELITIS

Acute poliomyelitis results from an acute viral infection, with localization in the anterior horn cells of the spinal cord and certain brain stem motor nuclei. It is caused by one of three polioviruses known as Brunhilde (type 1), Lansing (type 2), and Leon (type 3). Humans are the natural host for poliovirus, transmitting the disease by the oropharyngeal route. Each one of the polioviruses has varying virulence. Most poliovirus infections have an abortive course, with only mild gastrointestinal symptoms. Fewer than 1% of infections develop the paralytic form of the disease. Development of prophylactic vaccines has greatly reduced the incidence of polio, although the disease remains a major health problem in developing countries. Fewer than 10 cases occur in the United States annually, and these most commonly result from the use of the active oral polio vaccine (318,319).

Pathology

The poliovirus invades the body through the oropharyngeal route and multiplies in the gastrointestinal tract lymph nodes before spreading to the central nervous system by the hematogenous route. The incubation period ranges from 6 to 20 days. Motoneuron cells of the anterior horn cells of the spinal cord and brain stem are acutely attacked. In the spinal cord, the lumbar and cervical regions are particularly involved. The medulla, cerebellum, and midbrain may be involved also. Except for the motor areas, the white matter of the spinal cord and the cerebral cortex are uninvolved.

Damage to the anterior horn cells may be due directly to viral multiplication, toxic byproducts of the virus, or indirectly from ischemia, edema, and hemorrhage in the glial tissues surrounding the anterior horn cells. In addition to acute inflammatory cellular reaction, edema with perivascular mononuclear cuffing occurs.

The inflammatory response gradually subsides, and the necrotic ganglion cells are surrounded and partially dissolved by macrophages and neutrophils. After 4 months, the spinal cord is left with residual areas of gliosis and lymphocytic cell collections occupying the area of the destroyed motor cells. Evidence exists of continuous disease activity in spinal cord segments examined two decades after the onset of the disease. Histopathologic sections demonstrate a loss or atrophy of motor neurons, severe reaction gliosis, and mild-to-moderate perivascular interparenchymal inflammation, with sparing of corticospinal tracts. Skeletal muscle demonstrates gross atrophy and replacement by fat and connective tissue histologically. The percentage of motor units destroyed in an individual muscle varies markedly, and the resultant clinical weakness is proportionate to the number of lost motor units. Sharrard has stated that clinically detectable weakness is present only when more than 60% of the motor nerve cells supplying the muscle have been destroyed (320). Involved muscles can range from those of one extremity to those of all four extremities, the trunk, and the bulbar musculature.

Muscles innervated by the cervical and lumbar segments are most frequently involved. However, involvement occurs twice as frequently in the lower extremity than in the upper extremity muscles. Sharrard (321,322) combined clinical and histologic studies which demonstrated that muscles with short motor nerve cell columns often are severely paralyzed, whereas those with long motor cell columns are more frequently left paretic or weak. The quadriceps, tibialis anterior, medial hamstrings, and hip flexors are the lumbar innervated muscles most frequently involved. The deltoid, triceps, and pectoralis major are most frequently affected in the upper extremities. The sacral nerve roots are usually spared, resulting in the characteristic preservation of the intrinsic muscles of the foot (323).

Recovery of muscle function depends on return to function of those anterior horn cells damaged but not destroyed. Clinical recovery begins during the first month after the acute illness and is nearly complete by the sixth month, although there is limited potential for additional recovery through the second year. Sharrard has stated that the mean final grade of a muscle is two grades above its assessment at 1 month and one grade above it at 6 months (320).

Disease Stages

Management of poliomyelitis varies according to the stage of the disease process. These are designated acute, convalescent, and chronic stages. Because the acute and convalescent stages are rarely encountered in this country, orthopaedic management is usually confined to the chronic stage. Most pediatric orthopaedic programs see several children or more per year with poliomyelitis in the chronic stage. These children are usually adopted from nonindustrialized nations or from parents who have immigrated from such countries.

Acute Stage

Acute poliomyelitis may cause symptoms ranging from mild malaise to generalized encephalomyelitis with widespread paralysis. Diagnosis is based on clinical findings because there are no diagnostic laboratory tests. This phase generally lasts 7 to 10 days. The return to normal temperature for 48 h and the absence of progressive muscle involvement indicates the end of the acute phase. This phase is usually managed by pediatricians because there may be medical problems, especially respiratory, that may be life-threatening.

The orthopaedist should be familiar with the clinical signs of acute poliomyelitis. Meningismus is reflected in the characteristic flexor posturing of the upper and lower extremities. Involved muscles are tender, even to gentle palpation. Clinical examination can be difficult because of pain during the acute stage.

Orthopaedic treatment during this phase emphasizes prevention of deformity and comfort. This approach consists of physical therapy with gentle, passive range of motion exercises and splinting. Muscle spasms, which can lead to shortening and contractures, may respond to the application of warm, moist heat. This can relieve muscle sensitivity and discomfort. Sharrard (320) emphasized that rapid loss of elasticity, coupled with shortening of tendons, fascia, and ligaments, leads to contractures.

Convalescent Stage

The convalescent phase of poliomyelitis begins 2 days after the temperature returns to normal and progression of the paralytic disease ceases. The phase continues for 2 years, during which spontaneous improvement of muscle power occurs. The assessment of the rate of recovery in poliomyelitis is made by serial examination of the muscle strength. Muscle assessment should be performed monthly for 6 months and then at 3-month intervals during the remainder of the convalescent stage.

Johnson (324) demonstrated that an individual muscle demonstrating less than 30% of normal strength at 3 months should be considered to be permanently paralyzed. Muscles showing evidence of more than 80% return of strength require no specific therapy. He emphasized that muscles that fall between these two parameters retain the potential for useful function and that therapy should be directed toward recreating hypertrophy of the remaining muscle fibers.

The treatment goals during this phase include efforts to prevent contractures and deformity, restoration and maintenance of normal joint range of motion, and assisting individual muscles in achieving maximum recovery (316). Physical therapy and orthotics are the main treatment modalities. Physical therapy is directed toward having individual muscles assume maximum capability within their pattern of normal motor activity and not permitting adaptive or substitute patterns of associated muscles to persist. Hydrotherapy can also be helpful in achieving these goals. Orthoses, both ambulatory and nighttime, are necessary to support the extremity during this phase.

Chronic Stage

The chronic stage of poliomyelitis begins after 2 years, and it is during this stage that the orthopaedist assumes responsibility for the long-term management resulting from muscle imbalance.

The management goal during the chronic stage is to achieve maximal functional capacity. This is accomplished by restoring muscle balance, preventing or correcting soft tissue contractures, correcting osseous deformities, and directing allied personnel, such as physical therapists, occupational therapists, and orthotists.

Treatment

Soft Tissue Contractures

Flaccid paralysis, muscle imbalance, and growth all contribute to soft tissue contractures and fixed deformities in poliomyelitis. Contractures occur from increased mechanical advantage of the stronger muscles and continue the attenuation of their weaker antagonists. The greater the disparity in muscle balance, the sooner a contracture may develop.

Joint instability does not result in fixed deformity, except in cases in which it is allowed to occur over a period of years in a growing child. Static instability can be controlled readily and indefinitely by orthoses. Dynamic joint instabil-

ity readily produces a fixed deformity, and orthotic control is difficult. Deformities are initially confined to soft tissues, but later, bone growth and joint alignment may be affected.

The age at onset of poliomyelitis is important. The osseous growth potential of young children makes them more vulnerable to secondary osseous deformities. The worst deformities occur in young children and those with severe muscle imbalance. Release of soft tissue contractures and appropriate tendon transfers performed in a young child are important in preventing structural changes.

Tendon Transfers

Achievement of muscle balance in patients with dynamic instability effectively halts progression of paralytic deformity (326). Tendon transfers are performed when dynamic muscle imbalance is sufficient to produce deformity and when orthotic protection is required. Transfers should be delayed until the paralyzed muscle has been given adequate postural treatment to ensure that it has regained maximum strength and that the proposed tendon transfer is required. The objectives of tendon transfer are to provide active motor power to replace function of a paralyzed muscle or muscles, to eliminate the deformity caused by a muscle when its antagonist is paralyzed, and to produce stability through better muscle balance. The principles of tendon transfer have been well established (327,328).

The muscle to be transferred should rate good or fair before transfer and must have adequate strength to actively perform the desired function. On the average, one grade of motor power is lost after muscle transfer. The length and range of motion of the transferred muscle and that of the muscle being replaced must be similar. Loss of original function resulting from tendon transfers must be balanced against potential gains. Free passive range of motion is essential in the absence of deformity at the joint to be moved by the tendon transfer. A transfer as an adjunct to bony stabilization cannot be expected to overcome a fixed deformity (329). The smooth gliding channel for the tendon transfer is essential. Atraumatic handling of the muscle tissue can prevent injury to its neurovascular supply and prevent adhesions. The tendon should be rooted in a straight line between its origin and new insertion. Attachment of the tendon transfer should be under sufficient tension to correspond to normal physiologic conditions and should allow the transferred muscle to achieve a maximum range of contraction.

Osteotomies

Osseous deformities may produce joint deformities that impair extremity alignment and limit function. This most commonly occurs in the lower extremity. Osteotomies can be beneficial in restoring extremity alignment and improving function. Because of possible recurrence during subsequent growth, these procedures are usually postponed, if possible, until late childhood or early adolescence.

Arthrodeses

Arthrodeses are usually performed for salvage, except in the foot where a subtalar, triple, or pantalar arthrodesis may be useful in stabilization and realignment.

Treatment Guidelines

The basic treatment guidelines for chronic or postpoliomyelitis in children have been outlined by Watts (330). These guidelines include restoring ambulation, correcting factors that cause deformities with growth, correcting factors that obviate or reduce dependency on orthoses, correcting upper extremity problems, and treating spinal deformities. Understandably, these guidelines allow the child or adolescent to achieve maximum functional level. The specific methods to achieve each guideline are multiple, sometimes complex, and based on careful evaluation of the patient. Because children with previous poliomyelitis are infrequently encountered, specific details on the various procedures are not presented. Such information can be obtained from the references in the various sections.

The orthopaedist must establish a comprehensive plan for each child based on a thorough musculoskeletal examination—in particular, joint range of motion, existing deformities, and manual testing of the individual muscles of the extremities and trunk. The latter should be individually recorded on a worksheet so that it can be used for future reference. It is important to remember that a muscle normally loses one grade of power when transferred. To be functionally useful, a muscle grade of at least 4 is necessary, although a grade 3 muscle, when transferred, may be an effective tenodesis in preventing deformity by balancing an opposing muscle.

Upper Extremity

In polio upper extremity involvement tends to be less severe than in the lower extremity. A stable upper extremity, especially the shoulder, is necessary for support of the body weight with a walker or crutches. It is also necessary for transfers or shifting the trunk if wheelchair-bound. A functional elbow, wrist, and hand is necessary for maximum independent function.

Shoulder. Shoulder stability is essential for all upper extremity activities. Satisfactory level of function of the hand, forearm, and elbow is a prerequisite for any shoulder reconstructive surgery. The major problems affecting the shoulder are predominantly muscle paralysis of the deltoid, pectoralis major, subscapularis, supraspinatus, and infraspinatus muscles. Rarely are all muscles involved because of the multiple levels of innervation. Tendon transfers can occasionally be effective in restoring shoulder stability. When there is extensive weakness, shoulder arthrodesis may be helpful. It can also be indicated whether there is a painful subluxation or dislocation. A strong trapezius serratus anterior muscle is necessary to allow increased function after fusion.

Elbow. The major problem affecting the elbow is loss of flexion. When the biceps and brachialis are paralyzed, a tendon transfer may be helpful in restoring useful elbow flexion. Possible procedures include a Steindler flexorplasty, which transfers the origin of the wrist flexors to the anterior aspect of the distal humerus (331). The best functional results occur in patients whose elbow flexors are only partially paralyzed and whose fingers and wrist flexors are normal. Transfer of the sternal head of the pectoralis major also may be considered. Other possible procedures include transfer of the sternocleidomastoid, latissimus dorsi, and anterior transfer of the triceps brachii. Paralysis of the triceps brachii muscle may occur in poliomyelitis, but seldom interferes with elbow function because gravity passively extends the elbow. Triceps brachii function is necessary, however, in activities in which the body weight is shifted to the hands, such as in transferring from bed to wheelchair or in crutch walking.

Forearm. Fixed deformities of the forearm seldom create major functional disabilities in children and adolescents with poliomyelitis. Pronation contractures are the most common disability. Function can be improved with release of the pronator teres and transfer of the flexor carpi ulnaris muscle.

Hand. Tendon transfers and fusions to improve hand function can be considered in selected cases. The number of possible transfers is extensive, and each patient requires a careful evaluation to ensure maximum functional improvement. Carpal tunnel syndrome has also been reported as a long-term sequela of poliomyelitis (332). This is associated with prolonged use of crutches or cane.

Lower Extremity

Lower extremity problems are most common in poliomyelitis. They can have a significant impact on function, especially ambulation.

Leg-length Discrepancy. This is a common problem when there is asymmetrical neurologic involvement. If the discrepancy is greater than 2 cm, this can produce a great disturbance. An appropriately timed contralateral epiphysiodesis is the usual procedure of choice (see Chapter 28). Greater discrepancy may be treated orthotically. Lengthening is rarely a consideration. However, D'Souza and Shah recently demonstrated that circumferential periosteal sleeve resection of the distal femur and/or distal tibia can produce a transient growth stimulation that can be beneficial in mild discrepancies, usually 2 to 3 cm (325).

Hip. Hip problems in poliomyelitis include muscle paralysis, soft tissue contractures, internal or medial femoral torsion, coxa valga, and hip subluxation and dislocation. Periodic anteroposterior radiographs of the pelvis are necessary to assess growth and the relation between the femoral head and acetabulum. Function can be improved and subluxa-

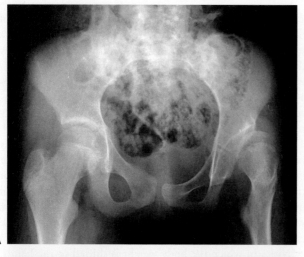

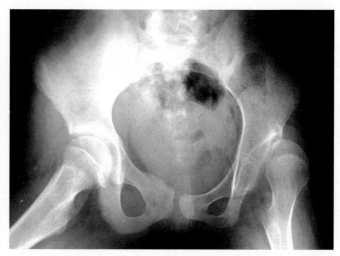

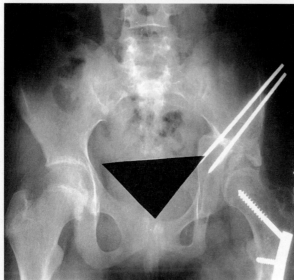

FIGURE 17-13. A: Anteroposterior radiograph of the pelvis of a 13-year-old Korean girl who had poliomyelitis. She has a painful subluxation of her left hip. The acetabulum is dysplastic, the center-edge angle is 6 degrees, and a coxa valga deformity of the proximal femur is present. **B:** Frog-leg or Lauenstein lateral. **C:** Two years after a proximal femoral varus derotation osteotomy and Chiari pelvic osteotomy there is markedly improved alignment of the left hip, and she is asymptomatic.

tion-dislocation prevented with appropriate soft tissue releases, tendon transfers, proximal femoral varus derotation osteotomy, and pelvic osteotomy (Fig. 17-13) (322,323). It is important that the procedures be coordinated to provide as balanced a musculature as possible so that hip stability can be maintained. Lau et al. (333) reported good or satisfactory results in 70% of patients with paralytic hip instability due to poliomyelitis. The key factors for success were muscle balance, the femoral neck shaft and anteversion angles, and the acetabular geometry.

Knee. Flexion contractures, extension contractures, genu valgum, and external rotation of the tibia are common knee deformities in poliomyelitis that can have an adverse effect on functional ambulation. Hamstring release, distal femoral extension osteotomy, proximal femoral extension osteotomy, and rotational tibial osteotomies are common procedures (334–337). One of the most common soft tissue procedures is that described by Yount, in which the distal iliotibial band, including the intermuscular septum, is re-

leased (80). This may be combined with an Ober release proximally if hip flexion contractures are also present (81). Shahcheraghi et al. recently reported that anterior hamstring tendon transfer significantly improved active knee extension and function in patients with paralysis of the quadriceps femoris muscle following poliomyelitis (338).

Foot and Ankle. Deformities of the foot and ankle are among the most common in adolescents with poliomyelitis. Drennan has discussed possible procedures to correct the deformities and improve muscle balance (339). This is again achieved with a combination of correction of soft tissue contractures, tendon transfers, and bone-stabilizing procedures, such as calcaneal osteotomy, subtalar arthrodesis, triple arthrodesis, and pantalar arthrodesis (340–345). The patient requires a careful evaluation to determine the appropriate procedures. Arthrodeses produce good long-term results with a low incidence of ankle-degenerative arthritis, due to lower functional demands and stresses of patients with poliomyelitis (302,340,342).

Spine

Scoliosis occurs in about one third of patients with poliomyelitis (346). The type and severity of the curvature depends on the extent of paralysis and residual muscle power of the involved trunk muscles and pelvic obliquity. The most common curve patterns are the double major thoracic and lumbar curves, followed by the long paralytic C-shaped thoracolumbar curve (347). Pelvic obliquity occurs in about 50% of cases of spinal deformity. Because of severe rotation, kyphosis in the lumbar spine and lordosis in the thoracic spine are also common.

The goals of treatment are to obtain a balanced vertical torso over a level pelvis. This permits stable sitting and hands-free activities. It also helps prevent decubiti and paralytic hip dislocation. In young children with curves between 20 and 40 degrees orthotic management with a TLSO can be tried. It rarely provides complete stability, but can be effective in slowing the rate of progression and allowing the child to reach a more suitable age for surgery. In severe cases in young children segmental spinal instrumentation without fusion may be considered. Eberle (348), however, reported failure of segmental spinal instrumentation in 15 of 16 children with poliomyelitis between 5 and 12 years of age. Thus, children who undergo instrumentation without fusion should be treated with TLSO and undergo fusion as soon as possible to prevent late complications. For adolescents with a supple spine and a curve of less than 60 degrees a posterior spinal fusion with segmental instrumentation, usually Luque rod instrumentation, provides stability and a low pseudarthrosis rate [➡2.5] (100,346,347,349). Other segmental systems (e.g., TSRH, Cotrel-Dubousset, Isola) should also be effective [➡2.9]. In severe curves of 60 to 100 degrees, a combined anterior and posterior spinal fusion is usually necessary. Anterior spinal instrumentation with a Dwyer or Zielke system may be used in thoracolumbar and lumbar curves [➡2.11]. Anterior discectomy and fusion is preferred for thoracic curves. The posterior spinal fusion and instrumentation may be performed the same day or performed 1 or 2 weeks later. Leong et al. (350) and others (349,351) have demonstrated that combined anterior and posterior spinal fusions provide excellent correction for postpoliomyelitis spinal deformity, including the associated pelvic obliquity (Fig. 17-14). Rarely is preoperative traction or traction between staged anterior and posterior procedures necessary for additional correction. Fusion to

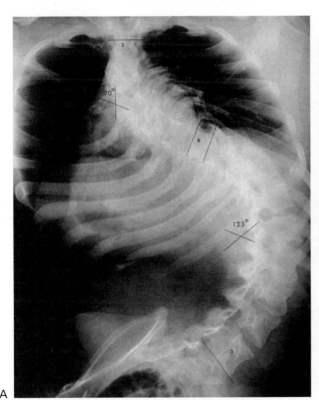 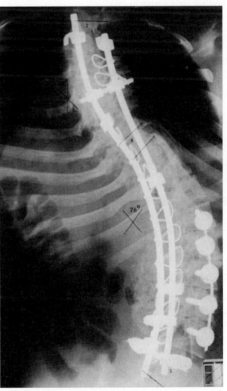

FIGURE 17-14. **A:** Anteroposterior sitting spinal radiograph of a 17-year-old girl from the Middle East who has a severe paralytic scoliosis. There is a 123-degree left thoracolumbar scoliosis and a 70-degree right thoracic scoliosis. She contracted poliomyelitis at the age of 2 years, which left her with flail lower extremities and essentially normal upper extremities. She is wheelchair-dependent and has pain from rib–pelvis impingement. **B:** Postoperative radiograph after staged anterior spinal fusion and Zielke instrumentation and posterior spinal fusion using Isola instrumentation from T3 to the sacrum. Pain relief was complete and sitting balance improved. The left thoracolumbar curve has been reduced to 70 degrees and the right thoracic curve to 47 degrees.

the pelvis or sacrum is usually necessary in patients with severe pelvic obliquity (346,352,353).

POSTPOLIOMYELITIS SYNDROME

Postpoliomyelitis syndrome is a true entity occurring in adults, and a sequela to previous poliomyelitis. Reactivation of the poliovirus has been confused with amyotrophic lateral sclerosis. Postpoliomyelitis syndrome is thought to be an overuse syndrome (354). Diagnosis is based on five criteria and is essentially a diagnosis of exclusion. The criteria include:

1. A confirmed history of previous poliomyelitis.
2. Partial to fairly complete neurologic and functional recovery.
3. A period of neurologic and functional stability of at least 15 years duration.
4. Onset of two or more of the following health problems since achieving a period of stability: unaccustomed fatigue, muscle and joint pain or both, new weakness in muscles previously affected or unaffected, functional loss, cold intolerance, and new atrophy.
5. No other medical diagnosis to explain the aforementioned health problems (170).

Postpoliomyelitis syndrome is more likely to develop in those with onset later than 10 years of age because older children are more likely to have severe poliomyelitis. Management of these patients is conservative and consists of muscle strengthening, decreasing the duration of effort, and orthotics (354). Reconstructive surgery is rarely indicated or necessary.

References

1. Read L, Galasko CS. Delay in diagnosing Duchenne muscular dystrophy in orthopaedic clinics. *J Bone Joint Surg Br* 1986;68:481.
2. Florence JM, Brocke MH, Carroll JE. Evaluation of the child with muscular weakness. *Ortho Clin North Am* 1978;9:409.

Diagnostic Studies

3. Shapiro F, Bresnan MJ. Current concepts review. Orthopaedic management of childhood neuromuscular disease. Part III: diseases of muscle. *J Bone Joint Surg Am* 1982;64:1102.
4. Shapiro F, Specht L. Current concepts review. The diagnosis and orthopaedic treatment of inherited muscular diseases of childhood. *J Bone Joint Surg Am* 1993;75:439.
5. Siegel IM. Diagnosis, management and orthopaedic treatment of muscular dystrophy. *AAOS Instr Course Lect* 1981;30:3.
6. Vignos PJ Jr. Diagnosis of progressive muscular dystrophy. *J Bone Joint Surg Am* 1967;49:1212.
7. Munsat TL, Baloh R, Pearson CM, et al. Serum enzyme alterations in neuromuscular disorders. *JAMA* 1973;226:1536.
8. Thomson WH, Leyburn P, Walton JN. Serum enzyme activity in muscular dystrophy. *Br Med J* 1960;2(5208):1276.

9. Zellweger H, Antonik A. Newborn screening for Duchenne muscular dystrophy. *Pediatrics* 1975;55:30.
10. Banker BQ. *Myology. Basic and clinical.* New York: McGraw-Hill, 1986:1527.
11. Dubowitz V. *Muscle biopsy,* 2nd ed. London: Bailliere Tindall, 1985.
12. Hurley ME, Davids JR, Mubarak SJ. Single-incision combination biopsy (muscle and nerve) in the diagnosis of neuromuscular disease in children. *J Pediatr Orthop* 1994;14:740.
13. Mubarak SJ, Chambers HG, Wenger DR. Percutaneous muscle biopsy in the diagnosis of neuromuscular disease. *J Pediatr Orthop* 1992;12:191.
14. Sanjal SK, Leung RK, Tierney RC, et al. Mitral valve prolapse syndrome in children with Duchenne's progressive muscular dystrophy. *Pediatrics* 1979;63:116.
15. Yazawa Y. Mitral valve prolapse related to geometrical changes of the heart in cases of progressive muscular dystrophy. *Clin Cardiol* 1984;7:198.
16. Emery AEH. X-linked muscular dystrophy with early contractures and cardiomyopathy [Emery-Dreifuss type]. *Clin Genet* 1987;32:360.
17. Seay AR, Ziter FA, Thompson JA. Cardiac arrest during induction of anesthesia in Duchenne muscular dystrophy. *J Pediatr* 1978;93:88.
18. Kurz LT, Mubarak SJ, Schultz P, et al. Correlation of scoliosis and pulmonary function in Duchenne muscular dystrophy. *J Pediatr Orthop* 1983;3:347.
19. Schreiber A, Smith WL, Ionasescu V, et al. Magnetic resonance imaging of children with Duchenne muscular dystrophy. *Pediatr Radiol* 1987;17:495.

Genetic and Molecular Biology Studies

20. Dietz FR, Mathews KD. Current concepts review. Update on genetic bases of disorders with orthopaedic manifestations. *J Bone Joint Surg Am* 1996;78:1583.
21. Specht LA. Molecular basis and clinical applications of neuromuscular disease in children. *Curr Opin Pediatr* 1991;3:966.

Sex-linked Muscular Dystrophies

22. Marsh GG, Munsat TL. Evidence for early impairment of verbal intelligence in Duchenne muscular dystrophy. *Arch Dis Child* 1974;49:118.
23. Sutherland DH, Olshen R, Cooper L, et al. The pathomechanics of gait in Duchenne muscular dystrophy. *Dev Med Child Neurol* 1981;23:3.
24. Sutherland DH. Gait analysis in neuromuscular diseases. *AAOS Instr Course Lect* 1990;39:333.
25. Hsu JD, Furumasu J. Gait and posture changes in the Duchenne muscular dystrophy child. *Clin Orthop* 1993;288:122.
26. Brooke MH, Fenichel GM, Griggs RC, et al. Duchenne muscular dystrophy. Patterns of clinical progression and effects of supportive therapy. *Neurology* 1989;39:475.
27. Emery AEH. *Duchenne muscular dystrophy,* 2nd ed. New York: Oxford University Press, 1988.
28. Rideau Y, Glorion B, Duport G. Prolongation of ambulation in the muscular dystrophies. *Acta Neurol* 1983;38:390.
29. Wilkins KE, Gibson DA. The patterns of spinal deformity in Duchenne muscular dystrophy. *J Bone Joint Surg Am* 1976;58:24.
30. Roses AD, Roses MJ, Miller SE, et al. Carrier detection in Duchenne muscular dystrophy. *N Engl J Med* 1976;294:193.
31. Kunkel LM, Monaco AP, Hoffman E, et al. Molecular studies of progressive muscular dystrophy (Duchenne). *Enzyme* 1987;38:72.

32. Slater GR. The missing link in Duchenne muscular dystrophy. *Nature* 1987;330:693.

33. Hoffman EP, Brown RH Jr, Kunkel LM. Dystrophin. The protein product of the Duchenne muscular dystrophy locus. *Cell* 1987;51:919.

34. Hoffman EP, Kunkel LM. Dystrophin abnormalities in Duchenne/Becker muscular dystrophy. *Neuron* 1989;2:1019.

35. Darras BT. Molecular genetics of Duchenne and Becker muscular dystrophy. *J Pediatr* 1990;117:1.

36. Uchino M, Araki S, Miike T, et al. Localization and characterization of dystrophin in muscle biopsy specimens for Duchenne muscular dystrophy and various neuromuscular disorders. *Muscle Nerve* 1989;12:1009.

37. Beggs AH, Hoffman EP, Snyder JR, et al. Exploring the molecular basis for variability among patients with Becker muscular dystrophy. Dystrophin gene and protein studies. *Am J Hum Genet* 1991;49:54.

38. Specht LA, Kunkel LM. Duchenne and Becker muscular dystrophies. In: Rosenberg RN, Prusiner SB, DiMauro S, et al., eds. *The molecular and genetic basis of neurological disease.* Boston: Butterworth-Heinemann, 1993:613.

39. Hoffman EP, Kunkel LM, Angelini C, et al. Improved diagnosis of Becker muscular dystrophy by dystrophin testing. *Neurology* 1989;39:1011.

40. Hoffman EP, Fischbeck KH, Brown RH, et al. Characterization of dystrophin in muscle-biopsy specimens from patients with Duchenne's or Becker's muscular dystrophy. *N Engl J Med* 1988;318:1363.

41. Specht LA, Beggs AH, Korf B, et al. Prediction of dystrophin phenotype by DNA analysis in Duchenne/Becker muscular dystrophy. *Pediatr Neurol* 1992;8:432.

42. Nicholson LVB, Johnson MA, Bushby KMD, et al. Functional significance of dystrophin positive fibres in Duchenne muscular dystrophy. *Arch Dis Child* 1993;68:632.

43. Gospe SM Jr, Lazaro RP, Lava NS, et al. Familial X-linked myalgia and cramps. A nonprogressive myopathy associated with a deletion in the dystrophin gene. *Neurology* 1989;39:1277.

44. Partridge TA. Invited review. Myoblast transfer. A possible therapy for inherited myopathies? *Muscle Nerve* 1991;14:197.

45. Partridge TA, Morgan JE, Coulton GR, et al. Conversion of mdx myofibres from dystrophin-negative to -positive by injection of normal myoblasts. *Nature* 1989;337:176.

46. Gussoni E, Pavlath GK, Lanctot AM, et al. Normal dystrophin transcripts detected in Duchenne muscular dystrophy patients after myoblast transplantation. *Nature* 1992;356:435.

47. Huard J, Bouchard JP, Roy R, et al. Human myoblast transplantation; preliminary results of 4 cases. *Muscle Nerve* 1992;15:550.

48. Karpati G, Ajdukovic D, et al. Myoblast transfer in Duchenne muscular dystrophy. Ann Neurol 1993;34:8.

49. Law PK, Goodwin TG, Fang Q, et al. Feasibility, safety and efficacy of myoblast transfer therapy on Duchenne muscular dystrophy boys. *Cell Transplant* 1992;1:235.

50. Mendell JR, Kissel JT, Amato AA, et al. Myoblast transfer in the treatment of Duchenne's muscular dystrophy. *N Engl J Med* 1995;333:832.

51. DeSilva S, Drachman D. Prednisone treatment in Duchenne muscular dystrophy. *Arch Neurol* 1987;44:818.

52. Heckmatt J, Rodillo E, Dubowitz V. Management of children. Pharmacological and physical. *Br Med Bull* 1989;45:788.

53. Dubowitz V. Prednisone in Duchenne dystrophy (editorial). *Neuromuscul Disord* 1991;1:161.

54. Fenichel GM, Florence JM, Pestronk A, et al. Long-term benefit from prednisone therapy in Duchenne muscular dystrophy. *Neurology* 1991;41:1874.

55. Mendell JR, Moxley RT, Griggs RC, et al. Randomized double-blind six-month trial of prednisone in Duchenne's muscular dystrophy. *N Engl J Med* 1989;320:1592.

56. Griggs RC, Moxley RT, Mendell JR, et al. Duchenne dystrophy: randomized, controlled trial of prednisone (18 months) and azathioprine (12 months). *Neurology* 1993;43:520.

57. Green NE. The orthopaedic care of children with muscular dystrophy. *AAOS Instr Course Lect* 1987;36:267.

58. Drennan JC. Neuromuscular disorders. In: Morrissy RT, ed. *Lovell and Winter's pediatric orthopaedics.* Philadelphia: JB Lippincott, 1990:381.

59. Johnson EW, Kennedy JH. Comprehensive management of Duchenne muscular dystrophy. *Arch Phys Med Rehabil* 1971;52:110.

60. Heckmatt JZ, Dubowitz V, Hyde SA, et al. Prolongation of walking in Duchenne muscular dystrophy with lightweight orthoses; review of 57 cases. *Dev Med Child Neurol* 1985;27:149.

61. Spencer GE Jr, Vignos PJ Jr. Bracing for ambulation in childhood progressive muscular dystrophy. *J Bone Joint Surg Am* 1962;44:234.

62. Spencer GE Jr. Orthopaedic care of progressive muscular dystrophy. *J Bone Joint Surg Am* 1967;49:1201.

63. Vignos PJ, Wagner MB, Karlinchak B, Katirji B. Evaluation of a program for long-term treatment of Duchenne muscular dystrophy. Experience at the University Hospitals of Cleveland. *J Bone Joint Surg Am* 1996;78:1844.

64. Chyatte SB, Long C, Vignos PJ. The balanced forearm orthosis in muscular dystrophy. *Arch Phys Med Rehabil* 1965;46:633.

65. Yasuda YL, Bowman K, Hsu JD. Mobile arm supports: criteria for successful use in muscle disease patients. *Arch Phys Med Rehabil* 1986;67:253.

66. Siegel IM, Miller JE, Ray RD. Subcutaneous lower limb tenotomies in treatment of pseudohypertrophic muscular dystrophy. *J Bone Joint Surg Am* 1968;50:1437.

67. Smith SE, Green NE, Cole RJ, et al. Prolongation of ambulation in children with Duchenne muscular dystrophy by subcutaneous lower limb tenotomy. *J Pediatr Orthop* 1993;13:331.

68. Bonnet I, Burgot D, Bonnard C, Glorion B. Surgery of the lower limbs in Duchenne muscular dystrophy. *Fr J Orthop Surg* 1991;5:160.

69. Bowker JH, Halpin PJ. Factors determining success in reambulation of the child with progressive muscular dystrophy. *Ortho Clin North Am* 1978;9:431.

70. Dubousset J, Queneau P. Place et indication de la chirurgie dans la dystrophie musculaire de Duchenne de boulogne a evolution rapide. *Rev Chir Orthop* 1983;69:207.

71. Hsu JD. The management of foot deformity in pseudohypertrophic muscular dystrophy (DMD). *Ortho Clin North Am* 1976;7:979.

72. Rideau Y, Duport G, Delaubier A. Premieres remissions reproductibles dans l'evolution de la dystrophie musculaire de Duchenne. *Bull Acad Natl Med* 1986;170:605.

73. Rodillo EB, Fernandez-Bermejo E, Heckmatt JZ, Dubowitz V. Prevention of rapidly progressive scoliosis in Duchenne muscular dystrophy by prolongation of walking with orthoses. *J Child Neurol* 1988;3:269.

74. Williams EA, Read L, Ellis A, et al. The management of equinus deformity in Duchenne muscular dystrophy. *J Bone Joint Surg Br* 1984;66:546.

75. Vulpius O, Stoffel A. Orthopaedische operationsiehre. 2nd ed. Stuttgart: Ferdinand Enke, 1920.

76. Greene WB. Transfer versus lengthening of the posterior tibial tendon in Duchenne's muscular dystrophy. *Foot Ankle* 1992;13:526.

77. Hsu JD, Hoffer MM. Posterior tibial tendon transfer through the interosseous membrane. A modification of the technique. *Clin Orthop* 1978;131:202.

78. Miller GM, Hsu JD, Hoffer MM, Rentfro R. Posterior tibial tendon transfer. A review of the literature and analysis of 74 procedures. *J Pediatr Orthop* 1982;2:363.

79. Melkonian GJ, Cristafaro RL, Perry J, et al. Dynamic gait electromyography study in Duchenne muscular dystrophy (DMD) patients. *Foot Ankle* 1983;1:78.

80. Yount CC. The role of the tensor fasciae femoris in certain deformities of the lower extremities. *J Bone Joint Surg Am* 1926; 8:171.

81. Ober FR. The role of the iliotibial band and fascia lata as a factor in the causation of low back disabilities and sciatica. *J Bone Joint Surg* 1936;18:105.

82. Soutter R. A new operation for hip contractures in poliomyelitis. *Boston Med Surg J* 1914;170:380.

83. Wagner MB, Vignos PJ Jr, Carlozzi C. Duchenne muscular dystrophy: a study of wrist and hand function. *Muscle Nerve* 1989;12:236.

84. Cambridge W, Drennan JC. Scoliosis associated with Duchenne muscular dystrophy. *J Pediatr Orthop* 1987;7:436.

85. Galasko CSB, Delaney C, Morris P. Spinal stabilisation in Duchenne muscular dystrophy. *J Bone Joint Surg Br* 1992;74:210.

86. Gibson DA, Wilkins KE. The management of spinal deformities in Duchenne muscular dystrophy. A new concept in spinal bracing. *Clin Orthop* 1975;108:41.

87. Hsu JD. The natural history of spine curvature progression in the nonambulatory Duchenne muscular dystrophy patient. *Spine* 1983;8:771.

88. Mubarak SJ, Miller LS. Muscular dystrophy. In: Weinstein SL, ed. *The pediatric spine. Principles and practice.* New York: Raven, 1994:1101.

89. Robin GC, Brief LP. Scoliosis in childhood muscular dystrophy. *J Bone Joint Surg Am* 1971;53:4666.

90. Siegel IM. Scoliosis in muscular dystrophy: some comments about diagnosis, observations on prognosis, suggestions for therapy *Clin Orthop* 1973;93:235.

91. Smith AD, Koreska J, Moseley CF. Progression of scoliosis in Duchenne muscular dystrophy. *J Bone Joint Surg Am* 1989;71: 1066.

92. Lord J, Behrman B, Varzos N, et al. Scoliosis associated with Duchenne muscular dystrophy. *Arch Phys Med Rehabil* 1990; 71:13.

93. Colbert AP, Craig C. Scoliosis management in Duchenne muscular dystrophy. Prospective study of modified Jewett hyperextension brace. *Arch Phys Med Rehabil* 1987;68:302.

94. Seeger BR, Sutherland AD, Clark MS. Orthotic management of scoliosis in Duchenne muscular dystrophy. *Arch Phys Med Rehabil* 1984;65:83.

95. Sussman MD. Advantage of early spinal stabilization and fusion in patients with Duchenne muscular dystrophy. *J Pediatr Orthop* 1984;4:532.

96. Swank SM, Brown JC, Perry RE. Spinal fusion in Duchenne's muscular dystrophy. *Spine* 1982;7:484.

97. Weimann RL, Gibson DA, Moseley CF, Jones DC. Surgical stabilization of the spine in Duchenne muscular dystrophy. *Spine* 1983;8:776.

98. Shapiro F, Sethna N, Colan S, et al. Spinal fusion in Duchenne muscular dystrophy: a multidisciplinary approach. *Muscle Nerve* 1992;15:604.

99. Heller KD, Forst R, Forst J, Hengstler K. Scoliosis in Duchenne muscular dystrophy: aspects of orthotic treatment. *Prosthet Orthot Int* 1997;21:202.

100. Boachie-Adjei O, Lonstein JE, Winter RB, et al. Management of neuromuscular spinal deformities with Luque segmental instrumentation. *J Bone Joint Surg Am* 1989;71:548.

101. Rideau Y, Glorion B, Delaubier A, et al. The treatment of scoliosis in Duchenne muscular dystrophy. *Muscle Nerve* 1984; 7:281.

102. Marchesi D, Arlet V, Stricker U, Aebi M. Modification of the original Luque technique in the treatment of Duchenne's neuromuscular scoliosis. *J Pediatr Orthop* 1997;17:743.

103. Miller F, Moseley CF, Koreska J. Spinal fusion in Duchenne muscular dystrophy. *Dev Med Child Neurol* 1992;34:775.

104. Oda T, Shimizu N, Yonenobu K, et al. Longitudinal study of spinal deformity in Duchenne muscular deformity. *J Pediatr Orthop* 1993;13:478.

105. Bridwell KH, O'Brien MF, Lenke LG, et al. Posterior spinal fusion supplemented with only allograft bone in paralytic scoliosis. Does it work? *Spine* 1994;19:2658.

106. Brook PD, Kennedy JD, Stern LM, et al. Spinal Fusion in Duchenne's muscular dystrophy. *J Pediatr Orthop* 1996;16:324.

107. Fox HJ, Thomas CH, Thompson AG. Spinal instrumentation for Duchenne's muscular dystrophy: experience of hypotensive anesthesia to minimize blood loss. *J Pediatr Orthop* 1997;17: 750.

108. Yazici M, Asher MA. Freeze-dried allograft for posterior spinal fusion in patients with neuromuscular spinal deformities. *Spine* 1997;22:1467.

109. Bridwell KH, Baldus C, Iffrig TM, et al. Process measures and patient/parent evaluation of surgical management of spinal deformities in patients with progressive flaccid neuromuscular scoliosis (Duchenne's muscular dystrophy and spinal muscular atrophy). *Spine* 1999;24:1300.

110. Ramirez N, Richards SB, Warren PD, Williams GR. Complications after posterior spinal fusion in Duchenne's muscular dystrophy. *J Pediatr Orthop* 1997;17:109.

111. Taddonio RF. Segmental spinal instrumentation in the management of neuromuscular spinal deformity. *Spine* 1982;7:305.

112. Broom MJ.

113. Lonstein JE. The Galveston technique using Luque or Cotrel-Dubousset rods. *Ortho Clin North Am.* 1994;25:311–320.

114. Allen BL Jr, Ferguson AL. The Galveston technique for L-rod instrumentation of the scoliotic spine. *Spine* 1982;7:119.

115. McCarthy RE, Bruffett WL, McCullough FL. S rod fixation to the sacrum in patients with neuromuscular spinal deformities. *Clin Orthop* 1999;364:26.

116. Mubarak SJ, Morin WD, Leach J. Spinal fusion in Duchenne muscular dystrophy—fixation and fusion to the sacropelvis? *J Pediatr Orthop* 1993;13:752.

117. Rice JJ, Jeffers BL, Devitt AT, McManus F. Management of the collapsing spine for patients with Duchenne muscular dystrophy. *Ir J Med Sci* 1998;167:242.

118. Jenkins JG, Bohn D, Edmonds JF, et al. Evaluation of pulmonary function in muscular dystrophy patients requiring spinal surgery. *Crit Care Med* 1982;10:645.

119. Rideau Y, Jankowski LW, Grellet J. Respiratory function in the muscular dystrophies. *Muscle Nerve* 1981;4:155.

120. Rideau Y, Delaubier A. Neuromuscular respiratory deficit. Setting back mortality. *Semin Orthop* 1987;2:203.

121. Smith PEM, Calverley PMA, Edwards RHT, et al. Practical problems in the respiratory care of patients with muscular dystrophy. *N Engl J Med* 1987;316:1197.

122. Kennedy JD, Staples AJ, Brook PD, et al. Effect of spinal surgery on lung function in Duchenne muscular dystrophy. *Thorax* 1995;50:1173.

123. Miller F, Moseley CF, Koreska J, et al. Pulmonary function and scoliosis in Duchenne dystrophy. *J Pediatr Orthop* 1988;8: 133.

124. Miller RG, Chalmers AC, Dao H, et al. The effects of spine fusion on respiratory function in Duchenne muscular dystrophy. *Neurology* 1991;41:38.

125. Granata C, Merlini L, Cervelatti S. Long-term results of spine surgery in Duchenne muscular dystrophy. *Neuromuscul Disord* 1996;6:61.

126. Noordeen MH, Hoddad FS, Muntoni F, et al. Blood loss in Duchenne muscular dystrophy: vascular smooth muscle dysfunction. *J Pediatr Orthop B* 1999;8:212.

127. Noordeen MHH, Lee J, Gibbons CER, et al. Spinal cord monitoring in operations for neuromuscular scoliosis. *J Bone Joint Surg Br* 1997;79:53.

128. Alexander MA, Johnson EW, Petty J, et al. Mechanical ventilation of patients with late stage Duchenne muscular dystrophy. Management in the home. *Arch Phys Med Rehabil* 1979;60:289.

129. Bach JR, O'Brien J, Krolenberg R, et al. Muscular dystrophy. Management of end stage respiratory failure in Duchenne muscular dystrophy. *Muscle Nerve* 1987;10:177.

130. Curran FJ. Night ventilation by body respirators for patients in chronic respiratory failure due to late stage Duchenne muscular dystrophy. *Arch Phys Med Rehabil* 1981;62:270.

131. Hilton T, Orr RD, Perkin RM, et al. End of life care in Duchenne muscular dystrophy. *Pediatr Neurol* 1993;9:165.

132. Stewart CA, Gilgoff Baydur A, Prentice W, et al. Gated radionuclide ventriculography in the evolution of cardiac function in Duchenne's muscular dystrophy. *Chest* 1988;94:1245.

133. Emery AEH, Watt MS, Clack ER. The effects of genetic counseling in Duchenne muscular dystrophy. *Clin Genet* 1972;3:147.

134. Becker PE. Two new families of benign sex-linked recessive muscular dystrophy. *Rev Can Biol* 1962;21:551.

135. Bradley WG, Jones MZ, Mussini JM, et al. Becker-type muscular dystrophy. *Muscle Nerve* 1978;1:111.

136. Daher YH, Lonstein JE, Winter RB, et al. Spinal deformities in patients with muscular dystrophy other than Duchenne. A review of 11 patients having surgical treatment. *Spine* 1985;10:614.

137. Dickey RP, Ziter FA, Smith RA. Emery-Dreifuss muscular dystrophy. *J Pediatr* 1984;104:555.

138. Miller RG, Layzer RB, Mellenthin MA, et al. Emery-Dreifuss muscular dystrophy with autosomal dominant transmission. *Neurology* 1985;35:1230.

139. Shapiro F, Specht L. Orthopedic deformities in Emery-Dreifuss muscular dystrophy. *J Pediatr Orthop* 1991;11:336.

140. Specht LA. Case records of the Massachusetts General Hospital. Case 34-1992. *N Engl J Med* 1992;327:548.

141. Merlini L, Granata C, Dominici P, et al. Emery-Dreifuss muscular dystrophy. Report of five cases in a family and review of the literature. *Muscle Nerve* 1986;9:481.

142. Goto I, Ishimoto S, Yamada T, et al. The rigid spine syndrome and Emery-Dreifuss muscular dystrophy. *Clin Neurol Neurosurg* 1986;88:293.

143. Consalez GG, Thomas NST, Stayton CL, et al. Assignment of Emery-Dreifuss muscular dystrophy to the distal region of Xq28. The results of a collaborative study. *Am J Hum Genet* 1991;48:468.

144. Thomas NS, Williams H, Elsas LJ, et al. Localization of the gene for Emery-Dreifuss muscular dystrophy to the distal long arm of the X-chromosome. *J Med Genet* 1986;23:596.

145. Hopkins LC, Jackson JA, Elsas LJ. Emery-Dreifuss humeroperoneal muscular dystrophy. An X-linked myopathy with unusual contractures and bradycardia. *Ann Neurol* 1981;10:230.

Autosomal Recessive Muscular Dystrophies

146. Arikawa E, Hoffman EP, Kaido M, et al. The frequency of patients with dystrophin abnormalities in a limb-girdle patient population. *Neurology* 1991;41:1491.

147. Bushby K. Report on the 12th ENMC sponsored international workshop—the 'limb-girdle' muscular dystrophies. *Neuromuscul Disord* 1992;2:3.

148. Beckman JS, Richard I, et al. A gene for limb-girdle muscular dystrophy maps to chromosome 15 by linkage. *C R Acad Sci III* 1991;312:141.

149. Speer MC, Yamaoka LH, Gilchrist JH, et al. Confirmation of genetic heterogeneity in limb-girdle muscular dystrophy: linkage of an autosomal dominant form to chromosome 5q. *Am J Hum Genet* 1992;50:1211.

150. Bailey RO, Marzulo DC, Hans MB. Muscular dystrophy. Infantile fascioscapulohumeral muscular dystrophy. New observations. *Acta Neurol Scand* 1986;74:51.

151. Carroll JE, Brooke MH. Infantile fascioscapulohumeral dystrophy. In: Serratrice G, Roux H, eds. *Peroneal atrophies and related disorders*. New York: Masson, 1978:305.

152. Korf BR, Bresnan MJ, Shapiro F, et al. Fascioscapulohumeral dystrophy presenting in infancy with facial diplegia and sensorineural deafness. *Ann Neurol* 1985;17:513.

153. Shapiro F, Specht L, Korf BR. Locomotor problems in infantile fascioscapulohumeral muscular dystrophy. Retrospective study of 9 patients. *Acta Orthop Scand* 1991;62:367.

154. Hanson PA, Rowland LP. Möbius syndrome and fascioscapulohumeral muscular dystrophy. *Arch Neurol* 1971;24:31.

Autosomal Dominant Muscular Dystrophies

155. Kazakov VM, Bogorodinsky DK, Znoyko ZV, et al. The fascioscapulo-limb (or the fascioscapulohumeral) type of muscular dystrophy. Clinical and genetic study. *Eur Neurol* 1974;11:236.

156. Fisher J, Upadhyaya M. Molecular genetics of fascioscapulohumeral muscular dystrophy (FSHD). *Neuromuscul Disord* 1997;7:55.

157. Wijmenga C, Frants RR, Brouwer OF, et al. Location of fascioscapulohumeral muscular dystrophy gene on chromosome 4. *Lancet* 1990;336:651.

158. Bodensteiner JB, Schochet SS. Fascioscapulohumeral muscular dystrophy. The choice of a biopsy site. *Muscle Nerve* 1986;9:544.

159. Bunch WH, Siegal IM. Scapulothoracic arthrodesis in fascioscapulohumeral muscular dystrophy. Review of seventeen procedures with three to twenty-one year follow-up. *J Bone Joint Surg Am* 1993;75:372.

160. Copeland SA, Howard RC. Thoracoscapular fusion for fascioscapulohumeral dystrophy. *J Bone Joint Surg Br* 1978;60:547.

161. Copeland SA, Levy O, Warner GC, et al. The shoulder in patients with muscular dystrophy. *Clin Orthop* 1999;368:80.

162. Jakab E, Gledhill RB. Simplified technique for scapulocostal fusion in fascioscapulohumeral dystrophy. *J Pediatr Orthop* 1993;13:749.

163. Ketenjian AY. Scapulocostal stabilization for scapular winging in fascioscapulohumeral muscular dystrophy. *J Bone Joint Surg Am* 1978;60:476.

164. Kocialkowski A, Frostick SP, Wallace WA. One-stage bilateral thoracoscapular fusion using allografts. A case report. *Clin Orthop* 1991;273:264.

165. Letournel E, Fardeau M, Lytle JO, et al. Scapulothoracic arthrodesis for patients who have fascioscapulohumeral muscular dystrophy. *J Bone Joint Surg Am* 1990;72:78.

166. Wosick WF, Alker G. CT manifestation of ocular muscular dystrophy. *Comput Radiol* 1984;8:391.

167. Olson W, Engel WK, Walsh GO, et al. Oculocraniosomatic neuromuscular disease with "ragged-red" fibers. *Arch Neurol* 1993;26:193.

168. Barbeau A. The syndrome of hereditary late onset ptosis and dysphagia in French Canada. In Kuhn E, ed. *Symposium uber*

Progressive Muskeldystrophie, Myotonie, Myasthenie. Berlin: Springer-Verlag, 1966;102.

169. Pratt MF, Meyers PK. Oculopharyngeal muscular dystrophy. Recent ultrastructural evidence for mitochondrial abnormalities. *Laryngoscope* 1986;96:368.

170. Dobrowski JM, Zajtchuck JT, LaPiana FG, et al. Oculopharyngeal muscular dystrophy. Clinical and histopathologic correlations. *Otolaryngol Head Neck Surg* 1986;95:131.

171. Duranceau A, Forand MD, Fautaux JP. Surgery in oculopharyngeal muscular dystrophy. *Am J Surg* 1980;139:33.

Myotonia

172. O'Brien TA, Harper PS. Course, prognosis and complications of childhood-onset myotonic dystrophy. *Dev Med Child Neurol* 1984;26:62.

173. Cook AW, Bird TD, Spence AM, et al. Myotonic dystrophy, mitral-valve prolapse and stroke. *Lancet* 1978;1:335.

174. Schonk D, Coerwinkel-Driessen M, van Dalen I, et al. Definition of subchromosomal intervals around the myotonic dystrophy gene region at 19q. *Genomics* 1989;4:384.

175. Bell DB, Smith DW. Myotonic dystrophy in the neonate. *J Pediatr* 1972;81:83.

176. Carroll JE, Brooke MH, Kaiser K. Diagnosis of infantile myotonic dystrophy. *Lancet* 1975;2:608.

177. Hanson PA. Myotonic dystrophy in infancy and childhood. *Pediatr Ann* 1984;13:123.

178. Vanier TM. Dystrophia myotonia in childhood. *Br Med J* 1960; 2(5208):1284.

179. Zellweger H, Ionasescu V. Early onset of myotonic dystrophy in infants. *Am J Dis Child* 1973;125:601.

180. Calderon R. Myotonic dystrophy. A neglected cause of mental retardation. *J Pediatr* 1966;68:423.

181. Speer MC, Pericak-Vance MA, Yamaoka L, et al. Presymptomatic and prenatal diagnosis in myotonic dystrophy by genetic linkage studies. *Neurology* 1990;40:671.

182. Bowen RS Jr, Marks HG. Foot deformities in myotonic dystrophy. *Foot Ankle* 1984;5:125.

183. Gross RH. The role of the Verebelyi-Ogston procedure: the management of the arthrogrypotic foot. *Clin Orthop* 1985;194:99.

184. Burnham R. Unusual causes of stiffness in two hocky players. *Clin J Sport Med* 1997;7:137.

185. Haig AJ. The complex interactions of myotonic dystrophy in low back pain. *Spine* 1991;16:580.

186. Weinberg J, Curl LA, Kuncl RW, et al. Occult presentation of myotonia congenita in a 15-year-old athlete. *Am J Sports Med* 1999;27:529.

187. Winters JL, McLaughlin LA. Myotonia congenita. *J Bone Joint Surg Am* 1970;52:1345.

188. Geschwind N, Simpson JA. Procaine amide in the treatment of myotonia. *Brain* 1955;78:81.

189. Kubisch C, Schmidt-Rose T, Fontaine B, et al. ClC-1 chloride channel mutations in myotonia congenita: variable penetrance of mutations shifting the voltage dependence. *Hum Mol Genet* 1998;7:1753.

190. Plassart-Schiss E, Gervais A, Eymard B, et al. Novel muscle chloride channel (ClCN1) mutations in myotonia congenita with various modes of inheritance including incomplete dominance and penetrance. *Neurology* 1998;50:1176.

Congenital Myopathies and Congenital Muscular Dystrophy

191. Brooke MH. *A clinician's view of neuromuscular diseases.* Baltimore: Williams & Wilkins, 1977.

192. Dubowitz V. *Muscle disorders in childhood.* Philadelphia: WB Saunders, 1978.

193. Zellweger H, McCormick WF, Mergner W. Severe congenital muscular dystrophy. *Am J Dis Child* 1967;114:591.

194. Banker BQ. *Myology. Basic and clinical.* vol. 2. New York: McGraw-Hill, 1986:1367.

195. Goebel HH. Congenital myopathies. In: Adachi M, Ser JH, eds. *Neuromuscular disorders.* New York: Igaku-Schoin, 1990:197.

196. Goebel HH. Congenital myopathies. *Semin Pediatr Neurol* 1996;3:152.

Congenital Myopathies

197. Gamble JG, Rinsky LA, Lee JH. Orthopaedic aspects of central core disease. *J Bone Joint Surg Am* 1988;70:1061.

198. Shuaib A, Paasuke RT, Brownell KW. Central core disease. Clinical features in 13 patients. *Medicine* 1987;66:389.

199. Armstrong RM, Koenigsberg R, Mellinger J, et al. Central core disease with congenital hip dislocation: study of two families. *Neurology* 1971;21:369.

200. Kumano K. Congenital non-progressive myopathy, associated with scoliosis: clinical, histological, histochemical and electron microscopic studies of seven cases. *Nippon Seikeigeka Gakkai Zasshi* 1980;54:381.

201. Ramsey PL, Hensinger RN. Congenital dislocation of the hip associated with central core disease. *J Bone Joint Surg Am* 1975;57:648.

202. Frank JP, Harati Y, Butler IJ, et al. Central core disease and malignant hyperthermia syndrome. *Ann Neurol* 1980;7:11.

203. Haan EA, Freemantle CJ, McCure JA, et al. Assignment of the gene for central core disease to chromosome 19. *Hum Genet* 1990;86:187.

204. Martinez BA, Lake BD. Childhood nemaline myopathy: a review of clinical presentation in relation to prognosis. *Dev Med Child Neurol* 1987;29:815.

205. Shimomura C, Nonaka I. Nemaline myopathy: comparative muscle histochemistry in the severe neonatal, moderate congenital and adult-onset forms. *Pediatr Neurol* 1989;5:25.

206. Shy GM, Engel WK, Somers JE, et al. Nemaline myopathy. A new congenital myopathy. *Brain* 1963;86:793.

207. Eeg-Olofsson O, Henriksson KG, Thornell LE, et al. Early infant death in nemaline (rod) myopathy. *Brain Dev* 1983;5:53.

208. Maayan C, Springer C, Armon T, et al. Nemaline myopathy as a cause of sleep hypoventilation. *Pediatrics* 1986;77:390.

209. McComb RD, Markesbery WR, O'Connor WN. Fatal neonatal nemaline myopathy with multiple congenital anomalies. *J Pediatr* 1979;95:47.

210. Cunliffe M, Burrows FA. Anesthetic implications of nemaline rod myopathy. *Can Anaesth Soc J* 1985;32:543.

211. Wallgren-Pettersson C, Clarke A, Samson F, et al. The myotubular myopathies: differential diagnosis of the X-linked recessive, autosomal dominant and autosomal recessive forms and present state of DNA studies. *J Med Genet* 1995;32:673.

212. Munsat TL, Thompson LR, Coleman RF. Centronuclear ("myotubular") myopathy. *Arch Neurol* 1969;20:120.

213. Spiro AJ, Shy GM, Gonatas NK. Myotubular myopathy. Persistence of fetal muscle in an adolescent boy. *Arch Neurol* 1966;14:1.

214. Darnsfors C, Larsson HEB, Oldfors A, et al. X-linked myotubular myopathy: a linkage study. *Clin Genet* 1990;37:335.

215. Cavanagh NPC, Lake BD, McMeniman P. Congenital fibre type disproportion myopathy. A histological diagnosis with an uncertain clinical outlook. *Arch Dis Child* 1979;54:735.

216. Brooke MH. A neuromuscular disease characterized by fiber

types disproportion. In: Kakulas BA, ed. *Proceedings of the Second International Congress on Muscle Diseases.* Perth, Australia, November 1971. Amsterdam: Excerpta Medica, 1973.

217. Gullotta F. Metabolic myopathies. *Pathol Res Pract* 1985;80: 10.
218. Cornelio F, DiDonato S. Myopathies due to enzyme deficiencies. *J Neurol* 1985;232:321
219. Kearns TP, Sayre GP. Retinitis pigmentosa, external ophthalmoplegia and complete heart block. *Arch Ophthalmol* 1958;60: 280.
220. Mechler F, Mastaglia FL, Serena M, et al. Mitochondrial myopathies. A clinico-pathological study of cases with and without extra-ocular muscle involvement. *Aust NZ J Med* 1986;16:185.

Congenital Muscular Dystrophy

221. Leyten QH, Gabreels FJ, Renier WO, et al. Congenital muscular dystrophy: a review of the literature. *Clin Neurol Neurosurg* 1996;98:267.
222. McManamin JB, Becker LE, Murphy EG. Congenital muscular dystrophy: a clinicopathologic report of 24 cases. *J Pediatr* 1982; 100:692.
223. Fukuyama Y, Osawa M, Suzuki H. Congenital progressive muscular dystrophy of the Fukuyama type—clinical, genetic and pathological considerations. *Brain Dev* 1981;3:1.
224. Fukuyama Y, Osawa M. A genetic study of the Fukuyama type congenital muscular dystrophy. *Brain Dev* 1983;6:373.
225. Hillaire D, Leclerc A, Faure S, et al. Localization of merosin-negative congenital muscular dystrophy to chromosome 6q2 by homozygosity mapping. *Hum Mol Genet* 1994;3:1657.
226. Philpot J, Sewry C, Pennock J, Dubowitz V. Clinical phenotype in congenital muscular dystrophy: correlation with expression of merosin in skeletal muscle. *Neuromuscul Disord* 1995;5:301.
227. Jones R, Kahn R, Hughes S, Dubowitz V. Congenital muscular dystrophy. The importance of early diagnosis and orthopaedic management in the long-term prognosis. *J Bone Joint Surg Br* 1979;61:13.

Spinal Muscular Atrophy

228. Gordon N. The spinal muscular atrophies. *Dev Med Child Neurol* 1991;33:930.
229. Iannaccone ST. Spinal muscular atrophy. *Sem Neurol* 1998;18: 19.
230. Russman BS, Melchreit R, Drennan, JC. Spinal muscular atrophy. The natural course of the disease. *Muscle Nerve* 1983;6: 179.
231. Shapiro F, Bresnan MJ. Current concepts review. Orthopaedic management of childhood neuromuscular disease. Part I. Spinal muscular atrophy. *J Bone Joint Surg Am* 1982;64:785.
232. Shapiro F, Specht L. Current concepts review. The diagnosis and orthopaedic treatment of childhood spinal muscular atrophy, peripheral neuropathy, Friedreich ataxia and arthrogryposis. *J Bone Joint Surg Am* 1993;75:1699.
233. Brzustowicz LM, Lehner T, Castilla LH, et al. Genetic mapping of chronic childhood-onset spinal muscular atrophy to chromosome 5q 11.2. *Nature* 1990;334:540.
234. Iannaccone ST, Browne RH, Samaha FJ, et al. Prospective study of spinal muscular atrophy before age 6 years. *Pediatr Neurol* 1993;9:187.
235. Schwentker EP, Gibson DA. The orthopaedic aspects of spinal muscular atrophy. *J Bone Joint Surg Am* 1976;58:32.
236. Brooke MH. *A clinician's view of neuromuscular diseases.* 2nd ed. Baltimore: Williams and Wilkins, 1986:36.
237. Pearn J. Classifications of spinal muscular atrophies. *Lancet* 1980;1:919.

238. Russman BS, Iannascone ST, Buncher CR, et al. Spinal muscular atrophy. New thoughts on the pathogenesis and classification schema. *J Child Neurol* 1992;7:347.
239. Burke SW, Jameson VP, Roberts JM, et al. Birth fractures in spinal muscular atrophy. *J Pediatr Orthop* 1986;6:34.
240. Gilgoff IS, Kahlstrom E, McLaughlin E, Keens TG. Long-term ventilatory support in spinal muscular atrophy. *J Pediatr* 1989; 115:904.
241. Evans GA, Drennan JC, Russman BS. Functional classification and orthopaedic management of spinal muscular atrophy. *J Bone Joint Surg Br* 1981;63:516.
242. Merlini L, Granata C, Bonfiglioli S, et al. Scoliosis in spinal muscular atrophy. Natural history and management. *Dev Med Child Neurol* 1989;31:301.
243. Gilliam TC, Brzustowicz LM, Castilla LH, et al. Genetic homogeneity between acute and chronic forms of spinal muscular atrophy. *Nature* 1990;345:823.
244. Melki J, Sheth P, Abdelhak S, et al. The French spinal muscular atrophy investigators. Mapping of acute (type 1) spinal muscular atrophy to chromosome 5q12 q14. *Lancet* 1990;336:271.
245. Melki J, Abdelhak S, Sheth P, et al. Gene for chronic proximal spinal muscular atrophies maps to chromosome 5q. *Nature* 1990;344:767.
246. Burlet P, Burglen L, Clermont O, et al. Large scale deletions of the 5q13 region are specific to Werdnig-Hoffman disease. *J Med Genet* 1996;33:281.
247. Stewart H, Wallace A, McGaughran J, et al. Molecular diagnosis of spinal muscular atrophy. *Arch Dis Child* 1998;78:531.
248. Miles JM. Diagnosis and discussion. Type I spinal muscular atrophy (Werdnig-Hoffman disease). *Am J Dis Child* 1993;147: 908.
249. Bowen JR, Forlin E. Spinal muscular atrophy. In: Weinstein SL, ed. *The pediatric spine. Principles and practice.* New York: Raven, 1994:1025.
250. Granata C, Cornelio F, Bonfiglioli S, et al. Promotion of ambulation of patients with spinal muscular atrophy by early fitting of knee-ankle-foot orthoses. *Dev Med Child Neurol* 1987;29: 221.
251. Thompson CE, Larsen LJ. Recurrent hip dislocation in intermediate spinal atrophy. *J Pediatr Orthop* 1990;10:638.
252. Brown CJ, Zeller JL, Swank SM, et al. Surgical and functional results of spine fusion in spinal muscular atrophy. *Spine* 1989; 14:763.
253. Granata C, Merlini L, Magni E, et al. Spinal muscular atrophy. Natural history and orthopaedic treatment of scoliosis. *Spine* 1989;14:760.
254. Phillips DP, Roye DP Jr, Farcy J-P, et al. Surgical treatment of scoliosis in a spinal muscular atrophy population. *Spine* 1990; 15:942.
255. Rodillo E, Marini ML, Heckmaht JZ, Dubowitz V. Scoliosis in spinal muscular atrophy. Review of 63 cases. *J Child Neurol* 1989;4:118.
256. Riddick MF, Winter RB, Lutter LD. Spinal deformities in patients with spinal muscle atrophy. A review of 36 patients. *Spine* 1982;7:476.
257. Aprin H, Bowen JR, MacEwen GD, et al. Spine arthrodesis in patients with spinal muscular atrophy. *J Bone Joint Surg Am* 1982;64:1179.
258. Hensinger RN, MacEwen GD. Spinal deformity associated with heritable neurological conditions. Spinal muscular atrophy. Friedreich's ataxia, familial dysautonomia, and Charcot-Marie-Tooth disease. *J Bone Joint Surg Am* 1976;58:13.
259. Piasecki JO, Mahinpour S, Lovine DB. Long-term follow-up of spinal fusion in spinal muscular atrophy. *Clin Orthop* 1986; 207:44.
260. Letts M, Rathbone D, Yamashita T, et al. Soft Boston orthosis

in management of neuromuscular scoliosis. *J Pediatr Orthop* 1992;12:470.

261. Furumasu J, Swank SM, Brown JC, et al. Functional activities in spinal muscular atrophy patients after spinal fusion. *Spine* 1989;14:771.

262. Askin GN, Hallett R, Hare N, Webb JK. The outcome of scoliosis surgery in the severely physically handicapped child. An objective and subjective assessment. *Spine* 1997;22:44.

263. Daher YH, Lonstein JE, Winter RB, Bradford DS. Spinal surgery in spinal muscular atrophy. *J Pediatr Orthop* 1985;5:391.

264. Liu GT, Specht LA. Progressive juvenile segmental spinal muscular atrophy. *Pediatr Neurol* 1992;9:54.

Friedreich Ataxia

265. Fujita R, Hanauer A, Vincent A, et al. Physical mapping of two loci (D9S5 and D9S15) tightly linked to Friedreich ataxia locus (FRDA) and identification of nearby CpG Islands by pulse-field gel electrophoresis. *Genomics* 1991;10:915.

266. Shapiro F, Bresnan MJ. Current concepts review. Orthopaedic management of childhood neuromuscular disease. Part II: peripheral neuropathies, Friedreich's ataxia and arthrogryposis multiplex congenita. *J Bone Joint Surg Am* 1982;64:949.

267. Geoffroy G, Barbeau A, Breton G, et al. Clinical description and roentgenologic evaluation of patients with Friedreich's ataxia. *Can J Neurol Sci* 1976;3:279.

268. Harding AE. Freidreich's ataxia. A clinical and genetic study of 90 families with an analysis of early diagnostic criteria and intrafamilial clustering of clinical features. *Brain* 1981;104:589.

269. Cady RB, Bobechko WP. Incidence, natural history and treatment of scoliosis in Friedreich's ataxia. *J Pediatr Orthop* 1984;4:673.

270. Daher YH, Lonstein JE, Winter RB, et al. Spinal deformities in patients with Freidreich ataxia. A review of 19 patients. *J Pediatr Orthop* 1985;5:553.

271. Filla A, DeMichele G, Caruso G, et al. Genetic data and natural history of Friedreich's disease. A study of 80 Italian patients. *J Neurol* 1990;237:345.

272. Labelle H, Beauchomp M, LaPierre Duhaime M, Allard P. Pattern of muscle weakness and its relation to loss of ambulatory function in Friedreich's ataxia. *J Pediatr Orthop* 1987;7:496.

273. Hewer RL. Study of fatal cases of Friedreich's ataxia. *Br Med J* 1968;3:649.

274. Chamberlain S, Shaw J, Rowland A, et al. Mapping of mutation causing Friedreich's ataxia to human chromosome 9. *Nature* 1988;334:248.

275. Campuzano V, Montermini L, Molto MD, et al. Friedreich's ataxia: autosomal recessive disease caused by an intronic GAA triplet repeat expansion. *Science* 1996;271:1423.

276. Hensinger RN, MacEwen GD. Spinal deformity associated with heritable neurological conditions. Spinal muscular atrophy, Friedreich's ataxia, familial dysautonomia, and Charcot-Marie-Tooth disease. *J Bone Joint Surg Am* 1976;58:13.

277. Labelle H, Tohme S, Duhaime M, et al. Natural history of scoliosis in Friedreich's ataxia. *J Bone Joint Surg Am* 1986;68:564.

278. Labelle H, Duhaime M, Allard P. Spinal deformities in Friedrieich's ataxia. In: Weinstein SL, ed. *The pediatric spine: principles of practice*. New York: Raven, 1994:999.

Hereditary Motor Sensory Neuropathies

279. Warner LE, Garcia CA, Lupski JR. Hereditary peripheral neuropathies: clinical forms, genetics, and molecular mechanisms. *Ann Rev Med* 1999;50:263.

280. Lupski JR, de Oca-Luna RM, Slaugenhaupt S, et al. DNA duplication associated with Charcot-Marie-Tooth disease type 1A. *Cell* 1991;66:219.

281. Vance JM, Nicholson GA, Yamaoka LH, et al. Linkage of Charcot-Marie-Tooth neuropathy type 1A to chromosome 17. *Exp Neurol* 1989;104:186.

282. Vance JM. Hereditary motor and sensory neuropathies. *J Med Genet* 1991;28:1.

283. Patel PI, Roa BB, Welcher AA, et al. The gene for the peripheral myelin protein pmp-22 is a candidate for Charcot-Marie-Tooth disease type 1A. *Nat Genet* 1992;1:159.

284. Timmerman V, Nelis E, Van Hul W, et al. The peripheral myelin protein gene pmp-22 is contained within the Charcot-Marie-Tooth disease type 1A duplication. *Nat Genet* 1992;1:171.

285. Valentijn LJ, Bolhuis PA, Zorn I, et al. The peripheral myelin gene PMP-22/GAS-3 is duplicated in Charcot-Marie-Tooth disease type IA. *Nat Genet* 1992;1:166.

286. Roa BB, Garcia CA, Suter U, et al. Charcot-Marie-Tooth disease type 1A. Association with a spontaneous point mutation in the PMP22 gene. *N Engl J Med* 1993;329:96.

287. Alexander TJ, Johnson KA. Assessment and management of pes cavus in Charcot-Marie-Tooth disease. *Clin Orthop* 1989;246:273.

288. Ghanem I, Zeller R, Seringe R. The foot in hereditary motor and sensory neuropathies in children. *Rev Chir Orthop Reparatrice Appar Mot* 1996;82:152.

289. Mann RA, Missirian J. Pathophysiology of Charcot-Marie-Tooth disease. *Clin Orthop* 1988;234:221.

290. McCluskey WP, Lovell WW, Cummings RJ. The cavovarus foot deformity. Etiology and management. *Clin Orthop* 1989;247:27.

291. Paulos L, Coleman SS, Samuelson KM. Pes cavovarus. Review of a surgical approach using selective soft-tissue procedures. *J Bone Joint Surg Am* 1980;62:942.

292. Sabir M, Lyttle D. Pathogenesis of Charcot-Marie-Tooth disease. Gait analysis and electrophysiologic, genetic, histopathologic, and enzyme studies in a kinship. *Clin Orthop* 1984;184:223.

293. Price AE, Maisel R, Drennan JC. Computed tomographic analysis of the pes cavus. *J Pediatr Orthop* 1993;13:646.

294. Bost FC, Schottstaedt ER, Larsen LJ. Plantar dissection. An operation to release the soft tissues in recurrent or recalcitrant talipes equinovarus. *J Bone Joint Surg Am* 1960;42:151.

295. Roper BA, Tibrewal SB. Soft tissue surgery in Charcot-Marie-Tooth disease. *J Bone Joint Surg Br* 1989;71:17.

296. Richardson EG. Neurogenic disorders. In: Crenshaw AH, ed. *Campbell's operative orthopaedics*. 8th ed, vol. 4. St. Louis: CV Mosby, 1992:2777.

297. Angus PD, Cowell HR. Triple arthrodesis. A critical long-term review. *J Bone Joint Surg Br* 1986;68:260.

298. Mann DC, Hsu JD. Triple arthrodesis in the treatment of fixed cavovarus deformity in adolescent patients with Charcot-Marie-Tooth disease. *Foot Ankle* 1992;13:1.

299. Gould N. Surgery in advanced Charcot-Marie-Tooth disease. *Foot Ankle* 1984;4:267.

300. Wetmore RS, Drennan JC. Long-term results of triple arthrodesis in Charcot-Marie-Tooth Disease. *J Bone Joint Surg Am* 1989;71:417.

301. Wukich DK, Bowen JR. A long-term study of triple arthrodesis for correction of pes cavovarus in Charcot-Marie-Tooth disease. *J Pediatr Orthop* 1989;9:433.

302. Saltzman CL, Fehrle MJ, Cooper RR, Spencer EC, Ponseti IV. Triple arthrodesis: twenty-five and forty-four-year average follow-up of the same patients. *J Bone Joint Surg Am* 1999;81:1391.

303. Hall JE, Calvert PT. Lambrinudi triple arthrodesis. A review with particular reference to the technique of operation. *J Pediatr Orthop* 1987;7:19.

304. Cole WH. The treatment of claw-foot. J Bone Joint Surg 1940; 22:895.

305. Pailthorpe CA, Benson MKD'A. Hip dysplasia in hereditary motor and sensory neuropathies. *J Bone Joint Surg Br* 1992;74: 538.

306. Walker JL, Nelson KR, Heavilon JA, et al. Hip abnormalities in children with Charcot-Marie-Tooth disease. *J Pediatr Orthop* 1994;14:54.

308. Kumar SJ, Marks HG, Bowen JR, MacEwen GD. Hip dysplasia associated with Charcot-Marie-Tooth disease in the older child and adolescent. *J Pediatr Orthop* 1985;5:511.

307. Fuller JE, DeLuca PA. Acetabular dysplasia and Charcot-Marie-Tooth disease in a family. A report of four cases. *J Bone Joint Surg Am* 1995;77:1087.

309. Osebold WR, Lester EL, Watson P. Dynamics of hip joint remodeling after Chiario steotomy. 10 patients with neuromuscular disease followed for 8 years. *Acta Orthop Scand* 1997;68: 128.

310. Trumble SJ, Mayo KA, Mast JW. The periacetabular osteotomy. Minium 2-year follow-up in more than 100 hips. *Clin Orthop* 1999;363:54.

311. Daher YH, Lonstein JE, Winter RB, Bradford DS. Spinal deformities in patients with Charcot-Marie-Tooth disease. A review of 12 patients. *Clin Orthop* 1986;202:219.

312. Hensinger RN, MacEwen GD. Spinal deformity associated with heritable neurological conditions. Spinal muscular atrophy, Friedreich's ataxia, familial dysautonomia, and Charcot-Marie-Tooth disease. *J Bone Joint Surg Am* 1976;58:13.

313. Walker JL, Nelson KR, Stevens DB, et al. Spinal deformity in Charcot-Marie-Tooth disease. *Spine* 1994;19:1044.

314. Krishna M, Taylor JF, Brown MC, et al. Failure of somatosensory-evoked-potential monitoring in sensorimotor neuropathy. *Spine* 1991;16:479.

315. Brown RE, Zamboni WA, Zook EG, Russell RC. Evaluation and management of upper extremity neuropathies in Charcot-Marie-Tooth disease. *J Hand Surg* 1992;17-A:523.

316. Miller MJ, Williams LL, Slack SL, Nappi JF. The hand in Charcot-Marie-Tooth disease. *J Hand Surg Br* 1991;16:191.

317. Mackin GA, Gordon MJ, Neville HE, Ringel SP. Restoring hand function in patients with severe polyneuropathy: the role of electromyography before tendon transfer surgery. *J Hand Surg Am* 1999;24:732.

Poliomyelitis

318. Gaebler JW, Kleiman MB, French ML, et al. Neurologic complications in oral polio vaccine recipients. *J Pediatr* 1986;108: 878.

319. Strebel PM, Sutter RW, Cochi SL, et al. Epidemiology of poliomyelitis in the United States one decade after the last reported case of indigenous wild virus-associated disease. *Clin Infect Dis* 1992;14:568.

320. Sharrard WJW. Muscle recovery in poliomyelitis. *J Bone Joint Surg Br* 1955;37:63.

321. Sharrard WJW. The segmental innervation of the lower limb musculature in man. *Ann R Coll Surg Engl* 1964;35:106.

322. Sharrard WJW. Posterior iliopsoas transplantation in the treatment of paralytic dislocation of the hip. *J Bone Joint Surg Br* 1964;46:426.

323. Kojima H, Furuta Y, Fujita M, et al. Onuf's motor neuron is resistant to poliovirus. *J Neurol Sci* 1989;93:85.

324. Johnson EW Jr. Results of modern methods of treatment of poliomyelitis. *J Bone Joint Surg* 1945;27:223.

325. D'Souze H, Shah NM. Circumferential periosteal sleeve resection: results in limb-length discrepancy secondary to poliomyelitis. *J Pediatr Orthop* 1999;19:215.

326. Schottsdaedt ER, Larsen LJ, Bost FC. Complete muscle transportation. *J Bone Joint Surg Am* 1955;37:897.

327. Herndon CH. Tendon transplantation of the knee and foot. *Instr Course Lect* 1961;18:145.

328. Mayer L. The physiologic method of tendon transplants. Review after forty years. *AAOS Instr Course Lect* 1956;13:116.

329. Kuhlmann RF, Bell JF. A clinical evaluation of tendon transplantations for poliomyelitis affecting the lower extremities. *J Bone Joint Surg Am* 1952;34:915.

330. Watts HG. Management of common third world orthopaedic problems. Paralytic poliomyelitis, tuberculosis of bones and joints, Hansen's disease (leprosy), and chronic osteomyelitis. *Instr Course Lect* 1992;41:471.

331. Liu T-K, Yang R-S, Sun J-S. Long-term results of the Steindler flexorplasty. *Clin Orthop* 1993;276:104.

332. Waring WP, Werner RA. Clinical management of carpal tunnel syndrome in patients with long-term sequelae of poliomyelitis. *J Hand Surg Am* 1989;14:865.

333. Lau JHK, Parker JC, Hsu LCS, Leong JCY. Paralytic hip instability in poliomyelitis. *J Bone Joint Surg Br* 1986;68:528.

334. Asirvatham R, Watts HG, Rooney RJ. Rotation osteotomy of the tibia after poliomyelitis. *J Bone Joint Surg Br* 1990;72: 409.

335. Asirvatham R, Rooney RJ, Watts HG. Proximal tibial extension medial rotation osteotomy to correct knee flexion contracture. *J Pediatr Orthop* 1991;11:646.

336. Mehta SN, Mukherjee AK. Flexion osteotomy of the femur for genu recurvatum after poliomyelitis. *J Bone Joint Surg Br* 1991; 73:200.

337. Men H-X, Bian C-H, Yang C-D, et al. Surgical treatment of the flail knee after poliomyelitis. *J Bone Joint Surg Br* 1991;73: 195.

338. Shahcheraghi GH, Jarid M, Zeighami B. Hamstring tendon transfer for quadriceps femoris transfer. *J Pediatr Orthop* 1996; 16:765.

339. Drennan JC. Poliomyelitis. In: Drennan JC, ed. *The child's foot and ankle.* New York: Rowen Press, 1992:305.

340. Adelaar RS, Dannelly EA, Meunier PA, et al. A long-term study of triple arthrodesis in children. *Orthop Clin North Am* 1996; 4:895.

341. Asirvatham R, Watts HG, Rooney RJ. Tendoachilles tenodesis to the fibula. A retrospective study. *J Pediatr Orthop* 1991;11: 652.

342. DeHeus JAC, Marti RK, Besselaar PP, et al. The influence of subtalar in triple arthrodesis on the tibiotalar joint. A long-term follow-up study. *J Bone Joint Surg Br* 1997;79:644.

343. El-Batonty MM, Aly El-S, El-Lakkany MR, et al. Triple arthrodesis for paralytic valgus; a modified technique: brief report. *J Bone Joint Surg Br* 1988;70:493.

344. Pandy AK, Pandy S, Prasnd V. Calcaneal osteotomy and tendon sling for the management of calcaneus deformity. *J Bone Joint Surg Am* 1989;71:1192.

345. Westin GW, Dingeman RD, Gausewitz SH. The results of tendodesis of the tendo achillis to the fibular for paralytic pes calcaneus. *J Bone Joint Surg Am* 1988;70:320.

346. Chen P-Q, Shen Y-S. Poliomyelitis scoliosis. In: Weinstein SL, ed. *The pediatric spine. Principles and practice.* New York: Raven, 1994:1069.

347. Mayer PJ, Edwards JW, Dove J, et al. Post-poliomyelitis paralytic scoliosis. A review of curve patterns and results of surgical treatment in 118 consecutive patients. *Spine* 1981;6:573.

348. Eberle CF. Failure of fixation after segmental spinal instrumentation without arthrodesis in the management of paralytic scoliosis. *J Bone Joint Surg Am* 1988;70:696.

349. DeWald RL, Faut M. Anterior and posterior spinal surgery for paralytic scoliosis. *Spine* 1979;4:401.

350. Leong JCY, Wilding K, Mok CD, et al. Surgical treatment of scoliosis following poliomyelitis: a review of 110 cases. *J Bone Joint Surg Am* 1981;63:726.

351. O'Brien JP, Yau ACMC, Gertzbien S, et al. Combined staged anterior and posterior correction of the spine in scoliosis following postmyelitis. *Clin Orthop* 1975;110:81.

352. Eberle CF. Pelvic obliquity and the unstable hip after poliomyelitis. *J Bone Joint Surg Br* 1982;64:300.

353. Gau YL, Lonstein JE, Winter RB, et al. Luque-Galveston procedure for correction and stabilization of neuromuscular scoliosis and pelvic obliquity. A review of 68 patients. *J Spinal Disord* 1991;4:399.

Postpoliomyelitis Syndrome

354. Perry J, Barnes G, Gronley JK. The postpolio syndrome. An overuse phenomenon. *Clin Orthop* 1988;233:145.

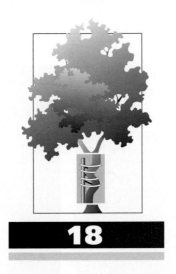

18

IDIOPATHIC AND CONGENITAL SCOLIOSIS

PETER O. NEWTON
DENNIS R. WENGER

CHILDHOOD AND ADOLESCENT SCOLIOSIS

"Idiopathic scoliosis" defines a common and potentially severe musculoskeletal disorder of unknown etiology, the diagnosis and treatment of which have been central in the development of orthopaedic surgery as a specialty. In its milder forms scoliosis may produce only trunk shape change, but when severe, can be markedly disfiguring as well as producing cardiac and pulmonary compromise (Fig. 18-1). The goal of this chapter is to present the key elements in diagnosis, natural history, and treatment of both idiopathic and congenital scoliosis.

P. O. Newton: Department of Orthopaedic Surgery, University of California–San Diego; Department of Orthopaedic Surgery, Children's Hospital and Health Center, San Diego, California 92123.
D. R. Wenger: Department of Orthopaedic Surgery, University of California–San Diego; Pediatric Orthopedics, Children's Hospital and Health Center, San Diego, California 92123.

The etiology of typical adolescent scoliosis remains unknown; thus, the term "idiopathic" remains appropriate. Scoliosis can also be classified based on associated conditions, since it occurs in many neuromuscular disorders (cerebral palsy, muscular dystrophy, and others) as well as in association with generalized diseases and syndromes (neurofibromatosis, Marfan syndrome, and bone dysplasia). Congenital scoliosis, caused by failure in vertebral formation or segmentation, causes a more mechanically understandable type of scoliosis.

The etiology of a scoliotic deformity (idiopathic, neuromuscular, syndrome related, and congenital) largely dictates its natural history, including the risk for and rate of curve progression, as well as the effect the curve will have on the cardiopulmonary function, mobility, and appearance. Although scoliosis includes both sagittal plane and torsional malalignment of the spinal column, the deformity is most readily noted as frontal plane deformity. Better understand-

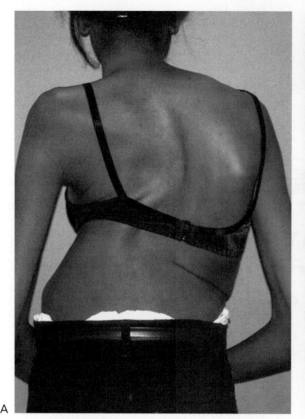
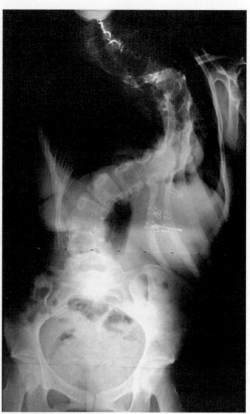

FIGURE 18-1. A: This 16-year-old female with severe scoliosis refused early surgical treatment and had severe curve progression. Her clinical examination demonstrates marked trunk and rib cage deformity, and she had reduced pulmonary function. **B:** The posteroanterior radiograph demonstrates a right thoracic curvature of 125 degrees.

ing of the three-dimensional nature of scoliosis has led to many recent advances in its treatment.

Definitions

The normal spine is straight in the frontal plane, but has sagittal plane contours including thoracic kyphosis averaging 30 to 35 degrees (range 10 to 50 degrees, T5–T12) and lumbar lordosis averaging 50 to 60 degrees (range 35 to 80 degrees, T12–S1) (1–3). The scoliotic spine deviates from midline in the frontal plane, and rotates maximally at the apex of the curve (4). The vertebral rotation toward the convexity of the curve, through the attached ribs, produces the typical chest wall prominence (Adams sign) that allows early diagnosis (5,6) (Fig. 18-2).

In the past, it was thought that the lateral curvature of scoliosis was also kyphotic (increased roundback). It is now understood that the apparent "hump" on the back is due to rib prominence secondary to the rotational deformity of the vertebrae and rib cage, and that most thoracic idiopathic scoliosis is associated with a *decrease* in normal thoracic kyphosis (7,8). Dickson and others have postulated that an early evolution to lordosis in the normally kyphotic thoracic spine leads to an unstable mechanical environment, leading

to rotational collapse (9,10) (Fig. 18-3). This is not to say that all thoracic scoliosis is hypokyphotic, since many congenital, neuromuscular, and a few idiopathic cases have a true kyphotic component.

In addition to global deformity of the spine and trunk, wedging of individual discs and vertebral bodies develops, due to the Hueter-Volkmann effect (suppression of growth on the concave side of the curve) (11) (Fig. 18-4). This includes asymmetric growth and/or remodeling of the vertebral bodies, pedicles, laminae, and facet joints, as well as the transverse and spinous processes.

Etiology

Although the etiology of idiopathic scoliosis remains unknown, substantial research has been performed with many theories proposed. These range from genetic factors to disorders of bone, muscles, and disc, as well as growth abnormalities and central nervous system causes.

Genetic Factors

Several studies have demonstrated an increased incidence of scoliosis in the family members of affected individuals,

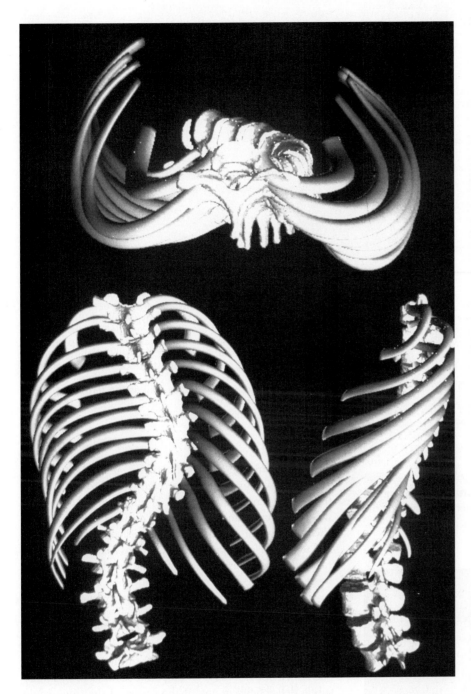

FIGURE 18-2. A three-dimensional reconstruction of the scoliotic spine and trunk demonstrates the three-plane deformity of the spine and attached ribs. The torsional deformity is maximal at the apex of the curvature. (Courtesy of St. Justine Hospital, Montreal, Canada.)

confirming a genetic etiologic component to the etiology of scoliosis (12–16). Risenborough and Wynne-Davies found scoliosis in 11.1% of first-degree relatives of 207 patients with idiopathic scoliosis (16). These familial studies suggest a polygenic inheritance pattern.

Examination of scoliosis in birth twins has led to further confirmation of genetic etiologic factors. In a meta-analysis of scoliosis in twins, Kesling and Reinker demonstrated 73% concordance in 37 pairs of monozygotic twins. They found that in 37 pairs of identical twins in which at least one twin was identified with scoliosis, 27 of the pairs had

both twins affected. However, only 36% of the 31 dizygotic twins were concordant. In addition, the severity of the scoliosis was statistically similar for the monozygotic twins, but not for the dizygotic twins (17). Inoue et al. demonstrated even greater concordance in twins. DNA fingerprinting confirmed the zygosity, and found concordance of idiopathic scoliosis in 92% of monozygotic and 63% of dizygotic twins (18). Despite this confirming evidence of a genetic etiology, the genes and gene products responsible for the development of idiopathic scoliosis remain unknown.

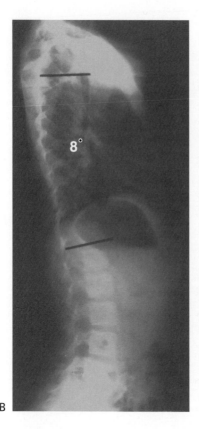
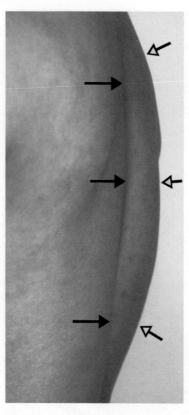

A,B

FIGURE 18-3. A: This standing lateral radiograph demonstrates the decreased kyphosis of the thoracic spine ("hypokyphosis"), commonly seen in thoracic curves in patients with idiopathic scoliosis common in adolescent idiopathic scoliosis. **B:** An oblique view clinical photograph of the patient demonstrates both the prominence of the rib cage due to the rotational deformity (*open arrows*), as well as the flattening of the thoracic kyphosis along the midline (*closed arrows*).

Tissue Deficiencies

Competing theories propose that the primary pathology of scoliosis is centered in each of the structural tissues of the spine (bone, muscle, ligament/disc). There are known con-

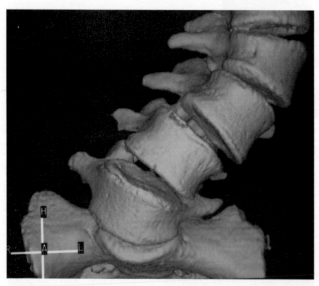

FIGURE 18-4. A three-dimensional CT scan in a patient with severe lumbar scoliosis demonstrates the wedging of both the discs and vertebral bodies, which occurs through asymmetric loading and growth (Hueter-Volkmann effect).

ditions in which each of these tissues are pathologic and associated with scoliosis. For example, fibrous dysplasia (bone collagen abnormality) resulting in dysplastic, misshapen vertebrae (19); muscle disorders such as Duchenne muscular dystrophy leading to a collapsing scoliosis; and soft tissue-collagen disorders, such as Marfan syndrome, each have a clear association with the development of scoliosis.

In Marfan syndrome there is a defective gene coding for fibrillin. Fibrillin is found in many soft tissues including ligament, cartilage, and periosteum (20). The fibrillin abnormality found in Marfan syndrome is associated with scoliosis in 55 to 63% of cases (21,22). Although fibrillin has been ruled out as a cause of idiopathic scoliosis (23), similar subtle deficiencies in any of the tissues of the spine could result in idiopathic scoliosis (24). For instance, several (25–27) have suggested that adolescent idiopathic scoliosis (AIS) may be related to osteopenia. They found the vertebral bone mineral density to be lower in girls ages 12 to 14 years with scoliosis compared to matched controls, with the density lower not only in the vertebrae, but also in the proximal femur (25). The mechanism by which osteopenia alone leads to scoliosis, however, remains undefined.

Vertebral Growth Abnormality Theories

Abnormalities of spinal growth mechanisms also provide an attractive etiology theory because scoliosis development and progression are temporally related to the time of rapid adolescent growth (28,29). Differential growth rates between the right and left sides of the spine could generate an asymmetry that would be accentuated with asymmetric biomechanical loading and the Heuter-Volkmann effect (11,30,31). Milner and Dickson (32), as well as others (10,31,33–35), have postulated that the etiology of scoliosis relates to the development of relative thoracic lordosis. Dickson believes that anterior spinal growth outpaces posterior growth, producing hypokyphosis with subsequent buckling of the vertebral column, leading to the rotational deformity of scoliosis; however, the cause for this theorized "mismatch" of anterior and posterior spinal column growth has not been presented, and may be secondary rather than primary. Interestingly, it has been documented that thoracic kyphosis tends to decrease in normal children during the normal adolescent growth spurt (36). Thus, irregularities in the changing sagittal shape of the spine during the rapid period of adolescent growth may be important in the development of scoliosis.

Several studies suggest that adolescents with scoliosis are taller than their peers (37–42). Increased levels of growth hormones (43,44) and characteristic body morphometry (thin, physically less developed appearance) (45–49) may also relate to scoliosis development.

Central Nervous System Theories

Clearly, disorders of the brain, spinal cord, and muscles may result in scoliosis with the role of the central nervous system in idiopathic scoliosis having been studied in detail (50–57). Goldberg et al. noted greater asymmetry of the cerebral cortices in scoliotic patients (55). Also, abnormalities in equilibrium and vestibular function have been noted in patients with scoliosis (50,58–63); however, it is difficult to know if these findings are primary or secondary (64). Woods et al. have suggested a neurologic etiology to scoliosis based on the surprising finding that hearing-impaired children seem to have a lower incidence of scoliosis (63). Syringomyelia is associated with an increased incidence of scoliosis (65,66) possibly due to direct pressure on the sensory or motor tracts of the spinal cord. Alternatively, there may be no relation to the dilation of the central canal, but instead, brain stem irritation from an associated Chiari malformation or enlargement of the fourth ventricle of the brain as the cause.

Recently, it has been postulated that melatonin and the pineal gland may be related to scoliosis. This is based on research of pinealectomy in chickens that resulted in a high incidence of severe scoliosis (67–69). In these studies, presumably melatonin deficiency led to scoliosis in the chicken (70). Melatonin receptors are located in the brainstem and spinal cord dorsal gray matter, areas associated with postural control. Subsequent studies of human melatonin levels have been conflicting and inconclusive. Machida et al. found lower than normal melatonin concentration in the serum of patients with progressive scoliosis compared to those with stable curves (71). In contrast, Hilibrand et al. (72) and Fagan et al. (73) found no difference in urine melatonin levels between patients with scoliosis and normal control subjects. In addition, Bagnall et al. found no difference in serum melatonin levels of patients with scoliosis (74). Thus confirmation that melatonin deficiency in humans is associated with scoliosis, as seen in chickens, is lacking.

Histologic analysis of paraspinous muscles has revealed denervation changes suggestive of a neuropathic cause (75), as well as ultrastructural changes in the sarcolemma at the myotendinous junction, supporting the concept of a primary muscle disorder (76). As in the findings relating to equilibrium, it is difficult to determine a causal relationship, and the findings in muscle could be secondary, reflecting the muscle's response to asymmetric spine loading (77).

In summary, the etiology of scoliosis remains puzzling. From a biomechanical standpoint the vertebral column is a naturally unstable construct, made of multiple mobile segments. As Stagnara has noted, one should not be surprised that a minor disturbance in the structure, support system, or growth of the spine could lead to scoliosis, particularly in a complex structure where the "normal" state includes multiple curves (sagittal plane), and is based on an oblique foundation (the sacrum) (78). There are likely several causes of idiopathic scoliosis, and active research continues in an attempt to find a unifying theory as to its cause.

Classification

Curve Location

Scoliotic deformities assume a variety of curve patterns, and several useful classification systems have been developed. The terminology committee of the Scoliosis Research Society (SRS) defines the following technical description of curve locations (this is in contrast to curve pattern descriptions developed for the purpose of planning surgical correction; see "Surgical Correction of Idiopathic Scoliosis"):

- Cervical: apex between C2 and C6
- Cervicothoracic: apex between C7 and T1
- Thoracic: apex between T2 and T11
- Thoracolumbar: apex between T12 and L1
- Lumbar: apex between L2 and L4
- Lumbosacral: apex at L5 or below

The apex of a curve defines its center, and is the most laterally deviated disc or vertebra of the curve. Usually a single vertebra can be defined, but in other cases a pair of vertebrae are at the apex (in this case the "apical disc" is used to define the level of the apex). The apical vertebra(e) are also the most horizontal. The end vertebrae of a curve define the proximal and distal extent of a curve, and are

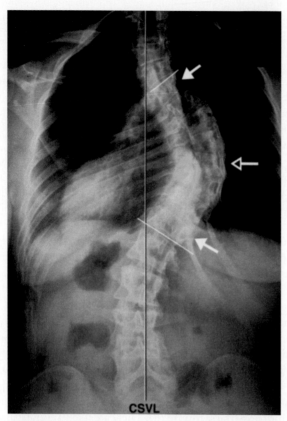

FIGURE 18-5. The end vertebrae (*solid arrows*), apical vertebra (*open arrow*), and central sacral vertical line (*CSVL*) are demonstrated on this upright film. The CSVL is commonly used to determine the distal-most extent of a spinal fusion that classically extends to the "stable vertebra." In this radiograph, the stable vertebra is arguably L1 or L2.

determined by locating the vertebrae most tilted from the horizontal (these vertebrae are used to make the Cobb measurement). The central sacral vertical line, a vertical line which bisects the sacrum, is used to assess the balance of the spine in relation to its base (the pelvis) (Fig. 18-5).

Age at Onset

Age at diagnosis is also used to define idiopathic scoliosis groups as follows:

- Infantile (ages 0 to 3 years)
- Juvenile (age 4 to 10 years)
- Adolescent (11 to 17 years)
- Adult (≥18 years)

The age when idiopathic scoliosis develops is one of the most important factors in determining the natural history of the disorder, with early onset cases more likely to be progressive. Scoliosis onset before the adolescent growth spurt is more likely to have an underlying spinal cord abnormality as the cause of the deformity with the incidence of

abnormality approximately 20% in the juvenile group and as high as 50% in the infantile group (79).

Primary and Secondary, Structural and Nonstructural Curves

Curves may also be described as primary or secondary. The primary curve is the first to develop; however, at times two or even three curves of equal severity exist that make the determination of a primary versus secondary curve difficult. Secondary or compensatory curves develop after formation of the primary curve as a means of balancing the head and trunk over the pelvis. Similar compensation occurs in the sagittal plane in which the typical lordotic thoracic curve may end both cranially and caudally with a junctional kyphosis. Sagittal plane abnormalities have only recently been well understood and considered when planning surgical correction.

The terms structural and nonstructural have also been used to describe the flexibility of scoliotic curves with structural curves being more rigid (i.e., do not correct well with side-bending). The degree of curve rigidity that differentiates a structural and nonstructural curve, however, has not been clearly defined.

Etiologic Classification

Classification of scoliosis by etiology may be broadly described as idiopathic (or idiopathic-like), neuromuscular, syndrome related, and congenital. It is important to consider a patient presenting with scoliosis as a patient presenting with a sign (i.e., scoliosis), rather than a diagnosis. Most scoliosis (approximately 80%) is idiopathic; however, the remaining cases are associated with a wide variety of disorders in which scoliosis is often the presenting complaint.

The SRS has classified scoliosis as associated with each of the diagnoses seen in Table 18-1. The scoliosis associated with these conditions is discussed in other chapters of this text. Neuromuscular disorders of either neuropathic or myopathic etiology make up a large proportion of the nonidiopathic causes of scoliosis in childhood. Intra- or extraspinal tumors or abnormalities must also be considered as a cause of scoliosis. Congenital scoliosis and kyphosis also may lead to progressive spine deformity. An awareness of each potentially associated condition helps when analyzing the various proposed etiologic factors in idiopathic scoliosis, and, more importantly, the diagnosis of idiopathic scoliosis requires the exclusion of these conditions.

Clinical Features

History

Understanding what prompted a physician visit for evaluation of scoliosis is key. For example, in North America, a

TABLE 18-1. CLASSIFICATION OF SCOLIOSIS

Idiopathic	Fiber-type disproportion	Osteochondrodystrophies
Infantile	Congenital hypotonia	Achondroplasia
Resolving	Myotonia dystrophica	Spondyloepiphyseal dysplasia
Progressive	Other	Diastrophic dwarfism
Juvenile	Congenital	Mucopolysaccharidoses
Adolescent	Failure of formation	Other
Muscular	Wedge vertebra	Tumor
Neuropathic	Hemivertebra	Benign
Upper motor neuron	Failure of segmentation	Malignant
Cerebral palsy	Unilateral bar	Rheumatoid disease
Spinocerebellar degeneration	Bilateral (fusion)	Metabolic
Friedreich disease	Mixed	Rickets
Charcot-Marie-Tooth disease	Associated with neural tissue defect	Juvenile osteoporosis
Roussy-Levy disease	Myelomeningocele	Osteogenesis imperfecta
Syringomyelia	Meningocele	Related to lumbosacral area
Spinal cord tumor	Spinal dysraphism	Spondylolysis
Spinal cord trauma	Diastematomyelia	Spondylolisthesis
Other	Other	Other
Lower motor neuron	Neurofibromatosis	Thoracogenic
Poliomyelitis	Mesenchymal	Postthoracoplasty
Other viral myelitides	Marfan syndrome	Postthoracotomy
Traumatic	Homocystinuria	Other
Spinal muscular atrophy	Ehlers-Danlos syndrome	Hysterical
Werdig-Hoffmann disease	Other	Functional
Kugelberg-Welander disease	Traumatic	Postural
Myelomeningocoele (paralytic)	Fracture or dislocation (nonparalytic)	Secondary to short leg
Dysautonomia (Riley-Day syndrome)	Postirradiation	Due to muscle spasm
Other	Other	Other
Myopathic	Soft tissue contractures	
Arthrogryposis	Postempyema	
Muscular dystrophy	Burns	
Duchenne (pseudohypertrophic)	Other	
Limb-girdle		
Fascioscapulohumeral		

screening examination (either in school or at a routine primary care visit) often leads to referral. History-taking should include questions about family history of scoliosis, recent growth, and the physical changes of puberty (onset of menses). When an affected sibling or parent has scoliosis, prevalence increases seven times (sibling) and three times (parent), respectively, compared to the general population (14). A record of height increases over the prior few years is important in predicting remaining spinal growth and the risk for curve progression (80). This information may be available from the primary care physician or, at times, from measurements on the wall/door marked in the family's home. The onset of menses forms an important maturational time point in females (81). The family history, as well as the review of systems, should identify disorders known to be associated with scoliosis (Table 18-1).

The presence or absence of severe back pain is important, because most idiopathic scoliosis patients have only mild discomfort. Patients seen after scoliosis has been diagnosed (in a screening setting) commonly develop "pain" that continues until the exact diagnosis, and particularly the prog-

nosis, have been clarified by an orthopaedic consultant who can provide reassurance. Despite the common belief that mild idiopathic scoliosis is not painful, a recent study suggests that adolescents with mild curves often report discomfort of a mild fatigue variety. Ramirez et al. noted back pain in 23% of 2,442 patients with "idiopathic" scoliosis. Only 9% of those with pain were subsequently found to have an underlying pathologic condition to explain it (diagnoses such as spondylolysis/spondylolisthesis, Scheuermann kyphosis, syringomyelia, herniated disc, tethered cord, and intraspinal tumor) (82).

In evaluating a child with scoliosis, a significant complaint of back pain is a clue that should raise one question, "Is this truly an idiopathic curve?" A child or adolescent who presents with *severe* back pain, and is subsequently found to have scoliosis requires a very careful history, physical examination, and radiographic study (a bone scan and MRI study may be required), because an underlying etiologic cause is more likely (82–84). However, the clinician must distinguish between "severe pain" (requiring further workup) and the mild fatigue pain (noted above) reported

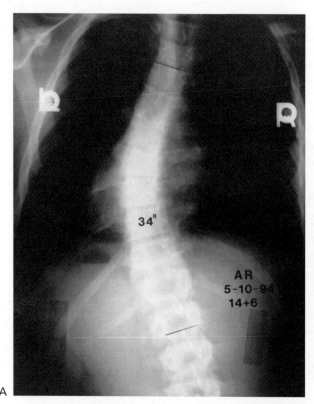

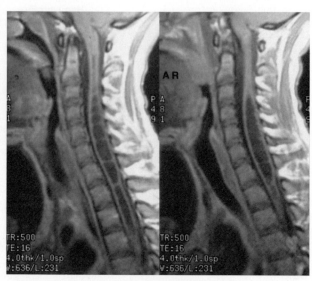

FIGURE 18-6. **A:** This 14-year-6-month-old male who presented with a 34 degree left thoracic scoliosis was asymptomatic with a normal physical examination, except for the absence of a left abdominal reflex. This finding, in addition to the presence of a left thoracic curve—an "abnormal" pattern for idiopathic scoliosis—was the indication for further evaluation with an magnetic resonance imaging (MRI) scan. **B:** The sagittal MRI scan showed a large cervical spinal cord syrinx.

by Ramirez et al. and others (82,85). During adolescence, activity-related musculoskeletal low back pain occurs at a frequency greater than in childhood, but less than in adults (86,87).

Age at onset, rate of curve progression, and the presence of neurologic symptoms and signs are the most useful findings in identifying nonidiopathic scoliosis. In younger patients (less than 10 years) with a neurologic cause, actual neurologic findings on physical examination are often absent, and often the spinal curvature itself must be considered the initial sign of a neural axis abnormality (79,88–90). The most common intraspinal abnormality found in this age group is syringomyelia (dilation of the central spinal canal) with an associated Chiari malformation (brain stem below the level of the foramen magnum) (Fig. 18-6).

Rapid development of a severe curve suggests a nonidiopathic type of scoliosis. Neurologic symptoms such as weakness, sensory changes, and balance/gait disturbance suggest intraspinal pathology (syringomyelia, tethered cord, tumor, etc.) as the cause of spinal curvature (83,89,90). The neurologic history should therefore focus on difficulties with walking, running, and stair-climbing. A history of radiating pain, numbness, and tingling in the limbs, and difficulties with bowel or bladder control, should also be sought.

Physical Examination

Physical examination of a scoliosis patient includes evaluation of trunk shape, trunk balance, the neurologic system, limb length, skin markings, and associated skeletal abnormalities. Assessment of pubertal development includes assessment of the stages of breast development and the presence of axillary/pubic hair (Tanner stages). This can be done discretely without fully undressing the patient. Examination of girls while dressed in a two-piece swimsuit (patient instructed at time of telephone appointment to wear a swimsuit for the examination) reduces anxiety and apprehension, yet allows assessment of breast development and axillary hair.

With the patient standing, the back and trunk are inspected for asymmetry of shoulder height, scapular position, and shape of the waist (Fig. 18-7) viewed from both behind and in front. Potential pelvic tilt, (an indicator of limb-length difference) is determined by palpating the iliac crests and posterior inferior iliac spines bilaterally in the standing patient with both hips and knees fully extended. Lateral translation of the head can be measured in centimeters of deviation from the gluteal cleft by dropping a plumb line from C7 (Fig. 18-8). Deviation of the chest cage (trunk

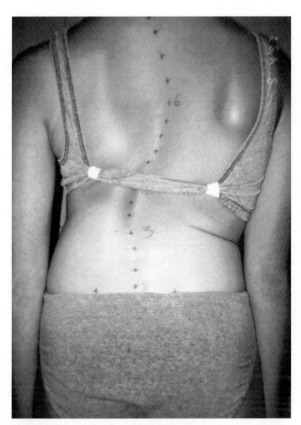

FIGURE 18-7. The clinical appearance of this 11-year-old female with right thoracic scoliosis demonstrates asymmetry of the waistline and scapulae as well as slight elevation of the right shoulder.

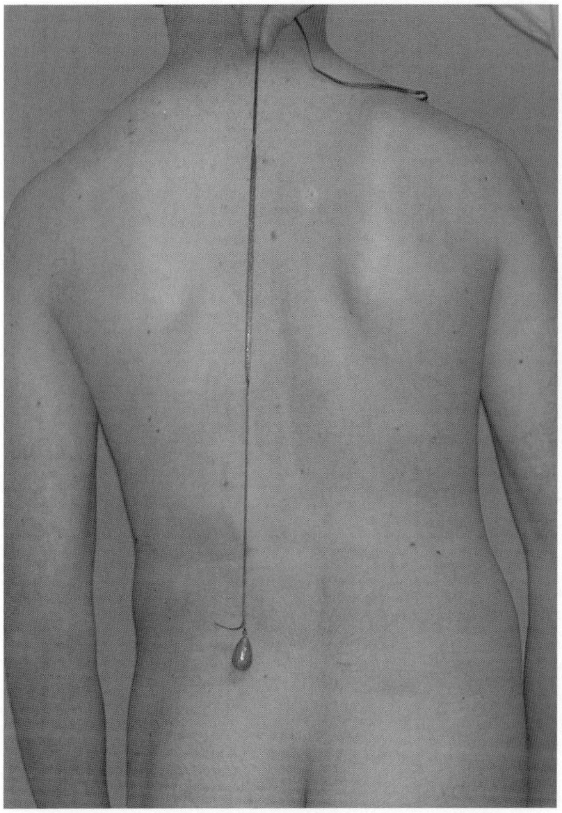

FIGURE 18-8. A small weight hanging from a string ("plumb bob") serves as a simple tool for quantifying trunk deviation. In this case, the plumb line is measured from C7 and quantified as a deviation in centimeters from the gluteal cleft below (5 cm).

shift) should also be assessed, since patients can have full head compensation (return of the head and neck back to midline), yet have marked lateralization of the trunk.

Forward-bend Test. The forward-bend test, first described by Adams in Britain (91), has the patient bend forward at the waist, with their knees straight and palms together. This examination should be performed from behind (to assess lower trunk rotation), from in front (to assess upper trunk rotation), as well as from the side (to assess kyphosis). Any asymmetry of the upper thoracic, midthoracic, thoracolumbar, and lumbar regions should be quantitated with a scoliometer (92) (angle of trunk rotation—ATR), or by measuring the height of the prominence in centimeters (Fig. 18-9). This prominence reflects the rotational deformity of the spine associated with scoliosis (93,94). Although not always exactly correlated, in general an angle of trunk rotation of 5 to 7 degrees is associated with a radiographic Cobb angle measurement of 15 to 20 degrees. (This is a guideline—occasionally patients have little trunk rotation yet have significant radiographic scoliosis, and vice versa (95)).

An inability to bend directly forward at the waist, or decreased range with forward/side bending, may be due to

pain, lumbar muscle spasm, and/or hamstring tightness; any of which should suggest underlying pathology. These findings, plus abnormalities in straight-leg–raise testing suggests irritation of the lumbar roots due to spondylolysis, disc herniation, infection, neoplasm, or other causes.

Skin, Limb Length. Additional components of a comprehensive scoliosis examination include inspection of the skin (both on the back and elsewhere) for cutaneous evidence of an associated disease. Café au lait spots and/or axillary freckles suggest possible neurofibromatosis, while dimpling or a hairy patch in the lumbosacral area may suggest an underlying spinal dysraphism. Excessive skin or joint laxity may be related to a connective tissue disorder, such as Marfan or Ehlers-Danlos syndrome.

Limb length should also be measured in the supine position if pelvic tilt is noted on the standing examination. A spinal curvature which results from a limb-length difference is usually compensatory and serves to rebalance the trunk over the pelvis. A short right leg results in a compensatory right lumbar curve. There is no rotational deformity of the spine with these curves, and in the lumbar region the rotational prominence noted on the forward-bend test is on the

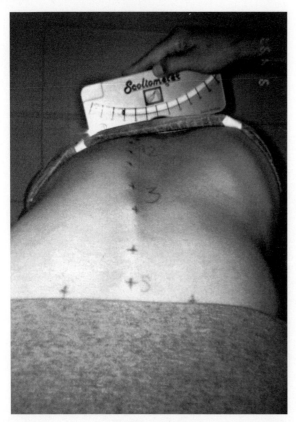

FIGURE 18-9. The Adams forward bend test is performed to detect small degrees of trunk rotation frequently associated with scoliosis. The scoliometer is used to quantify the angle of trunk rotation in degrees. This simple device is utilized in screening patients for scoliosis, as well as for quantifying the degree of trunk rotation in patients being followed clinically.

concave side of the curve (the long leg makes the iliac crest and lumbar spine more prominent on that side). This is the opposite of what is seen in true lumbar scoliosis, in which the rotational prominence noted on the bending test is found on the side of the curve convexity. Presence of the bending-test rotational prominence, on the "wrong" side in a lumbar curve, is almost always diagnostic of limb-length discrepancy spinal asymmetry, rather than true scoliosis. The prominence disappears if the pelvis is leveled with an appropriately sized block underneath the short leg.

Neurologic Examination

The neurologic examination should evaluate balance, motor strength in the major muscle groups of all four extremities, as well as sensation. Watching the patient walk, toe and heel walk, tandem walk, squat deeply, and single-leg hop allows rapid assessment of balance and motor strength. Reflex testing includes upper- and lower-extremity deep-tendon reflexes, as well as abdominal reflexes that are obtained by lightly stroking the abdominal wall with a blunt instrument (key, end of reflex hammer) adjacent to the umbilicus,

with the patient supine and relaxed. The expected brisk and symmetric unilateral contraction of the abdominal musculature, pulling the umbilicus toward the side being stroked, indicates normalcy. When persistently abnormal (reflex absent on one side and present on the other), intraspinal disorders, particularly syringomyelia, should be considered and an MRI study ordered (65,96).

Radiographic Assessment

The ideal screening radiograph for scoliosis is an upright (standing) posteroanterior (PA) projection of the entire spine exposed on a single cassette. In an adolescent, due to body size, this requires a three-foot length film to visualize the entire spine, as well as the head and pelvis on a single radiograph. Many radiology units do not have long cassettes and a chest-film–size cassette can be substituted, with the film centered on the area of maximal deformity (usually the thorax). If a lumbar curve is present, a separate film must be performed. Clearly, the child is better served if they can be referred to a center that uses long cassettes, allowing a single film.

The patient must be standing, since diagnostic and treatment standards developed over the years are based on upright films. In young patients, or those with severe neuromuscular involvement, sitting or even supine radiographs may be the only position possible. Curve magnitude is greater when the patient is upright (compared to supine), and is of particular importance in infantile and congenital curves with films taken before and after walking age. "Curve progression" may be noted with the first upright radiograph, compared to prior supine views, when in fact one has simply documented that gravity causes a curve to be more severe. A lateral film is not required as part of the initial x-ray screening of a thoracic curve, unless back pain or sagittal deformity are noted. A lateral view of the lumbosacral junction is often performed in lumbar scoliosis to assess for spondylolysis/spondylolisthesis as a possible cause (Fig. 18-10).

Radiographic techniques used to minimize radiation of sensitive organs (breast, thyroid, ovaries, bone marrow) include taking only the required number of x-rays, utilizing rare earth radiographic enhancing screens with fast film, and a posterior to anterior exposure (97–99). The lifetime risk for developing cancer of the breast and thyroid has been suggested to increase by 1 to 2% for patients exposed to multiple x-rays associated with scoliosis treatment; however, this rate was generated in the 1960s and 1970s, before new radiation reducing techniques were available. The greatest reduction to breast and thyroid exposure is associated with the posteroanterior exposure (compared to the anteroposterior), which reduces breast/thyroid exposure 3- to 7-fold (99). Shielding of the breasts with anteroposterior (AP) projection is possible, but not recommended, because of the increased thyroid exposure (shielding the thyroid obstructs the view of the upper spine) (Fig. 18-11). Wise doctors

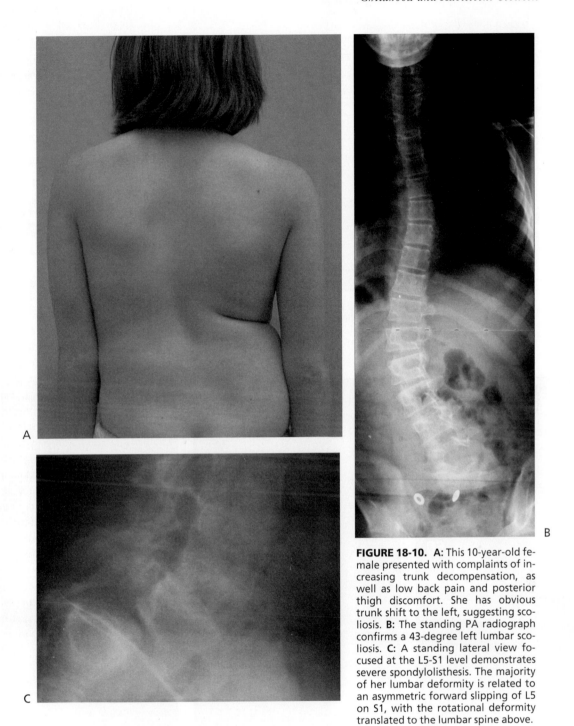

FIGURE 18-10. **A:** This 10-year-old female presented with complaints of increasing trunk decompensation, as well as low back pain and posterior thigh discomfort. She has obvious trunk shift to the left, suggesting scoliosis. **B:** The standing PA radiograph confirms a 43-degree left lumbar scoliosis. **C:** A standing lateral view focused at the L5-S1 level demonstrates severe spondylolisthesis. The majority of her lumbar deformity is related to an asymmetric forward slipping of L5 on S1, with the rotational deformity translated to the lumbar spine above.

counsel their patients by telling them that only the minimum number of x-rays required to treat the disorder correctly will be performed, and that the benefit of having the x-rays outweighs the risk of not knowing the type and severity of the scoliosis.

When surgical treatment is being considered, lateral-bend radiographs to assess curve flexibility as well as a standing lateral view are required. Side-bending radiographs allow one to determine curve flexibility, and to decide what levels

to include in the instrumented and fused segment. Controversy remains regarding the best method for obtaining bending films, with supine AP views (patient maximally bent to the right and left) being standard at many institutions (Fig. 18-12), whereas others believe that a standing bend film is a better indicator, particularly in the lumbar spine. Lateral bending over a bolster provides somewhat greater correction, and has been proposed as a more accurate predictor of the correction obtained with the more powerful modern surgi-

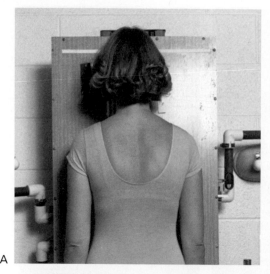
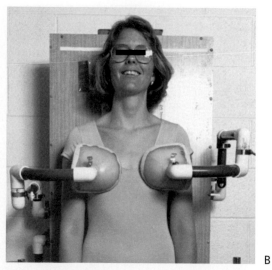

FIGURE 18-11. A: Positioning of a patient for a posteroanterior radiograph. **B:** Positioning of a patient for an anteroposterior radiograph with breast shielding.

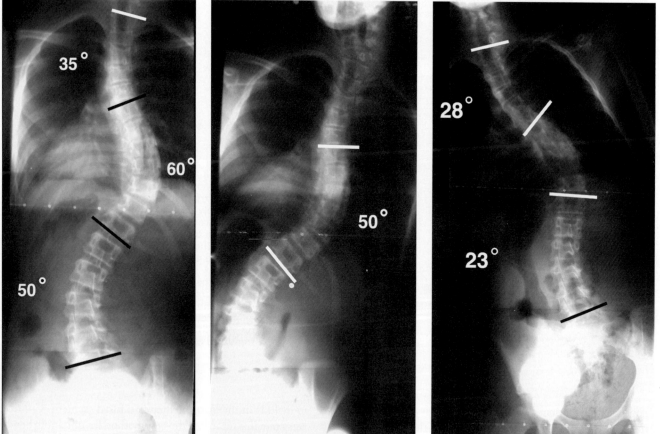

FIGURE 18-12. A: Standing PA radiograph of a premenarchal female demonstrating a 35-degree left upper thoracic scoliosis, 60-degree right thoracic scoliosis, and 50-degree left lumbar scoliosis. **B:** The bend film to the right is useful in determining the flexibility of the main right thoracic curve. In this case, the right thoracic curve decreased only to 50 degrees on supine side bending. **C:** The side-bending film to the left is useful in determining the curve flexibility of the left upper thoracic curve, which decreased to 28 degrees, and the left lumbar curve, which decreased to 23 degrees.

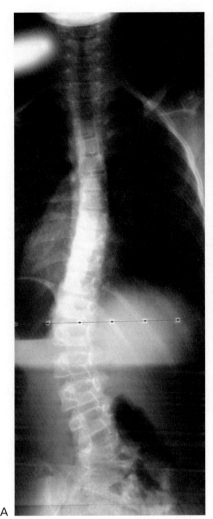

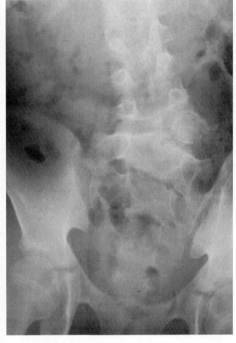

FIGURE 18-13. **A:** This adolescent patient presented with spinal deformity, with the standing PA radiograph demonstrating an obvious left thoracolumbar deformity. On more careful examination, an abnormality at the lumbosacral junction is suggested. **B:** A cone-down radiograph of the lumbosacral junction demonstrates a clear hemivertebra. This congenital malformation is the primary deformity, and the thoracolumbar deformity above is a compensatory curve.

cal instrumentation methods (100,101). In curves greater than 60 to 70 degrees, longitudinal traction films may also be helpful in evaluating curve flexibility (102,103).

The Stagnara oblique view, taken perpendicular to the rib prominence rather than in the PA direction, provides a more accurate picture of large curves with a large rotational component. Taken in this manner the true magnitude of the scoliosis can be measured (104).

Reading Scoliosis Films. Assessment of the standing PA film begins by looking for soft tissue abnormalities, congenital bony abnormalities (wedged vertebra, etc.), then by assessing curvature (coronal plane deviation). Bone assessment includes looking for wedged or hemivertebrae (Fig. 18-13), bar formation bridging a disc space, as well as midline irregularities, such as spina bifida or a bony spike suggesting diastematomyelia. The pedicles should be inspected to be certain that they are present bilaterally and that the interpedicular distance is not abnormally increased, suggesting an intraspinal mass (105,106). Absent pedicles or vertebral

body lucency are associated with lytic processes, such as tumor or infection. If a curve is noted, the symmetry and levelness of the pelvis are analyzed. A limb length discrepancy can be estimated by determining iliac wing and hip joint height differences, assuming the patient had both hips and knees fully extended when the film was exposed.

Curve measurement by the Cobb method (107) allows quantification of the curve. A protractor with single-degree demarcations that is not bent or warped allows more accurate measurements. The caudal and cranial end vertebrae to be measured are the vertebrae that are the most tilted, with the degree of tilt between these two vertebrae defining the Cobb angle (in a normal spine this angle is 0 degrees). One outlines the superior end plate of the cranial end vertebra and the inferior end plate of the caudal end vertebra, constructs a perpendicular to these lines, then measures the angle where the perpendicular lines cross. When more than one curve exists, a Cobb angle measurement is made for each curve (Fig. 18-14). When comparing serial radiographs of the same patient, the end vertebra chosen should gener-

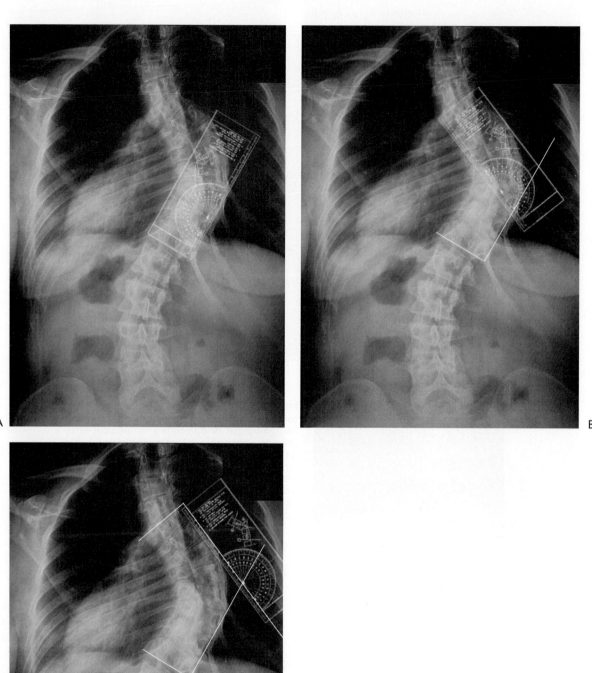

FIGURE 18-14. **A:** Measurement of the Cobb angle. The end vertebrae of a curve must be selected before any measurement can be made. The end vertebrae of a curve are those which are most tilted from the horizontal. **B:** The end plates of the superior and inferior end vertebrae are marked as seen in this figure. Perpendicular lines are then constructed at right angles to the mark on each of the end vertebra. **C:** The angle constructed by the two perpendicular lines is measured and defined as the Cobb angle.

ally remain constant; however, adjustments may be required over time, due to brace-influenced change or other curve pattern changes. The wide variation of inter- and intraobserver error (about 5 degrees for any curve measurement) should be understood by the surgeon and the anxious parents (and patient) (108–110). Carman et al. state that to be 95% certain that two measurements are truly different, a 10-degree change must be measured (111). A useful maneuver for both the neophyte and expert surgeon includes viewing the current film, the prior-visit film, and the original film side by side. (A good scoliosis clinic needs at least three long view boxes mounted side-by-side). Then, before making a Cobb measurement, one should use the "eyeball method" to see whether the radiographic curve appears to be getting worse. Patients and their parents often want to make this assessment with you. This type of exercise puts the Cobb measurement in perspective (and sometimes humbles you as to your accuracy and reproducibility in measurement).

Vertebral rotation, maximal at the apex of a curve, is demonstrated radiographically by asymmetry of the pedicles and a shift of the spinous processes toward the concavity. Two methods are available for quantifying it: Nash and Moe (112), and Perdriolle (113). Vertebral rotation is not routinely measured clinically, and both methods have substantial inaccuracies, which limit their usefulness (114).

Skeletal maturity should be assessed radiographically to estimate remaining spinal growth, an important predictor of risk for curve progression. The most widely used method in scoliosis patients is that of Risser (115), who noted that the iliac crest apophysis ossifies in a predictable fashion, from lateral to medial, and that its fusion to the body of the ilium mirrors the fusion of the vertebral ring apophysis, signifying completion of spinal growth. The lateral to medial ossification of the iliac crest apophysis occurs over a period of 18–24 months, finally capping the entire iliac wing. Risser classified the extent of apophyseal ossification in stages, with Risser 0 indicating absence of ossification in the apophysis and Risser 5 indicating fusion of the fully ossified apophysis to the ilium (spinal growth complete) (116). Risser 1 through 4 are assigned to the intermediate levels of maturity as seen in Fig. 18-15.

The status of the triradiate cartilage of the acetabulum also provides a landmark for assessing growth potential. The triradiate growth cartilage usually closes before the iliac apophysis appears (Risser 0) at about the time of maximal spinal growth (117,118). Skeletal age can also be measured using the Greulich and Pyle atlas to compare hand radiographs against illustrated standards, although these readings become less accurate (large standard deviations) in the adolescent age group (119).

Specialized Imaging Studies

Most idiopathic scoliosis cases do not require imaging beyond plain radiography. Specialized imaging methods that

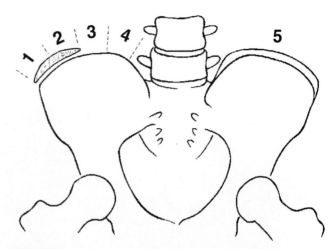

FIGURE 18-15. Risser sign. The iliac apophysis ossifies in a predictable manner, beginning laterally and progressing medially. This capping of the iliac wing is correlated with slowing and completion of spinal growth occurring over an 18- to 24-month period.

can be used to evaluate cases with unusual features include magnetic resonance imaging (MRI), computed tomography (CT), and bone scintigraphy, each with specific indications and advantages.

In the developed world, MRI has almost completely replaced myelography for the study of the neural elements in spine disorders. An exception is the patient who has had prior placement of stainless steel hardware (making MRI visualization nearly impossible) who has continued or new symptoms that require study.

MRI study of the spine is indicated for all infantile and juvenile idiopathic patients (79,120,121), as well as those with congenital bony anomalies, if surgical correction is planned (122,123). Left thoracic curves and scoliosis in boys have been shown to have an increased association with spinal cord anomalies and may be an indication for MRI study (120,124). Indications for routine MRI study in patients with typical idiopathic scoliosis prior to corrective surgery (and who have a normal clinical neurologic examination), remain unclear (125). At present there is no prospective study that confirms the efficacy of MRI screening for preoperative assessment (spine and brain) of all patients with idiopathic scoliosis, although a few centers have made this the routine for all operative cases. Clearly, patients with an abnormality in the neurologic examination (120), or with cutaneous findings (suggesting dysraphism or neurofibromatosis), should have an MRI study of the spine and/or brain. Severe angular and rotational deformities may be difficult to analyze with an MRI, because the spinal canal deviates into and out of the planar cuts of the sagittal and coronal images. CT myelography that produces a dye column may be better for revealing stenosis or an intraspinal filling defect in extremely severe cases of scoliosis.

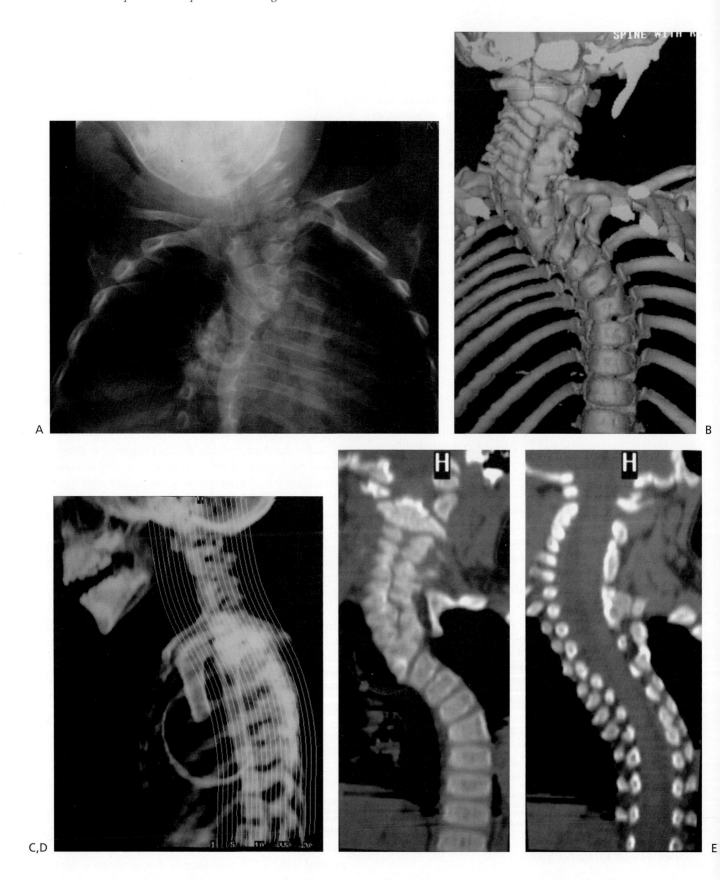

A

B

C,D

E

The workup of patients with substantial back pain with no obvious cause may require a bone scan to evaluate for possible tumor, infection, or spondylolysis. The bone scan is an excellent screening test for studying the painful scoliotic patient, allowing one to screen for conditions ranging from osteoid osteoma to hydronephrosis. A single proton emission computed tomography (SPECT) type bone scan (computerized tomographic enhancement) is very useful in identifying spondylolysis and its varying presentations (unilateral, bilateral, cold scan, hot scan, etc.). If an area of increased activity is noted on the bone scan, additional imaging (either MR or CT) may be required. CT studies can be performed with increasing sophistication, and provide the best method for imaging the bony anatomy in complex deformities and congenital anomalies. Standard two-dimensional transverse images are less helpful in scoliosis, compared to coronal, sagittal, and three-dimensional reformatted images. Additional multiplanar (curved along the deformity) reformatted coronal and sagittal images are particularly helpful in imaging the scoliotic spine when congenital anomalies are suspected (Fig. 18-16).

Imaging the kidneys and urologic collecting system is important in patients with congenital scoliosis (126,127), because identification of a congenital spinal deformity may be the first clue of an abnormality of the genitourinary (GU) system (which, if unrecognized, could lead to permanent kidney damage). An ultrasound study is the most practical screening test for detecting GU system abnormalities and should be obtained once a congenital spinal abnormality has been identified (126).

IDIOPATHIC SCOLIOSIS—DETAILS OF DIAGNOSIS AND TREATMENT

Idiopathic scoliosis makes up the largest subset of patients with spinal deformity, and because its etiology is unknown, this diagnosis is one of exclusion made only after a careful evaluation has ruled out other causes of scoliosis. Clinical features and treatment vary by age group (infantile, juvenile, adolescent), and are summarized below.

Prevalence and Natural History of Idiopathic Scoliosis

The prevalence of idiopathic scoliosis (with a curve of greater than 10 degrees) in a childhood and adolescent population has been reported to be from 0.5 to 3 per 100 (128–134). The reported prevalence of larger curves (greater than 30 degrees) ranges from 1.5 to 3 per 1,000 (135,136) (Table 18-2). Thus small to moderate curves are common, and severe (life threatening) curves are rare.

The percentage of cases seen in each age group demonstrates a strong predominance of adolescent curves, with a series of patients from Boston showing 0.5% infantile, 10.5% juvenile, and 89% adolescent (16). The natural history for each group varies substantially.

Although classically idiopathic scoliosis has been divided into three groups according to the age of onset (infantile, juvenile, adolescent), there is a movement in Britain to simplify this to early-onset scoliosis (before age 10 years) and late-onset scoliosis (typical adolescent scoliosis) (131). Dickson and Weinstein believe that only early-onset scoliosis has the potential for evolution to severe thoracic deformity with cardiac and pulmonary compromise (137). This simpler classification has not been fully evaluated, thus the traditional three–age-group division remains the standard in North America.

Infantile Idiopathic Scoliosis

Infantile idiopathic scoliosis (IIS) cases have been more commonly reported from Britain, compared to North America (16,138,139). More recent reports, however, have suggested a decrease in the frequency of infantile cases more closely paralleling the North American experience (140).

IIS presents as a left thoracic curve in approximately 90% of cases with a male : female ratio of 3 : 2 (138,139,141,142). The curvature is associated with plagiocephaly, hip dysplasia, congenital heart disease, and mental retardation (14, 143). The series from Britain suggests that the vast majority (up to 90%) of these curves are self-limited and resolve spontaneously (142); however, the few that are progressive can be difficult to manage (Fig. 18-17).

FIGURE 18-16. A: This 3-year-old patient presented with severe cervicothoracic scoliosis. The AP radiograph demonstrates a congenital etiology to the deformity; however, the details of the malformation are difficult to appreciate on the plain radiograph. **B:** A three-dimensional CT scan demonstrates much more clearly the anatomic deformities in the vertebral bodies. **C:** Frontal plane reformatted images are helpful in analyzing the size and number of hemivertebrae, as well as detecting unsegmented bars. The ability to obtain these images along a curved surface (produced with special software) is particularly useful in following the curvature of the spine in either the AP or lateral projections. Here the sagittal plane (lateral) curved scout film is seen. **D:** The anteroposterior reformatted images through the mid-portion of the vertebral bodies allows identification of the hemivertebrae and associated wedged vertebrae throughout the cervical and upper thoracic spine. **E:** An anteroposterior reformatted image, through the level of the pedicles, demonstrates two areas of an unsegmented bar in the concavity of the cervicothoracic deformity.

TABLE 18-2. PREVALENCE OF SCOLIOSIS

		(% of Patients with Curves of this Magnitude)			
Author (Ref)	No. Patients	>5 degrees	>10 degrees	>20 degrees	>30 degrees
Stirling et al. (131)	15,799	2.7	0.5		
Bruszewski & Kamza (130)	15,000	3.8	3.0	0.5	0.15
Rogala et al. (133)	26,947	5.3	2.2		
Shands & Eisberg (129)	50,000	1.9	1.4	0.5	0.29
Kane & Moe (128)	75,290				0.13
Huang (94)	33,596		1.5	0.2	0.04
Morais et al. (134)	29,195		1.8	0.3	
Soucacos et al. (171)	82,901		1.7	0.2	0.04

Prediction of Progression in Infantile Curves. Risk factors which predict a high likelihood for curve progression have been identified by Mehta who, in a study of 135 patients with infantile idiopathic scoliosis, determined radiographic prognostic factors: 1) rib vertebral angle difference (RVAD) and 2) phase of the rib head (144). The RVAD is the most commonly utilized measure, and is determined at the apical vertebra on an AP radiograph. The difference in the obliquity between the two ribs attaching to the apical vertebra (right versus left) is known as the RVAD. The ribs in the concavity of progressive infantile scoliosis are relatively horizontal, while those on the convex side are

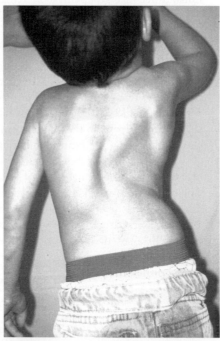

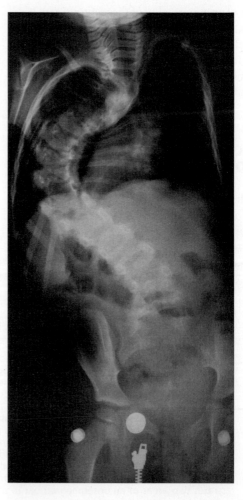

FIGURE 18-17. A: This 3-year-old male presented before 1 year of life with a 45-degree left thoracic scoliosis. An MRI evaluation of his brain and spinal cord was normal; therefore, he was diagnosed as having infantile idiopathic scoliosis. The initial PA radiograph demonstrated a severe left thoracic scoliosis with a rib–vertebral angle difference (RVAD) of 40 degrees. **B:** Progression was noted despite bracing and corrective casting and by age 2 years the curve was greater than 90 degrees.

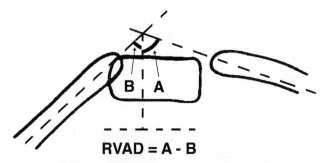

RVAD = A - B

FIGURE 18-18. In infantile idiopathic scoliosis the rib–vertebral angle difference (*RVAD*) helps in predicting curve progression. The RVAD is constructed by first determining the angle of the right and left ribs at the apical level of the deformity. The slope of the ribs relative to the transverse plane is measured for each rib. The difference in the angle between the right and left sides is the RVAD.

more vertically aligned (Fig. 18-18). Eighty-three percent of Mehta's reported cases resolved when the RVAD was less than 20 degrees compared to 84% progressing when the RVAD was greater than 20 degrees (144,145).

Juvenile Idiopathic Scoliosis

Juvenile idiopathic scoliosis (JIS), defined as scoliosis with an onset between the age of 4 to 10 years, makes up approximately 8 to 16% of the childhood idiopathic scoliosis (146–148), and in many respects, represents a transitional group between the infantile and adolescent groups. Curves with onset in this age group are often progressive with potential for trunk deformity and eventual cardiac and pulmonary compromise. Many patients who present in adolescence (previously undiagnosed and untreated), with severe thoracic curves requiring immediate surgery, have had the onset of their curve in the juvenile age period, making differentiation of the juvenile versus adolescent grouping problematic.

In JIS, boys seem to be affected earlier than girls (146,149). In a series of 109 patients evaluated by Robinson and McMaster, the boys presented at a mean age of 5 years 8 months, compared to an age of 7 years 2 months for the girls. The ratio of girls to boys was 1:1.6 for those younger than 6 years and 2.7:1 for those older than 6 years at presentation. Additionally, there were equal numbers of right- and left-sided curves in the younger group (less than 6 years), with a predominance of right sided curves (3.9:1) in the patients older than 6 years (146). When curves reach 30 degrees they are nearly always progressive if left untreated (150). The rate of progression is 1 to 3 degrees per year before age 10 years, and sharply increases to 4.5 to 11 degrees per year after that age (146). This is particularly true for thoracic curves, which despite brace treatment, require arthrodesis greater than 95% of the time (146,150). The surgical treatment of JIS is similar to that for adolescent

idiopathic scoliosis; however, anterior growth ablation (fusion), in addition to posterior instrumentation and fusion, is more commonly indicated to prevent "crankshaft" rotational growth following posterior fusion (see p. 729). In very young cases, instrumentation using a system that can be periodically lengthened is sometimes used (instrumentation without fusion-fusion only at proximal and distal hook sites).

Adolescent Idiopathic Scoliosis

This most common category of adolescent idiopathic scoliosis (AIS) theoretically develops a curve after the age of 10 years, associated with the rapid growth of adolescence. Again, the separation of adolescent and juvenile curves is somewhat arbitrary, since an 11-year-old girl who presented with a 70-degree scoliosis almost certainly had the onset of scoliosis in the juvenile age period. Thus the European view is that scoliosis should be considered either early-onset or late-onset. As noted previously, the prevalence data range between 0.5 and 3% for curves ≥10 degrees. These data have been collected from a variety of sources, including screening chest x-rays as well as school screening programs (Table 18-2). Roughly 2% of adolescents have a scoliosis of ≥10 degrees, but only 5% of these cases have progression of the curve to greater than 30 degrees. The ratio of boys to girls is equal for minor curves, yet is dominated by girls as the curve magnitude increases, reaching 1:8 for those requiring treatment (151).

Risk Factors for Progression

Knowledge of which curves will likely worsen and which will not is critical in deciding whom to treat. Risk factors for scoliosis progression that have been identified include gender, remaining skeletal growth, curve location, and curve magnitude with scoliosis progression being most rapid during peak skeletal growth (early infancy and adolescence). The peak growth velocity of adolescence averages 6 to 8 cm of overall height gain per year (28,118) with half of this growth coming from the trunk (spine) (152) (Fig. 18-19). Several determinants are useful in predicting the remaining growth. The age of the patient is obvious; however, substantial variation in skeletal growth exists for patients of the same chronologic age; therefore, bone age is a more consistent indicator (153). Menarchal status helps determine the growth spurt in females with the onset of menses generally following the most rapid stage of skeletal growth by approximately 12 months.

The Risser sign, associated with the stages of vertebral body end-plate growth, has been demonstrated to be a useful measure for assessing risk for curve progression. When the Risser sign is 1 or less, the risk for progression is up to 60 to 70%, while if the patient is Risser 3, the risk is reduced to less than 10% (29,154).

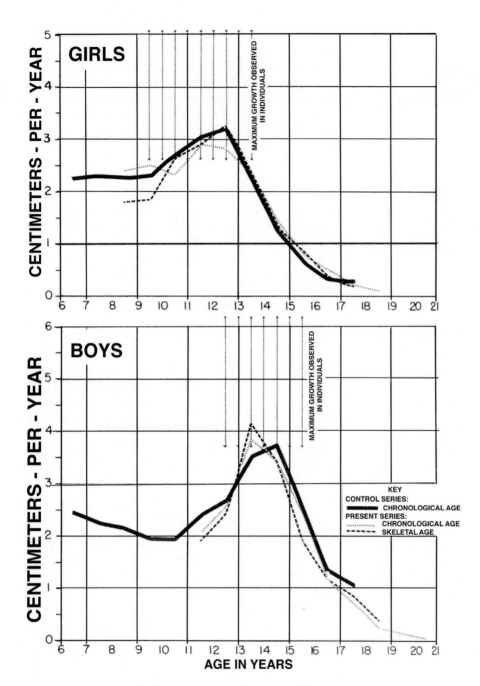

FIGURE 18-19. Increase in sitting height during the adolescent growth spurt for girls and boys is noted in this graph. The peak gain in trunk height ranges between 3 and 6 cm per year. (From ref. 152, with permission.)

Unfortunately many of the readily identified markers of maturity (menarchal status and Risser sign) are quite variable, and appear just after the adolescent growth spurt. It is therefore impossible to tell if a premenarchal, Risser 0 patient is approaching, in the midst of, or past the time of most rapid growth and risk for scoliosis progression, if there is no accurate record of prior growth. Recently, closure of the triradiate cartilage of the acetabulum has been identified as a radiographic sign which more closely approximates the time of peak growth velocity (118).

Curve pattern has also been identified as an important variable for predicting the probability of progression. Curves with an apex above T12 are more likely to progress than isolated lumbar curves (154). Curve magnitude at initial diagnosis appears to be a factor predicting progression (29,155) (Fig. 18-20). In a series of skeletally immature patients (Risser 0 or 1), curve progression occurred in 22% of cases with a curve at initial diagnosis of 5 to 19 degrees compared to 68% incidence of curve progression when the initial curve was 20 to 29

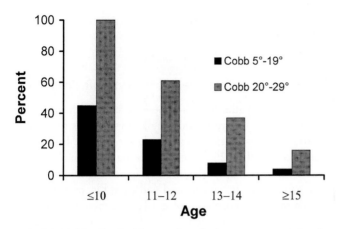

FIGURE 18-20. The incidence of scoliosis curve progression is greatest at a younger age and for larger curves. (From ref. 29, with permission.)

degrees (29). This rate increases to 90% when the initial curve is 30 to 59 degrees (156).

Natural History in Adulthood

The long-term effects of idiopathic scoliosis in adults should be understood when considering treatment in childhood and adolescence. The risk of curve progression is greatest during the rapid phases of growth as discussed above; however, not all curves stabilize after growth stops. In the long-term studies performed at the University of Iowa, greater than two-thirds of patients experienced curve progression following skeletal maturity. Curves of less than 30 degrees tended not to progress with the most marked progression occurring in curves that were between 50 and 75 degrees at the completion of growth (continuing at a rate of nearly 1 degree/year). Lumbar curves generally progressed if they were greater than 30 degrees at skeletal maturity (157,158). Several studies have been performed which provide insight into what the future holds for affected individuals. Early studies of untreated scoliosis patients, with up to 50-year follow-up, claimed a mortality rate twice that expected in the general population with cardiopulmonary problems as the most common cause of death (159,160). Disability and back pain were common in the living patients (160,161). Unfortunately the etiology of the scoliosis in these studies was mixed (idiopathic, congenital, neuromuscular), and the severity of the scoliosis was not known for many of the patients, making correlations to those with idiopathic scoliosis impossible.

In more recent studies in which only adolescent idiopathic scoliosis patients were included, the increased mortality rate reported previously has not been confirmed (162). Mortality from cor pulmonale and right heart failure was seen only in severe thoracic curves (>90 to 100 degrees) (162,163).

Pulmonary function becomes limited as thoracic scoliosis becomes more severe (>80 to 90 degrees curve) (162,164,165). Forced vital capacity (FVC) and forced expiratory volume in one second (FEV_1) decrease linearly with approximately a 20% reduction in predicted values with curves of 100 degrees (162) (Fig. 18-21). The associated deformity of the chest cavity causes restrictive lung disease. Thoracic lordosis also decreases lung volume and increases the deleterious effects of scoliosis on pulmonary function (166).

Estimates regarding the frequency of back pain and associated disability in adults with scoliosis vary, but most studies have demonstrated slightly higher rates of back pain compared to control groups (162,167–169). The 1,476 patients with AIS surveyed in Montreal had more frequent and more severe back pain than did 1,755 control subjects (167). Disability rates have been higher (160,167) in some series and similar in others (162).

The social impact of scoliosis varies with the individual and the cultural setting. Many current patients have substantial concern about the appearance of their back and seek medical treatment for correction of their deformity (170). The rate of marriage for females with scoliosis is lower in some studies implying a psychosocial effect of the deformity (159,160). Many modern parents are unwilling to accept significant deformity of any type in their child whether it be dental, dermatologic, or orthopedic, particularly if there is a reasonable and safe way to correct the condition.

School Screening for Scoliosis

School screening programs to detect scoliosis at an early stage have been instituted in many countries, with a goal of detecting childhood scoliosis early enough to allow brace treatment, rather than in its late stages, when surgical correc-

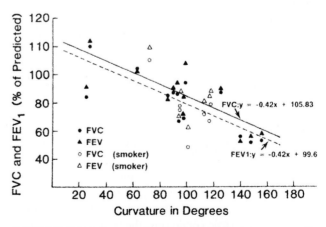

FIGURE 18-21. Pulmonary function as it relates to curve severity in both nonsmoking and smoking patients. (From ref. 162, with permission.)

tion and fusion would be needed (171–173). Screening programs for any disease are indicated if effective early treatment methods exist, and if the disorder is frequent enough to justify the cost. Although screening programs for scoliosis are widespread in North America, the variable sensitivity and specificity of the screening exam, and the borderline efficacy of brace treatment, have caused some to suggest that school screening is not justified (137,172,174–177).

Despite these concerns, scoliosis screening is commonly performed on school children between the fifth and sixth grades (age 10 to 12 years) (178). The Adams forward-bend test is employed in combination with scoliometer (179) measurement of the maximum angle of trunk rotation (ATR) (Fig. 18-9). A referral and radiograph are recommended when the ATR is >7 degrees (93,94,179,180). The 7-degrees ATR standard detects nearly all curves greater than 30 degrees, yet leads to a large number of patient referrals (2 to 3 per 100 children screened) (93,179) for radiographs in adolescents who have only spinal asymmetry (Cobb <10 degrees) or mild scoliosis (Cobb <25 degrees) not needing treatment. Overall, in screening programs the incidence of curves of >10 degrees (Cobb angle) is approximately 3%, and of curves >25 degrees, about 0.3%.

Both the Adams forward-bend test and measurement of the ATR with a scoliometer have been shown to have reasonable intraexaminer agreement (95,180–182). Although there is an overall linear correlation between the ATR and Cobb angles (95,183), precise prediction of the magnitude of deformity is not possible without a radiograph. The positive predictive value (the probability of having scoliosis with an abnormal screening test) of the forward-bend test is highly variable (94,134,174,176,184) and thought by many to be too low to warrant current scoliosis screening practices.

Despite the criticism leveled at school screening (cost and over-referral), many experts believe that the emphasis placed on screening for early diagnosis has greatly increased awareness of scoliosis, not only in the lay public, but also among primary care physicians. It appears that the combination of increased awareness plus the efficacy of screening programs has reduced the number of patients who do not see a physician until they have marked deformity (171,173,185,186). This remains controversial, and others have presented longitudinal data following the institution of a screening program which reject this idea (135,176).

Treatment of Idiopathic Scoliosis

Analysis of idiopathic scoliosis treatment is dependent on understanding the natural history of the condition in the untreated state compared to the outcome with intervention. As in many pediatric conditions, the short-term outcomes of treatment are reasonably well known; however, the long-term results are less well defined. Due to this lack of knowl-

edge, controversy continues regarding treatment choices in any individual patient.

Nonoperative Treatment of Idiopathic Scoliosis

Because most patients with idiopathic scoliosis have curves of less than 20 degrees, and only a few progress to require treatment, most patients are simply monitored. Idiopathic curves of less than 25 degrees should be monitored every 4 to 12 months (depending on the age and growth rate of the patient) with clinical and radiographic examination. Those in the rapid phases of growth are seen at more frequent intervals (every 4 to 6 months). Curves of greater than 30 degrees should be monitored for progression after skeletal maturity with radiographs obtained approximately every 5 years. Curve progression in the mature patient (when it occurs) is slow enough (approximately 1 degree per year) that more frequent follow-up is not indicated.

Indications for Orthotic (Brace) Treatment. In growing children, a spinal orthosis (brace) is generally indicated when a curve progresses to 25 to 30 degrees (187–189). Scoliosis braces of many different styles and corrective mechanical principles have been developed with each having in common the goal of modifying spinal growth by applying an external force. Because brace treatment depends on spinal growth modulation, treatment is prescribed only for patients with substantial spinal growth remaining (Risser 2–3 or less). The upper limit of curve magnitude amenable to brace treatment is approximately 45 degrees. Most studies have confirmed that, even in the most cooperative patients, the final result of brace treatment is maintenance of the curve at the degree of severity present at the onset of bracing. Correction may occur while in the brace, but when the brace is discontinued, the curve will generally settle to its pre-treatment severity (190–192). Scoliosis patients and their parents should be advised of this, because most anticipate that the brace will provide permanent correction, as is seen in orthodontic correction, a common point of reference for the layperson. In more severe curves with trunk deformity already present, this information may cause some patients and their parents to select surgical correction rather than brace maintenance.

In general, a brace is indicated for growing adolescents with a curve between 25 and 45 degrees. Most surgeons insist that curve progression of more than 5 degrees be documented before bracing curves of less than 30 degrees. These indications may need to be altered depending on the clinical circumstance; for example, a 10-year-old premenarchal female, with a curve that has increased from 14 to 22 degrees in the prior 6 months, should probably be braced before reaching 25 degrees. Early bracing may also be considered when a strong positive family history for progressive scoliosis exists (mother or sibling required treatment).

Brace Types. The Milwaukee brace, developed by Walter Blount at Milwaukee Children's Hospital in the 1940s, became the standard to which other designs were compared (193). This brace remained popular into the 1980s (194), and remains an option in selected situations. The original design provided longitudinal traction between the skull and pelvis with lateral translational forces directed through pads on the chest wall (Fig. 18-22). The brace uprights can be adjusted in length to accommodate growth—a feature useful in treating infantile and juvenile patients. In addition, it remains one of the few designs that has the potential to maintain upper thoracic curves.

Underarm braces (e.g., Boston (195,196) and Wilmington (197,198)) (Fig. 18-23) have replaced the Milwaukee brace in most centers due to increased acceptance by the patients. Because no upright or neckpiece is used, the brace is less conspicuous, a feature highly important to the adolescent. The stigma of wearing a visible scoliosis brace produces a negative self-image in many teenagers (199,200). Despite improvements in brace appearance (brace worn under clothes—no visible neckpiece), many teenagers will not cooperate with brace wear. Factors for failure include pain (201), poor fit, heat, family environment, and concerns

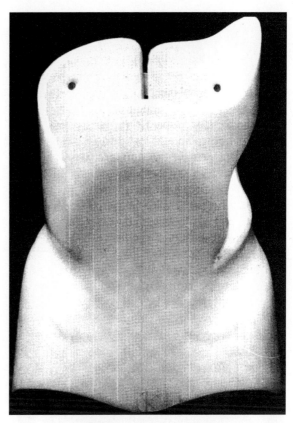

FIGURE 18-23. Boston brace.

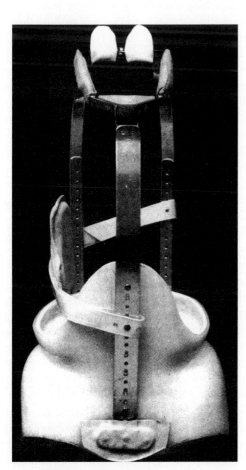

FIGURE 18-22. Milwaukee brace.

about self-esteem. The brace must be acceptable to the patient if it is to be worn and have any chance of limiting curve progression.

The Charleston nighttime bending brace (202), an alternative that attempts to create a more complete correction of the curve (Fig. 18-24), requires a trunk bend so severe that it precludes walking. This brace is therefore only prescribed for nighttime wear and is best suited for single curves that are more distal (thoracolumbar and lumbar curves).

Wearing Schedule. Correction by a brace is thought to be due to the constant corrective molding of the trunk and spine during growth. As such, full-time (23 h per day) brace wear was first advised by Blount, and continues to be recommended by many who prescribe scoliosis braces. About 15 years ago, certain centers began to treat patients for only 16 h per day, allowing the child to go to school without the brace, hoping that the abbreviated schedule would lead to greater patient compliance (197,203). This schedule is popular with many surgeons (and patients); however, one must question the biomechanical validity of the concept since the preponderance of brace wear is at night when the curve is least severe (patient supine). Alternatively, during daytime hours, when the curve is at its greatest (upright, forces of gravity), the curve is uncorrected. A metaanalysis

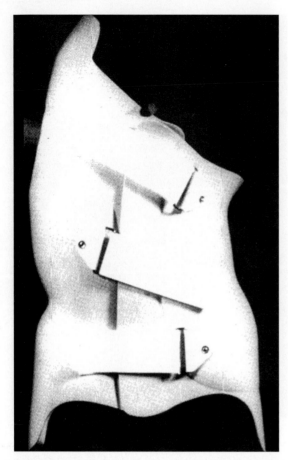

FIGURE 18-24. Charleston brace (nighttime bending brace).

performed by the Scoliosis Research Society Prevalence and Natural History Committee found a dose dependent relationship between the time per day in brace and success in preventing curve progression (204), suggesting that more hours of brace wear per day provides more effective correction. This contradicted a study of the Wilmington brace, which did not demonstrate a difference in efficacy between part-time and full-time bracing (197).

This recommendation for full-time brace wear is in sharp contrast to the Charleston nighttime bending brace philosophy, which attempts to produce hypercorrection. In a series reported by Price et al., the average curve correction while in the brace was 73% (205), and they postulated that less time per day of wear was required because of the marked correction while in the brace.

Brace Efficacy. The effectiveness of bracing for idiopathic scoliosis has been presumed for many years, yet controlled treatment trials with and without bracing had not been completed until recently (187,206). Earlier studies reporting high success rates for brace treatment were subsequently

noted to have included many patients who were at low risk for progression. Lonstein and Winter evaluated 1,020 patients treated with a Milwaukee brace, over half who were at substantial risk for progression, and for whom the natural history was known. In the group with an initial curve between 20 and 29 degrees, and at high risk for progression, the brace was found to be effective compared to natural history data (194). This is in contrast to the findings of Noonan et al. who have recently called into question the efficacy of the Milwaukee brace (207).

In 1995 the results of a prospective controlled study of bracing by the Scoliosis Research Society was published. The results in 286 patients age 10 to 15 years, with an initial curve of 25 to 35 degrees, treated with either observation alone (129 patients), an underarm brace (111 patients), or nighttime electrical stimulation (46 patients) were compared. Curve progression at the end of bracing (skeletal maturity) was limited to less than 5 degrees in 74% of those treated with a brace, compared to 34% of those followed without treatment. The group treated with electrical stimulation had a success rate of only 33% (187). Although critics (137) site flaws in this and other studies, most centers have accepted the results, and continue to advise brace treatment for progressive curves in skeletally immature adolescents.

Data regarding the efficacy of various brace designs are mixed with differing inclusion criteria making direct comparisons impossible (203,204). However, in two recent studies a full-time underarm brace was more successful than a nighttime Charleston bending brace both in preventing curve progression and in preventing surgery (188,208). Both of these studies were retrospective with potential biases, and no prospective comparison of various braces has been performed to confirm these conclusions. In the series from Dallas, the nighttime Charleston brace equaled the efficacy of a Boston brace for single lumbar and thoracolumbar curves (188).

For each of these braces correction of the curve should be maximized in the brace with careful fitting, and adjustment of the pads by an experienced orthotist with an interest in scoliosis treatment. Efficacy is increased when the in-brace radiographic Cobb angle is reduced by 20% or more, compared to the pre-brace Cobb measurement (207).

In summary, although brace treatment for progressive curves provide the standard of care in most of the developed world, the scientific basis for brace efficacy is not powerful. When to intervene remains problematic, because very mild curves are easier to control with a brace, yet wholesale adoption of this policy leads to many children being braced unnecessarily. Waiting until the curve reaches 30 degrees allows one to brace the least number of patients, yet the margin between a curve of 30 degrees (brace instituted) and 40 to 45 degrees (surgery required) is distressingly small. Finally, many adolescents strongly resist brace wear, and their resistance is understandable (209,210), particularly in teenage boys with scoliosis, who might have to wear a brace for as long as 5 years (skeletal maturity often age >18 years). Each of these factors make the brace treatment of scoliosis a continuing challenge.

Surgical Correction of Idiopathic Scoliosis

Introduction and Indications. Goals for surgical treatment of idiopathic scoliosis include improved spinal alignment/balance and prevention of subsequent curve progression. Corrective instrumentation plus arthrodesis (fusion) provides the best method for achieving lasting correction, and can be used either anteriorly or posteriorly to restore spinal alignment, as well as to provide postoperative stabilization while the fusion mass progressively solidifies. All current methods rely on the development of a stable bony fusion mass to maintain the correction over time with the rods serving as internal struts while fusion occurs. Application of a rod system without a bony fusion predictably leads to rod fracture and loss of correction.

The indications for surgical correction of scoliosis are based on curve magnitude, clinical deformity, risk for progression, skeletal maturity, and curve pattern. In general, thoracic curves of greater than 40 to 50 degrees (Cobb angle) in skeletally immature patients should have surgical correction, while in mature patients (i.e., risk of progression decreased), surgical correction is reserved for curves of 50 degrees or more. These Cobb angle ranges are meant as guidelines rather than absolute indications and are based on the natural history of untreated scoliosis in immature and mature patients. Factors other than Cobb angle should be considered when deciding between operative and nonoperative treatment. Trunk deformity (rotation), as well as trunk balance, are important factors in deciding when to advise surgical correction. A patient with a lumbar curve of 35 degrees may have such a severe lateral trunk shift that surgical correction is indicated. The curve pattern has a great impact on the cosmetic deformity associated with the scoliosis, with single curves producing a more noticeable unbalanced trunk, compared to double or triple curves (Fig. 18-25).

When recommending surgical treatment of scoliosis, it is implied that both early and long-term outcome will be

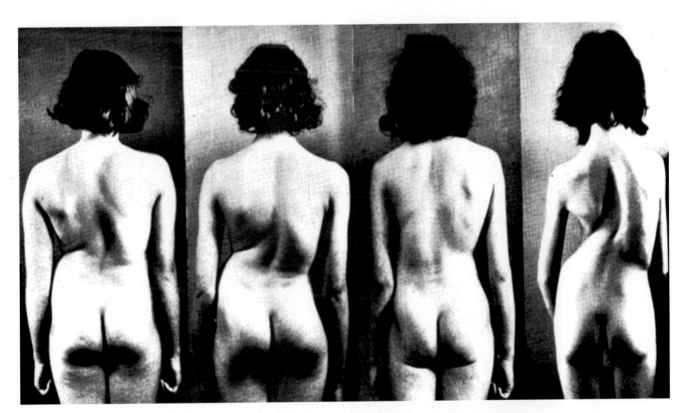

Lumbar   Thoracolumbar   Double Major   Thoracic

FIGURE 18-25. This classic series of photographs from J.I.P. James demonstrates the clinical appearance of four patients, each with a 70-degrees magnitude curvature, although with different curve patterns. The clinical deformity is greater in single curves, particularly in the thoracic curve. (From ref. 141, with permission.)

improved compared to the nonoperative treatment. The short-term results of surgical treatment are well known with a variety of surgical techniques having been studied for most curve types. Midterm (5 to 10 years) outcomes for modern corrective surgery are becoming available (211,212), but like all advancing technologies, the surgical methods tend to change faster than the results can be collected. The study by Dickson et al. of Harrington's surgically treated patients, with 20-year follow-up, showed good long-term results. Although the methods of Harrington (single distraction rod) have been replaced in many parts of the world, the fusion of patients with scoliosis in that era led to lasting stabilization in most cases (213).

Posterior Spinal Instrumentation. Paul Harrington of Houston introduced posterior spinal instrumentation in the early 1960s to make spine fusions more predictable (214). Prior to this, *in situ* fusions with body cast correction were performed (215) to correct the deformity and immobilize the spine while the fusion occurred. The addition of Harrington instrumentation improved scoliosis correction and greatly reduced the incidence of pseudarthrosis following scoliosis surgery.

Harrington Instrumentation. The Harrington instrumentation system consists of a ratcheted concave distraction rod with hooks at either end and a threaded compression rod attached to the transverse processes on the convex side of the curve [➔2.2]. Coronal plane improvement provided by the Harrington distraction rod was often gained at the expense of decreased thoracic kyphosis and flattening of the lumbar spine (so-called "flat-back deformity"), as noted in the sagittal plane (Fig. 18-26). Subsequent modifications of the Harrington concept included the use of sublaminar wires or a square-ended rod to allow rod contouring (in an attempt to maintain thoracic kyphosis and lumbar lordosis) while preventing rod rotation with distraction [➔2.3] (216).

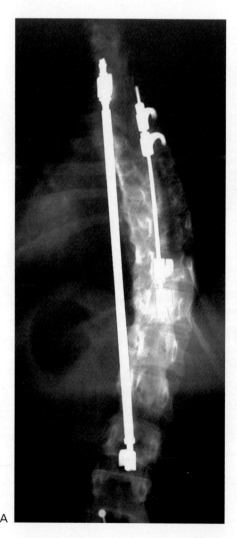

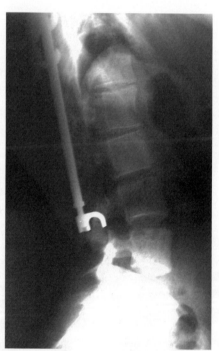

FIGURE 18-26. A: Harrington distraction rod can be seen on the left with the smaller threaded compression rod on the right. **B:** Distraction into the lumbar spine reduces lumbar lordosis creating a "flat-back" deformity.

The trend toward protecting normal lumbar contour was greatly advanced by Moe's clarification that most scoliosis (with apparent double curves) requiring surgical correction did *not* require fusion of the lumbar curve. He clarified that the lumbar curve is very often secondary, and does not require fusion (the so-called King-Moe type 2 curve). Application of the King-Moe curve classification is emphasized later in this chapter (217).

Cotrel-Dubousset and Other Double Rod, Multiple Hook Systems.

Nearly 20 years after the Harrington method was introduced, Cotrel and Dubousset (France) introduced a multi-hook system that allowed distraction and compression on the same rod (218). Sagittal plane contouring of the rods and segmental hook fixation improved curve correction, as well as postoperative stability. Many additional segmental fixation posterior instrumentation systems utilizing similar concepts are now available for surgical correction of scoliosis. Current options for attachment to the posterior spine include hooks (for attachment to the transverse processes, laminae, and pedicles), sublaminar wires (Luque), and pedicle screws [➥2.9].

The introduction of pedicle screw fixation into posterior scoliosis constructs distally, allows greater correction compared to distal hook constructs, and allows fewer levels to be instrumented caudally (219,220). The utility of pedicle screw attachment to vertebra was first recognized in Europe (221), and was initially quite controversial in North America because of an increased potential for neurologic injury associated with screw insertion. Pedicle screw attachment is highly effective, but the surgeon must have appropriate training and skill when using them to safely improve the stability of corrective scoliosis constructs. In North America they are generally used only in the lower thoracic and upper lumbar spine when used at all for scoliosis correction. The use of pedicle screws in mid and even upper thoracic vertebrae in scoliosis has been advocated by Suk et al., but this more demanding technique has not been widely adopted (222,223).

It must be emphasized that with all of these procedures the goal is to obtain fusion, and one must first perform careful subperiosteal exposure of the spine as well as meticulous facet excision [➥2.1]. The spine must also be decorticated prior to adding bone graft. The complexity of modern instrumentation sometimes causes surgeons to pay too little attention to the details required to obtain a successful fusion.

Mechanisms of Correction.

Several strategies can be utilized when implanting posterior instrumentation systems. Frontal plane realignment of the spine can be accomplished by translating the vertebra to the concave rod. This translational movement may be performed by connecting the concave rod, precontoured to the desired sagittal profile to each fixation site along the spine, then rotating the rod into the sagittal plane. This rod rotation maneuver, popularized by

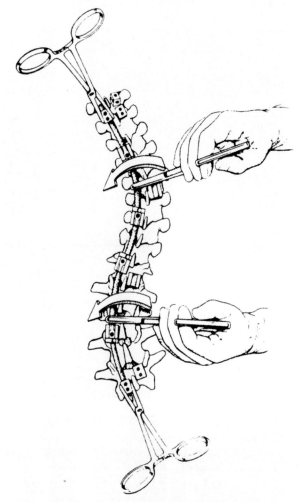

FIGURE 18-27. Example of the rod derotation maneuver popularized by Dubousset. The rod, first contoured to match the scoliosis, is then secured to the hooks and rotated 90 degrees to recreate thoracic kyphosis and lumbar lordosis.

Dubousset, remains an effective method for translating the apex of the curve into a more normal position (Fig. 18-27). Another method for translating the apex in space involves locking the concave rod into the position of anticipated correction, then sequentially (with hooks) or incrementally (with sublaminar wires) drawing the spine to the rod. Compression and distraction forces are then added to enhance both frontal and sagittal plane correction.

Distraction on the concave (usually left sided) rod in the thoracic spine increases thoracic kyphosis and decreases a right-sided scoliosis. Both are generally desired, given the frequent loss of normal thoracic kyphosis noted in idiopathic scoliosis. Similarly, *compression* applied on the same left-sided rod in the lumbar spine (of a double curve) corrects scoliosis and allows restoration/maintenance of lumbar lordosis. In most posterior instrumentation systems used to correct a right thoracic curve, the left-sided (concave) tho-

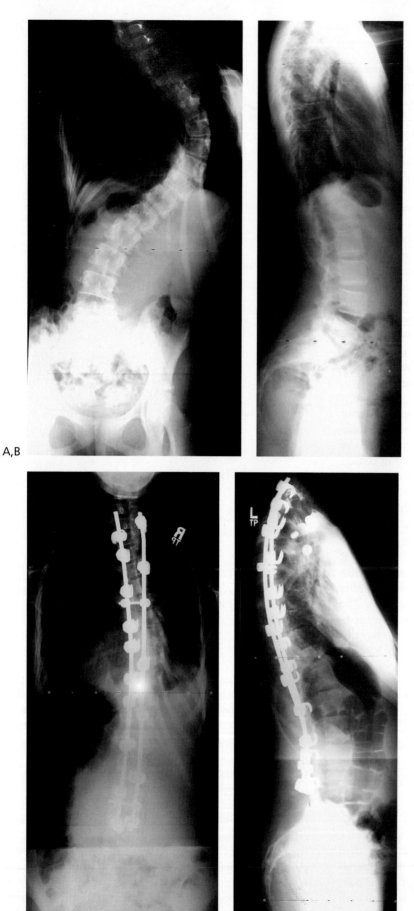

A,B

C,D

FIGURE 18-28. A: This adolescent female presented with a 90-degrees right thoracic scoliosis with marked trunk shift to the right. She corrected to 60 degrees on bending to the right. **B:** Preoperative lateral radiograph. **C:** Following thoracoscopic release and fusion the patient underwent a posterior spinal instrumentation and fusion, with correction of her deformity. A distraction was used through the concavity of the thoracic curve on the left rod with lumbar compression to restore trunk balance and maintain sagittal alignment through the lumbar spine. **D:** Postoperative lateral radiograph demonstrates maintenance of appropriate sagittal alignment.

racic rod that is placed first provides the majority of the deformity correction. The second rod, placed on the right side, primarily adds stability and resistance to fatigue failure. In most modern systems, the two rods are then cross-linked to improve stability.

Anterior Release and Fusion. Indications for a combined anterior and posterior approach in idiopathic scoliosis include patients with large (greater than 75 degrees), rigid (bend correction less than 50 degrees) curves, and those at risk for post-fusion crankshaft deformity. Curve flexibility is increased by anterior disc excision, allowing greater correction with posterior instrumentation, and the bone graft used anteriorly leads to a very stable fusion (anterior and posterior). The procedure involves anterior disc excision with release of the anterior longitudinal ligament, removal of the annulus fibrosis and nucleus pulposus, excision of the vertebral endplate cartilage, and occasionally (in severe cases), excision of the rib head (at the costovertebral joint) (Fig. 18-28).

The term "crankshaft deformity" (117,224–227) identifies a circumstance in which anterior spinal growth continues despite successful posterior fusion, resulting in worsening rotational deformity even after successful posterior fusion (Fig. 18-29). The problem occurs only in skeletally immature patients (Risser 1 or less, triradiate cartilage open). Defining and measuring crankshaft growth is difficult, and has been defined as an increase in the Cobb measurement of >10 degrees, or an increase in apical rotation despite successful posterior fusion. This largely axial rotational deformity is difficult to measure with routine radiog-

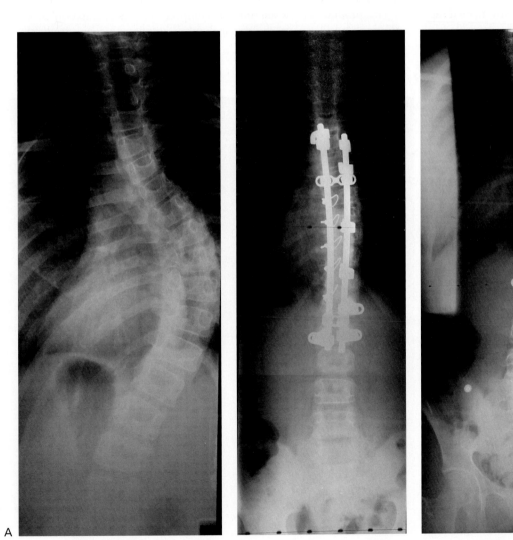

A   B,C

FIGURE 18-29. A: This 8-year, 9-month-old female (clearly skeletally immature) presented with a 60-degree right thoracic scoliosis. **B:** She underwent an isolated posterior instrumentation and fusion with correction to 22 degrees. **C:** Due to continued anterior spinal growth, a crankshaft deformity developed with curve progression, and the trunk decompensated despite a successful posterior fusion. One year postoperatively her curve measured 34 degrees. In this illustration (taken two years postoperatively), her curve has progressed to 43 degrees.

raphy. Recent reports suggest that anterior fusion arrests the anterior growth center and limits the development of this late deformity (228).

An additional advantage of anterior release and fusion is the increased area for the arthrodesis (vertebral end plates) presumably reducing the risk of pseudarthrosis. The thoracoscopic approach is being developed as a means of accomplishing anterior disc excision and fusion with minimally invasive methods (229–231).

Anterior Spinal Instrumentation. At the time of anterior disc excision and fusion, anterior corrective instrumentation with vertebral body screw fixation and a single or double anterolateral rod construct can be considered for some curve patterns [➡**2.11**]. The first anterior instrumentation systems, introduced by Dwyer (232) and then Zielke (233), were both flexible rod compression systems that generated kyphosis within the instrumented segments. This production of kyphosis may be desirable in the scoliotic thoracic

spine (that has become relatively lordotic), but is generally undesirable in the lumbar region.

Subsequently, more rigid solid-rod anterior systems were developed in an attempt to improve the sagittal alignment, particularly when used for thoracolumbar and lumbar curves. Scoliotic curve patterns that are amenable to corrective anterior instrumentation and fusion generally include those with a single structural deformity (thoracic, thoracolumbar, or lumbar).

The greatest experience with anterior scoliosis correction has been gained in the treatment of thoracolumbar and lumbar scoliosis (234–237). Direct access to the vertebral bodies and intervertebral discs is possible via an open anterior thoracoabdominal approach. Anterior disc excision creates mobility, which enhances correction in the frontal and axial planes, but decreases sagittal plane lordosis. Special attention to the sagittal plane is required when anterior compression instrumentation is used distal to the thoracolumbar junction to avoid production of an

A,B

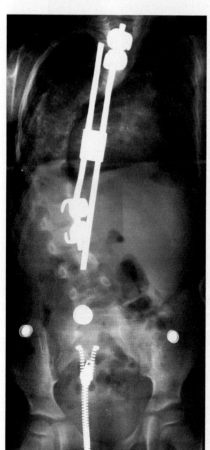 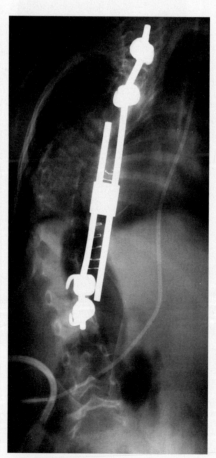 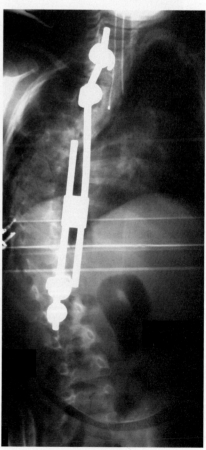

C

FIGURE 18-30. **A:** This patient with infantile idiopathic scoliosis (seen also in Fig. 18-17) underwent apical anterior and posterior hemiepiphysiodesis with posterior instrumentation at age 4 years. **B, C:** At the first repeat lengthening procedure, he achieved an increase in spine length of 2.5 cm. Additional lengthening procedures were performed every 6 months with a total length gain of 6 cm (some from deformity correction, some from growth of the spine) achieved 2½ years following the initial procedure.

iatrogenic flat-back deformity (due to loss of desired lordosis). Structural interbody support, by use of a structural bone graft or an interbody "cage," has been advocated as a means of maintaining sagittal alignment (238). Double-rod, double-screw anterior systems have also been introduced as a means of providing additional sagittal plane control (239,240). In most cases, anterior instrumentation can achieve similar or greater correction (than posterior instrumentation for the same curve) with fewer levels instrumented (241,242).

The selection of the most appropriate approach for correction of idiopathic scoliosis (anterior versus posterior) is dependent on the curve pattern, sagittal deformity, age of the patient, and experience of the surgeon. The selection of the fusion levels for any given patient is also dependent on several factors and remains a topic of much controversy. The fusion should be as short as possible, minimizing the changes in spinal mobility, yet be long enough to ensure optimal correction and lasting spinal balance (both coronal and sagittal).

Instrumentation without Fusion. Instrumentation without fusion, a technique utilized in young children with curves that progress relentlessly despite aggressive brace treatment, includes a subcutaneously positioned distraction construct that spans the deformity (243). At the proximal and distal hook sites, a limited fusion is performed to decrease the incidence of hook dislodgment. In the intervening segments, the spine is *not* stripped subperiosteally, since exposure alone may lead to spontaneous fusion in a young child (thus the concept of a "subcutaneous" rod). Sequential distraction is performed every 6 to 12 months during growth, until no further correction can be obtained. The height gained with these procedures is usually modest, and complications are common (243) (hook dislodgement, spontaneous fusion (244), and infection); therefore, these systems are presently used in children less than 5 to 6 years of age in whom there are few other options. The internal splint (spinal rods) requires external protection with a brace throughout the period of sequential rod distraction. Eventually, a formal instrumentation and fusion are performed. A short convex hemiepiphysiodesis (anterior and posterior) over the apical levels may also be included in the subcutaneous rod technique (224,245) (Fig. 18-30).

Surgical Correction According to Curve Pattern

Idiopathic scoliosis takes on several typical and distinct curve patterns with the most common being a right thoracic curve. To surgically correct scoliosis one must understand these curve patterns. The most widely used classification, developed by Moe as reported by King et al. (King-Moe

TABLE 18-3. CURVE PATTERNS OF THORACIC CURVES

Type I
Double thoracic and lumbar curves
Thoracic and lumbar prominences clinically
Both curves cross the midline
Lumbar curve may be larger than the thoracic curve
Both curves are structural with nearly equal flexibility on supine side bending
True double-major curve, both require fusion

Type II
Thoracic and lumbar curves
Minimal lumbar prominence clinically
Both curves cross the midline
Lumbar curve is more flexible on supine side-bending examination
False double-major pattern allowing selective fusion of the thoracic curve

Type III
Thoracic curve
Minimal or no decompensation
Lumbar curve does not cross the midline

Type IV
Long thoracic curve
Marked decompensation
Curve reaches the midline at L4, which tilts into the curve

Type V
Double thoracic curve
Positive tilt of T1 with prominent left neckline
High left and right thoracic prominences clinically
Upper left curve structural on side-bending examination

(From ref. 217, with permission.)

Classification) (Table 18-3, Fig. 18-31), was designed primarily to decide when to instrument the thoracic curve alone (in patients with apparent double curves), and when to instrument both the thoracic and lumbar curves. Despite the common use of this classification when planning surgery, the system was not designed as a comprehensive classification of idiopathic scoliosis curve patterns.

Primary lumbar and thoracolumbar curves, as well as triple curves, are not included in the King-Moe classification. Others have designed classification systems that are more comprehensive (246,247). The system proposed by Lenke et al. considers both frontal and sagittal plane deformity and is designed to guide surgical treatment decision-making for all curve patterns. This classification system is currently being evaluated at several scoliosis centers around the world with the practicality and usefulness of such a classification system yet to be proven (Fig. 18-32).

Right Thoracic Curve Pattern. The common idiopathic right thoracic curve pattern is most often corrected with posterior spinal instrumentation and fusion of the thoracic curve. Selection of the best cranial and caudal vertebrae to attach to is critical, with the goal to fuse as short as possible,

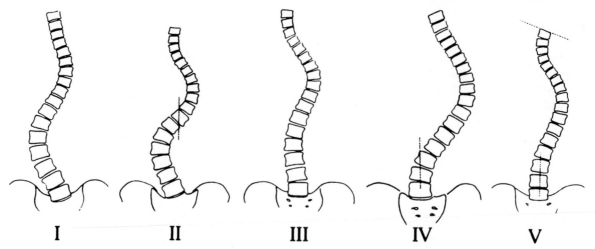

FIGURE 18-31. Diagrammatic representation of the King-Moe classification system for thoracic idiopathic scoliosis. (From ref. 217, with permission.)

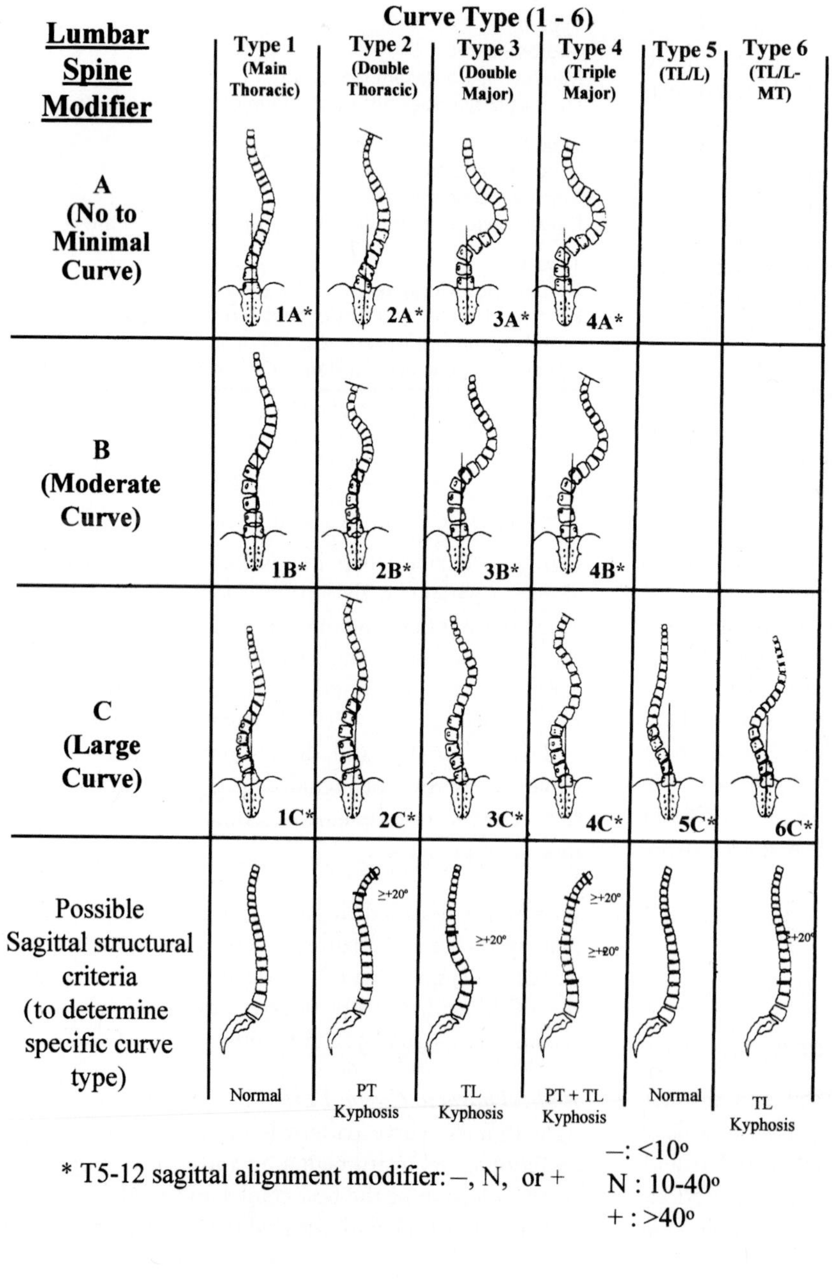

Lumbar Spine Modifier	Curve Type (1 - 6)					
	Type 1 (Main Thoracic)	Type 2 (Double Thoracic)	Type 3 (Double Major)	Type 4 (Triple Major)	Type 5 (TL/L)	Type 6 (TL/L-MT)
A (No to Minimal Curve)	1A*	2A*	3A*	4A*		
B (Moderate Curve)	1B*	2B*	3B*	4B*		
C (Large Curve)	1C*	2C*	3C*	4C*	5C*	6C*
Possible Sagittal structural criteria (to determine specific curve type)	Normal	≥+20° PT Kyphosis	≥+20° TL Kyphosis	≥+20° ≥+20° PT + TL Kyphosis	Normal	≥+20° TL Kyphosis

* T5-12 sagittal alignment modifier: −, N, or +

−: <10°
N : 10-40°
+ : >40°

FIGURE 18-32. A, B: This comprehensive scoliosis classification scheme has been proposed by Lenke et al. to classify all forms of adolescent idiopathic scoliosis. Each curve is given a type 1 to 6, as well as a lumbar spine modifier A to C, and a thoracic sagittal profile modifier −, N, +. *(continued)*

A

		Curve Type		
Type	**Proximal Thoracic**	**Main Thoracic**	**Thoracolumbar / Lumbar**	**Curve Type**
1	Non-Structural	Structural (Major)	Non-Structural	Main Thoracic (MT)
2	Structural	Structural (Major)	Non-Structural	Double Thoracic (DT)
3	Non-Structural	Structural (Major)	Structural	Double Major (DM)
4	Structural	Structural (Major)	Structural	Triple Major (TM)
5	Non-Structural	Non-Structural	Structural (Major)	Thoracolumbar / Lumbar (TL/L)
6	Non-Structural	Structural	Structural (Major)	Thoracolumbar / Lumbar - MT (TL/L-MT) (Lumbar Curve > Thoracic by ≥ 10°)

STRUCTURAL CRITERIA

Proximal Thoracic: - Side Bending Cobb ≥ 25°
- T2 - T5 Kyphosis ≥ +20°

Main Thoracic: - Side Bending Cobb ≥ 25°
- T10 - L2 Kyphosis ≥ 25°

Thoracolumbar / Lumbar: - Side Bending Cobb ≥ 25°
- T10 - L2 Kyphosis ≥ +20°
- > I Nash-Moe (Apical S.B.)

LOCATION OF APEX
(SRS definition)

CURVE	APEX
THORACIC	T2 - T11-12 DISC
THORACOLUMBAR	T12 - L1
LUMBAR	L1-2 DISC - L4

Modifiers

Lumbar Spine Modifier	CSVL to Lumbar Apex			
A	CSVL Between Pedicles			
B	CSVL Touches Apical Body(ies)			
C	CSVL Completely Medial	A	B	C

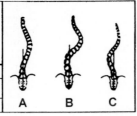

Thoracic Sagittal Profile T5 - T12		
-	(Hypo)	< 10°
N	(Normal)	10°- 40°
+	(Hyper)	> 40°

Curve Type (1-6) **+** Lumbar Spine Modifier (A, B, or C) **+** Thoracic Sagittal Modifier (-, N, or +)

Classification (e.g.1B+):_____

B

FIGURE 18-32. *(continued)*

yet long enough to minimize residual trunk imbalance or late curve progression. For typical correction of a thoracic curve the most distal hook is attached to the vertebra that is one level proximal to the stable vertebra (vertebra bisected by the central sacral vertical line). Multiple hooks or sublaminar wires on the concave side of the spine are used to draw up the apex of the curve from its lordoscoliotic position into a more normal kyphotic alignment. The concave (left-sided) rod is placed first; setting the hooks in distraction on the concavity provides both scoliosis correction and also aids in restoration of more normal kyphosis with posterior distraction. The convex (right-sided) rod is then added, and the two rods are connected with a cross-link (Fig. 18-33).

Thoracic curves can also be corrected by anterior instrumentation. This concept, more commonly used for thoracolumbar and lumbar curves in North America, has been regularly employed to also correct thoracic curves in multiple European centers for at least two decades. Advantages include greater correction, a shorter fusion, and ease of recreating normal kyphosis in the hypokyphotic thoracic spine. Most recently, several American centers have begun to correct thoracic cases with anterior instrumentation (241,248). The levels selected for fusion in anterior instrumentation to correct thoracic scoliosis include all vertebrae within the measured Cobb angle. The thoracotomy required for this approach, which results in at least a temporary decrease of pulmonary function, is a disadvantage of the method (Fig. 18-34). Also, in most systems only a single rod is used with the vertebral screw attached to the vertebral body, which is relatively more cancellous in nature compared to posterior fixation sites. This may increase the risk for screw–bone separation, especially at the cranial end of a thoracic curve, where the vertebral bodies are smaller.

Anterior thoracic corrective instrumentation is being developed for thoracoscopic implantation, and may be a future option for correction of thoracic scoliosis in patients with only moderately severe curves.

Right Thoracic, Left Lumbar Curve Pattern. The lumbar curve (usually convex to the left) that often presents in association with a right thoracic curve, may vary substantially in both magnitude (Cobb angle) and severity of rotation. Either the thoracic or lumbar curve may dominate such a double-curve pattern, although the thoracic curve is more often primary. In deciding on surgical treatment, one must determine which of the curves requires instrumentation and fusion (thoracic, lumbar, or both). When the thoracic curve is larger and/or more rigid than the lumbar curve (King II), selective fusion of the thoracic curve only should be considered (217,249) (Fig. 18-35). There are situations, however, in which the lumbar curve is large enough to require fusion if a well-balanced spine is to be achieved after correction.

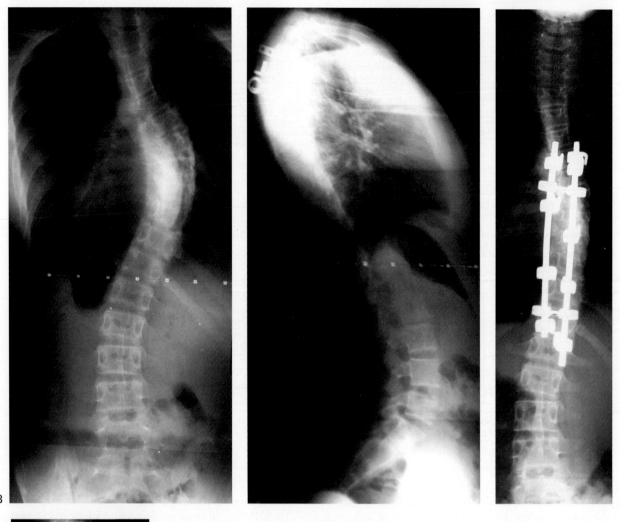

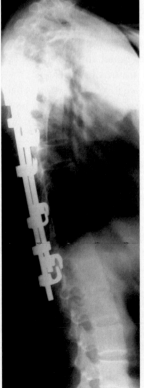

FIGURE 18-33. A, B: Preoperative radiographs (PA and lateral) of this 12-year-old female demonstrate a 45-degree right thoracic scoliosis. The stable vertebra (best bisected by a central vertical sacral line) is L2. The surgeon elected to perform a fusion extending distally only to T12 because of curve flexibility noted on bend films. **C, D:** PA and lateral views following posterior spinal instrumentation and fusion from T4 to T12. The trunk remains well balanced.

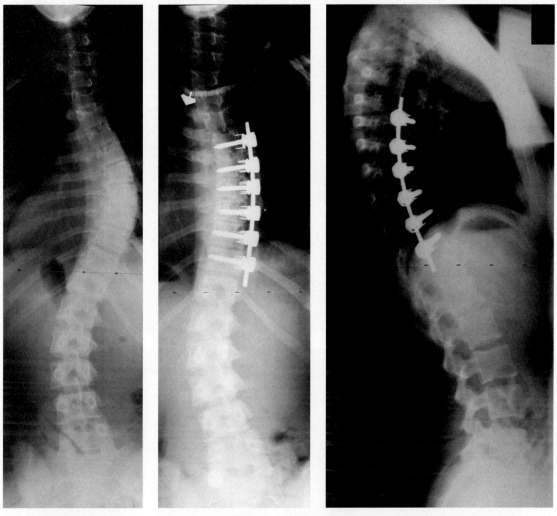

A   B, C

FIGURE 18-34. A: This 13-year-old female presented with a typical right thoracic curve. **B, C:** Postoperative PA and lateral radiographs demonstrate correction with limited anterior thoracic instrumentation and fusion from T6 to T11.

Several authors have provided criteria for selective fusion of the thoracic curve alone (249–251). Although universal agreement has not been reached, several factors should be understood. The instrumentation should not end inferiorly just above a "junctional kyphosis" (as noted on the lateral view). The junction between the thoracic and lumbar curves (approximately T12) may be focally kyphotic in the sagittal plane. A selective fusion of the thoracic spine in such a case will exaggerate the kyphosis at the thoracolumbar junction. When the lateral view demonstrates junctional kyphosis, the corrective instrumentation should extend distal to the kyphosis. If the lumbar curve is greater than 45 to 50 degrees, vigorous correction of only the thoracic curve with a posterior instrumentation system may result in postoperative truncal decompensation to the left (252,253). If selective fusion is elected in these cases, correction of the thoracic curve should be modest to minimize the chance of residual trunk imbalance (251).

When instrumentation of both the thoracic and the lumbar curves is required, the distal extent is usually to the L3 or L4 level (Fig. 18-36). Ideally, the distal extent of the fusion should be as proximal as possible to preserve lumbar motion segments, yet long enough to avoid creating trunk imbalance. Choosing between L3 and L4 can be difficult. The most predictable spinal balance occurs when the fusion/ instrumentation extends distally to the stable vertebra (the vertebra best bisected by the central sacral vertical line). In patients with limited remaining growth and a left-sided lumbar curve, fusion to L3 may be considered, if there is minimal axial rotation of L3 as noted on the bend film to the left, and L3 levels above the pelvis with side bending to the right. With posterior instrumentation, laminar hook, or pedicle screw, fixation can be used to attach to lumbar vertebrae. When required to achieve thoracic and lumbar curve balance, pedicle screws provide an option that allows greater control and correction of a lumbar curve. Again, the

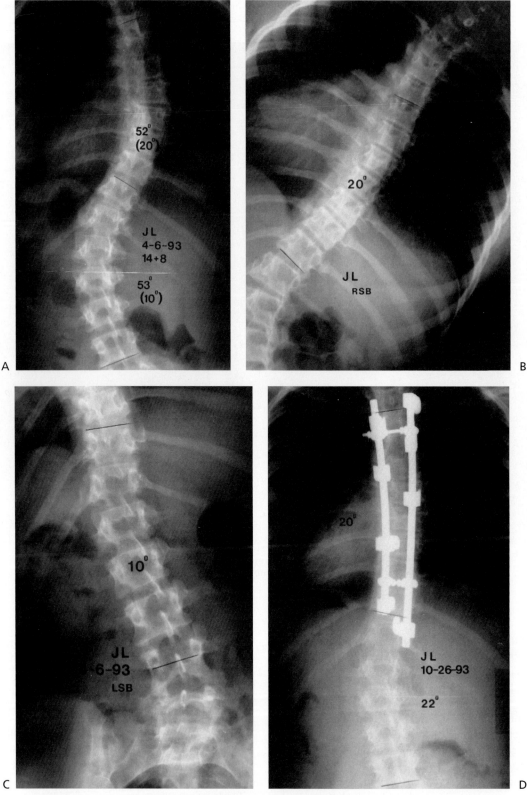

FIGURE 18-35. A: This 14-year-old female presented with idiopathic scoliosis and a right thoracic curve of 52 degrees and a left lumbar curve of 53 degrees. Clinically, she was balanced with level shoulders, and primarily a thoracic prominence on forward-bending. **B:** Supine-side bending to the right demonstrated correction of the right thoracic curve to 20 degrees. **C:** Supine side-bending to the left demonstrated lumbar curve correction to 10 degrees. Selective fusion of the thoracic curve alone is possible in this case, as long as there is not overcorrection of the right thoracic curve. The lower end vertebra of the curve (T11) is neutrally rotated and stable (bisected by the center sacral vertical line). **D:** Instrumentation and fusion were performed from T4 to T11. The thoracic curve was corrected to 20 degrees, and the lumbar curve spontaneously corrected to 22 degrees.

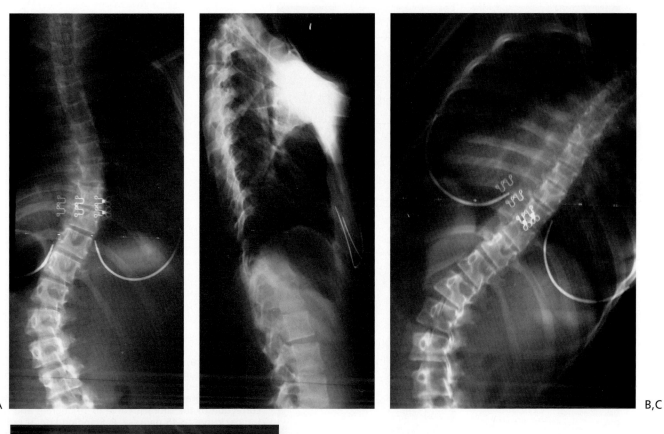

A   B,C

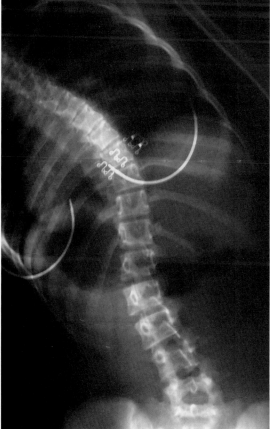

D

FIGURE 18-36. **A:** This 12-year-old female with a 43-degree right thoracic and 53-degree left lumbar curve pattern is seen. **B:** The lateral radiograph demonstrates relative loss of thoracic kyphosis. **C:** Side-bending radiograph to the right demonstrates L4 leveling above the pelvis with flexibility of the thoracic curve to 15 degrees. L3 remains with substantial rotational deformity on the side-bending radiograph as seen by the asymmetry of the pedicles. **D:** Side-bending to the left demonstrates flexibility of the lumbar curve. *(continued)*

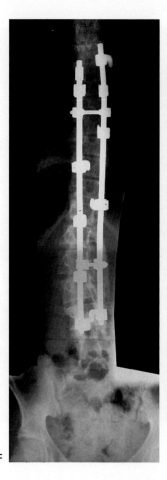
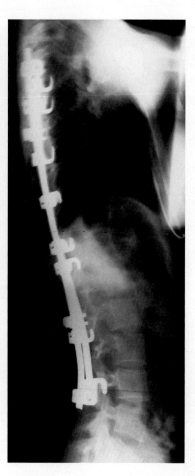

E,F

FIGURE 18-36. *(continued)* **E:** Given the magnitude of the lumbar curve relative to the thoracic curve, both curves required instrumentation and fusion. The standing PA radiograph 2 years postoperatively demonstrates correction of the thoracic curve to 10 degrees and the lumbar curve to 15 degrees. **F:** Standing lateral radiograph demonstrates maintenance of lumbar lordosis and slight improvement in the thoracic kyphosis.

surgical goal is to achieve improved spinal alignment with global truncal balance, with both C7 and the trunk well-centered over the pelvis in both the sagittal and coronal planes (Fig. 18-37).

Double Thoracic Curve Pattern. The double thoracic curve is recognized by the presence of an elevated left shoulder, whereas an isolated right thoracic curve is typically associated with an elevated right shoulder. If the left shoulder is higher, an upper thoracic curve to the left should be suspected. A left upper thoracic curve that is relatively rigid (reduces to >20 to 25 degrees on bend film) generally requires instrumentation beginning proximally at T1 or T2 (254). If the double pattern is not recognized, and the right thoracic curve alone is straightened, the left shoulder elevation is often worse following the surgery (255).

Left Lumbar or Thoracolumbar Curve Pattern. A primary lumbar or thoracolumbar curve pattern does not have a significant thoracic component and is usually convex to the left with a trunk shift to the left. In these cases, isolated fusion of a lumbar or thoracolumbar curve

is appropriate, and can be accomplished by either anterior or posterior methods. Correction with posterior hook constructs has not been as successful in achieving derotation of the lumbar curve, compared to anterior instrumentation. Limited anterior instrumentation of the apical 3 or 4 vertebrae has been proposed by Bernstein and Hall with satisfactory early outcomes in the majority of patients [➡2.11] (242). Longer anterior constructs (256) some with the use of bone graft or a structural cage in the disc space, have become popular in the treatment of these curves (Fig. 18-38). Pedicle screw fixation has allowed better control and correction of these curves when corrected with posterior instrumentation (Fig. 18-39). In severe cases, both anterior and posterior instrumentation may be indicated (Fig. 18-40).

Triple Curve Pattern. Not infrequently, a combined curve pattern includes curves in all three locations: left upper thoracic, right thoracic, left lumbar/thoracolumbar. Although it may not be necessary to surgically treat all three curves, each should be considered individually to determine if they are structural (relatively rigid), and treated accordingly

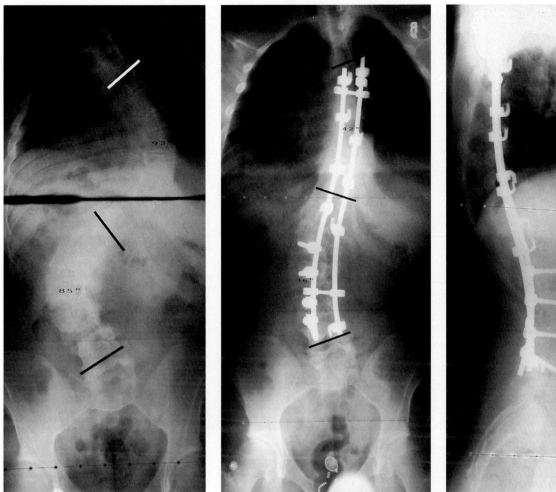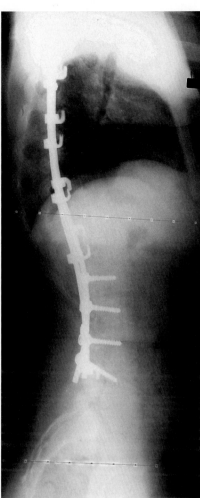

FIGURE 18-37. **A:** This 16-year-old male presented with severe double major scoliosis, with a right thoracic curve of 93 degrees and a left lumbar curve of 85 degrees. On side-bending radiographs to the right, the thoracic curve decreased to 68 degrees. On side-bending to the left the lumbar curve corrected to 52 degrees. **B:** The patient underwent a thoracoscopic anterior spinal release from T5 to T12, followed by a posterior spinal instrumentation and fusion of both curves. The lumbar curve was corrected to 36 degrees with pedicle screw fixation on the convex side of the curve. Coronal balance was maintained with correction of the thoracic curve to 42 degrees. **C:** The lateral radiograph demonstrates restoration of alignment in the sagittal plane.

(Fig. 18-41). In these triple curves the lower thoracic curve, if dominant, is certainly included in the arthrodesis. The inclusion criteria for the upper thoracic and lumbar curves are the same as those used for the corresponding double-curve patterns. For example, elevation of the left shoulder, in an upper thoracic curve with a curve that remains greater than 20 to 25 degrees on side-bending, should be considered for inclusion within the levels of fusion. Similarly, the lumbar curve should be instrumented when its Cobb angle magnitude is equal to or greater than the thoracic curve. The greater the difference in magnitude and rotation between the thoracic and lumbar curves (i.e., thoracic greater than lumbar), the more likely the lumbar curve can be spared from fusion (249,251).

Outcomes of Surgical Treatment

Given the relatively new methods used for surgical correction of adolescent idiopathic scoliosis (Harrington instrumentation in the 1960s, Cotrel-Dubousset instrumentation in the 1980s), very long-term outcome data are not yet available. Spinal instrumentation techniques continue to undergo modification and improvement almost faster than outcome studies can be performed. The Scoliosis Research Society has recently developed an outcomes instrument which will allow more careful functional outcomes analysis of patients treated with scoliosis (257).

Outcome after Posterior Surgery. The longest follow-up exists for patients treated with Harrington instrumentation

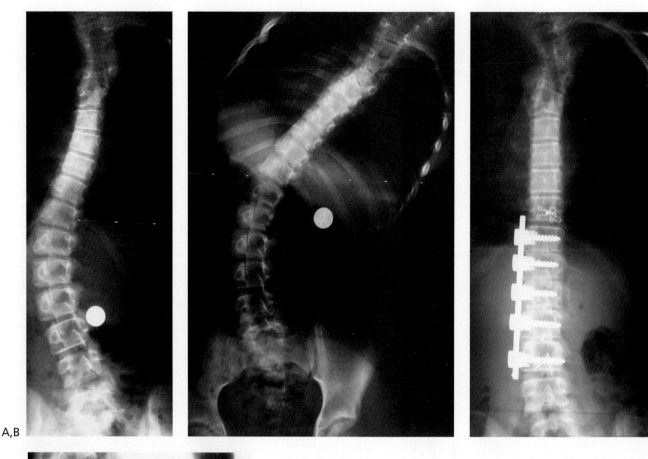

A,B

C

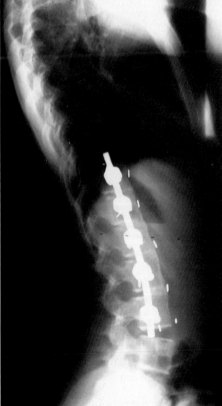

D

FIGURE 18-38. **A:** 12-year-old female who presented with a left lumbar scoliosis and trunk shift to the left. Of note, she also had a minor well-balanced congenital deformity of the upper thoracic spine. **B:** On side-bending to the right L3 leveled over the pelvis. Because this was the end vertebra of the curvature and it leveled on side-bending to the right, it was selected as the end-instrumented vertebra. **C:** The patient underwent anterior instrumentation and fusion with correction of the thoracolumbar curve. **D:** A lateral radiograph obtained 2 years postoperatively demonstrates solid arthrodesis and reasonable maintenance of lumbar lordosis.

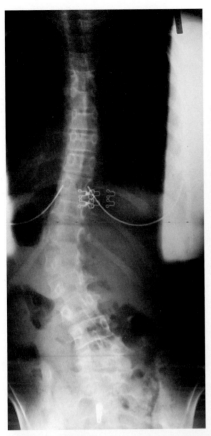
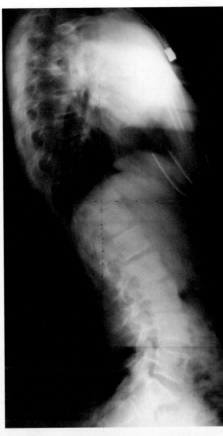

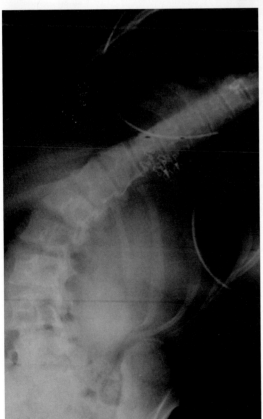
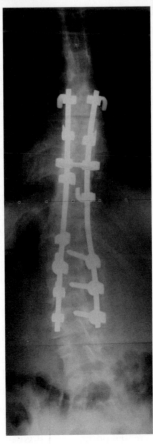
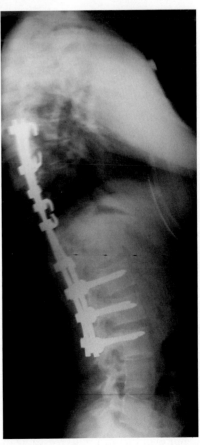

FIGURE 18-39. **A:** This 13-year-old female presented with a progressive left thoracolumbar scoliosis associated with trunk shift to the left. **B:** The lateral radiograph demonstrates maintenance of relatively normal sagittal alignment. **C:** Side-bending to the right demonstrates that L3 is level with the top of the pelvis. **D:** Posterior instrumentation and fusion were performed utilizing pedicle screw fixation through the apex of the lumbar spine at L1, L2, and L3 bilaterally. This provided correction of her lumbar deformity and improved her trunk shift, resulting in a balanced spine. **E:** Postoperative lateral radiograph demonstrates maintenance of lumbar lordosis in the instrumented segments.

A,B

C,D

E

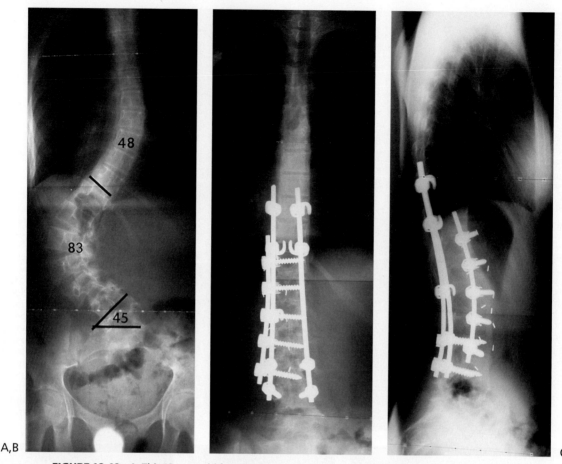

FIGURE 18-40. A: This 13-year-old female presented with previously untreated severe left lumbar scoliosis measuring 83 degrees. She had a flexible compensatory right thoracic deformity. **B:** Due to the severity of the lumbar curvature, an anterior disc excision with instrumentation was performed from T12 to L4. Following this procedure an additional posterior instrumentation was performed from T10 to L5, further correcting the inferior aspect of the lumbar spine with pedicle screw fixation. The patient has a sixth lumbar vertebra below the lowest instrumented level. **C:** Sagittal alignment has been restored and maintained with solid anterior and posterior arthrodesis seen 2 years postoperatively.

and fusion. An average coronal plane improvement of 48% of the Cobb angle has been reported (258). The long-term functional results of long posterior fusions have focused on the prevalence of late-onset low back pain. Conflicting results regarding the prevalence of pain and the correlation of pain with the caudal level of instrumentation have been reported. Moskowitz et al. (259) found no increase in pain or any correlation with the caudal level of arthrodesis. In contrast, Dickson et al. (168) found an increased incidence of back pain an average of 21 years after Harrington instrumentation compared with a control population. Cochran et al. (260) noted an increased frequency of pain in patients fused to L4 or L5 compared to those fused to L3 or above. Dickson et al. and Connolly et al. however, found no statistical correlation between the level of fusion and back pain (168,261).

Despite conflicting results regarding the increased poten-

tial for low back pain with more caudal levels of instrumentation and fusion, it seems intuitive that one should minimize the caudal extent of a fusion. Winter et al. demonstrated a significant loss of spinal motion when an arthrodesis included L4 compared to those only fused inferiorly to upper or midlumbar levels (262). Fusion to more caudal levels has also been associated with higher rates of radiographic degenerative changes in the unfused distal levels (spondylolisthesis, lateral olisthesis, disc narrowing, facet sclerosis) (261) (Fig. 18-42).

In addition to minimizing the caudal extent of the fusion, alignment in both the coronal and sagittal planes of the unfused segments should be optimized. It remains unclear whether the long-term functional results are better if the spine is fused to L4, with maintenance of lordosis and improved coronal position, compared to fusion to L3, with slightly greater residual deformity of the remaining caudal

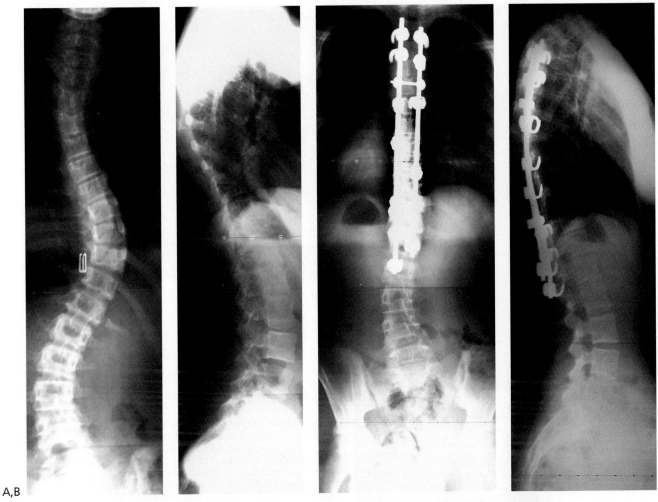

A,B   C,D

FIGURE 18-41. A: This premenarchal female had progressive scoliosis with a triple curve pattern. The left upper thoracic curve is seen with tilt of T1 and a 35-degree left upper thoracic deformity. The main right thoracic scoliosis measures 60 degrees and the left lumbar deformity 50 degrees. **B:** The lateral radiograph demonstrates hypokyphosis without a thoracolumbar junction kyphosis. The side-bending radiographs for this patient can be seen in Figure 18-12B and C. **C:** Given the clinical elevation of the left shoulder, it was elected to include the left upper thoracic curve in the instrumented segment to prevent further elevation of this shoulder. The main right thoracic deformity was larger than the left lumbar curve; therefore, the lumbar curve was not included in the instrumentation. Postoperative radiograph demonstrates spontaneous improvement of the lumbar curve with balance of C7 over the pelvis. The shoulders are now more level. **D:** The lateral radiograph demonstrates restoration of a more normal sagittal profile. Hook reversal at L1 on the left rod was used to initiate lumbar lordosis, as well as limit the risk of significant trunk decompensation.

levels. The relationship of alignment and degenerative changes to the development of low back pain requires additional follow-up and analysis.

The early (253,263) and midterm (212) (5 to 10-year follow-up) results of CD instrumentation suggest improved coronal and sagittal plane correction, compared to Harrington instrumentation (264). An average correction of 61% can be expected when considering all curve types (258). The segmental hook constructs have provided clear improvement in postoperative sagittal alignment (265), although little improvement in the axial rotation deformity

has been appreciated despite the early promise that systems such as the CD type would greatly derotate the spine by an intraoperative rotational maneuver as the instrumentation is applied (266–269). Postoperative immobilization has been minimal at most centers using the CD system, compared to Harrington instrumentation, yet the incidence of pseudarthrosis and loss of correction has been less with the newer system (212,264).

Early in the experience with CD instrumentation, truncal decompensation to the left was commonly noted in King type II curves when selective thoracic fusion was performed

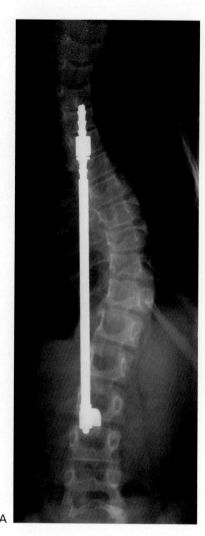

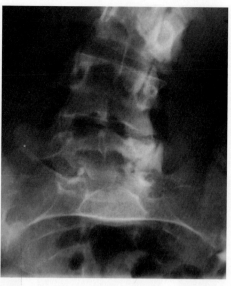

FIGURE 18-42. A: This 10-year-old female underwent posterior distraction instrumentation with a Harrington rod to L3. **B:** Eleven years postoperatively the degenerative changes in the remaining unfused lumbar spine has begun to be symptomatic. The facets have degenerated and become sclerotic, particularly at L5-S1 on the right side.

(250,253,270). Several techniques have been suggested to avoid this difficulty (249,252). The most important is to avoid over-correction of the thoracic spine beyond a degree that the unfused lumbar curve can adapt to. Also, hook reversal at the lower-most hook of the concave rod (most inferior hook upgoing) initiates coronal plane balance and lumbar lordosis, minimizing the risk for trunk decompensation (250,251,253) (Fig. 18-43).

Outcome after Anterior Surgery. Until recently, anterior correction of scoliosis has been primarily used for the correction of lumbar and thoracolumbar scoliosis. The percentage of frontal plane correction, with either Dwyer, Zielke, TSRH (Texas Scottish Rite Hospital) or Kaneda instrumentation, has been reported between 67 and 98% (234–238,242,271). Some authors have noticed a loss of sagittal plane lumbar lordosis with anterior compressive systems (272,273). Even solid ¼″ rod systems, such as the TSRH system have not been able to entirely preserve normal lordosis when used without anterior interbody structural

support (234). Sweet et al. have reported that sagittal alignment in the lumbar spine can be maintained if interbody structural support is added (238); however, even with this interbody support, if a pseudarthrosis develops eventual rod breakage and collapse into increased scoliosis and kyphosis will occur (Fig. 18-44). Two rod anterior systems also provide an option that may allow better maintenance of lumbar lordosis (240,256), although reported follow-up remains limited.

The results of anterior instrumentation in the thoracic spine are beginning to be reported with Betz et al. having made a nonrandomized comparison of anterior versus posterior thoracic instrumentation for thoracic idiopathic scoliosis. The anterior 3.2- or 4.0-mm threaded rods resulted in comparable coronal plane scoliosis correction, compared to posterior hook systems, but were associated with a 31% incidence of rod breakage. The distal level of fusion in the anterior fusion group was on average two segments proximal to the those in the posterior group (241). Lenke et al. have also reported a greater spontaneous improvement of the

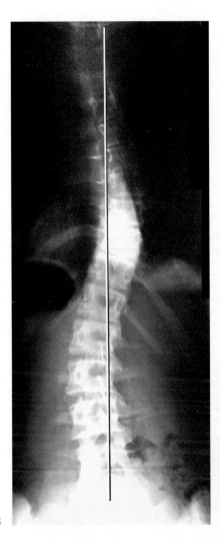 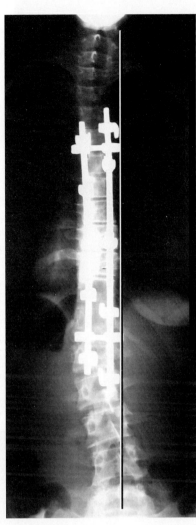

A,B

FIGURE 18-43. A: The preoperative PA radiograph demonstrates the stable vertebra to be at T12. **B:** The patient was instrumented posteriorly to L1 with a down-going hook at the distal end on the left side, resulting in decompensation to the left. This could have been prevented by either stopping the instrumentation at T12 or reversing the direction of the left-sided L1 hook to up-going.

uninstrumented portion of the lumbar spine when the thoracic instrumentation was anterior (and shorter), as compared to posterior in treating thoracic curves that had a compensatory lumbar curve pattern. At 2-year follow-up the thoracic curves were corrected 58% and the lumbar curves (uninstrumented) 56% in the anterior instrumentation group, compared to 38 and 37%, respectively, for the posterior instrumentation group (248). The rate of pseudarthrosis and rod breakage appears to be greatly reduced with the introduction of solid (nonthreaded) rods for thoracic curves, although proximal screw pull out can be more problematic as the rod stiffness is increased.

Complications

The complications of scoliosis surgery can be serious, although over the last 20 years these procedures have become much safer due to advances in anesthesia, blood loss management, instrumentation systems, and neurologic monitoring.

The remarkable corrective power of the new instrumentation methods, coupled with better surgical skills, spinal cord monitoring, and methods to minimize blood loss have changed how one advises patients regarding possible complications following scoliosis surgery. In the past, the surgeon focused on blood loss, hook dislodgment, infections, and paraplegia or other neurologic deficits. Although all potential complications must be mentioned in the current era, patients are more likely to experience problems such as postoperative trunk imbalance or a need for subsequent metal removal. Due to the size, complexity, and modularity of the implants, they are more likely to produce muscle irritation, bursitis, or even a late low-grade infection in the bursitic area (274–276).

Neurologic Injury

The risk for neurologic injury during idiopathic scoliosis surgery is not well documented in a large series, although data from the membership of the Scoliosis Research Society

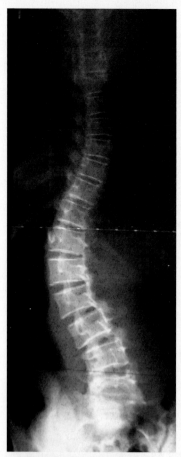
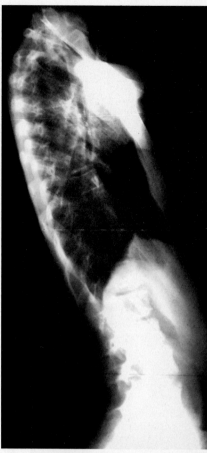

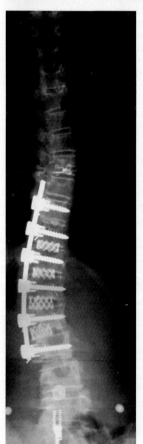
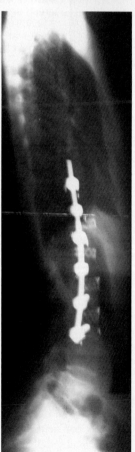
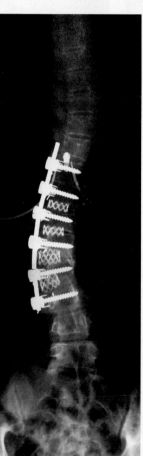
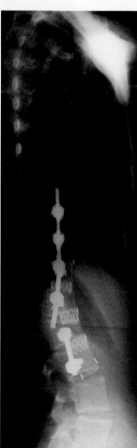

FIGURE 18-44. A: This 13-year-old female presented with a lumbar curve and trunk shift to the left. **B:** The preoperative lateral view demonstrates decreased lumbar lordosis. **C, D:** This was addressed with an anterior approach utilizing a single rod with interbody support to increase lumbar lordosis. **E, F:** She returned 1 year after the surgery asymptomatic but with loss of correction and fracture of the rod. This demonstrates that a single-rod anterior system may not always be strong enough to maintain correction while the bone graft is maturing, particularly in a very active patient.

A,B

C,D

E,F

is collected annually. In 1995 the reported incidence of neurologic injury after surgery was 1% in all types of scoliosis surgery in all ages. One of the 1,643 patients undergoing surgery for idiopathic scoliosis developed a complete spinal cord injury. The incidence of partial spinal cord and nerve root injury was 10 of 1,643 for the idiopathic scoliosis group, compared to 7 of 211 for the congenital scoliosis group. More than one-half of these patients had subsequent recovery of normal neurologic function. In a series of 1,090 patients undergoing spinal deformity correction by Bridwell et al., four patients developed a neurologic deficit postoperatively. However, only one of these patients had idiopathic scoliosis, and the total number of idiopathic scoliosis cases is not reported (277).

The etiology of spinal cord dysfunction can be classified as a result of direct trauma (contusion) to the cord, excessive traction to the neural elements produced by corrective instrumentation, and vascular insufficiency to the cord. The blood supply to the spinal cord is segmental and enters via the neural foramina. There has been some controversy as to the risk of vascular insufficiency to the cord associated with ligation of the anterior segmental blood vessels in anterior spine surgery. Winter et al. reported 1,197 cases in which segmental vessels were divided with no neurologic sequelae noted (278). There have, however, been other reports suggesting a possible vascular cause of spinal cord dysfunction postoperatively after segmental vessel ligation (279). Those at greatest risk appear to be patients with congenital malformations and hyperkyphosis (279–281). If an anterior procedure requires division of the segmental vessels, they should be ligated in the midvertebral body area rather than near the neural foramen. In high risk cases (congenital, kyphosis, revision surgery), temporary clamping of the vessels with concomitant spinal cord monitoring has been suggested by some as a means of detecting a potentially critical source of spinal cord blood supply (280).

Induced hypotension is a well-accepted standard in scoliosis to minimize operative blood loss; however, the mean arterial pressure must be maintained at a safe level to assure adequate blood flow to the spinal cord. In extremely complex corrections (kyphosis, osteotomies, revision surgery) in which the risk for cord ischemia is greater, the surgeon may elect to keep the blood pressure higher (even though blood loss will be greater) to assure cord perfusion (279).

Spinal Cord Monitoring

The wake-up test described by Stagnara was the first widely used method for monitoring spinal cord function after deformity correction. This technique includes decreasing the level of anesthesia intraoperatively to a level that allows the patient to follow commands. The patient is instructed to move their feet/toes, confirming the competency of the spinal cord motor tracts (282).

Subsequently, continuous electrical spinal cord monitoring has become almost standard in surgical correction of spine deformity. Monitoring of sensory and motor pathways is possible; however, from a technical standpoint sensory monitoring is simpler and more widely accepted. Somatosensory evoked potentials (SSEPs) are obtained by stimulating distally (legs) and measuring the response proximally (brain), and have been very reliable in detecting changes in spinal cord function, providing the surgeon relatively rapid feedback about any effect that deformity correction is having on neurologic function (283). The lag time between the insult to the spinal cord and the resulting monitoring changes may be 10 to 20 min. Other factors (besides injury to the cord that have been found to affect spinal cord monitoring) resulting in false-positive indications of injury include hypotension, hypothermia, and dislodgment of the monitoring leads, as well as other technical malfunctions in the system. If changes are noted these factors should be evaluated and corrected, and if the monitoring abnormalities persist, a wake-up test should be performed to confirm the findings. Loosening of the implants to remove any corrective forces, or complete removal of the implants, should be performed as soon as a deficit is confirmed. Institution of the methylprednisolone steroid spinal cord injury protocol (284) also seems warranted, although the efficacy in this specific group of spinal cord injury patients has not been carefully studied.

Blood Loss and Transfusion

Scoliosis surgery may be associated with blood loss requiring transfusion. This requires appropriate anticipation by the surgeon based on the type of deformity and the extent of the planned surgery. Preoperative autologous donation may be the most reliable way to avoid exposure to allogenic blood products, although this is not possible in all patients (too small, psychologic stress of donating too great, long distance to the blood bank, preoperative anemia, congenital heart disease, and/or expense). Alternatives to minimize allogenic blood exposure include intraoperative blood salvage, preoperative erythropoietin administration (285), intraoperative hemodilution (286), and (used with the precautions noted above) controlled hypotensive anesthesia (287).

Early Postoperative—In-hospital Complications

Complications in the early postoperative period include respiratory compromise, wound infection, and delayed neurologic injury. The incidence of respiratory complications in idiopathic scoliosis is approximately 1%, whereas wound infection occurs in approximately 2% of cases (childhood and adult surgery). The incidence for infection in childhood and adolescent surgery is probably lower (288). Delayed neurologic injury has been recognized with increasing frequency, and the importance of careful neurologic monitoring of lower-extremity function for the 48 h following cor-

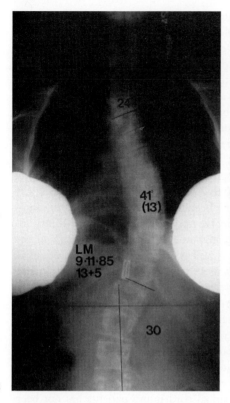
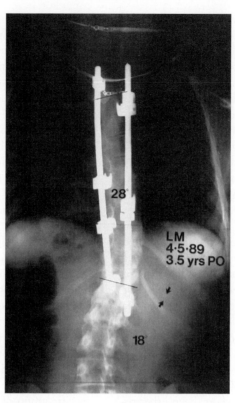

A,B

FIGURE 18-45. **A:** This 13-year-old female presented with a 41-degree right thoracic idiopathic scoliosis. The stable vertebra is probably L2. **B:** The patient was fused from T5 to T12. This radiograph 1 year postoperatively shows correction of the deformity to 13 degrees, but with acute angulation at T12-L1 and a 2-cm decompensation to the right. This case demonstrates the pitfalls of fusing too short.

rective surgery must be emphasized. Cases have been reported that confirmed intact neurologic function after the surgery with loss of motor and sensory function in the days following surgery (277,289,290). The etiology of delayed-onset paraplegia is unclear, and may be vascular due to postoperative hypotension, or mechanical resulting from a compressive hematoma.

Implant–Hardware Complications

Complications related to the hardware may present early or late in the postoperative period. Despite greatly improved implant systems, there is still a potential for early failure of the bone–hardware interface by either implant dislodgment or bony fracture. If a pseudarthrosis develops, late hardware failure can be anticipated. The time to hardware failure depends to some degree on the size and number of the rods used (Fig. 18-44). Small single-rod systems may fatigue and fracture in less than a year, compared to a double-rod system that may not fail for up to 5 years, if a pseudarthrosis is present. Rod fracture is diagnostic of pseudarthrosis; however, pseudarthrosis and rod failure may not be associated with any clinical problems. If pain or curve progression are noted revision surgery may be necessary.

Due to their prominence, the newer instrumentation systems have increased the need for late hardware removal, compared to the experience with Harrington rods. Another problem with new systems has been the development of

delayed infection and/or metal reaction (274–276). The cause of these problems likely relates to the bulk of the systems and their modularity. Loosening of any one component of the complex system can lead to formation of a bursa, which can then eventually become infected.

Late Alignment Problems

Postoperative spinal alignment may not match what was anticipated preoperatively. The problems and causes of trunk decompensation have been discussed above. The correction of spinal deformities should result in a harmonious transition from the instrumented to the noninstrumented regions of the spine. Abrupt changes in sagittal or coronal alignment may result in junctional problems (Fig. 18-45). Levels adjacent to a fused segment of spine are subjected to increased mechanical stresses, and this is likely increased if malalignment exists. The use of new multisegmental, powerfully corrective instrumentation has the potential for increasing the incidence of postsurgical trunk imbalance.

CONGENITAL SCOLIOSIS—DETAILS OF DIAGNOSIS AND TREATMENT

Definition

Congenital scoliosis is the result of abnormally formed vertebral elements with the altered vertebral shape producing deviations in spinal alignment. These deficiencies occur in the embryonic period of intrauterine development (before 48 days gestation), and are commonly associated with cardiac and urologic abnormalities that develop during the same period (126,127). The etiology is unknown in humans; however, in animal studies congenital scoliosis has been produced by transient exposure to toxic elements during the fetal period (291). Congenital deformities are classified broadly into failures of vertebral formation and failures of segmentation between the vertebrae. Congenital scoliosis, by definition, involves anomalous vertebral elements, and when these anomalies are identified, the curve should be classified as congenital, even if the scoliosis is not diagnosed until adolescence. Similarly, patients noted early in life to have scoliosis without abnormally formed vertebrae should not be diagnosed as having congenital scoliosis. Occasionally, in infants with significant curves with the vertebrae not yet fully ossified, differentiation between an idiopathic and a congenital curve can be difficult.

Classification

Congenital scoliosis classification (based on the developmental anomaly of the spine) includes deficiencies in vertebral formation, segmentation, or a combination of the two (mixed) (Fig. 18-46). Failures of formation and segmentation may occur on either the right or left side of the body resulting in "pure" scoliosis, or in the anterior and posterior elements resulting in "pure" kyphosis or lordosis, respectively. Combined deficiencies are common, and associated sagittal plane deformity is important to recognize (292) (Fig. 18-47).

In the classic failure of formation anomaly, hemivertebra (a triangular-shaped vertebra) forms on only one side, and can be subclassified into those that have disc and growth potential on: a) both the superior and inferior ends of the vertebra—*fully segmented*, b) either the superior or inferior end only—*semi-segmented*, or c) those that are fused to the vertebrae above and below—*nonsegmented* (Fig. 18-48).

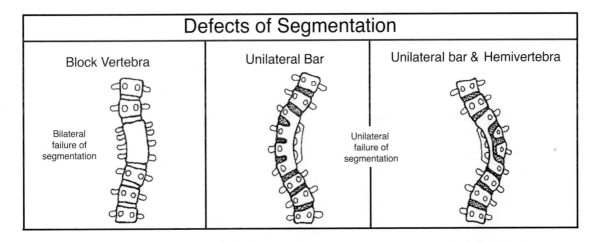

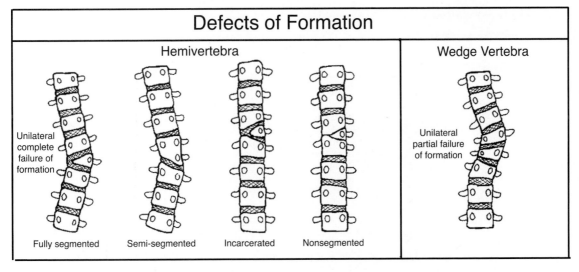

FIGURE 18-46. Diagrammatic representation of classification system of congenital scoliosis. (From ref. 294, with permission.)

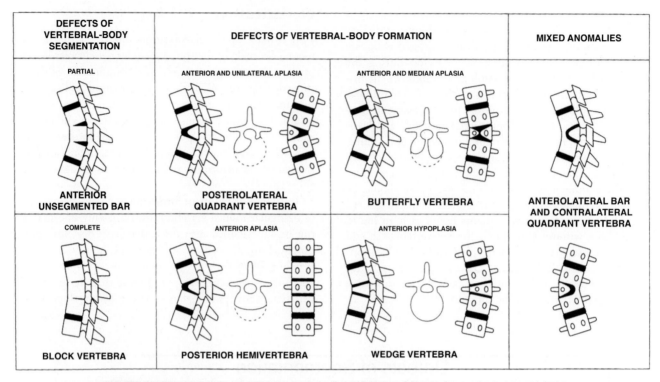

FIGURE 18-47. Diagrammatic representation of the failure of formation and segmentation in congenital kyphosis. (From ref. 292, with permission.)

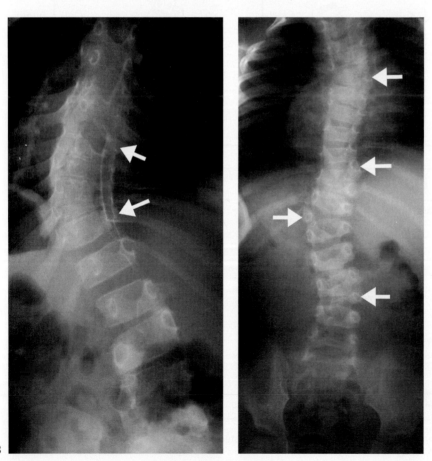

A,B

FIGURE 18-48. A: This radiograph demonstrates a long unilateral unsegmented bar (*arrows*). **B:** This radiograph demonstrates multiple hemivertebrae, both fully segmented and semi-segmented, as well as incarcerated and non-incarcerated varieties.

The degree of deficiency in unilateral formation is variable, and in the mildest form, a "wedge" vertebra develops. The vertebral width is normal, although the height of the vertebra is asymmetric on the right and left side. Rib deficiencies tend to match the vertebral deficiencies, and when the number of ribs on the right and left sides do not match, a hemivertebra or other congenital anomalies should be suspected.

Failure of normal segmentation of the vertebral column may occur on both sides of the spine symmetrically or unilaterally. Segmentation deficiencies result in inhibition of longitudinal growth, and result in little deformity if they occur circumferentially around the spine (block vertebra). A unilateral unsegmented bar, however, produces a growth tether that often results in marked scoliosis due to growth only on one side of the spine. Mixed deformities are common, and at times exact classification of congenital scoliosis is difficult.

Identifying a congenital malformation on the spinal radiographs requires careful assessment of the films. Asymmetry of the size or number of the pedicles may suggest a failure of formation, and an absent rib is often associated with a deficiency of the vertebral elements. An unsegmented bar is suggested when the corresponding ribs and/or pedicles are conjoined. Segmentation defects can also be presumed when the disc space is narrowed. A three-dimensional CT study often helps to clarify the diagnosis in an older child with a complex deformity (293) (see Fig. 18-16).

Natural History

The likelihood of any single case of congenital scoliosis developing progressive deformity is difficult to state with certainty. There are, however, known anomalies and curve locations that make some generalizations possible. McMaster and Ohtsuka reviewed 251 patients with congenital scoliosis, documenting curve progression during growth (292,294). Three-fourths of the patients' curves progressed substantially, and they were able to relate this to curve location and type. Those with a thoracic location progressed the greatest, and the curve types with the poorest prognosis were those with multiple hemivertebrae and a convex unilateral bar (failure of segmentation) opposite the hemivertebrae.

A summary of the median annual rate of curve progression is seen in Figure 18-49. Block and wedge vertebrae progressed <1 degree per year and generally did not require treatment. Hemivertebrae, however, increased between 1 degree and 2.5 degrees per year. Double hemivertebrae increased at roughly twice that rate. Unilateral unsegmented bars progressed at rates up to 6 to 9 degrees per year in the thoracolumbar junction, whereas the unilateral unsegmented bars with a contralateral hemivertebra were at the greatest risk of progression, at times exceeding 10 degrees per year (294) (Fig. 18-50).

Despite the information gained from the review of these patients, the growth potential of a curve may be difficult to classify and/or predict in any single case. Careful monitoring of radiographs is required to document and detect progression. The most likely times of increasing deformity match the phases of normally rapid spinal growth (the first 2 to 3 years of life and the adolescent years). Cobb angle measurement remains the method of following curves for progression, yet it is more difficult to apply in complex congenital curves (296), and the use of patient photographs can at times be helpful in addition.

Treatment

Nonoperative Treatment—Observation

The presence of a congenital spinal anomaly requires close monitoring of spinal growth until maturity. Initially, most

Site of curvature	Type of congenital anomaly					
	Block vertebra	Wedge vertebra	Hemivertebra		Unilateral unsegmented bar	Unilateral unsegmented bar and contralateral hemivertebrae
			Single	Double		
Upper thoaracic	<1°–1°	★–2°	1°–2	2°–2.5°	2°–4°	5°–6°
Lower thoracic	<1°–1°	2°–3°	2°–2.5°	2°–3°	5°–6.5°	6°–7°
Thoracolumbar	<1°–1°	1.5°–2°	2°–3.5°	5°–★	6°–9°	>10°–★
Lumbar	<1°–★	<1°–★	<1°–1°	★	>5°–★	★
Lumbosacral	★	★	<1°–1.5°	★	★	★

☐ No treatment required ■ May require spinal surgery ☐ Require spinal fusion ★ Too few or no curves

Ranges represent the degree of derotation before and after 10 years of age

FIGURE 18-49. The annual rates of curve progression for each of the congenital anomalies are shown. The shaded areas represent the likelihood of spinal fusion based on the predicted increase in deformity. (From ref. 294, with permission.)

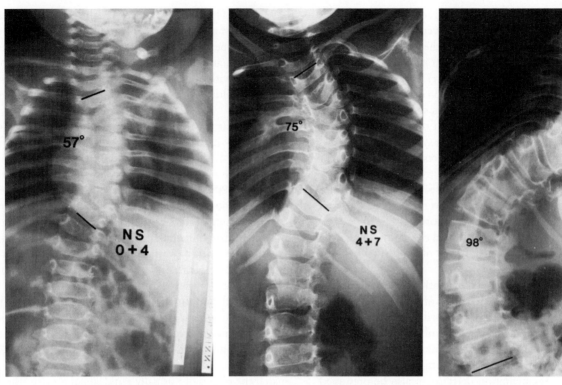

A,B   C

FIGURE 18-50. **A:** Four-month-old female presented with a 57-degree congenital right thoracic scoliosis. There is a hemivertebra on the right and a segmentation defect on the left (*unsegmented bar*). She did not receive treatment. **B:** At 4 years of age, the curve had progressed to 75 degrees. The congenital bar on the left is more easily seen, as well as the fusion between the ribs. **C:** By 12 years of age her curve progressed to 141 degrees with a 98-degree compensatory lumbar curve developing. (From ref. 295, with permission.)

curves are simply monitored, with radiographic assessment performed every 4 to 12 months, depending on the age of the patient and the suspicion (based on curve type) that progression is likely. Early in life, supine radiographs are the most reproducible; however, when old enough to cooperate (approximately age 2 years), upright radiographs should be taken. The landmarks used for Cobb angle determination are often difficult to mark, and Loder et al. found the interobserver error in Cobb angle measurement of congenital scoliosis curves to be as high as 10 degrees (296). Sequential analysis of trunk shift and Cobb measurement of the compensatory curves are also useful in determining if progression is occurring. Often, the compensatory curve which has no vertebral anomalies is easier to measure than is the congenital curve, and serves as an accurate "biomechanical indicator" about what is happening in the primary congenital curve.

In general, brace treatment has not been shown to be very effective in managing the primary curve in congenital scoliosis, because the curves tend to be short with little flexibility. Certain curves with a long flexible component may be amenable to orthotic management. On occasion, the compensatory curves which develop above or below a con-

genital deformity become problematic, and bracing to aid trunk balance may be helpful in these circumstances (297).

Surgical Treatment

Operative management is the standard treatment for progressive congenital scoliosis; however, because of the relative inflexibility of these curves, correction with instrumentation is less feasible than in idiopathic deformities. Because significant correction can usually not be obtained within the anomalous segments of the spine, surgical intervention is required earlier in the development of the curve (compared to surgery for idiopathic scoliosis). Surgical treatment options include: posterior fusion (*in situ* or with instrumentation), combined anterior and posterior fusion, convex hemiepiphysiodesis (anterior and/or posterior hemiarthrodesis), and hemivertebra excision. Each of these methods has its own indications, risks, and benefits, and the principles of each must be understood in order to optimize the outcome.

Preoperative Assessment. The most important aspect of preoperative documentation is sequential radiographs confirming progressive deformity. An exception is an unsegmented bar with a contralateral hemivertebra that has been suggested as an indication for surgery at the time of initial diagnosis (298). As discussed previously, the genitourinary system should be screened with an ultrasound examination, looking for a treatable cause of urinary tract outflow obstruction. Prior to undertaking surgical treatment of a congenital spinal deformity, an MRI of the entire spinal cord should be considered, especially if distraction instrumentation is planned. Associated intraspinal malformations, such as a diastematomyelia or a tethered cord, have been noted in cases of congenital scoliosis (298,299) (Fig. 18-51). A detethering procedure should be performed before a corrective spinal fusion procedure if neurologic symptoms are present. The treatment of asymptomatic patients with MRI findings only is more controversial. If there is a large compensatory curve (with normal motion segments) that will be straightened with instrumentation and included in the fusion, a prophylactic detethering procedure is indicated.

Goals of Surgery in Congenital Scoliosis. The goal for the variety of surgical procedures used in congenital scoliosis is to limit progression of a deformity that has been documented to be increasing with growth. Removing or modifying this growth potential in a young patient will limit curve progression, but may also affect ultimate spinal length. A recent study by Goldberg et al. has shown that children with congenital scoliosis are usually both small for their age and remain very small (compared to their peers) into adulthood, even if they do not require surgery. Discussion of surgical methods and their potential effect on final height must be tempered with the knowledge that final height may be limited by these poorly understood constitutional factors that are associated with congenital scoliosis (300). In addition, the surgeon and the parents must accept that growth of abnormally shaped vertebrae does not generate increased trunk height if deformity is allowed to progress. Trunk height will be greatest if a progressive curve is fused early, and the adjacent segments allowed to grow straight, rather than becoming part of a large compensatory curve.

Although the goal for most cases is limiting curve progression with the use of instrumentation or vertebral excision, one can surgically *reduce* the degree of deformity in some cases. These procedures carry somewhat greater risk for neurologic injury, the degree of which varies with the procedure, the curve pattern, flexibility, the location within the spine (cervical, thoracic, and lumbar), and the experience of the surgeon. It is for this reason that many patients with congenital scoliosis are treated with *in situ* fusion.

Posterior Fusion. Posterior *in situ* arthrodesis is the simplest approach to the surgical treatment of congenital scoliosis with the resultant large posterior fusion mass designed to limit progression of congenital curves (298,301,302). The fusion must include all of the vertebrae of the measured Cobb angle, and extend laterally to the transverse processes. Without instrumentation, a postoperative cast or vigorously worn rigid plastic jacket is required for 4 to 6 months after the procedure. The expected correction, by placement of a molded Risser cast, is generally modest in most congenital deformities; thus, the method is referred to as an *in situ* fusion. The neurologic risks associated with the technique are minimal.

The success of this procedure in preventing further deformity (increase in the Cobb angle or increase in the rotational deformity) depends on the nature of the malformation and the growth potential of the remaining unfused anterior vertebral bodies. Increased rotational deformity after a posterior spinal fusion (the "crankshaft phenomenon") (225), first described in idiopathic scoliosis, has also been documented to occur in skeletally immature patients with congenital (301,303) and neuromuscular scoliosis (227,303,304). Predicting which curves are likely to develop late crankshaft deformity is difficult, and relates to the curve pattern and anterior growth potential; however, understanding that congenital curves—fused posteriorly only— are at risk for it has led many surgeons to also perform anterior fusion in cases in which the risk for progression is perceived to be high.

Use of Posterior Instrumentation. The addition of instrumentation to a posterior arthrodesis can be considered in older children. Pediatric-sized instrumentation systems are available for children older than approximately age 3 years, which makes limited deformity correction possible in selected cases. Postoperative immobilization may be avoided in cases with secure internal fixation (juvenile and adolescent patients), whereas in the younger group, extended immobilization may be required to protect the instrumentation from dislodgment. The risk of neurologic injury increases with more aggressive attempts at instrumented deformity correction (302). The dimension of the spinal canal, as well as the blood supply to the spinal cord may also be congenitally deficient, both of which make the placement of hooks and distraction rods somewhat more dangerous than in typical idiopathic deformities. Careful spinal cord monitoring is required (see Idiopathic Scoliosis section).

Anterior Fusion. Anterior *in situ* arthrodesis may be required when substantial anterior vertebral growth is expected. Anterior growth potential in congenital deformities appears dependent both on the age of the patient (as in idiopathic scoliosis) and on the presence and orientation of anterior growth cartilage. The width of the disc space can be used to make inferences regarding growth potential. For example, a hemivertebra that is semisegmented (fused to one of the adjacent vertebra anteriorly) has less growth potential than one that is fully segmented with growth cartilage on both the superior and inferior end plates. Anterior fusion is usually combined with a posterior procedure (posterior

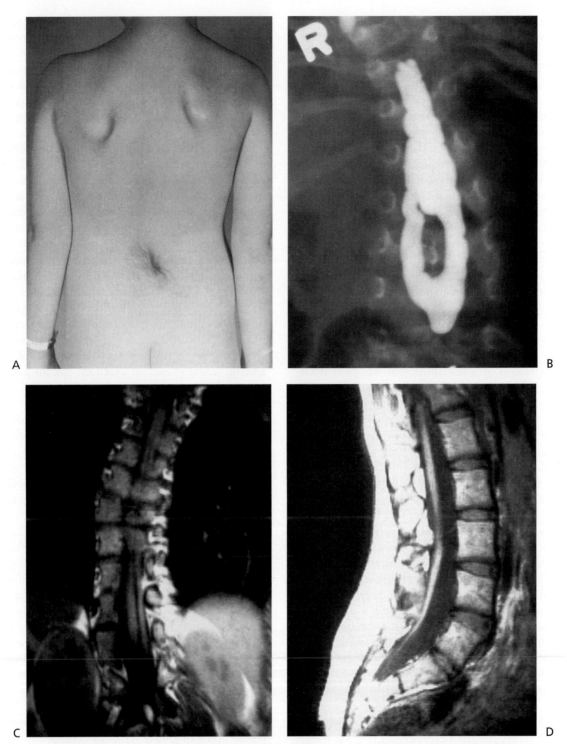

FIGURE 18-51. A: This patient presented with right thoracic scoliosis with a prominent right scapula and hair patch in the lumbar area. One foot was smaller than the other, and the ankle reflex was absent on that side. **B:** A myelogram demonstrates a diastematomyelia. **C:** Magnetic resonance imaging (MRI) scan also shows a diastematomyelia with a split in the spinal cord. **D:** On the sagittal MRI the cord extended to the sacral area with a tight filum terminale for each hemicord.

fusion with or without instrumentation), and is most commonly used for young patients with highly progressive deformities (e.g., hemivertebra and a contralateral bar). This gives the best chance for limiting growth in the circumstances known to be at greatest risk for rapid progressive deformity (305).

A fully segmented hemivertebra also may require an anterior fusion, because the additional growth centers of an anterior and laterally placed hemivertebra may generate substantial rotational deformity in the presence of a posterior fusion alone. The age at the time of surgery also plays a roll in this decision. Block vertebrae, semisegmented hemivertebrae, and wedge vertebrae are less likely to be progressive from the outset, and if they do progress, can often be treated with a posterior fusion alone.

Anterior procedures are designed primarily to limit growth of the vertebrae; however, some degree of flexibility may be obtained following discectomies in deformities which do not have a segmentation deficiency. The surgical exposure must allow for complete removal of the disc and end plate growth cartilage of the levels involved. The disc spaces are filled with autogenous rib or cancellous allograft bone to ensure an arthrodesis between the vertebrae. The risk of surgically related paralysis due to vascular insuffi-

ciency seems greatest in congenital scoliosis surgery (280) as compared to surgery on other curve types.

Partial Fusion, Growth Modulation, and Hemiepiphysiodesis. Methods for obtaining correction of a congenital deformity by modifying the growth of the involved levels have been proposed by many authors (306–310), with the principal of a Blount-type hemiepiphysiodesis (used to correct a long-bone deformity) applied to the spine. Convex hemiarthrodesis (hemiepiphysiodesis), a technique that includes performing a fusion only on the convex side of the curve, both anteriorly and posteriorly, has led to mixed results. Depending on the growth potential of the concave vertebral elements, the hemiarthrodesis may need to be extended one level above and below the measured curve. This technique has been most useful when utilized early in life (before age 5 years). Additionally, it should be employed when curves have proven to be progressive yet remain less than 50 degrees (Fig. 18-52). Beyond these levels, the results are less predictable. This procedure should not be used if a significant kyphotic component to the deformity exists, because the anterior fusion may lead to worsening of the kyphosis. It is similarly important to be certain that the anterior hemiarthrodesis component is extended posteriorly

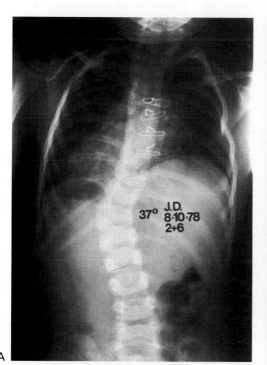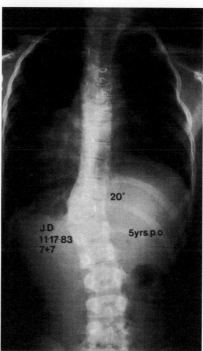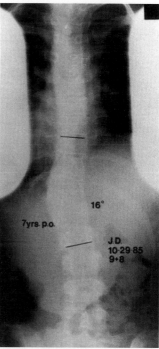

A   B,C

FIGURE 18-52. A: A 2-year, 6-month-old girl presented with progressive congenital thoracolumbar scoliosis caused by a hemivertebra. Treatment options included anterior and posterior fusion, epiphysiodesis, posterior fusion only, and hemivertebra excision. She underwent a convex anterior and posterior growth arrest (hemiepiphysiodesis). **B:** Five years after surgery the curve was 20 degrees. **C:** Seven years after surgery the curve was 16 degrees. Nine years after her surgery the curve was 10 degrees.

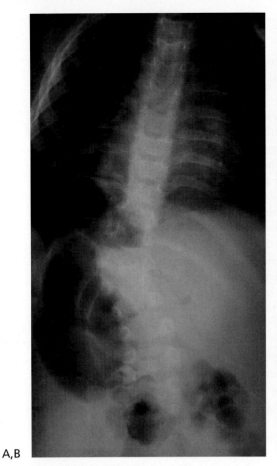
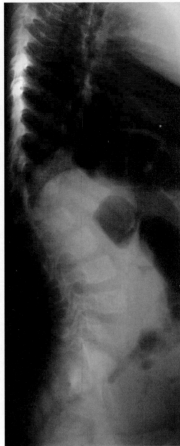

FIGURE 18-53. A: Preoperative radiograph in a 6-year-old male with progressive congenital scoliosis due to an apparent T12 hemivertebra. B: Lateral view demonstrates focal kyphosis centered at the T12 level. C: Anterior view on a three-dimensional CT study demonstrates that the hemivertebra may have a small "butterfly" component (small residual of body on the opposite side). The absence of body anteriorly is leading to severe kyphosis. D: Sagittal view on three-dimensional CT study. The cause of the kyphosis is clear. E: PA radiograph after vertebral body excision and corrective instrumentation. F: Lateral view after vertebral body excision and corrective instrumentation.

A,B

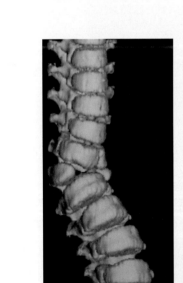
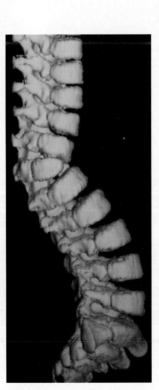
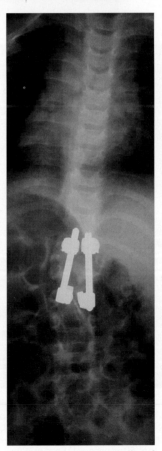
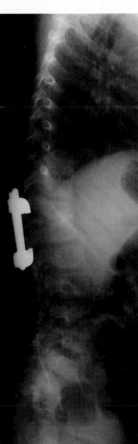

C,D

E,F

78. Stagnara P. *Spinal deformity*. Dove J., translator; Butterworth, 1988.

79. Gupta P, Lenke LG, Bridwell KH. Incidence of neural axis abnormalities in infantile and juvenile patients with spinal deformity. Is a magnetic resonance image screening necessary? *Spine* 1998;23:206.

80. Duval-Beaupere G, Lamireau T. Scoliosis at less than 30 degrees. Properties of the evolutivity (risk of progression). *Spine* 1985;10:421.

81. Soucacos PN, Zacharis K, Gelalis J, et al. Assessment of curve progression in idiopathic scoliosis. *Eur Spine J* 1998;7:270.

82. Ramirez N, Johnston CE, Browne RH. The prevalence of back pain in children who have idiopathic scoliosis. *J Bone Joint Surg Am* 1997;79:364.

83. Barnes PD, Brody JD, Jaramillo D, et al. Atypical idiopathic scoliosis: MR imaging evaluation. *Radiology* 1993;186:247.

84. Mehta MH. Pain provoked scoliosis. Observations on the evolution of the deformity. *Clin Orthop* 1978:58.

85. Fairbank JC, Pynsent PB, Van Poortvliet JA, et al. Influence of anthropometric factors and joint laxity in the incidence of adolescent back pain. *Spine* 1984;9:461.

86. Mierau D, Cassidy JD, Yong-Hing K. Low-back pain and straight leg raising in children and adolescents. *Spine* 1989;14:526.

87. Turner PG, Green JH, Galasko CS. Back pain in childhood. *Spine* 1989;14:812.

88. Lewonowski K, King JD, Nelson MD. Routine use of magnetic resonance imaging in idiopathic scoliosis patients less than eleven years of age. *Spine* 1992;17:S109.

89. Baker AS, Dove J. Progressive scoliosis as the first presenting sign of syringomyelia. Report of a case. *J Bone Joint Surg Br* 1983;65:472.

90. Citron N, Edgar MA, Sheehy J, et al. Intramedullary spinal cord tumours presenting as scoliosis. *J Bone Joint Surg Br* 1984;66:513.

91. Adams W. *Lectures on pathology and treatment of lateral and other forms of curvature of the spine*. London: Churchill Livingstone; 1865.

92. Bunnell WP. Outcome of spinal screening. *Spine* 1984;18:1572.

93. Grossman TW, Mazur JM, Cummings RJ. An evaluation of the Adams forward bend test and the scoliometer in a scoliosis school screening setting. *J Pediatr Orthop* 1995;15:535.

94. Huang S-C. Cut-off point of the scoliometer in school scoliosis screening. *Spine* 1997;22:1985.

95. Korovessis PG, Stamatakis MV. Prediction of scoliotic Cobb angle with the use of the scoliometer. *Spine* 1996;21:1661.

96. Yngve D. Abdominal reflexes. *J Pediatr Orthop* 1997;17:105.

97. Levy AR, Goldberg MS, Hanley JA, et al. Projecting the lifetime risk of cancer from exposure to diagnostic ionizing radiation for adolescent idiopathic scoliosis. *Health Phys* 1994;66:621.

98. Lescreve JP, Van Tiggelen RP, Lamoureux J. Reducing the radiation dosage in patients with a scoliosis. *Int Orthop* 1989;13:47.

99. Levy AR, Goldberg MS, Mayo NE, et al. Reducing the lifetime risk of cancer from spinal radiographs among people with adolescent idiopathic scoliosis. *Spine* 1996;21:1540.

100. Cheung KM, Luk KD. Prediction of correction of scoliosis with use of the fulcrum bending radiograph. *J Bone Joint Surg Am* 1997;79:1144.

101. Luk KD, Cheung KM, Lu DS, et al. Assessment of scoliosis correction in relation to flexibility using the fulcrum bending correction index. *Spine* 1998;23:2303.

102. Vaughan JJ, Winter RB, Lonstein JE. Comparison of the use of supine bending and traction radiographs in the selection of the fusion area in adolescent idiopathic scoliosis. *Spine* 1996;21:2469.

103. Takahashi S, Passuti N, Delecrin J. Interpretation and utility of traction radiography in scoliosis surgery. Analysis of patients treated with Cotrel-Dubousset instrumentation. *Spine* 1997;22:2542.

104. Stagnara P. Medical observation and tests for scoliosis. *Rev Lyon Med* 1968;17:391.

105. Papp T, Porter RW, Aspden RM. The growth of the lumbar vertebral canal. *Spine* 1994;15:2770.

106. Larsen JL. The lumbar spinal canal in children. Part II: the interpedicular distance and its relation to the sagittal diameter and transverse pedicular width. *Eur J Radiol* 1981;1:312.

107. Cobb J. Outline for the study of scoliosis. *Instr Course Lect* 1948;5:261.

108. Oda M, Rauh S, Gregory PB, et al. The significance of roentgenographic measurement in scoliosis. *J Pediatr Orthop* 1982;2:378.

109. Goldberg MS, Poitras B, Mayo NE, et al. Observer variation in assessing spinal curvature and skeletal development in adolescent idiopathic scoliosis. *Spine* 1988;13:1371.

110. Morrissy RT, Goldsmith GS, Hall EC, et al. Measurement of the Cobb angle on radiographs of patients who have scoliosis. Evaluation of intrinsic error. *J Bone Joint Surg Am* 1990;72:320.

111. Carman DL, Browne RH, Birch JG. Measurement of scoliosis and kyphosis radiographs. Intraobserver and interobserver variation. *J Bone Joint Surg Am* 1990;72:328.

112. Nash CL Jr, Moe JH. A study of vertebral rotation. *J Bone Joint Surg Am* 1969;51:223.

113. Perdriolle R. *La scoliose*. In: Maloine SA, ed; 1979.

114. Richards BS. Measurement error in assessment of vertebral rotation using the Perdriolle torsionmeter. *Spine* 1992;17:513.

115. Risser JC. The iliac apophysis: an invaluable sign in the management of scoliosis. *Clin Orthop* 1958;11:111.

116. Noordeen MH, Haddad FS, Edgar MA, et al. Spinal growth and a histologic evaluation of the Risser grade in idiopathic scoliosis. *Spine* 1999;24:535.

117. Sanders JO, Herring JA, Browne RH. Posterior arthrodesis and instrumentation in the immature (Risser-grade-0) spine in idiopathic scoliosis. *J Bone Joint Surg Am* 1995;77:39.

118. Sanders JO, Little DG, Richards BS. Prediction of the crankshaft phenomenon by peak height velocity. *Spine* 1997;22:1352.

119. Greulich W, Pyle S. *Radiographic atlas of skeletal development of the hand and wrist*. 2nd ed. Stanford CA: Stanford University Press; 1959.

120. Schwend RM, Hennrikus W, Hall JE, et al. Childhood scoliosis: clinical indications for magnetic resonance imaging. *J Bone Joint Surg Am* 1995;77:46.

121. Evans SC, Edgar MA, Hall-Craggs MA, et al. MRI of 'idiopathic' juvenile scoliosis. A prospective study. *J Bone Joint Surg Br* 1996;78:314.

122. Bradford DS, Heithoff KB, Cohen M. Intraspinal abnormalities and congenital spine deformities: a radiographic and MRI study. *J Pediatr Orthop* 1991;11:36.

123. McMaster MJ. Occult intraspinal anomalies and congenital scoliosis. *J Bone Joint Surg Am* 1984;66:588.

124. Mejia EA, Hennrikus WL, Schwend RM, et al. A prospective evaluation of idiopathic left thoracic scoliosis with magnetic resonance imaging. *J Pediatr Orthop* 1996;16:354.

125. Cheng JC, Guo X, Sher AH, et al. Correlation between curve severity, somatosensory evoked potentials, and magnetic resonance imaging in adolescent idiopathic scoliosis. *Spine* 1999;24:1679.

126. Drvaric DM, Ruderman RJ, Conrad RW, et al. Congenital

scoliosis and urinary tract abnormalities: are intravenous pyelograms necessary? *J Pediatr Orthop* 1987;7:441.

127. MacEwen GD, Winter RB, Hardy JH. Evaluation of kidney anomalies in congenital scoliosis. *J Bone Joint Surg Am* 1972;54:1451.

Idiopathic Scoliosis—Details of Diagnosis and Treatment

Prevalence and Natural History of Idiopathic Scoliosis

128. Kane WJ, Moe JH. A scoliosis-prevalence survey in Minnesota. *Clin Orthop* 1970;69:216.

129. Shands AR, Eisberg HB. The incidence of scoliosis in the State of Delaware. A study of 50,000 minifilms of the chest made during a survey for tuberculosis. *J Bone Joint Surg Am* 1955;37:1243.

130. Bruszewski J, Kamza A. Czestosc wystepowania Skolioz na Podstawie Anacizy Zdec maxoobrakowych. *Chir Narzadow Ruchu Ortop Pol* 1957;22:115.

131. Stirling AJ, Howel D, Millner PA, et al. Late-onset idiopathic scoliosis in children six to fourteen years old. A cross-sectional prevalence study. *J Bone Joint Surg Am* 1996;78:1330.

132. Dickson RA. Scoliosis in the community. *Br Med J* 1983;286:615.

133. Rogala EJ, Drummond DS, Gurr J. Scoliosis: incidence and natural history. A prospective epidemiological study. *J Bone Joint Surg Am* 1978;60:173.

134. Morais T, Bernier M, Turcotte F. Age and sex-specific prevalence of scoliosis and the value of school screening programs. *Am J Public Health* 1985;75:1377.

135. Montgomery F, Willner S. The natural history of idiopathic scoliosis. Incidence of treatment in 15 cohorts of children born between 1963 and 1977. *Spine* 1997;22:772.

136. Kane WJ. Scoliosis prevalence: a call for a statement of terms. *Clin Orthop* 1977:43.

137. Dickson RA, Weinstein SL. Bracing (and screening)—yes or no? *J Bone Joint Surg Br* 1999;81:193.

Infantile Idiopathic Scoliosis

138. James JIP, Lloyd-Roberts GC, Pilcher MF. Infantile structural scoliosis. *J Bone Joint Surg Br* 1959;41:719.

139. Scott JC, Morgan TH. The natural history and prognosis of infantile idiopathic scoliosis. *J Bone Joint Surg Br* 1955;37:400.

140. McMaster MJ. Infantile idiopathic scoliosis: can it be prevented? *J Bone Joint Surg Br* 1983;65:612.

141. James JIP. Idiopathic scoliosis: The prognosis, diagnosis, and operative indications related to curve patterns and the age of onset. *J Bone Joint Surg Br* 1954;36:36.

142. Lloyd-Roberts GC, Pilcher MF. Structural idiopathic scoliosis in infancy. *J Bone Joint Surg Br* 1965;47:520.

143. Hooper G. Congenital dislocation of the hip in infantile idiopathic scoliosis. *J Bone Joint Surg Br* 1980;62:447.

144. Mehta MH. The rib vertebral angle in the early diagnosis between resolving and progressive infantile scoliosis. *J Bone Joint Surg Br* 1972;54:230.

145. Ceballos T, Ferrer-Torrelles M, Castillo F, et al. Prognosis in infantile idiopathic scoliosis. *J Bone Joint Surg Am* 1980;62:863.

146. Robinson CM, McMaster MJ. Juvenile idiopathic scoliosis. Curve patterns and prognosis in one hundred and nine patients. *J Bone Joint Surg Am* 1996;78:1140.

147. Moe JH, Kettleson DN. Idiopathic scoliosis. Analysis of curve patterns and the preliminary results of Milwaukee-brace treatment in one hundred sixty-nine patients. *J Bone Joint Surg Am* 1970;52:1509.

148. Ponseti IV, Friedman B. Prognosis in idiopathic scoliosis. *J Bone Joint Surg Am* 1950;32:381.

149. Mannherz RE, Betz RR, Clancy M, et al. Juvenile idiopathic scoliosis followed to skeletal maturity. *Spine* 1988;13:1087.

150. Tolo VT, Gillespie R. The characteristics of juvenile idiopathic scoliosis and results of its treatment. *J Bone Joint Surg Br* 1978;60:181.

151. Bunnell WP. The natural history of idiopathic scoliosis. *Clin Orthop* 1988:20.

152. Anderson M, Hwang S-C, Green WT. Growth of the normal trunk in boys and girls during the second decade of life. Related to age, maturity, and ossification of the iliac epiphyses. *J Bone Joint Surg Am* 1965;47:1554.

153. Biondi J, Weiner DS, Bethem D, et al. Correlation of Risser sign and bone age determination in adolescent idiopathic scoliosis. *J Pediatr Orthop* 1985;5:697.

154. Peterson LE, Nachemson AL. Prediction of progression of the curve in girls who have adolescent idiopathic scoliosis of moderate severity. Logistic regression analysis based on data from The Brace Study of the Scoliosis Research Society. *J Bone Joint Surg Am* 1995;77:823.

155. Karol LA, Johnston CE 2nd, Browne RH, et al. Progression of the curve in boys who have idiopathic scoliosis. *J Bone Joint Surg Am* 1993;75:1804.

156. Nachemson A, Lonstein J, Weinstein S. Report of the Prevalence and Natural History Committee of the Scoliosis Research Society. Denver, CO: Annual Meeting of the Scoliosis Research Society, 1982.

157. Weinstein SL, Ponseti IV. Curve progression in idiopathic scoliosis. *J Bone Joint Surg Am* 1983;65:447.

Natural History in Adulthood

158. Weinstein SL. Idiopathic scoliosis. Natural history. *Spine* 1986;11:780.

159. Nachemson A. A long term follow-up study of non-treated scoliosis. *Acta Orthop Scand* 1968;39:466.

160. Nilsonne U, Lundgren KD. Long-term prognosis in idiopathic scoliosis. *Acta Orthop Scand* 1968;39:456.

161. Fowles JV, Sliman N, Nolan B, et al. The treatment of idiopathic scoliosis in Tunisia. A review of the first five years. *Acta Orthop Belg* 1978;44:416.

162. Weinstein SL, Zavala DC, Ponseti IV. Idiopathic scoliosis: long-term follow-up and prognosis in untreated patients. *J Bone Joint Surg Am* 1981;63:702.

163. Pehrsson K, Larsson S, Nachemson A, et al. A long term follow-up of patients with untreated scoliosis. A study of mortality, cause of death, and symptoms. Minneapolis, MN: Annual Meeting of the Scoliosis Research Society, 1991.

164. Pehrsson K, Bake B, Larsson S, et al. Lung function in adult idiopathic scoliosis: a 20 year follow up. *Thorax* 1991;46:474.

165. Upadhyay SS, Mullaji AB, Luk KD, et al. Relation of spinal and thoracic cage deformities and their flexibilities with altered pulmonary functions in adolescent idiopathic scoliosis. *Spine* 1995;20:2415.

166. Winter RB, Lovell WW, Moe JH. Excessive thoracic lordosis and loss of pulmonary function in patients with idiopathic scoliosis. *J Bone Joint Surg Am* 1975;57:972.

167. Mayo NE, Goldberg MS, Poitras B, et al. The Ste-Justine Adolescent Idiopathic Scoliosis Cohort Study. Part III: Back pain. *Spine* 1994;19:1573.

168. Dickson JH, Erwin WD, Rossi D. Harrington instrumentation and arthrodesis for idiopathic scoliosis. A twenty-one-year follow-up. *J Bone Joint Surg Am* 1990;72:678.

169. Collis DK, Ponseti IV. Long-term follow-up of patients with

idiopathic scoliosis not treated surgically. *J Bone Joint Surg Am* 1969;51:425.

170. Payne WK 3rd, Ogilvie JW, Resnick MD, et al. Does scoliosis have a psychological impact and does gender make a difference? *Spine* 1997;22:1380.

School Screening for Scoliosis

171. Soucacos PN, Soucacos PK, Zacharis KC, et al. School-screening for scoliosis. A prospective epidemiological study in north-western and central Greece. *J Bone Joint Surg Am* 1997;79:1498.

172. Pruijs JE, van der Meer R, Hageman MA, et al. The benefits of school screening for scoliosis in the central part of The Netherlands. *Eur Spine J* 1996;5:374.

173. Lonstein JE, Bjorklund S, Wanninger MH, et al. Voluntary school screening for scoliosis in Minnesota. *J Bone Joint Surg Am* 1982;64:481.

174. U.S. Preventive Services Task Force. Screening for adolescent idiopathic scoliosis. Policy statement. *JAMA* 1993;269:2664.

175. U.S. Preventive Services Task Force. Screening for adolescent idiopathic scoliosis. Review article. *JAMA* 1993;269:2667.

176. Goldberg CJ, Dowling FE, Fogarty EE, et al. School scoliosis screening and the United States Preventive Services Task Force. An examination of long-term results. *Spine* 1995;20:1368.

177. Morrissy RT. School screening for scoliosis. A statement of the problem. *Spine* 1988;13:1195.

178. Scoliosis Research Society. *Scoliosis: A handbook for patients.* Park Ridge, IL, 1986.

179. Bunnell WP. Outcome of spinal screening. *Spine* 1993;18: 1572.

180. Pruijs JE, Keessen W, van der Meer R, et al. School screening for scoliosis: the value of quantitative measurement. *Eur Spine J* 1995;4:226.

181. Murrell GA, Coonrad RW, Moorman CT, et al. An assessment of the reliability of the Scoliometer. *Spine* 1993;18:709.

182. Cote P, Kreitz BG, Cassidy JD, et al. A study of the diagnostic accuracy and reliability of the Scoliometer and Adam's forward bend test. *Spine* 1998;23:796; 803 (discussion).

183. Duval-Beaupere G. Threshold values for supine and standing Cobb angles and rib hump measurements: prognostic factors for scoliosis. *Eur Spine J* 1996;5:79.

184. Burwell RG, Dangerfield PH. Arthropometry. In: Findlay MD, Owens HJ, eds. *Surgery of the spine.* Oxford: Blackwell, 1992: 191.

185. Winter RB. The pendulum has swung too far. Bracing for adolescent idiopathic scoliosis in the 1990s. *Orthop Clin North Am* 1994;25:195.

186. Winter RB. Adolescent idiopathic scoliosis [editorial]. *N Engl J Med* 1986;314:1379.

Treatment of Idiopathic Scoliosis

187. Nachemson AL, Peterson LE. Effectiveness of treatment with a brace in girls who have adolescent idiopathic scoliosis. A prospective, controlled study based on data from the Brace Study of the Scoliosis Research Society. *J Bone Joint Surg Am* 1995; 77:815.

188. Katz DE, Richards BS, Browne RH, et al. A comparison between the Boston brace and the Charleston bending brace in adolescent idiopathic scoliosis. *Spine* 1997;22:1302.

189. Nash CL Jr. Current concepts review: scoliosis bracing. *J Bone Joint Surg Am* 1980;62:848.

190. Willers U, Normelli H, Aaro S, et al. Long-term results of Boston brace treatment on vertebral rotation in idiopathic scoliosis. *Spine* 1993;18:432.

191. Carr WA, Moe JH, Winter RB, et al. Treatment of idiopathic scoliosis in the Milwaukee brace. *J Bone Joint Surg Am* 1980; 62:599.

192. Mellencamp DD, Blount WP, Anderson AJ. Milwaukee brace treatment of idiopathic scoliosis: late results. *Clin Orthop* 1977: 47.

193. Blount W, Schmidt A. The Milwaukee brace in the treatment of scoliosis. *J Bone Joint Surg Am* 1957;37:693.

194. Lonstein JE, Winter RB. The Milwaukee brace for the treatment of adolescent idiopathic scoliosis. A review of one thousand and twenty patients. *J Bone Joint Surg Am* 1994;76:1207.

195. Emans JB, Kaelin A, Bancel P, et al. The Boston bracing system for idiopathic scoliosis. Follow-up results in 295 patients. *Spine* 1986;11:792.

196. Watts HG, Hall JE, Stanish W. The Boston brace system for the treatment of low thoracic and lumbar scoliosis by the use of a girdle without superstructure. *Clin Orthop* 1977:87.

197. Allington NJ, Bowen JR. Adolescent idiopathic scoliosis: treatment with the Wilmington brace. A comparison of full-time and part-time use. *J Bone Joint Surg Am* 1996;78:1056.

198. Piazza MR, Bassett GS. Curve progression after treatment with the Wilmington brace for idiopathic scoliosis. *J Pediatr Orthop* 1990;10:39.

199. Apter A, Morein G, Munitz H, et al. The psychosocial sequelae of the Milwaukee brace in adolescent girls. *Clin Orthop* 1978: 156.

200. MacLean WE Jr., Green NE, Pierre CB, et al. Stress and coping with scoliosis: psychological effects on adolescents and their families. *J Pediatr Orthop* 1989;9:257.

201. Ramirez N, Johnston CE 2nd, Browne RH, et al. Back pain during orthotic treatment of idiopathic scoliosis. *J Pediatr Orthop* 1999;19:198.

202. Price CT, Scott DS, Reed FR Jr, et al. Nighttime bracing for adolescent idiopathic scoliosis with the Charleston Bending Brace: long-term follow-up. *J Pediatr Orthop* 1997;17:703.

203. Green NE. Part-time bracing of adolescent idiopathic scoliosis. *J Bone Joint Surg Am* 1986;68:738.

204. Rowe DE, Bernstein SM, Riddick MF, et al. A meta-analysis of the efficacy of non-operative treatments for idiopathic scoliosis [see comments]. *J Bone Joint Surg Am* 1997;79:664.

205. Price CT, Scott DS, Reed FE Jr, et al. Nighttime bracing for adolescent idiopathic scoliosis with the Charleston bending brace. Preliminary report. *Spine* 1990;15:1294.

206. Fernandez-Feliberti R, Flynn J, Ramirez N, et al. Effectiveness of TLSO bracing in the conservative treatment of idiopathic scoliosis. *J Pediatr Orthop* 1995;15:176.

207. Noonan KJ, Weinstein SL, Jacobson WC, et al. Use of the Milwaukee brace for progressive idiopathic scoliosis. *J Bone Joint Surg Am* 1996;78:557.

208. Howard A, Wright JG, Hedden D. A comparative study of TLSO, Charleston, and Milwaukee braces for idiopathic scoliosis. *Spine* 1998;23:2404.

209. Climent JM, Sanchez J. Impact of the type of brace on the quality of life of adolescents with spine deformities. *Spine* 1999; 24:1903.

210. Wickers FC, Bunch WH, Barnett PM. Psychological factors in failure to wear the Milwaukee brace for treatment of idiopathic scoliosis. *Clin Orthop* 1977:62.

211. Edgar MA, Mehta MH. Long-term follow-up of fused and unfused idiopathic scoliosis. *J Bone Joint Surg Br* 1988;70:712.

212. Lenke LG, Bridwell KH, Blanke K, et al. Radiographic results of arthrodesis with Cotrel-Dubousset instrumentation for the treatment of adolescent idiopathic scoliosis. A five- to ten-year follow-up study. *J Bone Joint Surg Am* 1998;80:807.

213. Dickson JH, Mirkovic S, Noble PC, et al. Results of operative treatment of idiopathic scoliosis in adults. *J Bone Joint Surg Am* 1995;77:513.

214. Harrington PR. Treatment of scoliosis: correction and internal fixation by spine instrumentation. *J Bone Joint Surg Am* 1962; 44:591.

215. Hibbs RA. A report of fifty-nine cases of scoliosis treated by the fusion operation. By Russell A. Hibbs, 1924. *Clin Orthop* 1988:4.

216. Winter RB. Harrington instrumentation into the lumbar spine: technique for preservation of normal lumbar lordosis. *Spine* 1986;11:633.

217. King HA, Moe JH, Bradford DS, Winter RB. The selection of fusion levels in thoracic idiopathic scoliosis. *J Bone Joint Surg Am* 1983;65:1302.

218. Cotrel Y, Dubousset J, Guillaumat M. New universal instrumentation in spinal surgery. *Clin Orthop* 1988;227:10.

219. Barr SJ, Schuette AM, Emans JB. Lumbar pedicle screws versus hooks. Results in double major curves in adolescent idiopathic scoliosis. *Spine* 1997;22:1369.

220. Hamill CL, Lenke LG, Bridwell KH, et al. The use of pedicle screw fixation to improve correction in the lumbar spine of patients with idiopathic scoliosis. Is it warranted? *Spine* 1996; 21:1241.

221. Boos N, Webb JK. Pedicle screw fixation in spinal disorders: a European view. *Eur Spine J* 1997;6:2.

222. Suk SI, Lee CK, Min HJ, et al. Comparison of Cotrel–Dubousset pedicle screws and hooks in the treatment of idiopathic scoliosis. *Int Orthop* 1994;18:341.

223. Suk SI, Kim WJ, Kim JH, et al. Restoration of thoracic kyphosis in the hypokyphotic spine: a comparison between multiple-hook and segmental pedicle screw fixation in adolescent idiopathic scoliosis. *J Spinal Disord* 1999;12:489.

224. Andrew T, Piggott H. Growth arrest for progressive scoliosis. Combined anterior and posterior fusion of the convexity. *J Bone Joint Surg Br* 1985;67:193.

225. Dubousset J, Herring JA, Shufflebarger H. The crankshaft phenomenon. *J Pediatr Orthop* 1989;9:541.

226. Roaf R. Vertebral growth and its mechanical control. *J Bone Joint Surg Br* 1960;42:40.

227. Roberto RF, Lonstein JE, Winter RB, et al. Curve progression in Risser stage 0 or 1 patients after posterior spinal fusion for idiopathic scoliosis. *J Pediatr Orthop* 1997;17:718.

228. Lapinksy AS, Richards BS. Preventing the crankshaft phenomenon by combining anterior fusion with posterior instrumentation. Does it work? *Spine* 1995;20:1392.

229. Regan JJ, Mack MJ, Picetti GD 3rd. A technical report on video–assisted thoracoscopy in thoracic spinal surgery. Preliminary description. *Spine* 1995;20:831.

230. Newton PO, Wenger DR, Mubarak SJ, Meyer RS. Anterior release and fusion in pediatric spinal deformity. A comparison of early outcome and cost of thoracoscopic and open thoracotomy approaches. *Spine* 1997;22:1398.

231. Crawford AH, Wall EJ, Wolf R. Video-assisted thoracoscopy. *Orthop Clin North Am* 1999;30:367, viii.

232. Dwyer AF. Experience of anterior correction of scoliosis. *Clin Orthop* 1973;93:191.

233. Zielke K, Berthet A. [VDS—ventral derotation spondylodesis—preliminary report on 58 cases]. *Beitr Orthop Traumatol* 1978;25:85.

234. Turi M, Johnston CEd, Richards BS. Anterior correction of idiopathic scoliosis using TSRH instrumentation. *Spine* 1993; 18:417.

235. Suk SI, Lee CK, Chung SS. Comparison of Zielke ventral derotation system and Cotrel-Dubousset instrumentation in the treatment of idiopathic lumbar and thoracolumbar scoliosis. *Spine* 1994;19:419.

236. Kaneda K, Fujiya N, Satoh S. Results with Zielke instrumentation for idiopathic thoracolumbar and lumbar scoliosis. *Clin Orthop* 1986:195.

237. Luk KD, Leong JC, Reyes L, et al. The comparative results of treatment in idiopathic thoracolumbar and lumbar scoliosis using the Harrington, Dwyer, and Zielke instrumentations. *Spine* 1989;14:275.

238. Sweet FA, Lenke LG, Bridwell KH, et al. Maintaining lumbar lordosis with anterior single solid-rod instrumentation in thoracolumbar and lumbar adolescent idiopathic scoliosis. *Spine* 1999;24:1655.

239. Kaneda K, Shono Y, Satoh S, et al. Anterior correction of thoracic scoliosis with Kaneda anterior spinal system. A preliminary report. *Spine* 1997;22:1358.

240. Hopf CG, Eysel P, Dubousset J. Operative treatment of scoliosis with Cotrel-Dubousset-Hopf instrumentation. New anterior spinal device. *Spine* 1997;22:618; 627 (discussion).

241. Betz RR, Harms J, Clements DH 3rd, et al. Comparison of anterior and posterior instrumentation for correction of adolescent thoracic idiopathic scoliosis. *Spine* 1999;24:225.

242. Bernstein RM, Hall JE. Solid rod short segment anterior fusion in thoracolumbar scoliosis. *J Pediatr Orthop B* 1998;7:124.

243. Moe JH, Kharrat K, Winter RB, et al. Harrington instrumentation without fusion plus external orthotic support for the treatment of difficult curvature problems in young children. *Clin Orthop* 1984:35.

244. Fisk JR, Peterson HA, Laughlin R, et al. Spontaneous fusion in scoliosis after instrumentation without arthrodesis. *J Pediatr Orthop* 1995;15:182.

245. Marks DS, Iqbal MJ, Thompson AG, et al. Convex spinal epiphysiodesis in the management of progressive infantile idiopathic scoliosis. *Spine* 1996;21:1884.

246. Coonrad RW, Murrell GA, Motley G, et al. A logical coronal pattern classification of 2,000 consecutive idiopathic scoliosis cases based on the scoliosis research society–defined apical vertebra. *Spine* 1998;23:1380.

247. Lenke LG, Betz RR, Harms J, et al. A new comprehensive classification system of adolescent idiopathic scoliosis. Presented at: 32nd Annual Meeting of the SRS, 1997.

248. Lenke LG, Betz RR, Bridwell KH, et al. Spontaneous lumbar curve coronal correction after selective anterior or posterior thoracic fusion in adolescent idiopathic scoliosis. *Spine* 1999;24: 1663; 1672 (discussion).

249. Lenke LG, Bridwell KH, Baldus C, et al. Preventing decompensation in King type II curves treated with Cotrel–Dubousset instrumentation. Strict guidelines for selective thoracic fusion. *Spine* 1992;17:S274.

250. Thompson JP, Transfeldt EE, Bradford DS, et al. Decompensation after Cotrel-Dubousset instrumentation of idiopathic scoliosis. *Spine* 1990;15:927.

251. Bridwell KH, McAllister JW, Betz RR, et al. Coronal decompensation produced by Cotrel-Dubousset "derotation" maneuver for idiopathic right thoracic scoliosis. *Spine* 1991;16:769.

252. Richards BS. Lumbar curve response in type II idiopathic scoliosis after posterior instrumentation of the thoracic curve. *Spine* 1992;17:S282.

253. Richards BS, Birch JG, Herring JA, et al. Frontal plane and sagittal plane balance following Cotrel-Dubousset instrumentation for idiopathic scoliosis. *Spine* 1989;14:733.

254. Lenke LG, Bridwell KH, O'Brien MF, et al. Recognition and treatment of the proximal thoracic curve in adolescent idiopathic scoliosis treated with Cotrel-Dubousset instrumentation. *Spine* 1994;19:1589.

255. Winter RB. The idiopathic double thoracic curve pattern. Its recognition and surgical management. *Spine* 1989;14:1287.

256. Kaneda K, Shono Y, Satoh S, et al. New anterior instrumentation for the management of thoracolumbar and lumbar scoliosis.

Application of the Kaneda two-rod system. *Spine* 1996;21:1250; 1261 (discussion).

Outcomes of Surgical Treatment

257. Haher TR, Merola A, Zipnick RI, et al. Meta-analysis of surgical outcome in adolescent idiopathic scoliosis. A 35-year English literature review of 11,000 patients. *Spine* 1995;20:1575.

258. Stasikelis PJ, Pugh LI, Ferguson RL, et al. Distraction instrumentation outcomes in scoliosis. *J Pediatr Orthop B* 1998;7:106.

259. Moskowitz A, Moe JH, Winter RB, et al. Long-term follow-up of scoliosis fusion. *J Bone Joint Surg Am* 1980;62:364.

260. Cochran T, Irstam L, Nachemson A. Long-term anatomic and functional changes in patients with adolescent idiopathic scoliosis treated by Harrington rod fusion. *Spine* 1983;8:576.

261. Connolly PJ, Von Schroeder HP, Johnson GE, et al. Adolescent idiopathic scoliosis. Long-term effect of instrumentation extending to the lumbar spine. *J Bone Joint Surg Am* 1995;77:1210.

262. Winter RB, Carr P, Mattson H. A study of functional spinal motion in women after instrumentation and fusion for deformity or trauma. *Spine* 1997;22:1760.

263. Lenke LG, Bridwell KH, Baldus C, et al. Cotrel-Dubousset instrumentation for adolescent idiopathic scoliosis. *J Bone Joint Surg Am* 1992;74:1056.

264. Humke T, Grob D, Scheier H, et al. Cotrel-Dubousset and Harrington Instrumentation in idiopathic scoliosis: a comparison of long-term results. *Eur Spine J* 1995;4:280.

265. Bridwell KH, Betz R, Capelli AM, et al. Sagittal plane analysis in idiopathic scoliosis patients treated with Cotrel-Dubousset instrumentation. *Spine* 1990;15:921

266. Sawatzky BJ, Tredwell SJ, Jang SB, et al. Effects of three-dimensional assessment on surgical correction and on hook strategies in multi-hook instrumentation for adolescent idiopathic scoliosis. *Spine* 1998;23:201.

267. Labelle H, Dansereau J, Bellefleur C, et al. Preoperative three-dimensional correction of idiopathic scoliosis with the Cotrel–Dubousset procedure. *Spine* 1995;20:1406.

268. Aronsson DD, Stokes IA, Ronchetti PJ, et al. Surgical correction of vertebral axial rotation in adolescent idiopathic scoliosis: prediction by lateral bending films. *J Spinal Disord* 1996;9:214.

269. Willers U, Transfeldt EE, Hedlund R. The segmental effect of Cotrel-Dubousset instrumentation on vertebral rotation, rib hump and the thoracic cage in idiopathic scoliosis. *Eur Spine J* 1996;5:387.

270. Benli IT, Tuzuner M, Akalin S, et al. Spinal imbalance and decompensation problems in patients treated with Cotrel-Dubousset instrumentation. *Eur Spine J* 1996;5:380.

271. Kohler R, Galland O, Mechin H, et al. The Dwyer procedure in the treatment of idiopathic scoliosis. A 10-year follow-up review of 21 patients. *Spine* 1990;15:75.

272. Lowe TG, Peters JD. Anterior spinal fusion with Zielke instrumentation for idiopathic scoliosis. A frontal and sagittal curve analysis in 36 patients. *Spine* 1993;18:423.

273. Kostuik JP, Carl A, Ferron S. Anterior Zielke instrumentation for spinal deformity in adults. *J Bone Joint Surg Am* 1989;71:898.

Complications

274. Richards BS. Delayed infections following posterior spinal instrumentation for the treatment of idiopathic scoliosis. *J Bone Joint Surg Am* 1995;77:524.

275. Clark CE, Shufflebarger HL. Late-developing infection in instrumented idiopathic scoliosis. *Spine* 1999;24:1909.

276. Wimmer C, Gluch H. Aseptic loosening after CD instrumentation in the treatment of scoliosis: a report about eight cases. *J Spinal Disord* 1998;11:440.

277. Bridwell KH, Lenke LG, Baldus C, et al. Major intraoperative neurologic deficits in pediatric and adult spinal deformity patients. Incidence and etiology at one institution. *Spine* 1998;23:324.

278. Winter RB, Lonstein JE, Denis F, et al. Paraplegia resulting from vessel ligation. *Spine* 1996;21:1232.

279. Bridwell KH. Normalization of the coronal and sagittal profile in idiopathic scoliosis: options of treatment. *J Orthop Sci* 1998;3:125.

280. Apel DM, Marrero G, King J, et al. Avoiding paraplegia during anterior spinal surgery. The role of somatosensory evoked potential monitoring with temporary occlusion of segmental spinal arteries. *Spine* 1991;16:S365.

281. Glassman SD, Johnson JR, Shields CB, et al. Correlation of motor-evoked potentials, somatosensory-evoked potentials, and the wake-up test in a case of kyphoscoliosis. *J Spinal Disord* 1993;6:194.

282. Hall JE, Levine CR, Sudhir KG. Intraoperative awakening to monitor spinal cord function during Harrington instrumentation and spine fusion. Description of procedure and report of three cases. *J Bone Joint Surg Am* 1978;60:533.

283. Szalay EA, Carollo JJ, Roach JW. Sensitivity of spinal cord monitoring to intraoperative events. *J Pediatr Orthop* 1986;6:437.

284. Bracken MB. Methylprednisolone in the management of acute spinal cord injuries. *Med J Aust* 1990;153:368.

285. Vitale MG, Stazzone EJ, Gelijns AC, et al. The effectiveness of preoperative erythropoietin in averting allogenic blood transfusion among children undergoing scoliosis surgery. *J Pediatr Orthop B* 1998;7:203.

286. Olsfanger D, Jedeikin R, Metser U, et al. Acute normovolaemic haemodilution and idiopathic scoliosis surgery: effects on homologous blood requirements. *Anaesth Intensive Care* 1993;21:429

287. McNeill TW, DeWald RL, Kuo KN, et al. Controlled hypotensive anesthesia in scoliosis surgery. *J Bone Joint Surg Am Weekly* 1974;56:1167

288. Scoliosis Research Society. *Morbidity and Mortality Report.* 1995.

289. Johnston CE, Happel LT Jr, Norris R, et al. Delayed paraplegia complicating sublaminar segmental spinal instrumentation. *J Bone Joint Surg Am* 1986;68:556.

290. Mineiro J, Weinstein SL. Delayed postoperative paraparesis in scoliosis surgery. A case report. *Spine* 1997;22:1668.

Congenital Scoliosis—Details of Diagnosis and Treatment

291. Singh J, Aggison L Jr, Moore-Cheatum L. Teratogenicity and developmental toxicity of carbon monoxide in protein-deficient mice. *Teratology* 1993;48:149.

Classification

292. McMaster MJ, Singh H. Natural history of congenital kyphosis and kyphoscoliosis. A study of one hundred and twelve patients. *J Bone Joint Surg Am* 1999;81:1367.

293. Bush CH, Kalen V. Three-dimensional computed tomography in the assessment of congenital scoliosis. *Skeletal Radiol* 1999;28:632.

Natural History

294. McMaster MJ, Ohtsuka K. The natural history of congenital scoliosis. A study of two hundred and fifty-one patients. *J Bone Joint Surg Am* 1982;64:1128.

295. Winter RB. *Congenital deformities of the spine.* New York: Thieme-Stratton, 1983:55.

296. Loder RT, Urquhart A, Steen H, et al. Variability in Cobb angle measurements in children with congenital scoliosis. *J Bone Joint Surg Br* 1995;77:768.

Treatment

297. Winter RB, Moe JH. Orthotics for spinal deformity. *Clin Orthop* 1974;0:72.

298. McMaster MJ. Congenital scoliosis caused by a unilateral failure of vertebral segmentation with contralateral hemivertebrae. *Spine* 1998;23:998.

299. Winter RB, Haven JJ, Moe JH, Lagaard SM. Diastematomyelia and congenital spine deformities. *J Bone Joint Surg Am* 1974; 56:27.

300. Goldberg CJ, Moore DP, Fogarty EE, et al. Growth patterns in children with congenital vertebral anomalies. New York: Annual Meeting Scoliosis Research Society, 1998:58.

301. Terek RM, Wehner J, Lubicky JP. Crankshaft phenomenon in congenital scoliosis: a preliminary report. *J Pediatr Orthop* 1991; 11:527.

302. Winter RB, Moe JH, Lonstein JE. Posterior spinal arthrodesis for congenital scoliosis. An analysis of the cases of two hundred and ninety patients, five to nineteen years old. *J Bone Joint Surg Am* 1984;66:1188.

303. Lopez-Sosa F, Guille JT, Bowen JR. Rotation of the spine in congenital scoliosis. *J Pediatr Orthop* 1995;15:528.

304. Sanders JO, Evert M, Stanley EA, et al. Mechanisms of curve progression following sublaminar (Luque) spinal instrumentation. *Spine* 1992;17:781.

305. McMaster MJ, David CV. Hemivertebra as a cause of scoliosis. A study of 104 patients. *J Bone Joint Surg Br* 1986;68: 588.

306. Thompson AG, Marks DS, Sayampanathan SR, et al. Long-term results of combined anterior and posterior convex epiphysiodesis for congenital scoliosis due to hemivertebrae. *Spine* 1995; 20:1380.

307. Marks DS, Sayampanathan SR, Thompson AG, et al. Long-term results of convex epiphysiodesis for congenital scoliosis. *Eur Spine J* 1995;4:296.

308. Kieffer J, Dubousset J. Combined anterior and posterior convex epiphysiodesis for progressive congenital scoliosis in children aged < or = 5 years. *Eur Spine J* 1994;3:120.

309. King AG, MacEwen GD, Bose WJ. Transpedicular convex anterior hemiepiphysiodesis and posterior arthrodesis for progressive congenital scoliosis. *Spine* 1992;17:S291.

310. Winter RB, Lonstein JE, Denis F, et al. Convex growth arrest for progressive congenital scoliosis due to hemivertebrae. *J Pediatr Orthop* 1988;8:633.

311. Winter RB. Congenital scoliosis. *Orthop Clin North Am* 1988; 19:395.

312. Holte DC, Winter RB, Lonstein JE, et al. Excision of hemivertebrae and wedge resection in the treatment of congenital scoliosis. *J Bone Joint Surg Am* 1995;77:159.

313. Leatherman KD, Dickson RA. Two-stage corrective surgery for congenital deformities of the spine. *J Bone Joint Surg Br* 1979; 61:324.

314. Callahan BC, Georgopoulos G, Eilert RE. Hemivertebral excision for congenital scoliosis. *J Pediatr Orthop* 1997;17:96.

SUBJECT INDEX

Page numbers in *italics* denote figures; page numbers followed by "t" denote tables.